VARCAROLIS'S

# CANADIAN PSYCHIATRIC MENTAL HEALTH NURSING

## A Clinical Approach

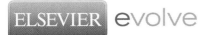
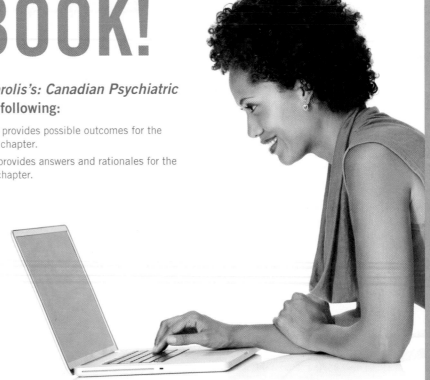

VARCAROLIS'S
# CANADIAN PSYCHIATRIC MENTAL HEALTH NURSING

## A Clinical Approach

### First Canadian Edition

**Margaret Jordan Halter, PMHCNS, PhD**
Associate Dean
Ashland University
Dwight Schar College of Nursing and Health Sciences
Mansfield, Ohio

*Canadian Editors*

**Cheryl L. Pollard, PN, RN, BScN, MN, PhD (Nursing)**
Assistant Professor
Faculty of Health and Community Studies, Nursing
MacEwan University
Edmonton, Alberta

**Susan L. Ray, RN, BScN, MScN, Post-Master's NP certificate, PhD**
Associate Professor
Arthur Labatt Family School of Nursing
Western University
London, Ontario
Associate Scientist
Mental Health Outcomes
Lawson Health Research Institute
London, Ontario

**Mary Haase, RN, RPN, BScN, PhD**
Faculty
Faculty of Health and Community Studies, Psychiatric Nursing
MacEwan University
Edmonton, Alberta

*Associate Editor*

**Sonya L. Jakubec, RN, BHScN, MN, PhD(c)**
Associate Professor
Faculty of Health & Community Studies, Nursing
Mount Royal University
Calgary, Alberta

ELSEVIER

ELSEVIER
SAUNDERS

Library and Archives Canada Cataloguing in Publication
ISBN 978-1-926648-33-0

**Library and Archives Canada Cataloguing in Publication**

Varcarolis's Canadian psychiatric mental health nursing: a clinical approach / [edited by] Margaret Jordan Halter, PMHCNS, PhD, Associate Dean, Ashland University, Dwight Schar College of Nursing and Health Sciences Mansfield, Ohio; Canadian editors, Cheryl L. Pollard, PN, RN, BScN, MN, PhD (Nursing), Assistant Professor, Faculty of Health and Community Studies, Nursing MacEwan University Edmonton, Alberta, Susan L. Ray, RN, BScN, MScN, Post-Master's NP certificate, PhD, Associate Professor, Arthur Labatt Family School of Nursing, Western University London, Ontario Associate Scientist Mental Health Outcomes, Lawson Health Research Institute, London, Ontario, Mary Haase, RN, RPN, BScN, PhD Faculty Faculty of Health and Community Studies, Psychiatric Nursing, MacEwan University, Edmonton, Alberta; associate editor, Sonya L. Jakubec, RN, BHScN, MN, PhD(c), Associate Professor, Faculty of Health & Community Studies, Nursing Mount Royal University, Calgary, Alberta.—First Canadian edition.

"Adapted from Varcarolis' Foundations of Psychiatric Mental Health Nursing: A Clinical Approach, seventh edition, by Margaret Jordan Halter, Copyright © 2014. Previous editions copyrighted 2010, 2006, 2002, 1998, 1994, 1990"—title page verso. Includes bibliographical references and index. ISBN 978-1-926648-33-0 (bound)

1. Psychiatric nursing—Canada.   2. Mental health—Canada.   I. Halter, Margaret J. (Margaret Jordan), author, editor of compilation   II. Title: Canadian psychiatric mental health nursing.

RC440.V37 2013                    616.89'0231                    C2013-905775-7

Vice President, Publishing: Ann Millar
Managing Editor: Roberta A. Spinosa-Millman
Publishing Services Manager: Deborah L. Vogel
Project Manager: John W. Gabbert
Substantive Editor: Cathy Witlox
Copy Editors: Cathy Witlox and Sherry Hinman
Proofreaders: Sherry Hinman and Wendy Thomas
Cover Image: solarseven
Book Designer: Maggie Reid
Printing and Binding: Transcontinental

Elsevier Canada
905 King Street West, 4th Floor, Toronto, ON, Canada M6K 3G9
Phone: 1-866-896-3331
Fax: 1-866-290-5590

Printed in Canada
2  3  4  5    17  16  15  14

Ebook ISBN: 978-1-926648-34-7

*The family legend of my dad losing his mother*
*to a brain tumour when he was five was not true.*
*In honour of my grandmother Edith (1882–1927), who lost*
*her life to depression before hope of recovery existed.*
*1-in-128 odds for seven female births in a row … to our dear daughters,*
*Elissa, Emily, and Monica, and their daughters, Kiran, Leela, Vivienne, and Violette.*
*My husband, Paul, is a loved man indeed!*
*And finally, to my twin sister, Anne, how subtle are the links that bind—what a bonus.*
**—Peggy Halter**

*For those who have shared*
*For those who will inspire*
*Showing your courage.*
**—Cheryl L. Pollard**

*In honour of the mental health clients who have shared their stories with me. Your stories
are of courage, strength, resilience, and hope. You have taught me much more than words
can express. Thank you for sharing your journey with me.*
*And to my daughters, Leanne and Jaclyn, with thanks for your love, patience, and
understanding through the years.*
**—Susan L. Ray**

*Throughout my years as a mental health nurse, patients have inspired me with their
strength, resilience, and drive to be well. A special acknowledgement goes out to all the
patients who allowed me into their lives and taught me so much. Thank you to my
husband, children, and grandchildren for enriching my life. And to those who
collaborated on this text, I thank you.*
**—Mary Haase**

*For those holding this text, the faculty looking to enliven teaching and practice, and the
students who already know mental health and practice in novel ways; for you to inspire
us in our shared responsibility for more compassionate and expanded experiences of
mental health in our daily lives, our communities, our practice, our politics, and in our
world. This text is also dedicated to those who have taught me about the power and
possibilities of listening, recovery, and inclusion—in particular to Fran, Elizabeth, and
Don: I am privileged to have worked alongside you all.*
**—Sonya L. Jakubec**

# CONTENTS

## UNIT 6    INTERVENTIONS FOR DISTINCT POPULATIONS

## UNIT 7   ADVANCED INTERVENTION MODALITIES

## APPENDIXES

# ACKNOWLEDGEMENTS

First, we would like to acknowledge the text from which this text has been adapted. To work from the years of work and expertise of Elizabeth Varcarolis and Margaret Halter and their contributors is to stand on the shoulders of giants. This adaptation was especially challenging, with its publication coinciding with a major revision that resulted in the fifth version of the American Psychiatric Association's *Diagnostic and Statistical Manual of Mental Disorders*. Clinical chapters were reorganized and updates were made throughout the text based on the most recent evidence available, including Canadian research and statistics, which provide a current perspective of mental health and mental health practice in Canada.

Our heartfelt appreciation also goes out to the talented group of writers who contributed to this first Canadian edition. Your contributions figuratively bind us together in this text, which is a collective source of current knowledge for Canadian practice. Special thanks go to those authors who created entirely new chapters and developed new content, in particular Karen Clements, who prepared the materials on Canadian Psychiatric Mental Health Nursing Standards of Practice, Code of Ethics, Beliefs, and Values, and Holly Symonds-Brown for her work on the historical overview of Canadian psychiatric mental health nursing. We have indeed sought the expertise of a talented pool of contributors. Their knowledge and passion has had a powerful influence on this edition. It has truly been a joy working with each of you.

Thanks for the countless hours—over several years—you spent researching, writing, and rewriting!

A huge debt of gratitude goes to the many educators and clinicians who reviewed the manuscript and offered valuable suggestions, ideas, opinions, and criticisms. All comments were appreciated; they helped refine and strengthen the individual chapters. In particular, we would like to thank Dr. Andrew Estefan at the University of Calgary for his thoughtful suggestions, which greatly strengthened the content and format of Chapter 19, "Substance Use and Addictive Disorders."

Throughout this project, a number of people at Elsevier provided superb, and patient, support and encouragement. Sincere thanks go to the Elsevier team: our Managing Editor, Roberta A. Spinosa-Millman, who held the project and us all together with the perfect combination of good organization and good humour; Cathy Witlox, our Substantive Editor and Copy Editor, who has lent clarity, currency, and perspective to the complex adaptation for this first Canadian edition; and finally to John Gabbert, our Project Manager, who has made our work shine.

A combined thank-you to the Canadian Editorial team. Everyone entered the project at different stages, presenting its own unique challenges, but with our combined dedication, creativity, and fortitude, we were able to complete this text, which will no doubt add to a critical dialogue about psychiatric mental health nursing in Canada.

# CANADIAN CONTRIBUTORS

**Karen Scott Barss, RPN, BHSc, MA**
Faculty
Nursing Division
Saskatchewan Institute of Applied Science &
    Technology (SIAST)
Saskatoon, Saskatchewan
Adjunct Undergraduate Professor
College of Nursing
University of Regina
Regina, Saskatchewan

**Karen Clements, RPN, BA, MA**
Assistant Professor
Department of Psychiatric Nursing, Faculty
    of Health Studies
Brandon University
Brandon, Manitoba

**Melodie B. Hull, RPN, BA, MSc, MEd,
    PID, TESOL**
Faculty
Nursing
College of the Rockies
Cranbrook, British Columbia
Open Learning Faculty—Nursing & Health
Thompson Rivers University
Kamloops, British Columbia

**Angela Hyden, RN, BScN, MN**
Professor
Sault College
Sault Ste. Marie, Ontario

**Wendy Kemp, RN, BN, MDE**
Nursing Tutor
Centre for Nursing and Health Studies
Athabasca University
Athabasca, Alberta

**Joanne Louis, MN, MSc, RN(EC)**
Lecturer
Lawrence S. Bloomberg Faculty of Nursing
University of Toronto
Toronto, Ontario

**Cyndee L. MacPhee, RN, BScN, MN**
Assistant Professor
Nursing Department
Cape Breton University
Sydney, Nova Scotia

**Robert J. Meadus, BN, BVocEd, MSc(N),
    PhD**
Associate Professor & Associate Dean,
    Undergraduate Programs Pro Tempore
School of Nursing
Memorial University
St. John's, Newfoundland

**Sherri Melrose, RN, MEd, PhD**
Associate Professor
Centre for Nursing and Health Studies
Athabasca University
Athabasca, Alberta

**Sandra Mitchell, RPN, ADPN, MScN,
    PhD(c)**
Nurse Educator
British Columbia Centre for Disease
    Control
Vancouver, British Columbia

**Sharon L. Moore, BA, RN, R Psych, MEd,
    PhD**
Professor
Centre for Nursing & Health Studies
Athabasca University
Athabasca, Alberta

**Elaine M. Mordoch, RN, BN, MN, PhD**
Assistant Professor
Faculty of Nursing
University of Manitoba
Winnipeg, Manitoba

**Wilma Schroeder, BN, MMFT**
Faculty
Faculty of Nursing
Red River College
Winnipeg, Manitoba

**Wendy Stanyon, RN, BN, MAEd, EdD**
Associate Professor
Faculty of Health Sciences
University of Ontario Institute of
    Technology
Oshawa, Ontario

**Beth Swart, BScN, MES**
Professor
Daphne Cockwell School of Nursing
Ryerson University
Toronto, Ontario

**Holly Symonds-Brown, BScN, MSN,
    PMHN(c)**
Faculty
Faculty of Health and Community Studies,
    Nursing
MacEwan University
Edmonton, Alberta

**Michel Andre Tarko, RPN, PhD**
President & CEO
Justice Institute of British Columbia
New Westminster, British Columbia

**Catherine A. Thibeault, RN, MN, PhD**
Assistant Professor
Trent/Fleming School of Nursing
Trent University
Peterborough, Ontario

**Ann-Marie Urban, RN, BScN, MN, PhD**
Assistant Professor
Faculty of Nursing
University of Regina
Regina, Saskatchewan

## SECTION EDITOR

**Melissa Watkins, BN, RN, RPN, GD
    PMHN, MN Mental Health**
Faculty
Clinical Coordinator
Faculty of Health and Community Studies,
    Psychiatric Nursing
MacEwan University
Edmonton, Alberta

# U.S. CONTRIBUTORS

## CONTRIBUTORS TO THE U.S. 6TH EDITION

**Leslie A. Briscoe, PMHNP-BC**
Psychiatric Nurse Practitioner
U.S. Department of Veterans Affairs
Cleveland, Ohio

**Verna Benner Carson, RN, PhD**
President of C&V Senior Care Specialist, Inc.
Associate Professor of Nursing
Towson University
Baltimore, Maryland

**Claudia A. Cihlar, PMHCNS-BC, PhD**
Coordinator of Behavioral Health Services
Center for Psychiatry
Akron General Medical Center
Akron, Ohio

**Avni Cirpili, RN, MSN**
Chief Nursing Officer
Department of Psychiatry
Ohio State University Harding Hospital
Columbus, Ohio

**Cherrill W. Colson, RN, BS, MA, EdD, CS**
Assistant Professor
Department of Nursing
Hostos Community College
City University of New York
New York, New York

**Charlotte Eliopoulos, RN, MPH, ND, PhD**
Executive Director
American Association for Long Term Care Nursing (AALTCN)
Cincinnati, Ohio

**Carissa R. Enright, RN, MSN, PMHNP-BC**
Associate Clinical Professor
Texas Woman's University
Psychiatric Consult Liaison
Presbyterian Hospital of Dallas
Dallas, Texas

**Elizabeth Hite Erwin, BC, APRN, PhD**
Assistant Professor
University of Virginia School of Nursing
Charlottesville, Virginia

**Mary A. Gutierrez, PharmD, BCPP**
Professor of Clinical Pharmacy and Psychiatry
Department of Pharmacotherapy and Outcomes Science
Loma Linda University School of Pharmacy
Loma Linda, California

**Edward A. Herzog, RN, BSN, MSN, CNS**
Lecturer
College of Nursing
Kent State University
Kent, Ohio

**Kathleen Ibrahim, APRN, BC, MA**
Assistant to the Director of Nursing
New York State Psychiatric Institute
New York, New York

**Mallie Kozy, PMHCNS-BC, PhD**
Associate Professor
Chair, Undergraduate Nursing Studies
College of Nursing
Lourdes University
Sylvania, Ohio

**Karyn I. Morgan, RN, MSN, CNS**
Instructor
University of Akron College of Nursing
Clinical Nurse Specialist
Intensive Outpatient Psychiatry
Summa Health System
Akron, Ohio

**John Raynor, PhD**
Professor
Borough of Manhattan Community College
City University of New York
New York, New York

**Judi Sateren, RN, MS**
Associate Professor Emerita
St. Olaf College
Northfield, Minnesota

**Nancy Christine Shoemaker, ARPN/PMH, BC**
Nurse Psychotherapist
Baltimore, Maryland

**Jane Stein-Parbury, RN, BSN, MEd, PhD, FRCNA**
Professor of Mental Health Nursing
Faculty of Health
University of Technology
Director
Area Professorial Mental Health Nursing Unit
South East Sydney Local Health District
Sydney, Australia

**Sylvia Stevens, APRN, MS, BC**
Professor of Nursing
Montgomery College
Silver Spring, Maryland
Psychotherapy Private Practice
Washington, District of Columbia

**Margaret R. Swisher, RN, MSN**
Assistant Professor of Nursing
Montgomery County Community College
Blue Bell, Pennsylvania

**Margaret Trussler, MS, APRN-BC**
Sleep Health Centers
Boston, Massachusetts
Clinical Faculty
University of Massachusetts
Worcester, Massachusetts

**Elizabeth M. Varcarolis, RN, MA**
Professor Emeritus
Formerly Deputy Chairperson
Department of Nursing
Borough of Manhattan Community College
Associate Fellow
Albert Ellis Institute for Rational Emotional Behavioral Therapy (REBT)
New York, New York

**Roberta Waite, EdD, RN, PMHCNS-BC**
Assistant Professor
College of Nursing and Health Professions
Drexel University
Philadelphia, Pennsylvania

**Evelyn Yap, BSN, ARPN-PMH, MScN**
Nurse, Advanced Practice
Psychiatry—Consultant
University of Maryland Rehabilitation & Orthopaedic Institute
Rehabilitation Research Center at Kernan
Baltimore, Maryland

## CONTRIBUTORS TO THE U.S. 7TH EDITION

**Lois Angelo, APRN, BC**
Assistant Professor of Nursing
Massachusetts College of Pharmacy and
    Health Sciences
Boston, Massachusetts

**Kimberly Gregg, PMHCNS-BC, MS, PhD(c)**
Psychiatric Mental Health Clinical Nurse
    Specialist
Hennepin County Medical Center
Minneapolis, Minnesota
Clinical Assistant Professor
University of North Dakota
Grand Forks, North Dakota

**Faye J. Grund, APRN, PMHNP-BC, PhD(c)**
Interim Dean
Dwight Schar College of Nursing and
    Health Sciences
Ashland University
Mansfield, Ohio

**Kathleen Wheeler, APRN-BC, PMHCNS, PMHNP, FAAN, PhD**
Professor
Fairfield University School of Nursing
Fairfield, Connecticut

**Rick Zoucha, APRN-BC, CTN-A, PhD**
Associate Professor
School of Nursing
Duquesne University
Pittsburgh, Pennsylvania

# CANADIAN REVIEWERS

**Anna Marie Alteen, RN, BN, MN, CPMHN(c)**
Nurse Educator
Western Regional School of Nursing
Corner Brook, Newfoundland

**Carrie Bullard, RN, MN, CPMHN(c)**
Assistant Clinical Professor
School of Nursing
McMaster University
Hamilton, Ontario
Clinical Nurse Specialist
Anxiety Treatment and Research Centre
St. Joseph's Healthcare Hamilton—Charlton Campus
Hamilton, Ontario

**Tanya Cheale, BScN, RN**
Instructor
Faculty of Nursing
Red River College
Winnipeg, Manitoba

**Sharon Chin, BSc (Hons), MHScN, CPMHN(c)**
Professor
Nursing
Nipissing University/Canadore College Collaborative BScN Program
North Bay, Ontario

**Kathryn Ellis, RN, BScN, MAEd**
Professor
Coordinator—Degree Nursing
School of Community and Health Studies—Centennial Site
Ryerson, Centennial, and George Brown Collaborative Nursing Degree
Toronto, Ontario

**Andrew Estefan, RPN, DipNSc, BN, MN, PhD**
Assistant Professor
Faculty of Nursing
The University of Calgary
Calgary, Alberta

**Pasquale Fiore, RN, BScN, MSc Health Adm, Cert Ed**
Faculty
Department of Nursing
Camosun College
Instructor
School of Nursing
University of Victoria
Victoria, British Columbia

**Suzanne Foster, MN, BN, RN**
Assistant Professor
School of Nursing
Dalhousie University
Halifax, Nova Scotia

**Lisa Giallonardo, RN, MScN**
Professor of Health Sciences, Nursing
Academic Advisor, Personal Support Worker Program
Faculty of Applied Health and Community Studies
Sheridan Institute of Technology & Advanced Learning
Oakville, Ontario

**Heather Gilfoy, BN, MN**
Instructor
Dalhousie School of Nursing—Yarmouth Site
Dalhousie University
Yarmouth, Nova Scotia

**Holly Graham-Marrs, RN, BA, BScN, MN, PhD, RD Psychologist (provisional)**
Assistant Professor
College of Nursing
University of Saskatchewan
Saskatoon, Saskatchewan

**Mary Haase, RN, RPN, BScN, PhD**
Faculty
Faculty of Health and Community Studies, Psychiatric Nursing
MacEwan University
Edmonton, Alberta

**Rae Harwood, RN, BN, MA, EdD (Counselling Psychology)**
Clinical Course Leader
Faculty of Nursing
University of Manitoba
Winnipeg, Manitoba

**Marilyn Hoffman, RN, BScN, MEd**
Clinical Instructor
Athabasca University
Athabasca, Alberta

**Angela Hyden, RN, BScN, MN**
Professor
Sault College
Sault Ste. Marie, Ontario

**Elsabeth Jensen, RN, BA, PhD**
Associate Professor
Graduate Program Director
Faculty of Health, School of Nursing
York University
Toronto, Ontario

**Susan Kagan, RN, BScN, CPMHN(c), EdD**
Professor
School of Nursing
Seneca College of Applied Arts & Technology
Coordinator, Forensic Health Studies Certificate Program
Toronto, Ontario

**Arlene E. Kent-Wilkinsin, RN, CPMHN(c), BSN, MN, PhD**
Associate Professor
College of Nursing
University of Saskatchewan
Saskatoon, Saskatchewan

**Ken Kustiak, RN, RPN, BScN, MN**
Faculty
Year 1 Coordinator
Faculty of Health and Community Studies, Psychiatric Nursing—Ponoka Site
MacEwan University
Edmonton, Alberta

**Annette M. Lane, PhD**
Assistant Professor
Faculty of Nursing
University of Calgary
Calgary, Alberta

**Cyndee L. MacPhee, RN, BScN, MN**
Assistant Professor
Nursing Department
Cape Breton University
Sydney, Nova Scotia

**Sherri Melrose, RN, MEd, PhD**
Associate Professor
Centre for Nursing and Health Studies
Athabasca University
Athabasca, Alberta

**Sharon L. Moore, BA, RN, R Psych, MEd, PhD**
Professor
Centre for Nursing & Health Studies
Athabasca University
Athabasca, Alberta

**Sue S. Myers, RPN, BSW, MVocTechEd**
Program Head
Psychiatric Nursing Program
Saskatchewan Institute of Applied Science
and Technology (SIAST)—Wascana
Campus
Regina, Saskatchewan

**Judy Osborne, RN, BN, MEd(c)**
Clinical Faculty
Mental Health
Fleming College
Peterborough, Ontario

**Geraldine Parsons, BScN**
Faculty
School of Health & Life Sciences and
Community Services
Conestoga College
Kitchener, Ontario

**J. Craig Phillips, RN, ARNP, ACRN,
PMHCNS-BC, LLM, PhD**
Assistant Professor
Faculty of Health Sciences, School of
Nursing
University of Ottawa
Ottawa, Ontario

**Ann Pottinger, BASc, BScN, MN**
Assistant Lecturer
Course Director, Mental Health
Faculty of Health, School of Nursing
York University
Toronto, Ontario
Advanced Practice Nurse
Professional Practice
Centre for Addiction and Mental Health
(CAMH)
Toronto, Ontario

**Elaine Santa Mina, RN, BA, BAAN, MSc,
PhD**
Associate Director
Daphne Cockwell School of Nursing
Ryerson University
Toronto, Ontario

**Wilma Schroeder, BN, MMFT**
Faculty
Faculty of Nursing
Red River College
Winnipeg, Manitoba

**Janis Seeley, RN, DNP, MScN, MEd**
Professor of Nursing
School of Health and Community Services
Confederation College
Thunder Bay, Ontario

**Debbie Shubat, RN, BScN, MScN**
Professor of Nursing (Retired)
Sault College
Sault Ste. Marie, Ontario

**Wendy Stanyon, RN, BN, MAEd, EdD**
Associate Professor
Faculty of Health Sciences
University of Ontario Institute of
Technology
Oshawa, Ontario

**Sharon Staseson, RN, BSN, MSN**
Faculty
Saskatchewan Collaborative Bachelor of
Science Nursing Program
Saskatchewan Institute of Applied Science &
Technology (SIAST)/University of
Regina
Regina, Saskatchewan

**Beth Swart, BScN, MES**
Professor
Daphne Cockwell School of Nursing
Ryerson University
Toronto, Ontario

**Lynne Theriault, MSHA, BScN, RN, PN**
Nursing Instructor
MacEwan University
Edmonton, Alberta

**Mary Jean Thompson, RN, BN, MHS,
MPC**
Nursing Faculty
Division of Health Studies
Medicine Hat College
Medicine Hat, Alberta

**Helen Timms, RPN, BA, MV/TEd**
Instructor
Nursing Division
Saskatchewan Institute of Applied Science
and Technology (SIAST)—Wascana
Campus
Regina, Saskatchewan

**Paula Tognazzini, RN, BSN, MSN**
Senior Instructor Emerita
School of Nursing
University of British Columbia
Vancouver, British Columbia

**Mark Welch, RPN, PhD**
Program Manager, Acute Mental Health
South Okanagan Region, Interior Health
Authority
Penticton Regional Hospital
Penticton, British Columbia

**Karen Wells, RN, BN, MN(c)**
Academic Assistant/Instructor
Faculty of Health Sciences, Nursing
University of Lethbridge
Lethbridge, Alberta

**Trish Whelan, PN, RN, BScN, MHS,
ENC(c)**
Assistant Professor
Faculty of Health & Community Studies,
Nursing
Mount Royal University
Calgary, Alberta

**Bernadine Wojtowicz, BN, RN, CPMHN**
Academic Assistant
School of Health Sciences
University of Lethbridge
Lethbridge, Alberta

# TO THE INSTRUCTOR

The role of the health care provider continues to become more challenging as federal cuts, lack of trained personnel, and the dictates of municipal, provincial and territorial, and federal governments compromise our health care system. We nurses and our patients are from widely diverse historical, cultural, religious, and socioeconomic contexts, bringing together a wide spectrum of knowledge, beliefs, and practices. An in-depth consideration and understanding of these contextual and social experiences are paramount in the administration of responsive and evidence-informed nursing care and are emphasized throughout this text.

We have made a concentrated effort to update diagnostic terms so they align with the new *Diagnostic and Statistical Manual of Mental Disorders, fifth edition*. However, note that we have decided to use the term *dementia* when referring to progressive degenerative neurocognitive disorders. Although the term *dementia* was dropped from the *DSM-5*, many current practitioners still frequently use it. Therefore, an editorial decision was made to include and use the term to ensure that readers using this text as a basis for clinical practice would be able to understand what is meant when *dementia* is used by more experienced health care providers.

We are living in an age of fast-paced research in neurobiology, genetics, and psychopharmacology that strives to find the most effective evidence-informed approaches for patients and their families. Legal issues and ethical dilemmas faced by the health care system are magnified accordingly. Given these myriad challenges, knowing how best to teach our students and serve our patients can seem overwhelming. With contributions from knowledgeable and experienced nurse educators with pan-Canadian perspectives, our goal is to bring to you the most current and comprehensive trends and evidence-informed practices in psychiatric mental health nursing.

## CONTENT NEW TO THIS EDITION

The following topics are at the forefront of nursing practice and, as such, are considered in detail in this first edition:

- Issues involving mental health parity and other current legislations (Chapter 8)
- Disaster preparedness (Chapter 24)
- Emphasis on the fact that we are all "from another culture" to encourage cultural awareness (Chapter 7)
- Neurotransmitter and immune stress responses, stress-inducing events and stress-reducing techniques, self-assessment of the nurse's stress level, and mindfulness (Chapter 12)
- Evidence-informed practices and an emphasis on health promotion, resiliency, and recovery in the disorders chapters (Unit 4)

- Depression screenings in children, adolescents, and older adults; vagus nerve stimulation; and additional subtypes of depression considered in the *DSM-5* (Chapters 14, 29, and 30)
- Emphasis throughout the text on recovery versus rehabilitation, victimization, social isolation and loneliness, unemployment and poverty, involuntary treatment, incarceration, wellness and recovery action plans, mental health first aid, interventions to promote adherence to treatment, and more
- A recognition of the increased prevalence and implications of sleep disturbances and sleep–wake disorders with a focus on their relationship to psychiatric illness and the nurse's role in assessment and management (Chapter 21)
- Sexual dysfunction and sexual disorders, including the complex issue of sexual behaviour and the knowledge of normal and abnormal sexuality necessary to conduct a sexual assessment, identify deviations from normal sexual behaviour, recognize nursing implications, and formulate interventions (Chapter 22)

Refer to the To the Student section of this introduction on pp. xxv for examples of thoroughly updated familiar features with a fresh perspective, including How a Nurse Helped Me boxes, Research Highlight boxes, Integrative Therapy boxes, Patient and Family Teaching boxes, Drug Treatment boxes, Considering Culture boxes, Key Points to Remember, Assessment Guidelines, and Vignettes, among others.

## ORGANIZATION OF THE TEXT

Chapters are grouped in units to emphasize the clinical perspective and facilitate location of information. All clinical chapters are organized in a clear, logical, and consistent format with the nursing process as the strong, visible framework. The basic outline for clinical chapters is as follows:

- Clinical Picture: Identifies disorders that fall under the umbrella of the general chapter name. Presents an overview of the disorder(s) and includes *DSM-5* criteria as appropriate.
- Epidemiology: Helps the student to understand the pattern of the problem and characteristics of those who would most likely be affected. This section provides information related to prevalence, lifetime incidence, age of onset, and gender differences.
- Co-Morbidity: Describes the most commonly associated co-morbid conditions. Knowing that co-morbid disorders are often part of the clinical picture of specific disorders helps students and clinicians understand how to better assess and treat their patients.
- Etiology: Provides current views of causation along with formerly held theories. It is based on the biopsychosocial

triad and includes biological, psychological, and environmental factors.

- Assessment:
  - General Assessment: Appropriate assessment for a specific disorder, including assessment tools and rating scales. Rating scales, for instance—used to gauge suicide risk, assess anxiety, or assess substance use problems—help to highlight important areas in the assessment. Because the ratings provided by patients are subjective in nature, experienced clinicians use these tools as a guide when planning care, in addition to their knowledge of their patients.
  - Self-Assessment: Discusses topics relevant to the nurse's self-reflection required to enhance self-growth and provide the best possible and most appropriate care to the patient.
  - Assessment Guidelines: Provides a summary of specific areas to assess by disorder.

Diagnosis: NANDA International–approved nursing diagnoses are used in all nursing process sections, and *DSM-5* (2013) taxonomy and criteria are used throughout.

- Outcomes Identification: *NIC* classifications for interventions and *NOC* classifications for outcomes are introduced in Chapter 1 and used throughout the text when appropriate.
- Planning
- Implementation: Interventions follow Canadian Standards of Psychiatric-Mental Health Nursing (2006) set by the Canadian Federation of Mental Health Nurses under the umbrella of the Canadian Nurses Association (CNA). These standards are incorporated throughout the chapters and are listed for easy reference in Appendix A, "Psychiatric Mental Health Nursing Standards of Practice, Code of Ethics, Beliefs, and Values."
- Evaluation

## TEACHING AND LEARNING RESOURCES

### For Instructors

**Instructor Resources on Evolve**, available at http://evolve.elsevier.com/Canada/Varcarolis/psychiatric/, provide a wealth of material to help you make your psychiatric nursing instruction a success. In addition to all of the Student Resources, the following are provided for Faculty:

- **Instructor's Manual** includes an expansive introduction with course preparation guidelines and teaching tips, Objectives and Key Terms from each chapter, annotated chapter outlines, Thoughts About Teaching the Topic, and Concept Maps.

- **PowerPoint Presentations** are organized by chapter, with approximately 525 slides for in-class lectures. These are detailed and include customizable text and image lecture slides to enhance learning in the classroom or in Web-based course modules. If you share them with students, they can use the Notes feature to help them with your lectures.
- **Audience Response Questions for i>clicker and other systems** are provided with two to five multiple-answer questions per chapter to stimulate class discussion and assess student understanding of key concepts.
- The **Test Bank** has more than 1100 test items, complete with correct answers, rationales, the cognitive level of each question, the corresponding step of the nursing process, appropriate NCLEX Client Needs labels, and text page reference(s).

### For Students

**Student Resources on Evolve**, available at http://evolve.elsevier.com/Canada/Varcarolis/psychiatric/, provide a wealth of valuable learning resources.

The Evolve Resources page near the front of the book gives login instructions and a description of each resource.

- The **Answer Key to Critical Thinking** questions provides possible outcomes for the Critical Thinking questions at the end of each chapter.
- The **Answer Key to Chapter Review** questions provides answers and rationales for the Chapter Review questions at the end of each chapter.
- **Case Studies and Nursing Care Plans** provide detailed case studies and care plans for specific psychiatric disorders to supplement those found in the textbook.
- The **Glossary** highlights psychiatric mental health nursing terms with definitions.
- **Examination Review Questions** provided for each chapter will help students prepare for course examinations and for the nursing licensure examination.
- **Pre-Tests and Post-Tests** provide interactive self-assessments for each chapter of the textbook, including instant scoring and feedback at the click of a button.

We are grateful to educators who send suggestions and provide feedback, and hope this first edition helps students learn and appreciate the scope of psychiatric mental health nursing practice.

Peggy Halter
Cheryl L. Pollard
Susan L. Ray
Mary Haase
Sonya L. Jakubec

# TO THE STUDENT

Psychiatric mental health nursing challenges us to understand the complexities of human behaviour. In the chapters that follow, you will learn about people with psychiatric mental health disorders and how to provide them with quality nursing care and promote their mental health. As you read, keep in mind these special features.

## READING AND REVIEW TOOLS

**1** **Key Terms and Concepts** and **2** **Objectives** introduce the chapter topics and provide a concise overview of the material discussed.

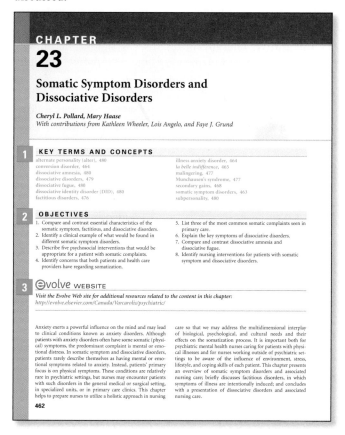

**Key Points to Remember** listed at the end of each chapter reinforce essential information.

**Critical Thinking** activities at the end of each chapter are scenario-based critical thinking problems to provide practice in applying what you have learned. **Answer Guidelines** can be found on the Evolve Web site.

Multiple-choice **Chapter Review** questions at the end of each chapter help you review the chapter material and study for exams. **Answers** with **rationales** are located on the Evolve Web site.

## ADDITIONAL LEARNING RESOURCES

Your **3** Evolve Resources at http://evolve.elsevier.com/Canada/Varcarolis/psychiatric/ offer more helpful study aids, such as additional Case Studies and Nursing Care Plans.

## CHAPTER FEATURES

**4** **How a Nurse Helped Me** boxes are patient accounts and narratives that introduce select chapters and invite exploration into the lived experiences of patients and families.

**5** **Considering Culture** boxes reinforce the importance of providing culturally competent care.

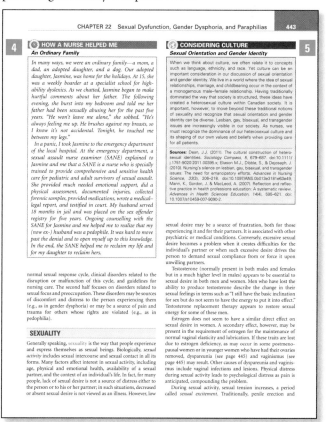

**6** **Vignettes** describe the unique circumstances surrounding individual patients with psychiatric disorders.

**7** **Assessment Guidelines** at the end of each Assessment section in most clinical chapters provide summary points for patient assessment.

*Illustrated on the next page:*

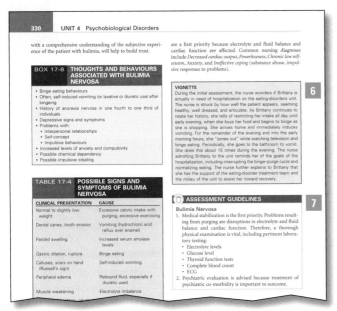

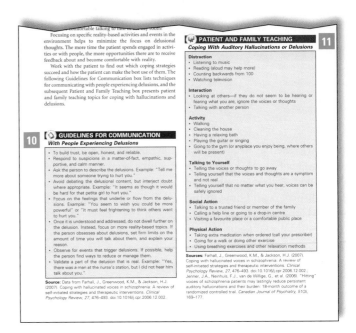

**8** **Research Highlight** boxes demonstrate how current research findings affect psychiatric mental health nursing practice and standards of care.

**9** **Self-Assessment** sections discuss topics relevant to a nurse's process of self-reflection needed to enhance self-growth and provide the best possible and most appropriate care to the patient.

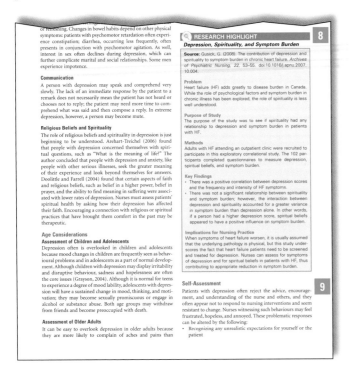

**10** **Guidelines for Communication** boxes provide tips for communicating therapeutically with patients and their families.

**11** **Patient and Family Teaching** boxes underscore the nurse's role in helping patients and families understand psychiatric disorders, treatments, complications, and medication adverse effects, among other important issues.

**12** **Drug Treatment** boxes present the latest information on medications used to treat psychiatric disorders.

**13** **Integrative Therapy** boxes discuss significant nursing considerations for complementary and alternative therapies and examine relevant study findings.

**Case Studies and Nursing Care Plans** present individualized histories of patients with specific psychiatric disorders following the steps of the nursing process. Interventions with rationales and evaluation statements are presented for each patient goal.

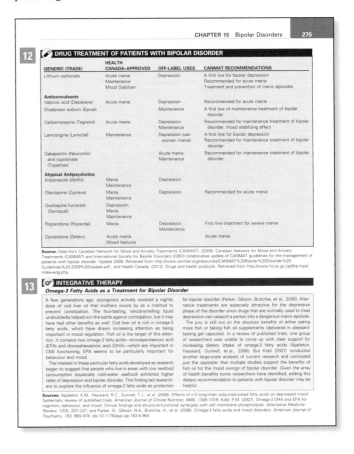

# Foundations in Theory

# 1

# Mental Health and Mental Illness

*Margaret Jordan Halter*
*Mary Haase*

## KEY TERMS AND CONCEPTS

## OBJECTIVES

1. Describe the two conceptualizations of mental health and mental illness.
2. Explore the role of resilience in the prevention of and recovery from mental illness, and consider your own resilience in response to stress.
3. Identify how culture influences our view of mental illnesses and behaviours associated with them.
4. Define and identify attributes of positive mental health.
5. Discuss the nature/nurture origins of psychiatric disorders.
6. Summarize the social determinants of health in Canada.
7. Explain how findings of epidemiological studies can be used to identify areas for medical and nursing interventions.
8. Identify how the *DSM-5* can influence a clinician to consider a broad range of information before making a diagnosis.
9. Describe the specialty of psychiatric mental health nursing.
10. Compare and contrast a *DSM-5* medical diagnosis with a NANDA nursing diagnosis.

## ⊖volve WEBSITE

*Visit the Evolve website for Flashcards, Case Studies, and additional testing resources related to
the content in this chapter: http://evolve.elsevier.com/Canada/Varcarolis/psychiatric/*   Pre-Test   interactive review

If you are a fan of vintage films, you may have witnessed a scene similar to the following: A doctor, wearing a lab coat and an expression of deep concern, enters a hospital waiting room and delivers the bad news to an obviously distraught gentleman who is seated there. The doctor says, "I'm afraid your wife has suffered a nervous breakdown." From that point on, the woman's condition is only vaguely hinted at. The husband visits her at a gated asylum, where staff members regard him with sad expressions. He may find his wife confined to her bed or standing by the window and staring vacantly into the middle distance or sitting motionless in the hospital garden. The viewer can only speculate about the nature of the problem but assumes she has had an emotional collapse.

## MENTAL HEALTH AND MENTAL ILLNESS

We have come a long way in acknowledging psychiatric disorders and increasing our understanding of them since the days

## HOW A NURSE HELPED ME

### When a Nurse Becomes a Patient

*I am a registered nurse working in the area of mental health. I always prided myself on my ability to give caring and compassionate care to all of my patients. Little did I know that one day I would be the patient. I was diagnosed with bipolar disorder when I was 34 years old. For many years, I struggled with devastating depressions and periods of acute mania. I felt stupid, shameful, and embarrassed about my behaviour during these times. Whenever I needed hospitalization, I begged the ambulance driver to take me to any hospital but the one I worked in. On one occasion, that did not happen, and I was admitted to the unit where I worked as a nurse. I thought I could have died of the deep shame I felt. Judy, the nurse assigned to me, seemed scared and embarrassed to come and speak with me, so I felt uncomfortable when I spoke with her. On about the fourth day of that admission, Brenda, another nurse I knew, was assigned to my care. Brenda started out by telling me that she would be my nurse for the shift and that she would make herself available to me for a one-on-one later in the day. When she came to speak with me, she said, "Let's talk about the elephant in the room, and then we can move into talking about how I can support you in getting well." We talked about my embarrassment and shame. I felt so relieved that she was willing to address my feelings about my mental illness. Over the next several weeks, we had many one-on-one sessions, and I was able to share my story with Brenda. Brenda helped me see that there was hope for my future and that I could learn to live well despite my diagnosis. I would love to say that I got well and stayed well, but actually, I have continued to struggle with my health. I can tell you that Brenda's acknowledgement of my feelings helped me deal with the stigma I felt about my illness. I no longer feel ashamed of having a mental illness.*

of "nervous breakdowns." In fact, the World Health Organization (WHO) (2009) maintains that a person cannot be considered healthy without taking into account mental as well as physical health. The WHO defines mental health as "a state of well-being in which each individual is able to realize his or her own potential, cope with the normal stresses of life, work productively and fruitfully, and make a contribution to the community" (World Health Organization, 2010). Our quality of life and our ability to enjoy life are enhanced by positive mental health and a sense of well-being (Mental Health Commission of Canada, 2009). Good mental health is associated with better physical health outcomes, improved educational attainment, increased economic participation, and rich social relationships

(Friedli & Parsonage, 2007). Mental health is described as more than merely the absence of mental disorders or disabilities (World Health Organization, 2010). The Public Health Agency of Canada (2003) offers the following definition of mental health: "the capacity of each and all of us to feel, think, and act in ways that enhance our ability to enjoy life and deal with the challenges we face. It is a positive sense of emotional and spiritual well-being that respects the importance of culture, equity, social justice, interconnections and personal dignity" (p. 2). Some of the attributes of positive mental health are presented in Figure 1-1.

Psychiatry's definition of *mental health* is continually evolving. It is shaped by the prevailing culture and societal values, and it reflects changes in cultural norms, society's expectations, and political climates. In the past, the term *mental illness* was applied to behaviours considered "strange" or "different"—behaviours that occurred infrequently and deviated from an established norm. Such criteria are inadequate because they suggest that mental health requires conformity. But there is a further problem in viewing people whose behaviour is unusual as mentally ill. Such a definition would mean nonconformists and independent thinkers like Abraham Lincoln, Mahatma Gandhi, and Socrates were mentally ill. And although the sacrifices of Mother Teresa or the dedication of Martin Luther King Jr. or Terry Fox is uncommon, virtually none of us would consider their much-admired behaviours to be signs of mental illness.

Alterations in cognition, mood, or behaviour that are coupled with significant distress and impaired functioning characterize mental illness (Health Canada, 2002). *Mental illness* refers to all mental disorders with definable diagnoses. Cognition may be impaired, as in Alzheimer's disease; mood may be affected, as in major depression; behaviour may change, as in schizophrenia; or a combination of the three types of symptoms may be apparent.

### Two Conceptualizations of Mental Health and Mental Illness

Published in 1988, *Mental Health for Canadians: Striking a Balance*, commonly called the "Epp Report," highlighted the importance of issues related to mental health and mental illness in Canada. It proposed seven guiding principles for the development of public policies to support mental health. Despite the forward thinking of this report, it was not until 2009 that Canada developed a mental health strategy framework (Mental Health Commission of Canada, 2009).

The Epp Report (1988) proposed two continua to depict the relationship between mental health and mental disorder. The Mental Disorder Continuum assigns one end point as maximal mental disorder while the opposite point is absence of mental disorder, allowing for a range of impairment and distress. For instance, a person with a severe clinical depression would be at the end point of maximal mental disorder, but as the depression subsided, he or she would move along the continuum toward absence of a mental disorder. The Mental Health Continuum assigns one pole as optimal mental health and the opposite pole as minimal mental health. On this scale, a person with optimal

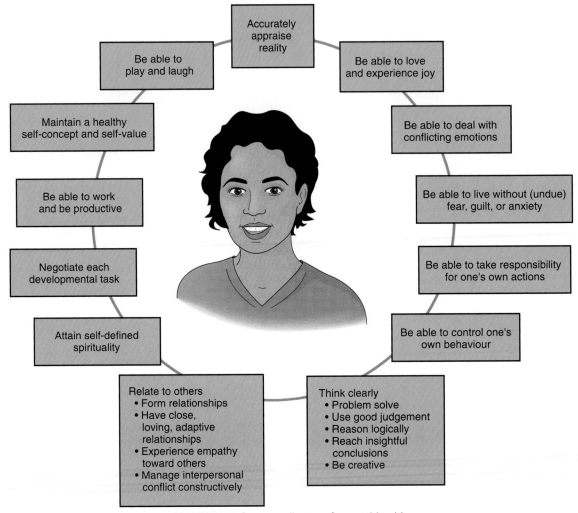

FIGURE 1-1 Some attributes of mental health.

mental health would demonstrate good coping skills and resilience when faced with stressors, and a person with minimal mental health may decompensate and not be able to cope with the stressors.

Considering the interaction between the continua suggested by Epp (see Figure 1-2) is interesting and could provide a basis for many research studies. For example, how can nurses increase health-related hardiness in people with schizophrenia?

This depiction of mental health and mental illness allows for four possible outcomes: (1) maximal mental disorder and optimal mental health; (2) optimal mental health and absence of mental disorder; (3) absence of mental disorder and minimal mental health; and (4) minimal mental health and maximal mental disorder. We will look at each outcome:

1. A person may have a severe mental disorder *and* optimal mental health. How could this be possible? Think of the person with a diagnosis of chronic schizophrenia who is stable on her medications, maintains contact with health care providers, has a social network, possibly works or volunteers, and follows a healthy diet and exercises. This person still has a mental disorder, yet she meets the criteria for optimal mental health.

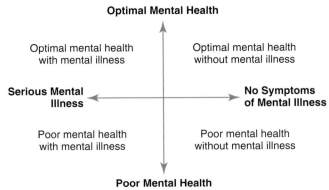

FIGURE 1-2 Continua from the "Epp Report." **Source:** Public Health Agency of Canada. (1988) *Mental health for Canadians: Striking a balance.* Reproduced with permission from the Minister of Health, 2013.

2. This quadrant is the one in which we would all like to be. Imagine a world with no mental illness and good mental health.

3. It is possible for a person to have poor coping skills and no resilience when faced with stressors and yet not have a mental disorder.

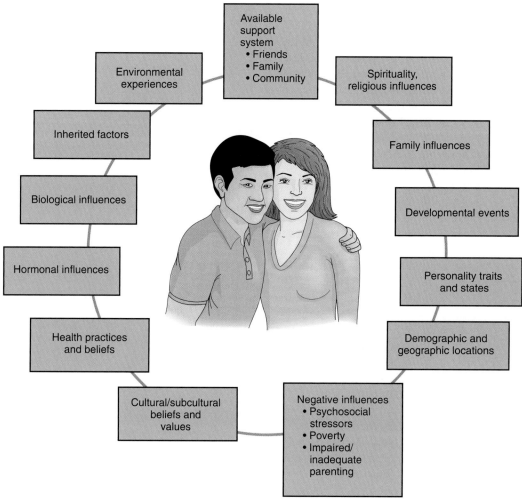

**FIGURE 1-3** Influences that can have an impact on an individual's mental health.

4. This quadrant is the one in which we would not like to be, yet many patients find themselves here. A person with borderline personality disorder would most likely be placed in this quadrant.

It is important to note it is possible to be anywhere along the continua, not just at one end.

## Contributing Factors

Many factors can affect the severity and progression of a mental illness, as well as the mental health of a person who does not have a mental illness (Figure 1-3). If possible, these influences need to be evaluated and factored into an individual's plan of care. In fact, the *Diagnostic and Statistical Manual of Mental Disorders, fifth edition (DSM-5)*, classifies around 350 mental disorders with evidence that suggests the symptoms and causes of a number of them are influenced by cultural and ethnic factors. The *DSM-5* is discussed in further detail later in this chapter.

## Resilience

Researchers, clinicians, and patients are all interested in actively facilitating mental health and reducing mental illness. A characteristic of mental health increasingly being promoted as essential to the recovery process is resilience. Canadian researcher Michael Ungar (2008) defines *resilience* as follows: "In the context of exposure to significant adversity, resilience is both the capacity of individuals to *navigate* their way to the psychological, social, cultural, and physical resources that sustain their well-being, and their capacity individually and collectively to *negotiate* for these resources to be provided in culturally meaningful ways" (p. 225). Ungar views resilience as a social construct that involves both a process and an outcome. Closely associated with the process of *adapting*, resilience helps people face tragedies, loss, trauma, and severe stress. We can see evidence of resilience in the wake of disasters such as the attack on the World Trade Center in 2001 and the 1998 airplane crash near Peggy's Cove, Nova Scotia. Being resilient does not mean being unaffected by stressors; rather, it means that instead of falling victim to negative emotions, resilient people recognize such feelings, readily deal with them, and learn from the experience.

Accessing and developing resilience assists people to recover from painful experiences and difficult events. It is characterized by optimism and a sense of mastery and competence. Research demonstrates that early experiences in mastering difficult or stressful situations enhance the prefrontal cortex's ability to cope with such situations later. According to Amat and colleagues (2006), when rats were exposed to uncontrollable stresses, their brains turned off mood-regulating cells, and they developed a syndrome much like major depression. However, rats that were given the chance to control a stressful situation were better able to respond to subsequent stress for up to a week following the success. In fact, when the successful rats were faced with uncontrollable stress, their brain cells responded as if they were in control.

You can get an idea of how good you are at regulating your emotions by taking the Resilience Factor Test in Box 1-1.

***Mental health recovery.*** According to the Substance Abuse and Mental Health Services Administration (SAMHSA) (2011), there are ten fundamental components of the recovery process:

1. Self-directed: Patients lead, control, exercise choice over, and determine their own path of recovery.
2. Individual- and person-centred: Recovery is based on unique strengths and resiliencies, as well as needs, preferences, experiences (including past trauma), and cultural backgrounds.
3. Empowering: Patients have the authority to choose from a range of options, participate in all decisions that will affect their lives, and be educated and supported in so doing.
4. Holistic: Recovery encompasses an individual's whole life, including mind, body, spirit, and community.
5. Nonlinear: Recovery is based on continual growth, occasional setbacks, and learning from experience.
6. Strengths-based: Recovery is focused on valuing and building on the multiple capacities, resiliencies, talents, coping abilities, and inherent worth of individuals.
7. Peer-supported: Patients encourage and engage with each other in recovery and provide a sense of belonging, supportive relationships, valued roles, and community.
8. Respect: Community, systems, and societal acceptance and appreciation of patients—including protecting their rights and eliminating discrimination and stigma—are crucial in achieving recovery.
9. Responsibility: Patients have a personal responsibility for their own self-care and recovery, for understanding and giving meaning to their experiences, and for identifying coping strategies and healing processes to promote their own wellness.
10. Hope: Recovery provides the essential motivating message of a better future: that people can and do overcome the barriers and obstacles that confront them. Hope is the catalyst of the recovery process.

---

**VIGNETTE**

Jeff is a mental health patient who has schizophrenia. Involvement in a recovery support group has changed his view of himself, and he has taken the lead role in his own recovery: "See, nobody knows your body better than you do, and some, maybe some mental health providers or doctors, think, 'Hey, I am the professional, and you're the person seeing me. I know what's best for you.' But technically, it isn't true. They only provide you with the tools to get better. They can't crawl inside you and see how you are."

---

## BOX 1-1   THE RESILIENCE FACTOR TEST

Use the following scale to rate each item listed below:
1 = Not true of me
2 = Sometimes true
3 = Moderately true
4 = Usually true
5 = Very true

1. Even if I plan ahead for a discussion with my spouse, my boss, or my child, I still find myself acting emotionally.
2. I am unable to harness positive emotions to help me focus on a task.
3. I can control the way I feel when adversity strikes.
4. I get carried away by my feelings.
5. I am good at identifying what I am thinking and how it affects my mood.
6. If someone does something that upsets me, I am able to wait until an appropriate time when I have calmed down to discuss it.
7. My emotions affect my ability to focus on what I need to get done at home, school, or work.
8. When I discuss a hot topic with a colleague or family member, I am able to keep my emotions in check.

| Add your score on the following items: | Add your score on the following items: |
|---|---|
| 3 _____ | 1 _____ |
| 5 _____ | 2 _____ |
| 6 _____ | 4 _____ |
| 8 _____ | 7 _____ |
| Positive total = _____ | Negative total = _____ |

Positive total minus negative total = _____

A score higher than 13 is rated as above average in emotional regulation.

A score between 6 and 13 is inconclusive.

A score lower than 6 is rated as below average in emotional regulation.

If your emotional regulation is below average, you may need to master some calming skills.

Here are a few tips:

- When anxiety strikes, your breathing may become shallow and quick. You can help control the anxiety by controlling your breathing. Inhale slowly through your nose, breathing deeply from your belly, not your chest. Exhale slowly with your lips pursed (as if whistling).
- Stress will make your body tight and stiff. Again, you can counter the effects of stress on the body and brain if you relax your muscles.
- Try positive imagery; create an image that is relaxing, such as visualizing yourself on a secluded beach.
- Resilience is within your reach.

**Source:** Excerpt from The Resilience Factor: Seven Essential Skills for Overcoming Life's Inevitable Obstacles by Karen Reivich, copyright © 2002 by Karen Reivich and Andrew Shatte. Used by permission of Broadway Books, an imprint of the Crown Publishing Group, a division of Random House LLC. All rights reserved. Any third party use of this material, outside of this publication, is prohibited. Interested parties must apply directly to Random House LLC for permission.

## Culture

There is no standard measure for mental health, in part because it is culturally defined and is based on interpretations of effective functioning according to societal norms (World Health Organization, 2007). One approach to differentiating mental health from mental illness is to consider what a particular culture regards as acceptable or unacceptable behaviour. In this view, mentally ill people are those who violate social norms and thus threaten (or make anxious) those observing them. For example, traditional Japanese may consider suicide to be an act of honour, and Middle Eastern "suicide bombers" are considered by some to be holy warriors or martyrs. Contrast these viewpoints with those in the West, where people who attempt or complete suicides are nearly always considered mentally ill.

Throughout history, people have interpreted health or sickness according to current views. A striking example of how cultural change influences the interpretation of mental illness is an old definition of *hysteria*. According to Webster's Dictionary (Porter, 1913), hysteria was "a nervous affection, occurring almost exclusively in women, in which the emotional and reflex excitability is exaggerated, and the will power correspondingly diminished, so that the patient loses control over the emotions, becomes the victim of imaginary sensations, and often falls into paroxysm or fits." Treatment for this condition often involved sexual outlets for afflicted women, whose condition was thought to be the result of sexual deprivation. According to some authors, this diagnosis fell into disuse as women gained rights, the family atmosphere became less restrictive, and societal tolerance of sexual practices increased.

Cultures differ not only in their views regarding mental illness but also in the types of behaviour categorized as mental illness. Culture-bound syndromes seem to occur in specific sociocultural contexts and are easily recognized by people in those cultures (Stern, Fricchione, Cassem, et al., 2010). For example, one syndrome recognized in parts of Southeast Asia is *running amok*, in which a person (usually a male) runs around engaging in furious, almost indiscriminate violent behaviour. *Pibloktoq*, an uncontrollable desire to tear off one's clothing and expose oneself to severe winter weather, is a recognized psychological disorder in parts of Greenland, Alaska, and the Arctic regions of Canada. In Canada, anorexia nervosa (see Chapter 17) is recognized as a psychobiological disorder that entails voluntary starvation. The disorder is well known in Europe, North America, and Australia but unheard of in many other parts of the world.

What is to be made of the fact that certain disorders occur in some cultures but are absent in others? One interpretation is that the conditions necessary for causing a particular disorder occur in some places but are absent in others. Another interpretation is that people learn certain kinds of abnormal behaviour by imitation. However, the fact that some disorders may be culturally determined does not prove that all mental illnesses are so determined. The best evidence suggests that schizophrenia (see Chapter 16) and bipolar disorders (see Chapter 15) are found throughout the world. The symptom patterns of schizophrenia have been observed among indigenous Greenlanders and West African villagers as well as in Western culture.

## Perceptions of Mental Health and Mental Illness

### Mental Illness Versus Physical Illness

People commonly make a distinction between mental illnesses and physical illnesses. It is an odd distinction, considering that *mental* refers to the brain, the most complex and sophisticated part of the body, the organ responsible for the higher thought processes that set us apart from other creatures. Surely the workings of the brain—the synaptic connections, the areas of functioning, the spinal innervations and connections—are *physical*. One problem with this distinction is that it implies that psychiatric disorders are "all in the head" and, therefore, under personal control and indistinguishable from a choice to indulge in bad behaviour. Although some physical disorders, such as a broken arm from skiing or lung cancer from smoking, are blamed on the victim, the majority of physical illnesses are considered to be beyond personal responsibility.

Perhaps the origin of this distinction between mental and physical illness lies in the religious and philosophical tradition of explaining the unexplainable by assigning a mystical or spiritual origin to cognitive processes and emotional activities. Despite many advances in understanding, mental illnesses continue to be viewed differently from illnesses that originate in other parts of the body.

Consider that people with epilepsy were once thought to be possessed by demons, under the attack of gods, or cursed; they were subjected to horrible "cures" and treatments. Today, most people would say that epilepsy is a disorder of the brain and not under one's personal control because epilepsy appears on brain scans as areas of overactivity and excitability. But there are no specific biological tests to diagnose most psychiatric disorders—for example, no blood test to diagnose obsessive-compulsive disorder (OCD). However, researchers are convinced that the root of most mental disorders lies in intercellular abnormalities, and they can now see clear signs of altered brain function in several mental disorders, including schizophrenia, OCD, stress disorders, and depression. Further details about these signs are discussed in Chapter 13.

### Nature Versus Nurture

For students learning about mental illness, one of its most intriguing aspects is its origins. Although for centuries people believed that extremely unusual behaviours were due to demonic forces, in the late 1800s, the mental health pendulum swung briefly to a biological focus with the "germ theory of diseases." Germ theory explained mental illness in the same way other illnesses were being described—that is, they were caused by a specific agent in the environment (Morgan, McKenzie, & Fearon, 2008). This theory was abandoned rather quickly since clinicians and researchers could not identify single causative factors for mental illnesses; there was no "mania germ" that could be viewed under a microscope and subsequently treated.

Although biological treatments for mental illness continued to be explored and ultimately dismissed as ineffective, over the next half century, psychological theories dominated and focused on the science of the mind and behaviour. These theories explained the origin of mental illness as faulty psychological processes that could be corrected by increasing personal insight and understanding. For example, a patient experiencing depression and apathy might be assisted to explore feelings left over from childhood, when his attempts at independence were harshly discouraged by overly protective parents.

This psychological focus was challenged in 1952, when chlorpromazine (Largactil) was found to have a calming effect on agitated, out-of-control patients. Imagine what this discovery must have been like for clinicians who had resorted to every biological treatment imaginable, including wet wraps, insulin shock therapy, and psychosurgery (in which holes were drilled in the head of a patient and probes inserted in the brain), in a futile attempt to change behaviour. Many began to believe that if psychiatric problems respond to medications that alter intercellular components, then the illness must be a disruption of intercellular components to begin with. At this point, the pendulum made steady and sure progress to a biological explanation of psychiatric problems and disorders.

Currently, the diathesis–stress model—in which diathesis represents biological predisposition, and stress represents environmental stress or trauma—is the most accepted explanation for mental illness. This nature-plus-nurture argument asserts that most psychiatric disorders result from a combination of genetic vulnerability and negative environmental stressors. While one person may develop major depressive disorder (MDD) largely as the result of an inherited and biological vulnerability that alters brain chemistry, another person with little vulnerability may develop depression from changes in brain chemistry caused by the insults of a stressful environment. MDD is discussed in Chapter 14.

### Social Influences on Mental Health Care
#### Self-Help Movement
In January 1918, the Canadian Mental Health Association (CMHA) was formed by Dr. Clarence M. Hincks and Clifford W. Beers to promote mental health. The CMHA is one of the oldest and most respected voluntary health organizations in Canada (Canadian Mental Health Association, Moose Jaw, n.d.). In the latter part of the twentieth century, the CMHA and other organizations and individuals expended tremendous energy on putting the notion of equality—treating people fairly and extinguishing stigmatizing labels—into widespread practice in Canada. In regard to mental illness, decades of institutionalization had created political and social concerns that gave rise to a mental health movement similar to the rights movements for women, people with disabilities, and the LGBT (lesbian, gay, bisexual, and transgender) communities. Groups of people with mental illnesses—or mental health patients—began to advocate for their rights and the rights of others with mental illness and to fight stigma, discrimination, and forced treatment.

#### Decade of the Brain
In 1990, President George H.W. Bush designated the last decade of the century the Decade of the Brain. This American initiative stimulated a worldwide growth of scientific research. Among the advances and progress made during the Decade of the Brain were the following:
- Understanding of the genetic basis of embryonic and fetal neural development

- Mapping of genes involved in neurological illness, including mutations associated with Parkinson's disease, Alzheimer's disease, and epilepsy
- Discovery that the brain uses a relatively small number of neurotransmitters but has a vast assortment of neurotransmitter receptors
- Uncovering of the role of cytokines (proteins involved in the immune response) in such brain disorders as depression
- Refinement of neuroimaging techniques, such as positron emission tomography (PET) scans, magnetic resonance imaging (MRI), magnetoencephalography, and event-related electroencephalography (EEG), which have improved our understanding of normal brain functioning, as well as areas of difference in pathological states
- Bringing together of computer modelling and laboratory research, which resulted in the new discipline of computational neuroscience.

### Mental Health for Canadians: Striking a Balance
*Mental Health for Canadians: Striking a Balance* (Epp, 1988) was one of the first government-generated reports that acknowledged the challenges of the mentally ill population. The purpose of the report was to assist Canadians engaged in developing and reviewing mental health–related policies and programs. Three challenges in mental health were identified: (1) reducing inequities, (2) increasing prevention, and (3) enhancing coping. These challenges continue. For example, recently, the Mental Health Commission of Canada (2012) identified similar challenges, which are reflected in its six strategic directions: (1) promoting mental health across the lifespan; (2) fostering recovery and well-being for people, while upholding their rights; (3) providing timely access to treatment and supports; (4) reducing disparities; (5) recognizing the distinct circumstances, rights, and cultures in addressing mental health needs of individuals and communities; and (6) ensuring effective leadership and collaboration across sectors, agencies, and communities.

### Human Genome Project
The Human Genome Project was a 13-year project (1990–2003) that was completed on the fiftieth anniversary of the discovery of the DNA double helix. The project has strengthened biological and genetic explanations for psychiatric conditions (Cohen, 2000). The goals of the project were to:
- Identify the approximately 20,000 to 25,000 genes in human DNA
- Determine the sequences of the three billion chemical base pairs that make up human DNA
- Store this information in databases
- Improve tools for data analysis
- Address the ethical, legal, and social issues that may arise from the project

Although researchers have begun to identify strong genetic links to mental illness (as you will see in the chapters on clinical disorders), it will be some time before we understand the exact nature of genetic influences on mental illness. What we do know is that most psychiatric disorders are the result of multiple mutated or defective genes, each of which in combination may contribute to the disorder.

### Changing Directions, Changing Lives: The Mental Health Strategy for Canada

In November 2009, the Mental Health Commission of Canada released a report titled *Toward Recovery & Well-Being: A Framework for a Mental Health Strategy for Canada*. Up to this time, Canada did not have a national plan for the development of a mental health strategy. Seven interconnected goals were identified to define what it would take to have a system oriented toward both enabling the recovery of people living with mental health problems and illnesses and fostering the mental health and well-being of everyone living in Canada (p. 19). This framework was the first phase in the development of a comprehensive Canadian mental health strategy. It put forward the vision and broad goals for the strategy that was released in 2012.

In May 2012, the Mental Health Commission of Canada released a report titled *Changing Directions, Changing Lives: The Mental Health Strategy for Canada*, which translated the visions described in *Toward Recovery & Well-Being* into recommendations for action. The aim of the strategy is to improve the mental health and well-being for all Canadians. Its authors strongly believe that we can create a mental health system that will meet the needs of people of all ages living with mental health problems and illnesses, and their families. Implementation of this strategy will help to ensure that people who experience mental health problems and illnesses, especially those with the most severe and complex ones, are treated with respect and dignity and enjoy the same rights as all Canadians. Six key strategic directions (see Box 1-2) were outlined in the report. Students are encouraged to access the full report to get an understanding of how health care providers, patients, families, and communities can work together to implement the strategies throughout Canada.

## EPIDEMIOLOGY OF MENTAL DISORDERS

Epidemiology, as it applies to psychiatric mental health, is the quantitative study of the distribution of mental disorders in human populations. Once the distribution of mental disorders has been determined quantitatively, epidemiologists can identify high-risk groups and high-risk factors associated with illness onset, duration, and recurrence. The further study of risk factors for mental illness may then lead to important clues about the causes of various mental disorders.

Two different but related words used in epidemiology are *incidence* and *prevalence*. Incidence refers to the *number of new cases* of mental disorders in a healthy population within a given period of time—for example, the number of Vancouver adolescents who were diagnosed with major depressive disorder between 2000 and 2012. Prevalence describes the *total number of cases*, new and existing, in a given population during a specific period of time, regardless of when the subjects became ill (e.g., the number of adolescents who screen positive for major depressive disorder in Toronto schools between 2000 and 2012). Each

---

### BOX 1-2 STRATEGIC DIRECTIONS IDENTIFIED IN CHANGING DIRECTIONS, CHANGING LIVES: THE MENTAL HEALTH STRATEGY FOR CANADA

**Strategic Direction 1: Promotion and Prevention**
Promote mental health across the lifespan in homes, schools, and workplaces, and prevent mental illness and suicide wherever possible. Reducing the impact of mental health problems and illnesses and improving the mental health of the population require promotion and prevention efforts in everyday settings where the potential impact is greatest.

**Strategic Direction 2: Recovery and Rights**
Foster recovery and well-being for people of all ages living with mental health problems and illnesses, and uphold their rights. The key to recovery is helping people to find the right combination of services, treatments, and supports, and eliminating discrimination by removing barriers to full participation in work, education, and community life.

**Strategic Direction 3: Access to Services**
Provide access to the right combination of services, treatments, and supports, when and where people need them. A full range of services, treatments, and supports includes primary health care, community-based and specialized mental health services, peer support, and supported housing, education, and employment.

**Strategic Direction 4: Disparities and Diversity**
Reduce disparities in risk factors and access to mental health services, and strengthen the response to the needs of diverse communities and Northerners. Mental health should be taken into account when acting to improve overall living conditions and addressing the specific needs of groups such as new Canadians and people in northern and remote communities.

**Strategic Direction 5: First Nations, Inuit, and Métis**
Work with First Nations, Inuit, and Métis to address their mental health needs, acknowledging their distinct circumstances, rights, and cultures. By calling for access to a full continuum of culturally safe mental health services, the *Mental Health Strategy for Canada* can contribute to truth, reconciliation, and healing from intergenerational trauma.

**Strategic Direction 6: Leadership and Collaboration**
Mobilize leadership, improve knowledge, and foster collaboration at all levels. Change will not be possible without a whole-of-government approach to mental health policy, without fostering the leadership roles of people living with mental health problems and illnesses, and their families, and without building strong infrastructure to support data collection, research, and human resource development.

**Source:** The Mental Health Commission of Canada. (2012). *Changing directions, changing lives: The mental health strategy for Canada.* Retrieved from strategy.mentalhealthcommission.ca/pdf/strategy-images-en.pdf.

level of investigation supplies information that can be used to improve clinical practice and plan public-health policies.

*A Report on Mental Illnesses in Canada*, a collaborative effort published in 2002, describes the major mental illnesses and reports their incidence and prevalence. The report includes the illness with the highest prevalence rate and greatest impact on individual health, society, and the health care system economics. Select highlights from the overview of the report include the following (Jacobs, Dewa, Lesage, et al., 2010):

- "Mental illnesses indirectly affect all Canadians through illness in a family member, friend, or colleague."
- "Twenty percent of Canadians will personally experience a mental illness during their lifetime."
- "Mental illnesses affect people of all ages, educational and income levels, and cultures."
- "Mental illnesses are costly to the individual, the family, the health care system, and the community."

Many individuals have more than one mental disorder at a time; this state is known as a co-morbid condition.

Some disorders may have a high incidence but a low prevalence and vice versa. A disease with a short duration, such as the common cold, tends to have a high incidence (many new cases in a given year) and a low prevalence (not many people suffering from a cold at any given time). Conversely, a chronic disease such as diabetes will have a low incidence, because a year (or whatever time increment is employed) after diagnosis, the person will be dropped from the list of new cases. Lifetime risk data, or the risk that one will develop a disease in the course of his or her lifetime, will be higher than both incidence and prevalence. Table 1-1 shows the prevalence of some psychiatric disorders in Canada.

Clinical epidemiology is a broad field that addresses what happens after people with illnesses are seen by clinical care providers. Using traditional epidemiological methods, studies are

### TABLE 1-1   PREVALENCE OF PSYCHIATRIC DISORDERS IN CANADA (OVER 12 MONTHS)

| DISORDER | PREVALENCE OVER 12 MONTHS (%) | COMMENTS |
|---|---|---|
| Schizophrenia | 0.2–2%; the accepted estimate is 1% at best | Affects men and women equally; onset is usually in early adulthood; about 52% of hospitalizations are for adults aged 25–44 years of age |
| **Mood Disorders** | | Leading cause of disability in Canada and established economies worldwide |
| Major (unipolar) depression (MDD) | 4.1–4.6% | Approximately 8% of adults will experience major depression at some time in their lives |
| Bipolar disorder | 0.2–0.6% | |
| Dysthymia | 0.8–3.1% | |
| Generalized anxiety disorder | 1.1% | Can begin across life cycle; risk is highest between childhood and middle age |
| Panic disorder | 0.7% | Typically develops in adolescence or early adulthood |
| Obsessive-compulsive disorder (OCD) | 1.8% | Symptoms begin in childhood or adolescence |
| Post-traumatic stress disorder (PTSD) | Canadian data unavailable | Can develop at any time |
| Social phobia | 7% | Typically begins in childhood or adolescence |
| Specific phobia | 8.7% | Begins in childhood |
| Personality disorders | Canadian data unavailable; US data suggests 6–9% | Symptoms typically begin in adolescence or early adulthood |
| **Eating Disorders** Anorexia | 0.7 % (women) 0.2% (men) | Approximately 3% of women will be affected by an eating disorder in their lifetime |
| Bulimia | 1.5% (women) 0.1 % (men) | |
| **Other** Suicidal behaviour (not classified as a mental illness but has significant impact) | In 1998, 3699 Canadians died as a result of suicide (Health Canada, 2002) | Suicide accounts for 24% of all deaths among 15- to 24-year-olds and 16% among 25- to 44-year-olds |

**Source:** Health Canada. (2002). *A report on mental illnesses in Canada.* Reproduced with permission from the Minister of Health, 2013.

conducted in groups usually defined by the illness or symptoms or by diagnostic procedures or treatments given to address the illness or symptoms. Clinical epidemiology includes the following:

- Studies of the natural history of an illness
- Studies of diagnostic screening tests
- Observational and experimental studies of interventions used to treat people with the illness or symptoms

Results of epidemiological studies are now routinely included in the *Diagnostic and Statistical Manual of Mental Disorders* (discussed below) to describe the frequency of mental disorders. Analysis of such studies can reveal the frequency with which psychological symptoms appear together with physical illness. For example, epidemiological studies demonstrate that depression is a significant risk factor for death in people with cardiovascular disease and for premature death in people with breast cancer.

## CLASSIFICATION OF MENTAL DISORDERS

### The Diagnostic and Statistical Manual

The first *Diagnostic and Statistical Manual of Mental Disorders* (*DSM*) was published by the American Psychiatric Association in 1952. Its purpose was to provide clinicians, educators, and researchers with a common framework to understand and communicate about mental disorders. With a common understanding about mental disorders, researchers and clinicians could work together in their attempts to improve care for people with mental illness.

Today, its fifth edition, the *DSM-5*, serves as the official guide for diagnosing psychiatric disorders. Listing over 350 diagnoses, this authoritative manual was influenced by psychiatrists, psychologists, licensed clinical social workers, licensed counsellors, licensed marriage and family therapists, and advanced-practice psychiatric mental health nurses. Consistent with the purposes of previous editions, the *DSM-5* also serves as a tool for collecting epidemiological statistics about the diagnosis of psychiatric disorders.

A common misconception is that a classification of mental disorders classifies *people*, when actually the *DSM-5* classifies *disorders* people have. For this reason, the *DSM-5* and this textbook avoid the use of expressions such as "a schizophrenic" or "an alcoholic." Viewing the person as a person and not an illness requires more accurate terms such as "an individual with schizophrenia" or "my patient has major depression."

### The DSM-5 Organizational Structure

The *DSM-5* (American Psychiatric Association, 2013) organizes diagnoses for psychiatric disorders on a developmental hierarchy, meaning that disorders that are usually seen in infancy, childhood, and adolescence are listed in the first chapter and neurodevelopmental disorders and disorders that occur later in life, such as the neurocognitive disorders, are further down the list. Also, within each chapter, specific disorders are listed based on the typical age of onset, from youngest to oldest. Diagnostic groups that are related to one another have been closely situated (for example, schizophrenia spectrum disorders are next to bipolar-related disorders, and feeding and eating disorders are next to elimination disorders).

Neurodevelopmental disorder
Schizophrenia spectrum disorder
Bipolar and related disorders
Depressive disorders
Anxiety disorders
Obsessive-compulsive disorders
Trauma and stressor disorders
Dissociative disorders
Somatic symptom disorders
Feeding and eating disorders
Elimination disorders
Sleep–wake disorders
Sexual dysfunctions
Gender dysphoria
Disruptive, impulse control, and conduct disorders
Substance and addictive disorders
Neurocognitive disorders
Personality disorders
Paraphilias
Other disorders

When making a diagnosis based on the *DSM-5*, clinicians and researchers need to consider presenting symptoms and how these symptoms are impacting the patient's life. Assessing the impact that the mental disorder is having on a person's day-to-day functioning requires the Disability Assessment Schedule II, a tool developed by the World Health Organization (see http://www.who.int/classifications/icf/whodasii/en/).

### The *ICD-10-CA*

The *International Classification of Diseases* (ICD) (World Health Organization, 2011) sets the global health information standard for mortality and morbidity statistics. Clinicians and researchers use this classification system to define diseases, study disease patterns, monitor outcomes and subsequently allocate resources based on the prevalence of disease. The *ICD* is used globally and has been translated into 43 different languages. An eleventh revision is expected in 2015.

The Canadian Institute for Health Information developed an enhanced version of the *ICD-10*, referred to as the *ICD-10-CA*. The *ICD-10-CA* goes beyond defining and classifying diseases to describe conditions and situations that are not diseases, including, for example, risk factors to health and psychosocial circumstances. Also, the *ICD-10-CA* better represents the social determinants of health than the *ICD-10* did. It has 23 different categories of diseases including diseases of the circulatory system, diseases of the nervous system, mental and behavioural disorders, certain conditions originating in the perinatal period, and factors influencing health status and contact with health services (Canadian Institute for Health Information, 2001). A complete listing of all the *ICD-10-CA* chapters can be found at http://www.cihi.ca/CIHI-ext-portal/internet/en/document/standards+and+data+submission/standards/classification+and+coding/codingclass_icd10head.

## PSYCHIATRIC MENTAL HEALTH NURSING

In all clinical settings, nurses work with people who are going through crises, including physical, psychological, mental, and spiritual distress. You will encounter patients who are experiencing feelings of hopelessness, helplessness, anxiety, anger, low self-esteem, or confusion. You will meet people who are withdrawn, suspicious, elated, depressed, hostile, manipulative, suicidal, intoxicated, or withdrawing from a substance. Many of you have already come across people who are going through difficult times in their lives. You may have handled these situations skillfully, but at other times, you may have wished you had additional skills and knowledge. Basic psychosocial nursing concepts will become central to your practice of nursing and increase your competency as a practitioner in all clinical settings. Whatever setting you choose to work in, you will have the opportunity to improve the lives of people who are experiencing mental illness as an additional challenge to their health.

Your experience in the mental health nursing rotation can help you gain insight into yourself and greatly increase your insight into the experiences of others. This part of your nursing education can also give you guidelines for and the opportunity to learn new skills for dealing with a variety of challenging behaviours. The following sections of this chapter present a brief overview of the work of professional psychiatric nurses, their scope of practice, and the challenges and evolving roles in the future health care environment.

## What Is Psychiatric Mental Health Nursing?

Psychiatric mental health nurses enrich the health and well-being of Canadians (Canadian Federation of Mental Health Nurses, 2006). They work with people throughout the lifespan and assist healthy people who are in crisis or who are experiencing life problems, as well as those with long-term mental illness. Their patients may include people with concurrent disorders (i.e., a mental disorder and a coexisting substance disorder), homeless people and families, people in jail, individuals who have survived abusive situations, and people in crisis. Psychiatric mental health nurses work with individuals, couples, families, and groups in every nursing setting: in hospitals, in patients' homes, in halfway houses, in shelters, in clinics, in storefronts, on the street—virtually everywhere.

Uniquely, Canada has two bodies that provide standards of practice for mental health nursing. In the four western provinces and the Yukon, registered psychiatric nurses follow the standards of practice issued by the Registered Psychiatric Nurses of Canada (RPNC). Registered nurses working in the specialty area of psychiatric mental health nursing follow the standards of practice issued by the Canadian Federation of Mental Health Nurses (CFMHN), an associate group of the Canadian Nurses Association (CNA).

## Classification of Nursing Diagnoses, Outcomes, and Interventions

To provide the most appropriate and scientifically sound care, the psychiatric mental health nurse uses standardized classification systems developed by professional nursing groups. The *Nursing Diagnoses: Definitions and Classification 2012–2014* of the North American Nursing Diagnosis Association International (NANDA-I) (Herdman, 2012) provides 216 standardized

diagnoses, more than 40% of which are related to psychosocial/psychiatric nursing care. These diagnoses provide a common language to aid in the selection of nursing interventions and ultimately lead to positive outcome achievement.

### DSM-5– and NANDA-I–Approved Nursing Diagnoses

A nursing diagnosis is "a clinical judgment about individual, family, or community responses to actual or potential health problems and life processes" (Herdman, 2012, p. 515). A well-defined nursing diagnosis provides the framework for setting priorities and identifying appropriate nursing interventions for dealing with the patient's reaction to the disorder. Those reactions might include confusion, low self-esteem, impaired ability to function in job or family situations, and so on, differing from the diagnoses that are made based on the criteria contained within the *DSM-5* that are used to label the patient's disorder.

Appendix B lists NANDA-I–approved nursing diagnoses, and the individual clinical chapters offer suggestions for potential nursing diagnoses for the behaviours and phenomena often encountered in association with specific disorders.

### Nursing Outcomes Classification (NOC)

The *Nursing Outcomes Classification (NOC)* provides "a comprehensive list of standardized outcomes, definitions, and measures to describe client outcomes influenced by nursing practice" (Moorhead, Johnson, Maas, et al., 2013, p. xx). Outcomes are organized into seven domains: functional health, physiologic health, psychosocial health, health knowledge and behaviour, perceived health, family health, and community health. The psychosocial health domain, which this text is most concerned with, includes four classes: psychological well-being, psychosocial adaptation, self-control, and social interaction.

### Nursing Interventions Classification (NIC)

The *Nursing Interventions Classification (NIC)* is another tool used to standardize, define, and measure nursing care. Bulechek and colleagues (2008) define a nursing intervention as "any treatment, based upon clinical judgment and knowledge, that a nurse performs to enhance patient/client outcomes" (p. xxi), including direct and indirect care through a series of nursing activities. There are seven domains: basic physiological, complex physiological, behavioural, safety, family, health system, and community. Two domains relate specifically to psychiatric nursing: behavioural, including communication, coping, and education; and safety, covering crisis and risk management.

### Evidence-Informed Practice

The nursing diagnosis classification systems mentioned have been extensively researched by nurses across a variety of treatment settings. They form a foundation for the novice or experienced nurse to participate in evidence-informed practice—that is, care based on the collection, interpretation and integration of valid, important, and applicable patient-reported, clinician-observed, and research-derived evidence. In the chapters that follow, you will see examples of the application of these classifications to specific patients in vignettes and case studies, along with brief descriptions of other relevant research in the Research Highlight boxes.

## Levels of Psychiatric Mental Health Clinical Nursing Practice

Registered nurses in Canada may choose to work in psychiatric mental health nursing settings without additional certifications. However, many will choose to write the Canadian Nurses Association's psychiatric/mental health nursing certification exam for the specialty. Registered psychiatric nurses (in the western provinces and Yukon) write national registration examinations.

Registered nurses and registered psychiatric nurses can further their education at a baccalaureate level or at the graduate level (master's, doctorate) and can become qualified to practise psychiatric mental health nursing at two levels—basic and advanced—depending on their educational preparation. Table 1-2 describes basic and advanced psychiatric nursing interventions.

## Future Challenges and Roles for Psychiatric Mental Health Nurses

There has been a great demand for psychiatric mental health nurses, and indications suggest this need will increase in the future. Four significant trends that will affect the future of psychiatric mental health nursing in Canada are the aging population, increasing cultural diversity, expanding technology, and an increased awareness of the impact of health determinants on mental illness.

## Aging Population

As the population of older adults grows, the prevalence of Alzheimer's disease and other dementias requiring the support of skilled and knowledgeable nurses will increase. Healthier older adults will need more services at home, in retirement communities, or in assisted-living facilities. For more information on the needs of older adults, refer to Chapters 18, 27, and 30.

## Increasing Cultural Diversity

Cultural diversity is steadily increasing in Canada. Recent immigrants represent about 16% of Canada's population (Ali, 2002). These new Canadians add to and form an important part of our social, cultural, and economic institutions. Potential immigrants to Canada are required to undergo health screening; those who do not meet the requirements for health are denied entry to the country. It is important for nurses to know how immigrants may be impacted by a mental illness. In the report *Mental Health of Canada's Immigrants* (Ali, 2002), cases of depression and alcohol dependence were examined and compared between immigrant and Canadian-born populations. The rate of depression in the Canadian-born population was 2.5%, compared to 6.2% for immigrants. Immigrants, however, had lower rates of alcohol dependence: 0.5%, compared to 2.5% for the Canadian-born population. The gap between the two groups increased for more recent immigrants than for those who had arrived earlier to Canada. Rates of depression and alcohol dependence for immigrants living in Canada for 10 to 14 years were on par with those of the Canadian-born population. Going forward, psychiatric mental health nurses will need

| TABLE 1-2 | BASIC-LEVEL AND ADVANCED-PRACTICE PSYCHIATRIC MENTAL HEALTH NURSING INTERVENTIONS | |
|---|---|
| **BASIC-LEVEL INTERVENTION** | **DESCRIPTION** |
| Coordination of care | Coordinates implementation of the nursing care plan and documents coordination of care |
| Health teaching and health maintenance | Provides individualized anticipatory guidance to prevent or reduce mental illness or enhance mental health (e.g., community screenings, parenting classes, stress management) |
| Milieu therapy | Provides, structures, and maintains a safe and therapeutic environment in collaboration with patients, families, and other health care clinicians |
| Pharmacological, biological, and integrative therapies | Applies current knowledge to assessing patients' response to medication; provides medication teaching; and communicates observations to other members of the health care team |
| **ADVANCED-PRACTICE INTERVENTION** | **DESCRIPTION** |
| *All of the above plus:* Medication prescription and treatment | Prescribes psychotropic medications, with appropriate use of diagnostic tests; has hospital admitting privileges |
| Psychotherapy | Provides individual, couple, group, or family therapy using evidence-informed therapeutic frameworks |
| Consultation | Shares clinical expertise with nurses or those in other disciplines to enhance their treatment of patients or address systems issues |

**Source:** Adapted from American Psychiatric Nurses Association, International Society of Psychiatric-Mental Health Nurses, & American Nurses Association. (2007). *Psychiatric-mental health nursing: Scope and standards of practice.* Silver Spring, MD: NurseBooks.org.

to increase their cultural competence—that is, their sensitivity to different cultural views regarding health, illness, and response to treatment.

## Expanding Technology

Genetic mapping from the Human Genome Project has resulted in a steady stream of research discoveries concerning genetic markers implicated in a variety of psychiatric illnesses. This information could be helpful in identifying at-risk individuals and in targeting medications specific to certain genetic variants and profiles. However, the legal and ethical implications of responsibly using this technology are staggering and generate questions such as:

- Would you want to know you were at risk for a psychiatric illness like bipolar disorder?
- Who should have access to this information—your primary care provider, future spouse, a lawyer in a child-custody battle?
- Who will regulate genetic testing centres to protect privacy and prevent twenty-first-century problems like identity theft and fraud?

Despite these concerns, the next decade holds great promise in the diagnosis and treatment of psychiatric disorders, and nurses will be central as educators and caregivers.

Scientific advances through research and technology are certain to shape psychiatric mental health nursing practice. Magnetic resonance imaging (MRI) research, in addition to comparing healthy people to people diagnosed with mental illness, is now focusing on the development of preclinical profiles of children and adolescents. The hope of this type of research is to be able to identify people at risk for developing mental illness, thereby allowing earlier interventions to try to decrease impairment.

Electronic health care services provided from a distance are gaining wide acceptance. In the early days of the Internet, patients were cautioned against the questionable wisdom of seeking advice through an unregulated medium. However, the Internet has transformed the way we approach our health care needs. It is used liberally by young and old alike, and men in particular seem to feel more comfortable researching online than seeking care in person (Ybarra & Suman, 2006). The Internet has empowered people to advocate for themselves and explore health problems and options related to treatment.

In an attempt to reach the population in rural and remote districts (25% of the population), Canada has been involved in the development of telepsychiatry (Urness, Weisser, Campbell, et al., 2003). Through the use of telepsychiatry, the mental health needs of these populations can be met with timely professional assessments and prescribed interventions.

## Twelve Key Social Determinants of Health

Psychiatric mental health nurses use the social determinants of health to facilitate their practice. An ever-increasing body of evidence that addresses what Canadians need to be healthy suggests that spending more on the treatment of illness and disease will not actually improve a person's health (Public Health Agency of Canada, 2003). Rather, it is suggested that factors such as income, social status, and education directly impact the health of individual Canadians. Psychiatric mental health nurses will be required to address patient needs related to disease prevention and health promotion, which are identified through the assessment of the social determinants of health. Twelve key social determinants of health have been identified. Each stands alone but is at the same time closely linked to the other determinants of health. The 12 determinants are as follows:

1. Income and social status
2. Social support networks
3. Education
4. Employment/working conditions
5. Social environments
6. Physical environments
7. Personal health practices and coping skills
8. Healthy child development
9. Biology and genetic endowment
10. Health services
11. Gender
12. Culture

For a brief explanation of each health determinant, see "Key Determinants" (Public Health Agency of Canada, 2003) at http://www.phac-aspc.gc.ca/ph-sp/determinants/index-eng.php#determinants.

## ■ KEY POINTS TO REMEMBER

- Resilience is a personal characteristic that aids people to recognize stressors and negative emotions, deal with them, and learn from the experience. This trait can be promoted and improved to strengthen patients' responses to stress.
- Mental health and mental illness exist along two distinct but intersecting continua.
- Culture influences behaviour, and symptoms may reflect a person's cultural patterns or beliefs. Symptoms, therefore, must be understood in terms of a person's cultural background.
- The study of epidemiology can help identify high-risk groups and behaviours, which can lead to a better understanding of the causes of some disorders. Incidence rates provide us with the number of new cases in a given period of time. Prevalence rates help us to identify the proportion of a population experiencing a specific mental disorder at a given time.
- Co-morbid conditions are those disorders that occur at the same time as another condition. For example, a person with schizophrenia may also have co-morbid diabetes, depression, and hypertension.
- Psychiatric mental health nurses work with a broad population of patients in diverse settings to promote optimal mental health.
- Due to social, cultural, scientific, and political factors, the future holds many challenges and possibilities for the psychiatric mental health nurse.

# CRITICAL THINKING

1. Amir, a 19-year-old first-year university student with a grade point average of 3.4, is brought to the emergency department after a suicide attempt. He has been extremely depressed since the death of his girlfriend five months previously, when the car he was driving crashed. His parents are devastated. They believe taking one's own life prevents a person from going to heaven. Amir has epilepsy and has had more seizures since the auto accident. He says he should be punished for his carelessness and does not care what happens to him. Over the past month, he has not been to school or shown up for his part-time job tutoring children in reading.
   a. What might be a possible NANDA nursing diagnosis for Amir? Before you plan your care, what are some other factors you would like to assess regarding aspects of Amir's overall health and other influences that can affect his mental health?
   b. Do you think that an antidepressant could help Amir through the grieving process? Why or why not? What additional care do you think Amir needs?
   c. Formulate at least two potential nursing interventions for Amir.
   d. Would the religious beliefs of Amir's parents factor into your plan of care? If so, how?

2. In a small study group, share experiences you have had with others from unfamiliar cultural, ethnic, religious, or racial backgrounds, and identify two positive learning experiences from these encounters.

3. Consider what it would be like working with a group of healthy women preparing for parenthood versus working with a group of depressed women in a mental health clinic. What do you feel are the advantages and disadvantages of working with each group?

4. Would you feel comfortable referring a family member to a mental health clinician? What factors make you feel that way?

5. How do basic-level and advanced-practice psychiatric mental health nurses work together to provide the highest quality of care?

6. Would you consider joining a professional group or advocacy group that promotes mental health? Why or why not?

# CHAPTER REVIEW

1. Resilience, the capacity to rebound from stressors via adaptive coping, is associated with positive mental health. Your friend has just been laid off from his job. Which of the following responses on your part would most likely contribute to his enhanced resilience?
   1. Using your connections to set up an interview with your employer
   2. Connecting him with a friend of the family who owns his own business
   3. Supporting him in arranging, preparing for, and completing multiple interviews
   4. Helping him to understand that the layoff resulted from troubles in the economy and is not his fault

2. Which of the following situations best supports the diathesis–stress model of mental illness development?
   1. The rate of suicide increases during times of national disaster and despair.
   2. A woman feels mildly anxious when asked to speak to a large group of people.
   3. A man with no prior mental health problems experiences sadness after his divorce.
   4. A man develops schizophrenia, but his identical twin remains free of mental illness.

3. Of the following statements about mental illness, identify all of the correct ones:
   1. About 20% of Canadians experience a mental disorder during their lifetime.
   2. Mental disorders and diagnoses occur very consistently across cultures.
   3. Most serious mental illnesses are psychological rather than biological in nature.
   4. The Mental Health Commission report *Changing Directions, Changing Lives* outlines the mental health strategy for Canada.

4. Jane is a 32-year-old mother of four. She is active with her family and in her community despite having a diagnosis of severe anxiety. Refer to the mental health/illness continuum shown in Figure 1-2 and consider where you would place Jane.
   1. Optimal mental health with mental illness
   2. Optimal mental health without mental illness
   3. Poor mental health with mental illness
   4. Poor mental health without mental illness

5. Which of the following actions represent the primary focus of psychiatric nursing for a basic-level registered nurse? Select all that apply.
   1. Determining a patient's diagnosis according to the *DSM-5*
   2. Ordering diagnostic tests such as EEGs or CT or MRI scans
   3. Identifying how a patient is coping with a symptom such as hallucinations
   4. Guiding a patient to learn and use a variety of stress-management techniques
   5. Helping a patient without personal transportation find a way to his or her treatment appointments
   6. Collecting petition signatures seeking the removal of stigmatizing images on television

# ⊖volve WEBSITE

Post-Test interactive review

*Visit the Evolve Web site for Chapter Review Answers and Rationales, Critical Thinking Answer Guidelines, and additional resources related to the content in this chapter:* http://evolve.elsevier.com/Canada/Varcarolis/psychiatric/

## REFERENCES

Ali, J. (2002). *Mental health of Canada's immigrants* (Catalogue 82-003) [Supplemental material]. *Health Reports, 13,* 1–12. Retrieved from http://www.statcan.gc.ca/pub/82-003-s/2002001/pdf/82-003-s2002006-eng.pdf.

Amat, J., Paul, E., Zarza, C., et al. (2006). Previous experience with behavioral control over stress blocks the behavioral and dorsal raphe nucleus activating effects of later uncontrollable stress: Role of the ventral medial prefrontal cortex. *Journal of Neuroscience, 26,* 13264–13272. doi:10.1523/JNEUROSCI.3630-06.2006.

Bulechek, G.M., Butcher, H.K., & Dochterman, J.M. (Eds.), (2008). *Nursing interventions classification (NIC)*. St. Louis, MO: Mosby.

Canadian Federation of Mental Health Nurses. (2006). *Standards of practice: Canadian standards for psychiatric-mental health nursing* (3rd ed.). Toronto: Author. Retrieved from http://cfmhn.ca/sites/cfmhn.ca/files/CFMHN%20standards%201.pdf.

Canadian Institute for Health Information. (2001). *Final report: The Canadian enhancement of ICD-10 (international statistical classification of diseases and related health problems, tenth revision)*. Ottawa: Author.

Canadian Mental Health Association, Moose Jaw. (n.d.). Retrieved from http://www.cmhamj.com/.

Cohen, J.I. (2000). Stress and mental health: A biobehavioural perspective. *Issues in Mental Health Nursing, 21,* 185–202. doi:10.1080/016128400248185.

Epp, J. (1988). *Mental health for Canadians: Striking a balance*. Ottawa: Minister of National Health and Welfare.

Friedli, L., & Parsonage, M. (2007). *Mental health promotion: Building an economic case*. Belfast, UK: Northern Ireland Association for Mental Health.

Health Canada. (2002). *A report on mental illnesses in Canada* (Cat. No. 0-662-32817-5). Ottawa: Health Canada Editorial Board Mental Illnesses in Canada.

Herdman, T.H. (Ed.), (2012). *NANDA International nursing diagnoses: Definitions and classification, 2012–2014*. Oxford, UK: Wiley-Blackwell.

Jacobs, P., Dewa, C., Lesage, A., et al. (2010). *The cost of mental health and substance abuse services in Canada*. Edmonton: Institute of Health Economics. Retrieved from http://www.ihe.ca/documents/Cost%20of%20Mental%20Health%20Services%20in%20Canada%20Report%20June%202010.pdf.

Mental Health Commission of Canada. (2009). *Toward recovery & well-being: A framework for a mental health strategy for Canada*. Retrieved from http://www.mentalhealthcommission.ca/SiteCollectionDocuments/boarddocs/15507_MHCC_EN_final.pdf.

Mental Health Commission of Canada. (2012). *Changing directions, changing lives: The mental health strategy for Canada*. Retrieved from strategy.mentalhealthcommission.ca/pdf/strategy-images-en.pdf.

Moorhead, S., Johnson, M., Maas, M.L., et al. (Eds.), (2013). *Nursing outcomes classification (NOC)*. St. Louis, MO: Mosby.

Morgan, C., McKenzie, K., & Fearon, P. (2008). *Society and psychosis*. London: Cambridge.

Porter, N. (Ed.), (1913). *Webster's revised unabridged dictionary*. Boston: Merriam.

Public Health Agency of Canada. (2003). *Determinants of health: What makes Canadians healthy or unhealthy*. Ottawa: Author. Retrieved from http://www.phac-aspc.gc.ca/ph-sp/determinants/index-eng.php#determinants.

Stern, T.A., Fricchione, G.L., Cassem, N.H., et al. (2010). *Handbook of general hospital psychiatry* (6th ed.). Philadelphia: Saunders.

Substance Abuse and Mental Health Services Administration. (2011). *Recovery support*. Retrieved from http://www.samhsa.gov/recovery/.

Ungar, M. (2008). Resilience across cultures. *British Journal of Social Work, 38,* 218–235. doi:10.1093/bjsw/bcl343.

Urness, D., Weisser, L., Campbell, R., et al. (2003). Telepsychiatry in Canada and the United States. In R. Wootton & P.Y. McLaren (Eds.), *Telepsychiatry and e-mental health* (pp. 97–111). London, UK: Royal Society of Medicine Press Ltd. Retrieved from http://www.medicine.mcgill.ca/ruis/Docs/telesante/Telepsychiatry_in_Canada_and_the_United_States.pdf.

World Health Organization. (2007). *International statistical classification of diseases and related health problems (10th rev.) (ICD-10)*. Geneva: Author.

World Health Organization. (2009). *Mental health: A state of well-being*. Retrieved from http://www.who.int/features/factfiles/mental_health/en/index.html.

World Health Organization. (2010). *Mental health: Strengthening our response* (Fact sheet no. 220). Retrieved from http://www.who.int/mediacentre/factsheets/fs220/en/index.html.

World Health Organization. (2011). *ICD 10: International statistical classification of diseases and related health problems (10th rev.). Instruction manual (vol. 2)*. Geneva, Switzerland: Author. Retrieved from http://www.who.int/classifications/icd/ICD10Volume2_en_2010.pdfs.

Ybarra, M., & Suman, M. (2006). Reasons, assessments, and actions taken: Sex and age differences in uses of Internet health information. *Health Education Research, 23,* 512–521. doi:10.1093/her/cyl062.

# Historical Overview of Psychiatric Mental Health Nursing

*Holly Symonds-Brown*

## KEY TERMS AND CONCEPTS

advanced-practice nursing (APN), 22

asylums, 17

Canadian Federation of Mental Health Nurses, 22

custodial care, 18

deinstitutionalization, 21

Dorothea Dix, 18

moral treatment, 18

Philippe Pinel, 18

Registered Psychiatric Nurses of Canada, 22

Weir Report, 20

William Tuke, 18

## OBJECTIVES

1. Identify the sociopolitical, economic, cultural, and religious factors that influenced the development of psychiatric mental health nursing.
2. Summarize the influence of psychiatric treatment trends on the role of the nurse.
3. Identify the factors that led to the separate designations of registered nurse and registered psychiatric nurse.
4. Analyze the factors that have enhanced and delayed the professionalization of psychiatric mental health nursing.
5. Consider the future potentials and challenges for psychiatric mental health nursing in Canada.

## ⊖volve WEBSITE

*Visit the Evolve website for Flashcards, Case Studies, and additional testing resources related to the content in this chapter: http://evolve.elsevier.com/Canada/Varcarolis/psychiatric/* Pre-Test interactive review

Exploring the history of nursing in Canada, and specifically psychiatric mental health nursing, can enrich our understanding of the factors that have shaped our profession in the past and that will shape it in the future. Throughout history, the evolution of the role of nursing has been affected by sociopolitical, economic, cultural, medical, and religious trends in Canada and around the world. While there has been much historical analysis of psychiatric mental health nursing in England, Holland, and the United States, Canadian nursing history has largely excluded the mental health field (McPherson, 1996). For many reasons, it is a convoluted history, unique to Canada, and separate from that of generalist registered nursing. Understanding it provides us with insight into the past challenges and accomplishments of psychiatric mental health

nursing and prepares us for the continuing development of the role (Leishman, 2005).

## EARLY MENTAL ILLNESS CARE

Trends in approaches to the treatment of mental illness have significantly contributed to the emergence and evolution of the role of psychiatric nursing. These trends stem largely from societal values, politics, culture, and economics.

Asylums, designed to be retreats from society, were built with the hope that, with early intervention and several months of rest, people with mental illness could be cured (Weir, 1932). Eighth-century Middle Eastern Islamic societies such as Baghdad and Cairo established the first asylums (Youssef,

Youssef, & Dening, 1996). Even that early, these treatment centres, guided by Islamic beliefs, provided a compassionate and peaceful environment in which to care for people with mental illnesses. In medieval Western Europe, however, strong religious influences inspired the belief that mental illness indicated demonic possession or sin. Unfortunately, mentally ill people without protective support systems were commonly subjected to torture or isolation from the community (Cellard & Thifault, 2006). By the fifteenth century, several asylums had been built across Europe, but attitudes had not evolved much. Patients in these settings were often chained or caged, and cruelty or neglect was not uncommon (Digby, 1983). This type of treatment reflected the societal view that people with mental illness were bestial or less human in nature and, therefore, required discipline and were immune to human discomforts such as hunger or cold (Digby, 1983).

In the late 1700s, Philippe Pinel, a French physician, along with other humanitarians, began to advocate for more humane treatment of people with mental illness by literally removing the chains of the patients, talking to them, and providing a calmer, soothing environment. Pinel and another reformer from England, William Tuke, described this use of social and psychological approaches to treatment as "moral treatment" (Digby, 1983). Critics such as French philosopher Michel Foucault argued that the asylum movement was little more than a shift from physical restraint to psychological and social control of people considered undesirable by societal norms (Foucault, 1971). Regardless, this revolutionary way of treating people with mental illness swept across Europe and influenced the design of early asylums in North America.

In Canada, the country's size, location, and history have played a significant part in how people with mental illness are treated. Canada's Aboriginal peoples had a variety of approaches to caring for people with mental illness. Most were holistic—treating mind, body, and soul—and included sweat lodges, animistic charms, potlatch, and Sundance (Kirkmayer, Brass, & Tait, 2000). In the sixteenth century, colonial settlers from France and, later, England brought with them their own approaches to mental illness care. As in their European homelands, much of the responsibility of caring for people with mental illness fell upon the family and the asylums established in the communities (Cellard & Thifault, 2006). Some Canadian religious orders, such as the Grey Nuns, were early providers of care for people with mental illness (Hardill, 2006). Those who could not be cared for in the community, however, often ended up in jails, where they received minimal shelter at best and abuse at worst (Moran, 1998). By the 1800s, migration to Canada increased, as did its urbanization. This relocation of families to cities or isolated settlements changed support systems and families' ability to care for people with mental illness (Cellard & Thifault, 2006). In Europe, the move to asylum care was well under way, and the Canadian colonies began to explore similar options.

## Early Canadian Asylums

Beauport, the first asylum in what would soon become Canada, was opened in Quebec in 1845 (Sussman, 1998). Soon, more asylums were established in Upper and Lower Canada, the Maritime colonies, and Canada's West. Despite the creation of asylums, early historical records demonstrate that most families of people with a mental illness maintained the care of those individuals themselves (Cellard & Thifault, 2006), so the asylums predominantly housed patients who were poor and had no family support. Many asylums were built in countrylike settings on large parcels of land that could provide opportunity for occupational therapies such as farming. Toward the end of the nineteenth century, asylum care became more acceptable, and, with family support systems becoming diluted due to urbanization and relocation, the inpatient population grew exponentially (Cellard & Thifault, 2006). While the moral treatment era had moved psychiatric treatment toward more humane treatment, the lack of success in treating mental illnesses combined with increased admissions to asylums led to overcrowding and less than humane conditions in many asylums. In most settings, a large population of people received only minimal custodial care—assistance in performing the basic daily necessities of life, such as dressing, eating, using a toilet, walking, and so on.

This situation caught the attention of many social reformers who, in the late nineteenth and early twentieth centuries, lobbied governments to create more humane environments of care for people with mental illness. Among them was Dorothea Dix, a retired school teacher from New England who became the superintendent of nurses during the American Civil War. Dix was educated in the asylum reform movements in England while she was there recuperating from tuberculosis. In 1841, during an encounter at a Boston jail, Dix was shocked to witness the degrading treatment of a woman with mental illness who was imprisoned there. Passionate about social reform, she began advocating for the improved treatment and public care of people with mental illness. Dix met with many politicians and

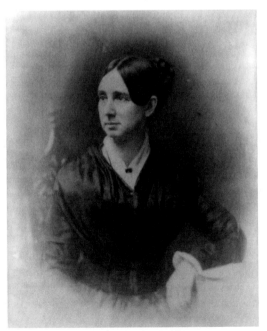

Dorothea Dix, advocate, 1802–1887. **Source:** Library of Congress Prints and Photographs Division. Washington, D.C., 20540, USA.

even the Pope to push her agenda forward. Ultimately, she was influential in lobbying for the first public mental hospital in the United States and for reform in British and Canadian institutions.

## EARLY PSYCHIATRIC TREATMENTS

By the end of the nineteenth century, the new field of psychiatry was being challenged to provide a medical cure for mental illness. Since there were few medications available other than heavily alcohol-based sedatives, doctors used many experimental treatments—for example, leeching (using bloodsucking worms), spinning (tying the patient to a chair and spinning it for hours), hydrotherapy (forced baths), and insulin shock treatment (injections of large doses of insulin to produce daily comas over several weeks). In the mid-twentieth century treatment choices expanded to include electroconvulsive therapy (see Chapter 14) and lobotomies, through which nerve fibres in the frontal lobe were severed. As treatments became more invasive, the need for patient monitoring beyond custodial care led many medical superintendents to recruit nurses to work in their institutions.

## THE INTRODUCTION OF NURSES TO ASYLUM CARE

In Canada, prior to the late 1800s, there were no nurses working in psychiatric settings; instead, asylums used predominantly male attendants to provide custodial care for patients. Changes in treatment approaches and the increased medicalization of psychiatry prompted a need for more specially trained providers, especially for female patients (Connor, 1996). In 1888, Rockwood Asylum in Kingston, Ontario, became the first psychiatric institution in Canada to open a training program for nurses (Kerrigan, 2011). The two-year program was overseen by the asylum's medical director and included one lecture a week combined with work experience training. The curriculum, taught by physicians, included courses in physiology, anatomy, nursing care of the sick, and nursing care of the insane (Legislature of the Province of Ontario, 1889). Consistent with societal beliefs of the time about women's innate caring capacity, the training was offered only to females. This exclusion of males from the program hindered the recognition of the importance of nursing knowledge and skills as well as lowered the status of male attendants at the time (Yonge, Boschma, & Mychajlunow, 2005). Both of these factors would greatly impact the future development of psychiatric mental health nursing in Canada.

Asylum-based training schools opened across Canada, and the training curriculum, similar to that of the hospital-based programs of generalist nurses, varied among institutions. Medical superintendents controlled the content and delivery of the programs, and hospital administrators valued highly the inexpensive labour provided by the female workforce, so much so that their cross-training in other medical settings was discouraged so as to maintain staffing supplies (Tipliski, 2004). The asylum-based programs were founded heavily on a medical model of training nurses to be obedient, orderly, and focused

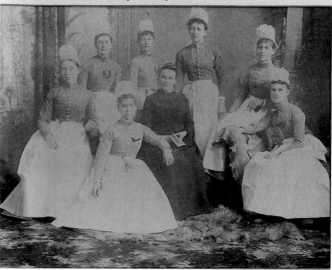

First graduating class of Rockwood Asylum Nursing School, Kingston, Ontario, 1890. **Source:** Providence Care Archives http://providencecarearchives.files.wordpress.com/2011/03/image2011-03-24-102507-1.jpg.

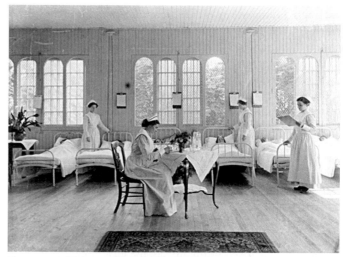

Nurses at Toronto Hospital for the Insane in 1910. **Source:** RG 10-276-2-0-8. Ministry of Health. Queen Street Mental Health Centre miscellaneous historical materials. Queen Street Mental Health Centre miscellaneous photographs. Female infirmary at the Hospital for the Insane, Toronto, ca. 1910. Archives of Ontario, I0018987.

on the discipline of the inpatients (Cowles, 1916). Nursing duties at the beginning of the twentieth century often included extensive cleaning, serving meals, counting cutlery after meals, and assisting patients with hygiene activities, as well as administering treatments such as the long baths referred to as "hydrotherapy," sedation with alcohol, and postoperative care (Forchuk & Tweedell, 2001). Nurses also played a key role in the care of patients in the infirmary. The custodial environment of asylums did not promote a sense of professional knowledge for nurses and limited their ability to question the treatment approaches being offered at the time (Leishman, 2005). Societal trends for women in the workforce reinforced nurses' lack of power in controlling their education programs and work environments (Anthony & Landeen, 2009).

## SHIFTS IN CONTROL OVER NURSING

In the early part of the twentieth century, nurses' lack of control over their own profession began to shift with changes to nursing education models and blossoming political advocacy by nursing groups across Canada, particularly with the formation of the Canadian National Association of Trained Nurses in 1908. This early group expanded, and by 1926, each province had an affiliate group, and the organization was renamed the Canadian Nurses Association (CNA). The CNA provided a united voice for nurses and increased advocacy for control over nursing by nurses (Canadian Nurses Association, 2011a). At this time, nursing training programs still varied by institution, but many had long hours of hospital ward service taking precedence over instructional hours for students. The Canadian Nurses Association's mandate included the professionalization of nursing, so it began to advocate for standardization of nursing education (Tipliski, 2004). This was a politically loaded issue for several reasons: physicians wanted control over nursing education; patriarchal society structures devalued nursing knowledge; nursing skills were seen as natural women's work; and hospitals relied on the economical service hours of nursing students (Anthony & Landeen, 2009). Some vocal physicians expressed concerns that giving nurses too much education may lead to their disobedience and boredom (Kirkwood, 2005).

In 1927, the Canadian Medical Association and the Canadian Nurses Association performed a joint study on the state of nursing education in Canada. The result, known as the "Weir Report," was released in 1932 and concluded that drastic changes were needed in nursing education programs, including standardization of curriculum, work hours, and instructor training, and that care of people with mental illnesses needed to be integrated into all generalist programs (Fleming, 1932). The uptake of the recommendations varied across Canada and even within regions. Since psychiatric hospitals and asylums had a harder time recruiting nurses, the idea of giving up their workforce so that students could complete an affiliation in general hospital settings was considered very costly. The medical superintendent psychiatrists were protective of their asylum-based training programs, which they felt developed specialized skills compared to general nursing skills (Tipliski, 2004). They argued that a 3- to 6-month affiliation in psychiatry was too short to learn the skills required in their institutions.

At the time, provincial legislation in the form of nursing acts was coming into existence and further formalizing the title and licensure of the registered nurse. There were provincial differences in government-legislated power over licensure and nursing education as well as variable interest in psychiatric training by provincial nursing associations (Tipliski, 2004). This, combined with the political influence of some medical superintendents from provincial psychiatric hospitals, led registered nursing associations in Manitoba, Saskatchewan, Alberta,

and British Columbia to be less inclusive of the psychiatric hospital–trained nurse than the associations in Eastern Canada were, leading to the exclusion of registered nurse licensure for graduates of asylum programs. This division of perspectives eventually resulted in a split between Western and Eastern Canada in training programs and the creation in the western provinces of the specialty-focused psychiatric nursing training programs and the registered psychiatric nurse designation.

### RESEARCH HIGHLIGHT

#### Reel Nursing: Psychiatric Nursing Care in Film

**Source:** Pollard, C.W. (2011). *Reel nursing: Psychiatric nursing care in film.* Saarbrucken, Germany: LAP Lambert Academic Publishing.

**Problem**
Inaccurate depictions of psychiatric or mental health nursing care in the media can result in a patient's delayed access to treatment and to self-stigmatization.

**Purpose of Study**
In this research, Dr. Pollard investigated the portrayal of psychiatric or mental health nursing care in the media.

**Methods**
Dr. Pollard critically analyzed movies and examined the depictions of nurses and the patients they cared for.

**Key Findings**
The media have constructed literally hundreds of thousands of images depicting nurses and the care they provide. These images typically encompassed two predominant facets: the role or function the nurses performed and the relationship they had with their patients. Regardless of the time period of the film, nurses were typically depicted as dominant and controlling over their patients. Within this discourse, concepts emerged related to the stigmatization, prejudice, domination, and marginalization of patients.

**Implications for Nursing Practice**
Dr. Pollard advocates for nurses to become more attentive to the messages disseminated by mass media since these images have consequences for the patients, their families, and the nurses working in this complex specialty area. Nurses can get involved in stigma-reducing activities such as public education, letter writing, and media policy advocacy.

### Eastern and Atlantic Canada

From the outset, the Registered Nurses' Association of Ontario (RNAO) accepted the asylum-based programs for licensing of prospective nurses who were affiliated with a general hospital (Tipliski, 2004). It also represented nurses working in asylum settings, providing them with advocacy and nursing leadership (Tipliski, 2004). With the support of nurse leaders like Nettie Fiddler and the publication of the "Weir Report," more generalist hospital programs began adding a psychiatry rotation to the curriculum. Also influential in the addition of a psychiatry rotation was the RNAO's addressing the nursing shortage in psychiatric settings and the care concerns of mentally ill patients at the organization's 1945 annual meeting (Tipliski, 2004). At this point, many psychiatric hospitals had large numbers of patients, inadequate staffing, and minimal enrollment of new students (Tipliski, 2004). The advocacy of nurse leaders, combined with the post–World War II mental hygiene movement, led to the addition of psychiatric nursing theory for all registered nurse education programs (Tipliski, 2004). Some asylum programs added training in general medical settings; however, by the 1950s, all of the psychiatric hospital training programs in Eastern Canada had closed. Nurses in psychiatric mental health were trained as generalist registered nurses with affiliations in psychiatry and the chance to specialize post-graduation.

### Western Canada

In the western provinces, where the population was much smaller and asylums were located in very rural settings, recruiting an adequate labour force was a major concern. In the early 1900s, British Columbia, Alberta, Saskatchewan, and Manitoba attempted different approaches to training nurses for psychiatric settings. Selkirk, Manitoba, opened the first asylum training school in Western Canada in 1920, followed closely by Brandon, Manitoba in 1921 (Hicks, 2011). Manitoba implemented several combination programs between general hospitals and psychiatric hospitals, but similar attempts at other institutions in the western provinces failed due to lack of investment from administrators and nurse leadership groups and difficulty enticing nurses to remain in the psychiatric settings after their graduation (Hicks, 2011; Tipliski, 2004).

In the 1930s, Saskatchewan's two provincial psychiatric hospitals began a training program for their attendants under the direction of superintendent James MacNeill. Unlike in the rest of Canada, this training was offered to both male and female attendants and, upon completion, gave graduates the title "nursing attendant." This program continued to evolve under the direction of superintendent Douglas McKerracher as he attempted to ensure the presence of adequately trained staff in Saskatchewan's provincial hospitals (Tipliski, 2004). However, the specialized training did not bestow upon graduates any professional title or licensure, so several attendants lobbied for the creation of the designation "psychiatric nurse." The movement for the designation of psychiatric nurse was supported by medical superintendents, unions, and politicians at the time, so despite opposition by provincial nursing leaders, the *Registered Psychiatric Nurses Act* was enacted in Saskatchewan in 1948 (Tipliski, 2004). This step toward professionalization of the role of the nurse in psychiatric hospitals was soon taken by other western provinces. At the same time, the Saskatchewan Registered Nurses' Association's leader, Kathryn Ellis, was also trying to address the nursing shortage in mental hospitals by convincing provincial hospitals to become more involved in training, but she was unable to negotiate satisfactory psychiatric or general hospital affiliations with McKerracher or his predecessor, MacNeill (Hicks, 2011; Tipliski, 2004).

Much of the professionalization movement was facilitated by the Canadian Council of Psychiatric Nurses (CCPN), an interprovincial organization of psychiatric nurses focused on increasing the standards and recognition of psychiatric nurse training (Hicks, 2011). The CCPN, along with the efforts of provincial psychiatrists, was successful in advocating for the registered psychiatric nurse specialty designation across the western provinces; subsequently, British Columbia passed its psychiatric nurses act in 1951; Alberta followed in 1955; and Manitoba, in 1960. To date, the separate designation has remained, resulting in both registered nurses and registered psychiatric nurses working in psychiatric mental health settings in the four western provinces and Yukon.

## DEINSTITUTIONALIZATION AND THE NURSING ROLE IN PSYCHIATRIC MENTAL HEALTH CARE

Psychiatric nursing continued to take place predominantly in hospital settings until the 1960s, when deinstitutionalization—the shift from caring for people with mental illness in institutions to caring for them in communities—began, significantly changing the role of the nurse. (See Chapter 6 for further discussion of deinstitutionalization.) The "pioneer" community mental health nurses set up many programs and frameworks for the delivery of psychiatric mental health care in the community (Boschma, 2012). The wide range of community-based mental health services that eventually developed (e.g., crisis management, consultation-liaison, primary care psychiatry) created new settings and skill requirements for psychiatric mental health nurses. The ability to assess and monitor clients and their environment changed nursing approaches toward mental health care. Assessment, autonomy, collaboration, crisis management, and resource finding became key skills for community-based nurses.

## UNIVERSITY-BASED NURSING CURRICULUM

In 1919, the University of British Columbia (UBC) launched the first university-based program in nursing. The program was a "sandwich model," with three years of hospital-based nursing sandwiched between the first and final year of university studies (Anthony & Landeen, 2009). At the time, the idea of a university program for nursing was considered so risky that UBC refused to fund or administer the middle years of the program. A leader in nursing education at the time, E. Kathleen Russell at the University of Toronto, supported by the Rockefeller Foundation, set up one of the first university-based training programs in public health nursing, leadership, and education. This revolutionary post-diploma certification program for registered nurses was attended internationally. Later, in 1928, Russell coordinated the first solely university-based nursing program at the University of Toronto; in 1942, it began granting bachelor of science degrees in nursing (BScN) (University of Toronto, 2011). These university programs initiated a critical change in nursing education: for the first time, education for nurses was separated from and prioritized over their service in the hospitals (Anthony & Landeen, 2009). Despite this revolution in nursing education, nursing programs remained under the control of medical faculties until 1962, when the University of Montreal set up the first independent nursing faculty (Anthony & Landeen, 2009).

Many other Canadian universities began to offer diploma programs in specialty areas such as public health. In the 1950s, the University of Saskatchewan became the first to offer one in advanced psychiatric nursing, a one-year diploma program done after completing registered nurse training (University of Saskatchewan, 2011).

The inception of university education for nurses led to the growth and formalization of nursing knowledge. The University of Western Ontario launched Canada's first graduate program in nursing in 1959, and the first PhD program in nursing began at the University of Alberta in 1991. The growth of graduate programs gave rise to increased research and theory in psychiatric nursing practice. The influence of nurse theorists such as American Hildegard Peplau, the first published nursing theorist since Florence Nightingale, contributed to the expansion of specialized nursing knowledge and related skills in the psychiatric mental health field. Much of Peplau's work focused on the role of the nurse in therapeutic relationships and anxiety management. The growth of academic study in nursing, in turn, influenced nursing in the practice setting: the Hamilton Psychiatric Hospital became the first health care institution in Canada to employ a clinical nurse specialist and to require theory-based nursing practice (Forchuk & Tweedell, 2001). Nursing research in mental health continues to expand through the works of nurse researchers such as Olive Yonge, Wendy Austin, Cheryl Forchuk, David Holmes, Mary Haase, Cheryl L. Pollard, Susan L. Ray, and Kimberley Ryan-Nicholls.

In Western Canada, the shift to the role of the registered psychiatric nurse and the increased range of practice settings (i.e., away from inpatient facilities and into primary care and community-based clinics) have also brought about changes in educational programs in the past 20 years. Registered psychiatric nursing programs have adjusted to ensure diversification of skills and knowledge base related to consumer-oriented primary health care and health promotion activities (Ryan-Nicholls, 2004). RPN training continued to be diploma-based across the western provinces until 1995, when Brandon University began its baccalaureate program in psychiatric mental health nursing. Registered Psychiatric Nurses of Canada (RPNC) issued a position statement in 2008 advocating for baccalaureate degree entry to practice for RPNs due to the increasingly complex needs and roles of the registered psychiatric nurse (Registered Psychiatric Nurses of Canada, 2008a). At this time, the RPNC also issued a position statement on the need for graduate programs for registered psychiatric nurses that could help to foster the professional development, research, and clinical training of baccalaureate registered psychiatric nursing students (RPNC, 2008b). The first graduate program in psychiatric nursing for registered psychiatric nurses began at Brandon University in January 2011.

## NATIONAL ORGANIZATIONS FOR PSYCHIATRIC MENTAL HEALTH NURSING AND CANADIAN NURSES ASSOCIATION CERTIFICATION

The division of Eastern and Western Canada in psychiatric nursing training and designation resulted in separate organizational groups. While having multiple organizations has led to some duplication and fragmentation of a voice for nurses in psychiatric settings, the groups have also worked collaboratively toward common goals. Since 1995, the Canadian Nurses Association has offered registered nurses certification in psychiatric mental health nursing; this certification exam is one of the most commonly written (CNA, 2011b). Under the umbrella of the CNA and with consumer input, the Canadian Federation of Mental Health Nurses, an organization of registered nurses across Canada who specialize in psychiatric mental health nursing, set the standards of practice for psychiatric mental health nursing (see http://cfmhn.ca/sites/cfmhn.ca/files/CFMHN standards 1.pdf). The RPNC has also published a code of ethics and standards of practice for RPNs, which in January 2013 were under review. Despite the separations in licensure and professional bodies, in workplaces in Western Canada, registered nurses and registered psychiatric nurses work closely together in mental health settings and have much opportunity for collaboration and advocacy for the people they serve.

## ADVANCED-PRACTICE NURSING IN PSYCHIATRIC MENTAL HEALTH CARE

Advanced-practice nursing (APN) includes the roles of nurse practitioner and clinical nurse specialist (CNA, 2008). Each province has its own regulations guiding the licensing and scope of practice for APN. The clinical nurse specialist (CNS) role has been well established in psychiatry since 1972, when Hamilton Psychiatric Hospital employed Pat Barry, a nurse with a graduate degree, to educate staff and increase theoretical-based nursing practice (Forchuk & Tweedell, 2001). CNSs can provide psychotherapy and have worked as consultants, educators, and clinicians in inpatient and outpatient psychiatry throughout Canada. Nurse practitioners, on the other hand, work as consultants or collaborative team members and can diagnose, prescribe and manage medications, and can also provide psychotherapy. While the role of psychiatric nurse practitioner has been well established in the United States, where specialized graduate programs and advanced certification exams are offered, the role has remained virtually nonexistent in Canada, likely because the nurse practitioner role itself is relatively new to Canada compared to the United States, where it has been well established and regulated since the 1970s.

There has been a recent attempt in Canada at standardizing the requirements for advanced practice nursing nationally through the use of exam certification. Currently, nurse practitioner certification falls under one of three areas of specialization: adult, family, or pediatric. All are focused more on physical health than mental health knowledge. Further differences in licensure for nurse practitioners exist among provinces due to hospital legislation and funding methodology for health care billing. Because of the strong need for psychiatric care throughout Canada and the lack of providers available, especially in rural areas, the role of the advanced-practice nurse in psychiatric mental health is expected to expand in the near future.

## THE FUTURE OF PSYCHIATRIC MENTAL HEALTH NURSING

As its history has shown, the role of the nurse in psychiatric mental health care will continue to evolve and be influenced by societal trends. The change in structure of health care delivery toward a primary health model and an integrative mental health care approach has led to new roles for nurses in psychiatric mental health, including shared-care roles in primary care and consultation-liaison psychiatry within the general hospital setting. The Association of Registered Nurses of Newfoundland and Labrador (2008) took some key steps in articulating the

range of competencies and role development required for community mental health nursing in its 2008 policy paper *Advancing the Role of the Psychiatric–Mental Health Nurse in the Community*. These competencies and role development are in line with the CNA 2020 vision statement, which has called for an increased role for nurses working in integrative mental health care roles and primary care (Villeneuve & MacDonald, 2006). Based on its success in the United States, the role of advanced-practice nurse in psychiatric mental health care is another one that is certain to develop in Canada in the near future. The changes in public perception of mental illness and decreases in stigma are beginning to increase the role of mental health promotion and illness prevention in schools and workplace settings. Evidence-informed approaches to treatment, such as concurrent treatment for people with mental illnesses and addictions or dialectical behavioural therapy for people with borderline personality disorder, have led to the creation of related nursing roles, education, and research.

## ■ KEY POINTS TO REMEMBER

- Early asylum care for people with mental illness predominantly focused on containment and sometimes punishment.
- Philippe Pinel and William Tuke were eighteenth-century reformers who introduced the moral treatment era of psychiatry, which attempted to focus on providing peaceful, nurturing environments for people with mental illness. Their theories influenced the rural, farmlike settings of early Canadian asylums.
- Nursing within asylums began in the late nineteenth century as a result of the increased medicalization of psychiatry.
- Psychiatric mental health nursing development in Canada was heavily influenced by societal values toward gender and toward mental illness, by politics, and by psychiatric care approaches.
- Early nursing roles in psychiatry were largely custodial until the introduction of new treatments such as electroconvulsive therapy, insulin shock therapy, and lobotomies.
- The division between western provinces and eastern provinces in the creation of the registered psychiatric nurse designation was largely related to differences in nursing leadership power, advocacy, and labour supply issues.

- The development of university-based programs in nursing in the 1920s was a key step in the professionalization of nursing and in the transition of nursing education from medical dominance to nursing-led knowledge development.
- Psychiatric mental health nursing led the way in reinforcing theory-based nursing practice with the use of clinical nurse specialists.
- Registered nurses work within psychiatric mental health settings across Canada.
- Registered psychiatric nurses work in psychiatric mental health settings in Manitoba, Saskatchewan, Alberta, British Columbia, and Yukon.
- The deinstitutionalization of patients in favour of community-based treatment led to the development of new nursing roles in psychiatric mental health care, including community mental health, crisis management, consultation-liaison, and primary care psychiatry.
- Advanced-practice nursing roles have had varied implementation in Canada. The clinical nurse specialist role has been well established, while the nurse practitioner role has had limited development.

## ■ CRITICAL THINKING

1. Consider the first students at Rockwood Asylum in 1888. What factors might have influenced their decision to enter into asylum nursing (a new program and role)?

2. How have educational programs for nurses evolved with the professionalization of nursing in Canada?

3. What are the potential implications of having two different designations and educational programs for nurses in

psychiatric mental health nursing in four Canadian provinces?

4. What traits and behaviours of nurses in the psychiatric setting are commonly portrayed in movies or TV shows that you have seen? How might these portrayals affect people with mental illness?

## CHAPTER REVIEW

1. Asylum care of people with mental illness in Canada began in which year?
   1. 1620
   2. 1932
   3. 1845
   4. 1798

2. The "Weir Report" was considered influential in which of the following areas?
   1. Asylum reform
   2. Nursing education curriculum reform
   3. Deinstitutionalization
   4. The establishment of the registered psychiatric nurse designation

3. Psychiatric mental health nursing in the community setting was influenced by which of the following factors?
   1. The "Weir Report"
   2. Deinstitutionalization
   3. The registered psychiatric nurse designation
   4. The increased medicalization of psychiatry

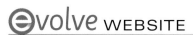 WEBSITE

Post-Test　interactive review

*Visit the Evolve Web site for Chapter Review Answers and Rationales, Critical Thinking Answer Guidelines, and additional resources related to the content in this chapter: http://evolve.elsevier.com/Canada/Varcarolis/psychiatric/*

## REFERENCES

Anthony, S.E., & Landeen, J. (2009). Evolution of Canadian nursing curricula: A critical retrospective analysis of power and caring. *International Journal of Nursing Education Scholarship, 69,* 1–14. doi:10.2202/1548-923X.1766.

Association of Registered Nurses of Newfoundland and Labrador. (2008). *Advancing the role of the psychiatric–mental health nurse in the community* (Policy paper). St. John's: Author.

Boschma, G. (2012). Community mental health nursing in Alberta, Canada: An oral history. *Nursing History Review, 20*(1), 103–135. doi:10.1891/1062-8061.20.103.

Canadian Nurses Association. (2008). *Advanced nursing practice: A national framework.* Ottawa: Author.

Canadian Nurses Association. (2011a). *History.* Retrieved from http://www.nurseone.ca/Default.aspx?portlet=StaticHtmlViewerPortlet&stmd=False&plang=1&ptdi=582.

Canadian Nurses Association (2011b). *CNA Certification.* Retrieved from http://www.nurseone.ca/Default.aspx?portlet=StaticHtmlViewerPortlet&plang=1&ptdi=153.

Cellard, A., & Thifault, M.C. (2006). The uses of asylums: Resistance, asylum propaganda and institutionalization strategies in turn of the century Quebec. In J. Moran (Ed.), *Mental illness and Canadian society: A historical perspective* (pp. 97–116). Montreal: McGill-Queen's University Press.

Connor, P. (1996). "Neither courage nor perseverance enough": Attendants at the Asylum for the Insane, Kingston 1877–1905. *Ontario History, 88*(4), 251–272.

Cowles, E. (1916). Training schools for nurses and the first school in McLean Hospital. In H. Hurd (Ed.), *The institutional care of the insane in the United States and Canada* (pp. 289–300). New York: Arno Press.

Digby, A. (1983). Changes in the asylum: The case of York, 1777–1815. *Economic History Review, 36,* 218–239. doi:10.1111/j.1468-0289.1983.tb01230.x.

Fleming, G. (1932). Survey on nursing education. *Canadian Medical Association Journal, 26*(4), 471–474.

Forchuk, C., & Tweedell, D. (2001). Celebrating our past. *Journal of Psychosocial and Mental Health Services, 39*(10), 16–24.

Foucault, M. (1971). *Madness and civilization: A history of insanity in the age of reason.* New York: Routledge.

Hardill, K. (2006). From the Grey Nuns to the streets: A critical history of outreach nursing in Canada. *Public Health Nursing, 24*(1), 91–97.

Hicks, B. (2011). Gender, politics, and regionalism: Factors in the evolution of registered psychiatric nursing in Manitoba, 1920–1960. *Nursing History Review, 19,* 103–126. doi:10.1891/1062-8061.19.103.

Kerrigan, M. (2011, March 11). *Providence Care family connection to Rockwood Nursing [Blog post].* Retrieved from http://providencecarearchives.wordpress.com/2011/03/25/providence-care-family-connection-to-rockwood-nursing/.

Kirkmayer, L.J., Brass, G.M., & Tait, C.L. (2000). The mental health of Aboriginal peoples: Transformations of identity and community. *The Canadian Journal of Psychiatry, 45*(7), 607–616.

Kirkwood, L. (2005). Enough but not too much: Nursing education in English language Canada. In C. Bates, D. Dodd, & N. Rousseau (Eds.), *On all frontiers: Four centuries of Canadian nursing* (pp. 183–196). Ottawa: University of Ottawa Press.

Legislature of the Province of Ontario. (1889). *Sessional papers. Volume xxi–Part 1.* Toronto: Queen's Printer.

Leishman, J. (2005). Back to the future: Making a case for including the history of mental health nursing in nurse education programmes. *The International Journal of Psychiatric Nursing Research, 10*(3), 1157–1164.

McPherson, K. (1996). *Bedside matters: The transformation of Canadian nursing, 1900–1990.* Toronto: Oxford University Press.

Moran, J. (1998). The ethics of farming-out: Ideology, the state, and the asylum in nineteenth-century Quebec. *Canadian Bulletin of Medical History, 15,* 297–316.

Registered Psychiatric Nurses of Canada. (2008a). *Position statement on baccalaureate preparation as entry to practice in psychiatric nursing.* Retrieved from http://www.rpnc.ca/sites/default/files/resources/pdfs/BACCAL_Prep_PositionStatement_2012.pdf.

Registered Psychiatric Nurses of Canada. (2008b). *Position statement on master's preparation in psychiatric nursing.* Retrieved from http://

www.rpnc.ca/sites/default/files/resources/pdfs/Masters_Preparation_PositionStatement_June2008.pdf.

Ryan-Nicholls, K.D. (2004). Impact of health reform on registered psychiatric nursing practice. *Journal of Psychiatric and Mental Health Nursing, 11,* 644–653. doi:10.1111/j.1365-2850.2004.00761.x.

Sussman, S. (1998). The first asylums in Canada: A response to neglectful community care and current trends. *Canadian Journal of Psychiatry, 43*(3), 260–264.

Tipliski, V.M. (2004). Parting at the crossroads: The emergence of education for psychiatric nursing in three Canadian provinces, 1909–1955. *Canadian Bulletin of Medical History, 21*(2), 253–279.

University of Saskatchewan. (2011). *History of the College of Nursing.* Retrieved from http://www.usask.ca/nursing/college/history.php.

University of Toronto. (2011). *Historic contributions.* Retrieved from http://bloomberg.nursing.utoronto.ca/about/history-of-the-faculty.

Villeneuve, M., & MacDonald, J. (2006). *Toward 2020: Visions for nursing.* Ottawa: Canadian Nurses Association.

Weir, G.M. (1932). *Survey of nursing education in Canada.* Toronto: University of Toronto Press.

Yonge, O., Boschma, G., & Mychajlunow, L. (2005). Gender and professional identity in psychiatric nursing practice in Alberta, Canada, 1930–1975. *Nursing Inquiry, 12,* 243–255. doi:10.1111/j.1440-1800.2005.00287.x.

Youssef, H.A., Youssef, F.A., & Dening, T.R. (1996). Evidence for the existence of schizophrenia in medieval Islamic society. *History of Psychiatry, 7,* 55–62.

# 3

# Relevant Theories and Therapies for Nursing Practice

*Margaret Jordan Halter, Verna Benner Carson*
*Adapted by Sherri Melrose and Sharon L. Moore*

## KEY TERMS AND CONCEPTS

automatic thoughts, 36
behavioural therapy, 34
biofeedback, 35
classical conditioning, 32
cognitive-behavioural therapy (CBT), 36
cognitive distortions, 36
conditioning, 32
conscious, 27
counter-transference, 28
defence mechanisms, 28
ego, 27
extinction, 33
id, 27

interpersonal psychotherapy, 31
milieu therapy, 40
negative reinforcement, 33
operant conditioning, 33
positive reinforcement, 33
preconscious, 27
psychodynamic therapy, 28
punishment, 33
reinforcement, 33
superego, 27
transference, 28
unconscious, 27

## OBJECTIVES

1. Evaluate the premises behind the various therapeutic models discussed in this chapter.
2. Describe the evolution of therapies for psychiatric disorders.
3. Identify ways each theorist has contributed to the nurse's ability to assess a patient's behaviours.
4. Drawing on clinical experience, provide the following:
   a. An example of how a patient's irrational beliefs influenced behaviour

   b. An example of counter-transference in your relationship with a patient
   c. An example of the use of behaviour modification with a patient
5. Identify Peplau's framework for the nurse–patient relationship.
6. Choose the therapeutic model that would be most useful for a particular patient or patient problem.

## ℮volve WEBSITE

*Visit the Evolve website for Flashcards, Case Studies, and additional testing resources related to the content in this chapter:* http://evolve.elsevier.com/Canada/Varcarolis/psychiatric/   Pre-Test | interactive review

Every professional discipline, from math and science to philosophy and psychology, bases its work and beliefs on theories. Most of these theories can best be described as explanations, hypotheses, or hunches, rather than testable facts.

Dealing with other people is one of the most universally anxiety-provoking activities we engage in. Psychological theories provide us with plausible explanations for various behaviour. In its position paper identifying core competencies in psychiatric mental health nursing for undergraduate nursing education, the Canadian Federation of Mental Health Nurses emphasized the importance of nurses' "understanding the models of care which effectively guide practice" (Tognazzini,

Davis, Kean, et al., 2009, p. 16). Our patients challenge us to understand stories that are complex and always unique. A broad base of knowledge about personality development, human needs, the ingredients of mental health, contributing factors to mental illness, and the importance of relationships can help to effectively guide our nursing practice.

This chapter will provide you with snapshot views of some of the most influential psychological theories. It will also provide an overview of the treatment, or therapy, they inspired and the contributions they have made to our practice of psychiatric mental health nursing.

## PSYCHOANALYTIC THEORIES AND THERAPIES

### Sigmund Freud's Psychoanalytic Theory

Sigmund Freud (1856–1939), an Austrian neurologist, revolutionized thinking about mental health disorders with his groundbreaking theory of personality structure, levels of awareness, anxiety, the role of defence mechanisms, and the stages of psychosexual development. Freud came to believe that the vast majority of mental health disorders were due to unresolved issues that originated in childhood. He arrived at this conclusion through his experiences treating people with hysteria—individuals who were experiencing physical symptoms despite the absence of an apparent physiological cause.

As part of his treatment, Freud initially used hypnosis, but this therapy provided mixed therapeutic results. He then changed his approach to talk therapy, known as the *cathartic method*. Today we refer to catharsis as "getting things off our chests." Talk therapy evolved to include "free association," which requires full and honest disclosure of thoughts and feelings as they come to mind. Freud (1961, 1969) concluded that talking about difficult emotional issues had the potential to heal the wounds causing mental illness. Viewing the success of these therapeutic approaches led Freud to construct his psychoanalytic theory.

### Levels of Awareness

Through the use of talk therapy and free association, Freud came to believe that there were three levels of psychological awareness in operation. He offered a topographic theory of how the mind functions, using the image of an iceberg to describe the levels of awareness (Figure 3-1).

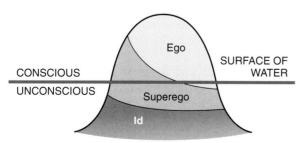

FIGURE 3-1 The mind as an iceberg.

**Conscious.** Freud described the conscious part of the mind as the tip of the iceberg. It contains all the material a person is aware of at any one time, including perceptions, memories, thoughts, fantasies, and feelings.

**Preconscious.** Just below the surface of awareness is the preconscious, which contains material that can be retrieved rather easily through conscious effort.

**Unconscious.** The unconscious includes all repressed memories, passions, and unacceptable urges lying deep below the surface. Freud believed that the memories and emotions associated with trauma are often "placed" in the unconscious because the individual finds it too painful to deal with them. The unconscious exerts a powerful yet unseen effect on the conscious thoughts and feelings of the individual. The individual is usually unable to retrieve unconscious material without the assistance of a trained therapist; however, with this assistance, unconscious material can be brought into conscious awareness.

### Personality Structure

Freud (1960) delineated three major and distinct but interactive systems of the personality: the id, the ego, and the superego.

**Id.** At birth we are all id. The id is the source of all drives, instincts, reflexes, needs, genetic inheritance, and capacity to respond, as well as all the wishes that motivate us. The id cannot tolerate frustration and seeks to discharge tension and return to a more comfortable level of energy. The id lacks the ability to problem-solve; it is not logical and operates according to the pleasure principle. A hungry, screaming infant is the perfect example of id.

**Ego.** The ego develops because the needs, wishes, and demands of the id cannot be satisfactorily met through primary processes and reflex action. The ego, which emerges in the fourth or fifth month of life, is the problem solver and reality tester. It is able to differentiate subjective experiences, memory images, and objective reality and attempts to negotiate a solution with the outside world. The ego follows the reality principle, which says to the id, "You have to delay gratification for right now," and then sets a course of action. For example, a hungry man feels tension arising from the id. His ego allows him not only to think about his hunger but to plan where he can eat and to seek that destination. This process is known as *reality testing* because the individual is factoring in reality to implement a plan to decrease tension.

**Superego.** The superego, the last portion of the personality to develop, represents the moral component of personality. The superego consists of the conscience (all the "should nots" internalized from parents) and the ego ideal (all the "shoulds" internalized from parents). The superego represents the ideal rather than the real; it seeks perfection, as opposed to seeking pleasure or engaging reason.

In a mature and well-adjusted individual, the three systems of the personality—the id, the ego, and the superego—work together as a team under the administrative leadership of the ego. If the id is too powerful, the person will lack control over impulses; if the superego is too powerful, the person may be self-critical and suffer from feelings of inferiority.

## Defence Mechanisms and Anxiety

Freud (1969) believed that anxiety is an inevitable part of living. The environment in which we live presents dangers, insecurities, threats, and satisfactions. It can produce pain and increase tension or produce pleasure and decrease tension. The ego develops defences, or defence mechanisms, to ward off anxiety by preventing conscious awareness of threatening feelings.

Defence mechanisms share two common features: (1) they all (except suppression) operate on an unconscious level, and we are not aware of their operation; and (2) they deny, falsify, or distort reality to make it less threatening. Although we cannot survive without defence mechanisms, it is possible for our defence mechanisms to distort reality to such a degree that we experience difficulty with healthy adjustment and personal growth. Chapter 13 offers further discussions of defence mechanisms.

## Psychosexual Stages of Development

Freud believed that human development proceeds through five stages from infancy to adulthood. From Freud's perspective, experiences that occur during the first five years of life determine an individual's lifetime adjustment patterns. In fact, Freud thought that personality is formed by the time a child enters school and that subsequent growth consists of elaborating on this basic structure. Freud's psychosexual stages of development are presented in Table 3-1.

## Implications for Psychiatric Mental Health Nursing

Freud's theory has relevance to nursing practice at many junctures. It offers a comprehensive explanation of complex human processes and suggests that the formation of a patient's personality is influenced by many diverse sources rooted in past events. Freud's theory of the unconscious is particularly valuable as a baseline for considering the complexity of human behaviour. By considering conscious and unconscious influences, a nurse can begin to think about meanings that might be behind certain behaviours. Freud emphasized the importance of individual talk sessions characterized by attentive listening, with a focus on underlying themes as an important tool of healing in psychiatric care.

## Classical Psychoanalysis

Classical psychoanalysis, as developed by Sigmund Freud, is seldom used today. Freud's premise that all mental illness is caused by early intrapsychic conflict—a mental struggle, often unconscious, between the id, ego, and superego—is no longer widely thought to be valid, and such therapy requires an unrealistically lengthy period of treatment, making it prohibitively expensive for most. However, there are two concepts from classic psychoanalysis that are important for all psychiatric nurses to know: transference and counter-transference (Freud, 1969).

Transference develops when the patient experiences feelings toward the nurse or therapist that were originally held toward significant others in his or her life. When transference occurs, these feelings become available for exploration with the patient. Such exploration helps the patient to better understand certain feelings and behaviours. Counter-transference is the health care worker's unconscious personal response to the patient. For instance, if the patient reminds you of someone you do not like, you may unconsciously react as if the patient were that individual. Counter-transference underscores the importance of maintaining self-awareness and seeking supervisory guidance as therapeutic relationships progress. Chapter 10 talks more about counter-transference and the nurse–patient relationship.

## Psychodynamic Therapy

Psychodynamic therapy follows the psychoanalytic model by using many of the tools of psychoanalysis, such as free association, dream analysis, transference, and counter-transference. However, the therapist has increased involvement and interacts with the patient more freely than in traditional psychoanalysis. The psychodynamic approach to therapy "understands that unconscious dynamics exist within normal human consciousness and that it is possible in therapy to engage many aspects of the human psyche in ways that are useful, creative, and healing" (Canadian Association for Psychodynamic Therapy, n.d., para. 2). Also, the therapy is oriented more to the here and now and makes less of an attempt to reconstruct the developmental origins of conflicts (Dewan, Steenbarger, & Greenberg, 2008). Psychodynamic therapy tends to last longer than other common therapeutic modalities and may extend for more than 20 sessions.

The best candidates for brief psychotherapy are relatively healthy and well-functioning individuals, sometimes referred to as the "worried well," who have a clearly circumscribed area of difficulty and are intelligent, psychologically minded, and well motivated for change. Patients with psychosis, severe depression, borderline personality disorders, and severe character disorders often are not appropriate candidates for this type of treatment. Supportive therapies, which are within the scope of practice of the basic-level psychiatric nurse, are useful for these patients. A variety of supportive therapies are described in chapters concerning specific disorders (see Chapters 13 to 23).

At the start of treatment, the patient and therapist agree on what the focus will be and concentrate their work on that focus. Sessions are held weekly, and the total number of sessions to be held is determined at the outset of therapy. There is a rapid, back-and-forth pattern between patient and therapist, with both participating actively. The therapist intervenes constantly to keep the therapy on track, either by redirecting the patient's attention or by interpreting deviations from the focus to the patient.

Brief therapies share the following common elements:
- Assessment tends to be rapid and early.
- Clear expectations are established for time-limited therapy with improvement demonstrated within a small number of sessions.
- Goals are concrete and focus on improving the patient's worst symptoms, improving coping skills, and helping the patient understand what is going on in his or her life.
- Interpretations are directed toward present life circumstances and patient behaviour rather than toward the historical significance of feelings.

| TABLE 3-1 | FREUD'S PSYCHOSEXUAL STAGES OF DEVELOPMENT | | | | |
|---|---|---|---|---|---|
| STAGE (AGE) | SOURCE OF SATISFACTION | PRIMARY CONFLICT | TASKS | DESIRED OUTCOMES | OTHER POSSIBLE PERSONALITY TRAITS |
| Oral (0–1 year) | Mouth (sucking, biting, chewing) | Weaning | Mastery of gratification of oral needs; beginning of ego development (4–5 months) | Development of trust in the environment, with the realization that needs can be met | Fixation at the oral stage is associated with passivity, gullibility, and dependence; the use of sarcasm; and the development of orally focused habits (e.g., smoking, nail-biting) |
| Anal (1–3 years) | Anal region (expulsion and retention of feces) | Toilet training | Beginning of development of a sense of control over instinctual drives; ability to delay immediate gratification to gain a future goal | Control over impulses | Fixation at the anal stage is associated with anal retentiveness (stinginess, rigid thought patterns, obsessive-compulsive disorder) or anal-expulsive character (messiness, destructiveness, cruelty) |
| Phallic (oedipal) (3–6 years) | Genitals (masturbation) | Oedipus and Electra | Sexual identity with parent of same sex; beginning of superego development | Identification with parent of same sex | Lack of successful resolution may result in difficulties with sexual identity and difficulties with authority figures |
| Latency (6–12 years) | — | — | Growth of ego functions (social, intellectual, mechanical) and the ability to care about and relate to others outside the home (peers of the same sex) | The development of skills needed to cope with the environment | Fixations can result in difficulty identifying with others and in developing social skills, leading to a sense of inadequacy and inferiority |
| Genital (12 years and beyond) | Genitals (sexual intercourse) | — | Development of satisfying sexual and emotional relationships with members of the opposite sex; emancipation from parents—planning of life goals and development of a strong sense of personal identity | The ability to be creative and find pleasure in love and work | Inability to negotiate this stage could result in difficulties in becoming emotionally and financially independent, lack of strong personal identity and future goals, and inability to form satisfying intimate relationships |

**Source:** Adapted from Gleitman, H. (1981). *Psychology*. New York: W.W. Norton.

- There is a general understanding that psychotherapy does not cure but that it can help troubled individuals learn to recognize that problems exist and can promote self-awareness as they deal with life's inevitable stressors.

## Erik Erikson's Ego Theory

Erik Erikson (1902–1994), an American psychoanalyst, was also a follower of Freud. However, Erikson (1963) believed that Freudian theory was restrictive and negative in its approach. He also stressed that more than the limited mother–child–father triangle influences an individual's development. According to Erikson, personality is not set in stone at age five but continues to develop throughout the lifespan and is influenced by culture and society.

Erikson described development as occurring in eight predetermined and consecutive life stages (psychosocial crises), each of which consists of two possible outcomes (e.g., industry versus inferiority). The successful or unsuccessful completion of each stage affects the individual's progression to the next (Table 3-2). For example, Erikson's crisis of industry versus inferiority occurs from the ages of 7 to 12. During this stage, the child's task is to gain a sense of personal abilities and competence and to expand relationships beyond the immediate family to include peers. The attainment of this task (industry) brings with it the virtue of confidence. The child who fails to navigate this stage successfully is unable to gain a mastery of age-appropriate tasks, cannot make a connection with peers, and will feel like a failure (inferiority).

| TABLE 3-2 | ERIKSON'S EIGHT STAGES OF DEVELOPMENT | | | |
|---|---|---|---|---|
| **APPROXIMATE AGE** | **DEVELOPMENTAL TASK** | **PSYCHOSOCIAL CRISIS** | **SUCCESSFUL RESOLUTION OF CRISIS** | **UNSUCCESSFUL RESOLUTION OF CRISIS** |
| Infancy (0–1½ years) | Forming attachment to mother, which lays foundations for later trust in others | Trust vs. mistrust | Sound basis for relating to other people; trust in people; faith and hope about environment and future "I'm confident that my son will arrange for me to stay with his family until I'm able to live on my own again." | General difficulties relating to people effectively; suspicion; trust–fear conflict; fear of future "I can't trust anyone; no one has ever been there when I needed them." |
| Early childhood (1½–3 years) | Gaining some basic control of self and environment (e.g., toilet training, exploration) | Autonomy vs. shame and doubt | Sense of self-control and adequacy; will power "I'm sure that with the proper diet and exercise program, I can achieve my target weight." | Independence/fear conflict; severe feelings of self-doubt "I could never lose the weight they want me to, so why even try?" |
| Late childhood (3–6 years) | Becoming purposeful and directive | Initiative vs. guilt | Ability to initiate one's own activities; sense of purpose "I like to help Mom by setting the table for dinner." | Aggression/fear conflict; sense of inadequacy or guilt "I know it's wrong, but I wanted the candy, so I took it." |
| School age (6–12 years) | Developing social, physical, and school skills | Industry vs. inferiority | Competence; ability to work "I'm getting really good at swimming since I've been taking lessons." | Sense of inferiority; difficulty learning and working "I can't read as well as the others in my class; I'm just dumb." |
| Adolescence (12–20 years) | Making transition from childhood to adulthood; developing sense of identity | Identity vs. role confusion | Sense of personal identity; fidelity "I'm homosexual, and I'm OK with that." | Confusion about who one is; submersion of identity in relationships or group memberships "I belong to the gang because without them, I'm nothing." |
| Early adulthood (20–35 years) | Establishing intimate bonds of love and friendship | Intimacy vs. isolation | Ability to love deeply and commit oneself "My husband has been my best friend for 25 years." | Emotional isolation; egocentricity "It's nearly impossible to find a man who is worth marrying." |
| Middle adulthood (35–65 years) | Fulfilling life goals that involve family, career, and society; developing concerns that embrace future generations | Generativity vs. self-absorption | Ability to give and to care for others "I've arranged for a 6-month leave of absence to stay with my mother now that her illness is terminal." | Self-absorption; inability to grow as a person "I've lived with this scar on my face for three years; it's worse than having cancer." |
| Later years (65 years to death) | Looking back over one's life and accepting its meaning | Integrity vs. despair | Sense of integrity and fulfillment; willingness to face death; wisdom "I've led a happy, productive life, and I'm ready to die." | Dissatisfaction with life; denial of or despair over prospect of death "I'm not ready to die; the doctors are wrong. You'll see they are wrong." |

**Source:** Altrocchi, J. (1980). *Abnormal psychology* (p. 196). New York: Harcourt Brace Jovanovich; and Erikson, E.H. (1963). *Childhood and society.* New York: W.W. Norton.

## Implications for Psychiatric Mental Health Nursing

Nurses use Erikson's developmental model as an important part of patient assessment. Analysis of behaviour patterns using Erikson's framework can identify age-appropriate or arrested development of normal interpersonal skills. A developmental framework helps the nurse know what types of interventions are most likely to be effective. For example, preschool and kindergarten-aged children in Erikson's initiative-versus-guilt stage of development respond best if they actively participate in imitative, imaginative, and dramatic play and ask questions in order to learn how to do things. Older adults respond to a life review strategy that focuses on the integrity of their life as a tapestry of experience. In the therapeutic encounter, individual responsibility and the capacity for improving one's functioning are addressed. Treatment approaches and interventions can be tailored to the patient's developmental level.

## INTERPERSONAL THEORIES AND THERAPIES

### Harry Stack Sullivan's Interpersonal Theory

Harry Stack Sullivan (1892–1949), an American-born psychiatrist, initially approached patients from a Freudian framework, but he became frustrated by dealing with what he considered unseen and private mental processes within the individual. He turned his attention to interpersonal processes that could be observed in a social framework. Sullivan (1953) defined *personality* as behaviour that can be observed within interpersonal relationships.

According to Sullivan, the purpose of all behaviour is to get needs met through interpersonal interactions and to decrease or avoid anxiety. He defined *anxiety* as any painful feeling or emotion that arises from social insecurity or that prevents biological needs from being satisfied (Sullivan, 1953). Sullivan coined the term *security operations* to describe measures the individual employs to reduce anxiety and enhance security. For example, a person might imagine him- or herself to be right, muster up anger to fuel this righteousness, and try to act to reduce anxiety. Collectively, the security operations an individual uses to defend against anxiety and ensure self-esteem make up the self-system.

There are many parallels between Sullivan's notion of security operations and Freud's concept of defence mechanisms. Both are unconscious processes, and both are ways we reduce anxiety. However, Freud's defence mechanism of repression is an intrapsychic activity, whereas Sullivan's security operations are interpersonal relationship activities that can be observed.

### Implications for Psychiatric Mental Health Nursing

Sullivan's theory is the foundation for Hildegard Peplau's nursing theory of interpersonal relationships that we examine later in this chapter. Believing that therapy should educate patients and assist them in gaining personal insight, Sullivan introduced the term *participant observer*, which underscores that professional helpers cannot be isolated from the therapeutic situation if they are to be effective. Sullivan would insist that the nurse interact with the patient as an authentic human being. Mutuality, respect for the patient, unconditional acceptance, and empathy, which are considered essential aspects of modern therapeutic relationships, were important aspects of Sullivan's theory of interpersonal therapy. Sullivan also demonstrated that a psychotherapeutic environment, characterized by an accepting atmosphere that provided numerous opportunities for practising interpersonal skills and developing relationships, is an invaluable treatment tool. Group psychotherapy, family therapy, and educational and skill training programs, as well as unstructured periods, can be incorporated into the design of a psychotherapeutic environment to facilitate healthy interactions. This method is used today in virtually all residential and day hospital settings.

### Interpersonal Psychotherapy

Interpersonal psychotherapy is an effective short-term therapy that originated with Adolph Meyer and Harry Stack Sullivan. The assumption is that psychiatric disorders are influenced by interpersonal interactions and the social context. The goal of interpersonal psychotherapy is to reduce or eliminate psychiatric symptoms (particularly depression) by improving interpersonal functioning and satisfaction with social relationships (Sadock & Sadock, 2008). Interpersonal psychotherapy has proved successful in the treatment of depression (Cuijpers, Geraedts, van Oppen, et al., 2011). Treatment is predicated on the notion that disturbances in important interpersonal relationships (or a deficit in one's capacity to form those relationships) can play a role in initiating or maintaining clinical depression. In interpersonal psychotherapy, the therapist identifies the nature of the problem to be resolved and then selects strategies consistent with that problem area. Four types of problem areas have been identified (Hollon & Engelhardt, 1997):

1. Grief—complicated bereavement following the death or loss of a loved one
2. Role disputes—conflicts with a significant other
3. Role transition—problematic change in life status or social or vocational role
4. Interpersonal deficit—an inability to initiate or sustain close relationships

### Hildegard Peplau's Theory of Interpersonal Relationships in Nursing

Hildegard Peplau (1909–1999) (Figure 3-2), influenced by the work of Sullivan and learning theory, developed the first systematic theoretical framework for psychiatric nursing in her groundbreaking book *Interpersonal Relations in Nursing*. Peplau (1952) not only established the foundation for the professional practice of psychiatric nursing but also continued to enrich

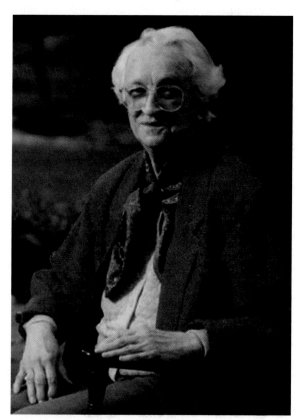

FIGURE 3-2 Hildegard Peplau. **Source:** Courtesy of Anne Peplau.

psychiatric nursing theory and work for the advancement of nursing practice throughout her career.

Peplau was the first nurse to identify psychiatric mental health nursing both as an essential element of general nursing and as a specialty area that embraces specific governing principles. She was also the first nurse theorist to describe the nurse–patient relationship as the foundation of nursing practice (Forchuk, 1991). In shifting the focus from what nurses do *to* patients to what nurses do *with* patients, Peplau (1989) engineered a major paradigm shift from a model focused on medical treatments to an interpersonal relational model of nursing practice. She viewed nursing as an educative instrument designed to help individuals and communities use their capacities to live more productively (Peplau, 1987). Her theory is mainly concerned with the processes by which the nurse helps patients make positive changes in their health care status and well-being and continues to influence our views of the nurse–patient relationship (Stockman, 2005). She believed that illness offered a unique opportunity for experiential learning, personal growth, and improved coping strategies and that psychiatric nurses play a unique role in facilitating this growth (Peplau, 1982a, 1982b).

Peplau identified stages of the nurse–patient relationship (see Chapter 10) and also taught the technique of *process recording* to help her students hone their communication and relationship skills (see Table 11-4). The skills of the psychiatric nurse include observation, interpretation, and intervention. The nurse observes and listens to the patient, developing impressions about the meaning of the patient's situation. By employing this process, the nurse is able to view the patient as a unique individual. The nurse's inferences are then validated with the patient for accuracy. Peplau believed it was essential for nurses to observe the behaviour not only of the patient but also of themselves and so proposed an approach in which nurses are both participants and observers in therapeutic conversations. This self-awareness on the part of the nurse is essential in keeping the focus on the patient, as well as keeping the social and personal needs of the nurse out of the nurse–patient conversation.

Peplau spent a lifetime illuminating the science and art of professional nursing practice, and her work has had a profound effect on the nursing profession, nursing science, and the clinical practice of psychiatric nursing (Haber, 2000). The art component of nursing consists of the care, compassion, and advocacy nurses provide to enhance patient comfort and well-being. The science component of nursing involves the application of knowledge to understand a broad range of human problems and psychosocial phenomena and intervening to relieve patients' suffering and promote growth (Haber, 2000). In her works, Peplau (1995) constantly reminds nurses to "care for the person as well as the illness" and "think exclusively of patients as persons" (p. 2).

### Implications for Psychiatric Mental Health Nursing

Perhaps Peplau's most universal contribution to the everyday practice of psychiatric mental health nursing is her application of Sullivan's theory of anxiety to nursing practice. She described the effects of different levels of anxiety (mild, moderate, severe,

and panic) on perception and learning. She promoted interventions to lower anxiety, with the aim of improving patients' abilities to think and function at more satisfactory levels. More on the application of Peplau's theory of anxiety and interventions is presented in Chapter 13. Table 3-3 lists select nursing theorists and summarizes their major contributions and the impact of these contributions on psychiatric mental health nursing.

## BEHAVIOURAL THEORIES AND THERAPIES

Behavioural theories also developed as a protest response to Freud's assumption that a person's destiny was carved in stone at a very early age. Behaviourists have no concern with inner conflicts but argue that personality simply consists of learned behaviours. Consequently, if behaviour changes, so does the personality.

The development of behavioural models began in the nineteenth century as a result of Ivan Pavlov's laboratory work with dogs. It continued into the twentieth century with John B. Watson's application of these models to shape behaviour and B.F. Skinner's research on rat behaviour. These behavioural theorists developed systematic learning principles that could be applied to humans. Behavioural models emphasize the ways in which observable behavioural responses are learned and can be modified in a particular environment. Pavlov's, Watson's, and Skinner's models focus on the belief that behaviour can be influenced through a process referred to as *conditioning*. Conditioning involves pairing behaviour with a condition that reinforces or diminishes the behaviour's occurrence.

### Ivan Pavlov's Classical Conditioning Theory

Ivan Pavlov (1849–1936) was a Russian physiologist. He won a Nobel Prize for his outstanding contributions to the physiology of digestion, which he studied through his well-known experiments with dogs. In incidental observation of the dogs, Pavlov noticed that the dogs were able to anticipate when food would be forthcoming and would begin to salivate even before actually tasting the meat. Pavlov labelled this process *psychic secretion*. He hypothesized that the psychic component was a learned association between two events: the presence of the experimental apparatus and the serving of meat.

Pavlov formalized his observations of behaviours in dogs in a theory of classical conditioning. Pavlov (1928) found that when a neutral stimulus (a bell) was repeatedly paired with another stimulus (food that triggered salivation), eventually the sound of the bell alone could elicit salivation in the dogs. An example of this response in humans would be an individual who became very ill as a child after eating spoiled coleslaw at a picnic and later in life feels nauseated whenever he smells coleslaw. It is important to recognize that classical conditioned responses are involuntary—not under conscious personal control—and are not spontaneous choices.

### John B. Watson's Behaviourism Theory

John B. Watson (1878–1958) was an American psychologist who rejected the unconscious motivation of psychoanalysis as

| TABLE 3-3 | SELECT NURSING THEORISTS, THEIR MAJOR CONTRIBUTIONS, AND THEIR IMPACT ON PSYCHIATRIC MENTAL HEALTH NURSING | |
|---|---|---|
| **NURSING THEORIST** | **FOCUS OF THEORY** | **CONTRIBUTION TO PSYCHIATRIC MENTAL HEALTH NURSING** |
| Patricia Benner | "Caring" as foundation for nursing | Benner encourages nurses to provide caring and comforting interventions. She emphasizes the importance of the nurse–patient relationship and the importance of teaching and coaching the patient and bearing witness to suffering as the patient deals with illness. |
| Dorothea Orem | Goal of self-care as integral to the practice of nursing | Orem emphasizes the role of the nurse in promoting self-care activities of the patient; this has relevance to the seriously and persistently mentally ill patient. |
| Sister Callista Roy | Continual need for people to adapt physically, psychologically, and socially | Roy emphasizes the role of nursing in assisting patients to adapt so they can cope more effectively with changes. |
| Betty Neuman | Impact of internal and external stressors on the equilibrium of the system | Neuman emphasizes the role of nursing in assisting patients to discover and use stress-reducing strategies. |
| Joyce Travelbee | Meaning in the nurse–patient relationship and the importance of communication | Travelbee emphasizes the role of nursing in affirming the suffering of the patient and in being able to alleviate that suffering through communication skills used appropriately throughout the stages of the nurse–patient relationship. |

**Source:** Benner, P., & Wrubel, J. (1989). *The primacy of caring: Stress and coping in health and illness.* Menlo Park, CA: Addison-Wesley; Leddy, S., & Pepper, J.M. (1993). *Conceptual bases of professional nursing* (3rd ed., pp. 174–175). Philadelphia: Lippincott; Neuman, B., & Young, R. (1972). A model for teaching total-person approach to patient problems. *Nursing Research, 21*(3), 264–269; Orem, D.E. (1995). *Nursing: Concepts of practice* (5th ed.). New York: McGraw-Hill; Roy, C., & Andrews, H.A. (1991). *The Roy adaptation model: The definitive statement.* Norwalk, CT: Appleton & Lange; and Travelbee, J. (1961). *Intervention in psychiatric nursing.* Philadelphia: F.A. Davis.

being too subjective. He developed the school of thought referred to as behaviourism, which he believed was more objective or measurable. Watson contended that personality traits and responses—adaptive and maladaptive—were socially learned through classical conditioning (Watson, 1919). In a famous (but terrible) experiment, Watson stood behind Little Albert, a 9-month-old who liked animals, and made a loud noise with a hammer every time the infant reached for a white rat. After this experiment, Little Albert became terrified at the sight of white fur or hair, even in the absence of a loud noise. Watson concluded that behaviour could be moulded by controlling the environment and that anyone could be trained to be anything, from a beggar man to a merchant.

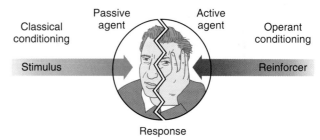

FIGURE 3-3 Classical versus operant conditioning. **Source:** From Carson, V.B. (2000). *Mental health nursing: The nurse–patient journey* (2nd ed., p. 121). Philadelphia: Saunders.

### B.F. Skinner's Operant Conditioning Theory

B.F. Skinner (1904–1990) represented the second wave of behavioural theorists. Skinner (1987) researched operant conditioning, in which voluntary behaviours are learned through consequences, and behavioural responses are elicited through reinforcement, which causes a behaviour to occur more frequently. A consequence can be a positive reinforcement, such as receiving a reward (getting high marks after studying hard all semester), or a negative reinforcement, such as the removal of an objectionable or aversive stimulus (walking freely through a park once the vicious dog is picked up by animal services).

Other techniques can cause behaviours to occur less frequently. One technique is an unpleasant consequence, or

punishment. Driving too fast may result in a speeding ticket, which—in mature and healthy individuals—decreases the chances that speeding will recur. Absence of reinforcement, or extinction, also decreases behaviour by withholding a reward that has become habitual. If a person tells a joke and no one laughs, for example, the person is less apt to tell jokes because his joke-telling behaviour is not being reinforced. Teachers employ this strategy in the classroom when they ignore acting-out behaviour that had previously been rewarded by more attention. Figure 3-3 illustrates the differences between classical conditioning (in which an involuntary reaction is caused by a stimulus) and operant conditioning (in which voluntary behaviour is learned through reinforcement).

### Implications for Psychiatric Mental Health Nursing

Skinner's behavioural model provides a concrete method for modifying or replacing behaviours. Behaviour management and modification programs based on his principles have proven to be successful in altering targeted behaviours. Programmed learning and token economies—in which tokens, or symbolic objects (e.g., check marks), can be exchanged for valued items, services, or privileges (e.g., food, passes out of the building, phone calls)—represent extensions of Skinner's thoughts on learning. Behavioural methods are particularly effective with children, adolescents, and individuals with many forms of chronic mental illness.

### Behavioural Therapy

Behavioural therapy is based on the assumption that changes in maladaptive behaviour can occur without insight into the underlying cause. This approach works best when it is directed at specific problems and the goals are well defined. Behavioural therapy is effective in treating people with phobias, alcoholism, schizophrenia, and many other conditions. Four types of behavioural therapy are discussed here: modelling, operant conditioning, systematic desensitization, and aversion therapy.

### Modelling

In modelling, the therapist provides a role model for specific identified behaviours, and the patient learns through imitation. The therapist may do the modelling, provide another person to model the behaviours, or present a video for the purpose. Bandura, Blahard, and Ritter (1969) were able to help people lessen their phobias about nonpoisonous snakes by having them first view close-ups of filmed encounters between people and snakes that had successful outcomes, and then view live encounters between people and snakes that also had successful outcomes. In a similar fashion, some behavioural therapists use role-playing in the consulting room. For example, a student who does not know how to ask a professor for an extension on a term paper would watch the therapist portray a potentially effective way of making the request. The clinician would then help the student practise the new skill in a similar role-playing situation.

### Operant Conditioning

Operant conditioning is the basis for behaviour modification and uses positive reinforcement to increase desired behaviours. For example, when desired goals are achieved or behaviours are performed, patients might be rewarded with tokens. These tokens can be exchanged for food, small luxuries, or privileges. This reward system is known as a token economy.

Operant conditioning has been useful in improving the verbal behaviours of mute, autistic, and developmentally disabled children. In patients with severe and persistent mental illness, behaviour modification has helped increase levels of self-care, social behaviour, group participation, and more.

We all use positive reinforcement in our everyday lives. A familiar case in point is the mother who takes her preschooler along to the grocery store, and the child starts acting out, demanding candy, nagging, crying, and yelling. Here are examples of three ways the child's behaviour can be reinforced:

| **Action** | **Result** |
|---|---|
| 1. The mother gives the child the candy. | The child continues to use this behaviour. This is positive reinforcement of negative behaviour. |
| 2. The mother scolds the child. | Acting out may continue, because the child gets what he really wants—attention. This positively rewards negative behaviour. |
| 3. The mother ignores the acting out but gives attention to the child when he is behaving appropriately. | The child gets a positive reward for appropriate behaviour. |

### Systematic Desensitization

Systematic desensitization is another form of behaviour modification therapy that involves the development of behavioural tasks customized to the patient's specific fears; these tasks are presented to the patient while using learned relaxation techniques. The process involves four steps:

1. The patient's fear is broken down into its components by exploring the particular stimulus cues to which the patient reacts. For example, certain situations may precipitate a phobic reaction, whereas others do not. Crowds at parties may be problematic, whereas similar numbers of people in other settings do not cause the same distress.
2. The patient is incrementally exposed to the fear. For example, a patient who has a fear of flying is introduced to short periods of visual presentations of flying—first with still pictures, then with videos, and finally in a busy airport. The situations are confronted while the patient is in a relaxed state. Gradually, over a period of time, exposure is increased until anxiety about or fear of the object or situation has ceased.
3. The patient is instructed in how to design a hierarchy of fears. For fear of flying, a patient might develop a set of statements representing the stages of a flight, order the statements from the most fearful to the least fearful, and use relaxation techniques to reach a state of relaxation as he or she progresses through the list.
4. The patient practises these techniques every day.

### Aversion Therapy

Today, aversion therapy (which is akin to punishment) is used widely to treat behaviours such as alcoholism, sexual deviation, shoplifting, violent and aggressive behaviour, and self-mutilation. Aversion therapy is sometimes the treatment of choice when other less drastic measures have failed to produce the desired effects. The following are three paradigms for using aversive techniques:

1. Pairing of a maladaptive behaviour with a noxious stimulus (e.g., pairing the sight and smell of alcohol with electric shock), so that anxiety or fear becomes associated with the once-pleasurable stimulus
2. Punishment (e.g., punishment applied after the patient has had an alcoholic drink)
3. Avoidance training (e.g., patient avoids punishment by pushing a glass of alcohol away within a certain time limit)

Simple examples of extinguishing undesirable behaviour through aversion therapy include painting foul-tasting substances on the fingernails of nail biters or the thumbs of thumb suckers. Other examples of aversive stimuli are chemicals that induce nausea and vomiting, noxious odours, unpleasant verbal stimuli (e.g., descriptions of disturbing scenes), costs or fines in a token economy, and denial of positive reinforcement (e.g., isolation).

Before initiating any aversive protocol, the therapist, treatment team, or society *must* answer the following questions:
- Is this therapy in the best interest of the patient?
- Does its use violate the patient's rights?
- Is it in the best interest of society?

If aversion therapy is chosen as the most appropriate treatment, those administering it must provide ongoing supervision, support, and evaluation.

### Biofeedback

Biofeedback is a form of behavioural therapy that uses sensitive instrumentation to acquire information about bodily functions such as muscle activity, brain waves, skin temperature, heart rate, and blood pressure. Biofeedback is successfully used today, especially for controlling the body's physiological response to stress and anxiety. This form of therapy is discussed in detail in Chapter 12.

## COGNITIVE THEORIES AND THERAPIES

While behaviourists focused on increasing, decreasing, or eliminating measurable behaviours, little attention was paid to the thoughts, or cognitions, that were involved in these behaviours. Rather than thinking of people as passive recipients of environmental conditioning, cognitive theorists proposed that there is a dynamic interplay between individuals and the environment. These theorists believe that thoughts come before feelings and actions and that thoughts about the world and our place in it are based on our own unique perspectives, which may or may not be based on reality. Two of the most influential theorists and their therapies are presented here.

### Rational-Emotive Behaviour Therapy

Rational-emotive behaviour therapy (REBT) was developed by Albert Ellis (1913–2007) in 1955. The aim of REBT is to eradicate core irrational beliefs by helping people recognize thoughts that are not accurate, sensible, or useful. These thoughts tend to take the form of *should*s (e.g., "I should always be polite."), *ought*s (e.g., "I ought to consistently win

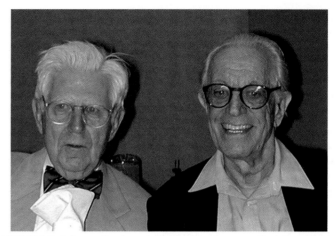

**FIGURE 3-4** Aaron Beck and Albert Ellis. **Source:** Fenichel, 2000.

my tennis games."), and *must*s (e.g., "I must be thin."). Ellis described negative thinking as a simple A-B-C process. *A* stands for the activating event, *B* stands for beliefs about the event, and *C* stands for the emotional consequence as a result of the event.

$$A \quad \rightarrow \quad B \quad \rightarrow \quad C$$

Activating Event      Beliefs      Emotional Consequence

Perception influences all thoughts, which in turn influence our behaviours. For example, imagine you have just received an invitation to a birthday party (activating event). You think, *I hate parties. Now I have to hang out with people who don't like me instead of watching my favourite television shows. They probably just invited me to get a gift* (beliefs). You will probably be miserable (emotional consequence) if you go. On the other hand, you may think, *I love parties!* (activating event). *This will be a great chance to meet new people, and it will be fun to shop for the perfect gift* (beliefs). You could have a delightful time (emotional consequence).

Although Ellis (Figure 3-4) admitted that the role of past experiences is instrumental in our current beliefs, the focus of rational-emotive behaviour therapy is on present attitudes, painful feelings, and dysfunctional behaviours. If our beliefs are negative and self-deprecating, we are more susceptible to depression and anxiety. Ellis noted that while we cannot change the past, we can change the way we are now. He was pragmatic in his approach to mental illness and colourful in his therapeutic advice: "It's too [darn] bad you panic, but you don't die from it! Get them over the panic about panic, you may find the panic disappears" (Ellis, 2000).

### Cognitive-Behavioural Therapy (CBT)

Aaron T. Beck (Figure 3-4), another follower of Sigmund Freud, was originally trained in psychoanalysis but is regarded as a neo-Freudian. When he attempted to study depression from a psychoanalytic perspective, he became convinced that people with depression generally had stereotypical patterns of negative and self-critical thinking that seemed to distort their ability to think and process information. Cognitive-behavioural therapy (CBT) is based on both cognitive psychology and behavioural theory. It is a commonly employed, effective, and well-researched therapeutic tool.

Beck's method (Beck, Rush, Shaw, et al., 1979), the basis for CBT, is an active, directive, time-limited, structured approach used to treat a variety of psychiatric disorders (e.g., depression, anxiety, phobias, pain problems). It is based on the underlying theoretical principle that how people feel and behave is largely determined by the way they think about the world and their place in it (Beck, 1967). Their cognitions (verbal or pictorial events in their stream of consciousness) are based on attitudes or assumptions developed from previous experiences. These cognitions may be fairly accurate, or they may be distorted. According to Beck, we all have schemata or unique assumptions about ourselves, others, and the world around us. For example, a person who has the schema "The only person I can trust is myself" will have expectations that everyone else has questionable motives, will lie, and will eventually hurt them. Other negative schemata include incompetence, abandonment, evilness, and vulnerability. We are typically not aware of such cognitive biases, but recognizing them as beliefs and attitudes based on distortions and misconceptions will help make apparent dysfunctional schemata underlying our thinking.

Rapid, unthinking responses based on schemata are known as automatic thoughts. These responses are particularly intense and frequent in psychiatric disorders such as depression and anxiety. Often, automatic thoughts, or cognitive distortions, are irrational and lead to false assumptions and misinterpretations. For example, if a person interprets all experiences in terms of whether he or she is competent and adequate, thinking may be dominated by the cognitive distortion "Unless I do everything perfectly, I'm a failure." Consequently, the person reacts to situations in terms of adequacy, even when these situations are unrelated to whether he or she is personally competent. Table 3-4 describes common cognitive distortions.

The therapeutic techniques of the cognitive therapist are designed to identify, reality-test, and correct distorted conceptualizations and the dysfunctional beliefs underlying them. Patients are taught to challenge their own negative thinking and substitute it with positive, rational thoughts. They are taught to recognize when thinking is based on distortions and misconceptions. Homework assignments play an important role in CBT. A particularly effective technique is the use of a four-column format to record the precipitating event or situation, the resulting automatic thought, the proceeding feeling(s) and behaviour(s), and, finally, a challenge to the negative thoughts based on rational evidence and thinking. The following is an example of the type of analysis done by a patient receiving CBT.

A 24-year-old nurse recently discharged from the hospital for severe depression presented this record (Beck, Rush, Shaw, et al., 1979):

| Event | Feeling | Cognitions | Other Possible Interpretations |
|---|---|---|---|
| While at a party, Jim asked me, "How are you feeling?" shortly after I was discharged from the hospital. | Anxious | Jim thinks I am a basket case. I must look really bad for him to be concerned. | He really cares about me. He noticed that I look better than before I went into the hospital and wants to know if I feel better too. |

Box 3-1 presents an example of cognitive-behavioural therapy, and Table 3-5 compares and contrasts psychodynamic, interpersonal, cognitive-behavioural, and behavioural therapies.

### Implications for Psychiatric Mental Health Nursing

Recognizing the interplay between events, negative thinking, and negative responses can be beneficial from both a patient-care standpoint and a personal one. Workbooks are available to aid in the process of identifying cognitive distortions. Personal benefits from this cognitive approach could help the nurse understand his or her own response to a variety of difficult situations. One example might be the anxiety that some students feel regarding the psychiatric nursing clinical rotation. Students may overgeneralize ("All psychiatric patients are dangerous.") or personalize ("My patient doesn't seem to be better; I'm probably not doing him any good.") the situation. The key to effectively using the CBT approach in clinical situations is to challenge the negative thoughts not based on facts and then replace them with more realistic appraisals.

## HUMANISTIC THEORIES

In the 1950s, humanistic theories arose as a protest against both the behavioural and psychoanalytic schools, which were thought to be pessimistic, deterministic, and dehumanizing. Humanistic theories focus on human potential and free will to choose life patterns that are supportive of personal growth. Humanistic frameworks emphasize a person's capacity for self-actualization. This approach focuses on understanding the patient's perspective as she or he subjectively experiences it. There are a number of humanistic theorists. We will explore Abraham Maslow and his theory of self-actualization.

### Abraham Maslow's Humanistic Psychology Theory

Abraham Maslow (1908–1970), considered the father of humanistic psychology, introduced the concept of a "self-actualized personality" associated with high productivity and enjoyment of life (Maslow, 1963, 1968). He criticized psychology for focusing too intently on humanity's frailties and not enough on its strengths. Maslow contended that the focus of psychology must go beyond experiences of hate, pain, misery, guilt, and conflict to include love, compassion, happiness, exhilaration, and well-being.

## TABLE 3-4   COMMON COGNITIVE DISTORTIONS

| DISTORTION | DEFINITION | EXAMPLE |
|---|---|---|
| All-or-nothing thinking | Thinking in black and white, reducing complex outcomes into absolutes | Although Marcia earned the second highest score in the provincial figure-skating competition, she consistently referred to herself as "a loser." |
| Overgeneralization | Using a bad outcome (or a few bad outcomes) as evidence that nothing will ever go right again | Marty had a minor traffic accident. She refuses to drive and says, "I shouldn't be allowed on the road." When asked why, she answers, "I'm a horrible driver; I could have killed someone!" |
| Labelling | Generalizing a characteristic or event so that it becomes definitive and results in an overly harsh label for self or others | "Because I failed the advanced statistics exam, I am a failure. I should give up. I may as well quit my nursing program." |
| Mental filter | Focusing on a negative detail or bad event and allowing it to taint everything else | René's boss evaluated his work as exemplary and gave him a few suggestions for improvement. He obsessed about the suggestions and ignored the rest. |
| Disqualifying the positive | Maintaining a negative view by rejecting information that supports a positive view as being irrelevant, inaccurate, or accidental | "I've just been offered the job I've always wanted. No one else must have applied." |
| Jumping to conclusions | Making a negative interpretation despite the fact that there is little or no supporting evidence | "My fiancé, Ryan, didn't call me for 3 hours, which just proves he doesn't love me anymore." |
| a. Mind-reading | Inferring negative thoughts, responses, and motives of others | "The grocery store clerk was grouchy and barely made eye contact, so I must have done something wrong." |
| b. Fortune-telling error | Anticipating that things will turn out badly as an established fact | "I'll ask her out, but I know she won't have a good time." |
| Magnification or minimization | Exaggerating the importance of something (such as a personal failure or the success of others) or reducing the importance of something (such as a personal success or the failure of others) | "I'm alone on a Saturday night because no one likes me. When other people are alone, it's because they want to be." |
| a. Catastrophizing | Magnifying to the extreme so that the very worst is assumed to be a probable outcome. | "If I don't make a good impression on the boss at the company picnic, she will fire me." |
| Emotional reasoning | Drawing a conclusion based on an emotional state | "I'm nervous about the exam. I must not be prepared. If I were, I wouldn't be afraid." |
| Should and must statements | Assuming rigid self-directives that presume an unrealistic amount of control over external events | "My patient is worse today. I should give better care so she will get better." |
| Personalization | Assuming responsibility for an external event or situation that was likely outside personal control. | "I'm sorry your party wasn't more fun. It's probably because I was there." |

**Source:** Adapted from Burns, D.D. (1989). *The feeling good handbook*. New York: William Morrow.

### Hierarchy of Needs

Maslow conceptualized human motivation as a hierarchy of dynamic processes or needs that are critical for the development of all humans. Central to his theory is the assumption that humans are active rather than passive participants in life, striving for self-actualization. Maslow (1968) focused on human need fulfillment, which he categorized into six incremental stages, beginning with physiological survival needs and ending

with self-transcendent needs (Figure 3-5). The hierarchy of needs is conceptualized as a pyramid, with the strongest, most fundamental needs placed on the lower levels. The more distinctly human needs occupy the top sections of the pyramid. When lower-level needs are met, higher needs are able to emerge.
- *Physiological needs*. The most basic needs are the physiological drives—food, oxygen, water, sleep, sex, and a constant

## BOX 3-1   EXAMPLE OF COGNITIVE-BEHAVIOURAL THERAPY

The patient was an attractive woman in her early 20s. Her depression of 18 months' duration was precipitated by her boyfriend's leaving her. She had numerous automatic thoughts that she was ugly and undesirable. These automatic thoughts were handled in the following manner:

**Therapist:** Other than your subjective opinion, what evidence do you have that you are ugly?

**Patient:** Well, my sister always said I was ugly.

**Therapist:** Was she always right in these matters?

**Patient:** No. Actually, she had her own reasons for telling me this. But the real reason I know I'm ugly is that men don't ask me out. If I weren't ugly, I'd be dating now.

**Therapist:** That is a possible reason why you're not dating. But there's an alternative explanation. You told me that you work in an office by yourself all day and spend your nights alone at home. It doesn't seem like you're giving yourself opportunities to meet men.

**Patient:** I can see what you're saying, but still, if I weren't ugly, men would ask me out.

**Therapist:** I suggest we run an experiment: that is, for you to become more socially active, stop turning down invitations to parties and social events, and see what happens.

After the patient became more active and had more opportunities to meet men, she started to date. At this point, she no longer believed she was ugly.

Therapy then focused on her basic assumption that one's worth is determined by one's appearance. She readily agreed this didn't make sense. She also saw the falseness of the assumption that one must be beautiful to attract men or be loved. This discussion led to her basic assumption that she could not be happy without love (or attention from men).

The latter part of treatment focused on helping her to change this belief.

**Therapist:** On what do you base this belief that you can't be happy without a man?

**Patient:** I was really depressed for a year and a half when I didn't have a man in my life.

**Therapist:** Is there another reason why you were depressed?

**Patient:** As we discussed, I was looking at everything in a distorted way. But I still don't know if I could be happy if no one was interested in me.

**Therapist:** I don't know either. Is there a way we could find out?

**Patient:** Well, as an experiment, I could not go out on dates for a while and see how I feel.

**Therapist:** I think that's a good idea. Although it has its flaws, the experimental method is still the best way currently available to discover the facts. You're fortunate in being able to run this type of experiment. Now, for the first time in your adult life, you aren't attached to a man. If you find you can be happy without a man, this will greatly strengthen you and also make your future relationships all the better.

In this case, the patient was able to stick to a "cold turkey" regimen. After a brief period of dysphoria, she was delighted to find that her well-being was not dependent on another person.

There were similarities between these two interventions. In both, the distorted conclusion or assumption was delineated, and the patient was asked for evidence to support it. An experiment to gather data was also suggested in both instances. However, to achieve the results, a contrasting version of the same experimental situation was required.

**Source:** Beck, A.T., Rush, A.J., Shaw, B.F., et al. (1979). *Cognitive therapy of depression.* New York: Guilford Press.

## TABLE 3-5   COMPARISON OF PSYCHODYNAMIC, INTERPERSONAL, COGNITIVE-BEHAVIOURAL, AND BEHAVIOURAL THERAPIES

|  | PSYCHODYNAMIC THERAPY | INTERPERSONAL THERAPY | COGNITIVE-BEHAVIOURAL THERAPY | BEHAVIOURAL THERAPY |
|---|---|---|---|---|
| **Treatment focus** | Unresolved past relationships and core conflicts | Current interpersonal relationships and social supports | Thoughts and cognitions | Learned maladaptive behaviour |
| **Therapist role** | Significant other transference object | Problem solver | Active, directive, challenging | Active, directive teacher |
| **Primary disorders treated** | Anxiety; depression; personality disorders | Depression | Depression; anxiety/panic; eating disorders | Post-traumatic stress disorder; obsessive-compulsive disorder; panic disorder |
| **Length of therapy** | 20+ sessions | Short term (12–20 sessions) | Short term (5–20 sessions) | Varies; typically fewer than 10 sessions |
| **Technique** | Therapeutic alliance; free association; understanding transference; challenging defence mechanisms | Facilitate new patterns of communication and expectations for relationships | Evaluating thoughts and behaviours; modifying dysfunctional thoughts and behaviours | Relaxation; thought stopping; self-reassurance; seeking social support |

**Source:** Dewan, M.J., Steenbarger, B.N., & Greenberg, R.P. (2008). Brief psychotherapies. In R.E. Hales, S.C. Yudofsky, & G.O. Gabbard (Eds.), *Textbook of psychiatry* (5th ed., pp. 1155–1170). Washington, DC: American Psychiatric Publishing.

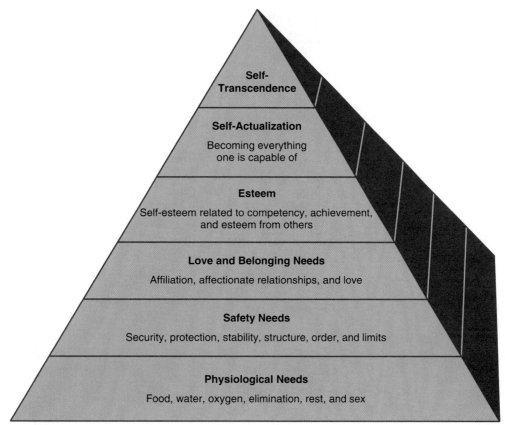

**FIGURE 3-5** Maslow's hierarchy of needs. **Source:** Adapted from Maslow, A.H. (1972). *The farther reaches of human nature.* New York: Viking.

body temperature. If all needs were deprived, this level would take priority over the rest.

- *Safety needs.* Once physiological needs are met, safety needs emerge. They include security; protection; freedom from fear, anxiety, and chaos; and the need for law, order, and limits. Adults in a stable society usually feel safe, but they may feel threatened by debt, job insecurity, or lack of insurance. It is during times of crisis, such as war, disasters, assaults, and social breakdown, that safety needs really take precedence. Children, who are more vulnerable and dependent, respond far more readily and intensely to safety threats.

- *Belongingness and love needs.* People have a need for intimate relationships, love, affection, and belonging and will seek to overcome feelings of aloneness and alienation. Maslow stresses the importance of having a family and a home and of being part of an identifiable group.

- *Esteem needs.* People need to have a high self-regard and have it reflected to them from others. If self-esteem needs are met, we feel confident, valued, and valuable. When self-esteem is compromised, we feel inferior, worthless, and helpless.

- *Self-actualization.* We are preset to strive to be everything we are capable of becoming. Maslow said, "What a man *can* be, he *must* be." What we are capable of becoming is highly individual—an artist must paint, a writer must write, and a healer must heal. The drive to satisfy this need is felt as a sort

of restlessness, a sense that something is missing. It is up to each person to choose a path that will bring about inner peace and fulfillment.

Although his early work included only five levels of needs, Maslow (1970) later took into account two additional factors: (1) cognitive needs (the desire to know and understand) and (2) the aesthetic needs. He describes the acquisition of knowledge (our first priority) and the need to understand (our second priority) as being hard-wired and essential; he identified the aesthetic need for beauty and symmetry as universal. How else, after all, do we explain the impulse to straighten a crooked picture?

Maslow based his theory on the results of clinical investigations of people who represented self-actualized individuals, who moved in the direction of achieving and reaching their highest potentials. Among those Maslow chose to investigate were historical figures such as Henry David Thoreau, Walt Whitman, and Ludwig von Beethoven, as well as others like Albert Einstein and Albert Schweitzer, who were living at the time they were studied. This investigation led Maslow (1963, 1970) to identify some basic personality characteristics that distinguish self-actualizing people from those who might be called "ordinary" (Box 3-2).

### Implications for Psychiatric Mental Health Nursing

The value of Maslow's model in nursing practice is twofold. First, an emphasis on human potential and the patient's

**SOME CHARACTERISTICS OF SELF-ACTUALIZED PERSONS (SAs)**

- Accurate perception of reality; not defensive in their perceptions of the world
- Acceptance of themselves, others, and nature
- Spontaneity, simplicity, and naturalness (SAs do not live programmed lives)
- Problem-centred rather than self-centred orientation (possibly the most important characteristic); SAs have a sense of a mission to which they dedicate their lives
- Enjoyment of privacy and detachment; pleasure in being alone; ability to reflect on events
- Freshness of appreciation; not taking life for granted
- Mystical or peak experiences (a moment of intense ecstasy, similar to a religious or mystical experience, during which the self is transcended)*
- Active social interest
- An unhostile sense of humour
- Democratic character structure; displaying little racial, religious, or social prejudice
- Creativity, especially in managing their lives
- Resistance to conformity (enculturation); autonomy, independence, and self-sufficiency

*More recently, Mihaly Csikszentmihalyi developed the term *flow experience* to describe times when people become so totally involved in what they are doing that they lose all sense of time and awareness of self.
**Source:** Adapted from Maslow, A.H. (1970). *Motivation and personality*. New York: Harper & Row.

strengths is key to successful nurse–patient relationships. Second, the model helps establish what is most important in the sequencing of nursing actions in the nurse–patient relationship. For example, to collect any but the most essential information when a patient is struggling with drug withdrawal is inappropriate. Following Maslow's model as a way of prioritizing actions, the nurse meets the patient's physiological need for stable vital signs and pain relief before further assessment.

## BIOLOGICAL THEORIES AND THERAPIES

### The Advent of Psychopharmacology

In 1950, a French drug firm synthesized chlorpromazine (Largactil)—a powerful antipsychotic medication—and psychiatry experienced a revolution. The advent of psychopharmacology presented a direct challenge to psychodynamic approaches to mental illness. The dramatic experience of observing patients freed from the bondage of psychosis and mania by powerful drugs such as chlorpromazine and lithium left witnesses convinced of the critical role of the brain in psychiatric illness.

Since the discovery of chlorpromazine, many other medications have proven effective in controlling psychosis, mania, depression, and anxiety. These medications greatly reduce the

need for hospitalization and dramatically improve the lives of people with serious psychiatric difficulties. Today we know that psychoactive medications exert differential effects on different neurotransmitters and help restore brain function, allowing patients with mental illness to continue living productive lives with greater satisfaction and far less emotional pain.

### The Biological Model

A biological model of mental illness focuses on neurological, chemical, biological, and genetic issues and seeks to understand how the body and brain interact to create emotions, memories, and perceptual experiences. This perspective views abnormal behaviour as part of a disease process or a defect and seeks to stop or alter it. The biological model locates the illness or disease in the body—usually in the limbic system of the brain and the synapse receptor sites of the central nervous system—and targets the site of the illness using physical interventions such as medications, diet, or surgery.

The recognition that psychiatric illnesses are as physical in origin as diabetes and coronary heart disease serves to decrease the stigma surrounding them. Just as people with diabetes or heart disease cannot be held responsible for their illness, patients with schizophrenia or bipolar affective disorder are not to blame for theirs. It often happens that one of the most helpful things we can tell those whose lives are affected by psychiatric illness is that they are not responsible or to blame.

### Implications for Psychiatric Mental Health Nursing

Historically, psychiatric mental health nurses always have attended to the physical needs of psychiatric patients. Nurses administer medications; monitor sleep, activity, nutrition, hydration, elimination, and other functions; and prepare patients for somatic therapies, such as electroconvulsive therapy. They have continued to do so with the advancement of the biological model, which has not altered the basic nursing strategies: focusing on the qualities of a therapeutic relationship, understanding the patient's perspective, and communicating in a way that facilitates the patient's recovery.

One of the risks in adopting a biological model to the exclusion of all other theoretical perspectives is that such a theory ignores the myriad other influences, including social, environmental, cultural, economic, spiritual, and educational factors, that play a role in the development and treatment of mental illness.

## ADDITIONAL THERAPIES

### Milieu Therapy

In 1948, Bruno Bettelheim coined the term milieu therapy to describe his use of the total environment to treat disturbed children. Bettelheim created a comfortable, secure environment (or milieu) in which psychotic children were helped to form a new world. Staff members were trained to provide 24-hour support and understanding for each child on an individual basis.

*Milieu* is sometimes a difficult concept to grasp. It is an all-inclusive term that recognizes the people, setting, structure, and emotional climate all as important to healing. Milieu therapy uses naturally occurring events in the environment as rich learning opportunities for patients. There are certain basic characteristics of milieu therapy, regardless of whether the setting involves treatment of psychotic children, patients in a psychiatric hospital, drug abusers in a residential treatment centre, or psychiatric patients in a day hospital. Milieu therapy, or a therapeutic community, has as its focus a living, learning, or working environment. Such therapy may be based on any number of therapeutic modalities, from structured behavioural therapy to spontaneous, humanistic-oriented approaches.

## Implications for Psychiatric Mental Health Nursing

Milieu therapy is a basic intervention in nursing practice. Although most commonly associated with inpatient treatment (Thibeault, Trudeau, d'Entremont, et al., 2010), other examples of milieu therapy include providing a safe environment for the suicidal patient or for a patient with a cognitive disorder (e.g., Alzheimer's disease), referring abused women to safe houses, and advocating for children suspected of being abused in their home environments.

You will be introduced to other therapeutic approaches later in the book. Crisis intervention (see Chapter 24) is an approach you will find useful, not only in psychiatric mental health nursing but also in other nursing specialties. Group therapy (see Chapter 35) and family interventions (see Chapter 36), which are appropriate for the basic-level practitioner, will also be discussed.

Table 3-6 lists additional theorists whose contributions influence psychiatric mental health nursing.

 **RESEARCH HIGHLIGHT**

### Recovery Narratives: A Mental Health Commission of Canada Pilot Project

**Source:** Jensen, J. (n.d.). *Brandon University develops unique program to reduce stigma.* Retrieved from http://www.mentalhealthcommission.ca/SiteCollectionDocuments/opening%20minds/Brandon_ENG.pdf.

#### Problem
Stigma remains an ongoing problem for individuals living with a major mental illness.

#### Purpose of Study
As part of the Mental Health Commission of Canada's ten-year anti-stigma initiative Opening Minds, a pilot project was initiated in which nurses came to know consumers of mental health services as "real people with real stories—people with feelings whose lives matter" (Jensen, n.d. para. 4).

#### Methods
In this project, graduate students were paired with an individual living with a mental illness. The students' assignment was to get to know the person in enough depth to write a recovery narrative.

#### Key Findings
A detailed personal account of the person's experiences with mental illness and treatment in the Canadian health care system was described in a recovery narrative. An extension of the pilot project is planned.

#### Implications for Nursing Practice
We can improve patient outcomes by viewing patients as real people with interesting stories to tell.

| TABLE 3-6 | ADDITIONAL THEORISTS WHOSE CONTRIBUTIONS INFLUENCE PSYCHIATRIC MENTAL HEALTH NURSING | | |
|---|---|---|---|
| **THEORIST** | **SCHOOL OF THOUGHT** | **MAJOR CONTRIBUTIONS** | **RELEVANCE TO PSYCHIATRIC MENTAL HEALTH NURSING** |
| Carl Rogers | Humanism | Developed a person-centred model of psychotherapy; emphasized the concepts of:<br>• Congruence—authenticity of the therapist in dealings with the patient<br>• Unconditional acceptance and positive regard—climate in the therapeutic relationship that facilitates change<br>• Empathic understanding—therapist's ability to apprehend the feelings and experiences of the patient as if these things were happening to the therapist | Encourages nurses to view each patient as unique; emphasizes attitudes of unconditional positive regard, empathic understanding, and genuineness that are essential to the nurse–patient relationship<br>*Example:* The nurse asks the patient, "What can I do to help you regain control over your anxiety?" |
| Jean Piaget | Cognitive development | Identified stages of cognitive development, including sensorimotor (0–2 years), preoperational (2–7 years), concrete operational (7–11 years), and formal operational (11 years–adulthood); these stages describe how cognitive development proceeds from reflex activity to application of logical solutions to all types of problems | Provides a broad base for cognitive interventions, especially with patients with negative self-views<br>*Example:* The nurse shows an 8-year-old all the equipment needed to start an intravenous when discussing the fact that he will need one prior to surgery. |

*Continued*

| TABLE 3-6 | ADDITIONAL THEORISTS WHOSE CONTRIBUTIONS INFLUENCE PSYCHIATRIC MENTAL HEALTH NURSING—cont'd | | |
|---|---|---|---|
| **THEORIST** | **SCHOOL OF THOUGHT** | **MAJOR CONTRIBUTIONS** | **RELEVANCE TO PSYCHIATRIC MENTAL HEALTH NURSING** |
| Lawrence Kohlberg | Moral development | Posited a six-stage theory of moral development | Provides nurses with a framework for evaluating moral decisions<br>*Example:* In Stage 5, the nurse views laws as social contracts that promote "the greatest good for the greatest number of people." The nurse would advocate access to universal health care. |
| Albert Ellis | Existentialism | Developed approach of rational-emotive behavioural therapy that is active and cognitively oriented; confrontation used to force patients to assume responsibility for behaviour; patients are encouraged to accept themselves as they are and are taught to take risks and try out new behaviours | Encourages nurses to focus on here-and-now issues and to help the patient live fully in the present and look forward to the future.<br>*Example:* The nurse encourages the patient to vacation with her family even though she will be in a wheelchair until her leg fracture heals. |
| Albert Bandura | Social learning theory | Responsible for concepts of modelling and self-efficacy—that is, a person's belief or expectation that he or she has the capacity to effect a desired outcome through his or her own efforts | Includes cognitive functioning with environmental factors, which provides nurses with a comprehensive view of how people learn.<br>*Example:* The nurse helps the teenage patient identify three negative outcomes of tobacco use. |
| Viktor Frankl | Existentialism | Developed "logotherapy," a future-oriented therapy offered to help people find their sense of self-respect and focused on their need to find meaning and value in living as their most important life task | Focuses the nurse beyond mere behaviours to understanding the meaning of these behaviours to the patient's sense of life meaning<br>*Example:* The nurse listens attentively as the patient describes what life has been like since her daughter died. |

**Source:** Bandura, A. (1977). *Social learning theory.* Englewood Cliffs, NJ: Prentice-Hall; Bernard, M.E., & Wolfe, J.L. (Eds.). (1993). *The RET resource book for practitioners.* New York: Institute for Rational-Emotive Therapy; Ellis, A. (1989). *Inside rational emotive therapy.* San Diego: Academic Press; Frankl, V. (1969). *The will to meaning.* Cleveland: New American Library; Kohlberg, L. (1986). A current statement on some theoretical issues. In S. Modgil & C. Modgil (Eds.), *Lawrence Kohlberg.* Philadelphia: Palmer; and Rogers, C.R. (1961). *On becoming a person.* Boston: Houghton Mifflin.

# ■ KEY POINTS TO REMEMBER

- Sigmund Freud advanced the first theory of personality development.
- Freud articulated levels of awareness (unconscious, preconscious, conscious) and demonstrated the influence of our unconscious behaviour on everyday life, as evidenced by the use of defence mechanisms.
- Freud identified three psychological processes of personality (id, ego, superego) and described how they operate and develop.
- Freud articulated one of the first modern develomental theories of personality, based on five psychosexual stages.
- Various psychoanalytic therapies have been used over the years. Currently a short-term, time-limited version of psychotherapy is common.

- Erik Erikson expanded on Freud's developmental stages to include middle age through old age. Erikson called his stages *psychosocial stages* and emphasized the social aspect of personality development.
- Harry Stack Sullivan proposed the interpersonal theory of personality development, which focuses on interpersonal processes that can be observed in a social framework.
- Hildegard Peplau, a nursing theorist, developed an interpersonal theoretical framework that has become the foundation of psychiatric mental health nursing practice.
- Abraham Maslow, the founder of humanistic psychology, offered the theory of self-actualization and human motivation that is basic to all nursing education today.

- Cognitive-behavioural therapy is the most commonly used, accepted, and empirically validated psychotherapeutic approach.
- A biological model of mental illness and treatment dominates care for psychiatric disorders.

- Milieu therapy is a philosophy of care in which all parts of the environment are considered to be therapeutic opportunities for growth and healing. The milieu includes the people (patients and staff), setting, structure, and emotional climate.

## CRITICAL THINKING

1. Consider the theorists and theories discussed in this chapter. The following questions address how they may impact your nursing practice.
   a. How do Freud's concepts of the conscious, preconscious, and unconscious affect your understanding of patients' behaviours?
   b. Do you believe that Erikson's psychosocial stages represent a sound basis for identifying disruptions in stages of development in your patients? Support your position with a clinical example.
   c. What are the implications of Sullivan's focus on the importance of interpersonal relationships for your interactions with patients?
   d. Peplau believed that nurses must exercise self-awareness within the nurse–patient relationship. Describe situations in your student experience in which this self-awareness played a vital role in your relationship(s) with patient(s).
   e. Identify someone you believe to be self-actualized. What characteristics does this person have that support your assessment?
   f. How do or will you make use of Maslow's hierarchy of needs in your nursing practice?
   g. What do you think about the behaviourist point of view that a change in behaviour results in a change in thinking? Can you give an example of this in your own life?

2. Which of the therapies described in this chapter do you think are or will be the most helpful to you in your nursing practice? Explain your choice.

3. How will you make use of the anti-stigma initiative presented in the RH box?

## CHAPTER REVIEW

1. The nurse is working with a patient who lacks the ability to problem-solve and seeks ways to self-satisfy without regard for others. Which system of the patient's personality is most pronounced?
   1. Id
   2. Ego
   3. Conscience (superego)
   4. Ego ideal (superego)

2. Which behaviour, seen in a 30-year-old patient, would alert the nurse to the fact that the patient is not in his appropriate developmental stage according to Erikson?
   1. States he is happily married
   2. Frequently asks to call his brother "just to check in"
   3. Looks forward to visits from a co-worker
   4. Says, "I'm still trying to find myself."

3. A patient has difficulty sitting still and listening to others during group therapy. The therapist plans to use operant conditioning as a form of behavioural modification to assist the patient. Which action would the nurse expect to see in group therapy?
   1. The therapist will act as a role model for the patient by sitting still and listening.
   2. The patient will receive a token from the therapist for each session in which she sits still and listens.
   3. The patient will be required to sit in solitude for 30 minutes after each session in which she does not sit still or listen.
   4. The therapist will ask that the patient sit still and listen for only 2 minutes at a time to begin with and will increase the time incrementally until the patient can sit and listen for ten minutes at a time.

4. The nurse is planning care for a patient with anxiety who will be admitted to the unit shortly. Which nursing action is most important?
   1. Consider ways to assist the patient to feel valued during his stay on the unit.
   2. Choose a roommate for the patient so that a friendship can develop.
   3. Identify a room where the patient will have comfortable surroundings, and order a balanced meal plan.
   4. Plan methods of decreasing stimuli that could cause heightened anxiety in the patient.

# Evolve WEBSITE

*Visit the Evolve Web site for Chapter Review Answers and Rationales, Critical Thinking Answer Guidelines, and additional resources related to the content in this chapter http://evolve.elsevier.com/Canada/Varcarolis/psychiatric/*

## REFERENCES

Bandura, A., Blahard, E.B., & Ritter, B. (1969). Relative efficacy of desensitization and modeling approaches for inducing behavioural, affective, and attitudinal changes. *Journal of Personality and Social Psychology, 13*, 173–199. doi:10.1037/h0028276.

Beck, A.T. (1967). *Depression: Clinical, experimental and theoretical aspects.* New York: Harper & Row.

Beck, A.T., Rush, A.J., Shaw, B.F., et al. (1979). *Cognitive therapy of depression.* New York: Guilford.

Canadian Association for Psychodynamic Therapy. (n.d.). About Canadian Association for Psychodynamic Therapy. Retrieved from http://psychodynamiccanada.org/about.

Cuijpers, P., Geraedts, A., van Oppen, P., et al. (2011). Interpersonal psychotherapy for depression: A meta-analysis. *American Journal of Psychiatry, 168*, 581–592. doi:10.1176/appi.ajp.2010.10101411.

Dewan, M.J., Steenbarger, B.N., & Greenberg, R.P. (2008). Brief psychotherapies. In R.E. Hales, S.C. Yudofsky, & G.O. Gabbard (Eds.), *Textbook of psychiatry* (5th ed., pp. 1155–1170). Washington, DC: American Psychiatric Publishing.

Ellis, A. (2000, August). *On therapy: A dialogue with Aaron T. Beck and Albert Ellis.* Symposium conducted at the American Psychological Association's 108th Convention, Washington, DC.

Erikson, E.H. (1963). *Childhood and society.* New York: W.W. Norton.

Forchuk, C. (1991). A comparison of the works of Peplau and Orlando. *Archives of Psychiatric Nursing, 5*, 38–45. doi:10.1016/0883-9417(91)90008-S.

Freud, S. (1960). *The ego and the id.* (J. Strachey, Trans.). New York: W.W. Norton.

Freud, S. (1961). *The interpretation of dreams.* (J. Strachey, Ed. & Trans.). New York: Scientific Editions.

Freud, S. (1969). *An outline of psychoanalysis.* (J. Strachey, Trans.). New York: W.W. Norton.

Haber, J. (2000). Hildegard E. Peplau: The psychiatric nursing legacy of a legend. *Journal of the American Psychiatric Nurses Association, 6*, 56–62. doi:10.1067/mpn.2000.104556.

Hollon, S.D., & Engelhardt, N. (1997). Review of psychosocial treatment of mood disorders. In D.L. Dunner (Ed.), *Current psychiatric therapy II.* Philadelphia: Saunders.

Maslow, A.H. (1963). Self-actualizing people. In G.B. Levitas (Ed.), *The world of psychology* (Vol. 2). New York: Braziller.

Maslow, A.H. (1968). *Toward a psychology of being.* Princeton, NJ: Van Nostrands.

Maslow, A.H. (1970). *Motivation and personality* (2nd ed.). New York: Harper & Row.

Pavlov, I. (1928). *Lectures on conditioned reflexes* (W.H. Grant, Ed. & Trans.). New York: International Publishers.

Peplau, H.E. (1952). *Interpersonal relations in nursing: A conceptual frame of reference for psychodynamic nursing.* New York: Putnam.

Peplau, H.E. (1982a). Therapeutic concepts. In S.A. Smoyak & S. Rouslin (Eds.), *A collection of classics in psychiatric nursing literature* (pp. 91–108). Thorofare, NJ: Slack.

Peplau, H.E. (1982b). Interpersonal techniques: The crux of psychiatric nursing. In S.A. Smoyak & S. Rouslin (Eds.), *A collection of classics in psychiatric nursing literature* (pp. 276–281). Thorofare, NJ: Slack.

Peplau, H.E. (1987). Interpersonal constructs for nursing practice. *Nursing Education Today, 7*, 201–208. doi:10.1016/0260-6917(87)90002-5.

Peplau, H.E. (1989). Future directions in psychiatric nursing from the perspective of history. *Journal of Psychosocial Nursing, 27*(2), 18–28.

Peplau, H.E. (1995). Another look at schizophrenia from a nursing standpoint. In C.A. Anderson (Ed.), *Psychiatric nursing 1946–94: The state of the art.* St. Louis, MO: Mosby.

Sadock, B.J., & Sadock, V.A. (2008). *Concise textbook of clinical psychiatry* (3rd ed.). Philadelphia: Lippincott, Williams & Wilkins.

Skinner, B.F. (1987). Whatever happened to psychology as the science of behavior? *American Psychologist, 42*, 780–786. doi:10.1037/0003-066X.42.8.780.

Stockman, C. (2005). A literature review of the progress of the psychiatric nurse–patient relationship as described by Peplau. *Issues in Mental Health Nursing, 26*, 911–919. doi:10.1080/01612840500248197.

Sullivan, H.S. (1953). *The interpersonal theory of psychiatry.* New York: W.W. Norton.

Thibeault, C.A., Trudeau, K., d'Entremont, M., et al. (2010). Understanding the milieu experiences of patients on an acute inpatient psychiatric unit. *Archives of Psychiatric Nursing, 24*, 216–226. doi:10.1016/j.apnu.2009.07.002.

Tognazzini, P., Davis, C., Kean, A., et al. (2009). *Canadian Federation of Mental Health Nurses core competencies in psychiatric mental health nursing for undergraduate nursing education: Position paper.* Toronto: Canadian Federation of Mental Health Nurses.

Watson, J.B. (1919). Psychology from the standpoint of a behaviourist. Philadelphia: Lippincott.

# Psychotropic Drugs

*Mary A. Gutierrez, John Raynor*
*Adapted by Beth Swart*

## KEY TERMS AND CONCEPTS

agonist, 61
antagonist, 61
antianxiety (anxiolytic) drugs, 58
anticholinesterase drugs, 70
atypical antipsychotics, 68
biopsychiatry, 46
circadian rhythms, 48
conventional antipsychotics, 67
hypnotic, 60
limbic system, 52
lithium carbonate, 65
metabolites, 58
monoamine oxidase inhibitors (MAOIs), 64

mood stabilizer, 65
neurons, 49
neurotransmitters, 48
pharmacodynamics, 58
pharmacogenetics, 58
pharmacokinetics, 58
receptors, 49
reticular activating system (RAS), 52
reuptake, 51
selective serotonin reuptake inhibitors (SSRIs), 61
synapse, 49
therapeutic index, 66
tricyclic antidepressants (TCAs), 63

## OBJECTIVES

1. Identify the functions of the brain and discuss how these functions can be altered by psychotropic drugs.
2. Describe how a neurotransmitter functions as a neuromessenger.
3. Identify the functions of the three major areas of the brain.
4. Explain how specific brain functions are altered in mental health disorders such as depression, anxiety, bipolar disorder, and schizophrenia.
5. Describe how imaging techniques are used to map brain structure and function in individuals with mental health disorders.
6. Describe the result of blockage of the muscarinic receptors and the $\alpha_1$ adrenergic receptors by the standard neuroleptic drugs.

7. Identify the main neurotransmitters affected by the following psychotropic drugs and their subgroups:
   a. Antianxiety drugs
   b. Sedative–hypnotic drugs
   c. Antidepressants
   d. Mood stabilizers
   e. Antipsychotic drugs
   f. Anticholinesterase drugs
8. Discuss dietary and drug restrictions for a patient taking a monoamine oxidase inhibitor.
9. Identify specific cautions for a patient taking natural health products and psychotropic drugs.
10. Explore the relevance of pharmacogenetics (i.e., variations in effects and therapeutic actions of medications among different ethnic groups) in the use of psychotrophic drugs.

## ⊖volve WEBSITE

*Visit the Evolve website for Flashcards, Case Studies, and additional testing resources related to the content in this chapter:* *http://evolve.elsevier.com/Canada/Varcarolis/psychiatric/*   Pre-Test  interactive review

One in every five Canadians will have a mental health problem at some point in their lives.

Biopsychiatry, sometimes referred to as the *biological approach*, is a theoretical approach to understanding mental health disorders as biological malfunctions of the nervous system. Implied in this approach is the idea that brain function is related to several factors, including genetics, neurodevelopmental factors, drugs, infection, psychosocial experience, or a combination of one or more of these factors that impact brain functioning. Clinicians using this approach believe that changes in the patient's behaviour and in mental and emotional experiences are caused by damage to the brain. For example, when the brain is damaged, the way it produces and responds to neurotransmitters, the "chemical messengers" of the nervous system, changes. These changes can result in depressive symptoms, symptoms of anxiety, symptoms of post-traumatic stress disorder, or any other combination of behavioural, emotional, or mental symptoms.

Medication is used to augment the effectiveness of the neurotransmitters. The primary goal of drug therapy is to restore "balance" to a malfunctioning brain. During recent years, there has been an explosion of information about the efficacy of psychotropic drugs (medication to treat mental illness) in reversing these alterations; however, a full understanding of how these drugs improve symptoms continues to elude investigators. Early theories, such as the dopamine theory of schizophrenia and the monoamine theory of depression, are currently seen as overly simplistic because a large number of other neurotransmitters, hormones, and co-regulators are now thought to play important and complex roles. Current researchers, therefore, are studying how to impact the brain's responses to neurotransmitters, hormones, and co-regulators, either by making more of the chemical available in the brain or by making the brain more sensitive to the chemical that is already there.

Included in this chapter is an overview of the major drugs used to treat mental health disorders and an explanation of how they work. Additional and detailed information regarding adverse and toxic effects, dosage, nursing implications, and teaching tools is presented in the appropriate clinical chapters (see Chapters 13 to 23).

Despite new knowledge about complex brain functions, there is still much to be clarified in understanding the complex ways in which the brain carries out its normal functions, is altered during disease, and is improved by pharmacological intervention. After reading this chapter, you should have a neurobiological framework into which you can place existing, as well as future, information about mental illness and its treatment.

## STRUCTURE AND FUNCTION OF THE BRAIN

### Functions and Activities of the Brain

Regulating behaviour and carrying out mental processes are important, but far from the only, responsibilities of the brain. Some of the major functions and activities of the brain are summarized in Box 4-1. Because these brain functions are carried out by similar mechanisms (interactions of neurons)

 **HOW A NURSE HELPED ME**
#### When the Adverse Effects Are Too Much to Take

*A patient with a mental health disorder faces numerous challenges during the search for the correct medication and treatment regimen. At 19, my brother was hearing voices and felt that others were talking about him or trying to watch him through windows. A number of factors were thought to contribute to his strange behaviours, among them, his being stressed over a recent breakup with a girlfriend and using marijuana. However, he was diagnosed with paranoid schizophrenia. It was an extremely stressful time for my family, who had difficulty understanding and coping with his seemingly irrational and illogical behaviours.*

*He was admitted to hospital and started on first-generation antipsychotics. After a psychiatric nurse met my parents, she assessed that they needed assistance in understanding my brother's illness. Specifically, she explained that my brother's behaviours were symptoms of his illness and also how the medications would help ease his symptoms. She also outlined the common adverse effects that he might experience as a consequence of taking the medication. As well, she listened to my parents' worries about the future.*

*My brother was started on fluphenazine decanoate, a medication administered by injection, and his symptoms improved. The drug was administered for two years, but then he stopped taking it because of the adverse effects he was experiencing. We learned that restlessness, dry mouth, fatigue, tremors, and dizziness are not uncommon for people who are being treated with this kind of medication. It has been 40 years now since my brother's diagnosis, and he has not been on any medications for treatment since. Unfortunately, without any medication, he has been homeless for many years.*

*If my brother resumes psychopharmacological treatment in the future, the nurse will need to identify what factors will impact his decision to continue to take the prescribed medication. The nurse will need to listen to my brother's preferences about when he takes the medication, and his level of tolerance for various adverse effects will need to be considered when making decisions about possible interventions. The treatment team will also have to examine ways to predict how my brother will respond to the medication so as to optimize initial treatment selections. It will be important to select the medication that will have the best effect on his schizophrenia and the one with the fewest adverse effects, because they may get only one more chance.*

## BOX 4-1  FUNCTIONS OF THE BRAIN

- Monitor changes in the external world
- Monitor the composition of body fluids
- Regulate the contractions of skeletal muscles
- Regulate the internal organs
- Initiate and regulate the basic drives: hunger, thirst, sex, aggressive self-protection
- Mediate conscious sensation
- Store and retrieve memories
- Regulate mood (affect) and emotions
- Think and perform intellectual functions
- Regulate the sleep cycle
- Produce and interpret language
- Process visual and auditory data

and often in similar locations, mental health disturbances are often associated with alterations in other brain functions, and the drugs used to treat mental disturbances can interfere with other activities of the brain.

### Maintenance of Homeostasis

The brain serves as the coordinator and director of the body's response to both internal and external changes. Appropriate responses require a constant monitoring of the environment, interpretation and integration of the incoming information, and control over the appropriate organs of response. The goal of these responses is to maintain homeostasis and thus to maintain life.

Information about the external world is relayed from various sense organs to the brain by the peripheral nerves. This information, which is at first received as gross sensation such as light, sound, or touch, must ultimately be interpreted into a picture, a train whistle, or a hand on the back. Interestingly, a component of major psychiatric disturbance (e.g., schizophrenia) is an alteration of sensory experience. Thus, the patient may experience a sensation that does not originate in the external world. For example, people with schizophrenia may hear voices talking to them (auditory hallucination).

To respond to external changes, the brain has control over the skeletal muscles. This control involves the ability not only to initiate contraction (e.g., to contract the biceps and flex the arm) but also to fine-tune and coordinate contraction so a person can, for example, guide the fingers to the correct keys on a piano. Unfortunately, both psychiatric disease and the treatment of psychiatric disease with psychotropic drugs are associated with movement disturbances. It is important to remember that the skeletal muscles controlled by the brain include the diaphragm, essential for breathing, and the muscles of the throat, tongue, and mouth, essential for speech. Therefore, drugs that affect brain function can, for example, stimulate or depress respiration or lead to slurred speech.

The brain not only monitors the external world but also keeps a close watch on internal functions. Information about blood pressure, body temperature, blood gases, and the chemical composition of the body fluids is continuously received by the brain, signalling it to send the responses required to

maintain homeostasis. Adjustments to changes within the body require that the brain exert control over the various internal organs. For example, if blood pressure drops, the brain must direct the heart to pump more blood and the smooth muscles of the arterioles to constrict. This increase in cardiac output and vasoconstriction allows the body to return blood pressure to its normal level.

### Regulation of the Autonomic Nervous System and Hormones

The autonomic nervous system and the endocrine system serve as the communication links between the brain and the cardiac muscle, smooth muscle, and glands of which the internal organs are composed (Figure 4-1). If the brain needs to stimulate the heart, it must activate the sympathetic nerves to the sinoatrial node and the ventricular myocardium. If the brain needs to bring about vasoconstriction, it must activate the sympathetic nerves to the smooth muscles of the arterioles.

The linkage between the brain and the internal organs that allows for the maintenance of homeostasis may also serve to translate mental health disturbances, such as anxiety, into alterations of internal function. For example, anxiety in some people can cause activation of parasympathetic nerves to the digestive tract, leading to hypermotility and diarrhea. Likewise, anxiety can activate the sympathetic nerves to the arterioles, leading to vasoconstriction and hypertension.

The brain also exerts influence over the internal organs by regulating hormonal secretions of the pituitary gland, which in turn regulates other glands. The hypothalamus is involved in several functions of the brain. It secretes hormones called *releasing factors*, which act on the pituitary gland to stimulate or inhibit the synthesis and release of pituitary hormones. Once in the general circulation, these hormones influence various internal activities. For example, when gonadotropin-releasing hormone is secreted by the hypothalamus at puberty, this hormone stimulates the release of two gonadotropins—follicle-stimulating hormone and luteinizing hormone—by the pituitary gland, which consequently activate the ovaries or testes.

The relationship between the brain, the pituitary gland, and the adrenal glands is particularly important in determining normal and abnormal mental function. Specifically, the hypothalamus secretes corticotropin-releasing hormone (CRH), which stimulates the pituitary to release corticotropin, which in turn stimulates the cortex of each adrenal gland to secrete the hormone cortisol. This system is activated as part of the normal response to a variety of mental and physical stresses. Among many other actions, all three hormones—CRH, corticotropin, and cortisol—influence the functions of the nerve cells of the brain. There is considerable evidence that in both anxiety and depression, this system is overactive and does not respond properly to negative feedback.

### Control of Biological Drives and Behaviour

To understand the neurobiological basis of mental disease and its treatment, it is helpful to distinguish between the various types of brain activity that serve as the basis of mental experience and behaviour. An understanding of these activities shows where to look for disturbed function and what to hope

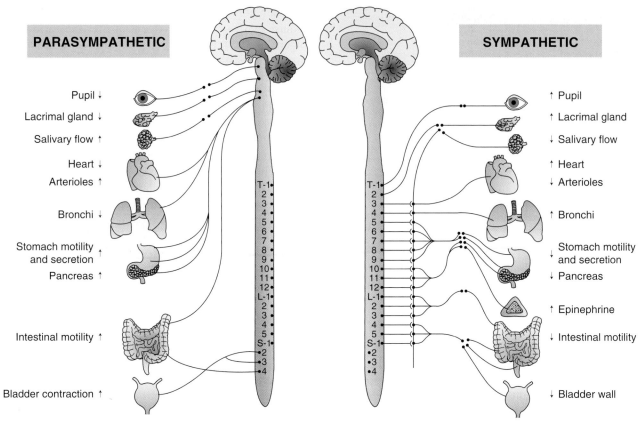

**PARASYMPATHETIC**

Pupil ↓
Lacrimal gland ↓
Salivary flow ↑
Heart ↓
Arterioles ↑
Bronchi ↓
Stomach motility and secretion ↑
Pancreas ↑
Intestinal motility ↑
Bladder contraction ↑

T-1
2
3
4
5
6
7
8
9
10
11
12
L-1
2
3
4
5
S-1
2
3
4

**SYMPATHETIC**

↑ Pupil
↑ Lacrimal gland
↓ Salivary flow
↑ Heart
↓ Arterioles
↑ Bronchi
Stomach motility and secretion ↓
↓ Pancreas
↑ Epinephrine
↓ Intestinal motility
↓ Bladder wall

**FIGURE 4-1** The autonomic nervous system has two divisions: the sympathetic and parasympathetic. The sympathetic division is dominant in stressful situations such as those that incite fear or anger—known as the *fight-or-flight response.*

for in treatment. The brain, for example, is responsible for the basic drives such as sex and hunger that play a strong role in moulding behaviour. Disturbances of these drives such as overeating or undereating and loss of sexual interest can be an indication of an underlying mental health disorder such as depression.

***Cycle of sleep and wakefulness.*** The entire cycle of sleep and wakefulness, as well as the intensity of alertness while the person is awake, is regulated and coordinated by various regions of the brain. Although the true homeostatic function of sleep is not well understood, sleep is known to be essential for both physiological and psychological well-being. Assessment of sleep patterns is part of what is required to determine a diagnosis of a mental health disorder.

Unfortunately, many of the drugs used to treat mental health problems interfere with the normal regulation of sleep and alertness. Drugs with a sedative–hypnotic effect can blunt the degree to which a person feels alert and focused and can cause drowsiness. Because of the sedative–hypnotic effect, caution is necessary in using these drugs while engaging in activities that require a great deal of attention, such as driving a car or operating machinery. One way of minimizing the danger is to take such drugs at night just before bedtime.

***Circadian rhythms.*** The cycle of sleep and wakefulness is only one aspect of circadian rhythms, the fluctuation of various physiological and behavioural parameters over a 24-hour cycle.

Other variations include changes in body temperature, secretion of hormones such as corticotropin and cortisol, and secretion of neurotransmitters—chemicals that transmit signals from one neuron to the next across synapses—such as norepinephrine and serotonin. Both norepinephrine and serotonin are thought to be involved in mood, and daily fluctuations of mood may be related in part to circadian variations in these neurotransmitters. There is evidence that the circadian rhythm of neurotransmitter secretion is altered in mental health disorders, particularly in those that involve mood.

### Conscious Mental Activity

All aspects of conscious mental experience and sense of self originate from the neurophysiological activity of the brain. Conscious mental activity can be a basic, meandering, stream-of-consciousness flow among thoughts of future responsibilities, memories, fantasy, and so on. Conscious mental activity can also be much more complex when it is applied to problem solving and the interpretation of the external world. Both the random stream of consciousness and the complex problem solving and interpretation of the environment can become distorted in mental health disorders. For instance, a person with schizophrenia may have chaotic and incoherent speech and thought patterns (e.g., a jumble of unrelated words known as *word salad* or unconnected phrases and topics known as *looseness of association*) and delusional interpretations of

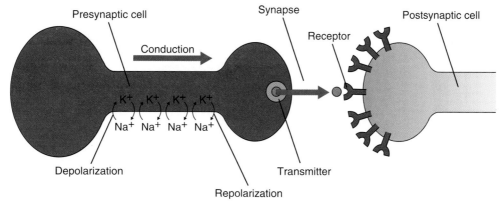

FIGURE 4-2 Activities of neurons. Conduction along a neuron involves the inward movement of sodium ions (Na⁺) followed by the outward movement of potassium ions (K⁺). When the current reaches the end of the cell, a neurotransmitter is released. The neurotransmitter crosses the synapse and attaches to a receptor on the postsynaptic cell. The attachment of neurotransmitter to receptor either stimulates or inhibits the postsynaptic cell.

personal interactions (e.g., beliefs about people or events that are not supported by data or reality).

### Memory

An extremely important component of mental activity is memory, the ability to retain and recall past experience. From both an anatomical and a physiological perspective, there is thought to be a major difference in the processing of short- and long-term memory. This can be seen dramatically in some forms of cognitive mental health disorders such as dementia, in which a person has no recall of the events of the previous eight minutes but may have vivid recall of events of decades earlier.

### Social Skills

An important and often neglected aspect of brain functioning involves the social skills that make interpersonal relationships possible. In almost all types of mental health disorders, from mild anxiety to severe schizophrenia, difficulties in interpersonal relationships are an important characteristic of the disorder, and improvements in these relationships are important gauges of progress. The connection between brain activity and social behaviour is an area of intense research and is believed to be influenced by a combination of genetic makeup and individual experience. There is evidence that positive, reward-based experiential learning and negative avoidance learning may involve different areas of the brain.

### Cellular Composition of the Brain

The brain is composed of approximately 100 billion neurons, nerve cells that conduct electrical impulses, as well as other types of cells that surround the neurons. Most functions of the brain, from regulation of blood pressure to the conscious sense of self, are thought to result from the actions of individual neurons and the interconnections between them. Although neurons come in a great variety of shapes and sizes, all carry out the same three types of physiological actions: (1) they respond to stimuli; (2) they conduct electrical impulses; and (3) they release chemicals called *neurotransmitters*.

An essential feature of neurons is their ability to conduct an electrical impulse from one end of a cell to the other. This electrical impulse consists of a change in membrane permeability that first allows the inward flow of sodium ions and then the outward flow of potassium ions. The inward flow of sodium ions changes the polarity of the membrane from positive on the outside to positive on the inside. Movement of potassium ions out of the cell returns the positive charge to the outside of the cell. Because these electrical charges are self-propagating, a change at one end of the cell is conducted along the membrane until it reaches the other end (Figure 4-2). The functional significance of this propagation is that the electrical impulse serves as a means of communication between one part of the body and another.

Once an electrical impulse reaches the end of a neuron, a neurotransmitter is released. Neurotransmitters are released from the axon terminal at the *presynaptic neuron* (the term for the neuron from which the neurotransmitter is released) on excitation. This neurotransmitter then diffuses across a space, or synapse, to an adjacent *postsynaptic neuron* (the neuron receiving the neurotransmitter), where it attaches to receptors (protein molecules embedded in a cell, to which one or more specific kinds of signalling molecules may attach) on the neuron's surface. This interaction from one neuron to another by way of a neurotransmitter and receptor allows the activity of one neuron to influence the activity of other neurons. Depending on the chemical structure of the neurotransmitter and the specific type of receptor to which it attaches, the postsynaptic cell will be rendered either more or less likely to initiate an electrical impulse. It is the interaction between neurotransmitter and receptor that is a major target of the drugs used to treat mental health disorders. Important neurotransmitters and the types of receptors to which they attach are identified in Table 4-1. Also identified are the mental health disorders associated with an increase or decrease in these neurotransmitters.

After attaching to a receptor and exerting its influence on the postsynaptic cell, the neurotransmitter separates from the

## TABLE 4-1 TRANSMITTERS AND RECEPTORS

| TRANSMITTERS | RECEPTORS | EFFECTS/COMMENTS | ASSOCIATION WITH MENTAL HEALTH DISORDERS |
|---|---|---|---|
| **MONOAMINES** | | | |
| Dopamine (DA) | $D_1$, $D_2$, $D_3$, $D_4$, $D_5$ | Involved in fine muscle movement<br>Involved in integration of emotions and thoughts<br>Involved in decision making<br>Stimulates hypothalamus to release hormones (sex, thyroid, adrenal) | *Decrease:*<br>Parkinson's disease<br>Depression<br>*Increase:*<br>Schizophrenia<br>Mania |
| Norepinephrine (NE) (noradrenaline) | $\alpha_1$, $\alpha_2$, $\beta_1$, $\beta_2$ | Causes changes in mood<br>Causes changes in attention and arousal<br>Stimulates sympathetic branch of autonomic nervous system for fight-or-flight in response to stress | *Decrease:*<br>Depression<br>*Increase:*<br>Mania<br>Anxiety states<br>Schizophrenia |
| Serotonin (5-HT) | 5-$HT_1$, 5-$HT_2$, 5-$HT_3$, 5-$HT_4$ | Plays a role in sleep regulation, hunger, mood states, and pain perception<br>Alters hormonal activity<br>Plays a role in aggression and sexual behaviour | *Decrease:*<br>Depression<br>*Increase:*<br>Anxiety states |
| Histamine | $H_1$, $H_2$ | Involved in alertness<br>Involved in inflammatory response<br>Stimulates gastric secretion | *Decrease:*<br>Sedation<br>Weight gain |
| **AMINO ACIDS** | | | |
| Gamma-aminobutyric acid (GABA) | $GABA_A$, $GABA_B$ | Plays a role in inhibition; reduces aggression, excitation, and anxiety<br>May play a role in pain perception<br>Has anticonvulsant and muscle-relaxing properties<br>May impair cognition and psychomotor functioning | *Decrease:*<br>Anxiety disorders<br>Schizophrenia<br>Mania<br>Huntington's disease<br>*Increase:*<br>Reduction of anxiety |
| Glutamate | N-methyl-D-aspartate (NMDA), α-amino-3-hydroxy-5-methyl-4-isoxazolepropionic acid (AMPA) | Is excitatory<br>AMPA plays a role in learning and memory | *Decrease (NMDA):* Psychosis<br>*Increase (NMDA):* Prolonged increased state can be neurotoxic<br>Neurodegeneration in Alzheimer's disease<br>*Increase (AMPA):* Improvement of cognitive performance in behavioural tasks |
| **CHOLINERGICS** | | | |
| Acetylcholine (ACh) | Nicotinic, muscarinic ($M_1$, $M_2$, $M_3$) | Plays a role in learning, memory<br>Regulates mood, mania, sexual aggression<br>Affects sexual and aggressive behaviour<br>Stimulates parasympathetic nervous system | *Decrease:*<br>Alzheimer's disease<br>Huntington's disease<br>Parkinson's disease<br>*Increase:*<br>Depression |
| **PEPTIDES (NEUROMODULATORS)** | | | |
| Substance P (SP) | SP | Has antidepressant and antianxiety effects in depression<br>Promotes and reinforces memory<br>Enhances sensitivity of pain receptors | Involved in regulation of mood and anxiety<br>Plays a role in pain management |
| Somatostatin (SRIF) | SRIF | Alters cognition, memory, and mood | *Decrease:*<br>Alzheimer's disease<br>Decreased levels of SRIF in spinal fluid of some depressed patients<br>*Increase:*<br>Huntington's disease |
| Neurotensin (NT) | NT | Has endogenous antipsychotic-like properties | Decreased levels in spinal fluid of schizophrenic patients |

## BOX 4-2 DESTRUCTION OF NEUROTRANSMITTERS

A full explanation of the various ways psychotropic drugs alter neuronal activity requires a brief review of the manner in which neurotransmitters are destroyed after attaching to the receptors. To avoid continuous and prolonged action on the postsynaptic cell, the neurotransmitter is released shortly after attaching to the postsynaptic receptor. Once released, the neurotransmitter is destroyed in one of two ways.

One way is the immediate inactivation of the neurotransmitter at the postsynaptic membrane. An example of this method of destruction is the action of the enzyme acetylcholinesterase on the neurotransmitter acetylcholine. Acetylcholinesterase is present at the postsynaptic membrane and destroys acetylcholine shortly after it attaches to receptors on the postsynaptic cell.

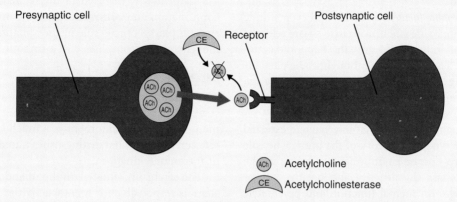

A second method of neurotransmitter inactivation is more complex. After interacting with the postsynaptic receptor, the neurotransmitter is released and taken back into the presynaptic cell, the cell from which it was released. This process, referred to as the *reuptake of neurotransmitter*, is a common target for drug action. Once inside the presynaptic cell, the neurotransmitter is either recycled or inactivated by an enzyme within the cell. The monoamine neurotransmitters norepinephrine, dopamine, and serotonin are all inactivated in this manner by the enzyme monoamine oxidase.

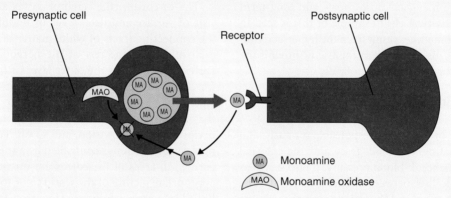

Before release, the neurotransmitter is stored within a membrane and is thus protected from and not destroyed by the *degradative enzyme* (an enzyme that breaks down the neurotransmitters). After release by the presynaptic neuron and reuptake by the postsynaptic neuron, the neurotransmitter is either destroyed by the enzyme or re-enters the membrane to be used again.

receptor and is destroyed. There are two basic mechanisms by which neurotransmitters are destroyed. Some neurotransmitters, such as acetylcholine (the neurotransmitter released by the postganglionic neurons of the parasympathetic nervous system) are destroyed by specific enzymes at the postsynaptic cell. The enzyme that destroys acetylcholine is called *acetylcholinesterase*. Other neurotransmitters, such as norepinephrine, are taken back into the presynaptic cell from which they were originally released, a process called cellular reuptake. Upon their return to these cells, the neurotransmitters are either reused or destroyed by intracellular enzymes. In the case of the monoamine neurotransmitters (e.g., norepinephrine, dopamine, serotonin), the destructive enzyme is called *monoamine*

*oxidase* (MAO). The process of neurotransmitter destruction is further described in Box 4-2.

Once the concentration of the neurotransmitter is strong enough, as a means of regulating this concentration at the postsynaptic receptors, many neurotransmitters attach to presynaptic receptors at the synapse, thereby inhibiting the further release of neurotransmitters.

Researchers have found that in many cases, neurons release more than one chemical at the same time. Neurotransmitters such as norepinephrine or acetylcholine—which have immediate effects on postsynaptic membranes—are often joined by larger molecules, neuropeptides, that may initiate long-term changes in the postsynaptic cells. These changes may involve basic cell functions, such as genetic expression, and lead to modifications of cell shape and responsiveness to stimuli. Ultimately, this means that the action of one neuron on another affects not only the immediate response of that neuron but also its sensitivity to future influence. The long-term implications of this for neural development, normal and abnormal mental health, and the treatment of mental health disorders are being investigated.

The communication between neurons at a synapse is not unidirectional. *Neurotrophic factors*—proteins and even simple gases, such as carbon monoxide and nitrous oxide—are released by postsynaptic cells and influence the growth, shape, and activity of presynaptic cells. These factors are thought to be particularly important during the development of the fetal brain, guiding the growing brain to form the proper neuronal connections. However, it is now apparent that the brain retains anatomical plasticity throughout life and that internal and external influences can alter the synaptic network of the brain. The role of altered genetic expression or environmental trauma in the action of these factors and the negative and positive consequences of these changes on mental function and psychiatric disease are areas of much research.

The development and responsiveness of neurons is dependent not only on chemicals released by other neurons but also on chemicals, particularly the steroid hormones, brought to the neurons by the blood. Estrogen, testosterone, and cortisol can bind to neurons, where they can cause short- and long-term changes in neuronal activity. A clear example of this is seen in the psychosis that can sometimes result from the hypersecretion of cortisol in Cushing's disease or from the use of prednisone in high doses to treat chronic inflammatory disease.

## Organization of the Brain
### Brain Stem
The central core of the brain stem is responsible for such vital functions as the regulation of blood gases and the internal organs and the maintenance of blood pressure. It also serves as a crucial psychosomatic link between higher brain activities, such as thought and emotion, and the functioning of the internal organs. The brain stem also functions as an initial processing centre for sensory information that is then sent on to the cerebral cortex. Through projections of the reticular activating system (RAS), the brain stem regulates the entire cycle of sleep and wakefulness and the ability of the cerebrum to carry out conscious mental activity.

Other ascending pathways, referred to as *mesolimbic* and *mesocortical pathways*, seem to play a strong role in modulating the emotional value of sensory material. These pathways project to those areas of the cerebrum—the hypothalamus, amygdala, and hippocampus, collectively known as the limbic system— that play a crucial role in emotional status and psychological function. The hypothalamus, a small area in the ventral superior portion of the brain stem, plays a vital role in such basic drives as hunger, thirst, and sex. They use norepinephrine, serotonin, and dopamine as their neurotransmitters. Much attention has been paid to the role of these pathways in normal and abnormal mental activity. For example, it is thought that the

release of dopamine from the *ventral tegmental pathway* plays a role in psychological reward and substance dependence. The neurotransmitters released by the neurons in the mesolimbic and mesocortical pathways are major targets of the drugs used to treat mental health disorders.

### Cerebellum
Located posteriorly to the brain stem, the cerebellum (Figure 4-3) is primarily involved in the regulation of skeletal muscle coordination and contraction and the maintenance of equilibrium. It plays a crucial role in coordinating contractions so that movement is accomplished in a smooth and directed manner.

### Cerebrum
The human brain stem and cerebellum are similar in both structure and function to these same structures in other mammals. The development of a much larger and more elaborate cerebrum is what distinguishes human beings from the rest of the animal kingdom.

The cerebrum, situated on top of and surrounding the brain stem, is responsible for mental activities and a conscious sense of being, including our conscious perception of the external world and our own body, emotional status, memory, and control of skeletal muscles that allows willful direction of movement. It is also responsible for language and the ability to communicate.

The cerebrum (the cerebral cortex and basal ganglia) consists of surface and deep areas of undulating grey matter and the connecting tracts of white matter that link these areas with each other and the rest of the nervous system. The cerebral cortex, which forms the outer layer of the brain, is responsible for conscious sensation and the initiation of movement. Specific areas of the cortex are responsible for specific sensations: the parietal cortex for touch, the temporal cortex for sound, the occipital cortex for vision, and so on. The initiation of skeletal muscle contraction is controlled by a specific area of the frontal cortex. All areas of the cortex are interconnected to enable an appropriate picture of the world to be formed and, if necessary, linked to a proper response (Figure 4-4).

Specialized areas of the cerebral cortex are responsible for language in both its sensory and motor aspects. Sensory language functions include the ability to read, understand spoken language, and know the names of objects perceived by the senses. Motor functions involve the physical ability to use muscles properly for speech and writing. In both neurological and psychological dysfunction, the use of language may become compromised or distorted. A change in linguistic ability may be a factor in determining a diagnosis.

The basal ganglia are located deep within the grey matter of the cerebrum; they are involved in the regulation of movement. Other structures, the amygdala and hippocampus, are involved in emotions, learning, memory, and basic drives. Significantly, there is an overlap of these various areas both anatomically and in the types of neurotransmitters employed. One consequence of this overlap is that drugs used to treat emotional disturbances may cause movement disorders, and drugs used to treat movement disorders may cause emotional changes.

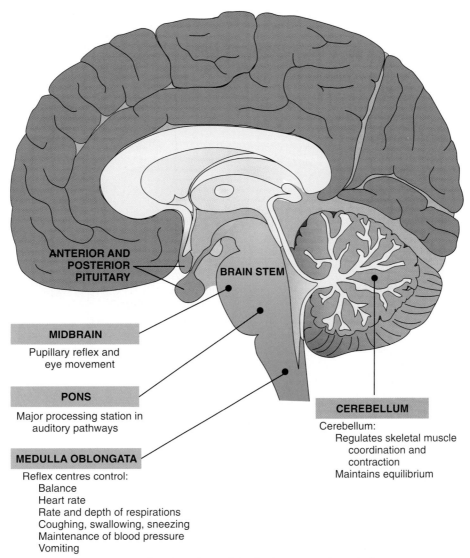

**ANTERIOR AND POSTERIOR PITUITARY**

**BRAIN STEM**

**MIDBRAIN**

Pupillary reflex and
eye movement

**PONS**

Major processing station in
auditory pathways

**MEDULLA OBLONGATA**

Reflex centres control:
Balance
Heart rate
Rate and depth of respirations
Coughing, swallowing, sneezing
Maintenance of blood pressure
Vomiting

**CEREBELLUM**

Cerebellum:
Regulates skeletal muscle
coordination and
contraction
Maintains equilibrium

**FIGURE 4-3** The functions of the brain stem and cerebellum.

## Visualizing the Brain

Various noninvasive imaging techniques are used to visualize brain structure, functions, and metabolic activity. Some common brain-imaging techniques and preliminary findings as they relate to psychiatry are identified in Table 4-2. There are basically two types of neuroimaging techniques: structural and functional. Structural imaging techniques, such as computed tomography (CT) and magnetic resonance imaging (MRI), identify gross anatomical changes in the brain. Functional imaging techniques, such as positron emission tomography (PET) and single-photon emission computed tomography (SPECT), reveal physiological activity in the brain.

PET scans are particularly useful in identifying physiological and biochemical changes as they occur in living tissue. Usually, a radioactive "tag" is used to trace compounds such as glucose. In the brain, glucose use is related to functional activity in certain areas. For example, in patients with untreated schizophrenia, PET scans may show a decreased use of glucose in the frontal lobes. Figure 4-5 shows lower brain activity in the frontal lobe of a twin diagnosed with schizophrenia than in that of the asymptomatic twin. The area affected in the frontal cortex of the twin with schizophrenia is an area associated with reasoning skills, which are greatly impaired in people with schizophrenia. Scans such as these suggest a location in the frontal cortex as the site of functional impairment in people with schizophrenia.

In people with obsessive-compulsive disorder (OCD), PET scans show that brain metabolism is increased in certain areas of the frontal cortex. Figure 4-6 shows increased brain metabolism in an individual with OCD as compared with a control, suggesting altered brain function in people with OCD.

PET scans of individuals with depression show decreased brain activity in the prefrontal cortex. Figure 4-7 shows the results of a PET scan taken after a form of radioactively tagged glucose was used as a tracer to visualize brain activity. The patient with depression has reduced brain activity compared with a control. Finally, shown in Figure 4-8 are three views of a PET scan of the brain of a patient with Alzheimer's disease.

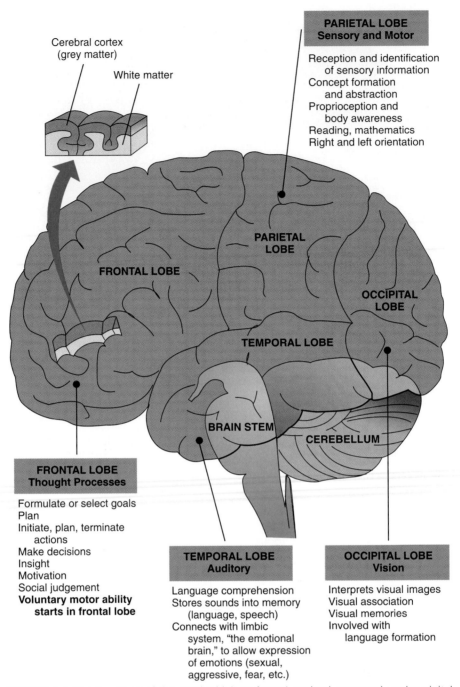

Cerebral cortex
(grey matter)

White matter

**PARIETAL LOBE**
**Sensory and Motor**

Reception and identification
of sensory information
Concept formation
and abstraction
Proprioception and
body awareness
Reading, mathematics
Right and left orientation

**PARIETAL LOBE**

**FRONTAL LOBE**

**OCCIPITAL LOBE**

**TEMPORAL LOBE**

**BRAIN STEM**

**CEREBELLUM**

**FRONTAL LOBE**
**Thought Processes**

Formulate or select goals
Plan
Initiate, plan, terminate
actions
Make decisions
Insight
Motivation
Social judgement
**Voluntary motor ability**
**starts in frontal lobe**

**TEMPORAL LOBE**
**Auditory**

Language comprehension
Stores sounds into memory
(language, speech)
Connects with limbic
system, "the emotional
brain," to allow expression
of emotions (sexual,
aggressive, fear, etc.)

**OCCIPITAL LOBE**
**Vision**

Interprets visual images
Visual association
Visual memories
Involved with
language formation

**FIGURE 4-4** The functions of the cerebral lobes: frontal, parietal, temporal, and occipital.

Modern imaging techniques have also become important tools in assessing molecular changes in mental health disorders and in marking the receptor sites of drug action. It is important to be able to understand where in the brain the various components of psychological activity take place and what types of neurotransmitters and receptors physiologically underlie this activity. Currently, the understanding of both of these questions is far from complete. However, it is thought that the limbic system—a group of structures that includes parts of the frontal cortex, the basal ganglia, and the brain stem—is a major locus of psychological activity. Within these areas, the monoamine neurotransmitters (norepinephrine,

dopamine, and serotonin), the amino acid neurotransmitters (glutamate and gamma-aminobutyric acid [GABA]), and the neuropeptides (CRH and endorphins), as well as acetylcholine, play a major role. Alterations in these areas appear to form the basis of psychiatric disease and are the target for pharmacological treatment.

## Disturbances of Mental Function

Most occurrences of mental health dysfunction are of unknown origin. Among known causes are drugs (e.g., lysergic acid diethylamide [LSD]), long-term use of prednisone, excess levels of hormones (e.g., thyroxine, cortisol), infection (e.g.,

| TABLE 4-2 | COMMON BRAIN-IMAGING TECHNIQUES | | |
|---|---|---|---|
| **TECHNIQUE** | **DESCRIPTION** | **DETECTION** | **PSYCHIATRIC RELEVANCE AND PRELIMINARY FINDINGS** |
| **STRUCTURAL: SHOW GROSS ANATOMICAL DETAILS OF BRAIN STRUCTURES** | | | |
| Computed tomography (CT) | A series of X-ray images of the brain is taken, and computer analysis produces "slices," providing a precise 3D-like* reconstruction of each segment | Lesions Abrasions Areas of infarct Aneurysm | *Schizophrenia:* Cortical atrophy Third ventricle enlargement Cognitive disorders: Abnormalities |
| Magnetic resonance imaging (MRI) | A magnetic field is applied to the brain; nuclei of hydrogen atoms absorb and emit radio waves that are analyzed by computer, providing 3D visualization of the brain's structure in sectional images | Brain edema Ischemia Infection Neoplasm Trauma | *Schizophrenia:* Enlarged ventricles Reduction in temporal lobe and prefrontal lobe |
| Functional magnetic resonance imaging (fMRI) | Functional imaging approach avoids exposure to ionizing radiation | (See MRI) | (See MRI) |
| **FUNCTIONAL: SHOW SOME ACTIVITY OF THE BRAIN** | | | |
| Positron emission tomography (PET) | Radioactive substance (tracer) injected, travels to the brain, and shows up as bright spots on the scan; data collected by detectors are relayed to a computer, which produces images of the activity and 3D visualization of CNS[†] | Oxygen utilization Glucose metabolism Blood flow Neurotransmitter/receptor interaction | *Schizophrenia:* Increased $D_2$, $D_3$ receptors in caudate nucleus Abnormalities in limbic system Mood disorders: Abnormalities in temporal lobes *Adult ADHD[‡]:* Decreased utilization of glucose |
| Single-photon emission computed tomography (SPECT) | Similar to PET but uses radionuclides that emit gamma radiation (photons); measures various aspects of brain functioning and provides images of multiple layers of the CNS (as does PET) | Circulation of cerebrospinal fluid Similar functions to PET | (See PET) |

*3D: three-dimensional
[†]CNS: central nervous system
[‡]ADHD: attention deficit hyperactivity disorder

encephalitis, acquired immunodeficiency syndrome [AIDS]), and physical trauma. Even when the cause is known, however, the link between the causative factor and the mental health dysfunction is far from understood.

Evidence suggests many people with psychiatric disorders are genetically predisposed to them. The incidence of both thought and mood disorders is higher in relatives of people with these diseases than in the general population. Evidence has also shown a strong concordance among identical twins, even when they are raised apart. *Concordance* refers to how often one twin will be affected by the same illness as the other. Psychosocial stress, either in the family of origin or in contacts with society at large, increases the likelihood of mental health problems, as does physical disease. Genetics and environment interact in complex ways so that some people are better able to cope with stress than others (Porcelli, Drago, Fabbri, et al., 2011).

Researchers ultimately want to be able to understand mental health dysfunction in terms of altered activity of neurons in specific areas of the brain. The hope is that such an understanding will lead to better treatments and possible prevention of mental disorders. Current interest is focused on certain neurotransmitters and their receptors, particularly those in the limbic system: norepinephrine, dopamine, serotonin, GABA, and glutamate, as mentioned.

Although the underlying physiology is complex, it is thought that a deficiency of norepinephrine or serotonin (or both) may serve as the biological basis of depression. As shown in Figure 4-9, an insufficient degree of transmission may be due to a deficient release of neurotransmitters by the presynaptic cell or to a loss of the ability of postsynaptic receptors to respond to the neurotransmitters. Changes in neurotransmitter release and receptor response can be both a cause and a consequence of intracellular changes in the neurons involved. Thought

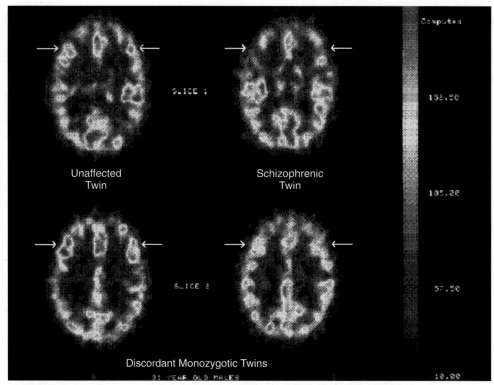

**FIGURE 4-5** PET scans of blood flow in identical twins, one of whom has schizophrenia, illustrate that individuals with this illness have reduced brain activity in the frontal lobes when asked to perform a reasoning task that requires activation of this area. Patients with schizophrenia perform poorly on the task. This suggests a site of functional impairment in schizophrenia. (From Karen Berman, MD, courtesy of National Institute of Mental Health, Clinical Brain Disorders Branch.)

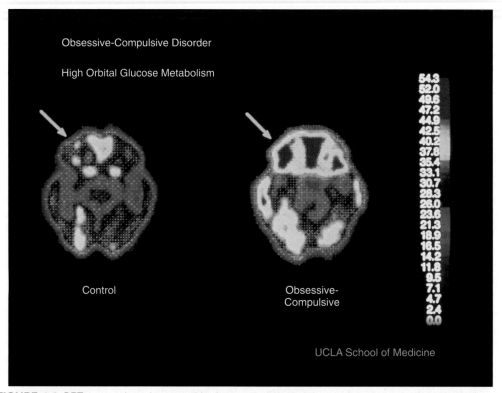

**FIGURE 4-6** PET scans show increased brain metabolism (brighter colours), particularly in the frontal cortex, in a patient with obsessive-compulsive disorder, compared with a control. This suggests altered brain function in OCD. (From Lewis Baxter, MD, UCLA.)

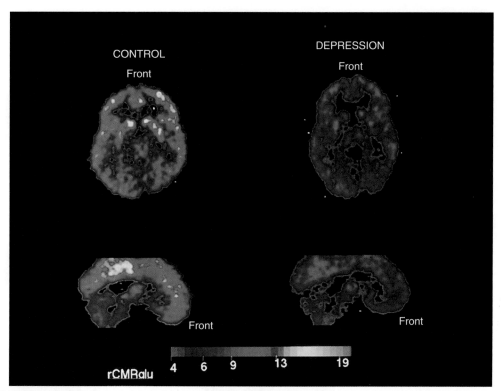

**FIGURE 4-7** PET scans of a patient with depression (right) and a person without depression (left) reveal reduced brain activity (darker colours) in depression, especially in the prefrontal cortex. A form of radioactively tagged glucose was used as a tracer to visualize levels of brain activity. (From Mark George, MD, courtesy National Institute of Mental Health, Biological Psychiatry Branch.)

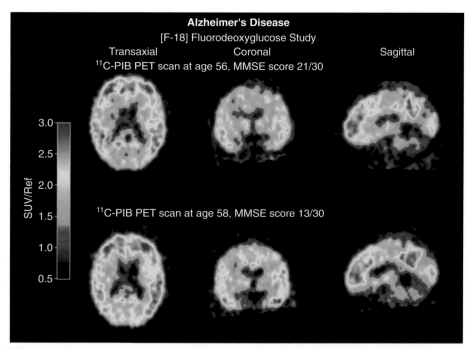

**FIGURE 4-8** A PET scan of a patient with Alzheimer's disease demonstrates a classic pattern for areas of hypometabolism in the temporal and parietal regions of the brain. Areas of reduced metabolism (dark blue and black regions) are very noticeable in the sagittal and coronal views. (From: "Positron emission tomography imaging and clinical progression in relation to molecular pathology in the first Pittsburgh Compound B positron emission tomography patient with Alzheimer's disease," by A. Kadir, A. Marutle, D. Gonzalez, M. Schöll, O. Almkvist, M. Mousavi, T. Mustafiz, T. Darreh-Shori, I. Nennesmo, A. Nordberg, 2011, *Brain 134; 301-317*. By permission of Oxford University Press.)

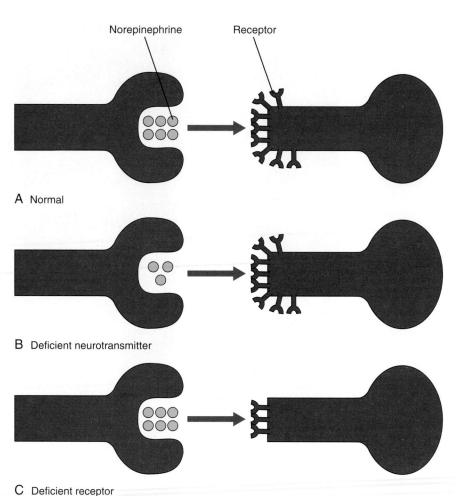

A  Normal

B  Deficient neurotransmitter

C  Deficient receptor

FIGURE 4-9 Normal transmission of neurotransmitters (A). Deficiency in transmission may be due to deficient release of neurotransmitter, as shown in B, or to a reduction in receptors, as shown in C.

disorders such as schizophrenia are associated physiologically with excess transmission of the neurotransmitter dopamine, among other changes. As illustrated in Figure 4-10, this change in dopamine transmission may be due to either an excess release of neurotransmitter or an increase in receptor responsiveness.

The neurotransmitter gamma-aminobutyric acid (GABA) seems to play a role in modulating neuronal excitability and anxiety. Not surprisingly, many antianxiety (anxiolytic) drugs act by increasing the effectiveness of this neurotransmitter, primarily by increasing receptor responsiveness.

It is important to keep in mind that the various areas of the brain are interconnected structurally and functionally by a vast network of neurons. This network serves to integrate the many and varied activities of the brain. A limited number of neurotransmitters are used in the brain, and thus, a particular neurotransmitter is often used by different neurons to carry out quite different activities. For example, dopamine is used by neurons involved not only in thought processes but also in the regulation of movement. Alterations in neurotransmitter activity due to a mental disturbance or to the drugs used to treat the disturbance can affect more than one area of brain activity. In other words, alterations in mental status, whether arising from disease or from medication, are often accompanied by changes in basic drives, sleep patterns, body movement, and autonomic functions.

## MECHANISMS OF ACTION OF PSYCHOTROPIC DRUGS

The concepts of pharmacodynamics and pharmacokinetics are important when studying drugs. Pharmacodynamics refers to the biochemical and physiological effects of drugs on the body, which include the mechanisms of drug action and its effect. Pharmacokinetics refers to the actions of the body on the drug and involves absorption (how much of the drug enters the circulation) and distribution of an administered drug; how long it takes for the drug action to begin and the duration of the effect; the way in which the drug is metabolized (broken down by the body); and the mode of excretion of the metabolites (the products that result from the body's breaking down the drug). Ultimately, pharmacokinetics determines the blood level of a drug and is used to guide the dosage schedule. It is also used to determine the type and amount of drug used in patients with liver and kidney disease.

The processes of pharmacokinetics and pharmacodynamics play an extensive role in how genetic factors give rise to variations in drug response among individuals and among ethnic groups. Pharmacogenetics is an approach to treatment that takes into consideration individual genetic differences when determining which and how much medication to prescribe (see Considering Culture box).

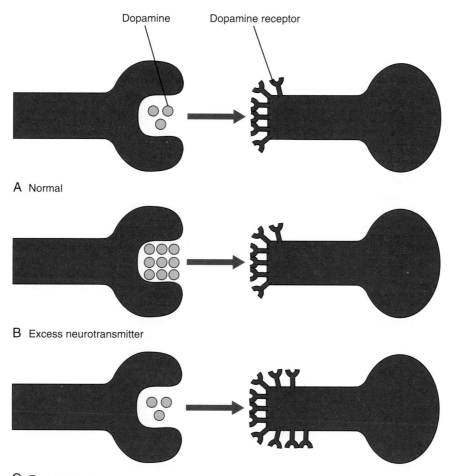

**A** Normal

**B** Excess neurotransmitter

**C** Excess receptors

**FIGURE 4-10** Causes of excess transmission of neurotransmitters. Excess transmission may be due to excess release of neurotransmitter, as shown in B, or to excess responsiveness of receptors, as shown in C.

## 🌐 CONSIDERING CULTURE

### *Pharmacogenetics*

Pharmacogenetic researchers are attempting to explain how genetic variations (metabolizer phenotypes) lead to clinical differences in drug responses for different individuals and ethnic groups (Zandi & Judy, 2010). For example, different metabolizer phenotypes have significant differences in drug metabolism rates due to variations in their cytochrome P450 (CYP450) liver enzymes (Bertilsson, 2007). Researchers have identified more than 50 different CYP450 enzymes in humans. Of these, seven metabolize greater than 90% of the clinically most important drugs. For example, CYP450 2D6 is involved in the metabolism of 25% to 30% of all prescribed drugs, while CYP450 2C19 is involved in metabolizing 15% of prescribed drugs (Lewis, 2004). Metabolism of many psychotropic drugs (e.g., risperidone) involves the CYP450 2D6 enzyme system. The people who poorly metabolize the drugs (about 5% to 10% of Caucasians) may experience more adverse effects from higher drug plasma levels. Comparatively, about 20% to 30% of Asian subgroups are poor drug metabolizers of CYP450 2C19 enzymes and, therefore,

typically experience more adverse effects from many of the psychotropic drugs.

In addition to adverse effects related to genetic factors, many other factors influence adherence to a medical regimen. For example, cultural and ethnic beliefs surrounding mental health disorders, attitudes toward the mental health system, and the cultural practices of an ethnic group all greatly impact a patient's degree of engagement with and adherence to the medical regimen. Adherence is discussed more fully in Chapter 6.

**Sources:** Bertilsson, L. (2007). Metabolism of antidepressant and neuroleptic drugs by cytochrome P450s: Clinical and interethnic aspects. *Clinical pharmacology and therapeutics, 82*(5), 606–609. doi:10.1038/sj.clpt.6100358; Lewis, D.F. (2004). 57 varieties: The human cytochromes P450. *Pharmacogenomics, 5*(3), 305–318. doi:10.1517/phgs.5.3.305.29827; and Zandi, P.P., & Judy, J.T. (2010). The promise and reality of pharmacogenetics in psychiatry. *Psychiatric Clinics of North America, 33*(1), 181–224.

Many drugs are transformed by the liver into active metabolites—chemicals that have pharmacological actions. This knowledge is used by researchers in designing new drugs that make use of the body's own mechanisms to activate a chemical for pharmacological use.

An ideal psychiatric drug would relieve the mental health disturbance of the patient without inducing additional cerebral (mental) or somatic (physical) effects. Unfortunately, in psychopharmacology—as in most areas of pharmacology—no drugs are both fully effective and free of unwanted adverse effects. Nevertheless, researchers are working toward developing medications that target the symptoms while producing no or few adverse effects.

As a result, many patients stop taking their psychotropic medications. Nonadherence to medications (i.e., primarily medication nonpersistence and the lack of consistency in adhering to the prescribed regimen) is a significant barrier to the successful treatment of mental health disorders in clinical practice. Poor adherence to medications significantly increases the risk of relapse. In addition, approximately 40% of patients fail to achieve clinical response with initial drug treatment, and 63% experience at least one adverse event during a course of treatment. Moreover, approximately 10% to 15% of patients discontinue treatment because of these adverse events (Gartlehner, Hansen, Morgan, et al., 2011).

Because all activities of the brain involve actions of neurons, neurotransmitters, and receptors, these parts are the targets of pharmacological intervention. Most psychotropic drugs act by either increasing or decreasing the activity of certain neurotransmitter–receptor systems. It is generally agreed that the dysfunctional neurotransmitter–receptor systems differ depending on a person's mental health condition. These differences offer more specific targets for drug action. In fact, much of what is known about the relationship between specific neurotransmitters and specific disturbances has been derived from knowledge of the pharmacology of the drugs used to treat these conditions. For example, most drugs that were effective in reducing the delusions and hallucinations of schizophrenia blocked the $D_2$ dopamine receptors. Consequently, it was concluded that delusions and hallucinations result from overactivity of dopamine at these receptors.

## Antianxiety and Hypnotic Drugs

Gamma-aminobutyric acid (GABA) is the major inhibitory (calming) neurotransmitter in the central nervous system (CNS). There are three major types of GABA receptors: $GABA_A$, $GABA_B$, and $GABA_C$ receptors. The various subtypes of $GABA_A$ ($\alpha_1$, $\alpha_2$, $\alpha_3$) receptors are the targets of benzodiazepines, barbiturates, and alcohol. Drugs that enhance $GABA_A$ receptors exert a sedative–hypnotic action on brain function. The most commonly used antianxiety drugs are the benzodiazepines and, more recently, the antidepressants selective serotonin reuptake inhibitors and serotonin–norepinephrine reuptake inhibitors.

### Benzodiazepines

Benzodiazepines promote the activity of GABA by binding to a specific receptor on the $GABA_A$ receptor complex. This binding results in inhibited cellular excitation because neurotransmitters cannot be released. If neurotransmitters cannot be released, the result is a calming effect. As shown in Figure 4-11, benzodiazepines, such as diazepam (Valium), clonazepam (Rivotril), and alprazolam (Xanax), bind to $GABA_A$ receptors. Alpha-2 subunits may be the most important for decreasing anxiety. These receptors are common in the limbic system, the brain's emotional centre.

At higher doses, all benzodiazepines can cause sedation. There are six benzodiazepines used in Canada for treatment of insomnia—lorazepam (Ativan), nitrazepam (Mogadon), oxazepam (Serax), temazepam (Restoril), triazolam (Halcion), and flurazepam (Dalmane)—with a predominantly hypnotic (sleep-inducing) effect. Used at lower doses, lorazepam (Ativan) and alprazolam (Xanax), can reduce anxiety without being as *soporific* (sleep-producing).

The fact that the benzodiazepines promote the ability of GABA to inhibit neurons probably accounts for their efficacy as anticonvulsants and for their ability to reduce the neuronal overexcitement of alcohol withdrawal. When used alone, even at high dosages, these drugs rarely inhibit the brain to the degree that respiratory depression, coma, and death result. However, when combined with other CNS depressants, such as alcohol, opiates, or tricyclic antidepressants (TCAs), the inhibitory actions of the benzodiazepines can lead to life-threatening CNS depression.

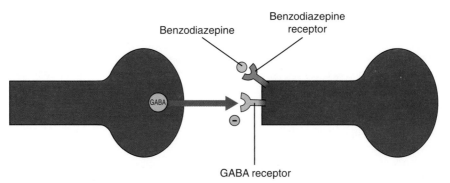

**FIGURE 4-11** Action of benzodiazepines. Drugs in this group attach to receptors adjacent to the receptors for the neurotransmitter gamma-aminobutyric acid (GABA). Drug attachment to these receptors strengthens the inhibitory effects of GABA. In the absence of GABA, there is no inhibitory effect of benzodiazepines.

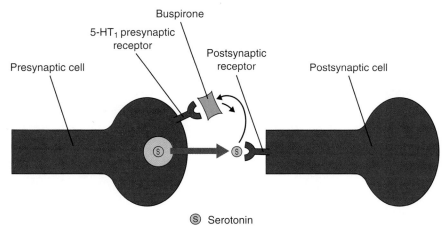

**FIGURE 4-12** Proposed mechanism of action of buspirone. Feedback inhibition by serotonin is blocked, leading to increased release of serotonin by the presynaptic cell. (5-HT$_1$ is a serotonin receptor.)

Any drug that inhibits electrical activity in the brain can interfere with motor ability, attention, and judgement. A patient taking benzodiazepines must be cautioned about engaging in activities that could be dangerous if reflexes and attention are impaired, including specialized activities such as working in construction and more common activities such as driving a car. In older adults, the use of benzodiazepines may contribute to falls and broken bones. Ataxia is a common adverse effect secondary to the abundance of GABA receptors in the cerebellum.

### Short-Acting Sedative–Hypnotic Sleep Drugs

Zopiclone (Imovane) is a newer class of hypnotic, termed a *Z-drug*, Structurally, it is unrelated to existing hypnotics; however, zopiclone also promotes GABA and inhibits the release of neurotransmitters. As a result, zopiclone has sedative effects as well as hypnotic, anxiolytic, anticonvulsant, and muscle-relaxant effects. The onset of action is faster than that of most benzodiazepines. It is important to inform patients taking non-benzodiazepine hypnotic drugs about the quick onset and advise them to take the drug only when they are ready to go to sleep.

Zopiclone has a short half-life (the amount of time it takes the body to eliminate half of the drug), with peak plasma concentration reached at two hours. Zopiclone also has the unique adverse effect of an unpleasant bitter taste upon awakening. Severe drowsiness or impaired coordination are signs of drug intolerance or excessive doses. Because of the potential for misuse, zopiclone should not be taken for more than seven to ten consecutive days and should be used with caution in those who misuse alcohol and other substances. All of the benzodiazepines are categorized as schedule IV to the *Controlled Drugs and Substances Act (CDSA)* and to the Benzodiazepines and Other Targeted Substances Regulations. Zopiclone is a Schedule F drug under the Food and Drug Regulations, which means that a prescription is required for its use.

### Buspirone Hydrochloride

Buspirone hydrochloride (Bustab) is an anxiolytic drug that is used for the short-term relief of excessive anxiety without having strong sedative–hypnotic properties. Because this drug

does not leave the patient sleepy or sluggish, it is often much better tolerated than the benzodiazepines. It is not a CNS depressant and so does not have as great a danger of interaction with other CNS depressants such as alcohol. Also, there is not the potential for dependence that exists with benzodiazepines.

Although, at present, the mechanism of action of buspirone hydrochloride is not clearly understood, one possibility is illustrated in Figure 4-12. Buspirone hydrochloride seems to moderately enhance the effects of serotonin. Therefore, it is referred to as a partial serotonin agonist. It also has a moderate affinity for dopamine-2 receptors, where it also stimulates release of this neurotransmitter and inhibits its destruction. Therefore, with dopamine-2 receptors, buspirone hydrochloride is both an antagonist, which blocks the effects of the neurotransmitter, and an agonist. Adverse effects include headache, dizziness, light-headedness, nausea, decreased concentration, and insomnia.

Refer to Chapter 13 for a discussion of adverse reactions, dosages, nursing implications, and patient and family teaching related to the antianxiety drugs.

### Treating Anxiety Disorders With Antidepressants

The symptoms, neurotransmitters, and circuits associated with anxiety disorders overlap extensively with those of depressive disorders (see Chapter 14), and many antidepressants have proven to be effective treatments for anxiety disorders (Stahl, 2008). Selective serotonin reuptake inhibitors (SSRIs), medications that increase both serotonin and norepinephrine, are often used to treat obsessive-compulsive disorder (OCD), social anxiety disorder (SAD), generalized anxiety disorder (GAD), panic disorder (PD), and post-traumatic stress disorder (PTSD). Venlafaxine hydrochloride (Effexor XR) is used to treat GAD, SAD, and PD. Duloxetine hydrochloride (Cymbalta) is approved for major depressive disorder (MDD), for GAD, and for neuropathic pain associated with peripheral neuropathy of diabetes, pain associated with fibromyalgia, and chronic low back pain.

### Antidepressant Drugs

Understanding of the neurophysiological basis of mood disorders is far from complete. However, a great deal of evidence

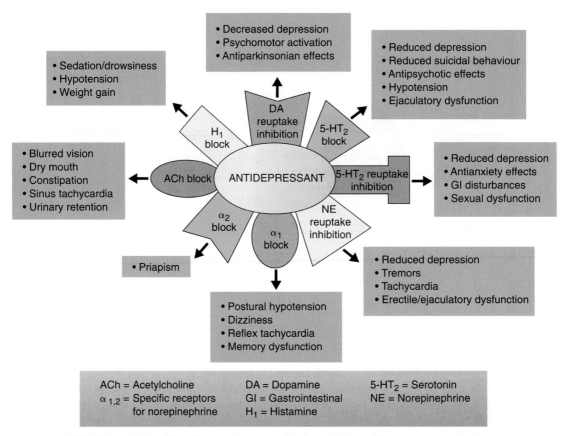

FIGURE 4-13 Possible effects of receptor binding of the antidepressant medications.

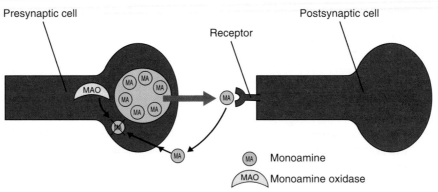

FIGURE 4-14 Normal release, reuptake, and destruction of the monoamine neurotransmitters.

seems to indicate that the neurotransmitters norepinephrine and serotonin play a major role in regulating mood. It is thought that a transmission deficiency of one or both of these monoamines within the limbic system underlies depression. One piece of evidence is that all of the drugs that show efficacy in the treatment of depression increase the synaptic level of one or both of these neurotransmitters (Chen, Gao, & Kemp, 2011). Identified in Figure 4-13 are the adverse effects of specific neurotransmitters' being blocked or activated. Illustrated in Figure 4-14 is the normal release, reuptake, and destruction of the monoamine neurotransmitters. A grasp of this underlying

physiology is essential for understanding the mechanisms by which the antidepressant drugs are thought to act.

Currently, three hypotheses of antidepressants' mechanism of action exist:

1. The *monoamine hypothesis of depression* suggests there is a deficiency in one or more of the three neurotransmitters—serotonin, norepinephrine, or dopamine. The theory is that increasing these neurotransmitters alleviates depression.
2. The *monoamine receptor hypothesis of depression* suggests that low levels of neurotransmitters cause postsynaptic receptors to be up-regulated (increased in sensitivity or

number). Increasing of neurotransmitters by antidepressants results in down-regulation (desensitization) of key neurotransmitter receptors (Stahl, 2008). Delayed length of time for down-regulation may explain why it takes so long for antidepressants to work, especially if they rapidly increase neurotransmitters.

3. Another hypothesis for the mechanism of antidepressant drugs is that they increase production of neurotrophic factors with prolonged use. These factors regulate the survival of neurons and enhance the sprouting of axons to form new synaptic connections (Stahl, 2008).

## Tricyclic Antidepressants

Tricyclic and heterocyclic antidepressants were widely used prior to the development of SSRIs. TCAs are no longer considered first-line treatment for depression since they have more adverse effects, take longer to reach an optimal dose, and are far more lethal in overdose. The tricyclic antidepressants (TCAs) are thought to act primarily by blocking the reuptake of norepinephrine for the secondary amines (e.g., nortriptyline hydrochloride [Aventyl, Norventyl]) and of both norepinephrine and serotonin for the tertiary amines (e.g., amitriptyline hydrochloride [Elavil, Levate], imipramine hydrochloride [Impril]). As shown in Figure 4-15, this blockage prevents norepinephrine from coming into contact with its degrading enzyme, MAO, and thus increases the level of norepinephrine at the synapse. Similarly, the tertiary TCAs block the reuptake and destruction of serotonin and increase the synaptic level of this neurotransmitter.

To varying degrees, many of the tricyclic drugs also block the muscarinic receptors that normally bind acetylcholine. This blockage leads to typical anticholinergic effects, such as blurred vision, dry mouth, tachycardia, urinary retention, and constipation. These adverse effects can be troubling to patients and may limit their adherence to the regimen.

Depending on the individual drug, these drugs can also block histamine-1 receptors in the brain. Blockage of these receptors by any drug causes sedation and drowsiness, an unwelcome adverse effect in daily use (Figure 4-13). People taking the TCAs often have adherence issues because of their adverse reactions. TCA overdose can be fatal, secondary to cardiac conduction disturbances from excessive sodium channel blockade.

## Selective Serotonin Reuptake Inhibitors

As the name implies, the selective serotonin reuptake inhibitors (SSRIs), such as fluoxetine hydrochloride (Prozac), paroxetine hydrochloride (Paxil), citalopram hydrobromide (Celexa), escitalopram oxalate (Cipralex), and fluvoxamine maleate (Luvox), preferentially block the reuptake and, therefore, the destruction of serotonin. Sertraline hydrochloride (Zoloft) also inhibits the neuronal reuptake of serotonin and has weak effects on norepinephrine and dopamine neuronal reuptake. SSRIs have less ability to block the acetylcholine muscarinic and histamine-1 receptors than do the TCAs. As a result of their more selective action, they seem to show comparable efficacy without the anticholinergic and sedating adverse effects that limit patient adherence to other drug regimens. However, SSRIs have other adverse effects: stimulation of various serotonin receptors may inhibit the spinal reflexes of orgasm, lead to apathy and low libido, and cause nausea or vomiting (Stahl, 2008). See Figure 4-16.

## Serotonin–Norepinephrine Reuptake Inhibitors

Serotonin–norepinephrine reuptake inhibitors (SNRIs) are medications that increase both serotonin and norepinephrine. Venlafaxine hydrochloride (Effexor XR) and its metabolite desvenlafaxine succinate (Pristiq) are potent inhibitors of neuronal serotonin and norepinephrine reuptake and weak inhibitors of dopamine reuptake. This SNRI has the flexibility of working as an SSRI at lower doses (75 mg/day), affecting the reuptake of serotonin, and as an SNRI at higher doses (150–225 mg/day). At doses above 350 mg/day, it also weakly blocks dopamine reuptake. Hypertension, induced in about 5% of patients, is a dose-dependent effect based on norepinephrine reuptake blockade. Doses higher than 150 mg/day can increase diastolic blood pressure about 7 to 10 mm Hg. Duloxetine hydrochloride (Cymbalta) has an equal balance of inhibitor effects of norepinephrine and serotonin reuptake. It also has a greater noradrenergic effect than does venlafaxine hydrochloride. This SNRI is indicated for acute and maintenance treatment of major depressive disorder, for acute treatment of generalized anxiety disorder, for managing neuropathic pain associated with

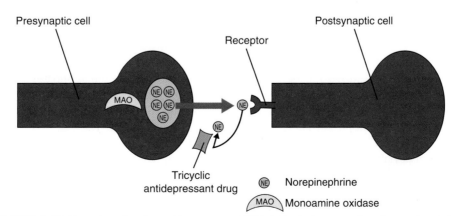

Presynaptic cell
Postsynaptic cell
Receptor
MAO
NE
Tricyclic antidepressant drug

NE Norepinephrine

MAO Monoamine oxidase

**FIGURE 4-15** How the tricyclic antidepressants (TCAs) block the reuptake of norepinephrine.

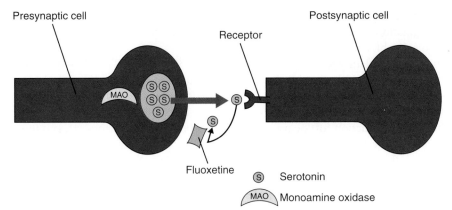

Presynaptic cell

Postsynaptic cell

Receptor

Fluoxetine

Ⓢ    Serotonin

MAO    Monoamine oxidase

**FIGURE 4-16** How the selective serotonin reuptake inhibitors (SSRIs) work.

diabetic peripheral neuropathy, and for managing fibromyalgia. As with the TCAs, many of the SNRIs also have therapeutic effects on neuropathic pain. The common underlying mechanism of *neuropathic pain* is nerve injury or dysfunction. The mechanism by which TCAs and SNRIs reduce neuropathic pain is through activation of the descending norepinephrine and serotonin pathways to the spinal cord, thereby limiting pain signals ascending to the brain.

### Serotonin and Norepinephrine Disinhibitors

The class of drugs described as serotonin and norepinephrine disinhibitors (SNDIs) is represented by only one drug, mirtazapine (Remeron). This unique drug increases norepinephrine, dopamine, and serotonin (5-HT) transmission by blocking central presynaptic $\alpha_2$ adrenergic inhibitory receptors. It may be that mirtazapine, because of its mixed neurotransmitter receptor effects, has a more rapid onset of effect than do single neurotransmitter antidepressant drugs. Mirtazapine is a potent antagonist of 5-HT$_2$ and 5-HT$_3$ receptors, which may account for its antianxiety and antidepressant effects. This antidepressant is also a potent histamine (H$_1$) receptor antagonist, which accounts for drowsiness and increased appetite resulting in weight gain being the most common adverse effects. Patients may also experience orthostatic hypotension and the occasional occurrence of anticholinergic adverse effects. As with all antidepressants—but more so at the beginning of treatment with SSRIs, SNRIs, or SNDIs—there is a chance that the medication may increase the risk of suicide or harm to others as a result of changing serotonin levels in the brain. It is hypothesized that the changes in serotonin may cause an increased amount of energy or severe agitation that creates this risk. This risk is greatest in patients less than 18 years of age; therefore, Health Canada has not authorized these drugs for use in children (Health Canada, 2011a). The advantages of using mirtazapine over other antidepressants are the lower incidence of sexual dysfunction and its antiemetic effects (for patients who suffer nausea).

When discontinuing use of any antidepressant, but particularly SSRIs or SNRIs, patients should be weaned gradually over several weeks rather than abruptly due to the risk of discontinuation symptoms such as dizziness, agitation, anxiety, sleeping difficulties, nausea, excessive sweating, and fatigue. These symptoms do not indicate that an addiction has developed. Most people taking antidepressants never develop a "craving" or feel the need to increase the dose. What these symptoms do indicate is that the brain is adapting to changes in the availability of neurotransmitters. These symptoms will typically resolve within four to six weeks after discontinuation. However, if the symptoms persist beyond this time frame, there is the potential that depression is still present and that the antidepressants are still needed.

### Monoamine Oxidase Inhibitors

Monoamine oxidase inhibitors (MAOIs) are a group of antidepressant drugs that prevent the destruction of monoamines by inhibiting the action of monoamine oxidase. MAOIs illustrate the principle that drugs can have a desired and beneficial effect in the brain, while at the same time having possibly dangerous effects elsewhere in the body. To understand the action of these drugs, keep in mind the following definitions:

- *Monoamines* are a type of organic compound and include the neurotransmitters norepinephrine, epinephrine, dopamine, and serotonin, as well as many different food substances and drugs.
- *Monoamine oxidase (MAO)* is an enzyme that destroys monoamines.
- *Monoamine oxidase inhibitors (MAOIs)* inhibit the action of MAO and thereby prevent the destruction of monoamines.

The monoamine neurotransmitters, as well as any monoamine food substance or drug, are destroyed by the enzyme MAO, which is located in neurons and in the liver. Antidepressant drugs such as phenelzine sulfate (Nardil), tranylcypromine sulfate (Parnate), and selegiline hydrochloride (Anipryl) are MAOIs that act by inhibiting the enzyme and interfering with the destruction of the monoamine neurotransmitters. This action, in turn, increases the synaptic level of the neurotransmitters and makes possible the antidepressant effects of these drugs (Figure 4-17).

The use of MAO-inhibiting drugs is complicated by the fact that MAO is also present in the liver and is responsible for destroying monoamine substances that enter the body via food or drugs. Of particular importance is the monoamine tyramine, which is present in many food substances, such as aged cheeses, pickled or smoked fish, chocolate, many types of beans, and

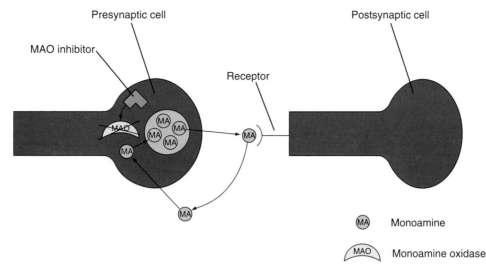

**FIGURE 4-17** Blocking of monoamine oxidase (MAO) by inhibiting drugs (MAOIs) and thereby preventing the breakdown of monoamine by MAO.

beer and wine. Tyramine poses a threat of hypertensive crisis. The displacement of norepinephrine from neuronal storage vesicles by acute tyramine ingestion is thought to cause the vasoconstriction and increased heart rate and blood pressure of the pressor response. In severe cases, adrenergic crisis can occur. Normally, this does not happen, because tyramine is destroyed by MAO as it passes through the liver before entering the general blood circulation. However, in the presence of MAOIs, tyramine is not destroyed by the liver and, in severe cases, can result in adrenergic crisis (extreme tachycardia and hypertension).

A substantial number of drugs are chemically monoamines. The dosages of these drugs are determined by the rate at which they are destroyed by MAO in the liver. In a patient taking MAOIs, the blood level of monoamine drugs can reach high levels and cause serious toxicity. Therefore, MAOIs are contraindicated with concurrent use of any other antidepressants or sympathomimetic drugs, those that affect the sympathetic nervous system. Concurrent use with some over-the-counter products with sympathomimetic properties (e.g., oral decongestants) should also be avoided.

Because of the serious dangers that result from inhibition of hepatic MAO, patients taking MAOIs *must* be given a list of foods high in tyramine and drugs that must be avoided. Chapter 14 contains a list of these foods, along with nursing measures and instructions for patient teaching.

### Other Antidepressants

Bupropion hydrochloride is effective both as an antidepressant (Wellbutrin) and for smoking cessation (Zyban). It seems to act as a dopamine–norepinephrine reuptake inhibitor and also inhibits nicotinic acetylcholine receptors to reduce the addictive action of nicotine. Since bupropion hydrochloride has no serotonin action, it does not cause sexual adverse effects. Adverse effects include insomnia, tremor, anorexia, and weight loss. Bupropion hydrochloride is contraindicated in patients with a seizure disorder, in patients with a current or prior diagnosis of bulimia or anorexia nervosa, and in patients undergoing abrupt

discontinuation of alcohol or sedatives (including benzodiazepines), owing to the increased seizure risk.

Trazodone hydrochloride (Oleptro, Trazodone, Trazorel) is a serotonin antagonist and reuptake inhibitor (SARI) and is not a first choice for antidepressant treatment. It is often given with another antidepressant drug because sedation, one of the common adverse effects, helps combat insomnia. Its antidepressant effects are seen only at high therapeutic doses. The common adverse effects are sedation and orthostatic hypotension: the sedative effect is from potent histamine-1 blockade, and orthostatic hypotension results from $\alpha_1$ adrenergic blockade. Its potent $\alpha_1$ blockade with minimal anticholinergic effects (e.g., constipation, dry mouth, tachycardia) can lead to another rare adverse effect: priapism (painful prolonged penile erection).

## Mood Stabilizers
### Lithium Carbonate

Although the efficacy of lithium carbonate (Carbolith, Lithane, Lithmax) as a mood stabilizer (drug used to treat mood disorders by balancing brain neurotransmitters) in patients with bipolar disorders has been established for many years ("Lithium Is Still," 2010), its mechanism of action is still far from understood. As a positively charged ion, similar in structure to sodium and potassium, lithium may well act by affecting electrical conductivity in neurons. As discussed earlier, an electrical impulse consists of the inward, depolarizing flow of sodium followed by an outward, repolarizing flow of potassium. These electrical charges are propagated along the neuron; if they are initiated at one end of the neuron, they will pass to the other end. Once they reach the end of a neuron, a neurotransmitter is released.

It may be that an overexcitement of neurons in the brain underlies bipolar disorders and that lithium carbonate interacts in some complex way with sodium and potassium at the cell membrane to stabilize electrical activity. Also, lithium carbonate may reduce the excitatory neurotransmitter glutamate and exert an antimanic effect. The other proposed mechanisms by which lithium carbonate works to regulate mood include the noncompetitive inhibition of the enzyme inositol monophosphatase. Inhibition of serotonin receptors by lithium is more related to the drug's antidepressant effects than to its antimanic effects (Shaldubina, Adam, & Belmaker, 2001).

While it is not known exactly how lithium works, it is certain that its adverse effects and toxicity result from its influence on electrical conductivity. By altering electrical conductivity, lithium represents a potential threat to all body functions regulated by electrical currents. Foremost among these functions is cardiac contraction; lithium can induce, although not commonly, sinus bradycardia. Overdose causes extreme alteration of cerebral conductivity, which can lead to convulsions. Changes in nerve and muscle conduction can commonly lead to tremor at therapeutic doses or more extreme motor dysfunction with overdose.

The fact that sodium and potassium play a strong role in regulating fluid balance and distribution in various body compartments explains the disturbances in fluid balance that lithium carbonate can cause, including polyuria (the output of large volumes of urine) and edema (the accumulation of fluid in the interstitial space). Long-term use of lithium carbonate can result in hypothyroidism in some patients by interfering with iodine molecules and affecting formation of and conversion to the active form of thyroid hormone, triiodothyronine (T3). In addition, hyponatremia can increase the risk of lithium carbonate toxicity because increased kidney reabsorption of sodium leads to increased reabsorption of lithium carbonate as well.

Primarily because of its effects on electrical conductivity, lithium has a low therapeutic index. The therapeutic index represents the ratio of the lethal dose to the effective dose and is a measure of overall drug safety regarding the possibility of overdose or toxicity. It can be expressed as therapeutic index equals median lethal dose/median effective dose. A low therapeutic index means that the drug blood level that can cause death is not far above the level required for drug effectiveness. This risk mandates that the blood level of lithium carbonate be monitored on a regular basis to ensure the drug is not accumulating and rising to dangerous levels. See Table 4-3 for a list of some of the adverse and toxic effects of lithium. Within Chapter 15 is a more in-depth discussion of lithium carbonate treatment and specific dose-related adverse and toxic effects, nursing implications, and the patient teaching plan.

| TABLE 4-3 | ADVERSE AND TOXIC EFFECTS OF LITHIUM |
|---|---|
| **SYSTEM** | **ADVERSE AND TOXIC EFFECTS** |
| Nervous and muscular | Tremor, ataxia, confusion, convulsions |
| Digestive | Nausea, vomiting, diarrhea |
| Cardiac | Arrhythmias |
| Fluid and electrolyte | Polyuria, polydipsia, edema |
| Endocrine | Goiter and hypothyroidism |

## Anticonvulsant Drugs

Valproate (available as sodium divalproex and valproic acid [Depakene]), carbamazepine (Tegretol), and lamotrigine (Lamictal) have demonstrated efficacy in the treatment of bipolar disorders. Their anticonvulsant properties derive from the alteration of electrical conductivity in membranes; in particular, they reduce the firing rate of very high frequency neurons in the brain. It is possible that this membrane-stabilizing effect accounts for the ability of these drugs to reduce the mood swings that occur in patients with bipolar disorders (Grunze, 2010). Other proposed mechanisms as mood stabilizers are glutamate antagonists and GABA agonists.

### Valproate

Valproate (Depakote, Depakene) is structurally different from other anticonvulsants and psychiatric drugs that show efficacy in the treatment of bipolar disorders. Divalproex is recommended for patients who have a rapid-cycling bipolar disorder. Common adverse effects include tremor, weight gain, and sedation. Occasional serious adverse effects are thrombocytopenia, pancreatitis, hepatic failure, and birth defects. Baseline levels are measured for liver function indicators and complete blood count (CBC) before an individual is started on this medication, and measurements are repeated periodically. In addition, the therapeutic blood level of the drug is monitored.

### Carbamazepine

Carbamazepine (Tegretol) is useful in preventing mania and in tempering episodes of acute mania (Williams, Ruekert, & Lum, 2011). It reduces the firing rate of overexcited neurons by reducing the activity of sodium channels. Common adverse effects include anticholinergic effects (e.g., dry mouth, constipation, urinary retention, blurred vision), orthostatic hypotension, sedation, and ataxia. Rash may occur in 10% of patients (Sadock & Sadock, 2008). Recommended baseline laboratory work includes liver function tests, CBC, electrocardiogram, and electrolyte levels. Blood levels are monitored to avoid toxicity (greater than 12 mcg/mL), but there are no established therapeutic blood levels for carbamazepine in the treatment of bipolar disorder.

### Lamotrigine

Lamotrigine (Lamictal) is perhaps the most effective drug for maintenance therapy of bipolar disorder, but it is not as effective in acute mania (Preston, O'Neal, & Talaga, 2005). Lamotrigine works well in treating the depression of bipolar disorder, with less incidence of switching the patient into mania than antidepressants (Lam, 2010). It modulates the release of glutamate and aspartate. Patients should promptly report any rashes, which could be a sign of life-threatening Stevens–Johnson syndrome. This risk can be minimized by slow titration to therapeutic doses.

### Other Anticonvulsants

Other anticonvulsants used as mood stabilizers are gabapentin (Neurontin), topiramate (Topamax), and oxcarbazepine

(Trileptal). None of them have Health Canada approval as mood stabilizers, and studies have not provided strong support for their use as primary treatments for bipolar disorders. However, they are used for their calming effects during mania. Chapter 15 offers a more detailed discussion of these medications.

## Antipsychotic Drugs

### Conventional Antipsychotics

First-generation antipsychotic drugs, or conventional antipsychotics (also called *typical* or *standard*), are strong antagonists at the $D_2$ dopamine receptors. By binding to these receptors and blocking the attachment of dopamine, they reduce dopaminergic transmission. It has been postulated that an overactivity of the dopamine system in certain areas of the mesolimbic system may be responsible for at least some of the symptoms of schizophrenia; thus, blockage of dopamine may reduce these symptoms—particularly the "positive" symptoms of schizophrenia, such as delusions (e.g., paranoid and grandiose ideas) and hallucinations (e.g., hearing or seeing things not present in reality). These drugs block not only dopamine but also receptors for acetylcholine and $\alpha_1$ adrenergic receptors for norepinephrine. See Chapter 16 for a more detailed discussion of schizophrenia and its symptoms.

Conventional antipsychotics are also antagonists, to varying degrees, of the muscarinic receptors for acetylcholine, $\alpha_1$ adrenergic receptors for norepinephrine, and histamine-1 receptors. Although it is unclear if this antagonism plays a role in the beneficial effects of the drugs, it is certain that antagonism is responsible for some of their major adverse effects (see Chapter 16).

The proposed mechanism of action of the conventional antipsychotics—which include the phenothiazines, thioxanthenes, butyrophenones, and pharmacologically related drugs—is illustrated in Figure 4-18. As summarized in Figure 4-19, many of the untoward adverse effects of these drugs can be understood as a logical extension of their receptor-blocking activity. Because dopamine in the basal ganglia plays a major role in the regulation of movement, it is not surprising that dopamine blockage can lead to drug-induced motor abnormalities (extrapyramidal adverse effects) such as parkinsonism, akinesia, akathisia, dyskinesia, and tardive dyskinesia. Anticholinergic drugs such as benzatropine or benzhexol hydrochloride are often prescribed to prevent or treat these antipsychotic-induced extrapyramidal symptoms. Benzatropine antagonizes the effect of acetylcholine, increasing the amount of available dopamine.

Nurses and physicians often monitor patients for evidence of involuntary movements after administration of the conventional antipsychotic drugs. One popular scale is called the Abnormal Involuntary Movement Scale (AIMS). See Chapter 16 for an example of AIMS and a discussion of the clinical use of antipsychotic drugs, adverse effects, specific nursing interventions, and patient teaching strategies.

An important physiological function of dopamine is that it acts as the hypothalamic factor that inhibits the release of prolactin from the anterior pituitary gland so that the blockage of dopamine transmission can lead to the increased pituitary secretion of prolactin. In women, this hyperprolactinemia can result in amenorrhea (absence of the menses) or galactorrhea (breast milk flow); in men, it can lead to gynecomastia (development of the male mammary glands).

Acetylcholine, as mentioned, is the neurotransmitter released by the postganglionic neurons of the parasympathetic nervous system. Through its attachment to muscarinic receptors, a type of acetylcholine receptor, on internal organs, it serves to help regulate internal function. Blockage of the muscarinic receptors by phenothiazines and a wide variety of other psychiatric drugs can lead to a constellation of untoward effects, which are predictable based on knowledge of the normal physiology of the parasympathetic nervous system. These adverse effects usually involve blurred vision, dry mouth, constipation, and urinary hesitancy. These drugs can also impair memory, since acetylcholine is important for memory function.

In addition to blocking dopamine and muscarinic receptors, many of the conventional antipsychotic drugs act as antagonists at the $\alpha_1$ adrenergic receptors for norepinephrine. These receptors are found on smooth muscle cells that contract in response to norepinephrine from sympathetic nerves. For example, the ability of sympathetic nerves to constrict blood vessels is dependent on the attachment of norepinephrine to $\alpha_1$ adrenergic receptors. Blockage of these receptors can bring about vasodilation and a consequent drop in blood pressure. Vasoconstriction mediated by the sympathetic nervous system is essential for maintaining normal blood pressure when the body is in the upright position; blockage of the $\alpha_1$ adrenergic receptors can lead to orthostatic hypotension.

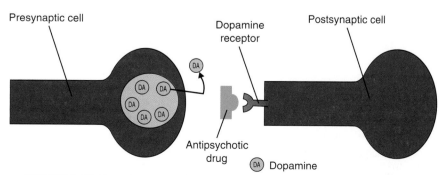

**FIGURE 4-18** How the conventional antipsychotics block dopamine receptors.

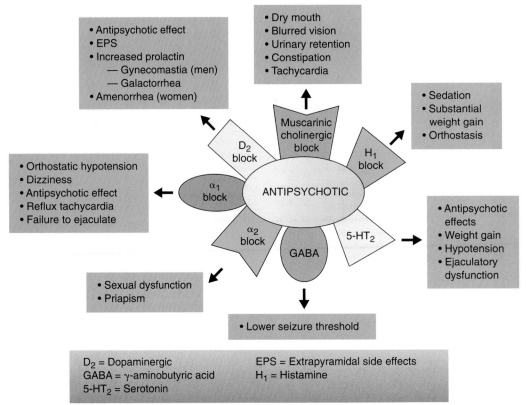

• Antipsychotic effect
• EPS
• Increased prolactin
   — Gynecomastia (men)
   — Galactorrhea
• Amenorrhea (women)

• Dry mouth
• Blurred vision
• Urinary retention
• Constipation
• Tachycardia

• Sedation
• Substantial
   weight gain
• Orthostasis

• Orthostatic hypotension
• Dizziness
• Antipsychotic effect
• Reflux tachycardia
• Failure to ejaculate

• Antipsychotic
   effects
• Weight gain
• Hypotension
• Ejaculatory
   dysfunction

• Sexual dysfunction
• Priapism

• Lower seizure threshold

$D_2$ block · Muscarinic cholinergic block · $H_1$ block · $\alpha_1$ block · ANTIPSYCHOTIC · $\alpha_2$ block · GABA · 5-HT$_2$

$D_2$ = Dopaminergic
GABA = γ-aminobutyric acid
5-HT$_2$ = Serotonin

EPS = Extrapyramidal side effects
$H_1$ = Histamine

**FIGURE 4-19** Adverse effects of receptor blockage of antipsychotic drugs. **Sources:** Lehne, R.A. (2001). *Pharmacology for nursing care* (4th ed.). Philadelphia: Saunders; Varcarolis, E. (2002). *Foundations of psychiatric mental health nursing* (4th ed.). Philadelphia: WB Saunders; and Keltner, N.L., & Folks, D.G. (2001). *Psychotropic drugs* (3rd ed.). St. Louis: Mosby.

The $\alpha_1$ adrenergic receptors are also found on the vas deferens and are responsible for the propulsive contractions leading to ejaculation. Blockage of these receptors can lead to a failure to ejaculate. Potent $\alpha_1$ adrenergic antagonists with few anticholinergic effects, such as trazodone hydrochloride, can lead to priapism, secondary to the inability for detumescence (subsidence of erection).

Finally, many of these conventional antipsychotic drugs, as well as a variety of other psychiatric drugs, block the histamine-1 receptors for histamine. The two most significant adverse effects of blocking these receptors are sedation and substantial weight gain. The sedation may be beneficial in severely agitated patients. Nonadherence to the medication regimen is a significant issue because of these troublesome adverse effects, and the atypical antipsychotic drugs have consequently become the drugs of choice.

### Atypical Antipsychotics

The second generation of antipsychotic drugs includes the atypical antipsychotics, which produce fewer extrapyramidal side effects (EPS) and target both the negative and positive symptoms of schizophrenia (see Chapter 16). These newer drugs are often chosen as first-line treatment over the conventional antipsychotics because of the lower risk of EPS (Leucht,

Corves, Arbter, et al., 2009). However, several of the available atypical antipsychotics can increase the risk of a metabolic syndrome, resulting in increased weight, blood glucose, and triglycerides. The simultaneous blockade of 5-HT$_{2C}$ and histamine-1 receptors is associated with weight gain due to increased appetite stimulation via the hypothalamic eating centres. Strong antimuscarinic properties at the M3 receptor on the pancreatic beta cells can cause insulin resistance, leading to hyperglycemia. The receptor responsible for elevated triglycerides is currently unknown (Stahl, 2008). Clozapine and olanzapine have the highest risk of causing metabolic syndrome; aripiprazole and ziprasidone hydrochloride monohydrate have the lowest risk.

The atypical antipsychotics are predominantly dopamine and serotonin antagonists. The blockade at the mesolimbic dopamine pathway is thought to decrease psychosis, similar to the mechanism by which the conventional antipsychotics work (Mackin & Thomas, 2011). Decreasing dopamine can reduce psychosis but cause adverse effects elsewhere, such as the movement effects of EPS, the worsening of cognitive and negative symptoms, and an increase in the hormone prolactin, leading to gynecomastia, galactorrhea, amenorrhea, and low libido (Stahl, 2008).

*Clozapine.* Clozapine (Clozaril), the first of the atypicals, is an antipsychotic drug that is relatively free of the motor adverse effects of the phenothiazines and other atypical antipsychotics. It is thought that clozapine preferentially blocks the dopamine receptors in the mesolimbic system, rather than those in the nigrostriatal area. This blockage allows clozapine to exert an antipsychotic action without leading to difficulties with EPS. Clozapine produces little or no prolactin elevation compared to the conventional antipsychotics. Although people who take clozapine are more likely to adhere to their medication regimen than those who are taking other atypical antipsychotics, it has the potential to suppress bone marrow and induce agranulocytosis. Because any deficiency in white blood cells renders a person prone to serious infection, regular measurement of white blood cell count is required. As a result of these risks, all patients taking clozapine must have weekly cell counts for the first six months, every other week for the next six months, and monthly thereafter. To ensure that these blood tests are completed, clozapine is dispensed at these same intervals. Due to the significant risk of agranulocytosis and seizure (in 5% of patients) associated with its use, clozapine should be limited to patients with treatment-resistant schizophrenia who are nonresponsive to, or intolerant of, conventional antipsychotic drugs.

Caution should be used with introducing other drugs that can increase the concentration of clozapine. There is also a potential for myocarditis that should be monitored, and fever, but the most common adverse effects of clozapine are drowsiness and sedation (39%), hypersalivation (31%), reflex tachycardia (25%), constipation (14%), and dizziness and vertigo (19%) (Health Canada, 2011a).

*Risperidone.* Risperidone (Risperdal) has a low potential for inducing agranulocytosis or convulsions. However, high therapeutic dosages (greater than 6 mg/day) may lead to motor difficulties. It has the highest risk of EPS among the atypical antipsychotics and may increase prolactin, which may lead to sexual dysfunction. Risperidone can cause orthostatic hypotension that can lead to falls, which are a serious problem among older adults. Weight gain, sedation, and sexual dysfunction are adverse effects that may affect adherence to the medication regimen and should be discussed with patients. It is notable that risperidone is the first atypical antipsychotic available as a long-acting injection. Risperdal Consta, administered every two weeks, provides an alternative to the depot form of conventional antipsychotics. A rare but serious adverse effect is an increased risk of stroke and transient ischemic attacks in older adults with dementia who are being treated for agitation (Lee, Gill, Freedman, et al., 2004).

*Quetiapine fumarate.* Quetiapine fumarate (Seroquel) has a broad receptor-binding profile. Its strong blockage of histamine-1 receptors accounts for the high sedation it can cause. The combination of histamine-1 and serotonin receptor blockage leads to the weight gain associated with use of this drug and also to a moderate risk for metabolic syndrome. It causes moderate blockage of $\alpha_1$ adrenergic receptors and associated orthostatic hypotension, dizziness, and syncope. Quetiapine fumarate has a low risk for EPS or prolactin elevation from low $D_2$ dopamine binding due to rapid dissociation at these receptors.

*Other atypical antipsychotics.* Other atypical antipsychotics include the following:

- Olanzapine (Zyprexa) is similar to clozapine in chemical structure. Adverse effects include sedation, weight gain, hyperglycemia with new-onset type 2 diabetes, and higher risk for metabolic syndrome.
- Ziprasidone hydrochloride monohydrate (Zeldox) is a serotonin–norepinephrine reuptake inhibitor. The main adverse effects are dizziness and moderate sedation. Ziprasidone is contraindicated in patients with a known history of QT interval prolongation, recent acute myocardial infarction, or uncompensated heart failure.
- Aripiprazole (Abilify) is a unique atypical antipsychotic known as a *dopamine system stabilizer*. In areas of the brain with excess dopamine, it lowers the dopamine level by acting as a receptor antagonist; however, in regions with low dopamine, it stimulates receptors to raise the dopamine level. It induces little sedation or weight gain. Adverse effects include insomnia and akathisia.
- Paliperidone (Invega) is the major active metabolite of risperidone. It has similar adverse effects to risperidone, such as EPS and prolactin elevation. Additional adverse effects are orthostasis and sedation. It is also available as paliperidone palmitate (Invega Sustenna), a prolonged-release injectable suspension.

The conventional and atypical antipsychotic drugs are discussed in detail in Chapter 15, including the indications for use, adverse reactions, nursing implications, and patient and family teaching.

## Drug Treatment for Attention Deficit Hyperactivity Disorder

Children and adults with attention deficit hyperactivity disorder (ADHD) show symptoms of short attention span, impulsivity, and overactivity. Paradoxically, the mainstay of treatment for this condition in children—and increasingly in adults—is the administration of psychostimulant drugs. Both methylphenidate hydrochloride (Biphentin, Concerta, Ritalin) and dextroamphetamines such as amphetamine aspartate monohydrate (Adderall XR) seem to show efficacy in these conditions. They are sympathomimetic amines and have been shown to function as direct and indirect agonists at adrenergic receptor sites. Psychostimulants act directly at the postsynaptic receptor, mimicking the effects of norepinephrine or dopamine. They block the reuptake of norepinephrine and dopamine into the presynaptic neuron and increase the release of these monoamines into the extraneuronal space. How this translates into clinical efficacy is far from understood, but it is thought that the monoamines may inhibit an overactive part of the limbic system.

Among many concerns with the use of these drugs are the adverse effects of agitation, exacerbation of psychotic thought processes, hypertension, and long-term growth suppression, as well as their potential for misuse. One nonstimulant medication available for the treatment of ADHD is atomoxetine hydrochloride (Strattera), a norepinephrine reuptake inhibitor approved for use in children 6 years and older, adolescents, and adults.

Common adverse effects include decreased appetite and weight loss, fatigue, and dizziness. Refer to Chapter 29 for more on these drugs.

## Drug Treatment for Alzheimer's Disease

The insidious and progressive loss of memory and other higher executive brain functions brought about by Alzheimer's disease is a tremendous individual, family, and social tragedy. Because the disease seems to involve progressive structural degeneration of the brain, there are two major pharmacological directions in its treatment. The first is to attempt to prevent or slow the structural degeneration. Although actively pursued, this approach has been unsuccessful so far. The second is to attempt to maintain normal brain function for as long as possible.

Much of the memory loss in this disease has been attributed to dysfunction of neurons that secrete acetylcholine. The anticholinesterase drugs (also called *cholinesterase inhibitors*) show some efficacy in slowing the rate of memory loss and, in some patients, may even improve memory. The drugs work by interfering with the action of acetylcholinesterase. Inactivation of this enzyme leads to less destruction of the neurotransmitter acetylcholine and, therefore, a higher concentration at the synapse. There are four drugs approved for the treatment of mild to moderate Alzheimer's disease in Canada, three of which are acetylcholinesterase inhibitors: donepezil hydrochloride (Aricept), galantamine hydrobromide (Reminyl), and rivastigmine hydrogen tartrate (Exelon). The fourth drug approved for treatment of Alzheimer's disease is memantine hydrochloride (Ebixa), a noncompetitive N-methyl-D-aspartate (NMDA) receptor antagonist. The glutamatergic neurotransmitter system plays an important role in memory formation. Amyloid plaques in the brain can lead to glutamatergic dysfunction and excess glutamate. When glutamate binds to NMDA receptors, calcium flows freely from the cell; overexposure to calcium results in cell degeneration. Memantine fills the NMDA receptor cites and reduces this degeneration. Memantine was shown to be effective in the treatment of moderate to severe Alzheimer's disease.

Refer to Chapter 18 for a more detailed discussion of these drugs, as well as their nursing considerations and patient and family teaching.

## Natural Health Products

The growing interest in natural health products is driven by a variety of factors. Many people believe that these products are safer because they are "natural" or that they may have fewer adverse effects than more costly traditional medications.

Natural health products have been researched in an effort to understand their mechanisms of action. They have also been studied in clinical trials to determine their safety and efficacy. This is especially true of kava kava and St. John's wort (Sarris & Kavanagh, 2009). Some natural health products have been found to be nontherapeutic, and others even deadly if taken over long periods of time or in combination with other chemical substances and prescription drugs (Preston, O'Neal, & Talaga, 2005). The risk of bleeding may be increased in patients taking ginkgo biloba and warfarin, and kava kava may increase the risk of hepatotoxicity at doses over 240 mg/day.

Among the major concerns of health care providers are the potential long-term effects of some natural health products (nerve, kidney, and liver damage) and the possibility of adverse chemical reactions when natural health products are taken in conjunction with other substances, including conventional medications.

St. John's wort can have serious interactions with a number of conventional medications (Howland, 2010). For example, taking St. John's wort with other serotonergic drugs (e.g., SSRIs, triptans) can result in serotonin syndrome (hyperserotonemia). Serotonin syndrome is a potentially life-threatening reaction that occurs when there is too much serotonin in the body. Symptoms include agitation, overactive reflexes (hyperreflexia), tremors, excessive sweating, racing heart, rapid changes in blood pressure, nausea, and loss of coordination (ataxia). It may also reduce the effectiveness of other medications by increasing their rate of metabolism and reducing blood levels of these medications. St. John's wort is a cytochrome P450 (CYP450) 3A4 enzyme inducer. Patients taking CYP450 3A4 metabolized medications (e.g., hormonal contraceptives, HIV protease inhibitors, HIV non-nucleoside reverse transcriptase inhibitors, the immunosuppressant drugs cyclosporine and tacrolimus, the antineoplastic drugs irinotecan and imatinib mesylate) concurrently with St. John's wort may experience increased metabolism and subtherapeutic drug levels (Alpert, 2008). Drugs with a narrow therapeutic index should be monitored more closely when St. John's wort is added or discontinued or when the dosage is changed.

Another key concern regarding the use of natural health products is the quality of natural health products that is available. Health Canada provides information on natural health products via the Licensed Natural Health Products Database. "Products with a licence have been assessed by Health Canada and found to be safe, effective and of high quality under their recommended conditions of use. Licensed natural health products have an eight-digit Natural Product Number (NPN) or Homeopathic Medicine Number (DIN-HM)" (Health Canada, 2011a). Health care providers, especially nurses, need to stay current, using unbiased sources of product information and passing this information on to patients taking alternative drugs. Recalls and warnings to stop use of certain brands are available at MedEffect Canada (Health Canada, 2011b).

It is important that nurses and other health care providers explore the patient's use of natural health products in a nonjudgemental manner by asking, "What over-the-counter medications or natural health products do you take to help your symptoms? Do they help? How much are you taking? How long have you been taking them?" Individuals taking medications or other natural health products should be made aware of drug or substance interactions and product safety. Such discussion should be part of the initial and ongoing interviews with patients. Complementary and integrative therapies are covered in more detail in Chapter 37.

# KEY POINTS

- All actions of the brain—sensory, motor, and intellectual—are carried out physiologically through the interactions of nerve cells. These interactions involve impulse conduction, neurotransmitter release, and receptor response. Alterations in these basic processes can lead to mental disturbances and physical manifestations.

- In particular, it seems that excess activity of dopamine is involved in the thought disturbances of schizophrenia, and deficiencies of norepinephrine, serotonin, or both underlie depression and anxiety. Insufficient activity of GABA also plays a role in anxiety.

- Pharmacological treatment of mental health disturbances is directed at the suspected neurotransmitter–receptor problem. Antipsychotic drugs decrease dopamine; antidepressant drugs increase synaptic levels of norepinephrine, serotonin, or both; and antianxiety drugs increase the effectiveness of GABA or increase 5-HT, norepinephrine, or both.

- Because the immediate target activity of a drug can result in many downstream alterations in neuronal activity, drugs with a variety of chemical actions may show efficacy in treating the same clinical condition. Thus, newer drugs with novel mechanisms of action are being used in the treatment of schizophrenia, depression, and anxiety.

- Unfortunately, drugs used to treat mental health disease can cause various undesired effects. Prominent among these can be sedation or excitement, motor disturbances, muscarinic blockage, $\alpha$ antagonism, sexual dysfunction, and weight gain. There is a continuing effort to develop new drugs that are effective, safe, and well tolerated.

# CRITICAL THINKING

1. No matter where you practise psychiatric mental health nursing, individuals under your care will be taking psychotropic drugs. Consider the importance of understanding normal brain structure and function as they relate to mental disturbances and psychotropic drugs by answering the following questions:
   a. How can you use the knowledge of normal brain function (control of peripheral nerves, skeletal muscles, the autonomic nervous system, hormones, and circadian rhythms) to better understand how a patient can be affected by psychotropic drugs or psychiatric illness?
   b. What information from the various brain imaging techniques can you use to understand and treat patients with mental disorders and provide support to their families? How might you use that information for patient and family teaching?

2. Based on your understanding of symptoms that may occur when the following neurotransmitters are altered, what specific information would you include in medication teaching?
   a. Dopamine $D_2$ (as with use of antipsychotic drugs)
   b. Blockage of muscarinic receptors (as with use of phenothiazines and other drugs)
   c. $\alpha_1$ receptors (as with use of phenothiazines and other drugs)
   d. Histamine (as with use of phenothiazines and other drugs)
   e. Monoamine oxidase (MAO) (as with use of a monoamine oxidase inhibitor [MAOI])
   f. Gamma-aminobutyric acid (GABA) (as with use of benzodiazepines)
   g. Serotonin (as with use of selective serotonin reuptake inhibitors [SSRIs] and other drugs)
   h. Norepinephrine (as with use of serotonin–norepinephrine reuptake inhibitors [SNRIs])

# CHAPTER REVIEW

1. Which patient statement would the nurse attribute to a neurobiological basis of mental disease?
   1. "I like to eat all day long."
   2. "I sleep seven hours nightly."
   3. "I have a number of close friends."
   4. "I enjoy solving word puzzles."

2. Which of the following medication orders would the nurse question?
   1. Buspirone hydrochloride—take in the morning
   2. Temazepam—take at bedtime
   3. Zopiclone—take early in the morning
   4. Flurazepam—take at bedtime

3. Which patient statement would require the nurse to provide further teaching?
   1. "I should report any unusual bleeding when I take gingko biloba."
   2. "I should not take St. John's wort with sertraline hydrochloride."
   3. "Natural health products are safe because they are made with all-natural ingredients."
   4. "I will tell my doctor that I am taking a natural health product."

4. The nurse is caring for a patient who is taking lithium. Which adverse effect would the nurse anticipate?
   1. Oliguria
   2. Confusion
   3. Constipation
   4. Hyperthyroidism

5. The nurse understands that norepinephrine is involved with the stimulation of which bodily process?
   1. The fight-or-flight response to stress
   2. The hypothalamus to release hormones
   3. Involvement in the inflammatory response
   4. The parasympathetic nervous system

## ⊖volve WEBSITE

Post-Test interactive review

*Visit the Evolve Web site for Chapter Review Answers and Rationales, Critical Thinking Answer Guidelines, and additional resources related to the content in this chapter:* http://evolve.elsevier.com/Canada/Varcarolis/psychiatric/

## REFERENCES

Alpert, J.E. (2008). Drug–drug interactions in psychopharmacology. In T.A. Stern, J.F. Rosenbaum, M. Fava, J. Biederman, & S.L. Rauch (Eds.), *Comprehensive clinical psychiatry* (pp. 687–704). Philadelphia: Elsevier.

Chen, J., Gao, K., & Kemp, D.E. (2011). Second-generation antipsychotics in major depressive disorder: Update and clinical perspective. *Current Opinion in Psychiatry, 24*(1), 10–17.

Gartlehner, G., Hansen, R.A., Morgan, L.C., et al. (2011). *Second-generation antidepressants in the pharmacologic treatment of adult depression: An update of the 2007 comparative effectiveness review (AHRQ Publication No. 12-EHC012-EF)*. Rockville, MD: Agency for Healthcare Research and Quality. Retrieved from http://www.effectivehealthcare.ahrq.gov/reports/final.cfm.

Grunze, H.C.R. (2010). Anticonvulsants in bipolar disorder. *Journal of Mental Health, 19*(2), 127–141.

Health Canada. (2011a). Drug product database. Retrieved from http://webprod.hc-sc.gc.ca/dpd-bdpp/info.do?lang=eng&code=67852.

Health Canada. (2011b). MedEffect Canada. Retrieved from http://www.hc-sc.gc.ca/dhpmps/medeff/advisories-avis/index-eng.php.

Howland, R.H. (2010). Psychopharmacology: Update on St. John's wort. *Journal of Psychosocial Nursing & Mental Health Services, 48*(11), 20–24.

Lam, Y.W.F. (2010). Raltegravir and lamotrigine. *Brown University Psychopharmacology Update, 21*(3), 2–3.

Lee, P.E., Gill, S.S., Freedman, M., et al. (2004). Atypical antipsychotic drugs in the treatment of behavioural and psychological symptoms of dementia: Systematic review. *British Medical Journal, 329*, 75. doi:10.1136/bmj.38125.465579.55.

Leucht, S., Corves, C., Arbter, D., et al. (2009). Second-generation versus first-generation antipsychotic drugs for schizophrenia: A meta-analysis. *Lancet, 373*(9657), 31–41.

Lithium is still a first-line option in the treatment of patients with bipolar disorder. (2010). *Drugs & Therapy Perspectives, 26*(3), 9–14.

Mackin, P., & Thomas, S.H.L. (2011). Atypical antipsychotic drugs. *British Medical Journal, 342*(7798), 650–654.

Porcelli, S., Drago, A., Fabbri, C., et al. (2011). Pharmacogenetics of antidepressant response. *Journal of Psychiatry & Neuroscience, 36*(2), 87–113.

Preston, J.D., O'Neal, J.H., & Talaga, M.C. (2005). *Handbook of clinical psychopharmacology for therapists* (3rd ed.). Oakland, CA.: New Harbinger.

Sadock, B.J., & Sadock, V.A. (2008). *Concise textbook of clinical psychiatry* (3rd ed.). Philadelphia: Lippincott, Williams & Wilkins.

Sarris, J., & Kavanagh, D.J. (2009). Kava and St. John's wort: Current evidence for use in mood and anxiety disorders. *Journal of Alternative & Complementary Medicine, 15*(8), 827–836.

Shaldubina, A., Adam, G., & Belmaker, R.H. (2001) The mechanism of lithium action: State of the art, ten years later. *Progress in Neuropsychopharmacology and Biological Psychiatry, 25*, 855–866.

Stahl, S.W. (2008). *Stahl's essential psychopharmacology* (3rd ed.). New York: Cambridge University Press.

Williams, K.L., Ruekert, L., & Lum, C. (2011). Treatment of bipolar disorder: A focus on medication therapy for mania. *Formulary, 46*(3), 82–97.

# Foundations for Practice

# Psychiatric Mental Health Nursing in Acute Care Settings

*Avni Cirpili, Margaret Swisher*
*Adapted by Karen Clements*

## KEY TERMS AND CONCEPTS

admission criteria, 76
clinical pathway, 77
elopement, 79

metabolic syndrome, 80
multidisciplinary treatment plan, 77
psychosocial rehabilitation, 82

## OBJECTIVES

1. Describe the population served by inpatient psychiatric care.
2. Identify key features of the Canadian health care system and funding structure.
3. List the criteria for admission to inpatient care.
4. Discuss the purpose of identifying the rights of hospitalized psychiatric patients.
5. Explain how the multidisciplinary treatment team collaborates to plan and implement care for the hospitalized patient.

6. Explain the importance of monitoring patient safety during hospitalization.
7. Describe the role of the nurse as advocate and provider of care for the patient.
8. Discuss the managerial and coordinating roles of nursing on an inpatient acute care unit.
9. Discuss the process for preparing patients to return to the community for ongoing care.

## Ɵvolve WEBSITE

*Visit the Evolve website for Flashcards, Case Studies, and additional testing resources related to the content in this chapter:* http://evolve.elsevier.com/Canada/Varcarolis/psychiatric    Pre-Test  interactive review

---

Mental illness is a significant problem faced by Canadians (20% will experience a mental illness during their life), and hospitalization continues to be a treatment option for some individuals with mental disorders and emotional crises (Health Canada, 2002). In fact, 3.8% of all general hospital admissions in 1999 had a mental disorder as the primary diagnosis (Health Canada, 2002, p. 19). Although most inpatient psychiatric treatment today takes place in the community or in general hospital psychiatric units, there continue to be provincial psychiatric hospitals serving individuals from some rural and northern catchment areas, as well as specialty populations such as forensic patients referred by the court for evaluation or treatment.

Inpatient psychiatric care has undergone significant change over the past half century. As discussed in Chapters 2 and 6,

treatment locales for mental health disorders shifted from provincial psychiatric hospitals to psychiatric units in general hospitals and to outpatient services offered in the community (Government of Canada, 2006). Two important Canadian reports—the *Royal Commission on Health Services* by Emmett Hall and *More for the Mind* by the Committee on Psychiatric Services of the Canadian Mental Health Association—had recommended that mental health care be delivered in community settings in the same manner as the delivery of physical health care (Kirby & Keon, 2004). Consequences of the deinstitutionalization shift have included a reduction in long-stay psychiatric beds (as these are concentrated in the provincial psychiatric hospitals) and an increase in the number of individuals with mental illness who are homeless or in the penitentiary system

## HOW A NURSE HELPED ME

### When Hope Fades

*I'm Amanda, just twenty-three years old, but I reached a dark place where my life seemed intolerably painful and without hope. I felt weighted down by problems in my home community in Nunavut. At the same time, I felt the incredible pressure of my community, my family, and my own dream to complete a medical degree at McGill University Faculty of Medicine so that I could contribute to the healing of my people.*

*It was so strange and lonely at university. I felt isolated and without supports. I started to have trouble finding enough energy to keep up with the relentless pace of my studies. I couldn't concentrate, couldn't sleep, and couldn't be bothered eating, so I lost weight. I was anxious and afraid. In order to cope with my anxiety, I started to drink alone in my residence. I wanted to give up and felt I had no option other than suicide. I ate a whole bottle of Tylenol and drank it down with a bottle of gin.*

*When I was admitted to an acute care psychiatric facility, I felt so ashamed, so hopeless, and so angry. I just wanted to scream, but instead I was polite and withdrawn because that is proper behaviour for an Inuk. Luckily, a nurse, Andrea, reached out and helped me change my life. How? I think mostly by listening respectfully—that's important where I come from. When I whispered, "You can't understand my life," she said, "I know, but maybe I can help you understand your life better."*

*Andrea listened, but she also taught me about the symptoms of and treatment for depression. Andrea and I made a plan to keep me safe while I explored some options to make my life seem livable again. She was very clear that she had a responsibility to keep me safe while in hospital and explained the suicide precautions needed. I felt safe. Andrea helped me identify my health priorities (like getting back to healthy eating and sleeping), and she also helped me identify some community supports. I didn't know there was an Inuk medical resident at McGill. It was a huge relief to talk with him about university. Andrea also helped me talk with my family when they came all the way from home to visit me. Gradually, I began to see hope for life again. Andrea helped me by listening and respecting me. I will always be grateful for her care.*

(Romanow, 2002; Sapers, 2010; Canadian Institute for Health Information, 2007). Between 1994 and 2003, the number of psychiatric hospital admissions and the lengths of stay (LOS) decreased; in 2003, the average LOS for general hospital psychiatric beds was 16.9 days and, for provincial psychiatric hospital beds, 148.5 days (Canadian Institute for Health Information 2006, pp. iii, vii). Shorter lengths of stay in acute care, however, are associated with an increased likelihood of readmission as well as shorter intervals before readmission for individuals with schizophrenia (Canadian Institute for Health Information, 2008). Fewer psychiatric beds means that acuity within psychiatric facilities has been increasing and that admission is commonly reserved for those people who are suicidal, homicidal, or extremely disabled and in need of short-term acute care (Simon & Shuman, 2008).

## FUNDING PSYCHIATRIC MENTAL HEALTH CARE

The Canadian mental health care system has areas of strength—for example, most citizens have equal access to mental health services—but it also has problematic gaps in access to care and in community services that offer care in acute psychiatric settings. Canada has a predominately publicly financed and administered health care system whereby all eligible residents have reasonable access to medically necessary hospital and physician services (referred to as "insured services") (Aglukkaq, 2010). Federal government and provincial and territorial government roles and responsibilities for health care are set out, primarily, in the *Medicare Act* (1966) and the *Canada Health Act* (1984). Provincial and territorial governments are responsible for health care within their jurisdictions. The federal government is responsible for transferring health care funds to the provincial and territorial governments and for ensuring that insured health care services are publicly funded and administered by the provinces and territories according to five basic principles: public administration, comprehensiveness, universality, portability, and accessibility. The federal government maintains health care responsibility for select populations (First Nations communities, armed forces, RCMP, individuals in federal penitentiaries, refugees) and select functions (such as health promotion, disease surveillance, drug regulation). For instance, the federal government operates Operational Stress Injury Social Support (OSISS) programs across Canada for military members, veterans, and their families to help them cope with the psychological effects of stress and trauma associated with warfare. (For more information on OSISS programs, you can visit http://www.osiss.ca/engraph/index_e.asp) The mental health strategy for Canada includes a First Nations, Inuit, and Métis advisory committee to promote mental health and wellness in Canadian Aboriginal individuals and communities (Mental Health Commission of Canada, 2012). Responsibility for health care services is further devolved from the provincial and territorial governments to regional organizations—for instance, regional health boards, regional health authorities, hospitals—the type depending on the province or territory (Canadian Institute for Health Information, 2000). This distribution of roles and responsibilities sets up unique tensions within the Canadian health care system and leaves gaps in services, impacting mental health care in general and, by extension, acute psychiatric care.

Although differences exist among the various provinces or territories, mental health and addiction services generally include inpatient and outpatient psychiatric hospital treatment, community-based treatment (such as that provided by mental health workers), crisis response and emergency services, psychiatrists, psychologists, counsellors, social workers, housing, self-help, vocational or educational services, and drug insurance plans (Canadian Institute for Health Information, 2000). Not all these services, however, are publicly funded. Canadians pay directly or indirectly for all health care: 71% through taxation, 11% through private or employment insurance plans, 16% out of pocket, and another 2% through other means (Romanow, 2002, p. 24). Individuals with mental health problems often have financial challenges related to their illness, which makes private or employment health insurance plans and out-of-pocket expenses difficult or impossible to access; these expenses may include medication costs, counselling, appropriate housing, re-entry to employment or education support, and dental care.

## INPATIENT PSYCHIATRIC MENTAL HEALTH CARE

### Entry to Inpatient Care

Although some patients are directly admitted based on a psychiatrist or primary care provider referral, the majority of patients (71% in 2004–2005) receiving inpatient acute psychiatric care are admitted through the emergency department (ED) (Canadian Institute for Health Information, 2005, p. 14). The average ED wait time for a patient in need of hospitalization is increasing—in some areas, the wait can be days. Nurses who work on psychiatric units should recognize that patients admitted from the ED may need additional patience and attention. They may have been deprived of medication, treatments, sleep, or proper food.

People with psychiatric symptoms are often isolated and ignored from the outset of their hospitalization. However, an increasing number of Canadian emergency departments are using nurses who have experience working with people with mental illness in the ED to assist with triage and care of patients with mental health problems.

In the ED, the patient is generally evaluated by an emergency department physician and a social worker, who will determine if the patient meets criteria to justify admission. The admission criteria to a hospital begin with the premise that the person is suffering from a mental illness and include evidence of one or more of the following:

- Imminent danger of harming self
- Imminent danger of harming others
- Inability to care for basic needs, placing individual at imminent risk of harming self

Patients who meet the admission criteria are then given the option of being admitted on a voluntary basis, which means that they agree with the need for treatment and hospitalization. The vast majority of patient admissions to psychiatric inpatient units are voluntary. If patients do not wish to be hospitalized but mental health care providers feel that admission is necessary, the patients can be admitted against their wishes—commonly known as an "involuntary admission." Involuntarily admitted patients still have rights: right to receive information on rights in a timely manner, right to retain counsel, and right

to an independent review of committal (O'Reilly, Chaimowitz, Brunet, et al., 2010). If the admission is contested, a mental health review board (or panel or tribunal, depending on the province or territory) reviews the committal decision on behalf of the patient (Liddle, Shone, & Gray, 2008). Chapter 8 discusses legal requirements for admissions, commitment, and discharge procedures in more detail.

> **VIGNETTE**
> Shane is a 22-year-old male who was brought to the emergency room by police after expressing thoughts of suicide. He reports having had difficulty sleeping and eating for the past several days and a weight loss of five pounds. He is restless and demanding. When approached, he becomes very irritable and threatening to the nurses and physicians, stating that he wants to leave and does not understand why he needs to be here. He states that he was tricked by his mother and brother, who are trying to have him admitted only so they can take his money. He is exhibiting poor judgement, insight, and impulse control. He has been nonadherent with his antipsychotic medication, risperidone, which he stopped taking three weeks ago because of adverse effects.
> Shane did not want to be admitted, and despite several attempts by the nursing staff, he continued to refuse hospitalization. The decision was made to involuntarily admit him to the locked psychiatric inpatient unit. On arrival to the inpatient unit, Shane was informed of his rights and the fact that he was involuntarily committed to the unit.

### Rights of the Hospitalized Patient

Patients admitted to any psychiatric unit retain rights as citizens, which vary from province to province to territory, and are entitled to certain privileges. Laws and regulatory standards require that patients' rights be explained in a timely fashion after an individual has been admitted to the hospital and that the treatment team always be aware of these rights. Any instances of physical restraint, seclusion, or administration of medications against a person's will must be documented, and actions must be justifiable. All mental health facilities provide a written statement of patients' rights, often with copies of applicable provincial laws attached. Box 5-1 provides a sample list of patients' rights, and Chapter 8 offers a more detailed discussion of this issue.

### Multidisciplinary Treatment Team

There are three regulated nursing professions in Canada: licensed practical nurses (LPN) or registered practical nurses (RPN), licensed registered nurses (RN), and licensed registered psychiatric nurses (RPN). The nursing mix in specific work situations is guided by the principle that higher acuity, greater complexity of needs, and more independence in practice require nursing professionals with higher levels of training in mental health.

Psychiatric mental health nurses are core members of the multidisciplinary treatment team, a group of professionals and nonprofessionals who work together to provide care (see Box 5-2). The full team generally meets within 72 hours of the patient's admission to formulate a full treatment plan. The

## BOX 5-1    PSYCHIATRIC INPATIENT RIGHTS

- Right to be treated with dignity and respect
- Right to express opinions and be heard
- Right to communication in language and manner you understand
- Right to participate in religious worship
- Right to clear explanation on the nature, risk, benefits, adverse effects, and alternatives of any treatment, and likely consequences of not having treatment
- Right to make decisions regarding admission and treatment if you are capable of doing so
- Right to be informed of the reasons for involuntary admission (and involuntary treatment as per provincial or territorial mental health act)
- Right to make decisions about your money and belongings if you are capable of doing so
- Right to appeal decisions regarding your person made under the provincial or territorial mental health act
- Right to advice and legal counsel
- Right to access and correct your personal health information as per provincial or territorial legislation
- Right to send and receive communication
- Right to vote
- Right to care and treatment consistent with professional conduct and codes of ethics
- Right to confidentiality in accordance with provincial or territorial legislation

**Source:** Adapted from Psychiatric Patient Advocate Office. (2008). *What are your rights as a psychiatric patient?* Retrieved from http://www.sse.gov.on.ca/mohltc/ppao/en/Pages/InfoGuides/MentalHealthActAdmissions_A.aspx?openMenu=smenu_MentalHealthActAdmissions.

nurse's role in this process often is to lead the planning meeting. This nursing leadership reflects the holistic nature of nursing, as well as the fact that nursing is the discipline that is represented on the unit at all times. Nurses are in a unique position to advocate on behalf of the patient and to contribute valuable information such as continuous assessment findings, the patient's adjustment to the unit, and any health concerns, psychoeducational needs, and patient self-care deficits.

The treatment plan will be the guideline for the patient's care during the hospital stay. It is based on goals for the hospitalization and defines how achievement of the goals will be measured. Input from the patient and family (if available and desirable) is critical in formulating goals. Incorporating the patient's feedback in developing the treatment plan goals increases the likelihood of the success of the outcomes.

Members of each discipline are responsible for gathering data and participating in the planning of care. Newly admitted patients may find meeting with so many people and answering similar questions from each of them extremely stressful or threatening; team members, therefore, must consider appropriate timing. The urgency of the need for data should be weighed against the patient's ability to tolerate assessment. Assessments, in particular suicide assessments, made by the nurse often provide the basis for initial care. In most settings, the psychiatrist must evaluate the patient and provide orders within a limited time frame. Physical medical problems are usually referred to a primary care physician or specialist, who assesses the patient and consults with the attending psychiatrist.

The plan of care reflects a nursing process–based or multidisciplinary path–based approach to care. The latter approach may be in the form of a multidisciplinary treatment plan—a plan of care that has been developed with input from all the treatment team members, including the patient. The multidisciplinary treatment plan is influenced by the clinical pathway (when available), which is a guideline that outlines the clinical standards—the usual care provided for a patient undergoing a certain procedure or for a patient who has a certain illness. Since all patients are unique, each person's care will be customized to meet his or her needs while keeping these guidelines in mind. The use of a clinical pathway is intended to improve patient care. The team composes the plan of care, which is often based on the appropriate clinical pathway, revising the plan along the way if the patient's progress differs from that expected. A reduction in overt symptoms and the development of an adequate outpatient plan signal that discharge is imminent.

> **VIGNETTE**
>
> Joelle is assigned as Shane's primary nurse, and Tazmine as his evening-shift nurse. Joelle met with the treatment team to plan Shane's care during his hospitalization. The physician's diagnosis was major depression with psychotic features. The major problems the team identified, based on reports of the past two days and nursing assessments, were safety, paranoia, nonadherence to medication regimes, and hypertension. Joelle identified that the nursing diagnoses were risk for self-directed violence, disturbed thought processes, noncompliance, and deficient knowledge. Along with the treatment team, Joelle identified the therapy and psychoeducation groups that Shane should participate in and recommended that suicide-precaution monitoring be maintained, owing to Shane's inability to promise that he would not harm himself on the unit or he would tell one of the staff members if his thoughts about committing suicide changed.

## Nursing Care
### Admission Assessment

Being admitted to a hospital is anxiety-provoking for anyone, but anxiety can be severe for patients admitted to a psychiatric unit. Especially for the first-time patient, admission often summons preconceptions about psychiatric hospitals and the negative stigma associated with them. Patients may experience shame, and families may be reluctant to be forthcoming with pertinent information. Psychiatric mental health nurses can be most effective when they are sensitive to both the patient and family during the admission process. In this initial encounter with the patient, nurses must try to provide reassurance and hope.

Upon admission, the nurse will assess the patient with the goals of gathering information that will enable the treatment team to develop a suitable plan of care; ensuring that safety concerns are identified and addressed; identifying the learning needs of the patient so the nurse can prioritize the information

## BOX 5-2 POTENTIAL MEMBERS OF THE MULTIDISCIPLINARY TREATMENT TEAM

**Registered psychiatric nurses:** Licensed professionals trained with an extensive focus on the knowledge and skills required for psychiatric mental health nursing (see the Registered Psychiatric Nurses of Canada Web site: http://www.rpnc.ca/pages/home.php).

**Registered nurses:** Registered nurses working in psychiatric mental health care do not necessarily have specific certification, but many have some specialty experience. Registered nurses in Canada can complete a specialty certificate in psychiatric mental health nursing (see the Canadian Nurses Association certification program: http://www.nurseone.ca/Default.aspx?portlet=StaticHtmlViewerPortlet&plang=1&ptdi=153). Among the responsibilities of a registered nurse are diagnosing and treating responses to psychiatric disorders, coordinating care, counselling, giving medication and evaluating responses, and providing education.

**Licensed practical nurses or registered practical nurses:** Provincial or territorial licensing or registration bodies regulate these professionals by determining entry-to-practice requirements and establishing and promoting standards for registration, practice, and professional conduct. These nurses are involved with the care of psychiatric patients by providing care within their scope of practice as determined by their provincial or territorial governing body.

**Psychiatric mental health advanced-practice nurses:** Psychiatric mental health advanced-practice nurses work as nurse therapists, clinical nurse specialists, or education specialists by virtue of advanced training (e.g., master's- or doctorate-prepared) or recognized advanced level of experience. These nurses may be involved in conducting therapy, case management, consulting, education, or research.

**Social workers:** Basic-level social workers help the patient prepare a support system that will promote mental health upon discharge from the hospital. They may help patients develop contacts with day treatment centres, employers, sources of financial aid, and landlords. Social workers can also undergo training in individual, family, and group therapies and function as primary care providers.

**Counsellors:** Counsellors prepared in disciplines such as psychology, rehabilitation counselling, nursing or psychiatric nursing, and addiction counselling may augment the treatment plan by co-leading groups, providing basic supportive counselling, or assisting in psychoeducational and recreational activities. Private counselling services in the community are not covered by medicare.

**Psychologists:** In keeping with their doctoral degree preparation, psychologists conduct psychological testing, provide consultation for the team, and offer direct services such as specialized individual, family, or marital therapies. Psychologists' services in the community are not covered by medicare.

**Occupational, recreational, art, music, and dance therapists:** Based on their specialist preparation, these therapists assist patients in gaining skills that help them cope more effectively, gain or retain employment, use leisure time to the benefit of their mental health, and express themselves in healthy ways.

**Psychiatrists:** Depending on their specialty of preparation, psychiatrists may provide in-depth psychotherapy or medication therapy or head a team of mental health providers functioning as a community-based service. Psychiatrists may be employed by the hospital or may hold practice privileges in the facility. Because psychiatry is a medical specialty, treatment and care by psychiatrists—with the exception of psychoanalysis—is covered by medicare. Because they have the legal power to prescribe and to write orders, psychiatrists often function as the leaders of the teams managing the care of patients individually assigned to them.

**Medical physicians:** Medical physicians provide medical diagnoses and treatments on a consultation basis. Medical physicians will also provide referrals to psychiatrists, mental health nurses, psychologists, and social workers when needed. Occasionally, a physician trained as an addiction specialist may play a more direct role on a unit that offers treatment for addictive disease.

**Health care aides:** Health care aides function under the direction and supervision of nurses. They provide assistance to patients in meeting basic needs and also help the community to remain supportive, safe, and healthy.

**Community mental health workers:** Community mental health workers are registered nurses or registered psychiatric nurses, social workers, or other trained professionals who offer case management and care in the community at various levels of intensity. Community mental health workers are sometimes involved in hospital-treatment-team and patient-discharge planning.

**Pharmacists:** In view of the intricacies of prescribing, coordinating, and administering combinations of psychotropic and other medications, the consulting pharmacist can offer a valuable safeguard. Physicians and nurses collaborate with the pharmacist regarding new medications, which are being introduced at a steady rate.

**Spiritual carers:** Spiritual advisors can play an important role in addressing the spiritual, and sometimes cultural, aspects of patients' lives and support spirituality as a coping resource.

needs; and initiating a therapeutic relationship between the nurse and the patient. Chapter 9 presents a more detailed discussion of how to perform an admission assessment, as well as a mental status examination.

### Ensuring Safety

Safety is one of the most important aspects of care in any inpatient setting. Protecting the patient is essential, but equally important is the safety of the staff and other patients. Nurses maintain safety primarily through collaborative teamwork, good patient assessment, respectful attention to patient concerns, and recognition and de-escalation of potentially dangerous situations.

Safety needs are identified and individualized interventions begin on admission. Staff should check all personal property and clothing to prevent any potentially harmful items from

## RESEARCH HIGHLIGHT

### Meaning of Caring for Canadian Nurses in Acute Inpatient Psychiatric Settings

**Source:** Reprinted from Chiovitti, R.F. (2008). Nurses' meaning of caring with patients in acute psychiatric hospital settings: A grounded theory study. *International Journal of Nursing Studies*, *45*, 203–223. doi:10.1016/j.ijnurstu.2006.08.018.

#### Problem
Caring is central but not exclusive to nursing. Articulating clearly the components of caring within nursing is important to making visible the intangible and abstract work of nurses. Research indicates that caring is conceptualized variously in different nursing specialties, but there has been a lack of research into what caring means in the context of psychiatric mental health nursing.

#### Purpose of Study
To develop a theory of caring from the perspective of nurses working in three Canadian acute inpatient psychiatric care settings.

#### Methods
A qualitative research method, grounded theory, was used to analyze interviews with 17 individual registered nurses working in acute care psychiatric settings in Ontario. Each nurse was interviewed twice: the first set of interviews was used to develop a tentative theoretical structure (themes and relationships between themes emerging from the nurses' interviews); the second set of interviews was used to verify the emergent theoretical structure.

#### Key Findings
- The basic social psychological process used by the nurses to describe caring with patients is one of "protective empowering."
- There are two antecedent and sustaining categories (with ten subcategories) that are necessary for protective empowering to occur: respecting the patient and not taking the patient's behaviour personally.
- There are four context categories (with 17 subcategories) involved in the nursing work of protective empowering: keeping the patient safe, encouraging the patient's health, authentic relating, and interactive teaching.
- The consequence of protective empowering is that patients are helped to "resume and sustain meaningful activities of daily living" (p. 209) and a healthy quality of life.

#### Implications for Nursing Practice
The theory of protective empowering balances patient safety with fostering autonomy and choice, seeks out the strengths and healthy aspects of patients even in illness, and encourages respect for the patient's view of quality of life. Balancing protection with empowerment and care with control is a fundamental challenge within psychiatric nursing. The caring work of nurses has been invisible and intangible and, therefore, difficult to document, acknowledge, teach, and reflect upon. The theory of protective empowering highlights nursing skills involved in caring and provides a theoretical framework nurses can use to evaluate and improve practice. One area of future research suggested by the researcher is to investigate patient perspectives on what constitutes caring within an acute care psychiatric setting.

---

being taken onto the unit (e.g., medication, alcohol, sharp objects). Some people are at greater risk of suicide than others, and nurses must be skillful in evaluating this risk through questions and observations. Understanding the types of precautions used in the hospital is one of the most important tasks a new staff member or nursing student can learn.

Accreditation Canada (2011) publishes required patient safety practices for Canadian hospitals (also see Brickell, Nicholls, Procyshyn, et al., 2009, for developing work on patient safety guidelines specific to mental health care in Canada). Box 5-3 lists important safety goals for care in mental health settings.

The nurse supervises the unit for overall safety. One of the most important interventions is tracking patients' whereabouts and activities. These checks are done periodically or continuously, depending upon patients' risk for a health crisis or self-harm. Visitors are another potential safety hazard. Although visitors can contribute to patients' healing through socialization, acceptance, and familiarity, visits may be overwhelming or distressing. Also, visitors may unwittingly or purposefully provide patients with unsafe items such sharp objects, glass, or drugs; bags and packages brought onto the unit should be inspected by unit staff. Sometimes unsafe items take the form of comfort foods from home or a favourite restaurant and should be monitored because they may be incompatible with prescribed diets or medications.

Intimate relationships between patients are generally discouraged or expressly prohibited. There are risks for sexually transmitted infections, pregnancy, and emotional distress at a time when patients are vulnerable and may lack the capacity for consent.

Aggression and violence are also a risk as a result of living in close quarters with reduced outlets for frustration. Aggression in the mental health workplace is an important concern (Clark, Griffith, & Brown, 2002). Psychiatric staff should have specialized training to minimize hostility while maintaining an atmosphere that promotes healthy and appropriate expression of anger and other feelings. Most psychiatric units are locked since some patients are hospitalized involuntarily, and elopement (absence from unit without leave) must be prevented in a way that avoids an atmosphere of imprisonment (see Chapter 5).

One of the most important safety aspects of a psychiatric unit's design is in patient rooms. The rooms are usually less institutional-looking than other hospital rooms and tend to

**BOX 5-3**  **PATIENT SAFETY GOALS IN MENTAL HEALTH CARE SETTINGS**

- Improve the accuracy of patient identification:
  - Use at least two ways, such as patient's name and date of birth, to identify patients.
- Improve the effectiveness of communication among caregivers:
  - Read back verbal orders.
  - Create a list of abbreviations and symbols that are not to be used.
  - Promptly report critical tests and critical results.
- Improve the safety of using medications:
  - Create a list of look-alike and sound-alike medications.
- Reduce the risk of health care–associated infections:
  - Follow hand-cleaning guidelines from the World Health Organization.
  - Record and report death or injury from infection.
- Accurately and completely reconcile medications across the continuum of care:
  - Compare current and newly ordered medications for compatibility.
  - Give a list of medications to the next provider and regular caregiver.
  - Provide a medication list to both the patient and family.
- Encourage patients' active involvement in their own care:
  - Encourage patients and families to report safety concerns.
- Identify safety risks inherent in the patient population:
  - Identify individuals at risk for suicide.

**Source:** Adapted from Accreditation Canada. (2012). *Qmentum program standards*.

resemble hotels. Closets should be equipped with "break-bars" designed to hold a minimal amount of weight; windows, with shatterproof glass, are locked; beds are often platforms rather than mechanical hospital beds, which can be dangerous because of their crushing potential; and showers should have non–weight-bearing shower heads.

## Physical Health Assessment

The nurse is in an excellent position to assess not only mental health but also physical health. Rates of metabolic syndrome, diabetes, and heart disease are all higher for individuals with mental health problems. Metabolic syndrome is a set of metabolic abnormalities (weight gain, hypertension, hyperlipidemia) indicative of increased risk for heart disease and diabetes (Park, Usher, & Foster, 2011). Nurses can play a key role in assessing for these problems and initiating patient teaching and supports for prevention and management (Brunero & Lamont, 2009).

Individuals with mental health problems may experience barriers to health care and healthy living practices necessary to maintain their health (Roberts & Bailey, 2011). Often, when patients with pre-existing or co-morbid conditions seek treatment in the ED for a physical medical condition, health care providers will downplay or attribute the patient's physical

complaints to the psychiatric condition. Patients also report reluctance to seek out health care providers, owing to the stigma they encounter when they reveal they are being treated for a co-morbid psychiatric illness. This reluctance to seek treatment not only adversely impacts the patient's quality of life but also contributes to a decreased life expectancy (Miller, Paschall, & Sevenson, 2006).

## Milieu Management

A well-managed milieu offers patients a sense of security and comfort. Structured aspects of the milieu include activities, unit rules, reality orientation practices, and unit environment. In addition to the structured components of the milieu, Peplau (1989) described other less tangible factors, such as the interactions that occur among patients and staff, patients and patients, patients and visitors, and so forth. This interactivity is quite different from the environment of medical units, where patients generally remain in their rooms, often with closed doors, and rarely interact with other patients or the milieu. On psychiatric units, patients are in constant contact with their peers and staff. These interactions help patients engage and can increase their sense of social competence and worth.

The therapeutic milieu can serve as a real-life training ground for learning about the self and practising communication and coping skills in preparation for a return to the community. Even events that seemingly distract from the program of therapies can be turned into valuable learning opportunities for the members of the milieu. Nurses can support the milieu and intervene when necessary. They usually develop an uncanny ability to assess the mood of the unit (e.g., calm, anxious, disengaged, or tense) and predict environmental risk. Nurses observe the dynamics of interactions, reinforce adaptive social skills, and redirect patients during negative interactions. Reports from shift to shift provide information on the emotional climate and level of tension on the unit.

## Structured Group Activities

On most mental health units, experienced psychiatric mental health nurses conduct specific, structured activities involving the therapeutic community, special groups, or families. Examples of these activities include morning goal-setting meetings and evening goal-review meetings. Community meetings may be held daily or at other scheduled times of the week. At these meetings, new patients are greeted, and departing patients are given farewells; ideas for unit activities are discussed; community problems or successes are considered; and other business of the therapeutic community is conducted.

Nurses also offer psychoeducational groups for patients and families on topics such as stress management, coping skills, grieving, medication management, healthy-living practices, and communication skills. Group therapy is a specialized therapy led by a mental health practitioner with advanced training. This therapy addresses communication and sharing, helps patients explore life problems and decrease their isolation and anxiety, and engages patients in the recovery process. Chapter 35 presents a more detailed discussion of therapeutic groups led by nurses.

## Documentation

Documentation of patient progress is the responsibility of the entire mental health team. Although communication among team members and coordination of services are the primary goals when choosing a system for charting, practitioners in the inpatient setting must also consider professional standards, legal issues, and accreditation by regulatory agencies. Information must also be in a format that is retrievable for quality-assurance monitoring, utilization management, peer review, and research. Chapter 9 gives an overview of documentation options.

## Medication Administration

The safe administration of medications and the monitoring of their effects is a 24-hour responsibility for psychiatric mental health nurses, who are expected to have detailed knowledge of psychoactive medications and the interactions and psychological adverse effects of other medications. Staff nurse reports regarding the patient's adherence to the medication regimen, the presence or absence of adverse effects, or changes in the patient's behaviours exert great influence on the physician's medication decisions. For example, feedback about excessive sedation or increased agitation may lead to a decrease or increase in the dosage of an antipsychotic medication.

Nurses often have numerous decisions to make about medications that are prescribed to be administered prn (as needed). These decisions must be based on a combination of factors: the patient's wishes, the team's plan, attempts to use alternative methods of coping, and the nurse's judgements regarding timing and the patient's behaviour. Documentation for administering each prn medication must include the rationale for its use and its effects.

*Medication adherence.* Medication adherence, or compliance, is a common challenge for psychiatric patients, often because of adverse effects, lack of understanding about the medications, and lack of sufficient patient consultation in treatment decisions (Colom & Lam, 2005). One of the nurse's goals during hospitalization is to assist the patient to learn the importance of medication adherence during and after hospitalization. Educating patients on how to recognize, report, and manage potential adverse effects can help empower patients and increase treatment success. This approach encourages the patient to seek out the nurse when it is time for medications to be administered and fosters responsibility and involvement in the treatment process.

*Pain management.* Just like others in the general population, psychiatric patients often suffer from medical problems that result in pain (e.g., neck, back, or spine problems, arthritis, migraine headaches). People with psychiatric conditions are often viewed as being unable to accurately assess their own sensations or are labelled "drug seeking," a situation that results in untreated or undertreated pain. Nurses can advocate for patients by stressing that relieving pain is a humanitarian consideration and that a patient in pain is less able to participate in formal activities on the unit and will have greater difficulty focusing on education. Psychological pain, which may manifest as anxiety, is equally distressing and can also decrease the ability of the individual to participate in activities of daily living and community life. Adequate assessment and treatment of pain within the psychiatric population may have a positive impact on the course of mental disorders.

## Crisis Management

*Medical crises.* Nurses anticipate, prevent, and manage emergencies and crises on the unit. These crises may be of a medical or behavioural nature. Mental health units must be able to assess and stabilize the condition of a patient who experiences a medical crisis. Mental health or addictive disease units that manage detoxification (withdrawal from alcohol or other drugs) must anticipate several common medical crises associated with that process. Mental health units, therefore, store crash carts containing the emergency medications used to treat shock and cardiorespiratory arrest. Nurses must maintain their cardiopulmonary resuscitation skills and be able to use basic emergency equipment. To be effective and practise at a high level of competency, nurses are advised to attend in-service sessions and workshops designed to teach and maintain skills. Nurses must also be able to alert medical support systems quickly and mobilize transportation to the appropriate medical facility.

*Behavioural crises.* Behavioural crises can lead to patient violence toward self or others and are usually, but not always, observed to escalate through fairly predictable stages. Crisis prevention and management techniques are practised by staff in most mental health facilities (see the Registered Nurses' Association of Ontario *Best Practice Guideline for Crisis Intervention*, http://rnao.ca/bpg/guidelines/crisis-intervention). Many psychiatric hospitals have special teams made up of nurses, psychiatric aides, and other professionals who respond to psychiatric emergencies. Each member of the team takes part in the team effort to defuse a crisis in its early stages. If preventive measures fail, each member of the team participates in a rapid, organized movement designed to immobilize, medicate, or seclude a patient. The nurse is most often this team's leader, not only organizing the plan but also timing the intervention and managing the concurrent use of prn medications. The nurse can initiate such an intervention in the absence of a physician but must secure a physician's order for restraint or seclusion within a specified time. The nurse also advocates for patients in crisis by ensuring that their legal rights are preserved, no matter how difficult to manage their behaviour may be. Refer to Chapters 8 and 26 for further discussions about and protocols for the use of restraints and seclusion.

Crises on the unit are upsetting and threatening to uninvolved patients as well. A designated staff member usually addresses their concerns and feelings. This person removes other patients from the area of the crisis and helps them express their fears. Patients may be concerned for their own safety or the welfare of the patient involved in the crisis. They may fear that they too might experience such a loss of control. The staff members of the code team and the patient in crisis all benefit from debriefing after these difficult situations.

### Preparation for Discharge to the Community

Discharge planning begins upon admission and is continually modified as required by the patient's condition until the time of discharge. The reduction of overt symptoms and the development of an adequate outpatient plan signal that discharge is imminent. As members of the multidisciplinary team, nurses assist patients and their families to prepare for independent or assisted living in the community. Community-based programs provide patients with psychosocial rehabilitation, which moves the mentally ill patient beyond stabilization toward recovery and a higher quality of life. This rehabilitation is especially important to health care system goals to reduce the length and frequency of hospital stays. Nurses, therefore, focus on the precipitating factors that led to the crisis and hospital admission. Patients are assisted to learn coping skills and behaviours that will help them avert future crises. Psychoeducational groups, individual exploration of options and supports, and on-the-spot instruction (such as during medication administration) offer the patient numerous learning opportunities. Nurses encourage patients to use their everyday experiences on the unit to practise newly learned behaviours.

The treatment plan or clinical pathway chosen for the patient should reflect this discharge-planning emphasis as early as the day of admission. The patient is expected to begin to progress toward a resolution of acute symptoms, assume personal responsibility, and improve interpersonal functioning. Patients with prolonged mental illness benefit most from a seamless transition to community services. Such a transition is facilitated through collaboration with community mental health services and through the intensive case-management programs available there. Readiness for community re-entry should include preparation by members of the patient's support system for their role in enhancing the patient's mental health. Poverty, stigma, unemployment, and lack of appropriate housing are identified as major barriers to recovery of mental health. The nurse needs to consider these gaps when planning discharge for patients from acute care settings as the gaps can delay discharge and increase the likelihood of readmission.

Chapter 6 has a more detailed discussion of the nurse's roles in the community setting.

---

**VIGNETTE**

Tazmine meets with Shane and his mother on the day of discharge to review the aftercare arrangements. Tazmine reviews the goals that were established by the treatment team and Shane's own goal for hospitalization. She reviews the accomplishments Shane made during his hospitalization; reinforces the importance of medication adherence; reviews each prescription, highlighting how and when the medication must be taken; and tells Shane when and where his aftercare appointment is. Tazmine answers Shane's and his mother's questions.

---

## ▌ KEY POINTS TO REMEMBER

- Inpatient care has increasingly become more acute and short term. Inpatient psychiatric care is guaranteed for all Canadians, with costs and delivery responsibilities shared by regional, provincial or territorial, and federal governments.
- Inpatient psychiatric mental health nursing requires strong skills in management, communication, and collaboration.
- The nurse plays a leadership role and also functions as a member of the multidisciplinary treatment team.
- The nurse advocates for the patient and ensures that the patient's rights are protected.
- Monitoring the environment and providing for safety are important components of good inpatient care. Psychiatric mental health nurses are skilled in protecting patients from suicidal impulses, aggressive behaviour, and psychological pain.

- Basic-level psychiatric mental health nursing interventions include admission, provision of a safe environment, psychiatric and physical assessments, milieu management, documentation, medication administration, and preparation for discharge to the community. Psychiatric mental health nurses also must have psychiatric intensive-care nursing skills.
- Documentation is an important form of communication to promote consistency in patient care and to justify the patient's stay in the hospital.
- Discharge planning begins on the day of admission and requires input from the treatment team and the community mental health care provider.

# CRITICAL THINKING

1. Imagine that you were asked for your opinion in regard to your patient's ability to make everyday decisions for himself. What sort of things would you consider as you weighed out safety versus autonomy and personal rights? How would you incorporate your knowledge of protective empowering?

2. If nurses function as equal members of the multidisciplinary mental health team, what differentiates the nurse from the other members of the team?

3. Identify gaps in community care that might impact patient discharge planning.

4. How might the community be affected when patients with serious mental illness live in group homes?

# CHAPTER REVIEW

1. A friend recognizes that his depression has returned and tells you he is suicidal and concerned he will harm himself. He is afraid that if he seeks help he will be involuntarily admitted to a psychiatric hospital, an idea that terrifies him. Which of the following responses best meets his immediate care needs?
    1. Provide emotional support and encourage him to contact his family.
    2. Express your concern for his safety, normalize psychiatric treatment as equal to treatment of any physical condition, and offer to accompany and support him through assessment at a nearby emergency department.
    3. Contact the police or a provincial/territorial magistrate to initiate involuntary assessment.
    4. Assist him to obtain an outpatient counselling appointment at an area community mental health centre, and call him frequently to ensure he is safe until his appointment occurs.

2. You are about to interview a newly admitted patient on your inpatient mental health unit. This is his first experience with psychiatric treatment. Which of the following interventions would be appropriate for this patient? Select all that apply.
    1. Discuss outpatient care options for after discharge.
    2. Anticipate and address possible increased anxiety and shame.
    3. Ensure that the individual understands his rights as a patient on your unit.
    4. Assess the patient for physical health needs that may have been overlooked.
    5. Carefully check all clothing and possessions for potentially dangerous items.

3. Which of the following nursing actions is appropriate in maintaining a safe therapeutic inpatient milieu? Select all that apply.

    1. Interact frequently with both individuals and groups on the unit.
    2. Ensure that none of the unit fixtures can be used for suicide by hanging.
    3. Initiate and support group interactions via therapeutic groups and activities.
    4. Stock the unit with standard hospital beds and other sturdy hospital furnishings.
    5. Provide and encourage opportunities to practise social and other life skills.
    6. Collaborate with housekeeping to provide a safe, pleasant environment.

4. A patient becomes agitated and hostile, threatening to smash a chair into the nurses' station door. Which of the following responses would be most appropriate for the student nurse to make?
    1. Maintain a safe distance, and attempt to de-escalate the patient verbally.
    2. When the response team arrives, assist in physically restraining the patient.
    3. Assist in promptly moving other patients to a safe distance or separate location.
    4. Meet with the patient immediately after the crisis to help him process what happened.

5. A student is considering a career in mental health nursing. Which of the following statements accurately reflects the role and expectations of mental health nurses in acute care settings?
    1. The primary role of the nurse is to monitor the patients from the nurses' station.
    2. Psychiatric patients rarely need medical care, so nurses do not need medical nursing skills.
    3. The close relationships developed with patients can lead to later romantic relationships.
    4. Mental health nursing requires a high degree of interpersonal comfort and therapeutic skill.

**ⓔvolve WEBSITE**                                                  Post-Test  interactive review

*Visit the Evolve Web site for Chapter Review Answers and Rationales, Critical Thinking Answer Guidelines, and additional resources related to the content in this chapter: http://evolve.elsevier.com/Canada/Varcarolis/psychiatric/*

# REFERENCES

Accreditation Canada. (2011). *Required organizational practices.* Ottawa: Author. Retrieved from http://www.accreditation.ca/uploadedFiles/ROP%20Handbook%20EN.pdf.

Aglukkaq, L. (2010). *Canada Health Act annual report 2009–2010.* Ottawa: Minister of Health. Retrieved from http://www.hc-sc.gc.ca/hcs-sss/pubs/cha-lcs/2010-cha-lcs-ar-ra/index-eng.php.

Brickell, T., Nicholls, T., Procyshyn, R., et al. (2009). *Patient safety in mental health.* Edmonton: Canadian Patient Safety Institute and Ontario Hospital Association. Retrieved from http://www.patientsafetyinstitute.ca/English/research/commissionedResearch/mentalHealthAndPatientSafety/Documents/Mental%20Health%20Paper.pdf.

Brunero, S., & Lamont, S. (2009). Systematic screening for metabolic syndrome in consumers with severe mental illness. *International Journal of Mental Health Nursing, 18,* 144–150. doi:10.1111/j.1447-0349.2009.00595.x.

Canadian Institute for Health Information. (2000). *Mental health and addiction services: Review of health information standards.* Retrieved from http://www.cihi.ca/CIHI-ext-portal/pdf/internet/HMDB_INDICATOR_MH_REV_EN.

Canadian Institute for Health Information. (2005). *Inpatient hospitalizations and average length of stay trends in Canada, 2003–2004 and 2004–2005.* Retrieved from https://secure.cihi.ca/free_products/hmdb_analysis_in_brief_e.pdf.

Canadian Institute for Health Information. (2006). *Hospital mental health services in Canada, 2003–2004.* Retrieved from https://secure.cihi.ca/free_products/HMHDB_2003-2004_e.pdf.

Canadian Institute for Health Information. (2007). *Improving the health of Canadians: Mental health and homelessness.* Retrieved from http://www.cpa.ca/cpasite/userfiles/Documents/Practice_Page/mental_health_homelessness_en.pdf.

Canadian Institute for Health Information. (2008). *Hospital length of stay and readmission for individuals diagnosed with schizophrenia: Are they related?* Retrieved from https://secure.cihi.ca/free_products/aib_los_and_readmission08_e.pdf.

Clark, D., Griffith, P., & Brown, A. (2002). *Aggression in the mental health workplace. Final report to the Workman's Compensation Board of Manitoba.* Winnipeg: Winnipeg Regional Health Authority.

Colom, F., & Lam, D. (2005). Psychoeducation: Improving outcomes in bipolar disorder. *European Psychiatry, 20,* 359–364. doi:10.1016/j.eurpsy.2005.06.002.

Government of Canada. (2006). *The human face of mental health and mental illness in Canada 2006* (Cat. No. HP5-19/2006E). Retrieved from http://www.phac-aspc.gc.ca/publicat/human-humain06/pdf/human_face_e.pdf.

Health Canada. (2002). *A report on mental illnesses in Canada* (Cat. No. 0-662-32817-5). Ottawa: Health Canada Editorial Board Mental Illnesses in Canada. Retrieved from http://www.phac-aspc.gc.ca/publicat/miic-mmac/.

Kirby, M., & Keon, J. (2004). *Mental health, mental illness and addiction: Overview of policies and programs in Canada.* Ottawa: The Standing Senate Committee on Social Affairs, Science and Technology.

Liddle, P., Shone, M., & Gray, J. (2008). *Canadian mental health law and policy* (2nd ed.) Toronto: LexisNexis Canada.

Mental Health Commission of Canada. (2012). *Changing directions, changing lives: The mental health strategy for Canada.* Calgary: Author.

Miller, B., Paschall, C., & Sevenson, D. (2006). Mortality and medical comorbidity among patients with serious mental illness. *Psychiatric Services 57*(10), 1482–1487. Retrieved from http://psychservices.psychiatryonline.org.berlioz.brandonu.ca/cgi/reprint/57/10/1482.

O'Reilly, R., Chaimowitz, G., Brunet, A., et al. (2010). Principles underlying mental health legislation [Position paper]. *Canadian Journal of Psychiatry, 55*(10), 1–5. Retrieved from http://publications.cpa-apc.org/media.php?mid=1037.

Park, T., Usher, K., & Foster, K. (2011). Description of a healthy lifestyle intervention for people with serious mental illness taking second-generation antipsychotics. *International Journal of Mental Health Nursing, 20,* 428–437. doi:10.1111/j.1447-0349.2011.00747.x.

Peplau, H.E. (1989). Interpersonal constructs for nursing practice. In A.W. O'Toole & S.R. Welt, (Eds.), *Interpersonal theory in nursing practice: Selected works of Hildegard E. Peplau* (pp. 42–55). New York: Putnam.

Roberts, S., & Bailey, E. (2011). Incentives and barriers to lifestyle interventions for people with severe mental illness: A narrative synthesis of quantitative, qualitative and mixed methods studies. *Journal of Advanced Nursing 67*(4), 690–708. doi:10.1111/j.1365-2648.2010.05546.x.

Romanow, R. (2002). *Building on values: The future of health care in Canada.* Ottawa: Commission on the Future of Health Care in Canada. Retrieved from http://dsp-psd.pwgsc.gc.ca/Collection/CP32-85-2002E.pdf.

Sapers, H. (2010). *Annual report of the Office of the Correctional Investigator 2009–2010.* Ottawa: The Correctional Investigator Canada. Retrieved from http://www.oci-bec.gc.ca/rpt/annrpt/annrpt20092010-eng.aspx.

Simon, R.I., & Shuman, D.W. (2008). Psychiatry and the law. In R. E. Hales, S.C. Yudofsky, & G.O. Gabbard, (Eds.), *Textbook of psychiatry* (pp. 1555–1659). Arlington, VA: American Psychiatric Publishing.

# Psychiatric Mental Health Nursing in Community Settings

*Avni Cirpili, Nancy Christine Shoemaker*
*Adapted by Holly Symonds-Brown*

## KEY TERMS AND CONCEPTS

assertive community treatment (ACT), 92
barriers to treatment, 94
biopsychosocial model, 88
case management, 89
continuum of psychiatric mental health treatment, 90

decompensation, 91
ethical dilemmas, 94
paternalism, 90
recovery, 87
serious mental illness, 86

## OBJECTIVES

1. Explain the evolution of the community mental health movement.
2. Identify elements of the nursing assessment that are critically important to the success of community treatment.
3. Explain the role of the nurse as the biopsychosocial care manager in the interprofessional team.
4. Discuss the continuum of psychiatric treatment.
5. Describe the role of the community psychiatric mental health nurse in disaster preparedness.
6. Describe the role of the psychiatric nurse in four specific settings: partial hospitalization program, psychiatric home care, assertive community treatment, and community mental health centre.
7. Identify two resources to assist the community psychiatric nurse in resolving ethical dilemmas.
8. Discuss barriers to mental health treatment.
9. Examine influences on the future of community psychiatric mental health nursing.

## ⊖volve WEBSITE

*Visit the Evolve website for Flashcards, Case Studies, and additional testing resources related to the content in this chapter:* *http://evolve.elsevier.com/Canada/Varcarolis/psychiatric/*  Pre-Test  interactive review

Psychiatric mental health nursing in the community began with nurses who specialized in community care, moved about within the community, were comfortable meeting with patients in their homes or in neighbourhood centres, were competent to act independently, used professional judgement in unanticipated situations, and possessed knowledge of community resources. The heritage of these nurses can be traced back to European women who cared for the sick at home and to Canadians such as the Grey Nuns, who organized religious and secular societies during the 1800s to visit the sick in their homes. By 1896, the Victorian Order of Nurses was established and trained public health nurses to provide care for and visit the

homes of the impoverished homesteaders in Western Canada (Hardill, 2006).

## THE EVOLUTION OF PSYCHIATRIC CARE IN THE COMMUNITY

Between 1960 and 1980, patients began to leave psychiatric hospitals in huge numbers. Several factors contributed to this shift, including financial pressures on the provincially funded psychiatric hospitals, changing societal values, and new mental health treatment philosophies (LaJeunesse, 2002; Sealy & Whitehead, 2004). Grassroots efforts, increased advocacy, and

**HOW A NURSE HELPED ME**

### Nurse Case Management to Meet Multiple Needs of a Client in the Community

*I am a 30-year-old woman who had been living in my parents' basement for all of my adult life. My parents were verbally abusive to me and had little tolerance for my obsessive-compulsive disorder and related hoarding behaviour that I'd had since adolescence. I rarely left the house as I was very fearful of people and contamination. When I did try to go to a doctor's appointment, frequently my parents would refuse to drive me to the appointment, and they would threaten to kick me out if I didn't give them all of my disability cheque.*

*One day, after I told my family doctor about my situation, she referred me to a community mental health nurse. The nurse came to see me in my home for the assessment, which was such a relief for me because it meant I didn't have to ask my parents for a drive. During the assessment, the nurse reviewed my history and current situation. She let me know that I was in an abusive situation, which was not helping my mental health problem. She also taught me about obsessive-compulsive disorder and offered to continue seeing me for cognitive-behavioural therapy. The nurse also coordinated referrals for me for housing, financial assistance, and psychiatry. After seeing a psychiatrist that the nurse brought to my home, I was started on medications, and I began doing cognitive-behavioural work with my nurse. She came weekly to see me and gradually encouraged me to leave my home for short periods of time, something I had not done for many years. I learned to navigate the bus system and began meeting my nurse at the local Tim Hortons. After several months, I decided I was ready to try to leave my abusive family. My nurse contacted Social Services to find extra housing funds and moving-expense coverage for me so that I could make the move. She also arranged for me to access subsidized housing.*

*On the day of the move, my nurse scheduled a visit to make sure I was coping with the stress. She even helped me unpack while we talked. I felt supported and excited to be gaining my independence. My transition to my new home took some time, but my nurse came for my regular appointments and made referrals for me to community agencies so I could get a food hamper and a washer and dryer. It's been four years now since I moved, and I am happy to say I am still in my apartment, I go to a support group, and I have a volunteer job!*

legal initiatives on behalf of people with mental illness and their right to humane care resulted in the provincial health care systems' looking for alternative treatment settings (LaJeunesse, 2002). Many hospitals were indeed grossly overcrowded, patients' rights were often disregarded, and seclusion and restraint were overused. Due to the largely custodial nature of inpatient treatment, patients were left with little incentive for growth or participation in their own care; this phenomenon became known as *institutionalization*.

In 1963, the Canadian Mental Health Association (CMHA) published *More for the Mind*, a report suggesting treatments for people with mental illnesses be in line with those for people with physical illnesses (Lurie, 2005). The report called for general hospital units to become the centre of community-based care for mental illness. This shift did occur, and it led to a phase of *transinstitutionalization* in many provinces as general hospitals opened up psychiatric units, and provincial psychiatric hospitals closed beds (Sealy & Whitehead, 2004).

However, policymakers came to believe that community care would be more humane and less expensive than hospital-based care, and the introduction of psychotropic drugs, beginning with chlorpromazine (Largactil), made community living a more realistic option for many people. Organizations like the CMHA opened up housing and support services for people living with mental illness in the community. From 1960 to 1980, all Canadian provinces implemented some type of deinstitutionalization of psychiatric services, although the timing and degree of bed closures varied greatly among regions (Sealy & Whitehead, 2004). For example, between 1965 and 1981, Canada saw a 70.6% decrease in psychiatry beds across the nation, but during that time, Saskatchewan had an 81.6% decrease and Prince Edward Island had only a 34.5% decrease (Sealy & Whitehead, 2004). A second pattern associated with deinstitutionalization was the change in duration of stay and admission rates to psychiatric inpatient beds. Days of care in inpatient units gradually shortened from the 1970s to the 1990s, with a drastic drop between 1994 and 1999 (Sealy & Whitehead, 2004).

Caring for patients with serious mental illness (chronic mental illness with ongoing symptoms) in the community presented many challenges in the early years after deinstitutionalization. At the time, few choices existed for outpatient treatment—usually a community mental health centre or therapy in a private office. Funding for community mental health centres began in the 1970s, but unfortunately, it was too limited for the level of system integration required to provide housing and case-management support for people with chronic mental illnesses (Lurie, 2005). Government promises to expand funding for community services were not kept, mental health funding continued to decline, and patients outnumbered resources. Many patients with serious mental illness resisted treatment with available providers, so providers began to use up scarce resources for the less mentally disabled but more committed population. While deinstitutionalization, in principle, was largely considered to have been a step toward improved care for people with mental illness, the lack of funding and available community supports negated many of the benefits. In reality, many people with mental illness were discharged to inadequate supports, a situation that led to increased homelessness and criminalization (LaJeunesse, 2002; Murphy, 1983).

Through the 1990s, advocacy by the CMHA and others continued. Increasing awareness resulted in increasing pressure on government to redesign the mental health system in Canada and to ensure adequate community supports. The 2006 senate report led by Michael Kirby and Wilbert Keon, *Out of the Shadows at Last*, was an optimistic step toward transforming the delivery system of mental health care. Subsequently, in 2007, the Mental Health Commission of Canada was formed, and, in 2009, it issued a mental health strategy for Canada focused on an underlying recovery principle for mental health care (Mental Health Commission of Canada, 2009).

Recovery is described as the ability of the individual to work, live, and participate in the community. It is a journey that provides patients with hope, empowerment, and confidence to take an active role in determining their own treatment paths. Ideally, recovery would be facilitated by interconnected community agencies that work in harmony to assist consumers of mental health care as they navigate an often confusing system. Realistically, funding has always been an issue in treating people with mental illness, and current economic realities have not improved the situation. Registered nurses and registered psychiatric nurses may be the answer to transforming an illness-driven and dependency-oriented system into a system that emphasizes recovery and empowerment. Nurses are adept at understanding the system and coordinating care as well as taking a health-oriented approach. They can work in a variety of roles, including direct care provider, crisis worker, case manager, community developer, program evaluator, educator, and advocate (Association of Registered Nurses of Newfoundland and Labrador, 2008).

Over the past 30 years—with advances in psychopharmacology and psychosocial treatments—psychiatric care in the community has become more sophisticated, with a continuum of care that provides more settings and options for people with mental illness. The role of the community psychiatric mental health nurse has grown to include service provision in a variety of these treatment settings, and nursing roles have developed outside traditional treatment sites.

For example, psychiatric needs among those in the criminal justice system and in the homeless population are well known. The number of individuals in the correctional systems who suffer from serious mental illness is growing, with self-reported admission data demonstrating that approximately 11% of individuals in federal prisons have a mental health diagnosis and 20% are prescribed psychiatric medications upon admission (Public Safety Canada Portfolio Corrections Statistics Committee, 2007). The community nurse's role is not only to provide care to individuals as they leave the criminal justice system and re-enter the community but also to educate police officers and justice staff in how to work with individuals entering the criminal system. Similarly, the percentage of homeless people with serious mental illness has been estimated to be as high as 15% (Folsom, Hawthorne, Lindamer, et al., 2005). The challenge to psychiatric mental health nurses is in making contact with these people, who are outside the system but desperately in need of treatment.

---

### BOX 6-1   POSSIBLE COMMUNITY MENTAL HEALTH PRACTICE SITES

**Primary Prevention**
Adult and youth recreational centres
  Schools
  Day care centres
  Churches, temples, synagogues, mosques
  Ethnic cultural centres

**Secondary Prevention**
Crisis centres
  Shelters (homeless, women subjected to domestic violence, adolescents)
  Correctional community facilities
  Youth residential treatment centres
  Partial hospitalization programs
  Chemical dependency programs
  Nursing homes
  Industry/work sites
  Early intervention psychosis programs
  Outreach treatment in public places
  Hospices and acquired immunodeficiency syndrome (AIDS) programs
  Assisted-living facilities

**Tertiary Prevention**
Community mental health centres
  Psychosocial rehabilitation programs

---

To support nursing interventions, the principles of the public health concept of prevention are useful. Primary prevention activities are directed at healthy populations and include providing information and teaching coping skills to reduce stress, with the goal of avoiding mental illness (e.g., a nurse may teach parenting skills in a well-baby clinic). Secondary prevention involves the early detection and treatment of psychiatric symptoms, with the goal of minimizing impairment (e.g., a nurse may conduct screening for depression at a work site). Tertiary prevention involves services that address residual impairments in psychiatric patients in an effort to promote the highest level of community functioning (e.g., a nurse may provide long-term treatment in a clinic). Box 6-1 presents examples of community practice sites for the psychiatric mental health nurse.

## COMMUNITY PSYCHIATRIC MENTAL HEALTH NURSING

Psychiatric mental health nursing in the community setting requires strong problem-solving and clinical skills, cultural sensitivity, flexibility, solid knowledge of community resources, and comfort with functioning more autonomously than acute care nurses do. Patients need assistance with problems related to individual psychiatric symptoms, family and support systems, and basic living needs, such as housing and financial support. Community treatment hinges on enhancing patients' strengths in the same environment in which they maintain their daily life, which makes individually tailored psychiatric care imperative.

Treatment in the community permits patients and those involved in their support to learn new ways of coping with symptoms or situational difficulties. The result can be one of empowerment and self-management for patients and their support systems.

## Roles and Functions

As noted in Chapter 1, psychiatric mental health nurses are educated at a variety of levels, including diploma, baccalaureate, master's, and doctoral. Perhaps the most significant distinction among the multiple levels of preparation is the extent to which the nurse acts autonomously and provides consultation to other providers, both inside and outside the particular agency. The health professions acts of individual provinces and territories grant nurses authority to practise, and the standards of practice—developed for registered nurses by the Canadian Federation of Psychiatric Mental Health Nurses (2006) and for registered psychiatric nurses by the Registered Psychiatric Nurses of Canada (2010)—guide nurses in their practice (see Chapter 9). Table 6-1 describes the roles of psychiatric mental health nurses according to level of education.

## Biopsychosocial Assessment

Assessment of the needs and capacities of patients living in the community requires expansion of the general psychiatric mental health nursing assessment (see Chapter 9). To be able to plan and implement effective treatment, the community psychiatric mental health nurse must also develop a comprehensive understanding of the patient's ability to cope with the demands of living in the community. The biopsychosocial model guides the nursing assessment and interventions in a holistic manner, taking a comprehensive view of clients, including their biology, social environment and skills, and psychological characteristics. Box 6-2 identifies the elements of a biopsychosocial assessment.

Key elements of this assessment are strongly related to the probability that the patient will experience successful outcomes in the community. Problems in any of the following areas

require immediate attention because they can seriously impair the success of other treatment goals:

- Housing adequacy and stability: A patient who faces daily fears of homelessness will not be able to focus on the treatment.
- Income and source of income: A patient must have a basic income—whether from an entitlement, a relative, or other

### BOX 6-2  ELEMENTS OF A BIOPSYCHOSOCIAL NURSING ASSESSMENT

Presenting problem and referring party
Psychiatric history, including symptoms, treatments, medications, and most recent usage of health services
Health history, including illnesses, treatments, medications, and allergies
Substance abuse history and current use
Family history, including health and mental health disorders and treatments
Psychosocial history, including:
- Developmental history
- School performance
- Socialization
- Vocational success or difficulty
- Interpersonal skills or deficits
- Income and source of income*
- Housing adequacy and stability*
- Family and support system*
- Level of activity
- Ability to care for needs independently or with assistance
- Religious or spiritual beliefs and practices
Legal history
Mental status examination
Strengths and deficits of the patient
Cultural beliefs and needs relevant to psychosocial care

*Strongly related to the probability that the patient will experience successful outcomes in the community.

### TABLE 6-1  COMMUNITY PSYCHIATRIC MENTAL HEALTH NURSING ROLES RELEVANT TO EDUCATIONAL PREPARATION

| ROLE | ADVANCED PRACTICE (MN, PHD) | BASIC PRACTICE (DIPLOMA, BSCN) |
| --- | --- | --- |
| Practice | Nurse practitioner or clinical nurse specialist; manage consumer care and prescribe or recommend interventions independently | Provide nursing care for consumer and assist with medication management as prescribed, under direct supervision |
| Consultation | Act as consultant to staff about plan of care, to consumer and family about options for care; collaborate with community agencies about service coordination and planning processes | Consult with staff about care planning and work with nurse practitioner or physician to promote health and mental health care; consult with consumer and family about options for care; collaborate with community agencies about service coordination and planning processes; collaborate with staff from other agencies |
| Administration | Assume administrative or contract consultant role within mental health agencies or mental health authority | Take leadership role within mental health treatment team |
| Research and education | Take on role as educator or researcher within agency or mental health authority | Participate in research at agency or mental health authority; serve as preceptor to undergraduate nursing students |

sources—to obtain necessary medication and meet daily needs for food and clothing.

- Family and support system: The presence of a family member, friend, or neighbour supports the patient's recovery and gives the nurse a contact person (with the patient's consent).
- Substance abuse history and current use: Often hidden or minimized during hospitalization, substance abuse can be a destructive force, undermining medication effectiveness and interfering with relationships, safety, community acceptance, and procurement of housing.
- Physical well-being: Factors that increase health risks and decrease life span for individuals with mental illnesses include decreased physical activity, smoking, adverse effects of medications, and absence of routine health exams.

Individual cultural characteristics are also very important to assess. For example, working with a patient who speaks a different language from the nurse requires the nurse to consider the implications of language and cultural background. In such a case, the use of a translator or cultural consultant from the agency or from the family is essential (see Chapter 7).

### Treatment Goals and Interventions

In the community setting, treatment goals and interventions are negotiated rather than imposed on the patient. To meet a broad range of patient needs, community psychiatric mental health nurses must approach interventions with flexibility and resourcefulness. Not unexpectedly, patient outcomes with

regard to mental status and functional level have been found to be more positive and achieved with greater cost effectiveness when the community psychiatric mental health nurse integrates case management into the professional role (Chan, Mackenzie, & Jacobs, 2000). Case management refers to the care coordination activities the nurse does with or for the patient and includes referrals, assistance with paperwork applications, connection to resources, and overall navigation of the health care system. The complexity of navigating the mental health and social service funding systems is often overwhelming to patients. The 1980s brought increased emphasis on case management as a core nursing function in treating the patient with serious mental illness.

In the private domain as well, case management, or care management, found a niche. The intent was to charge case managers with designing individually tailored treatment services for patients and tracking outcomes of care. The new case management included assessing patient needs, developing a plan for service, linking the patient with necessary services, monitoring the effectiveness of services, and advocating for the patient as needed. Newer models, particularly team concepts, have since been developed and will be discussed later in this chapter.

Differences in characteristics, treatment outcomes, and interventions between inpatient and community settings are outlined in Table 6-2. Note that all of these interventions fall within the practice domain of the basic-level registered nurse or registered psychiatric nurse.

| TABLE 6-2 | CHARACTERISTICS, TREATMENT OUTCOMES, AND INTERVENTIONS BY SETTING | |
|---|---|
| **INPATIENT SETTING** | **COMMUNITY MENTAL HEALTH SETTING** |
| **Characteristics** | |
| Unit locked by staff | Home locked by patient |
| 24-hour supervision | Intermittent supervision |
| Boundaries determined by staff | Boundaries negotiated with patient |
| Milieu with food, housekeeping, security services | Patient-controlled environment with self-care, safety risks |
| **Treatment outcomes** | |
| Stabilization of symptoms and return to community | Stable or improved level of functioning in community |
| **Interventions** | |
| Develop short-term therapeutic relationship | Establish long-term therapeutic relationship |
| Develop comprehensive plan of care, with attention to sociocultural needs of patient | Develop comprehensive plan of care for patient and support system, with attention to sociocultural needs |
| Enforce boundaries by seclusion or restraint as needed | Negotiate boundaries with patient |
| Administer medication | Encourage adherence to medication regimen |
| Monitor nutrition and self-care with assistance as needed | Teach and support adequate nutrition and self-care and provide referrals as needed |
| Provide health assessment and intervention as needed | Assist patient in self-assessment and self-management and provide referrals to meet health needs in community as needed |
| Offer structured socialization activities | Use creative strategies to refer patient to positive social activities |
| Plan for discharge to housing with family or significant other and plan for follow-up treatment | Communicate regularly with family or support system to assess and improve patient's level of functioning |

## Interprofessional Team Member

Interprofessional psychiatric nursing practice is one of the core mental health disciplines that work to the patient's benefit. In interprofessional team meetings, the individual and discipline-specific expertise of each member is recognized. Generally, the composition of the team reflects the availability of fiscal and professional resources in the area. Similar to the interprofessional team defined in Chapter 5, the community psychiatric team may include psychiatrists, nurses, social workers, psychologists, addictions specialists, recreational therapists, occupational therapists, and mental health workers.

The nurse is able to integrate a strong nursing identity into the team perspective. At the basic- or advanced-practice level, the community psychiatric mental health nurse holds a critical position to link the biopsychosocial and spiritual components relevant to mental health care. The nurse also communicates a discipline-specific expertise in a manner that the patient, significant others, and other members of the health care team can understand. In particular, the management and administration of psychotropic medications have become significant tasks the community nurse is expected to perform.

## Biopsychosocial Care Manager

The role of the community psychiatric mental health nurse includes coordinating mental health, physical health, spiritual health, social service, educational service, and vocational realms of care for the mental health patient. The reality of community practice in the new millennium is that few patients seeking treatment have uncomplicated symptoms of a single mental illness. The severity of illness has increased, and it is often accompanied by substance abuse, poverty, and stress. Repeated studies show that people with mental illnesses also have a higher risk for medical disorders than the general population (Robson & Gray, 2007).

The community psychiatric mental health nurse bridges the gap between the psychiatric and physical needs of the patient, meeting not only with the mental health treatment team but also with the patient's primary care team and serving as the liaison between the two. According to Griswold and colleagues (2005), integrating a nurse case manager to assist patients with primary care needs results in greater success with follow-up and attendance at appointments.

## Promoting Continuation of Treatment

A significant number of patients treated in the community struggle with continuing treatment and following through with prescribed treatments plans, particularly with taking medication. Traditionally, these problems have been called *noncompliance*. (Many people find this word objectionable since it implies a medical paternalism—that is, the patient is treated as a child who needs to be told what to do.) Deegan and Drake (2006), however, contend that there are actually two experts involved in the care of people with mental illnesses. One is the health care provider, who has advanced skills and training in psychiatric disorders, and the other is the consumer of care, who has intimate knowledge of the disorder and the response to treatment.

Shared decision making is the key to improving treatment adherence and success.

To take part in decision making, though, a patient must be knowledgeable about the illness and treatment options. Research demonstrates that people with mental illness want more than watered-down and simplistic information. (Imagine a pamphlet entitled *You and Your Mental Illness*.) To fully participate in the treatment plan, patients need current, evidence-informed information about their illness and treatment options (Tanenbaum, 2008).

A successful life in the community is more likely when medications are taken as prescribed. Nurses are in a position to help the patient manage medication, recognize adverse effects, and become aware of interactions among drugs prescribed for physical illness and mental illness. Patient and family education and coping strategies, in the context of a therapeutic relationship with the nurse, have been shown to significantly increase adherence to the medication regimen (Lacro & Glassman, 2004).

## Evolving Venues of Practice

Many community psychiatric mental health nurses originally practised on-site at community mental health centres, but practice locations have evolved because of financial, technological, health care, regulatory, cultural, and population changes. Nurses are now providing primary mental health care at therapeutic day care centres, schools, partial hospitalization programs, and shelters. In addition to these more traditional environments for care, psychiatric mental health nurses are entering forensic settings and drug and alcohol treatment centres.

Mobile mental health units have been developed in some service areas. In a growing number of communities, mental health programs are collaborating with other health or community services to provide integrated approaches to treatment. A prime example of this is the growth of concurrent disorder programming (programs that address the diagnosis of a mental illness and substance use disorder) at both mental health and chemical dependency clinics.

Technology has also contributed to changes in venues for providing community care. Telephone crisis counselling, telephone outreach, and the Internet are being used to enhance access to mental health services. Although face-to-face interaction is still preferred, technology has the potential to improve support, confidence, and health status among mental health care consumers (Akesson, Saveman, & Nilsson, 2007).

Over the course of a mental illness, patients may receive care from a range of psychiatric services. Figure 6-1 illustrates the continuum of psychiatric mental health treatment. A patient's movement along the continuum is fluid, from higher to lower levels of intensity of care, and changes are not necessarily made step by step. Upon discharge from acute hospital care or a 24-hour supervised crisis unit, many patients need intensive services to maintain their initial gains or to "step down" in care. Failure to follow up in outpatient treatment increases the likelihood of rehospitalization and other adverse outcomes (Kruse & Rohland, 2002).

Once a community treatment team has been established for a particular patient, that patient may return directly to his

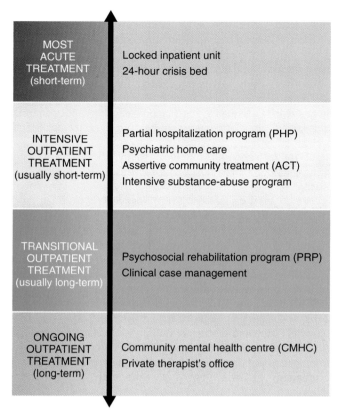

| | |
|---|---|
| **MOST ACUTE TREATMENT** (short-term) | Locked inpatient unit<br>24-hour crisis bed |
| **INTENSIVE OUTPATIENT TREATMENT** (usually short-term) | Partial hospitalization program (PHP)<br>Psychiatric home care<br>Assertive community treatment (ACT)<br>Intensive substance-abuse program |
| **TRANSITIONAL OUTPATIENT TREATMENT** (usually long-term) | Psychosocial rehabilitation program (PRP)<br>Clinical case management |
| **ONGOING OUTPATIENT TREATMENT** (long-term) | Community mental health centre (CMHC)<br>Private therapist's office |

**FIGURE 6-1** The continuum of psychiatric mental health treatment.

or her community mental health centre or psychosocial rehabilitation program. Homeless patients may be referred to a shelter with linkage to intensive case-management or assertive community treatment. Patients with a substantial substance-abuse problem may be transferred directly into a residential treatment program (see Chapter 19). It is also notable that patients may pass through the continuum of treatment in the reverse direction; that is, if symptoms do not improve, a lower-intensity service may refer the patient to a higher level of care in an attempt to prevent decompensation (deterioration of mental health) and hospitalization.

## COMMUNITY SETTINGS

The following sections describe four different community psychiatric settings and offer in each examples of basic-level nursing interventions—counselling, promotion of self-care activities, psychobiological interventions, health teaching, and case management:

- Counselling—assessment interviews, crisis intervention, problem solving in individual, group, or family sessions
- Promotion of self-care activities—fostering grooming, guidance in use of public transportation, instruction in budgeting (in home settings, the nurse may directly assist as necessary)
- Psychobiological interventions—medication administration, instruction in relaxation techniques, promotion of sound eating and sleep habits
- Health teaching—medication use, illness characteristics, coping skills, relapse prevention

- Case management—liaising with family, significant others, and other health care or community resource personnel to coordinate an effective plan of care

### Partial Hospitalization Programs

Partial hospitalization programs (PHPs) offer intensive, short-term treatment similar to inpatient care, except that the patient is able to return home each day. Criteria for referral to a PHP include serious symptoms that otherwise could lead to hospitalization or step-down from acute inpatient treatment, along with the presence of a responsible relative or caregiver who can assure the patient's safety (Shoemaker, 2000). Referrals come from inpatient or outpatient providers. Patients receive five to six hours of treatment daily, usually five days a week, although some programs operate on weekends. The average length of stay is approximately two to three weeks, depending on the program, and the interprofessional team consists of a psychiatrist, registered nurse or registered psychiatric nurse, social worker, occupational therapist, and recreational therapist.

The following vignette illustrates a typical day for a psychiatric mental health nurse in a PHP.

### Crisis Intervention Team

When psychiatric mental health care moved to a community setting, the need to address some of the acute mental health care concerns of individuals living in the community increased. Initially, the necessary response was left to local police departments, which often felt unprepared to deal effectively with mental health concerns. Crisis intervention teams were set up in many communities across Canada to address this issue and are now considered an essential part of comprehensive community mental health services (Bilsker, Moselle, Dick, et al., 2002). Various service-delivery models for crisis intervention teams are being used, but some commonalities among them exist, such as the use of an interprofessional team, mobile units, and collaborative partnerships with police (Forchuk, Jensen, Martin, et al., 2010). Often, the crisis intervention team is an interprofessional team made up of nurses, social workers, and psychologists. Psychiatrists often are used as consultants for the team. Crisis teams operate out of community clinics, emergency departments, or stand-alone offices.

Partnership with local police authorities has been found to be an extremely effective way of meeting the needs of individuals in acute psychiatric crisis and has led to decreased criminalization and improved access to services for people with severe chronic mental illness (Krupa, Stuart, Mathany, et al., 2010). When required, the interprofessional team may act as consultants to the police. Some crisis intervention models in Canada even include specially trained police members on the interprofessional team. Crisis services offer 24/7 phone support and in-person mental health assessments in homes, public places, and emergency rooms (Krupa, Stuart, Mathany, et al., 2010).

Nurses who work on crisis teams collaborate with other interprofessional members to assess patients in crisis, provide early intervention, provide crisis intervention counselling and support, offer short-term case management, including referrals

**VIGNETTE**

Michael Sanders is a nurse in a partial hospitalization program that is part of a general hospital's outpatient psychiatry department. Michael is the nurse member of the interprofessional team, and today his schedule is as follows:

**0830–0900:** Michael arrives at the PHP and meets with the team to review the patients expected to arrive in the program today. He prepares to meet with the patients who are scheduled for medication review with the psychiatrist. He also prepares the teaching outline for his daily psychoeducational groups.

**0900–1230:** Michael meets with a group of ten patients and teaches them goal setting, medication management, and relapse prevention. Throughout the sessions, Michael assesses each patient's mental status and any concerns that have arisen.

**1300–1400:** Michael conducts an intake interview with a newly admitted patient. Ms. Brown is a 50-year-old woman with a history of major depression who was hospitalized for two weeks after a drug overdose following an argument with her boyfriend. Michael completes the standardized interview form, paying extra attention to risk factors for suicide. When asked about substance abuse, Ms. Brown admits that she has been drinking heavily for the past two years, including the night she took the drug overdose. When the interview is completed, the patient is referred to the psychiatrist for a diagnostic evaluation.

**1400–1500:** Michael meets with four patients scheduled to see the psychiatrist. He reviews the cases with the psychiatrist and ensures that the patients understand any changes in their medication regimens.

**1500–1530:** Michael has a discharge meeting with Mr. Callaghan, a 48-year-old man with a diagnosis of schizophrenia. He was referred to the PHP by his clinic therapist to prevent hospitalization due to increasing paranoia and agitation. After two weeks in the PHP, he has restabilized and recognizes that he must adhere to his antipsychotic medication regimen. Michael finalizes Mr. Callaghan's medication teaching and confirms his aftercare appointments with his previous therapist and psychiatrist.

**1530–1600:** To ensure Ms. Brown's safety, Michael meets with her again before she goes home, assessing her suicide risk potential. Michael also shares the preliminary individual treatment plan and begins a discussion of resources for alcohol treatment, including Alcoholics Anonymous.

**1600–1700:** Michael meets with the team for daily rounds. He presents Ms. Brown, and the team develops an individual treatment plan for her. In this treatment plan, the team notes discharge planning needs for referrals to a community mental health centre and an alcohol treatment program. As a critical member of the treatment team, Michael reviews the remaining cases and makes needed adjustments to their treatment plans. He completes his notes and discharge summary. He also makes case-management telephone calls to arrange for community referrals, communicate with families, and report to any mental health referral programs to review how often the client has used the services.

to other resources, and advocate on behalf of families and patients.

The vignette on the following page describes a typical day of a nurse working on a crisis team.

## Assertive Community Treatment

Assertive community treatment (ACT) is an intensive type of case management developed in response to the community-living needs of people with serious, persistent psychiatric symptoms (Minzenberg, Yoon, & Carter, 2008). Patients with severe symptoms are referred to ACT teams by inpatient or outpatient providers because of a pattern of repeated hospitalizations, along with an inability to participate in traditional treatment.

ACT teams work intensively with patients in their homes or in agencies, hospitals, or clinics—whatever settings patients find themselves in. Creative problem solving and interventions are hallmarks of the care provided by mobile teams. The ACT concept takes into account that people need support and resources after 1700 hrs; teams are on call 24 hours a day. ACT teams are interprofessional and typically composed of psychiatric mental health nurses, social workers, psychologists, advanced-practice registered nurses, and psychiatrists. One of these professionals (often the nurse) serves as the case manager and may have a case load of up to ten patients who require visits three to five times per week. Length of treatment may extend to years, until the patient is ready to accept transfer to a less intensive site for care.

The vignette (page 94) illustrates a typical day for a psychiatric mental health nurse on an ACT team.

## Community Mental Health Centres

Community mental health centres were created in the late 1960s and have since become the main resource for those who require access to psychiatry services and counselling. The range of services available at these centres varies but generally includes emergency services and services for adults and children such as medication administration, individual therapy, group therapy, family therapy, psychoeducational services, and concurrent disorder treatment. A clinic may also be aligned with a psychosocial rehabilitation program that offers a structured day program, vocational services, and residential services. Some community mental health centres have an associated intensive case-management service to assist patients in finding housing or obtaining funding.

Community mental health centres also use interprofessional teams. The psychiatric mental health nurse may carry a caseload of 60 to 80 patients, each of whom is seen one to four times a month. Patients are either self-referred or referred by inpatient units or primary care providers for long-term or short-term follow-up. Patients may attend the clinic for years or be discharged when they improve and reach desired goals. Each clinic varies in design of service delivery; the nurse sees the majority of patients in the clinic but often will see patients in other settings such as primary care offices or their homes.

Walking into a person's home creates a different set of dynamics from those commonly seen in a clinical setting. Boundaries become important. The nurse may find it best to begin a visit informally by chatting about the patient's family events or by accepting refreshments offered. This interaction

**VIGNETTE**

Ben Thien is a nurse working on the mobile crisis team in a large urban setting; the following describes a typical evening shift.

**1500–1530:** Ben comes onto his shift and meets with the evening team to get a report from the day shift and plan for the evening shift. The team is told by day-shift staffers of any outstanding calls that have not been assessed and any updates regarding patients that are being case-managed by the team currently. The team decides that Ben and Officer George will go out at 1700 hrs to try to see a man whom a neighbour has called about today but who had not been at home when the day team went out earlier.

**1530–1630:** Ben takes the phones and receives a call from a woman who is feeling very sad and hopeless. Ben conducts a mental status exam over the phone and assesses the woman for risk. The woman appears to be suffering from depression but is not currently suicidal, so Ben offers her support and some psychoeducation about depression and its treatment. He gives her a phone number for the mental health clinic in her area, and she agrees to follow up. Ben asks for permission to fax a copy of his assessment to her family physician to ensure continuity of care, and the patient agrees. Ben completes his documentation and then faxes the report to the family physician.

**1630–1830:** Ben and his partner, Officer George, leave the office to follow up on the call from the day shift. They drive to the person's house in an unmarked police car. They both go to the door and ring the doorbell. A young man in his early 20s answers, and Ben explains who they are and that they would like to talk to him about how he has been feeling lately. The man agrees to speak to them. Officer George and Ben enter the house and assess it for any safety risks such as environmental issues, uncontrolled dogs, or other people present. Ben and George sit down at the kitchen table with the patient and begin the interview. The patient reports recent difficulties with his sleep and mood. He denies any history of mental illness or physical illness. He tells of his ability to control the weather and fear that perhaps people in the government are out to get him. He denies any risk for harm or self-harm, and he agrees that this is a recent change for him but does not feel the need to seek medical treatment. He does not demonstrate any impulsive behaviour during the interview, but Ben notices that many of the kitchen appliances are wrapped in tin foil. The patient vaguely refers to this as "anti-radar devices." At the completion of the interview, Ben concludes that while the patient seems to be showing signs of psychosis, he is not currently demonstrating risk and does not meet criteria under the mental health act for involuntary admission. Ben decides to try to engage the patient further so arranges a follow-up meeting for two days later. Prior to leaving, Ben ensures that the patient has adequate food supplies in his fridge and does some basic wellness teaching about sleep hygiene for the patient. Ben and George return to the office and document the visit.

**1830–2030:** George receives a call from a fellow police officer requesting an assessment of a person in the community who was reported for disturbing the peace at a bus shelter. Ben and George leave to drive to the scene. On the way to the scene, Ben takes a crisis call over the cellphone from a young man looking for resources for panic attacks. Upon arrival at the scene, Ben and George meet briefly with the police officers on-site, who bring them up to date on the situation. According to witnesses, the woman has been pacing at the bus stop for the past six hours, occasionally stepping into traffic. George and Ben go into the bus shelter and begin talking to the woman, who is dressed in shorts despite the cold weather, is pacing back and forth muttering to herself, and refuses to go to the hospital, stating, "I've had enough of all you FBI agents." Ben conducts the mental status and risk assessment and then, conferring with George, decides that this woman does meet the criteria of the mental health act for an involuntary assessment because she appears to have a mental illness, is at risk for self-harm (walking into traffic, continued exposure to the cold weather) and for further deterioration, and refuses to go to the hospital voluntarily. George and Ben explain that they need to take her to the hospital for an assessment. George puts her safely in the back of the police car, and Ben documents his assessment en route to the hospital. At the hospital, Ben informs the triage nurse of his assessment and arranges a secure room for the patient. Ben ensures that the patient is given food and fluids from the emergency staff and then discusses his assessment with the psychiatry resident on call. Ben and George then return to the office.

**2030–2230:** Ben continues to answer the phones and provide support, referrals, and assessments to callers. He arranges a home visit for the following day for a woman that is concerned about her father-in-law and his recent changes in behaviour.

**2230–2300:** Ben gets an update from the three other teams working the evening shift and then prepares his report for the night shift.

can be a strain for the nurse who has difficulty maintaining boundaries between the professional relationship and a personal one. However, there is great significance to the therapeutic use of self (i.e., the personality, insights, perceptions, and judgements of the nurse as part of the therapeutic process) in such circumstances to establish a level of comfort for the patient and family.

The vignette (page 95) illustrates the typical day for a nurse in a community mental health centre.

## DISASTER PREPAREDNESS

Educators now believe that all nurses need core competencies in emergency preparedness to be ready for natural and human-created disasters (Edwards, Williams, Scott, et al., 2007). Nurses who work in community mental health are often part of the intersectoral disaster response planning committee for the community in which they work. Following a disaster, the immediate goal is to ensure that those affected have shelter, food, and first aid as necessary. Then the community mental health nurse provides crisis management for victims and volunteers who are assisting in the relief efforts. After the crisis passes, the community psychiatric mental health nurse must find those individuals whose care was disrupted and help them to link back into the system. The nurse administers "psychological first aid" by assisting victims to meet basic needs, listening to individuals who need to share their stories, directing individuals to agencies that can help, and providing compassion and appropriate hope. In the United States, after Hurricane Katrina, survivors with mental illnesses often went untreated because of the disruption

Maria Restrepo is a nurse who works on an ACT team at a large, inner-city university medical centre. She had five years of inpatient experience before joining the ACT team, and she works with two social workers, two psychiatrists, and a mental health worker.

**0800–0930:** Maria starts the day at the clinic site with team rounds. Because she was on call over the weekend, she updates the team on three emergency-department visits: two patients were able to return home after she met with them and the emergency-department physician; one patient was admitted to the hospital because he made threats to his caregiver.

**0930–1030:** Maria's first patient is Mr. Zaman, a 35-year-old man with a diagnosis of bipolar disorder and alcohol dependence. He lives with his mother and has a history of five hospitalizations with nonadherence to outpatient clinic treatment. Except during his manic episodes, he isolates himself at home or visits a friend in the neighbourhood, at whose house he drinks excessively. Today he is due for his biweekly haloperidol decanoate (Haldol Decanoate) injection (a long-acting antipsychotic medication). Maria goes first to his house and learns that he is not at home. She speaks with his mother about his recent behaviour and an upcoming medical clinic appointment. Then she goes to the friend's house and finds Mr. Zaman playing cards and drinking a beer. He and his friend are courteous to her, and Mr. Zaman cooperates in receiving his injection. He listens as Maria repeats teaching about the risks of alcohol consumption. She encourages his attendance at an Alcoholics Anonymous meeting. He reports that he did go to one meeting yesterday. Maria praises him and encourages him and his friend to go again that night.

**1100–1300:** The next patient is Ms. Abbott, a 53-year-old single woman with a diagnosis of schizoaffective disorder and hypertension. She lives alone in a building for older adults and has no contact with family. Ms. Abbott was referred by her clinic team because she experienced three hospitalizations for psychotic decompensation over a period of a year despite receiving monthly decanoate injections. The ACT team is now the payee for her disability cheque. Today, Maria is taking Ms. Abbott out to pay her bills and to see her primary care physician for a checkup. Ms. Abbott greets Maria warmly at the door, wearing excessive makeup and inappropriate summer clothing. With gentle encouragement, she agrees to wear warmer clothes. She is reluctant to show Maria her medication box and briefly gets irritable when Maria points out that she has not taken her morning medications. As they stop by the apartment office to pay the rent, Maria talks with the manager briefly. This apartment manager is the team's only contact person and calls the team whenever any of the other residents report that Ms. Abbott is exhibiting unusual behaviour. Over the next hour and a half, Maria and Ms. Abbott drive to various stores and Ms. Abbott's medical appointment.

**1400–1630:** The last patient visit of the day is with Mr. Hahn, a 60-year-old widowed man diagnosed with schizophrenia and cocaine dependence. Mr. Hahn was referred by the emergency department last year after repeated visits due to psychosis and intoxication. Initially he was homeless, but he now lives in a recovery house shelter and has been clean of illegal substances for six months. He receives a monthly decanoate injection and is socially isolated in the house. Now that he receives disability support payments, he is seeking an affordable apartment. Maria has made appointments at two apartment buildings. After greeting him, Maria notes that he is wearing the same clothes he had on two days earlier, and his hair is uncombed. She suggests that he shower and change his clothes before they go out, and he agrees.

At the end of the day, Maria jots down information she will use to write her progress notes in patients' charts the next day when she returns to the clinic.

to existing services and the failure to reinitiate services (Wang, Gruber, Powers, et al., 2008). Chapter 24 offers a more detailed discussion of crisis and disaster.

## ETHICAL ISSUES

As community psychiatric mental health nurses assume greater autonomy and accountability for the care they deliver, ethical concerns become a more pressing issue. Ethical dilemmas are situations in which there are two choices to be made, neither of which resolves the situation in an absolutely ethical way. Weighing of the ethical principles and contextual issues is necessary. Ethical dilemmas are common in disciplines and specialties that care for the vulnerable and disenfranchised.

Psychiatric mental health nurses have an obligation to develop a model for assessing the ethical implications of their clinical decisions. Each incident requiring ethical assessment is somewhat different, and the individual nurse brings personal insights to each situation. The role of the nurse is to act in the best interests of the patient and of society, to the degree that this is possible.

Most organizations that employ nurses offer a designated resource for consultation regarding ethical dilemmas. For example, hospitals (with associated outpatient departments) are required by regulatory bodies to have an ethics committee to respond to clinicians' questions. Home care agencies or other independent agencies may have an ethics consultant in the administrative hierarchy of the organization. Professional nursing organizations and even boards of nursing can be used as resources by individual practitioners. Refer to Chapter 8 for an in-depth discussion of ethical guidelines for nursing practice.

## FUTURE ISSUES

### Barriers to Treatment

Despite the current availability and variety of community psychiatric treatments in Canada, many patients in need of services still do not receive them because of various barriers to treatment—factors that impede access to psychiatric care—including stigma, geographic challenges, financial limitations, policy issues, and system shortcomings. The *Canadian Community Health Survey*, Cycle 1.2, estimated that 2.6 million Canadians over age 15 have experienced mental health or substance-abuse problems in the previous year, but only 32% received treatment (Health Canada, 2002).

**VIGNETTE**

Nita Desai is a nurse at a community mental health centre. She is on the adult team and carries a caseload of patients diagnosed with chronic mental illness.

**0830–0900:** Upon arriving at the clinic, Nita receives a voice-mail message from Ms. DiTomasso, who is crying and says she is out of medication. Nita consults with the psychiatrist and calls Ms. DiTomasso to arrange for an emergency appointment later that day.

**0900–0930:** Nita's first patient is Mr. Enright, a 35-year-old man diagnosed with schizophrenia, who has been in treatment at the clinic for ten years. During their 30-minute counselling session, Nita assesses Mr. Enright for any exacerbation of psychotic symptoms (he has a history of grandiose delusions) and changes in eating and sleep habits or social functioning in the psychosocial rehabilitation program that he attends five days a week. Today, he presents as stable. Nita gives Mr. Enright his decanoate injection and schedules a return appointment for a month from now, reminding him of his psychiatrist appointment the following week.

**1000–1100:** Nita's second patient of the day is Susan, a 28-year-old mother with postpartum depression. Nita sees Susan weekly to assess her response to the antidepressant medication prescribed by her family physician and to work on anxiety coping strategies. She also spends time assessing Susan's attachment to her 6-month-old baby and provides education on any parenting questions that Susan may have. They discuss the idea of Susan attending a support group for postpartum depression as an adjunct to individual treatment. Susan is agreeable to the idea now that she is feeling less anxious and has more energy. Nita calls the group facilitator and arranges for Susan's intake for the following week.

**1100–1200:** Nita writes progress and medication notes, responds to telephone calls from patients and other agencies, such as home care and public-health nursing agencies, and prepares for the team conference.

**1200–1400:** All adult-team staff members attend the weekly intake meeting, at which new admissions are discussed and individual treatment plans are written with team input. Nita presents a patient in intake, reading from the standardized interview form. She also gives nursing input about treatment for the other five newly admitted patients. The new patient she presented is assigned to her, and she plans to call him later in the afternoon to set up a first appointment.

**1400–1500:** Nita co-leads a concurrent disorders therapy group with the addictions specialist, who is a social worker. The group is made up of seven patients who have concurrent diagnoses of substance abuse and a major psychiatric illness. The leaders take a psychoeducational approach, and today's planned topic is teaching about the physical effects of alcohol on the body. Nita focuses on risks associated with the interaction between alcohol and medications and answers the members' questions. Because this is an ongoing group, members take a more active role, and discussion may vary according to members' needs instead of following planned topics. After the session, the co-leaders discuss the group dynamics and write progress notes.

**1530–1600:** Nita meets with Ms. DiTomasso, who arrives at the clinic tearful and agitated. Ms. DiTomasso says that she missed her appointment this month because her son died suddenly. Nita uses crisis intervention skills to assess Ms. DiTomasso's status (e.g., any risks for her safety related to her history of suicidal ideation). After helping Ms. DiTomasso clarify a plan to increase support from her family, Nita notes that insomnia is a new problem. She takes Ms. DiTomasso to the psychiatrist covering "emergency prescription time" and explains the change in the patient's status. The psychiatrist refills Ms. DiTomasso's usual antidepressant and adds a medication to aid sleep. Nita makes an appointment for the patient to return to see her in one week instead of the usual one month and also schedules her to meet with her assigned psychiatrist that same day.

**1600–1630:** Nita completes all notes, makes necessary telephone calls to staff working with her patients in the psychosocial rehabilitation program, and phones her new patient to schedule an appointment.

Although the stigma of mental illness has lessened over the past 40 years—in part because mental illnesses are now recognized as biologically based and also because many well-known people have admitted to having received psychiatric treatment—many people still are afraid to disclose a psychiatric diagnosis. Instead, they seek medical care for vague somatic complaints from primary care providers, who too often fail to diagnose anxiety or depressive disorders.

In addition to stigma, as mentioned, geographic, financial, and systems factors can impede access to psychiatric care. Mental health services are scarce in some rural areas, and due to funding shortfalls, mental health treatment programs often have wait-lists. The 2006 Senate report, *Out of the Shadows at Last* (Kirby & Keon, 2006), identified national system and policy problems, including fragmented care for children and adults with serious mental illness, high unemployment and disability among those with serious mental illness, undertreatment of older adults, and lack of national priorities for mental health and suicide prevention. Provincial and other insurance plans do not reimburse for community mental health care at the same level that they cover other health care.

## Nursing Education

A baccalaureate degree is preferred in more autonomous community settings and will become increasingly in demand as the trend away from hospital-based acute care settings continues. However, educators believe that nonbaccalaureate-prepared nurses also should be educated to meet the challenges of providing community care. Clinical experiences in community settings are valuable for all nursing students; they increase cultural sensitivity, improve teaching skills, and foster an appreciation for building strong interprofessional teams (Sensenig, 2007).

Community psychiatric mental health nursing is a specialty area in transition. As this specialty area develops, competence-based position descriptions and scope-of-practice guidelines will be vital to ensuring that nurses with diverse levels of education (including licensed practical nurses) are performing appropriate tasks and functions (Kudless & White, 2007).

**Meeting Changing Demands**

As the population ages, nurses who elect to work with older psychiatric patients with increasingly complex health care needs will be in demand. As with other populations and other types of care, there will be pressure to expand the proportion of care allotted to community-based psychiatric care (Ryan, Garlick, and Happell, 2006). Community psychiatric mental health nurses may collaborate more with primary health care practitioners to fill the gap in existing community services. This need is particularly acute in rural areas where psychiatrists are scarce (Hanrahan & Hartley, 2008). Certainly, community psychiatric mental health nurses need to be committed to teaching the public about resources for mental health care, whether for long-term serious mental illness or for short-term situational stress.

## KEY POINTS TO REMEMBER

- Community psychiatric mental health nursing has historical roots dating to the 1800s and has been significantly influenced by public policies.
- Deinstitutionalization brought promise, as well as problems, for people with serious mental illness.
- The basic-level community psychiatric mental health nurse practises in many traditional and nontraditional sites.
- As part of the interprofessional team, the community psychiatric mental health nurse functions as a biopsychosocial care manager.
- The continuum of psychiatric treatment includes numerous community treatment alternatives with varying degrees of intensity of care.
- The community psychiatric mental health nurse needs access to resources to address ethical dilemmas encountered in clinical situations.
- Barriers to mental health care still exist, but the community psychiatric mental health nurse may be able to diminish them.

## CRITICAL THINKING

You are a nurse working at a local community mental health centre. While you are assessing a 45-year-old single male patient, he reports that he has not been sleeping and that his thoughts seem to be "all tangled up." Although he does not admit directly to being suicidal, he remarks, "I hope that this helps today because I don't know how much longer I can go on like this." He is dishevelled and has been sleeping in homeless shelters. He has little contact with his family and becomes agitated when you suggest that contacting them might be helpful. He reports a recent hospitalization and previous treatment at a concurrent disorders facility, yet he denies substance abuse. When asked about his physical condition, he says that he has tested positive for hepatitis C and is "supposed to take" multiple medications that he cannot name.

1. List your concerns about this patient in order of priority.

2. Which of these concerns must be addressed before he leaves the clinic today?

3. Do you feel there is an immediate need to consult with any other members of the interprofessional team about this patient?

4. Keeping in mind that the patient must always be an active part of his own care, how will you start to develop trust with the patient to gain his cooperation with the treatment plan?

## CHAPTER REVIEW

1. Which of the following factors contributed to the movement of patients out of large provincial institutions and into community-based mental health treatment? Select all that apply.
   1. Provinces wanted to save money by moving the patients to the community, where the cost of care would be less.
   2. The growing availability of generous mental health insurance coverage gave more patients the ability to seek private care in the community.
   3. Forward-thinking communities developed a system of coordinated and accessible community care that offered more effective treatment.
   4. The 1963 CMHA report *More for the Mind* advocated for community-based care.
   5. The advocacy work of families, patients, and other supporters demanded the right to treatment in the least restrictive setting.
   6. New psychotropic medications were created.

2. You are a community mental health nurse meeting with a patient who has just been discharged from the hospital, where he had received psychiatric care for the first time. Which of the following activities would you expect to undertake in your role as the nurse on the treatment team caring for this patient?
   1. Take medications to the patient's home each day and administer them.
   2. Solve day-to-day problems for the patient to minimize his exposure to stress.
   3. Refer the patient to counsellors or other providers when he indicates a need to talk with someone.
   4. Take a ride on the local bus system with the patient to help him learn routes and schedules.

3. A nurse providing in-home mental health care enjoys working with Mr. Moore, an older man suffering from depression since the loss of his wife and a recent below-knee amputation that has left him homebound. A fondness develops between the two, with the nurse reminding Mr. Moore of his daughter when she was young and the patient reminding the nurse of her grandfather. Mr. Moore begins to offer the nurse small statues and other trinkets that had belonged to his wife and seem of little monetary value. She tries to decline, but he persists with each visit and seems hurt when she does not accept the items. Which of the following responses is most appropriate and professional?
   1. Agree to accept one, and only one, small token gift to appease the patient
   2. Continue to decline the gifts while helping him find other ways to express his feelings
   3. Consult with her supervisor or designated ethics resource person about what to do next
   4. Identify Mr. Moore's efforts as a boundary violation and request not to be assigned to him

4. Mr. Laurent has been hospitalized twice in five years with a severe, chronic psychiatric disorder. He responds well to inpatient and community treatment and is usually stable, but he also has a history of becoming socially withdrawn and failing to provide for his self-care needs in the months following inpatient care. Hospital staff members feel he no longer needs inpatient care but do think that he needs a higher level of care than the typical periodic outpatient appointments at a community mental health centre. He is not homebound, has access to transportation and secure housing, and has a supportive family. Given these circumstances, which of the following programs would the nurse suggest for Mr. Laurent immediately after discharge?
   1. Crisis intervention team
   2. Partial hospitalization program
   3. Assertive community treatment
   4. Home-based mental health program

5. Mrs. Chan, a patient at the community mental health centre, tends to stop taking her medications at intervals, usually leading to decompensation. Which of the following interventions would most likely improve her adherence to her medications?
   1. Help Mrs. Chan to understand her illness and allow her to share in decisions about her care.
   2. Advise Mrs. Chan that if she stops her medications, her doctor will hospitalize her.
   3. Arrange for Mrs. Chan to receive daily home care so her use of medications is monitored.
   4. Discourage Mrs. Chan from focusing on adverse effects and other excuses for stopping her pills.

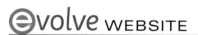 WEBSITE

Post-Test  interactive review

*Visit the Evolve Web site for Chapter Review Answers and Rationales, Critical Thinking Answer Guidelines, and additional resources related to the content in this chapter:* http://evolve.elsevier.com/Canada/Varcarolis/psychiatric/

## REFERENCES

Akesson, K.M., Saveman, B.I., & Nilsson, G. (2007). Health care consumers' experiences of information communication technology: A summary of literature. *International Journal of Medical Informatics, 76,* 633–645. doi:10.1016/j.ijmedinf.2006.07.001.

Association of Registered Nurses of Newfoundland and Labrador. (2008). *The role of the psychiatric mental health nurse working in the community: Position statement.* St. John's: Author.

Bilsker, D., Moselle, K., Dick, A., et al. (2002). *B.C.'s mental health reform best practices: Crisis response/emergency service.* British Columbia: Ministry of Health and Ministry Responsible for Seniors.

Canadian Federation of Psychiatric Mental Health Nurses. (2006). *Canadian standards of psychiatric mental health nursing* (3rd ed.). Retrieved from http://cfmhn.ca/sites/cfmhn.ca/files/CFMHN%20standards%201.pdf.

Canadian Mental Health Association. (1963). *More for the mind: A study of psychiatric services in Canada.* Toronto: Author.

Chan, S., Mackenzie, A., & Jacobs, P. (2000). Cost-effectiveness analysis of case management versus a routine community care organization for patients with chronic schizophrenia. *Archives of Psychiatric Nursing, 14,* 98–104. doi:10.1016/S0883-9417(00)80025-4.

Deegan, P.E., & Drake, R.E. (2006). Shared decision making and medication management in the recovery process. *Psychiatric Services, 57*(11), 1636–1639.

Edwards, D., Williams, L.H., Scott, M.A., et al. (2007). When disaster strikes: Maintaining operational readiness. *Nursing Management, 38*(9), 64–66.

Folsom, D.P., Hawthorne, W., Lindamer, L., et al. (2005). Prevalence and risk factors for homelessness and utilization of mental health services among 10,340 patients with serious mental illness in a large public mental health system. *American Journal of Psychiatry, 162*(2), 370–376.

Forchuk, C., Jensen, E., Martin, et al. (2010). Psychiatric crisis services in three communities [Special issue]. *Canadian Journal of Community Mental Health, 29*(5), 73–86.

Griswold, K., Servoss, T., Leonard, K., et al. (2005). Connections to primary care after psychiatric crisis. *Journal of the American Board of Family Practice, 18*(3), 166–172.

Hanrahan, N.P., & Hartley, D. (2008). Employment of advanced-practice psychiatric nurses stem rural mental health workforce shortages. *Psychiatric Services, 59*(1), 109–111.

Hardill, K. (2006). From the Grey Nuns to the streets: A critical history of outreach nursing in Canada. *Public Health Nursing, 24,* 91–97. doi:10.1111/j.1525-1446.2006.00612.x.

Health Canada. (2002). *A report on mental illnesses in Canada* (Cat. No. 0-662-32817-5). Ottawa: Health Canada Editorial Board Mental Illnesses in Canada. Retrieved from http://www.phac-aspc.gc.ca/publicat/miic-mmac/.

Kirby, M.L., & Keon, W.J. (2006). *Out of the shadows at last: Transforming mental health, mental illness and addiction services in Canada.* Ottawa: Standing Senate Committee on Social Affairs, Science and Technology. Retrieved from http://www.parl.gc.ca/39/1/parlbus/commbus/senate/com-e/soci-e/rep-e/pdf/rep02may06part1-e.pdf.

Krupa, T., Stuart, H., Mathany, A., et al. (2010). Evaluation of an integrated crisis-case management service [Special issue]. *Canadian Journal of Community Mental Health, 29*(5), 125–137.

Kruse, G.R., & Rohland, B.M. (2002). Factors associated with attendance at a first appointment after discharge from a psychiatric hospital. *Psychiatric Services, 53*(4), 473–476.

Kudless, M.W., & White, J.H. (2007). Competencies and roles of community mental health nurses. *Journal of Psychosocial Nursing, 45*(5), 36–44.

Lacro, J. & Glassman, R. (2004). Medication adherence. *Medscape Psychiatry & Mental Health 9*(1), 1–4. Retrieved from http://www.medscape.org.

LaJeunesse, R.A. (2002). *Political asylums.* Edmonton: Muttart Foundation.

Lurie, S. (2005). Comparative mental health policy: Are there lessons to be learned? *International Review of Psychiatry, 17*, 97–101. doi:10.1080/09540260500073356.

Mental Health Commission of Canada. (2009). Our history. Retrieved from http://www.mentalhealthcommission.ca/English/Pages/Background.aspx.

Minzenberg, M.J., Yoon, J.H., & Carter, C.S. (2008). Schizophrenia. In R.E. Hales, S.C. Yudofsky, & G.O. Gabbard (Eds.), *Textbook of psychiatry* (5th ed., pp. 407–456). Arlington, VA: American Psychiatric Publishing.

Murphy, R. (1983). *Backwards form the back-wards: The unmet needs of recovering psychiatric patients in Edmonton.* Edmonton: Boyle Street Community Services Co-Op.

Public Safety Canada Portfolio Corrections Statistics Committee. (2007). *Corrections and conditional release statistical overview: Annual report 2007.* (Catalogue No. PS1-3/2007E). Ottawa: Public Works and Government Services Canada.

Registered Psychiatric Nurses of Canada. (2010). *Standards of practice and code of ethics.* Edmonton: Registered Psychiatric Nurses of Canada.

Robson, D., & Gray, R. (2007). Serious mental illness and physical health problems: A discussion paper. *International Journal of Nursing Studies, 44*, 457–466. doi:10.1016/j.ijnurstu.2006.07.013.

Ryan, R., Garlick, R., & Happell, B. (2006). Exploring the role of the mental health nurse in community mental health care for the aged. *Issues in Mental Health Nursing, 27*(1), 91–105. doi:10.1080/01612840500312902.

Sealy, P., & Whitehead, P.C. (2004). Forty years of deinstitutionalization of psychiatric services in Canada: An empirical assessment. *Canadian Journal of Psychiatry, 49*(4), 249–257.

Sensenig, J.A. (2007). Learning through teaching: Empowering students and culturally diverse patients at a community-based nursing care center. *Journal of Nursing Education 46*(8), 373–379.

Shoemaker, N. (2000). The continuum of care. In V.B. Carson (Ed.), *Mental health nursing: The nurse–patient journey* (2nd ed., pp. 368–387). Philadelphia: Saunders.

Tanenbaum, S.J. (2008). Consumer perspectives on information and other inputs to decision-making: Implications for evidence-based practice. *Community Mental Health Journal, 44*(5), 331–335. doi:10.1007/s10597-008-9134-y.

Wang, P., Gruber, M., Powers, R., et al. (2008). Disruption of existing mental health treatments and failure to initiate new treatment after Hurricane Katrina. *American Journal of Psychiatry, 165*(1), 34–41.

# Cultural Implications for Psychiatric Mental Health Nursing

*Elaine M. Mordoch*

*With contributions from Rick Zoucha and Kimberly Gregg*

## KEY TERMS AND CONCEPTS

Aboriginal peoples, 99

acculturation, 108

assimilation, 108

colonization, 107

cultural competence, 109

culture, 100

cultural concepts of distress, 105

enculturation, 103

ethnicity, 100

ethnocentrism, 100

ethnopharmacology, 106

medicine wheel, 102

multiculturalism, 100

refugee, 108

social determinants of health, 100

somatization, 105

stereotyping, 103

Western tradition, 102

world view, 100

## OBJECTIVES

1. Discuss the development of cultural competence in the history of psychiatric mental health nursing.
2. Identify tensions that exist in the provision of culturally sensitive nursing care.
3. Compare and contrast dominant Western beliefs and values with the beliefs and values of nondominant diverse cultures.
4. Consider the world view and cultural beliefs of the First Nations people in Canada and their relation to mental health and mental illness.
5. Explain the unique mental health and mental illness issues of refugee and immigrant groups in Canada.
6. Identify culturally sensitive assessments that recognize inherent risk factors of nondominant cultural groups and barriers to culturally sensitive psychiatric mental health nursing care.
7. Develop culturally sensitive nursing care plans for people from diverse cultures.

## ⊖volve WEBSITE

*Visit the Evolve website for Flashcards, Case Studies, and additional testing resources related to the content in this chapter:* *http://evolve.elsevier.com/Canada/Varcarolis/psychiatric/* `Pre-Test` `interactive review`

In July 1988, Canada became the first country to pass a multiculturalism law, the *Multiculturalism Act*, with the intent of honouring cultural diversity, decreasing discrimination, increasing cultural awareness, and formulating federal government decisions in a culturally sensitive manner (Library of Parliament, 2006). Political pressures from Aboriginal peoples,

French Québécois, and other ethnic minorities prompted the recognition of Canadian multiculturalism. Historically, Canada has been composed of three main populations:

1. Aboriginal peoples, consisting of Inuit (4%), Métis (33%), and First Nations (around 60%). Aboriginal peoples, categorized as status or nonstatus, are governed by the *Indian Act*,

a comprehensive federal legislation now viewed as a colonialist and patriarchal document that has failed to recognize Aboriginal peoples' abilities to manage their own affairs (Kirmayer, Tait, & Simpson, 2009). Presently, there is serious contention between the Canadian government and Aboriginal groups.

2. The colonizing groups of English- and French-speaking people, known as the *Charter groups*.
3. Individuals with a non-French or non-English background. Recent robust immigration policies have resulted in high numbers of immigrants from Africa, Asia, the Middle East, the Caribbean, and Central and South America.

Multiculturalism refers to the presence of diverse racial and ethnic minorities who identify themselves as different and wish to remain so. In Canada, it is also a set of ideals, adopted at the federal, provincial, and municipal levels, celebrating the country's cultural diversity (Library of Parliament, 2006). Multiculturalism informs nursing practice and challenges nurses to educate themselves to deliver culturally sensitive, competent, holistic care, as required by nursing care standards at provincial and national governance levels. To meet this challenge, nurses must develop self-awareness, monitor their ethnocentrism (perception that one's own values, beliefs, and behaviours are superior), and be open to diverse world views and conceptualizations of mental health and illness, which will increasingly become part of their practice (Registered Nurses' Association of Ontario, 2007).

This chapter focuses on culture, its influence on the conceptualization of mental health and illness, and, ultimately, the care of patients and families who may be experiencing mental illness or mental health problems.

## CULTURAL COMPETENCE IN PSYCHIATRIC MENTAL HEALTH NURSING

Foundational theories derived from Western ideology have guided mental health service delivery and the formation of the Canadian mental health system. However, tensions exist between the divergent world views of the status quo delivering mental health services and those who use the services. Dr. Madeleine Leininger, a nurse anthropologist, identified the need for culturally sensitive nursing care. Leininger (1991) has advocated for culturally competent nursing practice in response to migration shifts and globalization. Cultural competence has since been included in nursing care standards, which now include cultural health information necessary for successful health outcomes. The Registered Nurses' Association of Ontario (2007), for example, has published *Embracing Cultural Diversity in Health Care: Developing Cultural Competence*, which clearly identifies nurses' responsibility to practise in a culturally safe and competent manner.

### Culture, Race, Ethnicity, and the Social Determinants of Health

All nurses and their clients with mental illness, whether from a dominant or nondominant cultural group, have an ethnic background and a culture influencing their perspectives and choices.

Culture comprises the shared beliefs, values, and practices that guide a group's members in patterned ways of thinking and acting and includes factors such as religion, geography, socioeconomic status, occupation, ability or disability, and sexual orientation. Culture can also be viewed as a blueprint for guiding actions that impact care, health, and well-being (Leininger & McFarland, 2006). *Cultural norms* define how group members make sense of the world and make decisions about how to relate and behave. Cultural norms prescribe what is "normal" and "abnormal" and influence the development of mental health and illness concepts. For example, in Western society, hearing voices and seeing visions is generally viewed as a sign of pathology and deviates from the cultural norms. In some Aboriginal cultures, however, vision quests, the seeking of visions, is honoured and valued and would not be viewed as pathological.

Ethnicity refers to the sharing of common traits, customs, and race. Ethnic groups have a common heritage, history, and world view. A world view is a major paradigm used to explain the world and its mysteries, inclusive of beliefs about health, illness, and the hereafter. Three major world views explaining health and illness are magic and religion, empirical science, and holistic health (Andrews & Boyle, 2008). Nurses need to be aware that basic concepts of mental health and illness may differ among ethnic groups, may clash with their own world view, and may affect how nursing care is received by a patient.

All culture exists within a societal context that has the potential to affect the mental well-being of individuals and of groups. The social determinants of health influence culture and its effects on mental health and mental illness. These determinants are identified as economic status, genetics, job security, employment opportunities, access to safe and affordable housing, child care availability, food security, and inclusion or exclusion from society (World Health Organization, 2008).

## DEMOGRAPHIC SHIFTS IN CANADA

In the latter years of the last century, the federal government developed a strong multiculturalism policy, which underlies nursing practice. As such, it is helpful for nurses to understand the development of this policy. See Table 7-1.

As well, six of the ten Canadian provinces have policies on multiculturalism to ensure social justice and cohesion within the changing Canadian society. Census data from 2006 indicates that the percentage of foreign-born people in Canada had reached 19.6%, representing one in five Canadians (Natural Resources Canada, 2009). Immigration patterns have changed, with Asian and Middle Eastern immigrants composing 59.4% of recent immigrants to Canada, decreasing numbers of European immigrants with the exception of Romanians, and an increase in African and South American immigrants. These rapid and massive shifts are concentrated in Toronto, Vancouver, and Montreal. In addition, Aboriginal peoples constitute an increasing proportion of the Canadian population, with 4.4% of the Canadian population identifying some form of Aboriginal ancestry (Library of Parliament, 2006). Their customs and unique perspectives are now more widely

## TABLE 7-1  DEVELOPMENT OF MULTICULTURAL POLICY

| YEARS | MULTICULTURALISM AS PUBLIC POLICY IN CANADA |
|---|---|
| 1947 | *Canadian Citizenship Act*: Previously, all citizens were British subjects with a focus on British identity<br>Influx of post–World War II immigrants from Europe |
| 1960s | Civil rights movements in the United States reflecting the growing dissatisfaction felt by Canadian racial minorities<br>Assertiveness of the Canadian First Nations people to reclaim their rights<br>Resentment of ethnic minorities related to their place in society<br>Royal Commission on Bilingualism and Biculturalism recognized the contribution of ethnic groups to society |
| 1970s | Beginning of an Integration Policy wherein cultural groups were given the right to identify with select elements of their cultural group<br>Work began to incorporate diverse cultural groups into the institutions of Canada |
| 1980s | Expanded multicultural policies; massive immigration; racist problems developed; anti-racism legislation was passed<br>Canadian Charter of Rights and Freedoms passed to uphold multiculturalism<br>*Multiculturalism Act* (1988) passed, honouring cultural identity and upholding equal participation in Canadian society |
| 1990s | Formation of a Department of Multiculturalism and Citizenship, emphasizing cross-cultural understanding<br>Review of multiculturalism policies with a renewed focus on identify, full participation in society, and social justice |
| 2002 | On November 13, 2002, the Government of Canada, by Royal Proclamation, designated June 27 of each year Canadian Multiculturalism Day. |

**Source:** Dewing, M. (1994, updated 2009). *Canadian multiculturalism* (Publication No. PRB 09-20E). Retrieved from http://publications.gc.ca/collections/collection_2010/bdp-lop/prb/prb0920-eng.pdf. Reproduced with the permission of the Library of Parliament, 2013.

## TABLE 7-2  TOP 10 COUNTRIES OF BIRTH OF RECENT IMMIGRANTS,* 1981 TO 2006

| RANK | 2006 CENSUS | 2001 CENSUS | 1996 CENSUS | 1991 CENSUS | 1981 CENSUS |
|---|---|---|---|---|---|
| 1 | People's Republic of China | People's Republic of China | Hong Kong | Hong Kong | United Kingdom |
| 2 | India | India | People's Republic of China | Poland | Viet Nam |
| 3 | Philippines | Philippines | India | People's Republic of China | United States |
| 4 | Pakistan | Pakistan | Philippines | India | India |
| 5 | United States | Hong Kong | Sri Lanka | Philippines | Philippines |
| 6 | South Korea | Iran | Poland | United Kingdom | Jamaica |
| 7 | Romania | Taiwan | Taiwan | Viet Nam | Hong Kong |
| 8 | Iran | United States | Viet Nam | United States | Portugal |
| 9 | United Kingdom | South Korea | United States | Lebanon | Taiwan |
| 10 | Colombia | Sri Lanka | United Kingdom | Portugal | People's Republic of China |

*"Recent immigrants" refers to landed immigrants who arrived in Canada within five years prior to a given census.
**Source:** Statistics Canada. (2008). Censuses of population, 1981 to 2006. Retrieved from http://www.statcan.gc.ca/pub/11-008-x/2008001/article/10556-eng.htm#2.

recognized and valued. This shifting Canadian demographic demands that nursing practice respond to the need for culturally sensitive and competent care in mental health service delivery.

Census data from 1981 to 2006 provide an overview of the changing demographics of Canadian society and highlights the need for nurses to maintain competency in mental health care provision (see Table 7-2).

## WORLD VIEWS AND PSYCHIATRIC MENTAL HEALTH NURSING

Psychiatric mental health nursing practice has historically been informed by borrowed theories from disciplines, such as psychology, that are grounded in the values and belief systems of the dominant Western culture. Nursing knowledge of psychology, human growth and development, and mental health and illness are based on traditions from Greek, Roman, and Judeo-Christian thought and the philosophy of Descartes's body–mind dualism. These predominant teachings often hinder nurses' understanding of other cultural groups' world views on mental health.

A group's world view outlines how its members explain and define their responses to life events, their position in the universe, and the phenomena of nature (Andrews & Boyle, 2008). World views shape perceptions about time, health and illness, rights and obligations in society, and acceptable ways of behaving in relation to others and nature. In Western tradition (biomedical, scientific traditions), identity arises from one's individuality, and personal accomplishments are underscored by the much-valued autonomy and self-reliance. Mind and body, viewed as separate entities, are treated by different practitioners. Disease has a specific, measurable, and observable cause, and treatment focuses on curing and eliminating the cause. Time is linear, moving forward, and waiting for no one. Success in life is obtained by preparing for the future (Kirmayer, Simpson, & Cargo, 2007).

Some other traditions view the family as central to one's identity, and family interdependence and group decision making are the norm. Body–mind–spirit is seen as a single entity (Chan, Ng, Ho, et al., 2006). For example, such ideas predominate in Eastern world views, prevalent in Asia and among many Asian immigrants, and are based on the ancient beliefs of Chinese and Indian philosophers and the spiritual traditions of Confucianism, Buddhism, and Taoism (Chiu, Ganesan, Clark, et al., 2005). Time is circular and recurring, hence a belief in reincarnation. One is born into an unchangeable fate and has a duty to comply. Similarly, the magico-religious view perceives illness as imposed by the gods or fates and, therefore, beyond individual control.

The traditional world views of Canadian Aboriginals concur with the holistic paradigm with overlap into the magico-religious view. Concepts of interconnectedness, balance, harmony, spirituality, and kinship are central to Aboriginal peoples' world views, as represented by the medicine wheel (see Figure 7-1). The medicine wheel is an ancient symbol that can be interpreted in many ways: the four directions, the four grandfathers, the four components of human nature (physical, mental, spiritual, and emotional). It represents a holistic world view of health and illness based on deep personal connections to the natural world and the tribe (Bopp, Bopp, Brown, et al., 1984).

Table 7-3 compares three world views' explanations of health and illness.

Psychiatric mental health nursing theories and methods originate within a cultural tradition. Consider how your assumptions about personality development, emotional expression, ego boundaries, and interpersonal relationships were formed and how they affect your clinical judgements. Nursing care is designed to promote verbalization of feelings, teach individually focused coping skills, and assist with behavioural and emotional self-control—all consistent with Western cultural ideals. However, all nurses are likely to come into contact with world views that differ from the philosophical traditions of

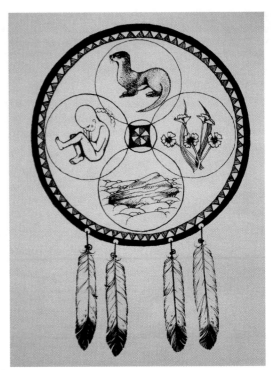

**FIGURE 7-1** "The medicine wheel is a symbolic tool that helps us to see interconnectedness of our being with the rest of creation." **Source:** Lane, P., Bopp, M., Bopp, J., et al. (2003) *The sacred tree* (3rd ed., p. 41). Lethbridge, AB: Four Worlds International Institute for Human and Community Development.

Western cultures, and these world views will influence nursing assessments and interventions. Being open to the rich diversity of world views and their impact on mental health and illness is fundamental to culturally competent nursing care. Failing to consider or attempt to understand the world view of the patient and the family will lead to a loss of meaningful communication and an inability to establish trust, the cornerstone of psychiatric mental health nursing. As nurses begin to acknowledge that many of the concepts and interventions enshrined in psychiatric mental health nursing are based on beliefs different from those of many clients and families, they will progress toward culturally sensitive and competent practice.

## CULTURE, MENTAL HEALTH, AND MENTAL ILLNESS

Cultures are dynamic, changing, and adjusting in relation to their histories and influences from the "outside" world. The pervasive experience of day-to-day cultural interactions shapes the mental health of both client and health care provider and influences how assessments and observations are conducted (Lo & Pottinger, 2007).

For all cross-cultural encounters, nurses must develop generic cultural competence inclusive of knowledge of the culture's values, locus of control, norms around emotional expression, and perspectives on time. Specific cultural competence is required to work with individual ethnocultural communities to ensure understanding of community norms (Lo & Pottinger,

| TABLE 7-3   WORLD VIEWS | SCIENTIFIC OR BIOMEDICAL | RELIGIOUS | HOLISTIC |
|---|---|---|---|
| General beliefs | Newest paradigm<br>Belief in human manipulation of chemical and physical processes<br>Reductionism: all life can be reduced to smaller components<br>Determinism: cause and effect can explain everything<br>Mechanism: life forms are viewed as parallel to machines | Belief in God or gods<br>Supernatural controls fate, illness, and health | Ancient viewpoint<br>Balance and harmony in individual and nature must be aligned for health<br>Natural laws are important to uphold<br>Concepts of the Aboriginal medicine wheel and Chinese yin and yang—ideas of balance of natural forces to promote harmony |
| Dominant cultures | The Western world embraces the biomedical model's explanations of disease and health | Many Latino, African, Caribbean, and Middle Eastern cultures support this view | Aboriginal and Asian peoples' traditional perspectives<br>Increasingly accepted in the Western world |
| Responsibility for health | Individual has responsibility for his or her health | Sense of community: one person's actions may have caused the illness or health of an individual | Mind, body, and spirit are considered so united that there may not be words to indicate them as distinct entities |
| Explaining illness | Does not consider mystical explanations | A belief in sorcery, breaking of taboos, *mal de ojo* (evil eye), God's will; illness may be a gift whereby one is given responsibility to accept the illness; health is a blessing | Considers explanation of disharmony and imbalance in the cosmos, resulting in illness |
| Prevention and cure | Science will cure or treat the disease | Prayer alone may change the health of the ill person<br>Techniques include laying on of hands and healing oils | Prevention and living well are the focus, not cure |

**Source:** Adapted from Andrews, M.M., & Boyle, J. (2008). *Transcultural concepts in nursing care* (5th ed.). New York: Lippincott.

2007). It is important to avoid stereotyping, the generalized conscious or unconscious conceptualization of a group of people that does not allow for individual differences within the group (Srivastava, 2007). For example, while many Aboriginal people are reconnecting with their traditional roots, other Aboriginal people may align themselves with Christian perspectives or have a mix of world views.

Diagnostic assessment of a mental illness is based on the interpretation of clinical behaviours and is guided by criteria from the *Diagnostic and Statistical Manual* (*DSM*), which historically has undervalued sociocultural interpretations of mental health and mental illness. Due to globalization, migration, and the international use of the *DSM-IV*, the new *DSM-5* has broadened the sociocultural considerations within assessment and diagnoses (Alarcon, Becker, Lewis-Fernandez, et al., 2009). This effort addresses the critiques of insensitivity to the context of people's lives and a lack of cultural awareness within previous editions (O'Mahony & Donnelly, 2007).

Understanding the cultural norms of ethnic groups is necessary to accurately assess behaviours, affect, and cognitions within the context of culture. For example, in Western culture, emotional expressiveness is valued, but some other cultures consider such expressiveness a sign of immaturity. In Western culture, independence and self-reliance are highly valued while the family interdependence valued by other cultures may be considered pathological enmeshment. Classic work by Kleinman (1980) and Kleinman, Eisenberg, and Good (1978) proposed that the environment and culture in which one lives determine the experience of health and illness and the value of treatment options. As such, nurses need to understand the perceptions and behaviours of patients and families within their cultural experience.

Each culture has different patterns of nonverbal communication (see Table 7-4), etiquette norms (see Box 7-1), beliefs, and values that shape the culture and influence how the culture understands health and illness.

Culture is transmitted to its members through a process called enculturation. Children learn from parents which behaviours, beliefs, values, and actions are "right" and which are "wrong." The culture outlines its acceptable range of options. Deviance from cultural expectations is problematic and frequently is labelled "illness." Mental health is perceived as the degree to which a person fulfills the expectations of the culture. The culture defines which differences are within the range of normal (mentally healthy) and which are outside the range of normal (mentally ill). The same thoughts and behaviours

## TABLE 7-4    SELECTED NONVERBAL COMMUNICATION PATTERNS

People perceive strong messages from nonverbal communication. The same nonverbal communication can be interpreted differently among cultures. In North American culture, eye contact is a sign of respectful attention. In other cultures, it may be considered arrogant and intrusive. Dr. Clare Brandt, the first Aboriginal psychiatrist in Canada, noted that often Aboriginal children's behaviours were erroneously assessed as pathological when judged within the dominant cultural norms. In reality, the children's behaviours were culturally appropriate (Brandt, 1990).

| NONVERBAL COMMUNICATION PATTERN | PREDOMINANT PATTERNS IN WESTERN SOCIETY | PATTERNS SEEN IN OTHER CULTURES |
|---|---|---|
| Eye contact | Associated with attentiveness, politeness, respect, honesty, and self-confidence | Associated with rudeness, arrogance, challenge, or sexual interest |
| Personal space | *Intimate space*: 0-0.5 m <br> *Personal space*: 0.5–1 m <br> Entering the intimate space of another person is perceived as aggressive, overbearing, and offensive. Staying more distant than expected is perceived as aloofness. | Personal space is significantly closer or more distant than in North American culture. <br> *Closer*—Middle Eastern, Southern European, and Latin American cultures <br> *Farther*—Asian cultures <br> When closer is the norm, standing close indicates acceptance of the other. |
| Touch | Moderate touch indicates personal warmth and conveys caring. <br> Often people will ask prior to touching an individual. | Touch norms vary. <br> *Low-touch cultures*—Touch may be considered an overt sexual gesture, a way of "stealing the spirit," or a taboo between women and men. <br> *High-touch cultures*—People frequently touch one another (e.g., linking arms when walking or holding a hand or arm when talking). |
| Facial expressions and gestures | A nod means "yes." <br> Smiling and nodding means "I agree." <br> Thumbs-up means "good job." <br> Rolling one's eyes while another is talking is an insult. | Raising eyebrows or rolling the head from side to side means "yes." <br> Smiling and nodding means "I respect you." <br> Thumbs-up is an obscene gesture. <br> Pointing one's foot at another is an insult. |

**Source:** Adapted from Narayan, M.C. (2004). Cultural implications for psychiatric mental health nursing. In E.M. Varcarolis & M.J. Halter (Eds.), *Foundations of psychiatric mental health nursing: A clinical approach* (Table 6-3, p. 105). St. Louis, MO: Saunders.

## BOX 7-1    NORMS OF ETIQUETTE

Rules for polite behaviour vary greatly from one culture to another. Unless aware of cultural differences in etiquette norms, nurses can infer rudeness from patients who may believe their behaviour to be respectful. Norms of etiquette that vary across cultures include the following:

- Expectation and importance of promptness
- Formality in addressing others
- Which people deserve recognition and honour, and how respect is shown
- Forms of appropriate social touch—for example, shaking hands
- Wearing shoes in the home
- Appropriate dress to be "modest"
- The meaning of acceptance or rejection of hospitality, such as food or drink
- The importance of and length of time that should be given to "small talk" prior to the business at hand
- The directness or subtlety of communication
- The tone of voice and pace of the conversation
- Taboo topics
- The treatment of children in the home—for example, can they be touched and admired?

considered mentally healthy in one culture can be considered mentally ill in another. For example, many religious traditions view "speaking in tongues" as mentally healthy and as a gift from God, whereas a different cultural group might perceive this activity as psychosis and a sign of mental illness.

Cultural interpretation of behaviours creates challenges for the nurse in conducting appropriate assessments and treatments. Professional socialization and ethnocentrism may cause nurses to unintentionally impose their own cultural norms on members of other cultural groups (Leininger & McFarland, 2006). Ongoing self-awareness can provide clarity about personal and professional beliefs and encourage openness to alternative cultural explanations.

## BARRIERS TO QUALITY MENTAL HEALTH SERVICES

Nurses may encounter various practice issues when providing care to culturally diverse clients and their families, including communication barriers, unique issues around stigma and discrimination, misdiagnosis of patients due to unrecognized cultural differences, and ethnic variations in pharmacodynamics.

## Communication Barriers

Therapeutic communication is key to nursing care, yet in Canada, nurses and clients and families often do not even speak the same language. In addition, emotional states can be difficult to accurately describe even in one's native tongue. In mental health nursing, communication and collateral data are important methods used to understand a client's situation. When a language barrier prevents understanding of what is happening, problems are likely to occur: for the client, hesitancy to seek out mental health services, and for the nurse, a tendency to avoid or stereotype certain patients. O'Mahony and Donnelly (2007) found, for example, that Asian immigrants underutilized health care services due to language barriers and cultural beliefs about health and treatment options.

The use of translators is one strategy for overcoming communication barriers. Several cautions apply when a professional translator is used. The translator should be informed that his or her role is to translate what the client or family state, not to apply meaning to the client's communication (O'Mahony & Donnelly, 2007). The translator should be matched to the patient as closely as possible in gender, age, social status, and religion. The translator alerts the nurse to the meaning of cultural norms and thus acts as a cultural broker, interpreting both language and culture. Translators should not be relatives or friends of the patient since the stigma of mental illness may prevent accurate portrayal of the situation (Srivastava, 2007). As well, informal translators may not have the language skills to meet the complex demands of translation in health care settings. Certain concepts may be so strongly culturally linked that an adequate translation is very difficult (Andrews & Boyle, 2008).

Nonverbal communication patterns are influenced by culture so also need to be interpreted within the context of the client's culture. For example, some Aboriginal cultures use silence to a far greater degree than the dominant Canadian culture does. This silence can be mistaken for belligerence or sullenness when, in fact, it is a common response to dealing with strangers, shows respect, and may be considered a sign of wisdom, as the patient is taking time to think things over (McCormick, 2009).

## Stigma and Discrimination

The ten-year anti-stigma campaign Opening Minds, initiated by the Mental Health Commission of Canada (MHCC) in 2009, recognizes that stigma and discrimination are a reality people with mental illness face (Corrigan & Wassel, 2008). Cultural beliefs, superstitions, and poor understanding of mental illness contribute to fear, stereotyping, and avoidance of people with mental illness. This stigma results in people concealing their illness and delaying or refusing treatment and follow-up care (Corrigan, Morris, Michaels, et al., 2012; Corrigan & Wassel, 2008). People with mental illness and their families face stigma and stigma by association because of mental illness. Stigma affects health determinants such as housing since discrimination limits consumers' abilities to secure safe and affordable housing. People with co-morbid mental illness and physical disability are doubly jeopardized by stigma from society and health care professionals (Bahm & Forchuk, 2008).

The reality of living with a mental illness is further complicated within a multicultural context. In cultural groups that emphasize the interdependence and harmony of the family, mental illness may be perceived as a failure of the family. In such groups, the pressures on both the individual with the mental illness and the family are increased since the illness reflects on the character of all family members. Stigma and shame impede health-seeking behaviour; therefore, members of these cultural groups may enter the mental health care system only at an advanced stage of illness, when the family has exhausted its ability to cope with the problem.

## Misdiagnosis

One reason for misdiagnosis of mental illness in culturally diverse people is the use of culturally inappropriate psychometric instruments and diagnostic tools. Most available tools have been validated using subjects of European origin. For instance, Kim (2002) stated that although there are over 40 validated depression scales, they tend to be "linguistically irrelevant and culturally inappropriate" (p. 110) for some groups. Kim argues that the current scales measure Western ways of expressing depression by focusing on the affective domain, whereas, for others, more attention needs to be given to the somatic domain. In cultures in which the body and mind are seen as one entity, or in cultures in which there is a high degree of stigma associated with mental illness, people frequently *somatize* their feelings of psychological distress. With somatization, psychological distress is experienced as physical problems instead of being perceived as emotional or affective pain. For example, a Cambodian woman may describe feelings of back pain, fatigue, and dizziness and say nothing about feelings of sadness or hopelessness (Henderson, Yeung, Fan, et al., 2008). Many cross-cultural mental health experts are skeptical about using the criteria of the *DSM* for diagnosing mental illness, because the criteria are based on studies that do not represent cultural diversity (Marsella, 2003). *DSM-5* has addressed some of these concerns.

The Glossary of Cultural Concepts of Distress in the *DSM-5* was an attempt to recognize cultural presentations of illness. Cultural Concepts of Distress are sets of signs and symptoms that are common in a limited number of cultures but virtually nonexistent in most other cultural groups (Henderson, Yeung, Fan, et al., 2008) (see Box 7-2).

Cultural concepts of distress or illnesses may seem irrational to Canadian-trained nurses as these illnesses are difficult to understand from a Western biomedical perspective. However, these illnesses are well understood by the cultural group who can name the problem, its etiology, its course, and its treatment. When treated in culturally prescribed ways, the remedies are frequently effective. Kleinman's classic work serves as a guide to how culture is interlinked with health, illness, and health care. Kleinman (1980) suggested that three sectors of influence—professional, popular (family, community, social network), and folk—interact. Negotiations between the client, family, and health care provider were critical and must consider the culture, history, and environment of the client. Some of the cultural concepts of distress appear to be mental health problems that manifest in somatic ways. For example, *Hwa-Byung* and

## BOX 7-2 EXAMPLES OF CULTURAL CONCEPTS OF DISTRESS

Following are examples of commonly recognized cultural concepts of distress:

- **Ataque de nervios**: Latin American. Characterized by a sudden attack of trembling, palpitations, dyspnea, dizziness, and loss of consciousness. Thought to be caused by an evil spirit and related to intolerable stress. Treated by an *espiritista* (spiritual healer) and by family and community support, which provides aid and considers the patient to be calling for help in a culturally acceptable way.
- **Ghost sickness**: Navajo. Characterized by "being out of one's mind," dyspnea, weakness, and bad dreams. Thought to be caused by an evil spirit. Treated by overcoming the evil spirit with a stronger spiritual force that the healer, a "singer," calls forth through a powerful healing ritual.
- **Being hit by bad medicine**: Aboriginal. Characterized by feelings of malaise (emotional, physical, psychological, and spiritual) caused by deliberate use of bad medicine by another; believed to be able to cause death (E.G. McGillivary, personal communication, January 7, 2012).
- **Hwa-Byung**: Korean. Characterized by epigastric pain, anorexia, palpitations, dyspnea, and muscle aches and pains. Thought to be caused by a lack of harmony and suppressed anger. Treated by re-establishing harmony.
- **Neurasthenia**: Chinese. Characterized by somatic symptoms of depression (e.g., anorexia, weight loss, fatigue, weakness, trouble concentrating, insomnia), although feelings of sadness or depression are denied. Thought to be related to a lack of yin–yang balance.
- **Susto**: Latin American. Characterized by a broad range of somatic and psychological symptoms. Thought to be related to a traumatic incident or fright that caused the patient's soul to leave the body. Treated by an *espiritista* (spiritual healer).
- **Wind illness**: Chinese, Vietnamese. Characterized by a fear of cold, wind, or drafts. Derived from the belief that yin–yang and hot–cold elements must be in balance or illness occurs. Treated by keeping very warm and avoiding foods, drinks, and herbs that are considered to have a cold quality, as well as "cold" colours, emotions, and activities. Also treated by pulling the "cold wind" out of the patient by coining (vigorously rubbing a coin over the body) or cupping (applying a heated cup to the skin, creating a vacuum).

neurasthenia have many similarities to depression (Park, Kim, Kang, et al., 2001), but because the somatic complaints are prominent, and patients deny feelings of sadness or depression, the symptoms may not fit the *DSM-5* diagnostic criteria for depression.

*Ataque de nervios* and ghost sickness are characterized by abnormal behaviours culturally understood as illness and are culturally acceptable ways to express overwhelming stress. *Susto*, or "soul loss," occurs after a traumatic incident (Lim, 2006). From a Western perspective, the client may be experiencing depression, anxiety, or post-traumatic stress disorder, but the patient believes he or she is experiencing the illness of soul loss. Similarly, some Aboriginal people will strongly believe that their symptoms are caused by "bad medicine" deliberately sent to harm them (E.G. McGillivary, personal communication, Personal communications are not put on the reference list (APA,

p. 179, 6.20) January 7, 2012). Some authors have suggested that anorexia nervosa and bulimia may be bound to European and North American cultural groups that place a high value on thinness (Marsella, 2003).

If culture is not considered in diagnosis and treatment, we are more likely to see culturally normal behaviour as "abnormal" instead of merely different. For example, what some may view as delusional or hallucinatory behaviour may be part of a vision quest from an Aboriginal perspective. Ross (1992) suggested that historical experiences of trauma were compounded by a loss of cultural traditions such as dance or song that would have helped Aboriginal people express and grieve their losses. Such historical experiences of many Aboriginal peoples may have made them more attuned to their senses and receptive to alternative ways of being. Nurses often work in environments that are steeped in biomedical perspectives, which may insidiously devalue cultural sensitivity and not sanction time to fully incorporate other potential perspectives. Nurses require ongoing education to understand alternative explanations for illness and to develop cultural competence in their practice (Registered Nurses' Association of Ontario, 2007).

### Ethnic Variation in Pharmacodynamics

There is a growing realization that the actions and effects of many drugs vary among diverse genetic–ethnic groups of people. For example, findings from drug studies performed with Euro-American subjects may not be valid for other ethnically diverse populations. Genetic variations in drug metabolism are documented for several drugs classifications, including antidepressants and antipsychotics (Henderson, Yeung, Fan, et al., 2008). The relatively new field of ethnopharmacology investigates the genetic and ethnic variations in drug pharmacokinetics. Many drugs are metabolized in part by the more than 20 cytochrome P-450 (CYP) enzymes present in human beings (Henderson, Yeung, Fan, et al., 2008). Genetic variations in enzymes, however, may alter drug metabolism and tend to be propagated through different racial and ethnic populations (Henderson, Yeung, Fan, et al., 2008). Some genetic variations result in rapid metabolism, resulting in minimization of the therapeutic effects; others may result in poor metabolism. With slow metabolism, serum levels become high, increasing intolerable adverse effects. Current practice requires that nurses be aware of ethnic variations in drug metabolism and monitor for unwanted adverse effects. Munoz and Hilgenberg (2005) have suggested the following interventions to minimize risk:

- Maintain a knowledge base on drugs likely to cause adverse responses in people from various ethnic groups.
- Monitor and document drug responses, and give the lowest possible safe dose.
- Carry out cultural assessments with all patients.
- Incorporate cultural context in nursing education to client and family.

## POPULATIONS AT RISK FOR MENTAL HEALTH PROBLEMS AND COMPROMISED CARE

Distinct cultural groups that are at risk for mental health problems and potentially compromised care are Aboriginal peoples

(First Nations peoples, Inuit, and Métis), immigrants, and refugees.

## Aboriginal Peoples

The residential school system enforced on Aboriginal populations and government assimilation policies have led to a history of oppression and contributed to the mental health problems of Aboriginal peoples. The residential school system began in Canada in the early seventeenth century, evolved to the modern residential schools of the 1880s, and finally began to be phased out in the 1960s, with the last Canadian government–operated school closing in 1996. The residential school system was created to assimilate First Nations children into the dominant Canadian European culture and to suppress indigenous values, which were considered inferior (Legacy of Hope Foundation, 2010a, 2010b). Children were removed from their homes and placed in schools often many miles away from their parents. They were forbidden to speak their languages and to practise their culture. Many children were physically, sexually, and emotionally abused (Legacy of Hope Foundation, 2010a, 2010b). These experiences have resulted in intergenerational trauma and a loss of parenting skill, resulting in a breakdown of family and community structures and social and economic problems within Aboriginal communities (Legacy of Hope Foundation, 2010a, 2010b).

While general psychiatric treatment focuses on individuals, the problems affecting the mental health of many Aboriginal people are problems relating with others, including family members, social networks, their communities, and governmental structures (Kirmayer, Brass, & Valaskakis, 2009). The impact of colonization—the process whereby a people are overcome by a more powerful group, and the views, philosophies, values, and beliefs of the powerful group are imposed on the original inhabitants of the land—has left a legacy of grief for many Aboriginal people, who live with historical oppression, the effects of post-colonization, and a lack of culturally appropriate and sensitive mental health therapies. This legacy of colonization contributes to the elevated rates of alcoholism, suicide, domestic violence, and community demoralization, in addition to the social problems experienced in many communities (Kirmayer, Tait, & Simpson, 2009). For example, the Inuit people of Nunavut face tremendous social problems with high incidences of suicide, domestic violence, and substance abuse, as well as overcrowding, unemployment, and legal difficulties. Societal changes, socio-economic conditions, and interpersonal problems contribute to increased mental health needs (Law & Hutton, 2007). Suicide rates of Aboriginal youth are three to six times the rate of that of the general Canadian population, and in some communities, these youth suicides have occurred in clusters (Niezen, 2009). High rates of family violence, sexual abuse, incarceration, and emotional distress underscore the significance of historical trauma on the current mental health and societal problems facing many Aboriginal people (Statistics Canada, 2006). The multiple traumas and revictimization that many Aboriginal people endure are linked to complex trauma responses, which require strong culturally sensitive intervention programs.

Despite a high proportion of mental health problems, mental health services are underused by Aboriginal people. Historical

| BOX 7-3 | KEY CONCEPTS OF ABORIGINAL TRADITIONAL WORLD VIEWS |
| --- | --- |

- Medicine wheel concept representing holism and interconnectedness
- Balance of emotional, physical, spiritual, and mental
- Interconnectedness in the web of life: all relations
- Four colours of the world's peoples: white, red, yellow, black
- Importance of ceremony: sweat lodges, sun dances, pow-wows, potlatch
- Connection to the land, Mother Earth, and Father Sky
- The four directions and their gifts
- Animal powers and metaphors
- Storytelling, dancing, and singing as healing guides
- Noninterference
- Honouring of ancestors, ancient wisdom, and oral histories
- Spirituality: belief in Creator, Manitou, and the supernatural—dreams, visions, and the afterlife
- Time: the impact of decisions and actions on seven generations

**Sources:** Blackstock, C., Bruyere, D., & Moreau, E. (2006). *Many hands, one dream: Principles for a new perspective on the health of First Nations, Inuit and Métis children and youth.* Ottawa: Canadian Paediatric Society; Bopp, J., Bopp, M., Brown, L., et al. (1984). *The sacred tree.* Lethbridge, AB: Four Worlds International Institute for Community and Human Development; and Ross, R. (1992). *Dancing with a ghost: Exploring Indian reality.* Toronto: Reed Books.

loss has caused anger, discomfort around White people, and mistrust of their intentions, which have impacted Aboriginal people's use of services dominated by Western ideologies and non-Aboriginal professionals (Kirmayer, Brass, & Valaskakis, 2009). Consideration of the impact of the collective identity and political situations of Aboriginal people is crucial for promoting healing (McCormick, 2009). However, most mental health services do not incorporate an Aboriginal understanding of mental health, illness, and healing.

While there is diversity among the many groups of Aboriginal peoples, some key traditional world views are shared (see Box 7-3).

## Immigrants

Eighteen percent of the Canadian population are immigrants. Generally, immigrants to Canada are more physically and mentally healthy and use the health care system less than the Canadian-born population. This reality may be because of strong entry-screening measures. Immigrants' health issues and health care system use align with those of the Canadian-born population as their length of residence increases (Statistics Canada, 2002).

While data on mental health problems and mental illness are sparse, certain factors may predispose immigrants to mental health problems. During their first ten years in Canada, 30% live in poverty, a known risk factor for developing mental health problems. Immigrants may experience acculturative stress in attempting to adapt to a new culture, negotiating new norms, and seeking meaningful employment (Samuel, 2009). For example, South Asian immigrant women in Atlantic Canada experienced acculturative stress in several ways: (1) self-perceived inability to adapt to the new country, (2) limited employment, (3) discrimination, (4) depression, and (5) inter-family and intergenerational conflicts (Samuel, 2009). In a study documenting the experiences of Chinese immigrant women in Canada, adverse life events related to employment and financial strain in the settlement period contributed to their sense of depression (Tang, Oatley, & Toner, 2007). Immigrant women are particularly vulnerable to mental illness and mental health problems due to their multiple social roles and limited autonomy (Reitmanova & Gustafson, 2009). In addition to assisting immigrants in a meaningful manner, services need to be language- and culturally sensitive and based on an understanding of the social context in which immigrants and refugees live (Chow, Law, & Andermann, 2009; Simich, Maiter, Moorlag, et al., 2009).

Immigrants and their families embark on a process of acculturation—learning and adopting the beliefs, values, and practices of their new cultural setting. Some immigrants adapt to the new culture quickly, absorbing the new world view, beliefs, values, and practices until these are more natural than the ones they learned in their homeland (assimilation). Others attempt to maintain their traditional cultural ways. Some become bicultural—able to move between their traditional culture and new culture, depending on where they are and with whom they associate. Some immigrants may suffer culture shock, finding the new norms disconcerting or offensive because they contrast so deeply with their traditional beliefs, values, and practices.

Children may assimilate into the new culture at a rapid pace while elders may maintain their traditional culture, predisposing families to intergenerational conflict. The hierarchical traditional status of elders may be challenged by children who are assimilating different values. Some children may feel caught between two cultures and unsure of where to place their cultural identity, similar to Aboriginal youth who feel a disconnect between traditional ways of living and modern society (Iarocci, Root, & Burack, 2009).

For immigrants, accessing mental health services may be problematic due to language barriers and stigma. Materials about mental illness and mental health care are needed in a variety of languages, in conjunction with strong outreach services (O'Mahony & Donnelly, 2007). Resources outside of formal medical services, such as social workers, health workers, and enhanced family support workers, may be better able to offer suitable services (Lai, 2007). Note that some Aboriginal people who do not speak English as a first language will experience some of the same issues related to accessing mental health services.

## Refugees

A refugee is a person who is seeking asylum in a new country due to threat of trauma or actual trauma and violation of human rights. Refugees have left their homeland to escape intolerable conditions. Refugee families, inclusive of their children, may require mental health assistance to adjust to their new surroundings and to feel a sense of safety and security.

## RESEARCH HIGHLIGHT
### Street-Involved Youth and Self-Esteem

**Source:** McCay, E., Langley, J., Beanlands, H, et al. (2010). Mental health challenges and strengths of street-involved youth: The need for a multi-determined approach. *Canadian Journal of Nursing Research, 42*(3), 31–49.

**Problem**
Street-involved youth have their own specific culture that helps them to survive on the street. Unfortunately, life on the streets often leads to a downward spiral of self-destructive behaviours, such as self-harm, drug abuse, and survival sex.

**Purpose of Study**
To understand illness symptoms, as well as resilience and self-esteem within street-involved youth.

**Methods**
This mixed-methods study (standardized questionnaires and two focus groups) included a convenience sample of 70 homeless youth.

**Key Findings**
While youth were found to have higher rates of mental illness symptomology, they also experienced moderately high levels of resilience and self-esteem. Self-esteem is a strong protective factor for street-involved youth, and programs delivering mental health services must include mental wellness strategies to promote strong self-esteem and resilience, as well as treatment of mental illness.

**Implications for Nursing Practice**
Research findings from this study encourage nurses to consider the strengths and resilience of street youth and to build on and use their strengths to make positive health changes. Youth involved in the street culture may be stereotyped and discriminated against. Findings from this research challenge nurses to look for strengths and reframe negative assumptions.

Many refugees from Southeast Asia, Central America, and Africa have been traumatized by war, genocide, torture, starvation, and other catastrophic events. Many have lost family members, a way of life, and a homeland to which they can never return. Refugees are at increased risk for post-traumatic stress disorder related to their past experiences (Statistics Canada, 2006).

## Culture of Poverty

Individuals and families living in poverty are vulnerable to a variety of disadvantages and limited opportunities for education and employment. Living in poverty subjects people to bias and discrimination that diminishes self-esteem and self-efficacy, contributing to exclusion and marginalization. *Relative poverty* refers to inequities in material resources across segments of the population—that is, between "the haves" and "the have-nots." In Canada, this gap is widening, which is cause for concern. The most impoverished group is Aboriginal women who use intravenous drugs, perform dangerous sex work, and have human immunodeficiency virus (HIV) or acquired immune deficiency syndrome (AIDS) (Elo, Mykyta, Margolis, et al., 2009).

## CULTURALLY COMPETENT CARE

As discussed, nurses require cultural competence to assist patients and their families to maintain and achieve mental health and well-being. With the changing demographics of Canadian society, the recognition of the legacy of residential schools, and the effects of poverty, nurses in community and acute psychiatric care environments will routinely encounter patients whose lived experiences challenge nurses to examine ethnocentric views and be open to alternative explanations of behaviours. But how, exactly, are psychiatric mental health nurses to practise culturally competent care?

Cultural competence is the ability of nurses to apply knowledge and skill appropriately in cross-cultural situations (Srivastava, 2007). Having cultural sensitivity or awareness is an essential component of cultural competence. Culturally competent care goes beyond culturally sensitive care by adapting care to meet the patient's cultural needs and preferences (Narayan, 2006).

Campinha-Bacote (2007, 2008) constructed a model, the Process of Cultural Competence in the Delivery of Healthcare Services, to assist nurses in providing culturally competent care. This model requires nurses to view themselves as becoming culturally competent and to see themselves as lifelong learners, open to learning from the immense cultural diversity of patients and families. The model consists of five constructs that promote the journey toward cultural competence:

1. Cultural awareness
2. Cultural knowledge
3. Cultural encounters
4. Cultural skill
5. Cultural desire

### Cultural Awareness

The culturally aware nurse recognizes the enormous impact culture makes on patients' health values and practices, how and when patients decide they are ill and need care, and what treatments they will seek when illness occurs. Cultural awareness encourages nurses to practise self-awareness and recognize that the norms of their own ethnic and professional cultures seem "right" (ethnocentrism) but only because these norms are what they know. Cultural awareness guides the nurse to examine all beliefs, values, and practices to ascertain which are cultural and which may be universally held (Campinha-Bacote, 2007). The process of cultural awareness and cultural humility guides the nurse to recognize ethnocentricity and remain respectful of each patient's cultural norms.

Nurses who examine their cultural definitions and underlying assumptions of mental health and illness, "healthy" self-concept, "healthy" family, and the "right way" to behave in society are practising cultural awareness. Assumptions and expectations about how people express psychological

distress require consideration in all assessments. Culturally biased assumptions may be the foundation of evidence-informed guidelines (derived from studies with dominant populations), so guidelines may thus require modification to address cultural diversity within nursing practice (Campinha-Bacote, 2002).

The Registered Nurses' Association of Ontario's (2007) document on cultural diversity suggests that four key concepts influence the delivery of culturally sensitive care within a culturally sensitive health care environment: globalization of society, human rights issues, workplace environment, and nursing shortages. Health care organizations are positively affected by a climate of diversity, group diversity (e.g., inclusion, communication, knowledge sharing), and individual characteristics related to cultural background, ethnicity, values, and beliefs.

### Cultural Knowledge

Nurses can enhance their cultural knowledge by attending cultural events and programs, developing friendships with members of diverse cultural groups, and participating in events at which members of diverse groups speak. Cultural knowledge may also be obtained by studying resources designed for health care providers. Cultural knowledge increases our awareness of diverse world views and values, alerts us to cultural differences, deepens our understanding of behaviours that might otherwise be misinterpreted. Cultural knowledge helps nurses establish rapport, ask the right questions, avoid misunderstandings, and identify cultural variables that may need to be considered when planning nursing care (Narayan, 2002).

### Cultural Encounters

Srivastava (2007) differentiates between stereotyping and the making of generalizations, noting that making generalizations that identify patterns of behaviour and knowledge related to a culture can be a helpful starting point for nurses. However, nurses need to be cautious about stereotyping people and acknowledge that there are individual variations within any culture. Individuals are a unique blend of the many ethnic, religious, socioeconomic, geographical, educational, and occupational cultures to which they belong. They have unique personalities, life experiences, and creative thoughts that contribute to their self-development and to the choices they make about which cultural norms to adopt or abandon.

Multiple cultural encounters enable nurses to personally experience diversity within cultural groups and help them understand that, although there are patterns that characterize a culture, individual members may adhere to the culture's norms in diverse ways. Through such encounters, nurses can develop confidence in cross-cultural interactions and skill at recognizing and avoiding the cultural pain that can occur when nursing care causes the patient discomfort or offence by failing to be culturally sensitive (Kavanagh, 2008). Nurses can become aware of signs of cultural pain (e.g., a patient's feeling of alienation) and recover trust and rapport by asking what has caused the offence, apologizing for insensitivity, and expressing willingness to provide culturally sensitive care.

BOX 7-4 **SOME CULTURAL CLINICAL GUIDELINES AND ASSESSMENT TOOLS**

- Giger and Davidhizar's Assessment of Family (in *Transcultural Nursing: Assessment and Intervention*, third edition, pages 10–11)
- Leininger's Inquiry Guide for Kinship and Social Factors (in *Transcultural Nursing: Concepts, Theories, Research and Practice*, third edition, page 137)
- Calgary Family Assessment Model (http://www.family nursingresources.com/dvds.htm)
- Nova Scotia Department of Health's *The Process of Cultural Competence in the Delivery of Health Care Services* (http://www.healthteamnovascotia.ca/cultural_competence/Cultural_Competence_guide_for_Primary_Health_Care_Professionals.pdf)
- Regional Health Authority Central Manitoba's *Culturally Appropriate Healing Services* (http://www.rha-central.mb.ca/service.php?id=178)
- College of Nurses of Ontario's *Practice Guideline: Culturally Sensitive Care* (http://www.cno.org/Global/docs/prac/41040_CulturallySens.pdf)
- Aboriginal Nurses Association of Canada's Cultural Competence and Cultural Safety in First Nations, Inuit and Métis Nursing Education (https://www.uleth.ca/dspace/bitstream/handle/10133/720/An_Integrated_Review_of_the_Literature.pdf?sequence=1)

## Cultural Skill

Cultural skill is the ability to perform a cultural assessment in a sensitive way (Campinha-Bacote, 2008). A nurse's first step should be to ensure that meaningful communication can occur. If there is a language barrier, a professional medical translator should be engaged.

Many cultural clinical guidelines and assessment tools are available to guide psychiatric mental health nurses in multicultural practice (see Box 7-4). For example, Kleinman, Eisenberg, and Good (1978) proposed the following questions as a useful mental health assessment tool:

- What do you call this illness? (diagnosis)
- When did it start? Why then? (onset)
- What do you think caused it? (etiology)
- How does the illness work? What does it do to you? (course)
- How long will it last? Is it serious? (prognosis)
- How have you treated the illness? How do you think it should be treated? (treatment)
- These questions allow the patient to feel heard and understood and elicit information about cultural concepts of distress. They can be expanded to include questions such as the following:
- What are the chief problems this illness has caused you?
- What do you fear most about this illness? Do you think it is curable?
- Do you know others who have had this problem? What happened to them? Do you think this will happen to you?

A conversational approach is generally more effective than using a direct, formal approach. One indirect technique is to ask the patient, "What does your family think is wrong? Why do they think it started? What do they think you should do about it?" After the patient describes what the family thinks, the nurse can ask in a nonjudgemental manner if the patient agrees.

Another technique for promoting openness is to make a declaratory statement before asking the questions. For instance, before asking about cultural treatments the patient has tried, the nurse can first say, "Everyone has remedies they find helpful when they are ill. Are there any special healers or treatments you have used or that you think might be helpful?"

Some areas that deserve special attention during an assessment interview are the following:

- Ethnicity, religious affiliation, and degree of acculturation to Western medical culture
- Spiritual practices important to preserving or regaining health
- Degree of proficiency in speaking and reading English
- Dietary patterns, including foods prescribed for sick people
- Attitudes about and experiences with pain in a Western medical setting
- Attitudes about and experience with Western medications
- Cultural remedies such as healers, herbs, and practices the patient may find helpful
- Who the patient considers "family," who should receive health information, and how decisions are made
- Cultural customs the patient feels are essential and is fearful will be violated in the mental health care setting

The purpose of a culturally sensitive assessment is to develop a therapeutic plan that is mutually agreeable, culturally acceptable, and potentially productive of positive outcomes. While gathering assessment data, nurses should identify cultural patterns that may support or interfere with the patient's health and recovery process. Nursing knowledge can then be used to categorize the patient's cultural norms into one of three different groups based on the Western medical perspective:

1. Those that facilitate the patient's health and recovery
2. Those that are neither helpful nor harmful
3. Those that are harmful to the patient's health and well-being

The first Canadian Aboriginal female psychiatrist, Corniela Wieman (2006), advised that Aboriginal clients will need time and opportunity to develop trust in a helping relationship. Further, some people will prefer traditional ways of healing.

A renegotiation of boundaries and the nurse's honouring the helpful components of traditional ways together with Western theories can form the basis of a culturally sensitive approach (Wieman, 2006). Including compatible culture-specific interventions assists nurses to build on the patient's coping and healing systems (see Box 7-4). For example, First Nations people with substance abuse problems may find ceremonies such as sweat lodges, sharing circles, and medicine wheel concepts more appropriate to their therapeutic program than standardized interventions. Finally, when cultural patterns are determined harmful, (e.g., if a patient is taking an herb that is contraindicated with the prescription medication), the nurse is responsible for alerting the patient and the mental health care team to these risks.

## Cultural Desire

The final construct in Campinha-Bacote's (2008) cultural competence model for psychiatric mental health nurses is cultural desire. Cultural desire indicates that the nurse is not acting out of a sense of duty but out of a genuine concern for the patient's welfare. Nurses exhibit cultural desire through patience, consideration, and empathy. Cultural desire enables the nurse to achieve good outcomes with culturally diverse patients.

## KEY POINTS TO REMEMBER

- Mental health and illness are biological, psychological, social, and cultural phenomena.
- With globalization, nurses will be caring for more people from diverse cultural groups.
- Nurses are challenged to deliver culturally competent care, inclusive of culturally congruent assessments and interventions.
- *Culture* is the shared beliefs, values, and practices of a group that shape their thinking and behaviour in patterned ways. Cultural groups share their norms with new members of the group through enculturation.
- A group's culture influences its members' world view, nonverbal communication patterns, etiquette norms, and ways of viewing the person, the family, and the "right" way to think and behave in society.
- The concept of mental health is formed within a culture, and deviance from cultural expectations can be defined as "illness" by other group members.
- Psychiatric mental health nursing is based on personality and developmental theories advanced by Europeans and Americans and grounded in Western cultural ideals and values.
- Nurses are influenced by their own professional and ethnic cultures, as are patients by their cultures. Nurses must guard against ethnocentric tendencies leading to cultural imposition.

- Barriers to quality mental health care include communication barriers, ethnic variations in psychotropic drug metabolism, and misdiagnoses caused by culturally inappropriate diagnostic tools.
- Colonization, including the residential school system and national assimilation policies, has resulted in intergenerational trauma of Canadian Aboriginal peoples, significantly contributing to their social and mental health problems.
- Living in poverty predisposes a person to mental health problems.
- Immigrants may experience acculturative stress related to resettlement. Refugees may develop post-traumatic stress because of past horrific experiences.
- Cultural competence consists of five constructs: cultural awareness, cultural knowledge, cultural encounters, cultural skill, and cultural desire.
- Through cultural awareness, nurses recognize their own cultural beliefs, values, and practices.
- Cultural knowledge is obtained by seeking cultural information from friends, attending cultural programs, immersing oneself in the culture, and consulting print and online sources.
- Cultural encounters help nurses avoid stereotyping individuals.
- Cultural desire is a genuine interest in the patient's perspective; it enables nurses to provide flexible and respectful care to patients of all cultures.

## CRITICAL THINKING

1. Describe the cultural factors that have influenced the development of Western psychiatric mental health nursing practice. Contrast these Western influences with the cultural factors that influence Aboriginal ways of healing.

2. Discuss the impact of assimilation policies such as the residential school system on the current mental health and social problems of Canadian Aboriginal peoples.

3. Analyze the effects cultural competence (or incompetence) can have on psychiatric mental health nurses, their patients, and patients' families.

4. How can barriers such as misdiagnosis and communication problems impede competent psychiatric mental health care? What can health care team members do to overcome such barriers?

5. Consider what types of programs might reinforce street youth's resilience and survival skills.

## CHAPTER REVIEW

1. Mr. Yeung, a recent immigrant from China, has been admitted to the observation unit for investigation of unspecified physical malaise. His family tells the nurse that Mr. Yeung began to exhibit certain behaviours when his import business declined and his creditors demanded money. He has subsequently made vague physical complaints for the past six weeks. Which patient behaviour would alert the nurse to the potential for somatization?

1. The patient states, "I am so sad that I don't know what to do."
2. The patient shows the nurse bottles of medication used to treat anxiety.
3. The patient presents with concerns involving back pain, dizziness, and fatigue.
4. The patient states, "My doctor diagnosed me with bipolar disorder."

2. Mr. Oliva has been admitted to the psychiatric ward for depression and substance abuse, mainly alcohol and recreational drugs. As you are explaining his diagnoses to him and the potential treatment plan, his wife and he state the problem is "ghost sickness," which came about when his mother died. What is the most therapeutic nursing response?
   1. "I have no idea what 'ghost sickness' is."
   2. "Please explain what you mean by 'ghost sickness.'"
   3. "There is not a disorder known as 'ghost sickness.'"
   4. "Why do you believe in evil spirits?"

3. You are a nurse in an outpatient well-baby clinic. You are planning care for a young First Nations Cree mother and her infant. The young mother has been identified as at risk for postpartum depression. Which intervention is most appropriate?
   1. Assess whether the patient follows traditional Cree beliefs
   2. Contact an elder from Aboriginal Services
   3. Discuss the medicine wheel concept of healing with the patient
   4. Contact a "singer" to provider a healing ritual within three days of admission

4. You are a nurse on a busy medical unit with a multicultural clientele. In your orientation to the unit, you learn that individualism is a concept closely aligned with North American values. When caring for clients with diverse cultural backgrounds, which general nursing action would be most appropriate?
   1. Maintain eye contact at all times
   2. Assume that personal space is significantly closer than the nurse's personal space
   3. State, "You can beat this diagnosis; you are in control of yourself"
   4. Ask if the family should be included in the decision-making process

5. You are a flight nurse who is bringing a young Inuit man from Nunavut for psychiatric assessment in a Winnipeg hospital. You assess the client as acutely suicidal. Which goal is appropriate?
   1. Patient will visit with a cultural leader from the Inuit community.
   2. Patient will experience rebalance of yin–yang by discharge.
   3. Patient will identify sources that increase "cold wind" within 24 hours of admission.
   4. Patient will be put on suicidal observation and assessment.

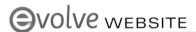 WEBSITE                                     Post-Test   interactive review

*Visit the Evolve Web site for Chapter Review Answers and Rationales, Critical Thinking Answer Guidelines, and additional resources related to the content in this chapter:* http://evolve.elsevier.com/Canada/Varcarolis/psychiatric/

## REFERENCES

Alarcon, R.D., Becker, A.E., Lewis-Fernandez, R., et al. (2009). Issues for DSM-V: The role of culture in psychiatric diagnosis. *The Journal of Nervous and Mental Disease, 197*(8), 559–560.

Andrews, M., & Boyle, J. (2008). *Transcultural concepts in nursing care* (5th ed.). Philadelphia: Lippincott.

Bahm, A., & Forchuk, C. (2008). Interlocking oppressions: The effect of a comorbid physical disability on perceived stigma and discrimination among mental health consumers in Canada. *Health and Social Care in the Community, 17*(1), 63–70. doi:10.1111/j.1365-2524.2008.00799.x.

Bopp, J., Bopp, M., Brown, L., et al. (1984). *The sacred tree.* Lethbridge, AB: Four Worlds International Institute for Community and Human Development.

Campinha-Bacote, J. (2002). *The process of cultural competence in the delivery of healthcare services* (4th ed.). Cincinnati: Transcultural C.A.R.E. Associates Press.

Campinha-Bacote, J. (2007). *The process of cultural competence in the delivery of healthcare services. The journey continues.* Retrieved from http://www.transculturalcare.net/Cultural_Competence_Model.htm.

Campinha-Bacote, J. (2008). Cultural desire: 'Caught' or 'taught'? *Contemporary Nurse: Advances in Contemporary Transcultural Nursing, 28*(1–2), 141–148.

Chan, C.L.W., Ng, S.M., Ho, R.T.H., et al. (2006). East meets West: Applying Eastern spirituality in clinical practice. *Journal of Clinical Nursing, 15*, 822–832.

Chiu, L., Ganesan, S., Clark, N., et al. (2005). Spirituality and treatment choices by South and East Asian women with serious mental illness. *Transcultural Psychiatry, 24*(4), 630–656.

Chow, W., Law, S., & Andermann, L. (2009). ACT tailored for ethnocultural communities of metropolitan Toronto. *Psychiatric Services, 60*(6), 847. doi:10.1176/appi.ps.60.6.847.

Corrigan, P.W., Morris, S.B., Michaels, P.J., et al. (2012). Challenging the public stigma of mental illness: A meta-analysis of outcome studies. *Psychiatric Services.* doi:10.1176/appi.ps.005292011.

Corrigan, P.W., & Wassel, A. (2008). Understanding and influencing the stigma of mental illness. *Journal of Psychosocial Nursing and Mental Health Services, 46*(1), 42–48.

Elo, I.T., Mykyta, L. Margolis, R., et al. (2009). Perceptions of neighborhood disorder: The role of individual and neighborhood characteristics. *Social Science Quarterly*, 90(5), 1298–1320.

Henderson, D.C., Yeung, A., Fan, X., et al. (2008). Culture and psychiatry. In T.A. Stern, J.F. Rosenbaum, M. Fava, et al. (Eds.), *Comprehensive clinical psychiatry* (pp. 907–916). Philadelphia: Mosby.

Iarocci, G., Root, R., & Burack, J.A. (2009). Social competence and mental health among Aboriginal youth: An integrative developmental perspective. In L.J. Kirmayer & G. Valaskakis (Eds.), *The mental health of Canadian Aboriginal peoples: Transformations of identity and community*. Vancouver: UBC Press.

Kavanagh, H.K. (2008). Transcultural perspectives in mental health nursing. In M.M. Andrews & J.S. Boyle (Eds.), *Transcultural concepts in nursing care* (5th ed., pp. 226–260). Philadelphia: Wolters.

Kim, M. (2002). Measuring depression in Korean Americans: Development of the Kim depression scale for Korean Americans. *Journal of Transcultural Nursing*, 13, 109–117. doi:10.1177/104365960201300203.

Kirmayer, L.J., Brass, G.M., & Valaskakis, G.G. (2009). Conclusion: Healing, intervention and tradition. In L.J. Kirmayer & G.G. Valaskakis (Eds.), *Healing traditions: The mental health of Aboriginal peoples in Canada* (pp. 440–480). Vancouver: UBC Press.

Kirmayer, L.J., Simpson, C., & Cargo, M. (2007). Healing traditions: Culture, community and mental health promotion with Canadian Aboriginal peoples. *Australasian Psychiatry*, 11(3), S15–S23.

Kirmayer, L.J., Tait, C., & Simpson, C. (2009). The mental health of Aboriginal peoples in Canada: Transformations of identity and community. In L.J. Kirkmayer & G.G. Valaskakis (Eds.), *Healing traditions: The mental health of Aboriginal peoples in Canada* (pp. 3–35). Vancouver: UBC Press.

Kleinman, A. (1980). Major conceptual and research issues for cultural (anthropological) psychiatry. *Culture Med Psychiatry*, 4(1), 3–13.

Kleinman, A., Eisenberg, L., & Good, B. (1978). Culture, illness and care: Clinical lessons from anthropologic and cross-cultural research. *Annals of Internal Medicine*, 88, 251–258.

Lai, D.W.L. (2007). For better or worse: Elderly Chinese immigrants living alone in Canada. *Hallym International Journal of Aging*, 92, 107–122.

Law, S., & Hutton, E. (2007). Community psychiatry in the Canadian Arctic: Reflections from a 1 year continuous consultation series in Iqaluit, Nunavut. *Canadian Journal of Community Mental Health*, 26(2), 123–140.

Legacy of Hope Foundation. (2010a). *About residential schools*. Retrieved from http://www.legacyofhope.ca.

Legacy of Hope Foundation. (2010b). *Where are the children?* Retrieved from http://www.legacyofhope.ca.

Leininger, M. (1991). *Culture care diversity and universality: A theory of nursing*. New York: National League for Nursing Press.

Leininger, M., & McFarland, M. (2006). *Culture care diversity and universality: A worldwide nursing theory* (2nd ed.). Sudbury, MA: Jones & Bartlett.

Library of Parliament. (2006). *Canadian multiculturalism*. Retrieved from http://www.parl.gc.ca/Content/LOP/ResearchPublications/prb0920-e.htm.

Lim, R.F. (2006). *Clinical manual of cultural psychiatry*. Arlington, VA: American Psychiatric Publishing.

Lo, H.T., & Pottinger, A. (2007). Mental health practice. In R.H. Srivastava (Ed.), *The health care professionals' guide to clinical cultural competence* (pp. 247–263). Toronto: Mosby Elsevier.

Marsella, A.J. (2003). Cultural aspects of depressive experience and disorders. In W.J. Lonner, D.L. Dinnel, S.A. Hayes, et al. (Eds.), *Online readings in psychology and culture* (Unit 9, Chapter 4). Retrieved from http://www.wwu.edu/culture/Vontress.htm.

McCormick, R. (2009). Aboriginal approaches to counselling. In L.J. Kirkmayer & G. Valaskakis (Eds.), *Healing traditions: The mental health of Aboriginal peoples in Canada* (pp. 337–353). Vancouver: UBC Press.

Munoz, C., & Hilgenberg, C. (2005). Ethnopharmacology. *American Journal of Nursing*, 105(8), 40–48.

Narayan, M.C. (2002). Six steps towards cultural competence: A clinician's guide. *Home Health Care Management and Practice*, 14, 378–386. doi:10.1177/1084822302014005010.

Narayan, M.C. (2006). Culturally relevant mental health nursing: A global perspective. In E.M. Varcarolis, V.B. Carson, & N.C. Shoemaker (Eds.), *Foundations of psychiatric mental health nursing: A clinical approach* (5th ed., pp. 99–113). Philadelphia: Saunders.

Natural Resources Canada. (2009). *The atlas of Canada*. Retrieved from http://atlas.nrcan.gc.ca/site/english/dataservices/wallmaps.html.

Niezen, R. (2009). Suicide as a way of belonging: Causes and consequences of cluster suicides in Aboriginal communities. In L.J. Kirmayer & G.G. Valaskakis (Eds.), *Healing traditions: The mental health of Aboriginal peoples in Canada* (pp. 178–194). Vancouver: UBC Press.

O'Mahony, J.M., & Donnelly, T.T. (2007). Health care providers' perspective of the gender influences on immigrant women's mental health care experiences. *Issues in mental health nursing*, 28(10), 1171–1188.

Park, Y., Kim, H., Kang, H., et al. (2001). A survey of Hwa-Byung in middle-age Korean women. *Journal of Transcultural Nursing*, 12, 115–122. doi:10.1177/104365960101200205.

Registered Nurses' Association of Ontario. (2007). *Embracing cultural diversity in health care: Developing cultural competence*. Retrieved from http://rnao.ca/bpg/guidelines/embracing-cultural-diversity-health-care-developing-cultural-competence.

Reitmanova, S., & Gustafson, D.J. (2009). Mental health needs of visible minority immigrants in a small urban center: Recommendations for policy makers and service providers. *Journal of Immigrant Minority Health*, 11, 46–56. doi:10.1007/s10903-008-9122-x.

Ross, R. (1992). *Dancing with a ghost: Exploring Indian reality*. Toronto: Reed Books.

Samuel, E. (2009). Acculturative stress: South Asian immigrant women's experiences in Canada's Atlantic provinces. *Journal of Immigrant & Refugee Studies*, 7, 16–34.

Simich, L., Maiter, S., Moorlag, E., et al. (2009). Taking culture seriously: Ethnolinguistic community perspectives on mental health. *Psychiatric Rehabilitation Journal*, 30, 208–214. doi:10.2975/32.3.2009.208.214.

Srivastava, R.H. (2007). *The health care professionals' guide to clinical cultural competence* Toronto: Elsevier.

Statistics Canada. (2002). *Canadian community health survey: Mental health and well-being*. Retrieved from http://www.statcan.gc.ca/pub/82-617-x/index-eng.htm.

Statistics Canada. (2006). *Immigration in Canada: A portrait of the foreign-born population, 2006 census: Immigrants came from many countries*. Retrieved from http://www12.statcan.gc.ca/census-recensement/2006/as-sa/97-557/p6-eng.cfm.

Tang, T.N., Oatley, K., & Toner, B.B. (2007). Impact of life events and difficulties on the mental health of Chinese immigrant women. *Journal of Immigrant and Minority Health*, 9(4), 281–290.

Wieman, C. (2006). Western medicine meets traditional healing. The experience of Six Nations Mental Health Services. *Cross Currents 10*(1), 10–11.

World Health Organization. (2008). *Commission on the Social Determinants of Health final report: Closing the gap in a generation: Health equity through action and the social determinants of health*. Retrieved from http://www.who.int/social_determinants/thecommission/finalreport/en/index.html.

# Ethical Responsibilities and Legal Obligations for Psychiatric Mental Health Nursing Practice

*Cheryl L. Pollard*

## KEY TERMS AND CONCEPTS

abandonment, 126
advance directives, 120
assault, 125
autonomy, 117
battery, 125
beneficence, 115
bioethics, 115
competency, 120
confidentiality, 123
consequentialist theory, 116
deontology, 115
duty to protect, 123
duty to warn, 123
engagement, 116
ethics, 115
false imprisonment, 125
guardianship, 121
implied consent, 120
informed consent, 120

intentional torts, 125
justice, 116
malpractice, 125
moral agent, 117
moral distress, 117
moral residue, 117
moral uncertainty, 117
negligence, 125
nonmaleficence, 115
relational ethics, 115
respect for autonomy, 115
right to privacy, 123
right to refuse treatment, 121
tort law, 124
unintentional torts, 125
utilitarianism, 116
virtue ethics, 116
virtues, 116

## OBJECTIVES

1. Identify the differences between ethical responsibilities and legal obligations within the practice of psychiatric mental health nursing.
2. Describe key elements of the common approaches that inform health care ethics.

3. Identify the ethical nursing responsibilities related to psychiatric mental health research.
4. Identify relevant legislation enacted to protect, promote, and improve the lives of Canadians with mental illness.

## ⊖volve WEBSITE

*Visit the Evolve website for Flashcards, Case Studies, and additional testing resources related to the content in this chapter:* *http://evolve.elsevier.com/Canada/Varcarolis/psychiatric/*    Pre-Test   interactive review

Every nurse will face dilemmas in which values, responsibilities, and obligations seem to conflict; in which there is no clear path to "doing good" or determining what is "most fitting." The purpose of this chapter is to help nurses think about the ethical responsibilities and the legal obligations of their practice. It is important to recognize that professional nursing ethical responsibilities and legal obligations are each distinct areas, but they often have overlapping influences on clinical practice. Nursing ethics is unique in that it is "an expression of the values and beliefs that guide nursing practice. Nursing is an applied discipline, so nursing ethics cannot be merely theoretical; ethics must guide action in real situations. In fact, ethics is the foundation of nursing practice, as 'doing it right' is what practice is all about. Ethics is a fundamental part of every nursing action" (Oberle & Bouchal, 2009, p. 3).

In contrast, legislation, the foundation of legal obligations, is a means used within society to meet objectives and consolidate values. For example, mental health legislation is designed to "protect, promote and improve the lives and mental well-being of citizens" (World Health Organization, 2005, p. 1). This legislation acknowledges the fundamental value of mental health and aims to ensure that the rights of individuals are protected. The type and form of legislative text varies from country to country and, within Canada between jurisdictions. Jurisdictions may organize their laws related to the protection of rights for people with mental illness within a single statute or within a variety of different legislative measures. In Canada, the laws are dispersed within a variety of legislative measures, which include the *Canada Health Act*, *Canadian Employment Equity Act*, and provincial/territorial legislation regarding social welfare and benefits, disability, guardianship, employment, housing, and involuntary admission and treatment of individuals with mental illness. Although the legislation that impacts the social determinants of health for people with mental illness is important, the focus of the legal implication discussion in this chapter will be related to the involuntary admission and involuntary treatment of people with mental illness.

## ETHICAL CONCEPTS

"Like other kinds of growth, moral development is more likely to occur in the right environment—one that provides models, mentors, heroes and antiheroes; support, guidance and correction; relevant experiences and time for healing, and reflection, and building" (Andre, 2000, p. 61).

Ethics are an expression of the values and beliefs that guide practice. Three types of moral theories have traditionally been used as a foundation for the development of nursing ethics: deontological theory, consequentialist theory, and virtue theory. More recently, the developing theory of relational ethics—a developing ethical theory with the core elements of mutual respect, engagement, embodied knowledge, interdependent environment, and uncertainty—has also impacted the application of ethics within nursing.

Deontology is a system of ethics with the central concepts of reason and duty: there is an obligation to act in accordance

with particular rules and principles. The Canadian Nurses Association (2008) code of ethics (Box 8-1), Canadian Federation of Mental Health Nurses (2006) standards of practice (Box 8-2) and the Registered Psychiatric Nurses of Canada (2010) code of ethics and standards of practice (Box 8-3) are written from this perspective. Immanuel Kant (1724–1804), a prominent deontologist, believed that people were free to make choices and that those choices should be based not on emotion but on reason alone. Within the paradigm of deontology, Beauchamp and Childress (2001) outlined several fundamental principles that are irreducible and must be balanced in clinical situations (referred to as bioethics). The basic principles are as follows:

1. Respect for autonomy—respecting the rights of others to make their own decisions (e.g., acknowledging the patient's right to refuse medication).
2. Nonmaleficence—the duty to minimize harm and do no wrong to the patient (e.g., by maintaining expertise in nursing skill through nursing education).
3. Beneficence—the duty to act to benefit or promote the good of others (e.g., spending extra time to help calm an extremely anxious patient).

## BOX 8-3   REGISTERED PSYCHIATRIC NURSES OF CANADA CODE OF ETHICS AND STANDARDS OF PRACTICE

Psychiatric nursing is regulated as a distinct profession in Canada by the provinces of Alberta, British Columbia, Manitoba, and Saskatchewan, as well as the territory Yukon. Registered psychiatric nurses provide services relating to mental, physical, and developmental health and engage in various roles providing health care services to individuals, families, groups, and communities. The practice of psychiatric nursing occurs within the domains of direct practice, education, administration, and research.

### The Code of Ethics
The code of ethics articulates four professional values that professional registered psychiatric nurses use to guide their practice:
1. Safe, competent, and ethical practice to ensure the protection of the public
2. Respect for the inherent worth, right of choice, and dignity of persons
3. Health, mental health, and well-being
4. Quality practice

### Standards of Psychiatric Nursing Practice
The standards provide a guide to the knowledge, skills, values, judgement, and attitudes that psychiatric nurses needed to practise safely. There are four standards of psychiatric nursing practice:
1. Registered psychiatric nurses establish professional, interpersonal, and therapeutic relationships with individual, groups, families, and communities.
2. Registered psychiatric nurses apply and integrate theory-based knowledge relevant to professional practice derived from psychiatric nursing education and continued lifelong learning.
3. Registered psychiatric nurses are accountable to the public for safe, competent, and ethical psychiatric nursing practice.
4. Registered psychiatric nurses understand, promote, and uphold the ethical values of the profession.

**Source:** Registered Psychiatric Nurses of Canada. (2010). *Code of ethics & standards of psychiatric nursing practice.* Edmonton: Author.

4. Justice—the duty to distribute resources or care equally, regardless of personal attributes (e.g., an intensive-care nurse devotes equal attention to someone who has attempted suicide as to someone who suffered a brain aneurysm).

Other pluralistic deontologists have identified two other principles to consider when making ethical decisions in clinical settings. These additional principles are:

5. Principle of impossibility—the principle that a right or obligation that cannot be met within the current situation is no longer an obligation (e.g., a person does not have a right to receive an MRI if an MRI is not available, or a person does not have a right to be cured of schizophrenia when there are currently no permanent cures).

6. Principle of fidelity or best action—maintaining loyalty and commitment to the patient to perform your duty in the best manner possible (e.g., if a patient requires a dressing change, it is your duty to use the greatest skill and care possible).

The consequentialist theory is based on the belief that every person in society has the right to be happy and that we have an obligation to make sure happiness results from our actions. Accordingly, this theory's central concept relates to bringing about the greatest good and the least harm for the greatest number of people (called utilitarianism). John Stuart Mill (1806–1873) referred to this idea as the *principle of utility*. This type of approach is used when decisions are based on the outcomes of a cost/benefit analysis.

Unlike deontology or utilitarianism, virtue theories are not fundamentally concerned with duties or obligations. The ancient philosopher Aristotle believed that virtuous people would make decisions that would maximize their own and others' well-being. Similarly, the central premise of virtue ethics is that good people will make good decisions. Virtues are attitudes, dispositions, or character traits (e.g., honesty, courage, compassion, generosity, fidelity, integrity, fairness, self-control) that enable us to be and to act in ways that develop ethical potential and ensure ethical outcomes. The most prevalent and most valued virtues in health care are compassion and care. Just as the ability to run a marathon develops through much training and practice, so too does our capacity to be fair, to be courageous, and to be compassionate. Virtues, fostered through learning, practice, and self-discipline, enable us to pursue the ideals we have adopted.

Relational ethics, an action-based ethic, requires nurses to appreciate the context in which an ethical issue arises. Context, though, is not a mathematical equation to be figured out, nor is it a black-and-white phenomenon to be described. Context is a dynamic and fluid interaction of the participants, and it is this interaction that inspires (requires) responsibility (Olthuis, 1997). This responsibility, in turn, evokes ethical action. From the perspective of relational ethics, the fulcrum for action (how to be and how to act) is the relationship (Austin, Bergum, & Dossetor, 2003). When using a relational ethics approach, the core question to be answered in an ethical situation is "What action/decision is most fitting?" Understanding the relationship and the actions to be taken requires knowledge of traditions, universal principles, rationality, our subjectivity, and our interconnectedness (Gadow, 1999; Rodney, Pauly, & Burgess, 2004). As researchers explored relational ethics, they found five core elements that were cornerstones for ethical action (Austin, Bergum, & Dossetor, 2003):

1. Mutual respect—an intersubjective experience arising from a nonoppositional perception of difference. There is a recognition that individuals are affected by how others view and react to them as well as by their attitudes toward themselves and others.

2. Engagement—the connection between the self and another. It is through this connection that nurses can develop a meaningful understanding of another person's experience, perspective, and vulnerability.

3. Embodied knowledge—our understanding of the other, incorporated with a scientific body of knowledge. Nursing knowledge and compassion are given equal weight; therefore, emotions and feelings are viewed to be as important as physical signs and symptoms.

4. Interdependent environment—the recognition that we are not separate entities but that we exist as part of a larger community, society, and system. We are not merely affected by our environment; each action we take affects the environment, too.

5. Uncertainty/vulnerability—a recognition that ethical dilemmas exist and, furthermore, that ethical deliberation and contemplation are difficult and at times unpleasant.

From a relational ethics perspective, the consequences of uncertainty/vulnerability are ethical dilemmas. An ethical dilemma results when a choice must be made between two mutually exclusive courses of action, each carrying favourable and unfavourable consequences. How we respond to these dilemmas is based partly on our own morals (beliefs of right and wrong) and values. The nurse is a moral agent who has the power and capacity "to direct his or her motives and actions to some ethical end; essentially, doing what is good and right" (Canadian Nurses Association, 2008, p. 26). Suppose you are caring for a pregnant woman with schizophrenia who wants to carry the baby to term but whose family insists she get an abortion. To promote fetal safety, her antipsychotic medication will need to be reduced, putting her at risk for exacerbation of the illness. Furthermore, there is a question as to whether she can safely care for the child. If you rely on the ethical principle of autonomy (the right to make decisions for oneself), you may conclude that she has the right to decide. Would other ethical principles be in conflict with autonomy in this case? At times, your personal values may be in conflict with the value system of the institution. This situation further complicates the decision-making process and necessitates careful consideration of the patient's desires. For example, you may experience a conflict of values in a setting where older adult patients are routinely tranquilized to a degree you do not feel comfortable with. Whenever one's value system is challenged, increased stress results.

Consequently, psychiatric mental health nurses may develop moral (or ethical) distress, moral uncertainty, moral residue, or a combination of these stressors. The Canadian Nurses Association (CNA) (2008) describes moral distress as arising "in situations where nurses know or believe they know the right thing to do, but for various reasons (including fear or circumstances beyond their control) do not or cannot take the right action or prevent a particular harm" (p. 6). This is in comparison to moral uncertainty, which occurs "when a nurse feels indecision or [has] a lack of clarity, or is unable to even know what the moral problem is, while at the same time feeling uneasy or uncomfortable" (Canadian Nurses Association, 2008, p. 6). However, should nurses "seriously compromise themselves or allow themselves to be compromised" (Canadian Nurses Association, 2008, p. 7), they will experience moral residue. "The moral residue that nurses carry forward from these kinds of situations can help them reflect on what they would do

differently in similar situations in the future" (Canadian Nurses Association, 2008, p. 7).

The last area of ethical consideration to be discussed in this chapter is research ethics. The codes of ethics of the Canadian Nurses Association (2008) and the Registered Psychiatric Nurses of Canada (RPNC) (2010) outline ethical standards of practice, among them, research. Actions and ethical responsibilities of the nurse can include ensuring that clients are informed of their rights with regard to research; however, the CNA code of ethics also comprises rules and regulations to ensure that nursing research is conducted legally and ethically. These rules and regulations apply to all areas of nursing and parallel the *Tri-Council Policy Statement: Ethical Conduct for Research Involving Humans* (Canadian Institutes of Health Research, Natural Sciences and Engineering Research Council of Canada, & Social Sciences and Humanities Research Council of Canada, 2010) core principles of respect for persons, concern for welfare, and justice. Research within a mental health setting raises unique ethical considerations. People with a mental illness are potentially very vulnerable. "Vulnerability is often caused by limited capacity, or limited access to social goods, such as rights, opportunities and power" (Canadian Institutes of Health Research, Natural Sciences and Engineering Research Council of Canada, & Social Sciences and Humanities Research Council of Canada, 2010, p. 10). There is a strong research tradition in Canada. As nurses continue to transform their practices using evidence-informed knowledge, they must be aware of the consequences of not adhering to ethical standards. An example is highlighted in the following Research Highlight.

Nurses must consider both the ethical and legal dimensions of practice—which are distinct. Ideally, the system of law would be completely compatible with both the CNA's and the RPNC's codes of ethics; however, there may be times that nurses will need to collaborate with others to change a law or policy that is incompatible with ethical practice. When this occurs, the relevant codes of ethics can guide and support nurses' actions as they advocate for changes to law, policy, or practice. These "code[s] can be powerful political instrument[s] for nurses when they are concerned about being able to practice ethically" (Canadian Nurses Association, 2008, p. 4).

## MENTAL HEALTH LEGISLATION

Canada is a society that respects and cares for its people. As a result, legislation that protects vulnerable citizens has been developed. "People with mental disorders are, or can be, particularly vulnerable to abuse and violation of rights" (World Health Organization, 2005, p. 1). Historically, in Canada, mental health legislation was developed to protect members of the public from so-called mentally deranged and dangerous patients. Legislation ensured that these "dangerous" individuals were isolated from the public, rather than ensuring that their rights as people and Canadian citizens were protected. Violation of human rights also occurred with legislation that permitted long-term custodial care for people who were deemed to be "a danger" and were unable to care for themselves. This type of legislation heightened the burden of stigma and discrimination

## RESEARCH HIGHLIGHT

### LSD: The Cure for Alcoholism!

**Source:** Dyck, E. (2005). Flashback: Psychiatric experimentation with LSD in historical perspective. *The Canadian Journal of Psychiatry, 50*(7), 381–388.

#### Problem

Psychoactive substances may have an impact on serotonin levels. To confirm this theory, research using psychoactive substances is being conducted. For example, the usefulness of the street drug "ecstasy" is being explored for the treatment of pain and as an adjunctive therapy for people with post-traumatic stress disorder. Historically, there have been ethical concerns related to experimentation with psychoactive substances.

#### Purpose of Study

Discuss potential current challenges of incorporating psychedelic drugs into neuropsychopharmacological practice through the analysis of previous d-lysergic acid diethylamide (LSD) experimentation.

#### Methods

A historical research method was used to systematically describe, analyze, and interpret the challenges associated with previous research that used psychedelic substances.

#### Key Findings

The Saskatchewan government provided financial support for the exploration of the effectiveness of administering mega doses of LSD to individuals being treated for alcoholism. Dr. Humphry Osmond and Dr. Abram Hoffer hypothesized that the LSD reaction was so similar to the experience of delirium tremens as described by patients with alcoholism that inducing this experience could be the catalyst for patients to seek help.

The political culture in Saskatchewan provided tremendous opportunities for initiating experimental theories and practices with political and local support for programs that reformed health care and attracted professionals to underserved rural communities. The region supported medical research that challenged contemporary assumptions about the classification of mental disorders, about treatment modalities, about professional authority, and about institutionalization. (Dyck, 2005, p. 387).

#### Implications for Nursing Practice

The principle of justice was violated when Osmond and Hoffer used the people in the psychiatric institutions in which they worked as the primary source of subjects for their experiments. The principle of concern for welfare was also violated, as there is no evidence in this research program that the subjects were provided with enough information to be able to adequately assess the risks and potential benefits of mega LSD dosing.

Although the intentions of researchers may well be beneficent, protecting research participants' rights is critical. Nurses must advocate for the rights of vulnerable populations.

### BOX 8-4   MENTAL HEALTH CARE LAW: TEN BASIC PRINCIPLES

These principles were developed from a comparative analysis of national mental health laws in 45 countries worldwide conducted by the World Health Organization. The selection of principles drew from the Principles for the Protection of Persons with Mental Illness and the Improvement of Mental Health Care adopted by the UN General Assembly Resolution 46/119 of December 17, 1991.

1. Promotion of mental health and prevention of mental disorders
2. Access to basic mental health care
3. Mental health assessments in accordance with internationally accepted principles
4. Provision of the least restrictive type of mental health care
5. Self-determination
6. Right to be assisted in the exercise of self-determination
7. Availability of review procedure
8. Automatic periodical review mechanism
9. Qualified decision-maker
10. Respect of the rule of law

**Source:** World Health Organization. (1996). *Mental health care law: Ten basic principles.* Geneva, Switzerland: Author.

recognized that individuals with mental illness are subjected to treatment that people with other illnesses are not and determined this treatment to be discriminatory (*Battlefords and District Co-operative Ltd. v. Gibbs,* 1996). Despite these historical legislative limitations, thoughtful and well-developed legislation "offers an important mechanism to ensure adequate and appropriate care and treatment, protection of human rights of people with mental disorders and promotion of the mental health of populations" (World Health Organization, 2005, p. 1). The United Nations Universal Declaration of Human Rights, written in 1948, and other international agreements provide the foundation for mental health legislation. The fundamental basis for mental health legislation is human rights, and the key rights and principles reflected are "equality and non-discrimination, the right to privacy and individual autonomy, freedom from inhuman and degrading treatment, the principle of least restrictive environment, and the rights to information and participation" (World Health Organization, 2005, p. 3). Many Canadian jurisdictions have used the *Mental Health Care Law: Ten Basic Principles* (World Health Organization, 1996) to guide the revision of old and the development of new mental health legislation. See Box 8-4.

Legislation consolidates fundamental principles, values, goals, and objectives of mental health policies and programs. It provides a legal framework to ensure that critical issues affecting the lives of people with mental disorders, in facilities and in the community, are addressed (World Health Organization, 1996). In Canada, there are 12 different mental health acts, all of which allow for the involuntary confinement of people with mental illness to protect them from themselves and others from them (Browne, 2010). Each of the provinces and territories has developed its mental health act from a perspective that prioritizes either the respect of persons (autonomy) or the concern for welfare (beneficence). As a result, the acts differ in many

faced by people with mental illness (World Health Organization, 2005). The Supreme Court of Canada has also recognized the disadvantages endured by people with mental illness. In *Battlefords and District Co-operative Ltd. v. Gibbs* (1996), the court recognized that it was discriminatory to differentiate between physical and mental disability. The court further

| TABLE 8-1 | PROVINCIAL AND TERRITORIAL MENTAL HEALTH ACTS |
|---|---|
| **PROVINCE OR TERRITORY** | **WEBSITE LINK** |
| Alberta | http://www.qp.alberta.ca/574.cfm?page=M13.cfm&leg_type=Acts&isbncln=0779748727 |
| British Columbia | http://www.bclaws.ca/EPLibraries/bclaws_new/document/ID/freeside/00_96288_01 |
| Manitoba | http://web2.gov.mb.ca/laws/statutes/ccsm/m110e.php |
| New Brunswick | http://laws.gnb.ca/en/ShowTdm/cs/M-10// |
| Newfoundland and Labrador | http://www.assembly.nl.ca/legislation/sr/statutes/m09-1.htm |
| Northwest Territories | http://www.justice.gov.nt.ca/PDF/ACTS/Mental%20Health.pdf |
| Nova Scotia | http://www.gov.ns.ca/health/mhs/ipta.asp |
| Nunavut | http://www.hss.gov.nu.ca/en/About%20Us%20Legislation.aspx |
| Ontario | http://www.e-laws.gov.on.ca/html/statutes/english/elaws_statutes_90m07_e.htm |
| Prince Edward Island | http://www.gov.pe.ca/law/statutes/pdf/m-06_1.pdf |
| Quebec | http://www2.publicationsduquebec.gouv.qc.ca/dynamicSearch/telecharge.php?type=2&file=/P_38_001/P38_001.html |
| Saskatchewan | http://www.qp.gov.sk.ca/documents/English/Statutes/Statutes/M13-1.pdf |
| Yukon | http://www.hss.gov.yk.ca/mental_health_act.php |

ways. However, there are three primary areas of difference: "(1) involuntary admission criteria, (2) the right to refuse treatment, and (3) who has the authority to authorize treatment" (Browne, 2010, p. 290). You are encouraged to review your province's or territory's act to better understand the legal climate in which you will practise (see Table 8-1).

Changes in the provincial/territorial acts over the years reflect a shift in emphasis from institutional care of people with mental illness to community-based care delivery models. Along with this shift in setting has come the more widespread use of psychotropic drugs in the treatment of mental illness—which has enabled many people to integrate more readily into the larger community—and an increasing awareness of the need to provide mentally ill patients with care that respects their human rights.

## Establishing Best Practice
### Standards of Practice
The standards of practice determined by professional associations differ from the minimal qualifications set forth by provincial/territorial licensure for entry into the profession of nursing because the primary purposes of each are different. The provinces' or territory's qualifications for practice provide consumer protection by ensuring that all practising nurses have successfully completed an approved nursing program and passed the national licensing examination, whereas the professional association's primary focus is to elevate the practice of its members by setting standards of excellence.

### Standards of Care
Nurses are held to a basic standard of care that is based on what other nurses who possess the same degree of skill or knowledge would do in the same or similar circumstances. Psychiatric patients, whether in a large, small, rural, or urban facility, have a right to the standard of care recognized by professional bodies governing nursing. Nurses must participate in continuing education courses to stay current with existing standards of care.

### Policies and Procedures
Hospital policies and procedures define institutional criteria for care, which may be introduced in legal proceedings to prove that a nurse met or failed to meet them. The weakness of individual institutions' setting such criteria is that a particular hospital's policy may be substandard. Substandard institutional policies, however, do not absolve the individual nurse of responsibility to practise on the basis of professional standards of nursing care.

### Traditional Practice Knowledge
Like hospital policies and procedures, traditional practice knowledge can be used as evidence of a standard of care. But using traditional practice knowledge to establish a standard of care may result in the same defect as using hospital policies and procedures: traditional practice knowledge may not comply with the laws, recommendations of the accrediting body, or other recognized standards of care. Traditional practice knowledge must be carefully and regularly evaluated to ensure that substandard routines have not developed.

## GUIDELINES FOR ENSURING ADHERENCE TO STANDARDS OF CARE

### Negligence, Irresponsibility, or Impairment
It is not unusual for a student or practising nurse to suspect negligence on the part of a peer. In most provinces and territories, nurses have a legal duty to report such risks for harm. It is also important for nurses to document the evidence clearly and accurately before making serious accusations against a peer. If

you question any regulated health professional's orders or actions, it is wise to communicate these concerns directly to the person involved. If the risky behaviour continues, you have an obligation to communicate your concerns to a supervisor, who should then intervene to ensure that the patient's rights and well-being are protected.

If you suspect a peer of being chemically impaired or of practising irresponsibly, you have an obligation to protect not only the rights of the peer but also the rights of all patients who could be harmed by this person. If the danger persists after you have reported suspected behaviour of concern to a supervisor, you have a duty to report the concern to someone at the next level of authority. It is important to follow the channels of communication in an organization, but it is also important to protect the safety of the patients. To that end, if supervisors' actions or inactions do not rectify the dangerous situation, you have a continuing duty to report the behaviour of concern to the appropriate authority, such as the provincial/territorial nursing college or association.

The Canadian Nurses Association, the Registered Psychiatric Nurses of Canada, and the Canadian Federation of Mental Health Nurses have on their Web sites useful information related to standards of practice.

## Unethical or Illegal Practices

The issues become more complex when a professional colleague's conduct (including that of a student nurse) is criminally unlawful. Specific examples include the diversion of drugs from the hospital and sexual misconduct with patients. Increasing media attention and the recognition of substance abuse as an occupational hazard for health professionals have led to the establishment of substance abuse programs for health care workers in many provinces or territories. These programs provide appropriate treatment for impaired professionals to protect the public from harm and to rehabilitate the professional.

The problem of reporting impaired colleagues becomes a difficult one, particularly when no direct harm has occurred to any patients. Concern for professional reputations, damaged careers, and personal privacy has generated among health professionals a code of silence regarding substance abuse. Chapter 19 deals more fully with issues related to the chemically impaired nurse.

## Self-Determination
### Consent

The principle of informed consent is based on a person's right to self-determination and the ethical principle of autonomy. Proper orders for specific therapies and treatments are required and must be documented in the patient's medical record. Consent for surgery, electroconvulsive treatment, or the use of experimental drugs or procedures must be obtained. Patients have the right to refuse participation in experimental treatments or research and the right to voice grievances and recommend changes in policies or services offered by the facility without fear of punishment or reprisal.

For consent to be effective, it must be informed. Generally, the informed consent of the patient must be obtained by the physician or other health care provider before a treatment or procedure is performed. Patients must be informed of the following:
- The nature of their problem or condition
- The nature and purpose of a proposed treatment
- The risks and benefits of that treatment
- The alternative treatment options
- The probability of success of the proposed treatment
- The risks of not consenting to treatment

It is important that psychiatric mental health nurses know that the presence of psychotic thinking does not mean that the patient is mentally incompetent or incapable of understanding; he or she is still able to provide or deny consent.

Competency is the capacity to understand the consequences of one's decisions. Patients must be considered legally competent until they have been declared incompetent through a legal proceeding. If found incompetent, the patient may be appointed a legal guardian or representative, who is legally responsible for giving or refusing consent for the patient while always considering the patient's wishes. Guardians are typically selected from among family members. The order of selection is usually (1) spouse, (2) adult children or grandchildren, (3) parents, (4) adult siblings, and (5) adult nieces and nephews. If a family member is either unavailable or unwilling to serve as guardian, the court may also appoint a court-trained and -approved social worker, representing the province or territory, or a member of the community.

Many procedures nurses perform have an element of implied consent attached. For example, if you approach the patient with a medication in hand, and the patient indicates a willingness to receive the medication, implied consent has occurred. The fact that you may not have a legal duty to be the person to inform the patient of the associated risks and benefits of a particular medical procedure, however, does not excuse you from clarifying the procedure to the patient and ensuring his or her expressed or implied consent.

### Advance Directives

Since the 1960s, the public's desire to participate in decision making about health care has increased. Most provinces and territories have passed legislation that establishes the right of a person to provide directions (advance directives) for clinicians to follow in the event of a serious illness. Such a directive indicates preferences for the types of medical care or extent of treatment desired. The directive comes into effect should physical or mental incapacitation prevent the patient from making health care decisions. Health care institutions are required to (1) provide to each patient at the time of admission written information regarding his or her right to execute advance health care directives and (2) inquire if the patient has made such directives. The patient's admission records should state whether such directives exist.

Patients concerned that they may be subject to involuntary admission can prepare an advance directive document that will express their treatment choices. The advance directive for mental health decision making should be followed by health care providers when the patient is not competent to make informed decisions. This document can clarify the patient's choice of a surrogate decision maker and instructions about hospital choices, medications, treatment options, provider preferences, and emergency interventions.

## Guardianship

A guardianship is an involuntary trust relationship in which one party, the *guardian*, acts on behalf of an individual, the *ward*. The law regards the ward as incapable of managing his or her own person or affairs. Through investigation and an evaluation process, probate court determines if guardianship is warranted. A physician's expert opinion indicating incompetence is required to initiate the proceeding. Many people with mental illness, mental retardation, traumatic brain injuries, and organic brain disorders such as dementia have guardians. It is important that health care providers identify patients who have guardians and communicate with the guardians when health care decisions are being made.

## The Nurse's Role in Decision Making

The nurse is often responsible for explaining the legal policies of the institution to both the patient and family and can help them understand advance directives. The nurse serves as an advocate and knowledgeable resource for the patient and family and encourages the patient to verbalize thoughts and feelings during this sensitive time of decision making.

Nurses must be knowledgeable about both the provincial/territorial regulations on advance directives and the potential obstacles in completing the directives for the province or territory in which they practise. Maintaining an open and continuing dialogue among patient, family, nurse, and physician is of principal importance. The nurse supports any surrogates appointed to act on the patient's behalf and seeks consultation for ethical issues the nurse feels unprepared to handle.

Nurses must prepare themselves to deal with the legal, ethical, and moral issues involved when counselling about advance directives. The law does not specify who should talk with patients about treatment decisions, but in many facilities, nurses are asked to discuss such issues with the patient. If the advance directive of a patient is not being followed, the nurse should intervene on the patient's behalf. If the problem cannot be resolved with the physician, the nurse must follow the facility's protocol providing for notification of the appropriate supervisor.

Although nurses may discuss options with their patients, they may not assist patients in writing advance directives because doing so is considered a conflict of interest. The existence of an advance directive serves as a guide to health care providers in advocating for the patient's rightful wishes in this process.

## Involuntary Admission Criteria

All the provinces and territories have written legislation that enables the legally sanctioned violation of human rights for a person with mental illness. This violation occurs when an individual is involuntarily admitted to a mental health facility. Every mental health act in Canada specifies the data, assessment

findings, or symptoms that must be present for an involuntary admission. For example, in Alberta, a person must be (1) suffering from a mental disorder, (2) likely to cause harm to him or herself or others or to suffer substantial mental or physical deterioration or serious physical impairment, and (3) unsuitable for admission to a facility other than as a formal patient (*Mental Health Act*: Revised Statutes of Alberta, 2000, 2010). However, in all provinces and territories, coupled with the criteria for the original involuntary commitment are safeguards for inappropriately detaining a person in hospital by mandating the completion of an independent examination by a second physician before the person can be kept in hospital. Many jurisdictions stipulate that this physician must be a psychiatrist.

## PATIENTS' RIGHTS UNDER THE LAW

### The Right to Refuse Treatment

Admission to the hospital, whether voluntary or involuntary, is not synonymous with the commencement of treatment. "In some jurisdictions, treatment can begin as soon as admission is deemed appropriate, that is, after the confirmation by the second physician. In others, it cannot begin until all the appeals have been exhausted" (Browne, 2010, pp. 292–293). At the core of the right to refuse treatment is a person's ability to understand and appreciate his or her condition. The importance of this right was highlighted in 2003 in the case of *Starson v. Swayze*, discussed in Box 8-5.

Community treatment orders (CTOs) are "legal mechanisms by which individuals with mental illness and a history of noncompliance can be mandated against their will to undergo psychiatric treatment in an outpatient setting" (Snow & Austin, 2009, p. 177). Community treatment orders can be used in most provinces in Canada but not in New Brunswick or any of the three territories (Rynor, 2010). There are several ethical implications related to the enactment of a CTO. The principles of respect for autonomy/paternalism, beneficence/nonmaleficence, and justice must be considered when working with an individual affected by a CTO. From a relational ethics perspective, this type of "forced treatment" or coercive relationship impacts the power dynamics between the nurse and the person with mental illness. Therefore, special consideration needs to be given to the aspects of engagement, mutual respect, the environment, and uncertainty.

### Authorization of Treatment

Two models of decision making are supported by legislation. The first, the state model, is used to build a system wherein the psychiatrists make the decisions (paternalism). The premise of this model is that the education and experience of a psychiatrist enable him or her to make better treatment decisions than the patient's family members would make. Thus, treatment can be started immediately and without delay. The second is the private model. Within this model, the patient or his or her family member is viewed as the most appropriate authority for making treatment decisions. In Canada, in physical medicine, the private model is used exclusively, based on a civil liberties perspective (Browne, 2010). However, legislation regarding

## BOX 8-5 FACTS: STARSON V. SWAYZE (2003)

From the age of 24, Scott Starson (Schutzman) had been in and out of psychiatric hospitals after being diagnosed with a severe form of bipolar disorder. When he was in a manic state, he had boundless energy and became psychotic. In this state, he would frequently utter death threats and would then be arrested. Often, after the arrests, he would be brought to a psychiatric hospital for assessment and treatment. Despite his bipolar disorder, Scott Starson was brilliant. He was obsessed with physics, and although he had no formal education and was often unemployed, he co-authored articles in physics and "his autodidact theories earned him a welcome among some academic scientists, who gave him the honorific of 'Professor'" (p. 53).

In 1998, he was once again arrested and taken to the Centre for Addiction and Mental Health in Toronto. His treatment plan included neuroleptic medication, which he refused. Because physicians felt strongly that Starson needed this medication, the issue was taken to the courts. In January 1999, the Ontario Consent and Capacity Board found the patient incapable to refuse medication. Starson appealed the decision and, later that same year, won his case in the Superior Court of Ontario, which deemed him capable. The physicians appealed that ruling, taking the case first to the Ontario Court of Appeal (2001) and ultimately to the Supreme Court of Canada (SCC) (p. 53).

### Decision of the Supreme Court of Canada

The SCC upheld Starson's decision to refuse treatment. The majority of the justices believed that Starson was an extraordinarily intelligent and unique man. They indicated that having a mental disorder need not be thought of solely in negative terms and that it is not synonymous with having an illness. As with any other disorder or illness, the patient is not required to comply with the treatment recommendations of the physician, nor is the patient required to believe the medical explanations about the causes of his or her disorder or illness. The decision to accept treatment is the patient's. "Nonetheless, if the patient's condition results in him being unable to recognize that he is affected by its manifestations, he will be unable to apply the relevant information to his circumstances, and unable to appreciate the consequences of his decision" (p. 66).

### Effects on Mr. Starson

With the SCC decision, Scott Starson continued to refuse treatment, and his condition declined markedly. On the premise that his nonexistent son would be tortured if he ate or drank, he nearly died and was found without capacity in 2005. His mother became his substitute decision maker and allowed him to be treated with neuroleptic medication. Once he was treated, his condition improved and he spent two years living in a community-based supportive housing setting while under a community treatment order. In April 2008, he appealed his incapacity finding, and treatment was suspended. His condition deteriorated, and he was again hospitalized involuntarily. Starson appealed his incapacity finding to the Ontario Superior Court. The court upheld the finding of incapacity.

**Source:** Dull, M.W. (2009). *Starson v. Swayze*, 2003–2008: Appreciating the judicial consequences. *Health Law Journal, 17*, 51–79.

authorization of treatment of mental illnesses has been developed using either a state or a private model, depending on the jurisdiction. Both models have consequences for the provision of mental health nursing care. Therefore, nurses need to reflect on the impact that the current legislation in use in their province or territory has on autonomy, beneficence, nonmaleficence, engagement, mutual respect, reciprocity, and an interdependent environment.

---

**VIGNETTE**

Elizabeth is a 50-year-old woman with a long history of admissions to psychiatric hospitals. During previous hospitalizations, she was diagnosed with paranoid schizophrenia. She has refused visits from her case worker and quit taking medication, and her young-adult children have become increasingly concerned about her behaviour. When they stop to visit, she is unkempt and smells bad, her apartment is filthy and filled with cats, there is no food in the refrigerator except for ketchup and an old container of yogurt, and she is not paying her bills. Elizabeth accuses her children of spying on her and of being in collusion with the government to get at her secrets of mind control and oil-rationing plans. Elizabeth is making vague threats to the local officials, claiming that the people who have caused the problems need to be "taken care of." Her daughter contacts her psychiatrist with this information, and a decision is made to begin emergency involuntary admission proceedings.

---

### Provision of the Least Restrictive Type of Mental Health Care

As previously mentioned, the use of the least restrictive means of restraint for the shortest duration is always the general rule. Using verbal interventions such as asking the patient for cooperation is the first approach, and medications are considered if verbal interventions fail. Chemical interventions (i.e., medications) are usually considered less restrictive than physical or mechanical interventions (e.g., restraints, seclusion), but they can have a greater impact on the patient's ability to relate to the environment because medication alters our ability to think and produces other effects. However, when used judiciously, psychopharmacology is extremely effective and helpful as an alternative to physical methods of restraint.

The history of using mechanical restraints and seclusion is marked by abuse, overuse, and even a tendency to use restraint as punishment, especially prior to the 1950s, when there were no effective chemical treatments. Most mental health acts in Canada now legislate that clinicians attempting to bring under control people with a mental illness who are a danger to themselves or others are to use a minimal amount of force or treatment in order to protect the patient and others. Nurses must know under which circumstances the use of seclusion and restraints is contraindicated (Box 8-6).

When in restraints, the patient must be protected from all sources of harm. The behaviour leading to restraint or seclusion and the time the patient is placed in and released from restraint must be documented. The patient in restraint must be assessed at regular and frequent intervals (e.g., every 5 to 15 minutes)

## BOX 8-6 CONTRAINDICATIONS TO SECLUSION AND RESTRAINT

- Extremely unstable medical and psychiatric conditions*
- Delirium or dementia leading to inability to tolerate decreased stimulation*
- Severe suicidal tendencies*
- Severe drug reactions or overdoses or need for close monitoring of drug dosages*
- Desire for punishment of patient or convenience of staff

*Unless close supervision and direct observation are provided.
**Source:** Simon, R.I., & Shuman, D.W. (2007). *Clinical manual of psychiatry and law* (Box 7-1, p. 125). Washington, DC: American Psychiatric Press.

for physical needs (e.g., food, hydration, toileting), safety, and comfort, and these observations must also be documented. The patient must be removed from restraints when safer and quieter behaviour is observed.

Agencies have continued to revise their policies and procedures regarding restraint and seclusion, further limiting these practices after recent changes in laws.

### Rights Regarding Confidentiality

Confidentiality (the right to privacy of information) of care and treatment is also an important right for all patients, particularly psychiatric patients. Any discussion or consultation involving a patient should be conducted discreetly and only with individuals who have a need and a right to know this privileged information.

The Canadian Nurses Association (2008) asserts that it is a duty of the nurse to protect confidential patient information (Box 8-1). The fundamental principle underlying the code on confidentiality is a person's right to privacy—the assurance that only those with a right to know will have access to privileged information. Failure to provide this protection may harm the nurse–patient relationship as well as the patient's well-being. However, the CNA's code of ethics clarifies that this duty is not absolute. In some situations, disclosure may be mandated to protect the patient, other persons, or public health. The following four situations warrant the violation of this right to privacy by the nurse:

1. There is the potential for suspected harm to another.
2. There is suspected harm to a child.
3. There is the potential for harm to the patient's self (suicide risk).
4. There is the presence of a reportable communicable disease.

### Duty to Warn and Protect Third Parties

Although the following event occurred in the United States, it also had an impact in Canada. The California Supreme Court, in its 1974 landmark decision *Tarasoff v. Regents of the University of California*, ruled that a psychotherapist has a duty to warn a patient's potential victim of potential harm. A university student who was in counselling at the University of California was despondent over being rejected by Tatiana Tarasoff, whom he had once kissed. The psychologist notified police verbally

and in writing that the young man might pose a danger to Tarasoff. The police questioned the student, found him to be rational, and secured his promise to stay away from his love interest. The student killed Tarasoff two months later.

The *Tarasoff* case acknowledged that generally there is no common-law duty to aid third persons, except when special relationships exist, and the court found the patient–therapist relationship sufficient to create a duty of the therapist to aid Ms. Tarasoff, the victim. It asserted that the duty to protect the intended victim from danger arises when the therapist determines—or, pursuant to professional standards, should have determined—that the patient presents a serious danger to another.

This case created much controversy and confusion in the psychiatric and medical communities over (1) breach of patient confidentiality and its impact on the therapeutic relationship in psychiatric care and (2) the ability of the therapist to predict when a patient is truly dangerous. Nevertheless, many jurisdictions have adopted or modified the California rule despite objections from the psychiatric community.

The California Supreme Court held a second hearing in 1976 in the case of *Tarasoff v. Regents of the University of California* (now known as *Tarasoff II*). It delivered a second ruling that broadened the earlier duty to warn: when a therapist determines that a patient presents a serious danger of violence to another, the therapist has the duty to protect that other person; in providing protection, it may be necessary for the therapist to call and warn the intended victim, the victim's family, or the police or to take whatever steps are reasonably necessary under the circumstances.

Most areas have similar laws regarding the duty to protect third parties of potential life threats. The duty to protect usually includes the following:

- Assessing and predicting the patient's danger of violence toward another
- Identifying the specific persons being threatened
- Taking appropriate action to protect the identified potential victims

As this trend toward the therapist's duty to warn third persons of potential harm continues to gain wider acceptance, it is important for nurses to understand its implications for nursing practice. Although none of these cases has dealt with nurses, it is fair to assume that in jurisdictions that have adopted the *Tarasoff* doctrine, the duty to warn third persons will be applied to advanced-practice psychiatric mental health nurses who engage in individual therapy in private practice. If a staff nurse—who is a member of a team of psychiatrists, psychologists, psychiatric social workers, and other nurses—does not report to other members of the team a patient's threats of harm against specified victims or classes of victims, this failure is considered substandard nursing care.

Failure to communicate and record relevant information from police, relatives, or the patient's old records may also be deemed negligent. Breach of patient–nurse confidentiality should not pose ethical or legal dilemmas for nurses in these situations, because a team approach to the delivery of psychiatric care presumes communication of pertinent information to other staff members to develop a treatment plan in the patient's best interest.

***Risk-of-violence assessment findings.*** The nurse's assessment of the patient's potential for violence must be documented and acted on if it suggests legitimate concern about a patient's discussing or exhibiting potentially violent behaviour. The psychiatric mental health nurse must communicate his or her observations to the medical staff when discharge decisions are being considered.

## Reporting of Abuse

All the provinces and territories have enacted child abuse reporting legislation. Although these statutes differ among provinces and territories, they generally include a definition of *child abuse*, a list of persons required or encouraged to report abuse, and the governmental agency designated to receive and investigate the reports. Most statutes include the consequences of failure to report. Many provinces and territories specifically require nurses to report cases of suspected abuse. Refer to Box 8-7 for a possible example of how to report abuse.

As incidents of abuse in society surface, some jurisdictions may require health care providers to report other kinds of abuse. A growing number of provinces and territories are enacting "protection for persons in care" legislation, which requires registered nurses and others to report cases of abuse of people who are receiving care or support services. Under most provincial/territorial laws, a person who is required to report suspected abuse, neglect, or exploitation of a person in care and willfully does not do so is guilty of a misdemeanour crime. Most provincial/territorial legislation provides protection to anyone who makes a report in good faith, ensuring immunity from civil liability in connection with the report. Because provincial/territorial laws vary, students are encouraged to become familiar with the requirements of their province or territory.

## Confidentiality and Communicable Diseases

All provinces and territories have enacted legislation in which health care providers must report suspected or confirmed cases of selected communicable diseases. Examples of these are Creutzfeldt-Jakob disease, human immunodeficiency virus (HIV), syphilis, tuberculosis, and West Nile virus infections.

---

### BOX 8-7 | HOW DOES A NURSE REPORT CHILD ABUSE?

Institutions usually have policies for reporting abuse. Often, the responsibility goes to social workers who have expertise in these matters and know how to navigate the system. However, if you are caring for a child covered in old and new bruises or who has a broken bone or decaying teeth, and you suspect abuse, it is your legal and ethical responsibility to make a report to your province's or territory's child welfare agency. You should also let the child's parents or guardians know that you are filing the report. Whether the physician or your peers agree with you or not, if you report suspected child abuse in good faith, you will be protected from criminal or civil liability. More important, you may save a child from further suffering.

---

Additionally, some provinces and territories have enacted mandatory or permissive legislation that directs health care providers to warn a spouse if a partner tests positive for HIV. Nurses must understand the laws in their jurisdiction of practice regarding privileged communications and warnings of infectious disease exposure.

## Confidentiality After Death

A person's reputation can be damaged even after death. Therefore, it is important after a person's death not to divulge information that you would not have been able to share legally before the death.

## Protection of Patients

A health care provider who believes that a patient is going to try to kill him- or herself has a duty to try to mitigate the risk for that person. For example, the nurse working on an inpatient unit would, in consultation with the other team members, develop a plan of care to mitigate the potential for the person to commit suicide. If a suicidal patient is left alone with a means of self-harm, the nurse who has a duty to protect the patient will be held responsible for the resultant injuries. For instance, leaving a suicidal patient alone in a room on the sixth floor with a window that opens demonstrates unreasonable judgement on the part of the nurse. Precautions to prevent harm also must be taken whenever a patient is restrained.

## Legal Duties and Responsibilities

Legal issues common in psychiatric mental health nursing relate to the failure to protect the safety of patients (Table 8-2). Miscommunications and medication errors are common in all facets of nursing, including psychiatric care. Another common area of liability in psychiatry is abuse of the therapist–patient relationship. Issues of sexual misconduct during the therapeutic relationship have become a source of concern in the psychiatric community. Diagnosing a patient—and avoiding misdiagnosing—also requires ethical, moral, and legal responsibility of the treatment team.

## Tort Law

Tort law is a law developed from obligations to another. Although these laws are not based on nurses' professional codes of ethics, they have many similarities. Both describe the nurse's obligations and responsibilities to the patient. The difference is that tort laws have a much broader applicability. They apply to all Canadians.

## Intentional Torts

Nurses in psychiatric settings may encounter provocative, threatening, or violent behaviour that may require the use of restraint or seclusion. However, such interventions must be carefully determined and used only in the most extreme situations. As discussed earlier in this chapter, restraint and seclusion historically were used with little regard to patients' rights, and overuse and abuses were common. Stories of patients restrained and left to lie in their own excrement or locked in seclusion for days for being annoying have resulted in strict laws. Accordingly, the nurse in the psychiatric setting should understand

| TABLE 8-2 | COMMON LIABILITY ISSUES |
|---|---|
| **ISSUE** | **EXAMPLES** |
| Patient safety | Failure to notice of or take action on suicide risks<br>Failure to use restraints properly or to monitor the restrained patient<br>Miscommunication<br>Medication errors<br>Violation of boundaries (e.g., sexual misconduct)<br>Misdiagnosis |
| Intentional torts | Voluntary acts intended to bring a physical or mental consequence<br>Purposeful acts<br>Recklessness<br>Not obtaining patient consent |
| Negligence/malpractice | Carelessness<br>Foreseeability of harm |
| Assault and battery | Reasonable belief that a person means to cause one harm (assault) through harmful or offensive<br>  touching (battery)<br>Threat to use force, along with opportunity and ability to carry out threat<br>Giving treatment without patient's consent |
| False imprisonment | Intent to confine to a specific area<br>Indefensible use of seclusion or restraints<br>Detention of voluntarily admitted patient, with no agency or legal policies to support detaining |
| Defamation of character:<br>• Slander (spoken)<br>• Libel (written) | Sharing private information with people who are not directly involved with care<br>Confidential documents shared with people who are not directly involved with care |
| Supervisory liability<br>  (vicarious liability) | Inappropriate delegation of duties<br>Lack of supervision of those supervising |

intentional torts, which are willful or intentional acts that violate another person's rights or property. Some examples of intentional torts include assault (reasonable belief that a person means to cause one harm), battery (offensive or harmful touching), and false imprisonment (detention of a patient with no agency or legal policies to support detention) (see Table 8-2).

Other types of intentional torts may hurt a person's sense of self or financial status. They include invasion of privacy and defamation of character. Invasion of privacy in health care has to do with breaking a person's confidences or taking photographs without explicit permission. Defamation of character includes slander (verbal), such as talking about patients on the elevator with others around, and libel (printed), such as sharing written information about the patient with people outside the professional setting.

## Unintentional Torts

Unintentional torts are unintended acts that produce injury or harm to another person. Negligence (carelessness) is a general tort for which anyone may be found guilty. For example, if you do not shovel the snow from your driveway, and a visitor falls and breaks a hip, you may be charged with negligence. Health care providers who fail to act in accordance with professional standards, or who fail to foresee consequences that other professionals with similar skills and education would foresee, can be liable for a tort of professional negligence, or malpractice. Malpractice is an act or omission to act that breaches the duty of due care and results in or is responsible for a person's injuries.

The five elements required to prove negligence are (1) duty, (2) breach of duty, (3) cause in fact, (4) proximate cause, and (5) damages. Foreseeability, or likelihood of harm, is also evaluated.

*Duty.* When nurses represent themselves as being capable of caring for psychiatric patients and accept employment, a duty of care has been assumed. As a psychiatric mental health nurse, you have the duty to understand the theory and medications used in the care of psychiatric patients whether they are being treated in a community clinic, general practitioner's office, medical unit, or psychiatric treatment unit. The staff nurse who is responsible for care delivery must be knowledgeable enough to assume a reasonable or safe duty of care for the patients.

The nurse's duty of care includes a duty to intervene when the safety or well-being of the patient or another person is obviously at risk. For example, a nurse who knowingly follows an incorrect or possibly harmful order is responsible for any harm that results to the patient. If you have information that leads you to believe that the physician's orders need to be clarified or changed, it is your duty to intervene and protect the patient. It is important that you communicate the concern to the physician who has ordered the treatment. If the treating physician does not appear willing to consider your concerns, you should carry out your duty to intervene through other appropriate channels. The following vignette illustrates two possible outcomes of a nurse's intervention in a medication issue.

The duty to intervene on the patient's behalf poses legal and ethical dilemmas for nurses in the workplace. Institutions

**VIGNETTE**

Monia is a new nurse on the crisis management unit. She completed the hospital and unit orientations two weeks ago and has begun to care for patients independently. As she prepares to give her 1700 hrs medications, Monia notices that Greg Thorn, a 55-year-old man admitted after a suicide attempt, has been given a new order for the antidepressant sertraline (Zoloft). Monia remembers that Mr. Thorn had been taking phenelzine (Nardil) before his admission and seems to recall something unsafe about mixing these two medications. She looks up the antidepressants in her drug guide and realizes that Nardil is a monoamine oxidase inhibitor (MAOI) and that adding this second antidepressant within two weeks of discontinuing the Nardil could result in severe adverse effects and possibly a lethal response.

After clarifying with Mr. Thorn that he had been on Nardil and discussing the issue with another nurse, Monia realizes she needs to put the medication on hold and contact Mr. Thorn's psychiatrist, Dr. Cruz. Monia phones him and begins by saying, "I see that Mr. Thorn has been ordered Zoloft. I am looking at his nursing admission assessment, and it says that he had been taking Nardil up until a few days ago. However, I don't see it listed on the medical assessment that was done by the resident."

**First Possible Outcome**

Dr. Cruz responds, "Thank you for calling that to my attention. When I make my rounds in the morning, I'll decide what to do with his medications. For now, please put a hold on the Zoloft." Monia clarifies what Dr. Cruz has said, writes the order, and documents what happened in the nurses' notes.

**Second Possible Outcome**

Dr. Cruz responds, "Are you telling me how to do my job? If it wasn't on the medical assessment, then he wasn't taking it. A nurse must have made a mistake—again. I wrote an order for Nardil, so give him the Nardil." He hangs up. Monia documents the exchange, determines that the safest and most appropriate response is to hold the medication for now, and contacts her nursing supervisor. The supervisor supports her decision and follows up with the chief of psychiatry.

with a chain-of-command policy or other reporting mechanisms offer some assurance that the proper authorities in the administration are notified of nursing concerns. Most patient-care issues regarding physicians' orders or treatments can be settled fairly early in the process through the nurse's discussion of concerns with the physician. However, if further intervention by the nurse is required to protect the patient, generally, the nurse would notify his or her immediate nursing supervisor, who would discuss the problem with the physician and subsequently, if necessary, the chief of staff of a particular service until a resolution is reached. If there is no time to resolve the issue through the normal process because of a life-threatening situation, the nurse has no choice but to act to protect the patient's life. It is important to follow agency policies and procedures for reporting differences of opinion. If you fail to intervene and the patient is injured, you may be partly liable for the injuries that result because of your failure to use safe nursing practice and good professional judgement.

***Breach of duty.*** Breach of duty is any conduct that exposes a patient to an unreasonable risk of harm, through either commission or omission of acts by the nurse. If you are not capable of providing the standard of care that other nurses would be expected to supply under similar circumstances, you have breached the duty of care. Or if you do not have the required education and experience to provide certain interventions, you have breached the duty by neglecting or omitting the provision of necessary care.

The legal concept of abandonment is another concern of nurses. When a nurse is given an assignment to care for a patient, he or she must provide the care or ensure that the patient is safely reassigned to another nurse, or abandonment occurs. Abandonment also takes place in the absence of accurate, timely, and thorough reporting and in the absence of follow-through of care on which the patient relies.

The same principles apply to the psychiatric mental health nurse working in a community setting. For example, if a suicidal patient refuses to go to the hospital for treatment, you must take the necessary steps to ensure the patient's safety. These actions may include enlisting the assistance of the law in involuntarily admitting the patient on a temporary basis.

***Cause in fact, proximate cause, damages, and foreseeability.*** Cause in fact may be evaluated by asking, "Would this injury have occurred without the nurse's actions?" If the answer is no, then the nurse is guilty of causing the injury.

Proximate cause, or legal cause, may be evaluated by determining whether any intervening actions or persons, other than the nurse, were, in fact, the cause of harm to the patient. If determined that the harm resulted from intervening persons or actions, the nurse is not guilty of proximate cause.

Damages include actual damages (e.g., loss of earnings, medical expenses, property damage), as well as pain and suffering. They also include incidental or consequential damages. For example, giving a patient the wrong medication may incur actual damage of a complicated hospital stay, but it also may result in permanent disability, which could require such needs as special education and special accommodations in the home. Furthermore, incidental damages may deprive others of the benefits of life with the injured person, such as losing a normal relationship with a husband or father.

Forseeability of harm evaluates the likelihood of the outcome under the circumstances. If the average, reasonable person could foresee that injury could result from the action or inaction, then the injury was foreseeable.

## DOCUMENTATION OF CARE

The purposes of the medical record are to provide accurate and complete information about the care and treatment of patients and to give health care personnel a means of communicating with each other, supporting continuity of care. A record's usefulness is determined by its accuracy and thoroughness in portraying the patient's behavioural status at the time it was written. For example, if a psychiatric patient describes to a nurse a plan to harm himself or another person and that nurse fails to document the information—including the need to protect the patient or the identified victim—the information will be lost when the nurse leaves work. If the patient's plan is carried out, the harm caused could be linked directly to the nurse's failure to communicate this important information. Even though documentation takes time away from the patient, the importance of communicating and preserving the nurse's memory through the medical record cannot be overemphasized.

Patients have the right to see their medical records, but records belong to the institution. Patients must follow appropriate protocol to view their records.

## Facility Use of Medical Records

The medical record has many uses aside from providing information on the course of the patient's care and treatment by health care providers. A retrospective medical record review can offer a facility valuable information on the quality of care given and on ways to improve that care. A facility may conduct reviews for risk-management purposes to determine areas of potential liability and to evaluate methods of reducing the facility's exposure to liability. For example, risk managers may review documentation of the use of restraints and seclusion for psychiatric patients, or a medical record may be used to evaluate care for quality assurance or peer review. Utilization review analysts use the medical record to determine appropriate use of hospital and staff resources consistent with reimbursement schedules. Insurance companies and other reimbursement agencies rely on the medical record in determining what payments they will make on the patient's behalf.

## Medical Records as Evidence

From a legal perspective, the medical record is a recording of data and opinions made in the normal course of the patient's hospital care. It is deemed to be good evidence because it is presumed to be true, honest, and untainted by memory lapses. Accordingly, the medical record finds its way into a variety of legal cases for a variety of reasons. Some examples of its use include determining (1) the extent of the patient's damages and pain and suffering in personal-injury cases, such as when a psychiatric patient attempts suicide while under the protective care of a hospital; (2) the nature and extent of injuries in child-abuse or elder-abuse cases; (3) the nature and extent of physical or mental disability in disability cases; and (4) the nature and extent of injury and rehabilitative potential in workers' compensation cases.

Medical records may also be used in police investigations, competency hearings, and involuntary-admission procedures. In provinces and territories that mandate mental health legal

services or a patients' rights advocacy program, medical-record audits may be performed to determine the facility's compliance with provincial/territorial laws or violation of patients' rights. Finally, medical records may be used in professional and hospital negligence cases.

During the initial, or discovery, phase of litigation, the medical record is a pivotal source of information for lawyers in determining whether a cause of action exists in a professional negligence or hospital negligence case. Evidence of the nursing care rendered will be found in what the nurse documented.

## Guidelines for Electronic Documentation

Accurate, descriptive, and legible nursing notes serve the best interests of the patient, the nurse, and the institution. Electronic documentation, now common, has created new challenges for protecting the confidentiality of records of psychiatric patients. While ensuring the appropriate sharing of information, institutions must, at the same time, protect against intrusions into patient-record systems. Sensitive information regarding treatment for mental illness can adversely impact patients who are seeking employment, insurance, or credit (Fung & Paynter, 2008).

Concerns for the privacy of patients' records have been addressed by provincial, territorial, and federal laws that provide guidelines for agencies that use electronic documentation. These guidelines include the recommendation that staff members be assigned individual passwords for entering patients' records to allow for the identification of persons who have accessed confidential information. Only health care providers who have a legitimate need for information about the patient are authorized to access a patient's electronic medical record. There are penalties, including termination of employment, for staff members who access a record without authorization. For this reason, it is important to keep your password private. You are responsible for all entries into records using your password. Various systems allow for specific time frames within which the nurse must make corrections if a documentation error is made.

Any documentation method that improves communication between health care providers should be encouraged. Courts assume that nurses and physicians read each other's notes on patient progress. Many courts take the attitude that if care is not documented, it did not occur. Your documentation also serves as a valuable memory refresher if the patient sues years after the care has been rendered. In providing complete and timely information on the care and treatment of patients, the medical record enhances communication among health care providers. Internal institutional audits of records can improve the quality of care rendered. Chapter 9 describes common documentation forms, gives examples, and gives the pros and cons of each.

## KEY POINTS TO REMEMBER

- Deontology, consequentialist theory, virtue ethics, and relational ethics have provided the foundation for nursing ethics and nursing standards of practice.
- Psychiatric mental health nurses frequently encounter ethical dilemmas.

- The provinces and territories have enacted laws (mental health acts) for public health and safety and for the care of those unable to care for themselves. Within these acts are provisions for involuntary admissions to a psychiatric hospital or unit.

- The principle of respect of persons provides the foundation for a person's right to self-determination.
- Provincial, territorial, and federal legislation provides the framework for the development of mental health policies and programs.
- The nurse's privilege to practise carries with it the responsibility to practise safely, competently, and according to provincial, territorial, and federal laws.

- Best practices are determined by standards of practice, standards of care, policies and procedures, and the use of traditional practice knowledge.
- Knowledge of the law, nursing codes of ethics, and the standards of practice for psychiatric mental health nursing are essential for providing safe, effective psychiatric mental health nursing care and will serve as a framework for decision making.

# CRITICAL THINKING

1. Noskye and Beth are nurses who have worked together on the psychiatric unit for two years. Beth confided to Noskye that her marital situation has become particularly difficult over the past six months. He expressed concern and shared his observation that she seems to be distracted and not as happy lately. Privately, Noskye concludes that this explains why Beth has become so irritable and distracted. As Noskye prepares the medication for the evening shift, he notices that two of his patients' medications are missing—both are bedtime lorazepam (Ativan). When he phones the pharmacy to request the missing medications, the pharmacist responds, "You people need to watch your carts more carefully because this has become a pattern." Shortly after, another patient complains to Noskye that he did not receive his 1700 hrs alprazolam (Xanax). On the medication administration record, Beth has recorded that she has given the drugs. Noskye suspects that Beth may be diverting the drugs.
   a. What action, if any, should Noskye take? Should he confront Beth with his suspicions?
   b. If Beth admits that she has been diverting the drugs, should Noskye's next step be to report Beth to their supervisor or to the board of nursing?
   c. When Noskye talks to the nursing supervisor, should he identify Beth, or should he state his suspicions in general terms?
   d. How does the nature of the drugs affect your responses? That is, if the drugs were to treat a "physical" condition such as hypertension, would you be more concerned?
   e. What does the nurse practice act in your province or territory mandate regarding reporting the illegal use of drugs by a nurse?

2. A 40-year-old man is admitted to the emergency department for a severe nosebleed and has both of his nostrils packed. Because of a history of alcoholism and the possibility for developing delirium tremens (withdrawal), the patient is transferred to the psychiatric unit. His physician has ordered a private room, restraints, continuous monitoring, and 15-minute checks of vital signs and other indicators. At the first 15-minute check, the nurse discovers that the patient has no pulse or respiration. He had apparently inhaled the nasal packing and suffocated.
   a. Does it sound as though the nurse was responsible for the patient's death?
   b. Was the order for the restraint appropriate for this type of patient?

c. What factors did you consider in making your determination in (b)?

3. Assume that there are no mandatory-reporting laws for impaired or incompetent colleagues in the following clinical situation. A 15-year-old boy is admitted to a psychiatric facility voluntarily at the request of his parents because of violent, explosive behaviour. This behaviour began after his father's recent remarriage after his parents' divorce. In group therapy, he has become incredibly angry in response to a discussion about weekend passes for Mother's Day. "Everyone has abandoned me. No one cares!" he screamed. Several weeks later, on the day before his discharge, he convinces his nurse to keep his plan to kill his mother confidential. Consider the CNA code of ethics on patient confidentiality, the principles of psychiatric nursing, and the duty to warn third parties in answering the following questions:
   a. Did the nurse use appropriate judgement in promising confidentiality?
   b. Does the nurse have a legal duty to warn the patient's mother of her son's threat?
   c. Is the duty owed to the patient's father and stepmother?
   d. Would a change in the admission status from voluntary to involuntary (based on an assessment determining that he is a danger to himself or others, has a mental disorder, and is unwilling to voluntarily remain in hospital) protect the patient's mother without violating the patient's confidentiality?
   e. What nursing action, if any, should the nurse take after this disclosure by the patient?

4. Patients admitted to an inpatient psychiatric unit are being recruited for research on a new drug that is hoped to have an impact on the negative symptoms of schizophrenia. The attending psychiatrists are all involved in the research. One of the patients asks a nurse about the experimental medication.
   a. Does the nurse have a responsibility to explain the research to the patient?
   b. Why are the patients involved in this research considered vulnerable?
   c. How can the nurse advocate for vulnerable patients?
   d. What are the documentation responsibilities of the nurses when they observe a medication adverse effect in one of the patients involved in the research?

## CHAPTER REVIEW

1. A patient with depression presents with her family in the emergency department. The family feels she should be admitted because "she might hurt herself." An assessment indicates moderate depression with no risk factors for suicide other than the depressed mood itself, and the patient denies any intent or thoughts of self-harm. The family agrees that the patient has not done or said anything to suggest that she might be a danger to herself. Which of the following responses is consistent with the concept of "least restrictive alternative" doctrine?
   1. Admit the patient as a temporary inpatient admission.
   2. Persuade the patient to agree to a voluntary inpatient admission.
   3. Admit the patient involuntarily to an inpatient mental health treatment unit.
   4. Arrange for an emergency outpatient counselling appointment the next day.

2. An advanced-practice nurse wishes to initiate treatment with an antipsychotic medication that, although very likely to benefit the patient, in a small percentage of patients may cause a dangerous adverse effect. The nurse explains the purpose, expected benefits, and possible risks of the medication. The patient readily signs a form accepting the medication, stating, "These pills will poison the demons inside of me." Although he has been informed of the risk of adverse effects, he is unable to state what these are and simply reports, "I won't have side effects because I am iron and cannot be killed." Which of the following responses would be most appropriate under these circumstances?
   1. Begin administration of the medications based on his signed permission because he has legally consented to treatment.
   2. Petition the court to appoint a guardian for the patient because of his being unable to comprehend the proposed treatment.
   3. Administer the medications even though consent is unclear because the patient is clearly psychotic and in need of the medications.
   4. Withhold the medication until the patient is able to identify the benefits and risks of both consenting and refusing consent to the medications.

3. A patient incidentally shares with you that he has difficulty controlling his anger when around children because their play irritates him, leading to resentment and fantasies about attacking them. He has a history of impulsiveness and assault, escalates easily on the unit, and has a poor tolerance for frustration. This weekend he has an overnight pass, which he will use to see his sister and her family. As you meet with the patient and his sister just prior to his getting the pass, the sister mentions that she has missed her brother because he usually helps her watch the children, and she has to work this weekend and needs him to babysit. The patient becomes visibly apprehensive upon hearing this. Which of the following responses would best reflect appropriate nursing practice relative to the conflict this situation presents between safety and the patient's right to confidentiality?
   1. Cancel the pass without explanation to the sister, and reschedule it for a time when babysitting would not be required of the patient.
   2. Suggest that the sister make other arrangements for child care, but withhold the information the patient shared regarding his concerns about harming children.
   3. Speak with the patient about the safety risk involved in babysitting, seeking his permission to share this information and advising against the pass if he declines to share the information.
   4. Meet with the patient's sister, sharing with her the patient's disclosure about his anger toward children and the resultant risk that his babysitting would present.

4. Mrs. Fujiwara was admitted for treatment of depression with suicidal ideation triggered by marital discord. She has spoken with staff about her fears that the marriage will end, has indicated that she does not know how she could cope if her marriage ended, and has a history of suicide attempts when the marriage has seemed threatened in the past. Her spouse visits one night and informs Mrs. Fujiwara that he has decided to file for divorce. Staff members, though aware of the visit and the husband's intentions regarding divorce, take no action, feeling that the 15-minute suicide checks Mrs. Fujiwara is already on are sufficient. Thirty minutes after the visit ends, staff make rounds and discover that Mrs. Fujiwara has hanged herself in her bathroom using hospital pyjamas she had tied together into a rope. Which of the following statements best describes this situation? Select all that apply.
   1. The nurses have created liability for themselves and their employer by failing in their duty to protect Mrs. Fujiwara.
   2. The nurses have breached their duty to reassess Mrs. Fujiwara for increased suicide risk after her husband's visit.
   3. Given Mrs. Fujiwara's history, the nurses should have expected an increased risk for suicide after the husband's announcement.
   4. The nurses correctly reasoned that suicides cannot always be prevented and did their best to keep Mrs. Fujiwara safe via the 15-minute checks.
   5. The nurses are subject to a tort of professional negligence for failing to increase the suicide precautions in response to Mrs. Fujiwara's increased risk.
   6. Had the nurses restricted Mrs. Fujiwara's movements or increased their checks on her, they would have been liable for false imprisonment and invasion of privacy, respectively.

# evolve WEBSITE

Post-Test   interactive review

*Visit the Evolve Web site for Chapter Review Answers and Rationales, Critical Thinking Answer Guidelines, and additional resources related to the content in this chapter:* http://evolve.elsevier.com/Canada/Varcarolis/psychiatric/

## REFERENCES

Andre, J. (2000). Humility reconsidered. In S.B. Rubin & L. Zoloth (Eds.), *Margin of error: The ethics of mistakes in the practice of medicine* (pp. 59–72). Hagerstown, MD: University Publishing Group.

Austin, W., Bergum, V., & Dossetor, J. (2003). Relational ethics. In V. Tshudin (Ed.), *Approaches to ethics* (pp. 45–52). Woburn, MA: Butterworth-Heinemann.

Battlefords and District Co-operative Ltd. v. Gibbs, 3 S.C.R. 566 (Canada Supreme Court, 1996).

Beauchamp, T., & Childress, J. (2001). *Principles of biomedical ethics* (5th ed.). Oxford, UK: Oxford University Press.

Browne, A. (2010). Mental health acts in Canada. *Cambridge Quarterly of Healthcare Ethics, 19*, 290–298. doi: 10.1017/S096318011000006X.

Canadian Federation of Mental Health Nurses. (2006). *Canadian standards of psychiatric mental health nursing practice* (3rd ed.). Toronto: Author.

Canadian Institutes of Health Research, Natural Sciences and Engineering Research Council of Canada, & Social Sciences and Humanities Research Council of Canada. (2010). *Tri-council policy statement: Ethical conduct for research involving humans.* Retrieved from http://www.pre.ethics.gc.ca/pdf/eng/tcps2/TCPS_2_FINAL_Web.pdf.

Canadian Nurses Association. (2008). *Code of ethics for registered nurses (2008 centennial edition).* Ottawa: Canadian Nurses Association.

Fung, M.Y.L., & Paynter, J. (2008). The impact of information technology in healthcare privacy. In P. Duquenoy, C. George, & K. Kimppa (Eds.), *Ethical, legal, and social issues in medical informatics* (pp. 186–227). Hershey, PA: Idea Group.

Gadow, S. (1999). Relational narrative: The postmodern turn in nursing ethics. *Scholarly Inquiry for Nursing Practice: An International Journal, 13*(1), 57–70.

Mental Health Act: Revised Statutes of Alberta 2000, Chapter M-13 (2010).

Oberle, K., & Bouchal, S.R. (2009). *Ethics in Canadian nursing practice: Navigating the journey.* Toronto: Pearson Education Canada.

Olthuis, J.H. (1997). Face-to-face: Ethical asymmetry or the symmetry of mutuality? In J.H. Olthuis (Ed.), *Knowing other-wise: Philosophy at the threshold of spirituality* (pp. 131–158). New York: Fordham University Press.

Registered Psychiatric Nurses of Canada. (2010). *Code of ethics & standards of psychiatric nursing practice.* Edmonton: Author.

Rodney, P., Pauly, B., & Burgess, M. (2004). Our theoretical landscape: A brief history on health care ethics. In J. Storch, P. Rodney, & R. Starzomski (Eds.), *Toward a moral horizon: Nursing ethics for leadership and practice* (pp. 77–97). Toronto: Pearson Education Canada.

Rynor, B. (2010). Value of community treatment orders remains at issue. *Canadian Medical Association Journal, 182*(8), E337–E338. doi:10.1503/cmaj.109-3237.

Snow, N., & Austin, W.J. (2009). Community treatment orders: The ethical balancing act in community mental health. *Journal of Psychiatric & Mental Health Nursing, 16*, 177–186. doi:10.1111/j.1365-2850.2008.01363.x.

Tarasoff v. Regents of the University of California, 529 P.2d 553, 118 Cal Rptr 129 (1974).

Tarasoff v. Regents of the University of California, 551 P.2d 334, 131 Cal Rptr 14 (1976).

World Health Organization. (1996). *Mental health care law: Ten basic principles.* Geneva, Switzerland: World Health Organization.

World Health Organization. (2005). WHO resource book on mental health, human rights and legislation. Geneva, Switzerland: Author.

# Psychosocial Nursing Techniques

# 9

# The Nursing Process and Standards of Care for Psychiatric Mental Health Nursing

*Elizabeth M. Varcarolis*
*Adapted by Karen Clements*

## KEY TERMS AND CONCEPTS

health teaching, 143

mental status examination (MSE), 136

outcome criteria, 141

psychosocial assessment, 137

self-care activities, 143

standards of nursing practice, 133

## OBJECTIVES

1. Compare the approaches you would consider when performing an assessment with a child, an adolescent, and an older adult.
2. Differentiate between the use of an interpreter and the use of a translator when performing an assessment with a non–English-speaking patient.
3. Understand the nursing-process steps used in psychiatric mental health nursing.
4. Conduct a mental status examination (MSE).
5. Perform a psychosocial assessment, including brief cultural and spiritual components.

6. Explain three principles a nurse follows in planning actions to meet agreed-upon outcome criteria.
7. Construct a plan of care for a patient with a mental or emotional health problem.
8. Identify two advanced-practice psychiatric mental health nursing interventions.
9. Demonstrate basic nursing interventions and evaluation of care.
10. Compare and contrast *Nursing Interventions Classification* (NIC), *Nursing Outcomes Classification* (NOC), and evidence-informed practice.

## Ǝvolve WEBSITE

*Visit the Evolve website for Flashcards, Case Studies, and additional testing resources related to*
*the content in this chapter: http://evolve.elsevier.com/Canada/Varcarolis/psychiatric/*  Pre-Test   interactive review

The nursing process is a six-step problem-solving approach intended to facilitate and identify appropriate, safe, culturally competent, developmentally relevant, and quality care for individuals, families, groups, or communities. The nursing process is not a linear but a continuous process of assessing, planning, implementing, and evaluating. Psychiatric mental health nursing practice bases nursing judgements and behaviours on this accepted theoretical framework (Figure 9-1). The most commonly used theories are developmental, psychodynamic, systems, holistic, cognitive, and biological.

Nursing care planning is a collaborative process undertaken with clients (individual patients, families, groups, or communities), working toward mutually agreed-upon definitions of problems, desired outcomes, and interventions. Engagement and collaboration in a client-centred, therapeutic relationship are fundamental to the practice of psychiatric mental health nursing. Each step in the nursing process includes collaboration with the patient:

- *Data gathering* is a transparent process (patient is aware of when, how, what, and why data is gathered about them).
- *Nursing diagnosis* is a process that includes the patient's definition of problems and patient education on the nursing perception of problems.

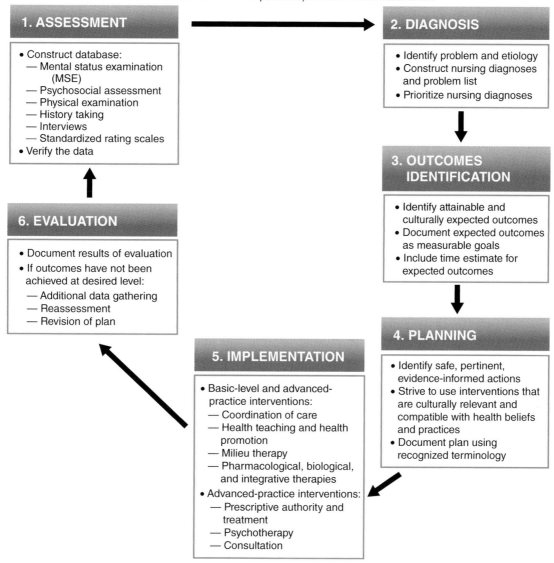

**FIGURE 9-1** The nursing process in psychiatric mental health nursing.

- *Outcome identification* is mutually negotiated and respects the patient's goals.
- *Planning* includes interventions to achieve goals and health teaching on best practice interventions.
- *Implementation* includes patient actions.
- *Evaluation* includes patient evaluation of progress toward goals.

(See O'Connor & Delaney, 2007, for a discussion of collaboration as inherent in evidence-informed practices aligned with recovery principles.)

The use of the nursing process in psychiatric mental health nursing is aligned with standards of nursing practice, as outlined in the *Code of Ethics and Standards of Psychiatric Nursing Practice* (Registered Psychiatric Nurses of Canada, 2010) and *Canadian Standards for Psychiatric-Mental Health Nursing* (Canadian Federation of Mental Health Nurses, 2006). Standards of practice are "authoritative statements that promote, guide, direct and regulate professional nursing practice" (College of Registered Nurses of Nova Scotia, 2012, p. 17). Both sets of standards of practice are provided on the inside back cover of this book.

## HOW A NURSE HELPED ME

### They Told Us He Has Schizophrenia

*My brother had lived next door to my parents for years. After Dad died, Mom said it was nice to have my brother so close so he could help her with the yardwork. Although I knew that my brother had some strange ideas and had always been a loner, he seemed to be doing okay. It was really only after Mom died that I fully understood that she had also been helping him.*

*My brother had been afraid of the police and the spies that, he was convinced, were tracking him. He had piled up old papers and magazines in front of his windows so no one could look in. Although he had been prescribed medication to help reduce these fears, he was not taking it. Soon, my brother also stopped eating because of his belief that his food was being poisoned. He was admitted to hospital. After several weeks, he was discharged and came to live with me and my family. He was not happy about this arrangement, and, frankly, neither was I. We soon moved him into an apartment a few blocks from my home. As part of the hospital discharge plan, my brother and I saw a nurse at our local community mental health office. She met with us and helped us understand what schizophrenia is and how it would impact our lives. The question she asked that was the most helpful was, "What action by your brother would let you know you didn't need to worry so much about him?" I told her his coming over for Sunday supper. My brother was surprised by my response. He thought that I was going to say his taking his medication. The nurse also helped my brother understand the purpose of the medication and how it would help reduce some of his worries; helped him get to his appointments; and also helped him plan his meals. But most important, the nurse helped my brother and me reconnect as brother and sister rather than as caregiver and a person who needed care.*

## ASSESSMENT

A view of the individual as a complex blend of many parts is consistent with nurses' holistic approach to care. Nurses who care for people with physical illnesses ideally maintain a holistic view that involves an awareness of psychological, social, cultural, and spiritual issues. Likewise, nurses who work in the psychiatric mental health field need to assess or have access to reports on past and present medical history, a recent physical examination, and any physical complaints, as well as document any observable physical conditions or behaviours (e.g., unsteady gait, abnormal breathing patterns, wincing as if in pain, doubling over to relieve discomfort). The assessment process begins with the initial patient encounter and continues throughout the duration of caring for the patient. To develop a basis for the plan of care and plan for discharge, every patient should have a thorough, formal nursing assessment upon entering treatment.

Subsequent to the formal assessment, data is collected continually and systematically as the patient's condition changes and, it is to be hoped, improves. For example, a patient may have come into treatment actively suicidal, and the initial focus of care was on protection from injury; through regular assessment, it may be determined that although suicidal ideation has diminished, negative self-evaluation is still certainly a problem.

Assessments are conducted by a variety of professionals, including nurses, psychiatrists, social workers, dietitians, and other therapists. Virtually all facilities have standardized nursing assessment forms to aid in organization and consistency among reviewers. These forms may be paper or electronic versions, according to the resources and preferences of the institution. The time required for the nursing interview—a standard aspect of the formal nursing assessment—varies, depending on the assessment form and the patient's response pattern (e.g., speaks at great length or rambles, is prone to tangential thought, has memory disturbances, or gives markedly slow responses). Refer to Chapter 11 for sound guidelines for setting up and conducting a clinical interview.

Emergency situations may require immediate intervention based on a minimal amount of data and the emergency sharing of personal health information. However, health care workers are required to adhere to legislation regulating the collection of, use of, and access to patient information. Protection of personal health information is a provincial and territorial legislative responsibility, as mandated by the federal *Personal Information Protection and Electronic Documents Act* (http://www.priv.gc.ca); therefore, each province and territory has specific health information legislation (see Table 9-1).

The nurse's primary source for data collection is the patient; however, there may be times when it is necessary to supplement or rely completely on another for the assessment information. These secondary sources can be invaluable when caring for a patient experiencing psychosis, muteness, agitation, or catatonia. Such secondary sources may include members of the family, friends, neighbours, police, health care workers, and medical records. It may be appropriate to conduct a nursing family assessment with the patient and his or her significant others in order to understand more fully the resources, supports, and problems in the patient's life (Wright & Leahey, 2009).

The best atmosphere in which to conduct an assessment is one of minimal anxiety. Therefore, if an individual becomes upset, defensive, or embarrassed regarding any topic, the topic should be abandoned. The nurse can acknowledge that the subject makes the patient uncomfortable and suggest within the medical record that the topic be discussed when the patient feels more comfortable. It is important that the nurse not probe, pry, or push for information that is difficult for the patient to discuss. However, it should be recognized that increased anxiety about any subject is data in itself and should be noted in the assessment even without obtaining any further information.

### Age Considerations

#### Assessment of Children

When assessing children, it is important to gather data from a variety of sources. Although the child is the best source for determining emotions, the caregivers (parents or guardians)

| TABLE 9-1 | PROVINCIAL AND TERRITORIAL HEALTH INFORMATION ACTS |
|---|---|
| **PROVINCE OR TERRITORY** | **WEBSITE LINK** |
| Alberta | http://www.health.alberta.ca/about/health-legislation.html |
| British Columbia | http://www.bclaws.ca/EPLibraries/bclaws_new/document/ID/freeside/00_03063_01 |
| Manitoba | http://www.gov.mb.ca/health/phia/ |
| New Brunswick | http://www.gnb.ca/0051/acts/index-e.asp |
| Newfoundland and Labrador | http://www.health.gov.nl.ca/health/PHIA/ |
| Northwest Territories | http://www.priv.gc.ca/resource/prov/index_e.asp#006 |
| Nova Scotia | http://novascotia.ca/dhw/phia/ |
| Nunavut | http://www.priv.gc.ca/resource/prov/index_e.asp#008 |
| Ontario | http://www.e-laws.gov.on.ca/html/statutes/english/elaws_statutes_04p03_e.htm |
| Prince Edward Island | http://www.healthpei.ca/index.php3?number=1020297&lang=E |
| Quebec | http://www.publicationsduquebec.gouv.qc.ca/fre/products/61184 |
| Saskatchewan | http://www.health.gov.sk.ca/hipa |
| Yukon | http://www.hss.gov.yk.ca/ (health privacy act under construction as of spring 2013) |

often can best describe the behaviour, performance, and attitude of the child. Caregivers also are helpful in interpreting the child's words and responses. However, an interview separate from caregivers is advisable when an older child is reluctant to share information, especially in cases of suspected abuse (Arnold & Boggs, 2007).

Developmental levels should be considered in the evaluation of children. One of the hallmarks of psychiatric disorders in children is the tendency to regress (i.e., return to a previous level of development). Although it is developmentally appropriate for toddlers to suck their thumbs, such a gesture in an older child is unusual.

Bernzweig, Takayama, Phibbs, and colleagues (1997) found that children felt more comfortable when their health care provider was the same gender. Waseem and Ryan (2005) indicated that although 60% of parents preferred their children be cared for by a man, 79% of the children studied, regardless of gender, requested a female physician. Age-appropriate communication strategies are perhaps the most important factor in establishing successful communication (Arnold & Boggs, 2007).

Assessment of children should be accomplished by a combination of interview and observation. Watching children at play provides important clues to their functioning. From a psychodynamic view, supported play (play encouraged to a level with which the child is comfortable) is a safe way for the child to act out thoughts and emotions and to release pent-up emotions—for example, having a child act out his or her story (or family's story) with the use of anatomically correct dolls. Asking the child to tell a story, draw a picture, or engage in specific therapeutic games can be useful assessment tools in determining critical concerns and painful issues a child may have difficulty expressing. Usually, a clinician with special training in child and adolescent psychiatry works with young children. Chapter 29 presents a more extensive overview of assessing children.

| BOX 9-1 | THE HEADSSS PSYCHOSOCIAL INTERVIEW TECHNIQUE |
|---|---|

**H**—Home environment (e.g., relationships with parents and siblings)
**E**—Education and employment (e.g., school performance)
**A**—Activities (e.g., sports participation, after-school activities, peer relations)
**D**—Drug, alcohol, or tobacco use
**S**—Sexuality (e.g., whether the patient is sexually active, practises safer sex, uses contraception)
**S**—Suicide risk or symptoms of depression or other mental health disorder
**S**—"Savagery" (e.g., violence or abuse in home environment or in neighbourhood)

### Assessment of Adolescents

Adolescents are especially concerned with confidentiality and may fear that anything they say to the nurse will be repeated to their parents. Lack of confidentiality can become a barrier of care with this population. Adolescents need to know that their records are private, and they should receive an explanation as to how information will be shared among the treatment team. The adolescent may be hesitant to answer questions related to such topics as substance use and sexual activity. Therefore, these must be asked in a nonjudgemental manner. If the answers to these questions do not indicate that the adolescent is at risk for harm, the answers may be handled confidentially (Arnold & Boggs, 2007). However, threats of suicide, homicide, sexual abuse, or behaviours that put the patient or others at risk for harm must be shared with other professionals, as well as with the parents. Because identifying risk factors is one of the key objectives when assessing adolescents, it is helpful to use a brief, structured interview technique such as the HEADSSS interview (Box 9-1). Chapter 29 offers more on assessment of adolescents.

## Assessment of Older Adults

As we get older, our five senses (taste, touch, sight, hearing, and smell) and brain function begin to diminish, but the extent to which this affects each person varies. Your patient may be a spry and alert 80-year-old or a frail and confused 60-year-old. Therefore, it is important not to stereotype older adults or expect them to be physically or mentally deficient. For example, the tendency may be to jump to the conclusion that someone who is hard of hearing is cognitively impaired, an assumption that should be avoided. However, it is true that many older adults need special attention. The nurse needs to be aware of any physical limitations—for example, any sensory condition (difficulty seeing or hearing), motor condition (difficulty walking or maintaining balance), or medical condition (back pain, cardiac or pulmonary deficits)—that could cause increased anxiety, stress, or physical discomfort for the patient during assessment of mental and emotional needs. It is wise to identify any physical deficits at the onset of the assessment and make accommodations for them. If the patient is hard of hearing, speak a little more slowly in clear, louder tones (but not too loud) and seat the patient close to you without invading his or her personal space. Often, a voice that is lower in pitch is easier for older adults to hear, and a higher-pitched voice may convey anxiety to some.

## Language Barriers

It is becoming more and more apparent that psychiatric mental health nurses can best serve their patients if they have a thorough understanding of the complex cultural and social factors that influence health and illness. Awareness of individual cultural beliefs and health care practices can help nurses minimize stereotyped assumptions that can lead to ineffective care and interfere with the ability to evaluate care. There are many opportunities for misunderstandings when assessing a patient from a different cultural or social background from your own, particularly if the interview is conducted in English or French, and the patient speaks a different language or a different form of English or French (Fontes, 2008).

To understand the patient's history and health care needs, health care providers often require a professional translator, as discussed in Chapter 7. Although there is no federal legislation mandating the use of trained translators for patients whose English or French proficiency is limited, Canadian health care organizations and providers recognize that language barriers compromise health and patient care; therefore, access to trained translators is considered a health care priority (see Hoen, Nielsen, & Sasso, 2006, for more on Canadian health care interpreter services). Unfortunately, professional translators are not always readily available in many health care facilities.

## Psychiatric Mental Health Nursing Assessment

The purposes of the psychiatric mental health nursing assessment are the following:
- Establish rapport
- Obtain an understanding of the current problem or chief complaint
- Review physical status and obtain baseline vital signs
- Assess for risk factors affecting the safety of the patient or others
- Perform a mental status examination
- Assess psychosocial status
- Identify mutual goals for treatment
- Formulate a plan of care

### Gathering Data

*Review of systems.* The mind–body connection is significant in the understanding and treatment of psychiatric disorders. Many patients who are admitted for treatment of psychiatric conditions also are given a thorough physical examination by a primary care provider. Likewise, most nursing assessments include a baseline set of vital statistics, a historical and current review of body systems, and a documentation of allergic responses.

Poole and Higgo (2006) point out that several medical conditions and physical illnesses may mimic psychiatric illnesses (Box 9-2). Therefore, physical causes of symptoms must be ruled out. Conversely, psychiatric disorders can result in physical or somatic symptoms such as stomach aches, headaches, lethargy, insomnia, intense fatigue, and even pain. When depression is secondary to a known physical medical condition, it often goes unrecognized and thus untreated. Therefore, all patients who come into the health care system need to have both a medical and mental health evaluation to ensure correct diagnoses and appropriate care.

Individuals with certain physical conditions may be more prone to psychiatric disorders such as depression. It is believed, for example, that the disease process of multiple sclerosis or other autoimmune diseases may actually bring about depression. Other physical diseases typically associated with depression are coronary artery disease, diabetes, and stroke. Individuals need to be evaluated for any medical origins of their depression or anxiety.

When evidence suggests the presence of mental confusion or organic mental disease, a mental status examination (MSE), discussed below, should be performed.

*Laboratory data.* Hypothyroidism may have the clinical appearance of depression, and hyperthyroidism may appear to be a manic phase of bipolar disorder; a simple blood test can usually differentiate between depression and thyroid problems. Abnormal liver enzyme levels can explain irritability, depression, and lethargy. People who have chronic renal disease often suffer from the same symptoms when their blood urea nitrogen and electrolyte levels are abnormal. A toxicology screen for the presence of either prescription or illegal drugs also may provide useful information.

*Mental status examination.* Fundamental to the psychiatric mental health nursing assessment is a mental status examination (MSE). In fact, an MSE is part of the assessment in all areas of medicine. The MSE in psychiatry is analogous to the physical examination in general medicine, and the purpose is to evaluate an individual's current cognitive, affective (emotional), and behavioural functioning. For acutely disturbed patients, it is not unusual for the mental health clinician to

## BOX 9-2   SOME MEDICAL CONDITIONS THAT MAY MIMIC PSYCHIATRIC ILLNESS

**Depression**

Neurological disorders:
- Cerebrovascular accident (stroke)
- Alzheimer's disease
- Brain tumour
- Huntington's disease
- Epilepsy (seizure disorder)
- Multiple sclerosis
- Parkinson's disease

Infections:
- Mononucleosis
- Encephalitis
- Hepatitis
- Tertiary syphilis
- Human immunodeficiency virus (HIV)

Endocrine disorders:
- Hypothyroidism and hyperthyroidism
- Cushing's syndrome
- Addison's disease
- Parathyroid disease

Gastrointestinal disorders:
- Liver cirrhosis
- Pancreatitis

Cardiovascular disorders:
- Hypoxia
- Heart failure

Respiratory disorders:
- Sleep apnea

Nutritional disorders:
- Thiamine deficiency
- Protein deficiency
- $B_{12}$ deficiency
- $B_6$ deficiency
- Folate deficiency

Collagen vascular diseases:
- Lupus erythematosus
- Rheumatoid arthritis

Cancer

**Anxiety**

Neurological disorders:
- Alzheimer's disease
- Brain tumour
- Stroke
- Huntington's disease

Infections:
- Encephalitis
- Meningitis

- Neurosyphilis
- Septicemia

Endocrine disorders:
- Hypothyroidism and hyperthyroidism
- Hypoparathyroidism
- Hypoglycemia
- Pheochromocytoma
- Carcinoid

Metabolic disorders:
- Low calcium
- Low potassium
- Acute intermittent porphyria
- Liver failure

Cardiovascular disorders:
- Angina
- Heart failure
- Pulmonary embolus

Respiratory disorders:
- Pneumothorax
- Acute asthma
- Emphysema

Drug effects:
- Stimulants
- Sedatives (withdrawal)

Lead, mercury poisoning

**Psychosis**

Medical conditions:
- Temporal lobe epilepsy
- Migraine headaches
- Temporal arteritis
- Occipital tumours
- Narcolepsy
- Encephalitis
- Hypothyroidism
- Addison's disease
- HIV

Drug effects:
- Hallucinogens (e.g., LSD)
- Phencyclidine
- Alcohol withdrawal
- Stimulants
- Cocaine
- Corticosteroids

administer MSEs every day. Box 9-3 provides an example of a basic MSE.

The MSE, by and large, aids in collecting and organizing objective data. The nurse observes the patient's physical behaviour, nonverbal communication, appearance, speech patterns, mood and affect, thought content, perceptions, cognitive ability, and insight and judgement.

***Psychosocial assessment.*** A psychosocial assessment provides additional information from which to develop a

plan of care. It includes the following information about the patient:

- Central or chief complaint (in the patient's own words)
- History of violent, suicidal, or self-mutilating behaviours
- Alcohol or substance abuse
- Family psychiatric history
- Personal psychiatric treatment, including medications and complementary therapies
- Stressors and coping methods

## BOX 9-3    MENTAL STATUS EXAMINATION

A. Appearance
  1. Grooming and dress
  2. Level of hygiene
  3. Pupil dilation or constriction
  4. Facial expression
  5. Height, weight, nutritional status
  6. Presence of body piercing or tattoos, scars, etc.
  7. Relationship between appearance and age
B. Behaviour
  1. Excessive or reduced body movements
  2. Peculiar body movements (e.g., scanning of the environment, odd or repetitive gestures, level of consciousness, balance and gait)
  3. Abnormal movements (e.g., tardive dyskinesia, tremors)
  4. Level of eye contact (keep cultural differences in mind; see Chapter 7)
C. Speech
  1. Rate: slow, rapid, normal
  2. Volume: loud, soft, normal
  3. Disturbances (e.g., articulation problems, slurring, stuttering, mumbling)
  4. Cluttering (e.g., rapid, disorganized, tongue-tied speech)
D. Mood
  1. Affect: flat, bland, animated, angry, withdrawn, appropriate to context, lability
  2. Mood: sad, euphoric, duration, degree, stability
E. Disorders of the Form of Thought
  1. Thought process (e.g., disorganized, coherent, flight of ideas, neologisms, thought blocking, circumstantiality)
  2. Thought content (e.g., delusions, obsessions)
F. Perceptual Disturbances
  1. Hallucinations (e.g., auditory, visual, tactile)
  2. Illusions
G. Cognition
  1. Orientation: time, place, person
  2. Level of consciousness (e.g., alert, confused, clouded, stuporous, unconscious, comatose)
  3. Memory: remote, recent, immediate
  4. Fund of knowledge (general knowledge as compared to the average person in a given society)
  5. Attention: performance on serial sevens (counting down from 100 by 7s), serial threes (counting down from 20 by 3s), digit span tests (recalling in order a series of digits)
  6. Abstraction: performance on tests involving similarities, proverbs
  7. Insight
  8. Judgement
H. Ideas of Harming Self or Others
  1. Suicidal or homicidal thoughts:
    a. Presence of a plan
    b. Lethality of means
    c. Means to carry out the plan
    d. Opportunity to carry out the plan

- Quality of activities of daily living
- Personal background
- Social background, including support system
- Weaknesses, strengths, and goals for treatment
- Racial, ethnic, and cultural beliefs and practices
- Spiritual beliefs or religious practices

The patient's psychosocial history is most often the subjective part of the assessment. The focus of the history is the patient's perceptions and recollections of current lifestyle and life in general (family, friends, education, work experience, coping styles, and spiritual and cultural beliefs).

A psychosocial assessment elicits information about the person's social functioning and the systems in which a person operates. To conduct such an assessment, the nurse should have fundamental knowledge of growth and development, basic cultural and religious practices, pathophysiology, psychopathology, and pharmacology. Box 9-4 provides a basic psychosocial assessment tool.

***Spiritual or religious assessment.*** Carson and Koenig (2004) stress the importance of a spiritual or religious assessment to a holistic nursing assessment. The idea that spirituality or religious involvement is recognized as an important influence on a person's health and behaviour has long been recognized (Miller & Thoresen, 2003). Spirituality and religious beliefs have the potential to exert a positive influence on patients' views of themselves and how they interact and respond to others (Mackenzie, Rajagopal, Meibohm, et al., 2000).

Baetz, Larson, Marcoux, and colleagues (2002) studied the level of religious commitment in Canadian psychiatric inpatients. They found that religious commitment in psychiatric inpatients was as high or higher than that of the general Canadian population and had a significant impact on depression, life satisfaction, hospital use, and alcohol use. Baetz and colleagues (2002) recommend addressing "the spiritual aspect of patients' lives whether positive, negative, or neutral in order to address the person as a whole" and to support spirituality or religious practices as coping mechanisms (p. 159).

Spirituality and religion are, however, quite different in their influences. *Spirituality* is more of an internal phenomenon, often understood as addressing universal human questions and needs (Anandarajab, 2008). Spirituality can be expressed as having three dimensions: (1) cognitive (beliefs, values, ideals, purpose, truth, wisdom), (2) experiential (love, compassion, connection, forgiveness, altruism), and (3) behavioural (daily behaviour, moral obligations, life choices, and medical choices) (Anandarajab, 2008). Spirituality can increase healthy behaviours, social support, and a sense of meaning, which are linked to decreased overall mental and physical illness (George, Larson, Koenig, et al., 2000).

*Religion*, on the other hand, is an external system that includes beliefs, patterns of worship, symbols, and requirements of membership (Koenig, 2001; Miller & Thoresen, 2003). Although religion is often concerned with spirituality, religious groups are social entities and are often characterized by other goals as well (cultural, economic, political, social) (Miller & Thoresen, 2003). Religious involvement is associated with better physical health, better mental health, and longer survival (George, Ellison, & Larson, 2002). Belonging to a religious community can provide support during difficult times, and prayer can be a source of hope, comfort, and support in healing.

Delgado (2007) notes that nurses and other health care providers may be uncomfortable with assessing for or discussing spiritual and religious issues with patients, even though their

## BOX 9-4  PSYCHOSOCIAL ASSESSMENT

A. Previous hospitalizations

B. Educational background

C. Occupational background

   1. Employed? Where? What length of time?

   2. Special skills

D. Social patterns

   1. Describe family.

   2. Describe friends.

   3. With whom does the patient live?

   4. To whom does the patient go in times of crisis?

   5. Describe a typical day.

E. Sexual patterns

   1. Sexually active? Practises safer sex? Practises birth control?

   2. Sexual orientation?

   3. Sexual difficulties?

F. Interests and abilities

   1. What does the patient do in his or her spare time?

   2. What sport, hobby, or leisure activity is the patient good at?

   3. What gives the patient pleasure?

G. Substance use and abuse

   1. What medications does the patient take? How often? How much?

   2. What herbal or over-the-counter medications does the patient take (e.g., caffeine, cough medicines, St. John's wort)? How often? How much?

   3. What psychotropic medications does the patient take? How often? How much?

   4. How many drinks of alcohol does the patient have per day? Per week?

   5. What recreational drugs does the patient use (e.g., club drugs, marijuana, psychedelics, steroids)? How often? How much?

   6. Does the patient overuse prescription medications (benzodiazepines, pain medications)?

   7. Does the patient identify the use of drugs as a problem?

H. Coping abilities

   1. What does the patient do when he or she gets upset?

   2. To whom can the patient talk?

   3. What usually helps to relieve stress?

   4. What did the patient try this time?

I. Spiritual assessment

   1. What importance does religion or spirituality have in the patient's life?

   2. Do the patient's religious or spiritual beliefs relate to the way the patient takes care of himself or herself or the illness? How?

   3. Does the patient's faith help the patient in stressful situations?

   4. Whom does the patient see when he or she is medically ill? Mentally upset?

   5. Are there special health care practices within the patient's culture that address his or her particular mental problem?

proximity to patients and intimate patient needs gives them a unique opportunity to develop spiritual care theory and practices.

The following questions may be included in a spiritual or religious assessment:

- Who or what supplies you with strength and hope?
- Do you have a religious affiliation?
- Do you practise any spiritual activities (yoga, tai chi, meditation, prayer)?
- Do you participate in any religious activities?
- What role does religion or spiritual practice play in your life?
- Does your faith help you in stressful situations?
- Has your illness affected your religious or spiritual practices?
- Would you like to have someone from your church, synagogue, or temple or from our facility visit?

***Cultural and social assessment.*** Canada is rich in cultural diversity. Canada's official policy of multiculturalism means that cultural diversity is respected, and privilege of one culture over another is challenged (Racher & Annis, 2007). One consequence of Canadian multiculturalism is an increased responsibility for nurses to "move beyond the superficial knowledge of a culture to seek and consider the personal meanings that individuals ascribe to their own ethnicity" (Racher & Annis, 2007, p. 263). Cultural safety is a concept that moves beyond understanding cultural differences toward an understanding of the power differentials in society and therefore also in health care. Respectful nursing care of

individuals, families, and communities from diverse cultural backgrounds requires consciousness of one's own cultural world view, an understanding of the political or economic inequalities in Canadian society, and the engagement of the advocacy role of nurses (Browne & Varcoe, 2006; Hart-Wasekeesikaw, 2009).

Kirmayer, Simpson, and Cargo (2003) outline the key issues of Aboriginal Canadian mental health and healing traditions. Healing traditions and cultural identity construction are used by many Aboriginal peoples in positive ways to bring about community, family, and individual healing; however, Aboriginal Canadians come from a wide range of cultural groups and vary as to how much they identify with Aboriginal culture. To assume that all members of a cultural group have the same characteristics, beliefs, goals, and problems is stereotyping and disrespectful of the individual. Chapter 7 offers a detailed discussion of the cultural implications for psychiatric mental health nursing and information for conducting a cultural and social assessment.

Some questions we can ask to help with a cultural and social assessment are:

- What is your primary language? Would you like a translator?
- How would you describe your cultural background?
- Who are you close to?
- Who do you seek in times of crisis?
- Who do you live with?
- Who do you seek when you are medically ill? Mentally upset or concerned?

- What do you do to get better when you have physical problems?
- What are the attitudes toward mental illness in your culture?
- How is your current problem viewed by your culture? Is it seen as a problem that can be fixed? A disease? A taboo? A fault or curse?
- Are there special foods that you eat?
- Are there special health care practices within your culture that address your particular mental or emotional health problem?
- Are there any special cultural beliefs about your illness that might help me give you better care?

After the cultural and social assessment, it is useful to summarize pertinent data with the patient. This summary provides patients with reassurance that they have been heard and gives them the opportunity to clarify any misinformation. The patient should be told what will happen next. For example, if the initial assessment takes place in the hospital, you should tell the patient who else he or she will be seeing. If you believe a referral is necessary, discuss this recommendation with the patient.

### Validating the Assessment

To gain an even clearer understanding of your patient, it is helpful to look to outside sources. Emergency department records can be a valuable resource in understanding an individual's presenting behaviour and problems. Police reports may be available in cases in which hostility and legal altercations occurred. Old medical records, most now accessible by computer, are a great help in validating information you already have or in adding new information to your database. If the patient was admitted to a psychiatric unit in the past, information about the patient's previous level of functioning and behaviour gives you a baseline for making clinical judgements. Check with your provincial or territorial personal health information act to find out when signed consent of the patient or an appropriate relative is necessary to obtain access to records. All personal health information legislation requires nurses to obtain verbal consent from patients before discussing confidential information and treatment with their families; however, nurses have the skills and a responsibility to facilitate the involvement of families where appropriate.

### Using Rating Scales

A number of standardized rating scales are useful for psychiatric evaluation and monitoring. Rating scales are often administered by a clinician, but many are self-administered. Table 9-2 lists some that are in common use. Many of the clinical chapters in this book include a rating scale.

## NURSING DIAGNOSIS

A nursing diagnosis is a clinical judgement about a patient's response, needs, actual and potential psychiatric disorders, mental health problems, and potential co-morbid physical illnesses. A well-chosen and well-stated nursing diagnosis is the basis for selecting therapeutic outcomes and interventions

| TABLE 9-2 | STANDARDIZED RATING SCALES* |
|---|---|
| **USE** | **SCALE** |
| Depression | Beck Inventory |
| | Brief Patient Health Questionnaire (Brief PHQ) |
| | Geriatric Depression Scale (GDS) |
| | Hamilton Depression Scale |
| | Zung Self-Report Inventory |
| | Patient Health Questionnaire-9 (PHQ-9) |
| Anxiety | Brief Patient Health Questionnaire (Brief PHQ) |
| | Generalized Anxiety Disorder–7 (GAD-7) |
| | Modified Spielberger State Anxiety Scale |
| | Hamilton Anxiety Scale |
| Substance use disorders | CAGE† (see Ewing, 1984; O'Brien, 2008) |
| | Addiction Severity Index (ASI) |
| | Recovery Attitude and Treatment Evaluator (RAATE) |
| | Brief Drug Abuse Screen Test (B-DAST) |
| Obsessive-compulsive behaviour | Yale-Brown Obsessive-Compulsive Scale (Y-BOCS) |
| Mania | Mania Rating Scale |
| Schizophrenia | Scale for Assessment of Negative Symptoms (SANS) |
| | Brief Psychiatric Rating Scale (BPRS) |
| Abnormal movements | Abnormal Involuntary Movement Scale (AIMS) |
| | Simpson Neurological Rating Scale |
| General psychiatric assessment | Brief Psychiatric Rating Scale (BPRS) |
| | Global Assessment of Functioning Scale (GAF) |
| Cognitive function | Mini-Mental State Examination (MMSE) |
| | St. Louis University Mental Status Examination (SLUMS) |
| | Cognitive Capacity Screening Examination (CCSE) |
| | Alzheimer's Disease Rating Scale (ADRS) |
| | Memory and Behavior Problem Checklist |
| | Functional Assessment Screening Tool (FAST) |
| | Global Deterioration Scale (GDS) |
| Family assessment | McMaster Family Assessment Device |
| Eating disorders | Eating Disorders Inventory (EDI) |
| | Body Attitude Test |
| | Diagnostic Survey for Eating Disorders |

*These rating scales highlight important areas in psychiatric assessment. Because many of the answers are subjective, experienced clinicians use these tools as a guide when planning care and also draw on their knowledge of their patients and their patients' perception of their own experience.
†This acronym helps the clinician remember to ask questions about **c**utting down, **a**nnoyance by criticism related to substance use, feelings of **g**uilt related to substance use, and if the substance is needed to "get going" in the morning—the **e**ye opener.

## TABLE 9-3 EXAMPLES OF LONG- AND SHORT-TERM GOALS FOR A SUICIDAL PATIENT

| LONG-TERM GOALS OR OUTCOMES | SHORT-TERM GOALS OR OUTCOMES |
|---|---|
| 1. Patient will remain free from injury throughout the hospital stay. | a. Patient will state he or she understands the rationale and procedure of the unit's protocol for suicide precautions shortly after admission.<br>b. Patient will sign a "no-suicide" contract for the next 24 hours, renewable at the end of every 24-hour period (if approved for use by the mental health facility).<br>c. Patient will seek out staff when feeling overwhelmed or self-destructive during hospitalization. |
| 2. By discharge, patient will state he or she no longer wishes to die and has at least two people to contact if suicidal thoughts arise. | a. Patient will meet with social worker to find supportive resources in the community before discharge and work on trigger issues (e.g., housing, job).<br>b. By discharge, patient will state the purpose of medication, time and dose, adverse effects, and who to call with questions or concerns.<br>c. Patient will have the written name and telephone numbers of at least two people to turn to if feeling overwhelmed or self-destructive.<br>d. Patient will have a follow-up appointment to meet with a mental health professional by discharge. |

(Herdman, 2012). Refer to Appendix B for a list of NANDA-I–approved nursing diagnoses.

A nursing diagnosis has three structural components:
1. Problem (unmet need)
2. Etiology (probable cause)
3. Supporting data (signs and symptoms)

The *problem*, or unmet need, describes the state of the patient at present. Problems that are within the nurse's domain to treat are termed *nursing diagnoses*. The nursing diagnostic title states what should change. Example: Hopelessness.

*Etiology*, or probable cause, is linked to the diagnostic title with the words *related to*. Stating the etiology or probable cause tells what needs to be addressed to effect the change and identifies causes the nurse can treat through nursing interventions. Example: Hopelessness related to multiple losses.

*Supporting data*, or signs and symptoms, state what the patient's condition is like at present. It may be linked to the diagnosis and etiology with the words *as evidenced by*. Supporting data (defining characteristics) that validate the diagnosis may include:
• The patient's statement (e.g., "It's no use; nothing will change.")
• Lack of involvement with family and friends
• Lack of motivation to care for self or environment

The complete nursing diagnosis might be *Hopelessness related to multiple losses, as evidenced by lack of motivation to care for self.*

## OUTCOMES IDENTIFICATION

Outcome criteria are the hoped-for outcomes that reflect the maximal level of patient health that can realistically be achieved through nursing interventions. Whereas nursing diagnoses identify problems, outcomes reflect desired changes. The expected outcomes provide direction for continuity of care (American Nurses Association [ANA], American Psychiatric Nurses Association, & International Society of Psychiatric

Mental Health Nurses, 2007). Outcomes should take into account the patient's culture, values, ethical beliefs, and personal goals. Specifically, outcomes are stated in attainable and measurable terms and include a time estimate for attainment (ANA et al., 2007). Moorhead, Johnson, Maas, and colleagues (2008) have compiled a standardized list of nursing outcomes in the *Nursing Outcomes Classification* (NOC) (see Chapter 1). *NOC* includes a total of 385 standardized outcomes that provide a mechanism for communicating the effect of nursing interventions on the well-being of patients, families, and communities. Each outcome has an associated group of indicators used to determine patient status in relation to the outcome. Whether nursing outcomes are derived from *NOC*, a psychiatric mental health nursing care plan text, best practice research, or other sources, it is important that criteria are individualized and documented as obtainable goals.

It is helpful to use long- and short-term outcomes, often stated as goals, when assessing the effectiveness of nursing interventions. The use of long- and short-term outcomes or goals is particularly helpful for teaching and learning purposes. It is also valuable for providing guidelines for appropriate interventions. The use of goals guides nurses in building incremental steps toward meeting the desired outcome. All outcomes (goals) are written in positive terms. Table 9-3 shows how specific outcome criteria might be stated for a suicidal individual with a nursing diagnosis of *Risk for suicide related to depression.*

## PLANNING

The nurse considers the following specific principles when planning care:
• *Safe*—Interventions must be safe for the patient, as well as for other patients, staff, and family.
• *Compatible and appropriate*—Interventions must be compatible with other therapies and with the patient's personal goals and cultural values, as well as with institutional rules.

- *Realistic and individualized*—Interventions should be (1) within the patient's capabilities, given the patient's age, physical strength, condition, and willingness to change; (2) based on the number of staff available; (3) reflective of the actual available community resources; and (4) within the student's or nurse's capabilities.
- *Evidence-informed*—Interventions should be based on scientific evidence and principles when available.

DiCenso (2003) defines evidence-informed nursing care as "methodologically sound, clinically relevant research about the effectiveness and safety of nursing interventions, the accuracy and precision of nursing assessment measures, the power of prognostic indicators, the strength of casual relationships, the cost-effectiveness of nursing interventions and the meaning of illness or patient experiences" (p. 21). While empirical evidence is an important aspect of nursing practice, the Canadian Nurses Association promotes the use of the term *evidence-informed decision making* in nursing practice because it includes other elements impacting clinical decision making such as professional clinical judgement, client preference, and collaboration with other key health stakeholders (Canadian Nurses Association, 2010). Box 9-5 lists several online resources for evidence-informed decision making and nursing practice. Keep in mind that whatever interventions are planned must be acceptable and appropriate to the individual patient. Psychiatric mental health nurses must also keep the principles of psychosocial rehabilitation in mind when planning care; as noted in a British Columbian mental health best practice document, the principles of psychosocial rehabilitation form the foundation for all best practices in mental health (Calsaferri, Treherne, & van der Leer, 2002).

The *Nursing Interventions Classification* (*NIC*) (Bulechek, Butcher, & Dochterman, 2008) is a research-based, standardized listing of 542 interventions reflective of current clinical practice the nurse can use to plan care (see Chapter 1). Nurses in all settings can use *NIC* to support quality patient care and incorporate evidence-informed nursing actions. Although many safe and appropriate interventions may not be included in *NIC*, it is a useful guide for standardized care. Individualizing interventions to meet a patient's special needs, with patient input, should always be part of the planning.

When choosing nursing interventions from *NIC*, psychiatric nursing care plan texts, or other sources, the nurse uses not just those that fit the nursing diagnosis (e.g., risk for suicide) but interventions that match the defining data. Although the outcome criteria might be similar or the same (e.g., suicide self-restraint), the safe and appropriate interventions may be totally different because of the defining data. For example, consider the nursing diagnosis *Risk for suicide related to feelings of despair, as evidenced by two recent suicide attempts and repeated statements that "I want to die."* The planning of appropriate nursing interventions might include the following:

- Initiate suicide precautions (e.g., ongoing observations and monitoring of the patient, provision of a protective environment) for the person who is at serious risk for suicide.
- Search the newly hospitalized patient and personal belongings for weapons or potential weapons during the inpatient admission procedure, as appropriate.
- Use protective interventions (e.g., area restriction seclusion, physical restraints) if the patient lacks the restraint to refrain from harming self, as needed.
- Assign the hospitalized patient to a room located near the nursing station for ease of observation, as appropriate.

However, if the defining data are different, the appropriate interventions will be as well—for example: *Risk for suicide related to loss of spouse, as evidenced by lack of self-care and statements evidencing loneliness.* The nurse might choose the following interventions for this patient's plan of care:

- Determine the presence and degree of suicide risk.
- Facilitate support of the patient by family and friends.
- Consider strategies to decrease isolation and opportunity to act on harmful thoughts.
- Assist the patient in identifying a network of supportive personnel and resources within the community (e.g., support groups, clergy, care providers).
- Provide information about available community resources and outreach programs.

Chapter 25 addresses assessment of and interventions for suicidal patients in more depth.

## IMPLEMENTATION

The therapeutic interpersonal relationship is recognized as the first standard of practice by both the Registered Psychiatric Nurses of Canada (2010) and the Canadian Federation of Mental Health Nurses (2006), emphasizing the critical importance of this fundamental competency. The basic implementation skills are accomplished through the nurse–patient relationship and therapeutic interventions. The nurse implements the plan using evidence-informed practice whenever

---

**BOX 9-5**  **USEFUL EVIDENCE-INFORMED DECISION MAKING AND NURSING PRACTICE WEBSITES**

- Canadian Best Practices Portal:
  http://cbpp-pcpe.phac-aspc.gc.ca/
- Evidence-Informed Decision-Making:
  http://www.nurseone.ca/Default.aspx?portlet=StaticHtmlViewerPortlet&plang=1&ptdi=866
- Evidence-Based Practice in Mental Health:
  http://ktclearinghouse.ca/cebm/syllabi/mental/intro
- Center for Research and Evidence Based Practice:
  http://www.son.rochester.edu/son/research/centers/research-evidenced-based-practice
- Academic Center for Evidence-Based Practice (ACE):
  http://www.acestar.uthscsa.edu
- The Cochrane Collaboration:
  http://www.cochrane.org
- The Joanna Briggs Institute:
  http://www.joannabriggs.edu.au

possible, uses community resources, and collaborates with nursing colleagues. Recent graduates and practitioners new to the psychiatric setting practise at the "entry to practice" level with the guidance and support of more experienced health care providers. The College of Registered Psychiatric Nurses of Manitoba (then called the Registered Psychiatric Nurses' Association of Manitoba) (1993) states in its psychiatric nursing competency document that the level at which the psychiatric nurse functions and the types of activities in which the psychiatric nurse engages depend on the prescribed legal limits of practice, the qualifications of the individual psychiatric nurse (education, work experience, certification), and the practice setting as well as personal competence and initiative.

## Basic-Level Interventions
### Coordination of Care
The psychiatric mental health nurse coordinates the implementation of the plan and provides documentation.

### Health Teaching and Health Promotion
Psychiatric mental health nurses use a variety of health teaching methods, which they adapt to the patient's needs (e.g., age, culture, ability to learn, readiness), integrating current knowledge and research and seeking opportunities for feedback and effectiveness of care. Health teaching includes identifying the health education needs of the patient and teaching basic principles of physical and mental health, such as giving information about coping, interpersonal relationships, social skills, mental health disorders, the treatments for such illnesses and their effects on daily living, relapse prevention, problem-solving skills, stress management, crisis intervention, and self-care activities. The last of these, self-care activities, assists the patient in assuming personal responsibility for activities of daily living (ADL) and focuses on improving the patient's mental and physical well-being.

### Milieu Therapy
Milieu therapy requires managing the environment in which treatment takes place so that patients feel comfortable, safe, and respected (see Chapter 3). Milieu management includes orienting patients to their rights and responsibilities, selecting specific activities that meet patients' physical and mental health needs, and ensuring that patients are maintained in the least restrictive environment safety permits. It also includes informing patients about the need for limits and the conditions necessary to set limits in a culturally competent manner (see Chapter 7).

### Pharmacological, Biological, and Integrative Therapies
Nurses need to know the intended action, therapeutic dosage, adverse reactions, and safe blood levels of medications being administered and must monitor them when appropriate (e.g., blood levels for lithium). The nurse is expected to discuss and provide medication teaching tools to the patient and family regarding drug action, adverse effects, dietary restrictions, and drug interactions and to provide time for questions. The nurse's assessment of the patient's response

to psychobiological interventions is communicated to other members of the multidisciplinary mental health team. Interventions are also aimed at alleviating untoward effects of medication.

### Advanced-Practice Interventions
Some registered nurses and registered psychiatric nurses are educationally and clinically prepared to conduct advanced interventions such as offering psychotherapy to individuals, couples, groups, and families and providing consultation to other disciplines using evidence-informed psychotherapeutic frameworks and nurse–patient therapeutic relationships. Refer to Chapter 3 for an overview of various psychotherapies, Chapter 35 for a discussion of therapeutic groups, Chapter 36 for a discussion of family interventions, and Chapter 37 for a discussion of integrative therapies.

## EVALUATION
Unfortunately, evaluation of patient outcomes is often the most neglected part of the nursing process. Evaluation of the individual's response to treatment should be systematic, ongoing, and criteria-based. Supporting data are included to clarify the evaluation. Ongoing assessment of data allows for revisions of nursing diagnoses, changes to more realistic outcomes, or identification of more appropriate interventions when outcomes are not met.

## DOCUMENTATION
Documentation could be considered the seventh step in the nursing process. Keep in mind that medical records are legal documents and may be used in a court of law. (Chapter 8 provides further information of the various purposes and guidelines for use of medical records.) Besides the evaluation of stated outcomes, the medical record should include changes in patient condition, informed consents (for medications and treatments), reaction to medication, documentation of symptoms (verbatim when appropriate), concerns of the patient, and any untoward incidents in the health care setting. Documentation of patient progress is the responsibility of the entire mental health team.

Although communication among team members and coordination of services are the primary goals when choosing a system for documentation, practitioners in all settings must also consider professional standards, legal issues, and accreditation by regulatory agencies.

Information also must be in a format that is retrievable for quality-assurance monitoring, utilization management, peer review, and research. Electronic medical records are increasingly used in both inpatient and outpatient settings. Whatever format is used, documentation must be focused, organized, and pertinent and must conform to certain legal and other generally accepted principles (Box 9-6). The College of Registered Nurses of British Columbia (2011) and the College of Registered Nurses of Nova Scotia (2005) have each published nursing documentation guidelines.

## BOX 9-6 LEGAL CONSIDERATIONS FOR DOCUMENTATION OF CARE

**Do:**
- Chart in a timely manner all pertinent and factual information.
- Be familiar with the nursing documentation policy in your facility, and make your charting conform to this standard. The policy generally states the method, frequency, and pertinent assessments, interventions, and outcomes to be recorded. If your employer's policies and procedures do not encourage or allow for quality documentation, bring the need for change to the administration's attention.
- Chart legibly in ink.
- Chart facts fully, descriptively, and accurately.
- Chart what you see, hear, feel, and smell.
- Chart pertinent observations: psychosocial observations, physical symptoms pertinent to the medical diagnosis, and behaviours pertinent to the nursing diagnosis.
- Chart follow-up care provided when a problem has been identified in earlier documentation. For example, if a patient has fallen and injured a leg, describe how the wound is healing.
- Chart fully the facts surrounding unusual occurrences and incidents.
- Chart all nursing interventions, treatments, and outcomes (including teaching efforts and patient responses) and safety and patient-protection interventions.
- Chart the patient's expressed subjective feelings.
- Chart each time you notify a physician, and record the reason for notification, the information that was communicated, the accurate time, the physician's instructions or orders, and the follow-up activity.

- Chart when nursing supervisors are consulted or informed about the patient, record reason for notification, information communicated, time, and any instructions or follow-up.
- Chart when family are notified of occurrences.
- Chart physicians' visits and treatments.
- Chart discharge medications and instructions given for use, as well as all discharge teaching performed, and note which family members were included in the process.

**Don't:**
- Do not chart opinions that are not supported by facts.
- Do not defame patients by calling them names or making derogatory statements about them (e.g., "an unlikeable patient who is demanding unnecessary attention").
- Do not chart before an event occurs.
- Do not chart generalizations, suppositions, or pat phrases (e.g., "patient in good spirits").
- Do not obliterate, erase, alter, or destroy a record. If an error is made, draw one line through the error, write "mistaken entry," the date, and initial. Follow your employer's guidelines closely.
- Do not leave blank spaces for chronological notes. If you must chart out of sequence, chart "late entry." Identify the time and date of the entry and the time and date of the occurrence.
- If an incident report is filed, do not note in the chart that one was filed. This form is generally a privileged communication between the hospital and the hospital's attorney. Describing it in the chart may destroy the privileged nature of the communication.

## ■ KEY POINTS TO REMEMBER

- The nursing process is a six-step problem-solving approach to patient care.
- The primary source of assessment is the patient. Secondary sources of information include family members, neighbours, friends, police, and other members of the health care team.
- A professional translator often is needed to prevent serious misunderstandings during assessment, treatment, and evaluation with non–English- or non–French-speaking patients.
- The assessment interview includes gathering objective data (mental or emotional status) and subjective data (psychosocial assessment).
- Medical examination, history, and systems review round out a complete assessment.
- Assessment tools and standardized rating scales may be used to evaluate and monitor a patient's progress.
- Determination of the nursing diagnosis (NANDA-I) defines the practice of nursing, improves communication between staff members, and assists in accountability of care.
- A nursing diagnosis consists of (1) an unmet need or problem, (2) an etiology or probable cause, and (3) supporting data.
- Outcomes are variable, measurable, and stated in terms that reflect a patient's actual state. Planning involves determining desired outcomes.

- Behavioural goals support outcomes. Goals are short, specific, and measurable; indicate the desired patient behaviour(s); and include a set time for achievement.
- Planning nursing actions (using *NIC*, psychiatric nursing care plan texts, evidence-informed practice, or other sources) to achieve outcomes includes the use of specific principles. The plan should be (1) safe, (2) compatible with and appropriate for implementation with other therapies, (3) realistic and individualized, and (4) evidence-informed whenever possible.
- Psychiatric mental health nursing practice includes four basic-level interventions: (1) coordination of care, (2) health teaching and health promotion, (3) milieu therapy, and (4) pharmacological, biological, and integrative therapies.
- Advanced-practice interventions (e.g., psychotherapy consulting work) are carried out by a nurse with advanced education or experience.
- The evaluation of care is a continual process of determining to what extent the outcome criteria have been achieved. The plan of care may be revised based on the evaluation.
- Documentation of patient progress through evaluation of the outcome criteria is crucial. The medical record is a legal document and should accurately reflect the patient's condition, medications, treatment, tests, responses, and any untoward incidents.

# CRITICAL THINKING

1. Martin Redbird, a 47-year-old Cree man, arrived by ambulance from a supermarket, where he had fallen. On his arrival to the emergency department (ED), his breath smells "fruity." He appears confused and anxious, saying that "they put a curse on me, they want me to die … they are yelling, they are yelling … no, no, I'm not bad. Oh God, don't let them get me!" Martin is from a reserve community 700 kilometres north of the city in which he is being treated. When his nephew (closest next of kin) is contacted by the ED by phone, he tells the staff that Martin has diabetes and a diagnosis of paranoid schizophrenia and that this happens when he doesn't take his medications or eat properly. In a group or in collaboration with a classmate, respond to the following:

   a. A number of nursing diagnoses are possible in this scenario. Given the above information, formulate at least two nursing diagnoses (problems); include *related to* and *as evidenced by*.
   b. For each of your nursing diagnoses, write out one long-term outcome (the problem, what should change, etc.). Include a time frame, desired change, and three criteria that will help you evaluate whether the outcome has been met, not met, or partially met.
   c. What specific needs might you take into account when planning nursing care for Mr. Redbird?
   d. Formulate an initial nurse's note for Mr. Redbird.

# CHAPTER REVIEW

1. The nurse is assessing a 6-year-old patient. When assessing a child's perception of a difficult issue, which methods of assessment are appropriate? Select all that apply.
   1. Engage the child in a specific therapeutic game.
   2. Ask the child to draw a picture.
   3. Provide the child with an anatomically correct doll to act out a story.
   4. Allow the child to tell a story.

2. Which are the purposes of a thorough mental health nursing assessment? Select all that apply.
   1. Establish a rapport between the nurse and patient.
   2. Assess for risk factors affecting the safety of the patient or others.
   3. Allow the nurse the chance to provide counselling to the patient.
   4. Identify the nurse's goals for treatment.
   5. Formulate a plan of care.

3. The nurse is performing a spiritual assessment on a patient. Which patient statement would indicate to the nurse that there is an experiential concern in the patient's spiritual life?
   1. "I really believe that my spouse loves me."
   2. "My sister will never forgive me for what I did."
   3. "I try to find time every day to pray, even though it's not easy."
   4. "I am happy with my life choices, even if my mother is not."

4. The nurse is caring for a patient who states he has "given up on life." His wife left him, he was fired from his job, and he is four payments behind on his mortgage, meaning he will soon lose his house. Which nursing diagnosis is appropriate?
   1. Anxiety related to multiple losses
   2. Defensive coping related to multiple losses
   3. Ineffective denial related to multiple losses
   4. Hopelessness related to multiple losses

5. The nurse is documenting. Which statement is appropriate to include in the patient's chart?
   1. "Patient states, 'I am going to kill myself.'"
   2. "Patient is in good spirits today."
   3. "Patient has been nasty to the nursing staff this afternoon."
   4. "Patient is demanding and uncooperative."

# Evolve WEBSITE

Post-Test interactive review

*Visit the Evolve Web site for Chapter Review Answers and Rationales, Critical Thinking Answer Guidelines, and additional resources related to the content in this chapter:* http://evolve.elsevier.com/Canada/Varcarolis/psychiatric/

# REFERENCES

American Nurses Association (ANA), American Psychiatric Nurses Association, & International Society of Psychiatric Mental Health Nurses. (2007). *Psychiatric mental-health nursing: Scope and standards of practice.* Washington, DC: Nursesbooks.org.

Anandarajab, G. (2008). The 3 H and BMSEST models for spirituality in multicultural whole-person medicine. *Annals of Family Medicine, 6*(5), 448–458.

Arnold, E.C., & Boggs, K.U. (2007). *Interpersonal relationships: Professional communication skills for nurses* (5th ed.). St. Louis, MO: Saunders.

Baetz, M., Larson, D., Marcoux, G., et al. (2002). Canadian psychiatric inpatient religious commitment: An association with mental health. *Canadian Journal of Psychiatry, 47*(2), 159–166. Retrieved from http://www.ebscohost.com.

Bernzweig, J., Takayama, J.I., Phibbs, C., et al. (1997). Gender differences in physician–patient communication. *Archives of Pediatric and Adolescent Medicine, 151*(6), 586–591. doi:10.1001/archpedi.1997.02170430052011.

Browne, A., & Varcoe, C. (2006). Critical cultural perspectives and health care involving Aboriginal peoples. *Contemporary Nurse, 22*(2), 155–167. Retrieved from http://www.galegroup.com.

Bulechek, G.M., Butcher, H.K., & Dochterman, J.M. (2008). *Nursing interventions classification (NIC)* (5th ed.). St. Louis, MO: Mosby.

Calsaferri, K., Treherne, T., & van der Leer, G. (2002). *B.C's mental health reform best practices: Psychosocial rehabilitation and recovery.* Victoria, BC: Ministry of Health. Retrieved from http://www.health.gov.bc.ca/library/publications/year/2000/MHABestPractices/bp_psychosocial_rehab.pdf.

Canadian Federation of Mental Health Nurses. (2006). *Canadian standards for psychiatric-mental health nursing* (3rd ed.). Toronto: Author. Retrieved from http://cfmhn.ca.

Canadian Nurses Association. (2010). *Position statement. Evidence-informed decision-making and nursing practice.* Ottawa: Author.

Carson, V.B., & Koenig, H.G. (2004). *Spiritual caregiving as a ministry.* Philadelphia: Templeton.

College of Registered Nurses of British Columbia. (2011). *Documentation in nursing practice [Interactive learning modules].* Vancouver: Author. Retrieved from https://www.crnbc.ca/Lists/Flash%20Modules/Documentation/player.html.

College of Registered Nurses of Nova Scotia. (2005). *Documentation guidelines for registered nurses.* Halifax: Author. Retrieved from http://www.crnns.ca/documents/DocumentationGuidelines.pdf.

College of Registered Nurses of Nova Scotia. (2012). *Standards of practice for registered nurses.* Halifax: Author. Retrieved from http://www.crnns.ca.

Delgado, C. (2007). Meeting clients' spiritual needs. *Nursing Clinics of North America, 42,* 279–293. doi:10.1016/j.cnur.2007.03.002.

DiCenso, A. (2003). Evidence-based nursing practice: How to get there from here. *Nursing Leadership, 16*(4), 20–26. Retrieved from http://www.longwoods.com/content/16257.

Fontes, L.A. (2008). *Interviewing across cultures.* New York: The Guilford Press.

George, L.K., Ellison, C.G., & Larson, D.B. (2002). Explaining the relationships between religious involvement and health. *Psychological Inquiry, 13*(3), 190–200.

George, L.K., Larson, D.B., Koenig, H.G., et al. (2000). Spirituality and health: What we know, what we need to know. *Journal of Social and Clinical Psychology, 19,* 102–116. doi:10.1521/jscp.2000.19.1.102.

Hart-Wasekeesikaw, F. (2009). *Cultural competence and cultural safety in nursing education. A framework for First Nations, Inuit, and Métis nursing.* Ottawa: Aboriginal Nurses Association of Canada. Retrieved from http://www.anac.on.ca.

Herdman, T.H. (Ed.). (2012). *NANDA International nursing diagnoses: Definitions & classification, 2012–2014.* Oxford, UK: Wiley-Blackwell.

Hoen, B., Nielsen, K., & Sasso, A. (2006). *Health care interpreter services: Strengthening access to primary health care. National report: An overview of the accomplishments, outcomes, and learning of the SAPHC Project.* Ottawa: SAPHC Project. Retrieved http://criticallink.org/wp-content/uploads/2011/02/SAPHCNationalReport.pdf.

Kirmayer, L., Simpson C., & Cargo, M. (2003). Healing traditions: Culture, community and mental health promotion with Canadian Aboriginal peoples. *Australasian Psychiatry, 11,* S15–S23. doi:10.1046/j.1038-5282.2003.02010.x.

Koenig, H.G. (2001). *Handbook of religion and mental health.* New York: Oxford Press.

Mackenzie, E., Rajagopal, D., Meibohm, M., et al. (2000). Spiritual support and psychological well-being: Older adults' perceptions of the religion and health connection. *Alternative Therapies in Health and Medicine, 6*(6), 37–45.

Miller, W.R., & Thoresen, C.E. (2003). Spirituality, religion, and health: An emerging research field. *American Psychological Association, 58,* 24–35. doi:10.1037/0003-066X.58.1.24.

Moorhead, S., Johnson, M., Maas, M.L., et al. (2008). *Nursing outcomes classification (NOC)* (4th ed.). St. Louis: Mosby.

O'Connor, F., & Delaney, K. (2007). The recovery movement: Defining evidence-based processes. *Archives of Psychiatric Nursing, 21,* 172–175. doi:10.1016/j.apnu.2007.02.007.

Poole, R., & Higgo, R. (2006). *Psychiatric interviewing and assessment.* Liverpool, UK: Cambridge University Press.

Racher, F., & Annis, R. (2007). Respecting culture and honoring diversity in community practice. *Research and Theory for Nursing Practice, 21*(4), 255–270. Retrieved from http://www.ebscohost.com.

Registered Psychiatric Nurses' Association of Manitoba. (1993). *Psychiatric nursing competencies.* Winnipeg: Author. Retrieved from http://www.crpnm.mb.ca/psychiatric-nursing/entry-level-competencies/.

Registered Psychiatric Nurses of Canada. (2010). *Code of Ethics & Standards of Psychiatric Nursing Practice.* Edmonton: Author. Retrieved from http://www.rpnc.ca/.

Waseem, M., & Ryan, M. (2005). "Doctor" or "doctora": Do patients care? *Pediatric Emergency Care, 21*(8), 515–517.

Wright, L., & Leahey, M. (2009). Nurses and families: A guide to family assessment and intervention (5th ed.). Philadelphia: F.A. Davis.

# Therapeutic Relationships

*Elizabeth M. Varcarolis*
*Adapted by Michel Andre Tarko*

## KEY TERMS AND CONCEPTS

## OBJECTIVES

1. Compare and contrast the three phases of the nurse–patient relationship and the dimensions of the helping relationship.
2. Compare and contrast a social relationship and a therapeutic relationship in terms of purpose, focus, communications style, and goals.
3. Identify at least four patient behaviours a psychiatric nurse may encounter in the clinical setting.
4. Explore qualities that foster a therapeutic nurse–patient relationship and qualities that contribute to a nontherapeutic psychiatric nursing interactive process.
5. Define and discuss the microcommunication skills of empathy, genuineness, and positive regard in a nurse–patient relationship.

6. Identify two attitudes and four actions that may reflect the nurse's positive regard for a patient.
7. Analyze what is meant by boundaries and the influence of transference and counter-transference on boundary blurring.
8. Understand the use of nonverbal behaviour or body language in the context of the psychiatric nurse–patient relationship of attending behaviours.
9. Discuss the influences of disparate values and cultural beliefs on the therapeutic relationship.

## ⊝volve WEBSITE

*Visit the Evolve website for Flashcards, Case Studies, and additional testing resources related to*
*the content in this chapter: http://evolve.elsevier.com/Canada/Varcarolis/psychiatric/*   `Pre-Test` `interactive review`

Psychiatric mental health nurses practise in a variety of contexts providing care to individuals, groups, families, and communities. Psychiatric nursing care is both an art and a science. Knowledge of anatomy, physiology, microbiology, and chemistry is the basis for providing safe and effective physiological nursing care. Knowledge of pharmacology—a medication's mechanism of action, indications for use, and adverse effects, based on evidence-informed studies and trials—is central to safe and competent psychiatric nursing practice. However, it is the nurse–patient relationship and the development of the interpersonal skills needed to enhance and maintain such a therapeutic relationship that comprise the art of psychiatric nursing.

### HOW A NURSE HELPED ME

**Dan's Story: "Our Friend Is Really a Well-Put-Together Guy!"**

*Our friend Dan was staying at our rural cottage for a long weekend. He had been increasingly stressed in his management job at an engineering firm in the city, where he was responsible for making big decisions that affected a number of employees. We knew Dan had not been sleeping or eating well and was finding his work increasingly difficult, so we offered our place as a sort of retreat while we were away.*

*When we returned on the Sunday afternoon, it was clear that Dan was in a very bad mental state. He recognized us, but he had not bathed or showered and could not really respond sensibly to any questions—it was almost as though he was speaking another language! My wife and I immediately drove Dan to our regional hospital's emergency department, where a psychiatric mental health nurse met with him. Dan could barely speak at this stage, so my wife and I were included in the interview. We had brought his belongings in with us and discovered he had been taking a strong herbal sleep aid that, in the end, was found to have contributed to the extreme changes—I guess it was a sort of drug reaction.*

*We were terribly frightened by the whole thing. We had never seen Dan like this before! Throughout the interview, the nurse paused often, spoke in a relaxed way, breathed, and made sure we took breaks to eat at mealtimes. She*
*asked Dan questions directly, even though he was not really taking it all in. When he was unable to answer, the nurse would invite my wife and me to think about our own possible responses. It was the most calming way of helping us all.*

*At the start of the interview, the nurse told us that "sometimes any number of things can create difficulties in the mood, behaviour, and thinking of people who are normally well put together." I remember my wife and I both spoke at the same time: "You are exactly right. Dan is normally the most well-put-together guy. This is something very out of the ordinary—please help sort it out!" This simple respect for Dan's dignity and acknowledgement of how seriously we took the situation allowed us to establish a good relationship with the nurse, helped get to the root of the problem, and started Dan's treatment in a way that made this complicated mess seem manageable. We felt Dan was in a good position to recover from the acute drug reaction and also his poor sleep and other stress-related troubles. Despite it being a very bad time for Dan—and us, as his friends—we will never forget how the nurse showed us all so much respect and dignity. What could have been an even more stressful as well as embarrassing experience for Dan ended up, well, okay.*

Quinlan (1996) stated, "The development of that very human relationship allows a place for caring and healing to occur. This use of the essential humanness of the nurse as a person is the most critical part of the way nurses make themselves available to both patients and colleagues" (p. 7). Quinlan goes on to say that how this relationship is achieved remains the domain of the individual nurse.

## CONCEPTS OF THE NURSE–PATIENT RELATIONSHIP

The nurse–patient relationship is the basis of all psychiatric mental health nursing care, regardless of the specific goals of patient care (Forchuk, 1993; Peplau, 1952). The very first connections between the psychiatric nurse and the patient are to establish an understanding that the nurse is safe, discreet, reliable, and consistent and that the relationship will be conducted within appropriate and clear boundaries (LaRowe, 2004).

It is argued that many psychiatric disorders—for example, schizophrenia, bipolar disorder, and major depression—have strong biochemical and genetic elements of origin. However, many accompanying emotional problems, such as altered self-concept and self-image, low self-esteem, and difficulties with adherence to a treatment regimen, can be significantly

improved through a therapeutic nurse–patient relationship (LaRowe, 2004). All too often, patients entering psychiatric treatment have exhausted their familial and social resources and find themselves isolated and in need of emotional and spiritual support.

The psychiatric nurse–patient relationship is a creative process unique to each nurse and patient. The notion of therapeutic use of self is rooted within one's individual, genuine ways of being with another person based upon one's personal values and beliefs of humanity and enhanced by the application of microcommunication skills (such as warmth, respect, and empathy) to guide the process of developing, maintaining, and terminating a therapeutic relationship. Travelbee (1971) defined therapeutic use of self as "the ability to use one's personality consciously and in full awareness in an attempt to establish relatedness and to structure nursing interventions" (p. 19). It is important to note that the efficacy of this therapeutic use of self has been scientifically substantiated as an evidence-informed intervention. A review of randomized clinical trials that studied patients with various psychiatric disorders (e.g., mood, eating, personality disorders) across a wide range of therapeutic modalities repeatedly found that the development of a therapeutic relationship (alliance) was an important and consistent predictor of a positive outcome in therapy (Butler Center for Research, 2006).

## RESEARCH HIGHLIGHT

### Constituents of a Therapeutic Relationship

**Source:** Dziopa, F., & Ahern, K. (2009). What makes a quality therapeutic relationship in psychiatric/mental health nursing: A review of the research literature. *Internet Journal of Advanced Nursing Practice, 10*(1). doi:10.5580/1060.

#### Problem

A therapeutic relationship is highly correlated to patient outcomes. Learning about the particular constituents of such a relationship can guide nursing practice and improve outcomes.

#### Purpose of Study

The study was undertaken to illuminate the constituents of a therapeutic relationship in advanced mental health nursing practice.

#### Methods

Dziopa and Ahern conducted a systematic review of the available research on therapeutic relationships.

#### Key Findings

The researchers uncovered nine general attributes of the therapeutic relationship: (1) conveyance of understanding and empathy, (2) acceptance of individuality, (3) provision of support, (4) availability, (5) genuineness, (6) promotion of equality, (7) demonstration of respect, (8) maintenance of clear boundaries, and (9) self-awareness.

#### Implications for Nursing Practice

Nurses can foster a relationship of equality by relating to patients as equal human beings and by minimizing their own visibility, accomplished through making assessments in a subtle and unobtrusive manner within the context of ordinary conversations and by being sensitive to power issues (e.g., a community mental health nurse not carrying a briefcase when conducting home visits). Recommendations from the literature review included incorporating these aspects of the therapeutic relationship into psychiatric mental health nursing curricula, in-service education, and reflective practice strategies.

Therapeutic success is thought to be as much a result of the quality and characteristics of the therapeutic relationship as of the particular medical treatment choices or processes (Korn, 2001). Evidence suggests that psychotherapy (talk therapy) within a therapeutic relationship actually changes brain chemistry in much the same way as medication. Many, therefore, believe that the best treatment for most psychological stressors is a combination of medication and psychotherapy (less so in the case of psychotic disorders). Cognitive-behavioural therapy, in particular, has met with great success in the treatment of depression, phobias, obsessive-compulsive disorders, and others.

Establishing a therapeutic relationship with a patient takes time. Competency in relationship building is developed from a basis in communication theory within the context of the nurse–patient relationship. With experience and mentoring from experts, nurses will develop expertise along the communication continuum from novice to expert (Benner, 2000).

## Goals and Functions

The nurse–patient relationship is often loosely defined. However, a therapeutic relationship has specific goals and functions, including the following:

- Facilitating verbal expression of distressing thoughts and feelings
- Assisting patients to develop self-awareness and insight into their thoughts, feelings, and behaviours in order for them to better manage the activities of daily living
- Helping patients examine self-defeating behaviours and test alternatives
- Promoting self-care and independence

## Social Versus Therapeutic

A relationship is an interpersonal process that involves two or more people. Throughout life, we meet people in a variety of settings and share a variety of experiences. With some individuals, we develop long-term relationships; with others, the relationship lasts only a short time. Naturally, the kinds of relationships we enter vary from person to person and from situation to situation. Generally, relationships can be defined as intimate, social, or therapeutic. Intimate relationships occur between people who have an emotional commitment to each other. Within intimate relationships, mutual needs are met, and intimate desires and fantasies are shared. For our purposes in this chapter, we will limit our exploration to the aspects of social and therapeutic relationships.

## Social Relationships

A social relationship can be defined as a relationship that is initiated primarily for the purpose of friendship, socialization, enjoyment, or accomplishment of a task. Mutual needs are met during social interaction (e.g., participants share ideas, feelings, and experiences). Communication skills may include giving advice, such as relationship advice, and, sometimes, meeting basic dependency needs, such as offering a listening ear or material support needed during a stressful time. Often, the content of the communication remains superficial. During social interactions, roles may shift. Within a social relationship, there is little emphasis on the evaluation of the interaction, as seen in the following example of two friends at a shopping mall:

*Friend A:* "Oh, gosh, I just hate to be alone. It's getting me down, and sometimes it hurts so much."

*Friend B:* "I know just how you feel. I don't like it either. What I do is get a friend and go to a movie or something. Do you have someone to do that sort of stuff with?" *(With this response, B is minimizing A's feelings and giving advice prematurely.)*

*Friend A:* "No, not really, but often, I don't even feel like going out. I just sit at home feeling scared and lonely."

*Friend B:* "Most of us feel like that at one time or another. Maybe if you took a class or joined a group, you could meet more people. I know of some great groups you could join. It's not good to be stuck in the house by yourself all the time." *(Again, B is not "hearing" A's distress and is minimizing her pain and isolation. B goes on to give A unwanted and unhelpful advice, thus closing off A's feelings and experience.)*

## Therapeutic Relationships

In a therapeutic relationship, the psychiatric nurse maximizes his or her communication skills, understanding of human behaviours, and personal strengths to enhance the patient's growth. The focus of the relationship is on the patient's ideas, experiences, feelings, and personal issues introduced during the clinical interview, with the development of personal insight as a desired outcome. The nurse and the patient identify areas that need exploration and periodically evaluate the degree of change in the patient's understanding of the stressors and pinpoint strategies to manage them differently.

Although the psychiatric nurse may assume a variety of roles (e.g., teacher, counsellor, socializing agent, liaison), the relationship is consistently focused on the patient's problem and needs. The psychiatric nurse's needs must be met outside the relationship. When psychiatric nurses begin to want the patient to "like them," "do as they suggest," "be nice to them," or "give them recognition," the needs of the patient cannot be adequately met, and the interaction transitions from being therapeutic to being detrimental (nontherapeutic) to the patient.

Working under clinical supervision (i.e., being evaluated, receiving feedback, and gradually gaining autonomy and responsibility) is an excellent way for a psychiatric nurse's focus and boundaries to remain clear. Communication skills and knowledge of the stages and phenomena in a therapeutic relationship are critical tools in the formation and maintenance of the therapeutic relationship. Within the context of a therapeutic relationship, the following occur:

- The needs of the patient are identified and explored.
- Clear boundaries are established.
- Alternative problem solving approaches are taken.
- New coping skills may be developed.
- Insight is developed, and behavioural change is encouraged.

Just like on-staff nurses, nursing students may struggle with the boundaries between social and therapeutic relationships initially because there is a fine line between the two. In fact, students often feel more comfortable "being a friend" because it is a more familiar role, especially with people close to their own age. However, before a social relationship takes root, the psychiatric nurse or student needs to make it clear (to him- or herself and the patient) that the relationship is a therapeutic one. This does not mean that the nurse is not friendly toward the patient, and it does not mean that talking about everyday topics (television, weather, children's pictures) is forbidden. It does mean, however, that the nurse must follow the prior stated guidelines regarding a therapeutic relationship: essentially, the focus is on the patient, and the relationship is not designed to meet the psychiatric nurse's needs. The patient's problems and concerns are explored, potential solutions are discussed by both patient and psychiatric nurse, and solutions are implemented by the patient, as in the following example:

> *Patient:* "Oh, gosh, I just hate to be alone. It's getting me down, and sometimes it hurts so much."
> *Nurse:* "Loneliness can be painful. Tell me what is going on now that you are feeling so alone."

> *Patient:* "Well, my mom died two years ago, and last month, my—oh, I am so scared." (Takes a deep breath, looks down, and looks as though she might cry)
> *Nurse:* (Sits in silence while the patient recovers) "Go on … tell me more."
> *Patient:* "My boyfriend left for Afghanistan. I haven't heard from him, and they say he's missing. He was my best friend, and we were going to get married, and if he dies, I don't want to live."
> *Nurse:* "Have you thought of wanting to end your life?"
> *Patient:* "Well, if he dies, I will. I can't live without him."
> *Nurse:* "Have you ever felt like this before?"
> *Patient:* "Yes, when my mom died. I was depressed for about a year until I met my boyfriend."
> *Nurse:* "It sounds as though you are worried, scared, and uncertain whether your boyfriend is alive because you have not heard from him. Perhaps you and I can talk some more and come up with some ways for you to feel less anxious, scared, and overwhelmed. Let's take some time to talk more about this together."

The ability of the psychiatric nurse to engage in interpersonal interactions in a goal-directed manner to assist patients with their emotional, spiritual, or physical health needs is the foundation of the therapeutic psychiatric nurse–patient relationship. The following are necessary behaviours of health care workers, including nurses:

- Accountability—Psychiatric nurses assume responsibility for their conduct and the consequences of their actions.
- Focus on patient needs—The interest of the patient, rather than that of the nurse, other health care workers, or the institution, is given first consideration. The psychiatric nurse's role is that of patient advocate.
- Clinical competence—The criteria on which the nurse bases his or her conduct are principles of knowledge and the most appropriate actions for specific situations. This knowledge and action involve awareness and incorporation of the latest knowledge available from research (evidence-informed practice).
- Delaying judgement—Ideally, nurses refrain from judging patients and avoid inflicting their own values and beliefs on others.
- Supervision—Supervision by a more experienced clinician or team is essential to developing one's competence in establishing therapeutic psychiatric nurse–patient relationships.

Nurses interact with patients in a variety of settings: emergency departments, medical-surgical units, obstetric and pediatric units, clinics, community settings, schools, forensic milieus, correctional facilities, psychiatric assessment units, and patients' homes. Nurses who are empathic to patients' experiences and have effective holistic assessment and communication skills can significantly help patients confront current stressors and anticipate future choices.

Sometimes the type of relationship that occurs may be informal and short-lived, such as when the psychiatric nurse and patient meet for only a few sessions. However, even though it is brief, the relationship may be substantial, useful, and important for the patient. This limited relationship is often referred to as

| TABLE 10-1 | PATIENT AND NURSE BEHAVIOURS THAT REFLECT BLURRED BOUNDARIES | |
|---|---|---|
| **WHEN THE PSYCHIATRIC NURSE IS OVERLY INVOLVED** | **WHEN THE PSYCHIATRIC NURSE IS NOT INVOLVED** | |
| More frequent requests for assistance by the patient, which causes increased dependency on the psychiatric nurse | Patient's increased verbal or physical expression of isolation (depression) | |
| Inability of the patient to perform tasks that he or she is known to have been capable of prior to the psychiatric nurse's help, which causes regression | Lack of mutually agreed-upon goals | |
| Unwillingness on the part of the patient to maintain performance or progress in the psychiatric nurse's absence | Lack of progress toward goals | |
| Expressions of anger by other staff who do not agree with the psychiatric nurse's interventions or perceptions of the patient | Psychiatric nurse's avoidance of spending time with the patient | |
| Psychiatric nurse's keeping of secrets about the psychiatric nurse–patient relationship | Failure of the psychiatric nurse to follow through on agreed-upon interventions | |

**Source:** Reprinted with permission from SLACK Incorporated: Pilette, P.C., Berck, C.B., & Achber, L.C. (1995). Therapeutic management of helping boundaries. *Journal of Psychosocial Nursing and Mental Health Services, 33*(1), 40–47.

a therapeutic encounter. When the nurse shows genuine concern for another's circumstances (empathy and compassion), even a short encounter can have a powerful effect.

At other times, the encounters may be longer and more formal, such as in inpatient settings, mental health units, crisis centres, and mental health facilities. This longer time span allows the therapeutic nurse–patient relationship to be more fully developed.

## Relationship Boundaries and Roles

### Establishing Boundaries

According to Fox (2008), boundaries can be thought of in terms of the following:

- Physical boundaries: general environment, office space, treatment room, conference room, corner of the day room, and other such places
- The contract: set time, confidentiality, agreement between nurse and patient as to roles and responsibilities of all involved in the therapeutic relationship (nurse, patient, and family)
- Personal space: physical space, emotional space, space set by roles, and so forth

### Blurring of Boundaries

A trusting therapeutic nurse–patient relationship is based upon clear boundaries that facilitate the sharing of the patient's ideas, thoughts, feelings, and behaviours, thus providing the opportunity to develop insight and explore barriers to achieving patient goals (Crawford & Tarko, 2004). Theoretically, the psychiatric nurse's role in the therapeutic relationship can be stated rather simply as follows: the patient's needs are separated from the nurse's needs, and the patient's role is different from that of the nurse; therefore, the boundaries of the relationship are well defined. However, boundaries are constantly at risk of blurring, and a shift in the psychiatric nurse–patient relationship may lead to nontherapeutic dynamics. Two common circumstances in which boundaries are blurred are (1) when the relationship is allowed to slip into a social context and (2) when the

psychiatric nurse's needs (for attention, affection, or emotional or spiritual support) are met at the expense of the patient's needs.

Boundaries are necessary primarily to protect the patient. The most egregious boundary violations are those of a sexual nature (Wheeler, 2008). This type of violation results in malpractice actions and the loss of professional licensure on the part of the nurse. Other boundary issues are not as obvious. Table 10-1 illustrates some examples of patient and psychiatric nurse behaviours that reflect blurred boundaries.

### Blurring of Roles

The blurring of roles in the psychiatric nurse–patient relationship is often a result of unrecognized transference or counter-transference.

*Transference.* Transference, originally identified by Sigmund Freud when he used psychoanalysis to treat patients, occurs when the patient unconsciously and inappropriately displaces (transfers) onto the nurse his or her feelings and behaviours related to significant figures in the patient's past (see Chapter 3). The patient may even say, "You remind me of my (mother, sister, father, brother, or so on)."

> *Patient:* "Oh, you are so high and mighty. Did anyone ever tell you that you are a cold, unfeeling machine, just like others I know?"
>
> *Nurse:* "Tell me about one person who is cold and unfeeling toward you." (In this example, the patient is experiencing the nurse in the same way he experienced a significant other or others during his formative years. In this case, the patient's mother was very aloof, leaving him with feelings of isolation, worthlessness, and anger.)

Although transference occurs in all relationships, it seems to be intensified in relationships of authority. One theory is that transference may occur in therapeutic relationships because parental figures were the original figures of authority. Physicians, nurses, and social workers are all potential objects of transference. This transference may be positive or negative. If a patient is motivated to work with you, completes assignments between sessions, and shares feelings openly, the patient may be experiencing positive transference (Wheeler, 2008).

Whereas positive transference does not need to be addressed with the patient, negative transference that threatens the nurse–patient relationship may need to be explored.

Common forms of transference include the desire for affection or respect and the gratification of dependency needs. Other transferential feelings are hostility, jealousy, competitiveness, and love.

Sometimes patients experience positive or negative thoughts, feelings, and reactions that are realistic and appropriate and not a result of transference onto the health care provider. For example, if a nurse makes promises to the patient that are not kept (e.g., not showing up for a scheduled meeting), the patient may feel resentment for and mistrust toward the nurse.

**Counter-transference.** Counter-transference occurs when the nurse unconsciously and inappropriately displaces feelings and behaviours related to significant figures in his or her past onto the patient. Frequently, the patient's transference evokes counter-transference in the psychiatric nurse. For example, it is normal to feel angry when attacked persistently, annoyed when frustrated unreasonably, or flattered when idealized. A nurse might feel extremely important when depended on exclusively by a patient.

If the nurse does not recognize his or her own omnipotent feelings as counter-transference, he or she may minimize encouragement of independent growth in the patient; the therapeutic relationship may stall; and patients may be disempowered by the nurse's experience of them not as individuals but as extensions of themselves. Recognizing counter-transference, on the other hand, maximizes nurses' ability to empower patients. For example:

**Patient:** "Yeah, well I decided not to go to that dumb group. 'Hi, I'm so-and-so, and I'm an alcoholic.' Who cares?" (Sits slumped in a chair chewing gum, nonchalantly looking around)

**Nurse:** (In a very impassioned tone) "You always sabotage your chances. You need AA to get in control of your life. Last week you were going to go, and now you've disappointed everyone." (*Here the nurse is reminded of his mother, who was an alcoholic. He had tried everything to get his mother into treatment and took it as a personal failure and deep disappointment that his mother never sought recovery. After the psychiatric nurse sorts out his thoughts and feelings and realizes the frustration and feelings of disappointment and failure belonged with his mother and not the patient, he starts out the next session with the following approach.*)

**Nurse:** "Look, I was thinking about last week, and I realize the decision to go to AA or find other help is solely up to you. It's true that I would like you to live a fuller and more satisfying life, but it's your decision. I'm wondering, however, what happened to change your mind about going to AA."

A nurse's feeling either a strongly positive or a strongly negative reaction to a patient most often signals counter-transference. One common sign of counter-transference is overidentification with the patient. In this situation, the nurse may have difficulty recognizing or objectively seeing patient problems that are similar to his or her own problems. For example, a nurse who is struggling with an alcoholic family member may feel uninterested in, cold toward, or disgusted by an alcoholic patient. Other indicators of counter-transference are the nurse's becoming involved in power struggles, competition, or arguments with the patient. Table 10-2 lists some common counter-transference reactions.

Identifying and working through various transference and counter-transference issues is central to working therapeutically with the patient if we are to achieve professional and clinical growth and allow for positive change in the patient. Transference and counter-transference, as well as numerous other issues, are best dealt with through the use of supervision by either the peer group or therapeutic team. Besides helping with boundary issues, supervision supplies practical and emotional support, education, and guidance regarding ethical issues. Regularly scheduled supervision sessions provide the psychiatric nurse with the opportunity to increase self-awareness, clinical skills, and growth, as well as allow for continued growth of the patient.

## TABLE 10-2   COMMON COUNTER-TRANSFERENCE REACTIONS

As a nurse, you will sometimes experience counter-transference feelings. Once you are aware of them, use them for self-analysis to understand those feelings that may inhibit productive nurse–patient communication.

| REACTION TO PATIENT | BEHAVIOURS CHARACTERISTIC OF THE REACTION | SELF-ANALYSIS | SOLUTION |
|---|---|---|---|
| Boredom (indifference) | Showing inattention<br>Frequently asking the patient to repeat statements<br>Making inappropriate responses | Is the content of what the patient presents uninteresting? Or is it the style of communication? Does the patient exhibit an offensive style of communication?<br>Have you anything else on your mind that may be distracting you from the patient's needs?<br>Is the patient discussing an issue that makes you anxious? | Redirect the patient if he or she provides more information than you need or goes "off track"<br>Clarify information with the patient<br>Confront ineffective modes of communication |

*Continued*

| TABLE 10-2 | COMMON COUNTER-TRANSFERENCE REACTIONS—cont'd | | |
|---|---|---|---|
| **REACTION TO PATIENT** | **BEHAVIOURS CHARACTERISTIC OF THE REACTION** | **SELF-ANALYSIS** | **SOLUTION** |
| Rescue | Reaching for unattainable goals<br>Resisting peer feedback and supervisory recommendations<br>Giving advice | What behaviour stimulates your perceived need to rescue the patient?<br>Has anyone evoked such feelings in you in the past?<br>What are your fears or fantasies about failing to meet the patient's needs?<br>Why do you want to rescue this patient? | Avoid secret alliances<br>Develop realistic goals<br>Do not alter the meeting schedule<br>Let the patient guide interaction<br>Facilitate patient problem solving |
| Overinvolvement | Coming to work early, leaving late<br>Ignoring peer suggestions, resisting assistance<br>Buying the patient clothes or other gifts<br>Accepting the patient's gifts<br>Behaving judgementally at family interventions<br>Keeping secrets<br>Calling the patient when off duty | What particular patient characteristics are attractive?<br>Does the patient remind you of someone? Who?<br>Does your current behaviour differ from your treatment of similar patients in the past?<br>What are you getting out of this situation?<br>What needs of yours are being met? | Establish firm treatment boundaries, goals, and nursing expectations<br>Avoid self-disclosure<br>Avoid calling the patient when off duty |
| Overidentification | Having a special agenda, keeping secrets<br>Increasing self-disclosure<br>Feeling omnipotent<br>Experiencing physical attraction | With which of the patient's physical, emotional, cognitive, or situational characteristics do you identify?<br>Recall similar circumstances in your own life. How did you deal with the issues now being created by the patient? | Allow the patient to direct issues<br>Encourage a problem-solving approach from the patient's perspective<br>Avoid self-disclosure |
| Misuse of honesty | Withholding information<br>Lying | Why are you protecting the patient?<br>What are your fears about the patient learning the truth? | Be clear in your responses and aware of your hesitation; do not hedge<br>If you can provide information, tell the patient and give your rationale<br>Avoid keeping secrets<br>Reinforce the interdisciplinary nature of treatment |
| Anger | Withdrawing<br>Speaking loudly<br>Using profanity<br>Asking to be taken off the case | What patient behaviours are offensive to you?<br>What dynamic from your past may this patient be re-creating? | Determine the origin of the anger (nurse, patient, or both)<br>Explore the roots of patient anger<br>Avoid contact with the patient if you do not understand the roots of the anger |
| Helplessness or hopelessness | Feeling sadness | Which patient behaviours evoke these feelings in you?<br>Has anyone evoked similar feelings in the past? Who?<br>What past expectations were placed on you (verbally and nonverbally) by this patient? | Maintain therapeutic involvement<br>Explore and focus on the patient's experience rather than on your own |

**Source:** Aromando, L. (1995). *Mental health and psychiatric nursing* (2nd ed.). Springhouse, PA: Springhouse.

## NURSING BOUNDARY INDEX SELF-CHECK

Please rate yourself according to the frequency with which the following statements reflect your behavior, thoughts, or feelings within the past 2 years while providing patient care.*

| | | | | |
|---|---|---|---|---|
| 1. Have you ever received any feedback about your behavior being overly intrusive with patients and their families? | Never _____ | Rarely _____ | Sometimes _____ | Often _____ |
| 2. Do you ever have difficulty setting limits with patients? | Never _____ | Rarely _____ | Sometimes _____ | Often _____ |
| 3. Do you ever arrive early or stay late to be with your patient for a longer period? | Never _____ | Rarely _____ | Sometimes _____ | Often _____ |
| 4. Do you ever find yourself relating to patients or peers as you might to a family member? | Never _____ | Rarely _____ | Sometimes _____ | Often _____ |
| 5. Have you ever acted on sexual feelings you have for a patient? | Never _____ | Rarely _____ | Sometimes _____ | Often _____ |
| 6. Do you feel that you are the only one who understands the patient? | Never _____ | Rarely _____ | Sometimes _____ | Often _____ |
| 7. Have you ever received feedback that you get "too involved" with patients or families? | Never _____ | Rarely _____ | Sometimes _____ | Often _____ |
| 8. Do you derive conscious satisfaction from patients' praise, appreciation, or affection? | Never _____ | Rarely _____ | Sometimes _____ | Often _____ |
| 9. Do you ever feel that other staff members are too critical of "your" patient? | Never _____ | Rarely _____ | Sometimes _____ | Often _____ |
| 10. Do you ever feel that other staff members are jealous of your relationship with your patient? | Never _____ | Rarely _____ | Sometimes _____ | Often _____ |
| 11. Have you ever tried to "match-make" a patient with one of your friends? | Never _____ | Rarely _____ | Sometimes _____ | Often _____ |
| 12. Do you find it difficult to handle patients' unreasonable requests for assistance, verbal abuse, or sexual language? | Never _____ | Rarely _____ | Sometimes _____ | Often _____ |

*Any item that is responded to with "Sometimes" or "Often" should alert the nurse to a possible area of vulnerability. If the item is responded to with "Rarely," the nurse should determine whether it is an isolated event or a possible pattern of behavior.

**FIGURE 10-1** Nursing Boundary Index Self-Check. **Source:** Reprinted with permission from SLACK Incorporated: Pilette, P., Berck, C., & Achber, L. (1995). Therapeutic management. *Journal of Psychosocial Nursing and Mental Health Services, 33*(1), 45.

No matter how objective clinicians may try to be in examining their interactions, professional support and help from an experienced supervisor are essential to good practice (Fox, 2008).

### Self-Check on Boundaries

It is useful for all of us to take time out to be reflective and aware of our thoughts and actions with patients, as well as with colleagues, friends, and family. Figure 10-1 is a helpful boundary self-test you can use throughout your career, no matter what area of nursing you choose.

## VALUES, BELIEFS, AND SELF-AWARENESS

Values are abstract standards that represent an ideal, either positive or negative. It is crucial that we have an understanding of our own values and attitudes so we may become aware of the beliefs or attitudes we hold that may interfere with establishing positive therapeutic relationships with patient groups.

When working with patients, it is important for nurses to understand that their values and beliefs are not necessarily "right" and certainly are not right for everyone. It is helpful to realize that our values and beliefs (1) reflect our own culture/ subculture, (2) are derived from a range of choices, and (3) are those we have chosen for ourselves from a variety of influences and role models. These chosen values (religious, cultural, societal) guide us in making decisions and taking actions that we hope will make our lives meaningful, rewarding, and fulfilling.

Interviewing others whose values, beliefs, cultures, or lifestyles are radically different from our own can be a challenge (Fontes, 2008). Several topics that cause controversy in society in general—including religion, gender roles, abortion, war, politics, money, drugs, alcohol, sex, and corporal punishment—also can cause conflict between nurses and patients (Fontes, 2008).

Although we emphasize that the patient and nurse should identify outcomes together, what happens when the psychiatric nurse's values, beliefs, and interpretive system are very different from those of a patient? Consider the following examples of possible conflicts:

- The patient wants an abortion, and abortion goes against the nurse's values.
- The psychiatric nurse believes the patient, who was raped, should get an abortion, but the patient refuses.

- The patient engages in unsafe sex with multiple partners, which goes against the nurse's values.
- The psychiatric nurse cannot understand a patient who refuses medications on religious grounds.
- The patient puts material gain and objects far ahead of loyalty to friends and family, in direct contrast to the nurse's values.
- The nurse is deeply religious, whereas the patient is a non-believer who shuns organized religion.
- The patient's lifestyle includes taking illicit drugs, an action that goes against the nurse's values.

How can nurses develop working relationships and help patients solve problems when patients' values, goals, and interpretive systems are so different from their own? Self-awareness requires that we understand what we value and the beliefs that guide our own behaviour. It is critical that as nurses we not only understand and accept our own values and beliefs but also are sensitive to and accepting of the unique and different values and beliefs of others. Supervision by an experienced colleague can prove invaluable in helping us develop this sensitivity.

## PEPLAU'S MODEL OF THE NURSE–PATIENT RELATIONSHIP

Hildegard Peplau introduced the concept of the nurse–patient relationship in 1952 in her groundbreaking book *Interpersonal Relations in Nursing*. This model of the nurse–patient relationship is well accepted in the United States and Canada (Registered Nurses' Association of Ontario, 2002) and has become an important tool for all nursing practice. A professional nurse–patient relationship includes a nurse who has skills and expertise and a patient who wants to alleviate suffering, find solutions to problems, explore different avenues to an improved quality of life, find an advocate, or do any combination of the above (Fox, 2008).

Peplau (1952) proposed that the nurse–patient relationship "facilitates forward movement" for both the nurse and the patient (p. 12). This interactive nurse–patient process is designed to assist in the patient's boundary management, independent problem solving, and decision making that promotes autonomy (Haber, 2000).

Peplau (1952, 1999) described the nurse–patient relationship as evolving through distinct interlocking and overlapping phases, generally recognized as follows:
1. Orientation phase
2. Working phase
3. Termination phase

An additional preorientation phase, during which the nurse prepares for the orientation phase—for instance, familiarizing him- or herself with the patient's background or engaging in self-reflection and other learning—has also since been identified. Most likely, you will not have time to develop all phases of the nurse–patient relationship in a brief student practice experience. However, it is important to be aware of these phases in order to recognize and consciously engage in them in your nursing practice and in the patient's experience with the treatment team. It is also important to remember that any contact that is caring, respectful, and demonstrative of concern for the situation of another person can have an enormous positive impact, as illustrated by Dan's story earlier in this chapter (see How a Nurse Helped Me on page 148).

### Preorientation Phase

Even before the first meeting, the psychiatric nurse may have many thoughts and feelings related to the first clinical session. Novice health care providers typically experience concerns and anxiety on their first practice days. These universal concerns include being afraid of people with psychiatric problems, saying "the wrong thing," and not knowing what to do in response to certain patient behaviours. Table 10-3 identifies common patient behaviours (e.g., crying, asking the nurse to keep a secret, threatening to commit suicide, giving a gift, wanting physical contact with the nurse) and gives examples of possible reactions by the nurse and suggested responses.

Talking with an instructor and participating in supervised peer group discussion will promote confidence and produce feedback and suggestions to prepare students for clinical practice. To prepare you for your first clinical day, your instructor will set the ground rules for safety. For example, do not go into a patient's room alone, know if there are any patients not to engage, stay in an open area where other people are around, and know the signs and symptoms of escalating anxiety. You should always trust your own instincts. If you feel uncomfortable for any reason, excuse yourself for a moment and discuss your feelings with your instructor or a staff member. In addition to getting reassurance and support, students can often provide valuable information about the patient's condition by sharing their perceptions.

Most experienced psychiatric mental health nursing faculty and staff are able to skillfully assess the unit atmosphere and behaviours that may indicate escalating tension. They are trained in crisis intervention, and formal security is often available on-site to give the staff support. There are actions a psychiatric nurse can take if a patient's anger begins to escalate, many of which are presented in Table 10-4. Chapter 26 offers a more detailed discussion of maintaining personal safety, recognizing potential agitation, and intervening with angry or aggressive patients. Refer to Chapter 11 for a detailed discussion of communication strategies used in clinical practice.

### Orientation Phase

The orientation phase can last for a few meetings or extend over a longer period. It marks the first time the nurse and the patient meet and is the phase during which the nurse conducts the initial interview (see Chapter 11). When strangers meet, they interact according to their own backgrounds, standards, values, and experiences. The fact that each person has a unique frame of reference underlies the need for self-awareness on the part of the nurse. The initial interview includes the following aspects:
- An atmosphere is established in which rapport can grow.
- The nurse's role is clarified, and the responsibilities (parameters) of both the patient and the nurse are defined.
- The contract containing the time, place, date, and duration of the meetings is discussed.

| TABLE 10-3 | COMMON PATIENT BEHAVIOURS, POSSIBLE NURSE REACTIONS, AND SUGGESTED NURSE RESPONSES |
|---|---|

| POSSIBLE REACTIONS | USEFUL RESPONSES |
|---|---|
| **If the Patient Threatens Suicide ...**<br>The nurse may feel overwhelmed or responsible for "talking the patient out of it."<br>The nurse may pick up some of the patient's feelings of hopelessness. | The nurse assesses whether the patient has a plan and the lethality of the plan.<br>The nurse tells the patient that this situation is serious, that the nurse does not want harm to come to the patient, and that this information needs to be shared with other staff:<br>"This is very serious, Mr. Lamb. I don't want any harm to come to you. I'll have to share this with the other staff."<br>The nurse can then discuss with the patient the feelings and circumstances that led to this decision. (Refer to Chapter 25 for strategies for suicide intervention.) |
| **If the Patient Asks the Nurse to Keep a Secret ...**<br>The nurse may feel conflict because he or she wants the patient to share important information but is unsure about making such a promise. | The nurse cannot make such a promise. The information may be important to the health or safety of the patient or others: "I cannot make that promise. It might be important for me to share the information with other staff."<br>The patient then decides whether to share the information |
| **If the Patient Asks the Nurse a Personal Question ...**<br>The nurse may think that it is rude not to answer the patient's question.<br>A new psychiatric nurse might feel relieved to put off having to start the interview.<br>The nurse may feel put on the spot and want to leave the situation.<br>New nurses are often manipulated by a patient into changing roles, thereby keeping the focus off the patient and preventing the building of a relationship. | The nurse may or may not answer the patient's query. If the nurse decides to answer a natural question, he or she answers in a word or two, then returns the focus to the patient:<br>**Patient:** Are you married?<br>**Nurse:** Yes. Do you have a spouse?<br>**Patient:** Do you have any children?<br>**Nurse:** This time is for you. Tell me about yourself.<br>**Patient:** You can just tell me if you have any children.<br>**Nurse:** This is your time to focus on your concerns. Tell me something about your family. |
| **If the Patient Makes Sexual Advances ...**<br>The nurse feels uncomfortable but may feel conflicted about "rejecting" the patient or making him or her feel "unattractive" or "not good enough." | The nurse needs to set clear limits on expected behaviour: "I'm not comfortable having you touch (kiss) me. This time is for you to focus on your problems and concerns."<br>Frequently restating the nurse's role throughout the relationship can help maintain boundaries. If the patient does not stop the behaviour, the nurse might say: "If you can't stop this behaviour, I'll have to leave. I'll be back at [time] to spend time with you then."<br>Leaving gives the patient time to gain control. The nurse returns at the stated time. |
| **If the Patient Cries ...**<br>The nurse may feel uncomfortable and experience increased anxiety or feel somehow responsible for making the person cry. | The nurse should stay with the patient and reinforce that it is all right to cry. Often, it is at that time that feelings are closest to the surface and can be best identified:<br>"You seem ready to cry."<br>"You are still upset about your brother's death."<br>"Tell me what are you thinking right now."<br>The psychiatric nurse offers tissues when appropriate. |

*Continued*

| TABLE 10-3 | COMMON PATIENT BEHAVIOURS, POSSIBLE NURSE REACTIONS, AND SUGGESTED NURSE RESPONSES—cont'd |

| POSSIBLE REACTIONS | USEFUL RESPONSES |
|---|---|
| **If the Patient Leaves Before the Session is Over ...** | |
| The nurse may feel rejected, thinking it was something that he or she did. The nurse may experience increased anxiety or feel abandoned by the patient. | Some patients are not able to relate for long periods without experiencing an increase in anxiety.<br>Some patients may be testing the nurse: "I'll wait for you here for 15 minutes, until our time is up."<br>During this time, the nurse does not engage in conversation with any other patient or even with the staff.<br>When the time is up, the nurse approaches the patient, says the time is up, and restates the day and time of their next meeting. |
| **If the Patient does not Want to Talk ...** | |
| The nurse new to this situation may feel rejected or ineffectual. | At first, the nurse might say something to this effect: "It's all right. I would like to spend time with you. We don't have to talk."<br>The nurse might spend short, frequent periods (e.g., five minutes) with the patient throughout the day: "Our five minutes is up. I'll be back at 10 o'clock and stay with you five more minutes."<br>This response gives the patient the opportunity to understand that the nurse means what he or she says and consistently returns on time. It also gives the patient time between visits to assess how he or she feels, to formulate thoughts about the nurse, and perhaps to feel less threatened. |
| **If the Patient Gives the Nurse a Present ...** | |
| The nurse may feel uncomfortable when offered a gift.<br>The meaning needs to be examined. Is the gift (1) a way of getting better care, (2) a way to maintain self-esteem, (3) a way of making the nurse feel guilty, (4) a sincere expression of thanks, or (5) a cultural expectation? | Possible guidelines:<br>If the gift is expensive, the only policy is to graciously refuse.<br>If it is inexpensive, then (1) if it is given at the end of hospitalization when a relationship has developed, graciously accept; (2) if it is given at the beginning of the relationship, graciously refuse and explore the meaning behind the present: "Thank you, but it is our job to care for our patients. Are you concerned that some aspect of your care will be overlooked?"<br>If the gift is money, it is always graciously refused. |
| **If Another Patient Interrupts During Time With Your Current Patient ...** | |
| The nurse may feel a conflict: he or she does not want to appear rude. Sometimes the nurse tries to engage both patients in conversation. | The time the nurse had contracted with a selected patient is that patient's time. By keeping his or her part of the contract, the nurse demonstrates commitment and conviction that the sessions are important: "I am with Mr. Rob for the next 20 minutes. At 10 o'clock, after our time is up, I can talk to you for five minutes." |

- Confidentiality is discussed and assumed.
- The terms of termination are introduced (these are also discussed throughout the orientation phase and beyond).
- The nurse becomes aware of transference and countertransference issues.
- Patient problems are articulated, and mutually agreed-upon goals are established.

## Establishing Rapport

A major emphasis during the first few encounters with the patient is on providing an atmosphere in which trust and understanding, or rapport, can grow. As in any relationship, rapport can be nurtured by demonstrating genuineness and empathy, developing positive regard, showing consistency, and offering assistance in problem solving and providing support.

### Parameters of the Relationship

The patient needs to know about the psychiatric mental health nurse (who the nurse is and the nurse's background) and the purpose of the meetings. For example, a student might provide the following information:

*Student:* "Hello, Mrs. Almodovar. I am Jim Thompson from the university. I am in my psychiatric rotation and will be coming here for the next six Thursdays. I would like to spend time with you each Thursday while you are here. I'm here to be a support person for you as you work on your treatment goals."

| TABLE 10-4 | GUIDELINES FOR MAINTAINING SAFETY WHEN A PATIENT'S ANGER ESCALATES |
|---|---|

| NURSING INTERVENTION | RATIONALE |
|---|---|
| Pay attention to angry and aggressive behaviour. Respond as early as possible. | Minimization of angry behaviours and ineffective limit setting are the most frequent factors contributing to the escalation of violence. |
| Assess for and provide for personal safety. Pay attention to the environment: Leave door open or use hallway. Interact with the patient in a quiet place that is visible to staff. Have a quick exit available. The more angry the patient, the more space he or she will need to feel comfortable. Never turn your back on an angry patient. Leave immediately if there are signs behaviour is escalating out of control or if you are uncomfortable. State, "I am leaving now. I will be back in ten minutes," and seek out your clinical instructor or another staff member right away. | Exercising basic caution is essential to protecting yourself. Although the risk for violence may be minimal, it is easier to prevent a problem than to get out of a bad situation. These precautions are similar to using universal precautions (gloves, masks, gowns, etc.) on medical floors. |
| Appear calm and in control. | The perception that someone is in control can be comforting and calming to an individual whose anxiety is beginning to escalate. |
| Speak softly in a nonprovocative, nonjudgemental manner. | When tone of voice is low and calm and the words are spoken slowly, anxiety levels in others may decrease. |
| Demonstrate genuineness and concern. | Even the most psychotic individual with schizophrenia may respond to nonprovocative interpersonal contact and expressions of concern and caring. |
| If patient is willing, both the psychiatric nurse and patient should sit at a 45-degree angle. Do not tower over or stare at the patient. | Sitting at a 45-degree angle puts you both on the same level but allows for frequent breaks in eye contact. Towering over or staring at someone can be interpreted as threatening or controlling by paranoid individuals. |
| When patient begins to talk, listen. Use clarification techniques. | Active listening allows the patient to feel heard and understood, helps build rapport, and can productively channel energy. |

## Formal or Informal Contract

A contract emphasizes the patient's participation and responsibility because it shows that the psychiatric nurse does something *with* the patient rather than *for* the patient. The contract, either stated or written, contains the place, time, date, and duration of the meetings. During the orientation phase, the patient may begin to express thoughts and feelings, identify problems, and discuss realistic goals. Mutual agreement about those goals is also part of the contract. Students also make this contract with patients they interact with.

> **Student:** "Mrs. Almodovar, we will meet at 10 o'clock each Thursday in the consultation room at the clinic for 45 minutes. We can use that time for further discussion of your feelings of loneliness and anger and explore some strategies you could use to make the situation better for yourself."

## Confidentiality

The patient has a right to know (1) that specific information may be shared with others on the treatment team and (2) who else will be given the information (e.g., a clinical supervisor, the physician, the staff, or, if the nurse is in training, other students in conference). The patient also needs to know that the

information will not be shared with relatives, friends, or others outside the treatment team, except in extreme situations. Extreme situations include (1) child or elder abuse, (2) threats of self-harm or of harm to others, and (3) intention not to follow through with the treatment plan.

If information must be shared with others, it is usually the physician who will share it, according to legal guidelines (see Chapter 8). The psychiatric nurse must be aware of the patient's right to confidentiality and must not violate that right. Safeguarding the privacy and confidentiality of patients is not only an ethical obligation but a legal responsibility as well (Erickson & Miller, 2005). For example, a student may say the following:

> **Student:** "Mrs. Almodovar, I will be sharing some of what we discuss with my nursing instructor, and at times I may discuss certain concerns with my peers in conference or with the staff. However, I will not be sharing this information with your husband or any other members of your family or anyone outside the hospital without your permission."

## Planning for Terms of Termination

Termination is that last phase in Peplau's model, but planning for termination actually begins in the orientation phase. It also may be mentioned, when appropriate, during the working phase if the nature of the relationship is time limited (e.g., six or nine sessions). The date of the termination should be clear from the beginning. In some situations, the nurse–patient contract may be renegotiated once the termination date has been reached. In other situations, when the therapeutic psychiatric nurse–patient relationship is an open-ended one, the termination date is not known.

> **Student:** "Mrs. Almodovar, as I mentioned earlier, our last meeting will be on October 25. We will have three more meetings after today."

## Working Phase

The development of a strong working relationship can provide support and safety for the patient, who may experience increased levels of anxiety and demonstrate dysfunctional behaviours while trying out new and more adaptive coping behaviours. In 1988, Moore and Hartman identified specific tasks of the working phase of the nurse–patient relationship that remain relevant in current practice:

- Maintain the relationship.
- Gather further data.
- Promote the patient's problem-solving skills, self-esteem, and use of language.
- Facilitate behavioural change.
- Overcome resistance behaviours.
- Evaluate problems and goals, and redefine them as necessary.
- Promote practice and expression of alternative adaptive behaviours.

During the working phase, the psychiatric nurse and patient together identify and explore areas that are causing problems in the patient's life. Often, the patient's present ways of handling situations stem from earlier means of coping devised to survive in a chaotic and dysfunctional family environment. Although certain coping methods may have worked for the patient at an earlier age, they now interfere with the patient's interpersonal relationships and prevent attainment of current goals. The patient's dysfunctional behaviours and basic assumptions about the world are often defensive, and the patient is usually unable to change the dysfunctional behaviour at will. Therefore, most of the problem behaviours or thoughts continue because of unconscious motivations and needs that are beyond the patient's awareness.

The psychiatric nurse can work with the patient to identify unconscious motivations and assumptions that keep the patient from finding satisfaction and reaching potential. Describing, and often re-experiencing, old conflicts generally awakens high levels of anxiety. Patients may use various defences against anxiety and displace their feelings onto the nurse. Therefore, during the working phase, intense emotions such as anxiety, anger, self-hate, hopelessness, and helplessness may surface. Defence mechanisms, such as acting out anger inappropriately, withdrawing, intellectualizing, manipulating, and denying are to be expected.

During the working phase, the patient may unconsciously transfer strong feelings about or for significant others from the past into the present and onto the nurse (transference). The emotional responses and behaviours of the patient may also awaken strong counter-transference feelings in the psychiatric nurse. The nurse's awareness of these personal feelings and of reactions to the patient are vital for effective interaction with the patient.

## Termination Phase

The termination phase is the final, integral phase of the nurse–patient relationship. Termination is discussed during the first interview and again during the working stage at appropriate times. Termination occurs when the patient is discharged. The tasks of termination are as follows:

- Summarizing the goals and objectives achieved in the relationship
- Discussing ways for the patient to incorporate into daily life any new coping strategies learned
- Reviewing situations that occurred during the nurse–patient relationship
- Exchanging memories, which can help validate the experience for both the nurse and the patient and facilitate closure of the relationship

Termination can stimulate strong feelings in both the nurse and the patient. Termination of the relationship signifies a loss for both, although the intensity and meaning of termination may be different for each. If a patient has unresolved feelings of abandonment, loneliness, being unwanted, or rejection, these feelings may be reawakened during the termination process. This process can be an opportunity for the patient to express these feelings, perhaps for the first time.

Important reasons for the nurse to engage consciously in the termination phase of the therapeutic relationship include the following:

- Feelings are aroused in both the patient and the nurse about the experience they have had; when these feelings are recognized and shared, patients learn that it is acceptable to feel sadness and loss when someone they care about leaves.
- Termination can be a learning experience; patients can learn that they are important to at least one person, and psychiatric nurses learn continually from each clinical experience and patient encounter.
- By sharing the termination experience with the patient, the psychiatric nurse demonstrates genuineness and caring for the patient.
- This encounter may be the first successful termination experience for the patient.

If a psychiatric nurse has been working with a patient for a while, it is important for the nurse to bring into awareness any feelings or reactions the patient may be experiencing related to separations. If a patient denies that the termination is having an effect (assuming the nurse–patient relationship was strong), the nurse may say something like "Goodbyes are difficult for people. Often they remind us of other goodbyes. Tell me about another separation in your past." If the patient appears to be displacing anger, either by withdrawing or by being overtly angry at the nurse, the nurse may use generalized statements such as "People may experience anger when saying goodbye. Sometimes they are angry with the person who is leaving. Tell me how you feel about my leaving."

New practitioners and students in a psychiatric nursing setting need to give serious thought to their final clinical experience with a patient and work with their supervisor or instructor to facilitate communication during this time. A common response of beginning practitioners and of students is feeling guilty about terminating the relationship. These feelings may, in rare cases, be manifested by the student's giving the patient his or her telephone number, making plans to get together for coffee after the patient is discharged, continuing to see the patient afterward, or exchanging emails or other communications. Often, such actions are in response to the student's need to feel less guilty for using the patient to meet learning needs, to maintain a feeling of being important to the patient, or to sustain the illusion that the student is the only one who understands the patient, among other student-centred rationales. Maintaining contact with a patient after discharge, however, is not acceptable and is in opposition to the goals of a therapeutic relationship.

Indeed, part of the termination process may be to explore—after discussion with the patient's case manager—the patient's plans for the future: where the patient can go for help, which agencies to contact, and which people may best help the patient find appropriate and helpful resources.

## WHAT HINDERS AND WHAT HELPS THE NURSE–PATIENT RELATIONSHIP

Not all nurse–patient relationships follow the classic phases outlined by Peplau. Some start in the orientation phase and move to a mutually frustrating phase and finally to mutual withdrawal (Figure 10-2).

Forchuk, Westwell, Martin, and colleagues (2000) conducted a qualitative study of the nurse–patient relationship. They examined the phases of both therapeutic and nontherapeutic relationships. From this study, they identified certain behaviours that were beneficial to the progression of the nurse–patient relationship, as well as those that hampered its development. The study emphasized that consistent, regular, and private interactions with patients are essential to the development of a therapeutic relationship. Nurses in this study stressed the importance of consistency, pacing, and listening. Specifically,

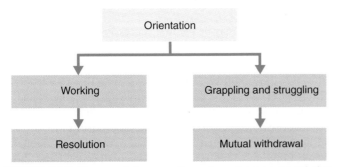

**FIGURE 10-2** Phases of therapeutic and nontherapeutic relationships. **Source:** Forchuk, C., Westwell, J., Martin, M., et al. (2000). The developing nurse–client relationship: Nurses' perspectives. *Journal of the American Psychiatric Nurses Association, 6*(1), 3–10, copyright © 2000 by SAGE Publications. Reprinted by Permission of SAGE Publications. doi:10.1177/107839030000600102.

the study found evidence that the following factors enhanced the nurse–patient relationship, allowing it to progress in a mutually satisfying manner:

- Consistency—ensuring that a nurse is always assigned to the same patient and that the patient has a regular routine for activities. Interactions are facilitated when they are frequent and regular in duration, format, and location. The importance of consistency extends to the nurse's being honest and consistent (congruent) in what is said to the patient.
- Pacing—letting the patient set the pace and letting the pace be adjusted to fit the patient's moods. A slow approach helps reduce pressure; at times, it is necessary to step back and realize that developing a strong relationship may take a long time.
- Listening—letting the patient talk when needed. The nurse becomes a sounding board for the patient's concerns and issues. Listening is perhaps the most important skill for nurses to master. Truly listening to another person (i.e., attending to what is behind the words) is a learned skill.
- Initial impressions, especially positive initial attitudes and preconceptions, are significant considerations in how the relationship will progress. Preconceived negative impressions and feelings toward the patient (e.g., the nurse's feeling that the patient is "interesting" or a "challenge") usually bode poorly for the positive growth of the relationship. In contrast, an inherent positive regard for the patient as a person is usually a favourable sign for the developing therapeutic relationship.
- Promoting patient comfort and balancing control usually reflect caring behaviours. *Control* refers to keeping a balance in the relationship: not too strict and not too lenient.
- Patient factors that seem to enhance the relationship include trust on the part of the patient and the patient's active participation in the nurse–patient relationship.

In relationships that did not progress to therapeutic levels, there seemed to be two major factors that hampered the development of positive relationships: inconsistency and unavailability (e.g., lack of contact, infrequent meetings, meetings in the hallway) on the part of the nurse, patient, or both. When nurse and patient are reluctant to spend time together, and meeting times become sporadic or superficial, the term *mutual avoidance* is used. This is clearly a lose–lose situation.

The nurse's personal feelings and lack of self-awareness are major elements that contribute to the lack of progression toward a positive relationship. Negative preconceived ideas and feelings (e.g., discomfort, dislike, fear, avoidance) about the patient seem to be a constant in relationships that end in frustration and mutual withdrawal. Sometimes these feelings are known, and sometimes the nurse is only vaguely aware of them.

## FACTORS THAT ENCOURAGE AND PROMOTE PATIENTS' GROWTH

Rogers and Truax (1967) identified three personal characteristics of the nurse that help promote change and growth in patients—factors still valued today as vital components for establishing a therapeutic relationship: genuineness, empathy, and positive regard. These are some of the intangibles that are at the heart of the art of nursing.

## Genuineness

Genuineness, or self-awareness of one's feelings as they arise within the relationship and the ability to communicate them when appropriate, is a key ingredient in building trust. When a person is genuine, one gets the sense that what the person displays is congruent with his or her internal processes. Genuineness is conveyed by listening to and communicating with patients without distorting their messages and being clear and concrete in communications. Being genuine in a therapeutic relationship implies the ability to use therapeutic communication tools in an appropriately spontaneous manner, rather than rigidly or in a parrotlike fashion.

## Empathy

Empathy is a complex multidimensional concept in which the helping person attempts to understand the world from the patient's perspective. It does not mean that the nurse condones or approves of the patient's actions but rather is nonjudgemental or uncritical of the patient's choices (Arkowitz, Westra, Miller, et al., 2008). Essentially, it means "temporarily living in the other's life, moving about in it delicately without making judgments" (Rogers, 1980, p. 142).

Therefore, empathy signifies a central focus and feeling with and in the patient's world. According to Mercer and Reynolds (2002), it involves:

- Accurately perceiving the patient's situation, perspective, and feelings
- Communicating one's understanding to the patient and checking with the patient for accuracy
- Acting on this understanding in a helpful (therapeutic) way toward the patient

## Empathy Versus Sympathy

There is much confusion regarding empathy versus sympathy. A simple way to distinguish them is to recognize that in empathy, we *understand* the feelings of others; in sympathy, we *feel* the feelings of others. When a helping person is feeling sympathy for another, objectivity is lost, and the ability to assist the patient in solving a personal problem ceases. Furthermore, sympathy is associated with feelings of pity and commiseration. Although these are considered nurturing human traits, they may not be particularly useful in a therapeutic relationship. When people express sympathy, they express agreement with another, which in some situations may discourage further exploration of a person's thoughts and feelings.

The following examples are given to clarify the distinction between empathy and sympathy. A friend tells you that her mother was just diagnosed with inoperable cancer. Your friend then begins to cry and pounds the table with her fist.

*Sympathetic response:* "I feel so sorry for you. I know exactly how you feel. My mother was hospitalized last year, and it was awful. I was so depressed. I still get upset just thinking about it." *(You go on to tell your friend about the incident.)*

Sometimes when psychiatric nurses try to be sympathetic, they are apt to project their own feelings onto the patient's, which can limit the patient's range of responses. A more useful response might be as follows:

*Empathic response:* "It sounds as though you are feeling upset and angry having learned about your mother's inoperable cancer diagnosis. Tell me what thoughts and feelings you are having." *(You continue to stay with your friend and listen to his or her thoughts and feelings.)*

Empathy is not a technique but rather an attitude that conveys respect, acceptance, and validation of the patient's strengths. In the practice of psychotherapy or counselling, empathy is one of the most important factors in building a trusting and therapeutic relationship (Wheeler, 2008).

## Positive Regard

Positive regard implies respect. It is the ability to view another person as being worthy of being cared about and as someone who has strengths and achievement potential. Positive regard is usually communicated indirectly by attitudes and actions rather than directly by words.

## Attitudes

One attitude through which a nurse might convey positive regard, or respect, is willingness to work with the patient. That is, the nurse takes the patient and the relationship seriously. The experience is viewed not as a job, part of a course, or time spent talking but as an opportunity to work with patients to help them develop personal resources and actualize more of their potential in living.

## Actions

Some actions that manifest an attitude of respect are attending, suspending value judgements, calling the individual by his or her first or last name, and helping patients develop their own resources.

*Attending.* Attending behaviour is the foundation of interviewing. To be effective, psychiatric nurses must pay attention to their patients in culturally and individually appropriate ways (Sommers-Flanagan & Sommers-Flanagan, 2003). *Attending* is a special kind of listening that refers to an intensity of presence, or of being with the patient. At times, simply being with another person during a painful time can make a difference.

Posture, eye contact, and body language are nonverbal behaviours that reflect a person's degree of attending and are highly influenced by culture. Refer to Chapter 11 for a more detailed discussion of the cultural implications of the clinical interview.

*Suspending value judgements.* Although we will always have personal opinions, nurses are more effective when they guard against using their own value systems to judge patients' thoughts, feelings, or behaviours. For example, if a patient is taking drugs or is involved in risky sexual behaviour, the nurse may recognize that these behaviours are hindering the patient from living a more satisfying life, posing a potential health threat, or preventing the patient from developing satisfying relationships. However, labelling these activities as bad or good is not useful. Rather, the nurse should focus on exploring the behaviour and work toward identifying the thoughts and feelings that influence this behaviour. Judgement on the part of the nurse will most likely interfere with further exploration.

The first steps in eliminating judgemental thinking and behaviours are to (1) recognize their presence, (2) identify how or where you learned these responses to the patient's behaviour, and (3) construct alternative ways to view the patient's thinking and behaviour. Denying judgemental thinking will only compound the problem.

> *Patient:* "I guess you could consider me an addictive personality. I love to gamble when I have money and spend most of my time in the casino. It seems as though I'm hooking up with a different woman every time I'm there, and it always ends in sex. This has been going on for at least three years."

A judgemental response would be:

> *Nurse A:* "So your compulsive gambling and promiscuous sexual behaviours really haven't brought you much happiness, have they? You're running away from your problems and could end up with sexually transmitted infections and no money."

A more helpful response would be:

> *Nurse B:* "So your sexual and gambling activities are part of the picture also. You make it sound as though these activities are not making you happy."

In this example, nurse B focuses on the patient's behaviours and the possible meaning they might have to the patient. This nurse does not introduce personal value statements or prejudices regarding promiscuous behaviour, as nurse A does. Empathy and positive regard are essential qualities in a successful nurse–patient relationship.

***Helping patients develop resources.*** The nurse becomes aware of patients' strengths and encourages patients to work at their optimal level of functioning. This support can be seen as one form of collaboration with the patient. The psychiatric nurse does not act for patients unless absolutely necessary, and then only as a step toward helping them act on their own. It is important that patients remain as independent as possible to develop new resources for problem solving. The following are examples of helping the patient develop independence:

> *Patient:* "This medication makes my mouth so dry. Could you get me something to drink?"
>
> *Nurse:* "There is juice in the refrigerator. I'll wait here for you until you get back" *or* "I'll walk with you while you get some juice from the refrigerator."
>
> *Patient:* "Could you ask the doctor to let me have a pass for the weekend?"
>
> *Nurse:* "Your doctor will be on the unit this afternoon. I'll let her know that you want to speak with her."

Consistently encouraging patients to use their own resources helps minimize the patients' feelings of helplessness and dependency and validates their potential for change.

## ■ KEY POINTS TO REMEMBER

- The nurse–patient relationship is well defined, and the roles of the nurse and the patient must be clearly stated.
- It is important that the nurse be aware of the differences between a therapeutic relationship and a social or intimate relationship. In a therapeutic psychiatric nurse–patient relationship, the focus is on the patient's needs, thoughts, feelings, and goals. The psychiatric nurse is expected to meet personal needs outside this relationship.
- Although the boundaries and roles of the nurse–patient relationship generally are clearly defined, they can become blurred; this blurring can be insidious and may occur on an unconscious level. Usually, transference and counter-transference phenomena are operating when boundaries are blurred.

- It is important to have a grasp of common counter-transferential feelings and behaviours and of the psychiatric nursing actions to counteract these phenomena.
- Supervision aids in promoting both the professional growth of the psychiatric nurse and of the psychiatric nurse–patient relationship, allowing the patient's goals to be worked on and met.
- The phases of the psychiatric nurse–patient relationship include preorientation, orientation, working, and termination.
- Genuineness, empathy, and positive regard are personal strengths of effective helpers who are able to foster growth and change in others.

## ■ CRITICAL THINKING

1. On your first clinical day, you are assigned to work with an older adult, Mrs. Schneider, who is depressed. Your first impression is, "Oh my, she looks like my nasty aunt Helen. She even sits like her." You approach her with a vague feeling of uneasiness and say hello. Mrs. Schneider responds, "Who are you, and how can you help me?" You answer by providing your name and telling her that you are a nursing student and will be working with her today. She tells you that "a student" could never understand what she is going through. She then says, "If you really want to help me, you would get me a good job after I leave here."

   a. Identify transference and counter-transference issues in this situation. What is your most important course of action?

   b. How could you best respond to Mrs. Schneider's question about who you are? What other information will you give her during this first clinical encounter? Be specific.

   c. What are some useful responses you could give Mrs. Schneider regarding her legitimate questions about ways you could be of help to her?

   d. Analyze Mrs. Schneider's request that you find her a job. Keeping in mind the aim of Peplau's interactive nurse–patient process, describe some useful ways you could respond to this request.

e. Consider how your response and ongoing discussions with Mrs. Schneider can convey key characteristics of a therapeutic relationship: respect, positive regard, genuineness, and empathy.

2. You are interviewing Tom Stone, a 17-year-old who was admitted to a psychiatric unit after a suicide attempt. How would you best respond to each of the following patient requests and behaviours?

a. "I would feel so much better if you would sit closer to me and hold my hand."

b. "I will tell you if I still feel like killing myself, but you have to promise not to tell anyone else. If you do, I just can't trust you, ever."

c. "I don't want to talk to you. I have absolutely nothing to say."

d. "I will be going home tomorrow, and you have been so helpful and good to me. I want you to have my watch to remember me by."

e. Tom breaks down and starts sobbing.

## CHAPTER REVIEW

1. Which of the following actions best represents the basis or foundation of all other psychiatric nursing care?
   1. The nurse assesses the patient at regular intervals.
   2. The nurse administers psychotropic medications.
   3. The nurse spends time sitting with a withdrawn patient.
   4. The nurse participates in team meetings with other professionals.

2. A male patient frequently inquires about the female student nurse's boyfriend, social activities, and school experiences. Which of the following initial responses by the student best addresses the issue raised by this behaviour?
   1. The student requests assignment to a patient of the same gender as the student.
   2. The student points out to the patient that he is making social inquiries and explores this behaviour.
   3. The student tells the patient that she cannot talk about her personal life and returns the focus to his issues.
   4. The student explains that if the patient persists in focusing on her, she cannot work with him.

3. Mary, a patient in the psychiatric unit, had a very rejecting and abusive father and a difficult childhood, but from age 10 on was raised by a very warm and supportive grandmother who recently passed away. Mary frequently comments on how hard her nurse, Jessa, works and on how other staff do not seem to care as much about their patients as Jessa does. Jessa finds herself agreeing with Mary and appreciating her insightfulness, recalling to herself that except for her former head nurse, other staff do not seem to appreciate how hard she works and seem to take her for granted. Jessa enjoys the time she spends with Mary and seeks out opportunities to interact with her. What phenomenon is occurring here, and which response by Jessa would most benefit her and the patient?
   1. Mary is experiencing transference; Jessa should help Mary to understand that she is emphasizing in Jessa those qualities that were missing in her father.

2. Jessa is idealizing Mary, seeing in her strengths and abilities that Mary does not really possess; Jessa should temporarily distance herself somewhat from Mary.

3. Mary is overidentifying with Jessa, seeing similarities that do not in reality exist; Jessa should label and explore this phenomenon in her interactions with Mary.

4. Jessa is experiencing counter-transference in response to Mary's meeting Jessa's needs for greater appreciation; Jessa should seek clinical supervision to explore these dynamics.

4. Which of the following statements would be appropriate during the orientation phase of the nurse–patient relationship? Select all that apply.
   1. "My name is Sarah, and I am a student nurse here to learn about mental health."
   2. "I will be here each Thursday from 8 a.m. until noon if you would like to talk."
   3. "Tell me about what you think would best help you to cope with the loss of your wife."
   4. "Let's talk today about how our plan for improving your sleep has been working."
   5. "We will meet weekly for one hour, during which we will discuss how to meet your goals."
   6. "Being home alone while your wife was hospitalized must have been very difficult for you."

5. A student nurse exhibits the following behaviours or actions while interacting with her patient. Which of these are appropriate as part of a therapeutic relationship?
   1. Sitting attentively in silence with a withdrawn patient until the patient chooses to speak.
   2. Offering the patient advice on how he or she could cope more effectively with stress.
   3. Controlling the pace of the relationship by selecting topics for each interaction.
   4. Limiting the discussion of termination issues so as not to sadden the patient unduly.

**ꞒVolve WEBSITE**

**Post-Test** interactive review

*Visit the Evolve Web site for Chapter Review Answers and Rationales, Critical Thinking Answer Guidelines, and additional resources related to the content in this chapter: http://evolve.elsevier.com/Canada/Varcarolis/psychiatric/*

# REFERENCES

Arkowitz, H., Westra, H.A., Miller, W.R., et al. (2008). *Motivational interviewing in the treatment of psychosocial problems*. New York: Guilford Press.

Benner, P. (2000). *From novice to expert: Excellence and power in clinical nursing practice, Commemorative edition*. Upper Saddle River, NJ: Prentice-Hall.

Butler Center for Research. (2006). *Therapeutic alliance: Improving treatment outcome. Research update*. Retrieved from http://www.hazelden.org/web/public/document/bcrup_1006.pdf.

Crawford, J.A., & Tarko, M.A. (2004). Family communication. In P.J. Bomar (Ed.), *Promoting health in families: Applying family research and theory to nursing practice* (pp. 162–185). Philadelphia: Saunders.

Erickson, J.I., & Miller, S. (2005). Caring for patients while respecting their privacy: Renewing our commitment. *Online Journal of Issues in Nursing 10*(2), 77–94. Retrieved from http://nursingworld.org.

Fontes, L.A. (2008). *Interviewing clients across cultures*. New York: Guilford Press.

Forchuk, C. (1993). *Hildgarde E. Peplau: Interpersonal nursing theory*. Newbury Park, CA: Sage Publications.

Forchuk, C., Westwell, J., Martin, M., et al. (2000). The developing nurse–client relationship: Nurses' perspectives. *Journal of the American Psychiatric Nurses Association, 6*(1), 3–10. doi:10.1177/107839030000600102.

Fox, S. (2008). *Relating to clients*. Philadelphia: Jessica Kingsley Publishers.

Haber, J. (2000). Hildegard E. Peplau: The psychiatric nursing legacy of a legend. *Journal of the American Psychiatric Nurses Association, 6*(2), 56–62. doi:10.1067/mpn.2000.104556.

Korn, M.L. (2001). *Cultural aspects of the psychotherapeutic process*. Retrieved from http://www.medscape.org/viewarticle/418608.

LaRowe, K. (2004). *The therapeutic relationship*. Retrieved from http://compassion-fatigue.com/.

Mercer, S.W., & Reynolds, W. (2002). Empathy and quality of care. *British Journal of General Practice, 52*(Suppl.), S9–S12.

Moore, J.C., & Hartman, C.R. (1988). Developing a therapeutic relationship. In C.K. Beck, R.P. Rawlins, & S.R. Williams (Eds.), *Mental health–psychiatric nursing*. St. Louis, MO: Mosby.

Peplau, H.E. (1952). *Interpersonal relations in nursing: A conceptual frame of reference for psychodynamic nursing*. New York: Putnam.

Peplau, H.E. (1999). *Interpersonal relations in nursing: A conceptual frame of reference for psychodynamic nursing*. New York: Springer.

Quinlan, J.C.F. (1996). *Co-creating personal and professional knowledge through peer support and peer approval in nursing* (Doctorial dissertation). Retrieved from http://people.bath.ac.uk/mnspwr/doc_theses_links/j_quinlan.html.

Registered Nurses' Association of Ontario. (2002). *Nursing best practice guidelines: Establishing therapeutic relationships*. Toronto: Author. Retrieved from http://rnao.ca/bpg/guidelines/establishing-therapeutic-relationships.

Rogers, C.R. (1980). *A way of being*. Boston: Houghton Mifflin.

Rogers, C.R., & Truax, C.B. (1967). The therapeutic conditions antecedent to change: A theoretical view. In C.R. Rogers (Ed.), *The therapeutic relationship and its impact*. Madison, OH: University of Wisconsin Press.

Sommers-Flanagan, J., & Sommers-Flanagan, R. (2003). *Clinical interviewing* (3rd ed.). Hoboken, NJ: Wiley.

Travelbee, J. (1971). *Interpersonal aspects of nursing* (2nd ed.). Philadelphia: F.A. Davis Co.

Wheeler, K. (2008). *Psychotherapy for the advanced practice psychiatric nurse*. St. Louis, MO: Mosby.

# Communication and the Clinical Interview

*Elizabeth M. Varcarolis*
*Adapted by Michel Andre Tarko*

## KEY TERMS AND CONCEPTS

active listening, 171
closed-ended questions, 172
cultural filters, 177
double messages, 169
double-bind messages, 169
feedback, 166

nontherapeutic communication techniques, 172
nonverbal behaviours, 168
nonverbal communication, 168
open-ended questions, 172
therapeutic communication skills and strategies, 170
verbal communication, 168

## OBJECTIVES

1. Identify three personal and two environmental factors that can impede communication.
2. Discuss the differences between verbal and nonverbal communication, and identify five examples of nonverbal communication.
3. Identify two attending behaviours the psychiatric nurse might focus on to increase communication skills.
4. Compare and contrast the range of verbal and nonverbal communication of different cultural groups in the areas of communication style, eye contact, and touch.

5. Relate problems that can arise when nurses are insensitive to cultural aspects of patients' communication styles.
6. Demonstrate the use of four techniques that can enhance communication, highlighting what makes them effective.
7. Demonstrate the use of four techniques that can obstruct communication, highlighting what makes them ineffective.
8. Identify and give rationales for suggested setting, seating, and methods for beginning the psychiatric nurse–patient interaction.
9. Explain the importance of clinical supervision.

## ⊝volve WEBSITE

*Visit the Evolve website for Flashcards, Case Studies, and additional testing resources related to the content in this chapter: http://evolve.elsevier.com/Canada/Varcarolis/psychiatric/*  Pre-Test  interactive review

Humans have a built-in need to relate to others, and our advanced ability to communicate contributes to the substance and meaning in our lives. Our need to express ourselves to others is powerful; it is the foundation on which we form happy and productive relationships in our adult lives. At the same time, stress and negative feelings within a relationship are often the result of ineffective communication. All our actions, words, and facial expressions convey meaning to others. It has been said that we cannot not communicate. Even silence can convey acceptance, anger, or thoughtfulness.

In the provision of psychiatric nursing care, communication takes on a new emphasis. Just as social relationships

are different from therapeutic relationships (see Chapter 10), *basic communication* is different from professional, patient-centred, goal-directed, and scientifically based *therapeutic communication*.

The ability to form therapeutic relationships is fundamental and essential to effective psychiatric nursing care, and therapeutic communication is central to the formation of a therapeutic relationship. Determining levels of pain in the postoperative patient, listening as parents express feelings of fear concerning their child's diagnosis, or understanding, without words, the needs of the intubated patient in the intensive care unit are essential skills in providing quality nursing care.

Research about psychiatric patients' perspectives of their therapeutic relationships with nurses revealed that the nurses' verbal and nonverbal communication shaped the development or deterioration of these relationships (Coatsworth-Puspoky, Forchuk, & Ward-Griffin, 2006). Ideally, therapeutic communication is a professional skill you learn and practise early in your nursing curriculum. But in psychiatric mental health nursing, communication skills take on a different and new emphasis. Psychiatric disorders cause not only physical responses (fatigue, loss of appetite, insomnia) but also emotional responses (sadness, anger, hopelessness, euphoria) that affect a patient's ability to relate to others.

It is often during a psychiatric nursing practice experience that students discover the utility of therapeutic communication and begin to rely on techniques they once considered artificial. For example, restating may seem like a funny thing to do. Using it in a practice session between students ("I felt sad when my dog ran away." "You felt sad when your dog ran away?") can derail communication and end the seriousness with laughter. Yet in the clinical setting, restating can become a powerful and profound communication strategy in building a therapeutic alliance:

> **Patient:** "At the moment they told me my daughter would never be able to walk like her twin sister, I felt as though I couldn't go on."
>
> **Nurse:** (After a short silence) "You felt uncertain that you could go on when you learned your daughter would never be able to walk like her twin sister."

The technique, and the empathy it conveys, is appreciated in such a situation. Developing therapeutic communication skills takes time, and with continued practice, you will develop your own style and rhythm. Eventually, these communication skills and strategies will become a part of the way you instinctively communicate with others in the clinical setting and in your personal life as you integrate them into your way of being with others.

Beginning psychiatric practitioners are often concerned that they may say the wrong thing, especially when learning to apply therapeutic techniques. Will you say the wrong thing? Yes, you probably will, but that is how we all learn to find more useful and effective ways of helping individuals reach their goals. The challenge is to recover from your mistakes and use them for learning and growth (Sommers-Flanagan & Sommers-Flanagan, 2003).

One of the most common concerns students have is that they will say the one thing that will "push the patient over the edge," or maybe even be the cause for the patient to give up on living. This is highly unlikely. Consider that behaviours associated with psychiatric disorders, such as irritability, agitation, negativity, disinterest in communication, and being hypertalkative, often frustrate and alienate friends and family. It is likely that the interactions the patient has had to date have not always been pleasant and supportive. Patients often see a well-meaning person who conveys genuine acceptance, respect, empathy, and concern for their well-being as a gift. Even if mistakes in communication are made or the "wrong thing" is said, there is little chance that the comments will do actual harm. With reflection and supervision, mistakes in communication can be corrected

and repaired. When a nurse explains his or her errors in communication and repairs the miscommunication, this show of humility and genuineness may even strengthen the therapeutic relationship.

## THE COMMUNICATION PROCESS

Communication is an interactive process between two or more people who send and receive messages to one another. The following is a simplified model of communication (Berlo, 1960):

1. One person has a need to communicate with another (*stimulus*) for information, comfort, or advice.
2. The person sending the message (*sender*) initiates interpersonal contact.
3. The *message* is the information sent or expressed to another. The clearest messages are those that are well organized and expressed in a manner familiar to the receiver.
4. The message can be sent through a variety of media, including auditory (hearing), visual (seeing), tactile (touch), smell, or any combination of these.
5. The person receiving the message (*receiver*) then interprets the message and responds to the sender by providing feedback (communication of impressions of and reactions to the sender's actions or verbalizations). Validating the accuracy of the sender's message is extremely important. The nature of the feedback often indicates whether the meaning of the message sent has been correctly interpreted by the receiver. An accuracy check may be obtained by simply asking the sender, "Is this what you mean?" or "I notice you turn away when we talk about your going back to college. Is there a conflict there?"

Figure 11-1 shows this simple model of communication, along with some of the many factors that affect it.

Effective communication in therapeutic relationships depends on nurses' knowing what they are trying to convey (the purpose of the message), communicating to the patient what is really meant, and comprehending the meaning of what the patient intentionally or unintentionally conveys (Arnold & Boggs, 2011). A systematic review of Peplau (1952) identified two main principles that can guide the communication process during the nurse–patient interview (which is discussed in detail later in this chapter): (1) clarity, which ensures that the meaning of the message is accurately understood by both parties in an ongoing mutual effort, and (2) continuity, which promotes the connections among relevant ideas and encourages a shared understanding of the activities, emotions, and context of those ideas. Maintaining this clarity and continuity requires particular concentration and attention when patients are acutely mentally ill and possibly experiencing symptoms impairing their communication.

## FACTORS THAT AFFECT COMMUNICATION

### Personal Factors

Personal factors that can impede accurate transmission or interpretation of messages include emotional factors (e.g., mood, responses to stress, personal bias), social factors (e.g., previous experience, cultural differences, language differences), and

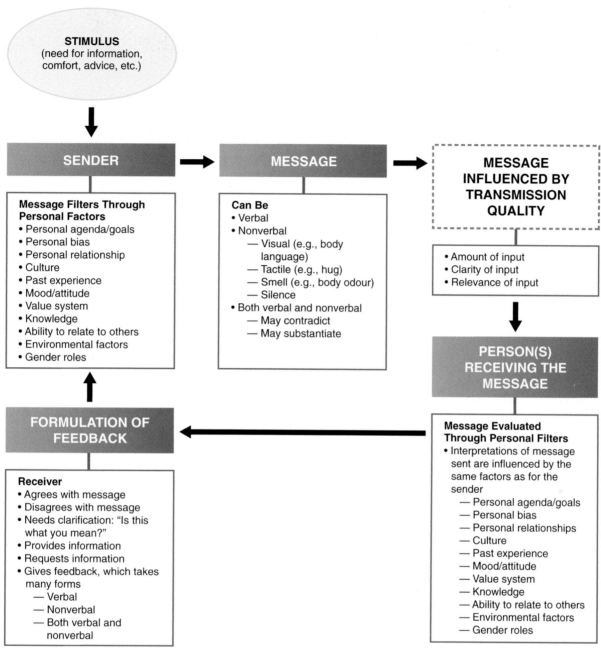

**FIGURE 11-1** Operational definition of *communication*. **Source:** Data from Ellis, R., & McClintock, A. (1990). *If you take my meaning.* London, UK: Arnold.

cognitive factors (e.g., problem-solving ability, knowledge level, language use).

## Environmental Factors

Environmental factors that may affect communication include physical factors (e.g., background noise, lack of privacy, uncomfortable accommodations) and societal determinants (e.g., sociopolitical, historical, and economic factors; the presence of others; expectations of others).

## Relationship Factors

Relationship factors refer to the status of individuals in terms of social standing, power, roles, responsibilities, age, and so on. Communication is influenced by all these factors. Consider how you would describe your day in the clinical setting to your instructor, compared to how you would describe it to your friend. The fact that your instructor has more education than you and is in an evaluative role would likely influence how much you share and your choice of words.

Now think about the relationship between you and your patient. Your patient may be older or younger than you are, more or less educated, richer or poorer, successful at work or unemployed. These factors play into the dynamics of the communication, whether at a conscious or an unconscious level, and recognizing their influence is important. It may be difficult for you to work with a woman your mother's age or one your own age, or you may feel impatient with a patient who is unemployed and abuses alcohol.

**Source:** Cleary, M., Hunt, G.E., Horsfall, J., et al. (2012). Nurse–patient interaction in acute adult inpatient mental health units: A review and synthesis of qualitative studies. *Issues in Mental Health Nursing, 33*(2), 66–79. doi:10.3109/01612840.2011.622428.

## RESEARCH HIGHLIGHT

### A Review of Nursing Communication With Patients in Acute Psychiatric Units

**Problem**

Communication can be challenging during the mental-status fluctuations of people experiencing acute mental illness.

**Purpose of Study**

This study set out to explore current notions of nursing communication with patients in acute care inpatient psychiatric settings.

**Methods**

The study used a systematic review method to identify, analyze, and synthesize research focused on nurse–patient interaction in acute care adult psychiatric nursing units. Electronic databases were searched to identify English-language research published from 1999 to present—a total of 18 research studies reported in 23 research papers.

**Key Findings**

The review revealed that nurses interact with patients in meaningful ways without appearing to be assessing, history-taking, or providing specific therapy. Findings were grouped into the following six categories: (1) sophisticated communication, (2) subtle discriminations, (3) managing security parameters, (4) ordinary communication, (5) reliance on colleagues, and (6) personal characteristics. These studies revealed that nurse communication involves interpersonal approaches and modalities that exemplify highly developed communication and personal skills designed specifically for this challenging setting.

This expanded notion of communication reflected the multiple demands on nurses' time, the variety and complexity of patients (e.g., new admissions and fragile or impulsive patients), and the presence of numerother caregivers or security guards in an acute care unit. These studies refute claims that acute care mental health nurses are not engaging adequately in therapeu-communication. If we consider only direct therapy as valuable nursing communication, then there is a dismissal of all the many more subtle elements of communication required for patient care.

**Implications for Nursing Practice**

Alternative categories of therapeutic communication identified in the systematic review demonstrate the importance of a broader perspective and expanded definitions of communication between psychiatric nurses and patients beyond traditional therapy, highlighting the importance of communicating at subtle interpersonal and institutional levels.

It is sometimes difficult for students to grasp or remember that patients, regardless of these relationship factors, are in a position of vulnerability. Wearing a hospital identification band or stepping through the door of a community mental health clinic formally indicates a need for care, and as a caregiver, you are viewed to be in a role of authority. Part of the art of therapeutic communication is in finding a balance between your role as a professional and your role as a human being who has been socialized into complex patterns of interactions based, at least in part, on status.

Students sometimes fall back into time-tested and comfortable roles. As such, one of the most common responses of nursing students to nurse–patient relationships is treating the patient as a buddy. Imagine a male nursing student walking onto the unit, seeing his assigned patient, and saying, "Hey, how's it going today?" while giving the patient a high-five. Or consider the female nursing student assigned to the 60-year-old woman who used to work as a registered nurse. This relationship has the potential to become unbalanced and nontherapeutic if the patient shifts the focus away from his or her own concerns and onto the student nurse's interests and concerns (see Chapter 10).

## VERBAL AND NONVERBAL COMMUNICATION

### Verbal Communication

Verbal communication consists of all the words a person speaks. We live in a society of symbols, and our main social symbols are words. Talking is our most common activity. It is our public link to one another, the primary instrument of instruction, a need, an art, and one of the most personal aspects of our private lives. When we speak, we:

- Communicate our beliefs and values
- Communicate perceptions and meanings
- Convey interest and understanding or insult and judgement
- Convey messages clearly or convey conflicting or implied messages
- Convey clear, honest feelings or disguised, distorted feelings

Words are culturally perceived; therefore, clarifying the intent of certain words is very important. Even if the nurse and patient have a similar cultural background, the mental image that each has for a given word may not be exactly the same. Although they believe they are talking about the same thing, the nurse and patient may actually be talking about two quite different things. While they produce mental images, words are also symbols for emotions.

### Nonverbal Communication

Nonverbal communication (often called *cues*) are those messages expressed through directly observable behaviours such as physical appearance, facial expressions, body posture, amount of eye contact, eye cast (i.e., emotion expressed in the eyes), hand gestures, sighs, fidgeting, and yawning. A person's tone of voice, emphasis on certain words, and pacing of speech are also examples of nonverbal behaviours. Sometimes these

| TABLE 11-1 | **NONVERBAL BEHAVIOURS** | |
|---|---|---|
| **BEHAVIOUR** | **POSSIBLE NONVERBAL CUES** | **EXAMPLE** |
| Body behaviours | Posture, body movements, gestures, gait | The patient is slumped in a chair, puts her face in her hands, and occasionally taps her right foot. |
| Facial expressions | Frowns, smiles, grimaces, raised eyebrows, pursed lips, licking of lips, tongue movements | The patient grimaces when speaking to the nurse; when alone, he smiles and giggles to himself. |
| Eye cast | Angry, suspicious, and accusatory looks | The patient's eyes harden with suspicion. |
| Voice-related behaviours | Tone, pitch, level, intensity, inflection, stuttering, pauses, silences, fluency | The patient talks in a loud singsong voice. |
| Observable autonomic physiological responses | Increase in respirations, diaphoresis, pupil dilation, blushing, paleness | When the patient mentions discharge, she becomes pale, her respirations increase, and her face becomes diaphoretic. |
| Personal appearance | Grooming, dress, hygiene | The patient is dressed in a wrinkled shirt, his pants are stained, his socks are dirty, and he is unshaven. |
| Physical characteristics | Height, weight, physique, complexion | The patient is grossly overweight, and his muscles appear flabby. |

behaviours operate outside of the awareness of the person exhibiting the behaviours—or unconsciously. It is often said that "it's not what you say but how you say it." In other words, it is the nonverbal behaviours that may be communicating the "real" message (see Table 11-1). Nonverbal behaviours must be observed and interpreted in light of a person's culture, class, gender, age, sexual orientation, and spiritual beliefs. Cultural influences on communication are addressed later in this chapter.

### Interaction of Verbal and Nonverbal Communication

Shawn Shea (1998), a nationally renowned psychiatrist and communication workshop leader, suggests that communication is roughly 10% verbal and 90% nonverbal. Our interpretation of feelings and attitudes may account for the high percentage of communication attributed to nonverbal behaviours. While it would be difficult to watch a foreign film and understand 90% of its meaning based solely on body language and vocal tones, nonverbal behaviours and cues do influence communication to a surprising degree in nurse–patient interactions. Communication thus involves two radically different but highly interdependent kinds of symbols: verbal and nonverbal.

Spoken words can be straightforward or may distort, conceal, deny, or disguise true feelings. Whereas spoken words represent our public selves, nonverbal behaviours (e.g., how a person listens and uses silence and sense of touch) can convey important information about the private self that is not available from conversation alone, especially in consideration of cultural norms.

Some elements of nonverbal communication, such as facial expressions, seem to be inborn and are similar across cultures. Matsumoto (2006) cited studies that found a high degree of agreement in spontaneous facial expressions or emotions across ten different cultures. However, some cultural groups (e.g., Japanese) may control their facial expressions in public. Other types of nonverbal behaviours, such as how close people stand to each other when speaking, depend on cultural conventions.

Some nonverbal communication is formalized and has specific meanings (e.g., the military salute, the Japanese bow).

Messages are not always simple; they can appear to be one thing when, in fact, they are another (Ellis, Gates, & Kenworthy, 2003). Often, people have greater conscious awareness of their verbal messages than of their nonverbal behaviours. The verbal message is sometimes referred to as the *content* of the message (what is said), and the nonverbal behaviour is called the *process* of the message (nonverbal cues a person gives to substantiate or contradict the verbal message). When the content is congruent with the process, the communication is more clearly understood and is considered healthy. For example, a student's saying "It's important that I get good grades in this class" is content. The student's having bought the books, taking good notes, and working with a study buddy is process. The content and process in this example are congruent and straightforward, and there is a "healthy" message. If, however, the verbal message is not reinforced or is in fact contradicted by the nonverbal behaviour, the message is confusing. For example, the student's not having the books, skipping several classes, and not studying is also process, but in this case, the student is sending two different messages.

Messages are sent to create meaning but also can be used defensively to hide what is actually going on, create confusion, and attack relatedness (Ellis, Gates, & Kenworthy, 2003). Conflicting messages are known as double messages or *mixed messages*. One way a nurse can respond to verbal and nonverbal incongruity is to reflect and validate the patient's feelings. For example, the nurse could say to the student, "You say you are upset you did not pass this semester, but I notice you look more relaxed and less conflicted than you have all term. What do you see as some of the pros and cons of not passing the course this semester?"

Bateson, Jackson, Haley, and colleague (1956) coined the term double-bind messages. A double-bind message is a contradictory mix of content and process that communicates both nurturing and hurtful expressions. The following vignette gives an example of a double-bind message.

---

**VIGNETTE**

A 21-year-old female who lives at home with her chronically ill mother wants to go out for an evening with her friends. She is told by her frail but not helpless mother: "Oh, go ahead, have fun. I'll just sit here by myself, and I can always call 911 if I don't feel well, but you go ahead and have fun." The mother says this while looking sad, eyes downcast, slumped in her chair, and letting her cane drop to the floor.

---

The recipient of this double-bind message is caught inside contradictory statements, so she cannot decide what is right. If she goes, the implication is that she is being selfish by leaving her sick mother alone. But if she stays, the mother could say, "I told you to go have fun." If she does go, the chances are she will not have much fun because of concern for the mother. The daughter is trapped in a no-win situation of which she may not be fully aware.

With experience, nurses become increasingly aware of patients' verbal and nonverbal communication and compare the two to gain important clues about the real message. What individuals do may either express and reinforce or contradict what they say. So, as in the saying "Actions speak louder than words," actions often reveal the true meaning of a person's intent, whether the intent is conscious or unconscious.

## COMMUNICATION SKILLS FOR NURSES

### Therapeutic Communication Strategies

Peplau emphasized the art of communication to highlight the importance of nursing interventions in facilitating achievement of quality patient care and quality of life (Haber, 2000). The nurse must establish and maintain a therapeutic relationship in which the patient will feel safe and hopeful that positive change is possible.

Once a therapeutic relationship is established, specific needs and problems can be identified, and the nurse can work with the patient on increasing self-awareness, developing insight and problem-solving skills, learning new coping behaviours, and experiencing more appropriate and satisfying ways of relating to others. To do this, the nurse must have a sound knowledge of communication theory and skills. Therefore, nurses must become more aware of their own interpersonal methods, eliminating obstructive, nontherapeutic communication techniques and strategies and developing additional responses that maximize the nurse–patient interactions and increase the use of therapeutic communication skills and strategies (i.e., skills such as warmth, respect, and empathy and strategies such as using silence, recognizing strengths, and making observations). Helpful tools for nurses when communicating with their patients are silence, active listening, and clarifying techniques.

### Silence

Silence can sometimes intimidate both interviewers and patients (Sommers-Flanagan & Sommers-Flanagan, 2003). In the United States, there is an emphasis on action and a high level of verbal activity. Students and practising nurses alike may find that when the flow of words stops, they become uncomfortable. They may rush to fill the void with "questions or chatter," thus cutting off potentially important thoughts and feelings the patient might be taking time to think about before articulating. Silence is not the absence of communication but a specific channel for transmitting and receiving messages; therefore, the practitioner needs to understand that silence is a significant means of influencing and being influenced by others.

Talking is a highly individualized practice. Some people find the telephone a nuisance, whereas others believe they cannot live without their cellphones on hand at all times. In the initial interview, patients may be reluctant to speak because of the newness of the situation, the fact that the nurse is a stranger, or feelings of distrust, self-consciousness, embarrassment, or shyness. The nurse must recognize and respect individual differences in styles and tempos of responding. People who are quiet, those who have a language barrier or speech disorder, older adults, and those who lack confidence in their ability to express themselves may communicate a need for support and encouragement through their silence.

Although there is no universal rule concerning how much silence is too much, silence has been said to be worthwhile only as long as it is serving some function and not frightening the patient. Knowing when to speak during the interview depends largely on one's perception about what is being conveyed through the silence. Icy silence may be an expression of anger and hostility; being ignored or given "the silent treatment" is recognized as an insult and is a particularly hurtful form of communication.

Silence may provide meaningful moments of reflection for both participants, giving an opportunity to contemplate thoughtfully what has been said and felt, weigh alternatives, formulate new ideas, and gain a new perspective on the matter under discussion. If the nurse waits to speak and allows the patient to break the silence, the patient may share thoughts and feelings that would otherwise have been withheld. Nurses who feel compelled to fill every void with words often do so because of their own anxiety, self-consciousness, and embarrassment. This action, however, prioritizes the nurse's need for comfort over the needs of the patient.

It is crucial to recognize that for some individuals living with a psychiatric disorder, such as major depression or schizophrenia, medications may cause an overall slowing of thought processes. This slowing may be so severe, it may seem like an eternity before the patient responds. Patience and gentle prompting (e.g., "You were saying that you would like to get a pass this weekend to visit your niece") can help patients gather their thoughts.

Silence is not always therapeutic. Prolonged and frequent silences by the psychiatric nurse may hinder an interview that requires verbal articulation. Although a less talkative nurse may be comfortable with silence, this mode of communication may make the patient feel like a fountain of information to be drained dry. Moreover, without feedback, patients have no way of knowing whether or not what they said was understood. Additionally, children and adolescents in particular tend to feel uncomfortable with silence.

## Active Listening

People want more than just a physical presence in human communication. Most people want the other person to be there for them psychologically, socially, emotionally, and spiritually. Active listening in the nurse–patient relationship includes the following aspects:

- Observing the patient's nonverbal behaviours
- Understanding and reflecting on the patient's verbal message
- Understanding the patient in the context of the social setting of the patient's life
- Detecting "false notes" (e.g., inconsistencies or things the patient says that need more clarification)
- Providing constructive feedback about the patient of which he or she might not be aware

Effective interviewers learn to become active listeners not only when the patient is talking but also when the patient becomes silent. During active listening, psychiatric nurses carefully note verbal and nonverbal patient responses and monitor their own nonverbal responses. Using silence effectively and learning to listen actively—both to the patient and to your own thoughts and reactions——are key ingredients in effective communication. Both skills take time to develop but can be learned; you will become more proficient with guidance and practice.

Some important principles of active listening include the following (Mohl, 2003):

- The answer is always inside the patient.
- Objective truth is never as simple as it seems.
- Everything you hear is modified by the patient's filters.
- Everything you hear is modified by your own filters.
- It is okay to feel confused and uncertain.
- Listen to yourself too.

Active listening helps strengthen the patient's ability to solve problems. By giving the patient undivided attention, the nurse communicates that the patient is not alone. This kind of intervention enhances self-esteem and encourages the patient to direct energy toward finding ways to deal with problems. Serving as a sounding board, the nurse listens as the patient tests thoughts by voicing them aloud. This form of interpersonal interaction often enables the patient to clarify thinking, link ideas, and tentatively decide what should be done and how best to do it (Collins, 1983).

***Listening with empathy.*** Wheeler (2008) identifies empathy as the most important element in therapeutic communication. Research indicates that the connectedness that results from empathy actually improves brain function by increasing brain plasticity. Wheeler describes the empathic process as the nurse's entering and feeling the patient's world, the patient's perceiving his or her own understanding of the world, and the patient's experiencing acceptance and confirmation of himself or herself.

It is not enough for the nurse to feel empathy; an important part of this process is the communication of empathy to the patient. Egan (2005) suggested that the communication of empathy is achieved by connecting to the emotions, experiences, and thoughts of our patients and, to this end, proposed two forms of empathic statements, demonstrated through these examples:

1. "You feel _____ (name the emotion) because _____ (describe the <u>experiences</u>, thoughts, and behaviours)."
2. "Your _____ (name the emotion) is an outcome of _____ (describe the <u>context</u> of the experiences)."

If we plug in a scenario to the first statement, emphasizing the experience, it could sound something like this: "You feel like a failure because you have let your father down by joining the Canadian Armed Forces rather than becoming a lawyer." Now try composing an empathic statement to the same scenario that will encompass the emotion in light of a particular context.

It is not always easy to be empathic and communicate a connection to the experiences, emotions, thoughts, behaviours, and contexts of our patients. Patients may describe experiences of brutal physical or sexual abuse, feelings of torment watching a loved one die, hate and anger toward another person, or acts of violence or hurtful inconsideration they have committed. When people are self-pitying, critical, angry, sarcastic, or demeaning, the nurse's ability to connect to these experiences and communicate empathy may also be challenged. Chapter 10 offers a more detailed discussion of empathy.

## Clarifying Techniques

Understanding depends on clear communication, which is aided by the nurse's verifying his or her interpretation of the patient's messages. The nurse can request feedback on the accuracy of the message received from verbal and nonverbal cues. The use of clarifying techniques helps both participants identify major differences in their frame of reference, giving them the opportunity to correct misperceptions before they cause any serious misunderstandings. The patient who is asked to elaborate on or clarify vague or ambiguous messages needs to know that the purpose is to promote mutual understanding.

***Paraphrasing.*** To clarify, the nurse might use *paraphrasing*, or explaining in different (often fewer) words the basic content of a patient's message (Sommers-Flanagan & Sommers-Flanagan, 2003). Using simple, precise, and culturally relevant terms, the nurse may readily confirm interpretation of the patient's previous message before the interview proceeds. By prefacing statements with a phrase such as "I'm not sure I understand" or "In other words, you seem to be saying ...," the nurse helps the patient form a clearer perception of what may be a bewildering mass of details. After paraphrasing, the nurse must validate the accuracy of the restatement and its helpfulness to the discussion. The patient may confirm or deny the perceptions through nonverbal cues or by direct response to a question from the nurse, such as "Was I correct in saying ...?" As a result, the patient is made aware that the interviewer is actively involved in the search for understanding.

***Restating.*** In *restating*, the nurse mirrors the patient's overt and covert messages, so the technique may be used to echo feeling as well as content or context. Restating differs from paraphrasing in that it involves repeating the same key words the patient has just spoken. If a patient remarks, "My life is empty … it has no meaning," additional information may be gained by restating, "Your life has no meaning?" The purpose of this technique is to explore more thoroughly subjects that may be significant.

Too frequent and indiscriminate use of restating, however, may be interpreted by patients as inattention or disinterest. It is easy to overuse this tool so that its application becomes mechanical. As well, parroting or mimicking what another has said may be perceived as poking fun at the person; therefore, the use of this nondirect approach can become a definite barrier to communication. To avoid overuse of restating, the nurse can combine restatements with direct questions that encourage descriptions: "What is lacking in your life?" "What are you missing in your life?" "Describe a day in your life that felt empty to you."

**Reflecting.** *Reflection* is a means of assisting people to better understand their own thoughts and feelings. Reflecting may take the form of a question or a simple statement that conveys the nurse's observations of the patient when sensitive issues are being discussed. The nurse might then describe briefly to the patient the apparent meaning of the emotional tone of the patient's verbal and nonverbal behaviour. For example, to reflect a patient's feelings about his or her life, a good beginning might be, "You sound as if you have had many disappointments."

Sharing observations with a patient shows that you accept him or her and that the patient has your full attention. When you reflect, you make the patient aware of inner feelings and encourage the patient to own them. For example, you may say to a patient, "You look sad." Perceiving your concern may allow the patient to spontaneously share feelings. The use of a question in response to the patient's question is another reflective technique (Arnold & Boggs, 2011). For example:

**Patient:** "Nurse, do you think I really need to be hospitalized?"

**Nurse:** "What do you think, Jane?"

**Patient:** "I don't know—that's why I'm asking you."

**Nurse:** "I'll be willing to share my impression with you at the end of this first session. However, you've probably thought about hospitalization and have some feelings about it. I wonder what they are."

**Exploring.** A technique that enables the nurse to examine important ideas, experiences, or relationships more fully is *exploring*. For example, if a patient tells you he does not get along well with his wife, you will want to further explore this area. Possible openers include:

"*Tell me more* about your relationship with your wife."

"*Describe* your relationship with your wife."

"*Give me an example* of how you and your wife don't get along."

Asking for an example can greatly clarify a vague or generic statement made by a patient.

**Patient:** "No one likes me."

**Nurse:** "Give me an example of one person who doesn't like you."

or

**Patient:** "Everything I do is wrong."

**Nurse:** "Give me an example of one thing you do that you think is wrong."

Table 11-2 lists more examples of therapeutic communication techniques.

### Asking Questions and Eliciting Patient Responses

*Open-ended questions.* Many of the questions cited as examples above and in Table 11-2 are open-ended. Open-ended questions and comments encourage lengthy responses and facilitate expression of thoughts, feelings, and information about experiences, perceptions, or responses to a situation. For example:

- "What do you perceive as your biggest problem right now?"
- "Give me an example of some of the stresses you are under right now."
- "Tell me more about your relationship with your wife."

Since open-ended questions are not intrusive and do not put the patient on the defensive, they help the clinician elicit information, especially at the beginning of an interview or when a patient is guarded or resistant to answering questions. They are particularly useful when establishing rapport with a person.

*Closed-ended questions.* Nurses are usually urged to ask open-ended questions to elicit more than a "yes" or "no" response. However, closed-ended questions, when used sparingly, can give you specific and needed information. Closed-ended questions (those requiring only a "yes" or "no" response) are most useful during an initial assessment or intake interview, to obtain concrete responses to specific assessment data such as a suicide risk assessment, or to determine outcomes of interventions (e.g., "Are the medications helping you?" "When did you start hearing voices?" "Did you seek therapy after your first suicide attempt?") Care needs to be exercised with this technique. Frequent use of closed-ended questions with a patient leaves the patient feeling interrogated and can close an interview down rapidly, especially in the case of patients who are guarded or resist engaging in interactions.

## Nontherapeutic Communication Techniques

Although people may use "nontherapeutic," or ineffective, communication techniques in their daily lives, these techniques can cause problems for nurses because they tend to impede or shut down nurse–patient interaction. Table 11-3 describes nontherapeutic communication techniques and suggests more helpful responses.

### Excessive Questioning

Excessive questioning—asking multiple questions (particularly closed-ended questions) consecutively or very rapidly—casts the nurse in the role of an interrogator who demands information without respect for the patient's willingness or readiness to respond. This approach conveys a lack of respect for and sensitivity to the patient's needs. Excessive questioning controls the range and nature of the responses, can easily result in a therapeutic stall, or may completely shut down an interview. It is a controlling tactic and may reflect the interviewer's lack of security in letting the patient tell his or her own story. It is better

## TABLE 11-2  THERAPEUTIC COMMUNICATION TECHNIQUES

| THERAPEUTIC TECHNIQUE | DESCRIPTION | EXAMPLE |
|---|---|---|
| Using silence | Gives the person time to collect thoughts or think through a point | Encouraging a person to talk by waiting for the answers |
| Accepting | Indicates that the person has been understood; an accepting statement does not necessarily indicate agreement but it is nonjudgemental (The nurse should not imply understanding when he or she does not understand.) | "Yes." "Uh-huh." "I follow what you say." |
| Giving recognition | Indicates awareness of change and personal efforts; does not imply good or bad, right or wrong | "Good morning, Mr. James." "You've combed your hair today." "I see you've eaten your whole lunch." |
| Offering self | Offers presence, interest, and a desire to understand; is not offered to get the person to talk or behave in a specific way | "I would like to spend time with you." "I'll stay here and sit with you awhile." |
| Offering general leads | Allows the other person to take direction in the discussion; indicates interest in what comes next | "Go on." "And then?" "Tell me about it." |
| Giving broad openings | Clarifies that the lead is to be taken by the patient; however, the nurse discourages pleasantries and small talk | "Where would you like to begin?" "What are you thinking about?" "What would you like to discuss?" |
| Placing the events in time or sequence | Puts events and actions in better perspective; notes cause-and-effect relationships and identifies patterns of interpersonal difficulties | "What happened before?" "When did this happen?" |
| Making observations | Calls attention to the person's behaviour (e.g., trembling, nail biting, restless mannerisms); encourages patient to notice the behaviour and describe thoughts and feelings for mutual understanding; helpful with mute and withdrawn people | "You appear tense." "I notice you're biting your lips." "You appear nervous whenever John enters the room." |
| Encouraging description of perception | Increases the nurse's understanding of the patient's perceptions; talking about feelings and difficulties can lessen the need to act them out inappropriately | "Tell me, what do these voices seem to be saying?" "What is happening now?" "Tell me when you feel anxious." |
| Encouraging comparison | Brings out recurring themes in experiences or interpersonal relationships; helps the person clarify similarities and differences | "Has this ever happened before?" "Is this how you felt when ...?" "Was it something like ...?" |
| Restating | Repeats the main idea expressed; gives the patient an idea of what has been communicated; if the message has been misunderstood, the patient can clarify it | *Patient:* "I can't sleep. I stay awake all night." *Nurse:* "You have difficulty sleeping?" *or* *Patient:* "I don't know ...he always has some excuse for not coming over or keeping our appointments." *Nurse:* "You think he no longer wants to see you?" |
| Reflecting | Directs questions, feelings, and ideas back to the patient; encourages the patient to accept his or her own ideas and feelings; acknowledges the patient's right to have opinions and make decisions and encourages the patient to think of self as a capable person | *Patient:* "What should I do about my husband's affair?" *Nurse:* "What do you think you should do?" *or* *Patient:* "My brother spends all of my money and then has the nerve to ask for more." *Nurse:* "You feel angry when this happens?" |
| Focusing | Concentrates attention on a single point; especially useful when the patient jumps from topic to topic; if a person is experiencing a severe level of anxiety, the nurse should not persist until the anxiety lessens | "This point you are making about leaving school seems worth looking at more closely." "You've mentioned many things. Let's go back to your thinking of 'ending it all.'" |

*Continued*

| TABLE 11-2 | THERAPEUTIC COMMUNICATION TECHNIQUES—cont'd | |
|---|---|---|
| **THERAPEUTIC TECHNIQUE** | **DESCRIPTION** | **EXAMPLE** |
| Exploring | Examines certain ideas, experiences, or relationships more fully; if the patient chooses not to elaborate by answering no, the nurse does not probe or pry but instead respects the patient's wishes | "Tell me more about that." "Would you describe it more fully?" "Could you talk about how you learned your mom was dying of cancer?" |
| Giving information | Makes available facts the person needs; supplies knowledge from which decisions can be made or conclusions drawn—for example, the patient needs to know the role of the nurse; the purpose of the nurse–patient relationship; and the time, place, and duration of the meetings | "My purpose for being here is ..." "This medication is for ..." "The test will determine ..." |
| Seeking clarification | Helps patients clarify their own thoughts and maximizes mutual understanding between nurse and patient | "I am not sure I follow you." "What would you say is the main point of what you just said?" "Give an example of a time you thought everyone hated you." |
| Presenting reality | Indicates what is real; the nurse does not argue or try to convince the patient but just describes personal perceptions or facts in the situation | "That was Dr. Todd, not a man from the Mafia." "That was the sound of a car backfiring." "Your mother is not here; I am a nurse." |
| Voicing doubt | Undermines the patient's beliefs by not reinforcing the exaggerated or false perceptions | "Isn't that unusual?" "Really?" "That's hard to believe." |
| Seeking consensual validation | Clarifies that both the nurse and patient share mutual understanding of communications; helps the patient see more clearly what he or she is thinking | "Tell me whether my understanding agrees with yours." |
| Verbalizing the implied | Puts into concrete terms what the patient implies, making the patient's communication more explicit | *Patient:* "I can't talk to you or anyone else. It's a waste of time." *Nurse:* "Do you perceive that no one understands?" |
| Encouraging evaluation | Aids the patient in considering people and events from the perspective of the patient's own set of values | "How do you feel about ...?" "What did it mean to you when he said he couldn't stay?" |
| Attempting to translate into feelings | Responds to the feelings expressed, not just the content; often termed *decoding* | *Patient:* "I am dead inside." *Nurse:* "Are you saying that you feel lifeless? Does life seem meaningless to you?" |
| Suggesting collaboration | Emphasizes working with the patient, not doing things for the patient; encourages the view that change is possible through collaboration | "Perhaps you and I can discover what produces your anxiety." "Perhaps by working together, we can come up with some ideas that might improve your communications with your spouse." |
| Summarizing | Brings together important points of discussion to enhance understanding; also allows the opportunity to clarify communications so that both nurse and patient leave the interview with the same ideas in mind | "Have I got this straight?" "You said that ..." "During the past hour, you and I have discussed ..." |
| Encouraging formulation of a plan of action | Allows the patient to identify alternative actions for interpersonal situations the patient finds disturbing (e.g., when anger or anxiety is provoked) | "What could you do to let anger out harmlessly?" "The next time this comes up, what might you do to handle it?" "What are some other ways you can approach your boss?" |

**Source:** Adapted from Hays, J.S., & Larson, K. (1963). *Interacting with patients.* New York: Macmillan.

| TABLE 11-3 | NONTHERAPEUTIC COMMUNICATION TECHNIQUES | | |
|---|---|---|---|
| **NONTHERAPEUTIC TECHNIQUE** | **DESCRIPTION** | **EXAMPLE** | **MORE HELPFUL RESPONSE** |
| Giving premature advice | Assumes the nurse knows best and the patient can't think for self; inhibits problem solving and fosters dependency | "Get out of this situation immediately." | *Encouraging problem solving:* "What are the pros and cons of your situation?" "What were some of the actions you thought you might take?" "What are some of the ways you have thought of to meet your goals?" |
| Minimizing feelings | Indicates that the nurse is unable to understand or empathize with the patient; the patient's feelings or experiences are being belittled, which can cause the patient to feel small or insignificant and devalued | *Patient:* "I wish I were dead." *Nurse:* "Everyone gets down in the dumps." "I know what you mean." "You should feel happy you're getting better." "Things get worse before they get better." | *Empathizing and exploring:* "You must be feeling very upset. Are you thinking of hurting yourself?" |
| Falsely reassuring | Under-rates a person's feelings and belittles a person's concerns; may cause the patient to stop sharing feelings if he or she expects to be ridiculed or not taken seriously | "I wouldn't worry about that." "Everything will be all right." "You will do just fine—you'll see." | *Clarifying the patient's message:* "What specifically are you worried about?" "What do you think could go wrong?" "What are you concerned might happen?" |
| Making value judgements | Prevents problem solving; can make the patient feel guilty, angry, misunderstood, not supported, or anxious to leave | "Why do you still smoke when your wife has lung cancer?" | *Making observations:* "I notice you are still smoking even though your wife has lung cancer. Is this a problem?" |
| Asking "why" questions | Implies criticism; often has the effect of making the patient feel a need to justify behaviour and leaves the patient feeling defensive | "Why did you stop taking your medication?" | *Asking open-ended questions; giving a broad opening:* "Tell me some of the events that led up to your not taking your medications." |
| Asking excessive questions | Results in the patient's not knowing which question to answer and possibly being confused about what is being asked | *Nurse:* "How's your appetite? Are you losing weight? Are you eating enough?" *Patient:* "No." | *Clarifying:* "Tell me about your eating habits since you've been depressed." |
| Giving approval, agreeing | Implies the patient is doing the right thing—and that not doing it is wrong; may lead the patient to focus on pleasing the nurse or clinician; denies the patient the opportunity to change his or her mind or decision | "I'm proud of you for applying for that job." "I agree with your decision." | *Making observations:* "I noticed that you applied for that job. What factors might contribute to your choice one way or the other?" *Asking open-ended questions; giving a broad opening:* "What led to that decision?" |
| Disapproving; disagreeing | Can make a person defensive | "You really should have shown up for the medication group." "I disagree with that." | *Exploring:* "What was going on with you when you decided not to come to your medication group?" "That's one point of view. How did you arrive at that conclusion?" |
| Changing the subject | May invalidate the patient's feelings and needs; can leave the patient feeling alienated and isolated and increase feelings of hopelessness | *Patient:* "I'd like to die." *Nurse:* "Did you go to Alcoholics Anonymous like we discussed?" | *Validating and exploring:* *Patient:* "I'd like to die." *Nurse:* "This sounds serious. Have you thought of harming yourself?" |

**Source:** Adapted from Hays, J.S., & Larson, K. (1963). *Interacting with patients.* New York: Macmillan.

to ask more open-ended questions and follow the patient's lead. For example:

*Excessive questioning:* "Why did you leave your wife? Did you feel angry at her? What did she do to you? Are you going back to her?"

*More therapeutic approach:* "Tell me about the situation between you and your wife."

## Giving Approval or Disapproval

"You look great in that dress." "I'm proud of the way you controlled your temper at lunch." "That's a great quilt you made." What could be bad about giving someone a pat on the back once in a while? Nothing, if it is done without conveying a positive or negative judgement. We often give our friends and family approval when they do something well. However, in a nurse–patient relationship, giving praise and approval becomes much more complex.

A patient may be feeling overwhelmed, experiencing low self-esteem, feeling unsure of where his or her life is going, or desperately seeking recognition, approval, and attention. Yet when people are feeling vulnerable, a value comment may be misinterpreted. For example, the nurse may say, "You did a great job in group telling John just what you thought about how rudely he treated you." This message implies that the nurse was pleased by the manner in which the patient talked to John. The patient then sees such a response as "doing the right thing" and as a way to please the nurse. To continue to please the nurse (and get approval), the patient may continue the behaviour. The behaviour may indeed be useful for the patient, but when done to please another person, it is not coming from the individual's own volition or conviction. Also, when the person the patient needs to please is not around, the motivation for the new behaviour may not be either. Thus, the new response really is not a change in behaviour as much as a ploy to win approval and acceptance from another.

Giving approval also cuts off further communication. A more therapeutic approach may be to say, "I noticed that you spoke up to John in group yesterday about his rude behaviour. How did it feel to be more assertive?" This response opens the way for finding out if the patient was scared, was comfortable, wants to work more on assertiveness, and so on. It also suggests that this behaviour was a self-choice made by the patient. While the patient is recognized for the change in behaviour, the topic is also opened for further discussion.

Giving disapproval (e.g., "You really should not cheat, even if you think everyone else is doing it") implies that the nurse has the right to judge the patient's thoughts or feelings. Again, an observation should be made instead (e.g., "Can you give me two examples of how cheating could negatively affect your goal of graduating?").

## Giving Advice

Although we ask for and give advice all the time in daily life, giving advice to a patient is rarely helpful. Often when we ask for advice, our real motive is to discover whether we are thinking along the same lines as someone else or if they would agree with us. When a nurse gives advice or offers solutions to a patient, the nurse is interfering with the patient's ability to make personal decisions. The patient may eventually begin to think the nurse does not view him or her as capable of making effective decisions. People often feel inadequate when they are given no choices over decisions in their lives. Not only can giving advice to patients undermine the patient's sense of competence and adequacy; it can also foster dependency ("I'll have to ask the nurse what to do about …").

However, people do need information and time to reflect in order to make informed decisions. Often, you can help a patient define a problem and identify what information might be needed to come to an informed decision. A useful approach would be to ask, "What do you see as some possible actions you can take?" It is much more respectful and ultimately constructive to encourage problem solving by the patient than simply to provide solutions. Sometimes, though, you might suggest several alternatives a patient could consider (e.g., "What are your thoughts of telling your friend about the incident?"). When you open up the conversation in this way, the patient is free to express his or her thoughts and feelings about such a disclosure, giving the nurse an opportunity to explore other potential alternatives and to support the patient in his or her decision.

## Asking "Why" Questions

"Why did you come late?" "Why didn't you go to the funeral?" "Why didn't you study for the exam?" Very often, "why" questions imply criticism. We may ask our friends or family such questions, and in the context of a solid relationship, the "why" may be understood more as "What happened?" With people we do not know—especially those who may be anxious or overwhelmed—a "why" question from a person in authority (e.g., nurse, psychiatrist, teacher) can be perceived as intrusive and judgemental, serving only to make the person feel the need to justify behaviour and respond defensively.

It is much more useful to ask *what* is happening than *why* it is happening. Questions that focus on who, what, where, and when often elicit important information that can facilitate problem solving and further the communication process. See Table 11-3 for additional ineffective communication techniques, as well as statements that would better facilitate interaction and patient comfort.

## Cultural Considerations

Canada is becoming increasingly culturally diverse, and health care providers need to be familiar with the verbal and nonverbal communication characteristics of a multicultural national population. The nurse's awareness of cultural meanings of certain verbal and nonverbal communications in initial face-to-face encounters with a patient can lead to the formation of a positive therapeutic relationship (Kavanaugh, 2003).

Unrecognized differences in cultural identities can result in assessment and interventions that are not optimally respectful of the patient and can be inadvertently biased or prejudiced. Health care workers need to have not only knowledge of various patients' cultures but also awareness of their own cultural identities. Especially important are nurses' attitudes and beliefs toward those from cultures other than their own, because these will affect their relationships with patients (Kavanaugh, 2003). Four areas that may prove problematic for the nurse trying to interpret specific verbal and nonverbal messages of the patient include:

1. Communication style
2. Use of eye contact
3. Perception of touch
4. Cultural filters

Further information about working with people of various cultures is presented in Chapter 7.

### Communication Style

People may communicate in an intense and highly emotional manner. Some may consider it normal to use dramatic body language when describing emotional problems, and others may perceive such behaviour as being out of control or reflective of some degree of pathology. For example, within the Hispanic community, intensely emotional styles of communication often are culturally appropriate and expected (Kavanaugh, 2003). Similarly, French and Italian Canadians typically use animated facial expressions and expressive hand gestures during communication, which can be misinterpreted by others.

In other cultures, a calm façade may mask severe distress. For example, in many South Asian cultures, expression of positive or negative emotions is a private affair, and open expression of them is considered to be in bad taste and possibly a weakness. A quiet smile by a South Asian Canadian may express joy, an apology, stoicism, or even anger. German and British Canadians also tend to value highly the concept of self-control and may show little facial emotion in the presence of great distress or emotional turmoil.

### Eye Contact

Fontes (2008) warned that the presence or absence of eye contact should not be used to assess attentiveness, judge truthfulness, or make assumptions about the degree of engagement one has with a patient. Cultural norms often dictate a person's comfort or lack of comfort with direct eye contact. Some cultures consider direct eye contact disrespectful and improper. For example, Aboriginal individuals have traditionally been taught to avoid eye contact with authority figures, including nurses, physicians, and other health care providers; avoidance of direct eye contact is seen as a sign of respect to those in authority, but it could be misinterpreted as a lack of interest or even as a lack of respect.

In Japanese culture, making direct eye contact is also considered a lack of respect and a personal affront; the preference is for shifting or downcast eyes or a focus on the speaker's neck. For many Chinese people, gazing around and looking to one side when listening to another is considered polite. In some Middle Eastern cultures, a woman's making direct eye contact with a man may imply a sexual interest or even promiscuity. On the other hand, most Canadians of European descent maintain eye contact during conversation and may interpret avoidance of eye contact by another person as a lack of interest, a show of dishonesty, or avoiding the sharing of important information.

### Touch

The therapeutic use of touch is a basic aspect of the nurse–patient relationship and is generally considered a gesture of warmth and friendship; however, the degree to which a patient is comfortable with the use of touch is often culturally determined. People from some cultures—Aboriginal people, for example—are accustomed to frequent physical contact. Holding an Aboriginal patient's hand in response to a distressing situation or giving the patient a reassuring pat on the shoulder may be experienced as supportive and thus help facilitate openness (Kavanaugh, 2003). People from Italian or French backgrounds may also be accustomed to frequent touching during conversation, and in the Russian culture, touch is an important part of nonverbal communication used freely with intimate and close friends (Giger & Davidhizar, 2008).

However, in other cultures, personal touch within the context of an interview may be perceived as an invasion of privacy or as patronizing, intrusive, aggressive, or sexually inviting. Among German, Swedish, and British Canadians, touch practices are infrequent, although a handshake may be common at the beginning and end of an interaction. Chinese Canadians may not like to be touched by strangers.

Even among people from similar cultures, the use of touch has different interpretations and rules regarding gender and class. Nurses and nursing students are urged to find out if their facility has a "no touch" policy, particularly with adolescents and children who have experienced inappropriate touch and may not know how to interpret therapeutic touch from the health care provider.

### Cultural Filters

It is important to recognize that it is impossible to listen to people in an unbiased way. In the process of socialization, we develop cultural filters through which we listen to ourselves, others, and the world around us (Egan, 2009). Cultural filters are a form of cultural bias or cultural prejudice that determine what we pay attention to and what we ignore. Egan (2009) stated that we need these cultural filters to provide structure for our lives and help us interpret and interact with the world. However, these cultural filters also unavoidably introduce various forms of bias into our communication, because they are bound to influence our personal, professional, familial, and sociological values and interpretations.

We all need a frame of reference to help us function in our world, but at the same time, we must understand that other people use other frames of reference to help them function in their worlds. Acknowledging that everyone views the world differently and understanding that these various views impact each person's beliefs and behaviours can go a long way toward minimizing our personal distortions in listening. Building acceptance and understanding of cultural diversity is a skill that can be learned. Chapter 7 has a more in-depth discussion of cultural considerations in nursing.

### Evaluation of Communication Skills

After you have had some introductory clinical experience, you may find the facilitative skills checklist in Figure 11-2 useful for evaluating your progress in developing interviewing and assessment skills. Note that some of the items might not be relevant for some of your patients (e.g., numbers 11 through 13 may not be possible when a patient is experiencing psychosis [disordered

**FACILITATIVE SKILLS CHECKLIST**

*Instructions:* During your clinical experience, periodically use this checklist to identify areas where growth is needed and progress has been made. Think of your clinical client experiences. Indicate the extent of your agreement with each of the following statements by marking the scale: *SA,* strongly agree; *A,* agree; *NS,* not sure; *D,* disagree; *SD,* strongly disagree.

| | | | | | |
|---|---|---|---|---|---|
| 1. I maintain good eye contact. | SA | A | NS | D | SD |
| 2. Most of my verbal comments follow the lead of the other person. | SA | A | NS | D | SD |
| 3. I encourage others to talk about feelings. | SA | A | NS | D | SD |
| 4. I am able to ask open-ended questions. | SA | A | NS | D | SD |
| 5. I can restate and clarify a person's ideas. | SA | A | NS | D | SD |
| 6. I can summarize in a few words the basic ideas of a long statement made by a person. | SA | A | NS | D | SD |
| 7. I can make statements that reflect the person's feelings. | SA | A | NS | D | SD |
| 8. I can share my feelings relevant to the discussion when appropriate to do so. | SA | A | NS | D | SD |
| 9. I am able to give feedback. | SA | A | NS | D | SD |
| 10. At least 75% or more of my responses help enhance and facilitate communication. | SA | A | NS | D | SD |
| 11. I can assist the person to list some alternatives available. | SA | A | NS | D | SD |
| 12. I can assist the person to identify some goals that are specific and observable. | SA | A | NS | D | SD |
| 13. I can assist the person to specify at least one next step that might be taken toward the goal. | SA | A | NS | D | SD |

**FIGURE 11-2** Facilitative Skills Checklist. **Source:** Adapted from Myrick, D., & Erney, T. (2000). *Caring and sharing* (2nd ed., p. 168). Minneapolis: Educational Media Corporation.

thought, delusions, and/or hallucinations]). Self-evaluation of clinical skills is a way to focus on therapeutic improvement. Role-playing can help prepare you for clinical experience and provide practice in using effective and professional communication skills.

## THE CLINICAL INTERVIEW

Ideally, the content and direction of the clinical interview are decided and led by the patient. The nurse employs communication skills and active listening to better understand the patient's situation.

### Preparing for the Interview
#### Pace
Helping a person with an emotional or medical problem is rarely a straightforward task, and the goal of assisting a patient to regain psychological or physiological stability can be difficult to achieve. Extremely important to any kind of counselling is permitting the patient to set the pace of the interview, no matter how slow or halting the progress may be (Arnold & Boggs, 2011).

#### Setting
Effective communication can take place almost anywhere. However, the quality of the interaction—whether in a clinic, a clinical unit, an office, or the patient's home—depends on the degree to which the nurse and patient feel safe; establishing a setting that enhances feelings of security is important to the therapeutic relationship. A health care setting, a conference room, or a quiet part of the unit that has relative privacy but is within view of others is ideal, but when the interview takes place in the patient's home, the nurse has a

valuable opportunity to assess the patient in the context of everyday life.

#### Seating
In all settings, chairs should be arranged so conversation can take place in a normal tone of voice, and eye contact can be comfortably maintained or avoided. A nonthreatening physical environment for both nurse and patient would involve:
- Assuming the same height, either both sitting or both standing
- Avoiding a face-to-face stance when possible; a 90- to 120-degree angle or side-by-side position may be less intense, and the patient and nurse can look away from each other without discomfort
- Providing safety and psychological comfort in terms of exiting the room—the patient should not be positioned between the nurse and the door, nor should the nurse be positioned in such a way that the patient feels trapped in the room
- Avoiding a desk barrier between the nurse and the patient

#### Introductions
In the orientation phase, nurses introduce themselves to their patients, describe the purpose of the meeting, and explain for how long and at what times they will be meeting with the patient. The issue of confidentiality is brought up during the initial interview. Remember that all health care providers must respect the private, personal, and confidential nature of the patient's communication, except in the specific situations outlined earlier (e.g., harm to self or others, child abuse, elder abuse). What is discussed with fellow staff and your clinical group in conference should not be discussed outside with others, no matter who they are (e.g., patient's relatives, news media, friends, etc.). The patient

needs to know that whatever is discussed will stay confidential unless permission is given for it to be disclosed. Refer to Chapter 10 to review the nurse's responsibilities in the orientation phase.

Ask the patient how he or she would like to be addressed. This question conveys respect and gives the patient direct control over an important ego issue. (Some patients like to be called by their last names; others prefer being on a first-name basis with the nurse) (Arnold & Boggs, 2011).

### Initiating the Interview

Once introductions have been made, you can turn the interview over to the patient by using one of a number of open-ended questions or statements:

- "Where should we start?"
- "Tell me a little about what has been going on with you."
- "What are some of the stresses you have been coping with recently?"
- "Tell me a little about what has been happening in the past couple of weeks."
- "Perhaps you can begin by letting me know what some of your concerns have been recently."
- "Tell me about your difficulties."

Communication can be facilitated by appropriately offering leads (e.g., "Go on"), making statements of acceptance (e.g., "Uh-huh"), or otherwise conveying interest.

### Tactics to Avoid

Certain behaviours are counterproductive and should be avoided (Moscato, 1988). For example:

| Do Not: | Try To: |
|---|---|
| Argue with, minimize, or challenge the patient | Keep focus on facts and the patient's perceptions |
| Give false reassurance | Make observations of the patient's behaviour (e.g., "Change is always possible.") |
| Interpret situations for the patient or speculate on interpersonal dynamics | Listen attentively, use silence, and try to clarify the patient's problems |
| Question or probe patients about sensitive topics they do not wish to discuss | Pay attention to nonverbal communication; strive to keep the patient's anxiety to a minimum |
| Try to sell the patient on accepting treatment | Encourage the patient to look at pros and cons |
| Join in attacks patients launch on their mates, parents, friends, or associates | Focus on facts and the patient's perceptions; be aware of nonverbal communication |
| Participate in criticism of another nurse or any other staff member | Focus on facts and the patient's perceptions; check out serious accusations with the nurse or staff member; have the patient meet with the nurse or staff member in question in the presence of a senior staff member and clarify perceptions |

### Helpful Guidelines

Meier and Davis (2001) offer some guidelines for conducting the initial interview:

- Speak briefly.
- When you do not know what to say, say nothing.
- When in doubt, focus on feelings.
- Avoid giving advice.
- Avoid relying on questions.
- Pay attention to nonverbal cues.
- Keep the focus on the patient.

### Attending Behaviours: The Foundation of Interviewing

Engaging in attending behaviours and actively listening are two key principles of counselling on which almost everyone can agree (Sommers-Flanagan & Sommers-Flanagan, 2003). Positive attending behaviours serve to open up communication and encourage free expression, whereas negative attending behaviours are more likely to inhibit expression. All behaviours must be evaluated in terms of cultural patterns and past experiences of both the interviewer and the interviewee. There are no universals; however, there are guidelines students can follow.

### Eye Contact

As previously discussed, cultural and individual variations influence a patient's comfort with eye contact. For some patients and interviewers, sustained eye contact is normal and comfortable. For others, it may be more comfortable and natural to make brief eye contact but look away or down much of the time. Sommers-Flanagan and Sommers-Flanagan (2003) state that in most situations, it is appropriate for nurses to maintain more eye contact when the patient speaks and less constant eye contact when the nurse speaks.

### Body Language

Body language involves two elements: kinesics and proxemics. *Kinesics* is associated with physical characteristics, such as body movements and postures. Facial expressions; eye contact or lack thereof; the way someone holds the head, legs, and shoulders; and so on convey a multitude of messages. A person who slumps in a chair, rolls the eyes, and sits with arms crossed in front of the chest can be perceived as resistant and unreceptive to what another wants to communicate. On the other hand, a person who leans in slightly toward the speaker, maintains a relaxed and attentive posture, makes appropriate eye contact, makes hand gestures that are unobtrusive and smooth while minimizing the number of other movements, and whose facial expressions match his or her feelings or the patient's feelings can be perceived as open to and respectful of the communication.

*Proxemics* refers to the study of personal space and the significance of the physical distance between individuals. Proxemics takes into account that these distances may be different for different cultural groups. Intimate distance in Canada is 0 to 45 centimetres and is reserved for those we trust most and with whom we feel most safe. Personal distance (45 to 120 centimetres) is for personal communications such as those with friends or colleagues. Social distance (120 to 360 centimetres, or approximately 3.5 metres) applies to strangers or acquaintances, often in public places or formal social gatherings. Public distance (3.5 metres) relates to public space (e.g., public speaking). In public space, one may hail another, and the parties may move about while communicating.

## Vocal Quality

Vocal quality, or *paralinguistics*, encompasses voice loudness, pitch, rate, and fluency. Sommers-Flanagan and Sommers-Flanagan (2003) say that "effective interviewers use vocal qualities to enhance rapport, communicate interest and empathy, and to emphasize special issues or conflicts" (p. 56). Paralinguistics provides a perfect example of "It's not what you say but how you say it." Speaking in soft and gentle tones is apt to encourage a person to share thoughts and feelings, whereas speaking in a rapid, high-pitched tone may convey anxiety and create it in the patient. Consider, for example, how tonal quality can affect communication in a simple sentence like "I will see you tonight."

1. "*I* will see you tonight." (I will be the one who sees you tonight.)
2. "I *will* see you tonight." (No matter what happens, or whether you like it or not, I will see you tonight.)
3. "I will see *you* tonight." (Even though others are present, it is you I want to see.)
4. "I will see you *tonight*." (It is definite—tonight is the night we will meet.)

## Verbal Tracking

Verbal tracking is just that: tracking what the patient is saying. Individuals cannot know if you are hearing or understanding what they are saying unless you provide them with cues. Verbal tracking offers neutral feedback in the form of simply restating or summarizing what the patient has already said without personal or professional opinions, judgements, or comments (Sommers-Flanagan & Sommers-Flanagan, 2003). For example:

*Patient:* "I don't know what the fuss is about. I smoke marijuana to relax, and everyone makes a fuss."

*Nurse:* "Do you see the use of marijuana as a problem for you?"

*Patient:* "No, I don't. It doesn't affect my work … well, most of the time, anyway. I mean, of course, if I have to think things out and make important decisions, then obviously it can get in the way. But most of the time, I'm cool."

*Nurse:* "So when important decisions have to be made, then it interferes; otherwise, you don't see it affecting your functioning."

*Patient:* "Yeah, well, most of the time, I'm cool."

Meier and Davis (2001) stated that verbal tracking involves checking one's understanding with the patient by restating—as much as possible, in one's own words—in order to confirm the patient's speech content (as well as to clarify the meaning of speech volume and tone, as discussed earlier). It can be difficult to know which leads to follow if the patient introduces many topics at once. When this happens, the nurse can summarize what he or she has heard; reflect the emotions, experiences, thoughts, and contexts as much as possible; and help the patient focus on and explore a specific topic or goal. "With everything going on in your life recently, you must really feel overwhelmed. You're $2000 in debt and don't have a job, you've gained 30 pounds in six months, and your wife is frustrated with your drinking. Let's talk more about what is going on with your wife and her concerns about alcohol."

## Clinical Supervision

Communication and interviewing techniques are acquired skills. You will learn to improve these abilities through practice and clinical supervision. With clinical supervision, the focus is on the nurse's behaviour in the nurse–patient relationship; nurse and supervisor have opportunities to examine and analyze the nurse's feelings and reactions to the patient and the way they affect the relationship.

The importance of clinical supervision was stressed in Chapter 10. Farkas-Cameron (1995) wrote that "the nurse who does not engage in the clinical supervisory process stagnates both theoretically and clinically, while depriving him- or herself of the opportunity to advance professionally" (p. 44). She observed that clinical supervision can be a therapeutic process for the nurse, during which feelings and concerns about the developing nurse–patient relationship are ventilated. The opportunity to examine interactions, obtain insights, and devise alternative strategies for dealing with various clinical issues enhances clinical growth and minimizes frustration and burnout. Clinical supervision is a necessary professional activity that fosters professional growth and helps minimize the development of nontherapeutic nurse–patient relationships.

## Process Recordings

The best way to improve communication and interviewing skills is to review your clinical interactions exactly as they occur. This process offers the opportunity to identify themes and patterns in both your own and your patients' communications. As students, clinical review helps you learn to deal with the variety of situations that arise in the clinical interview.

Process recordings are written records of a segment of the nurse–patient session that reflect as closely as possible the verbal and nonverbal behaviours of both patient and nurse. Process recordings have some disadvantages because they rely on memory and are subject to distortions. However, they can be a useful tool for identifying communication patterns. Sometimes an observing clinician takes notes during the interview, but this practice also has disadvantages in that it may be distracting for both interviewer and patient. Some patients (especially those with a paranoid disorder) may resent or misunderstand the observer's intent.

It is usually best to write notes verbatim (word for word) in a private area immediately after the interaction has taken place. You can carefully record your words and the patient's words, identify whether or not your responses are therapeutic, and recall your thinking and emotions at the time.

Videotaped simulations with professional actors may also provide the student nurse with an opportunity to analyze his or her communication skills through the use of a process recording.

Table 11-4 gives an example of a process recording.

| TABLE 11-4 | EXAMPLE OF A PROCESS RECORDING | | |
|---|---|---|---|

| NURSE | PATIENT | COMMUNICATION TECHNIQUE | NURSE'S THOUGHTS AND FEELINGS |
|---|---|---|---|
| "Good morning, Mr. Long." | | **Therapeutic.** Giving recognition. Acknowledging a patient by name can enhance self-esteem and communicates that the nurse views the patient as an individual. | I was feeling nervous. He had attempted suicide, and I didn't know if I could help him. Initially I was feeling somewhat overwhelmed. |
| | "Who are you, and where the devil am I?" (Gazes around with a confused look on his face—quickly sits on the edge of the bed) | | |
| "I am Ms. Rossi. I am your nurse, and you are at St. Paul's Hospital. I would like to spend some time with you today." | | **Therapeutic.** Giving information. Informing the patient of facts needed to make decisions or come to realistic conclusions. **Therapeutic.** Offering self. Making oneself available to the patient. | |
| | "What am I doing here? How did I get here?" (Spoken in a loud, demanding voice) | | I felt a bit intimidated when he raised his voice. |
| "You were brought in by your wife last night after swallowing a bottle of aspirin. You had to have your stomach pumped." | | **Therapeutic.** Giving information. Giving needed facts so that the patient can orient himself and better evaluate his situation. | |
| | "Oh ... yeah." (Silence for two minutes; shoulders slumped, Mr. Long stares at the floor and drops his head and eyes) | | I was uncomfortable with the silence, but since I didn't have anything useful to say, I stayed with him in silence for the two minutes. |
| "You seem upset, Mr. Long. What are you thinking about?" | | **Therapeutic.** Making observations. **Therapeutic.** Giving broad openings in an attempt to get at his feelings. | I began to feel sorry for him; he looked so sad and helpless. |
| | "Yeah, I just remembered. ...I wanted to kill myself." (Said in a low tone almost to himself) | | |
| "Oh, Mr. Long, you have so much to live for. You have such a loving family." | | **Nontherapeutic.** Defending **Nontherapeutic.** Introducing an unrelated topic. | I felt overwhelmed. I didn't know what to say—his talking about killing himself made me nervous. I could have said, "You must be very upset" (verbalizing the implied) or "Tell me more about this" (exploring). |
| | "What do you know about my life? You want to know about my family? My wife is leaving me, that's what." (Faces the nurse with an angry expression on his face and speaks in loud tones) | | Again, I felt intimidated by his anger, but now I linked it with his wife's leaving him, so I didn't take it as personally as I did the first time. |
| "I didn't know. You must be terribly upset by her leaving." | | **Therapeutic.** Reflective. Observing the angry tone and content of the patient's message and reflecting the patient's feelings. | I really felt for him, and now I thought that encouraging him to talk more about this could be useful for him. |

# KEY POINTS TO REMEMBER

- Knowledge of communication and interviewing techniques is the foundation for development of any nurse–patient relationship. Goal-directed professional communication is referred to as *therapeutic communication*.
- Communication is a complex process. Berlo's (1960) communication model has five parts: stimulus, sender, message, medium, and receiver.
- Feedback is a vital component of the communication process for validating the accuracy of the sender's message.
- A number of factors can minimize, enhance, or otherwise influence the communication process: culture, language, knowledge level, noise, lack of privacy, presence of others, and expectations.
- There are verbal and nonverbal elements in communication; the nonverbal elements often play the larger role in conveying a person's message. Verbal communication consists of all words a person speaks. Nonverbal communication consists of the behaviours displayed by an individual, outside of the actual content of speech.
- Communication has two levels: the content level (verbal speech) and the process level (nonverbal behaviour). When content is congruent with process, the communication is said to be healthy. When the verbal message is not reinforced by the communicator's actions, the message is ambiguous and incongruent; this is called a double (or mixed) message.
- Cultural background (as well as individual differences) has a great deal to do with what nonverbal behaviour means to different individuals. The degree of eye contact and the use of touch are two nonverbal behaviours that can be misunderstood by individuals of different cultures.
- There are a number of therapeutic communication techniques nurses can use to enhance their nursing practices (see Table 11-2).
- There are also a number of nontherapeutic communication techniques that nurses can learn to avoid to enhance their effectiveness with people (see Table 11-3).
- Most nurses are most effective when they use nonthreatening and open-ended communication techniques.
- Effective communication is a skill that develops over time and is integral to the establishment and maintenance of a therapeutic relationship.
- The clinical interview is a key component of psychiatric mental health nursing, and the nurse must establish a safe setting and plan for appropriate seating, introductions, and initiation of the interview.
- Attending behaviours (e.g., eye contact, body language, vocal qualities, verbal tracking) are key elements in effective communication.
- A meaningful therapeutic relationship is facilitated when values and cultural influences are considered. It is the nurse's responsibility to seek to understand the patient's perceptions.

# CRITICAL THINKING

1. Keep a written log of a conversation you have with a patient. In your log, identify the therapeutic and nontherapeutic techniques you noticed yourself using. Then rewrite the nontherapeutic communications and replace them with statements that would better facilitate discussion of thoughts and feelings. Share your log and discuss the changes you are working on with one classmate.

2. Role-play with a classmate at least five nonverbal communications, and have your partner identify the message he or she received.

3. With the other students in your class watching, plan and role-play a nurse–patient conversation that lasts about three minutes. Use both therapeutic and nontherapeutic techniques. When you are finished, have your other classmates try to identify the techniques that you used. Discuss ways that a reliance on colleagues or other subtle institutional concerns might factor in to the communication.

4. Demonstrate how the nurse would use touch and eye contact when working with patients from three different cultural groups.

# CHAPTER REVIEW

1. You have been working closely with a patient for the past month. Today, he tells you he is looking forward to meeting with his new psychiatrist but frowns and avoids eye contact while reporting this to you. Which of the following responses would most likely be therapeutic?
   1. "A new psychiatrist is a chance to start fresh. I'm sure it will go well for you."
   2. "You say you look forward to the meeting, but you appear anxious or unhappy."
   3. "I notice that you frowned and avoided eye contact just now—don't you feel well?"
   4. "I get the impression you don't really want to see your psychiatrist—can you tell me why?"

2. Which behaviour is consistent with therapeutic communication?
   1. Offering your opinion when asked in order to convey support
   2. Summarizing the essence of the patient's comments in your own words
   3. Interrupting periods of silence before they become awkward for the patient
   4. Telling the patient he did well when you approve of his statements or actions

3. Which statement about nonverbal behaviour is accurate?
   1. A calm expression means that the patient is experiencing low levels of anxiety.
   2. Patients respond more consistently to therapeutic touch than to verbal interventions.
   3. The meaning of nonverbal behaviours varies with cultural and individual differences.
   4. Eye contact is a reliable measure of the patient's degree of attentiveness and engagement.

4. A nurse stops in to interview a patient on a medical unit and finds the patient lying supine in her bed with the head elevated at ten degrees. Which initial response would most enhance the chances of achieving a therapeutic interaction?
   1. Apologize for the differential in height and proceed while standing to avoid delay
   2. If permitted, raise the head of the bed and, with the patient's permission, sit on the bed
   3. If permitted, raise the head of the bed to approximate the nurse's height while standing
   4. Sit in whatever chair is available in the room to convey informality and increase comfort

5. A patient with schizophrenia approaches staff arriving for day shift and anxiously reports, "Last night, demons came to my room and tried to rape me." Which response would be most therapeutic?
   1. "There are no such things as demons; what you saw were hallucinations."
   2. "It is not possible for anyone to enter your room at night; you are safe here."
   3. "You seem very upset; please tell me more about what you experienced last night."
   4. "That must have been very frightening, but we'll check on you at night, and you'll be safe."

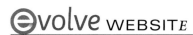 WEBSIT*E*

Post-Test interactive review

*Visit the Evolve Web site for Chapter Review Answers and Rationales, Critical Thinking Answer Guidelines, and additional resources related to the content in this chapter:* http://evolve.elsevier.com/Canada/Varcarolis/psychiatric/

## REFERENCES

Arnold, E., & Boggs, K.U. (2011). *Interprofessional relationships: Professional communication skills for nurses* (6th ed.). St. Louis, MO: Saunders.

Bateson, G., Jackson, D., Haley, J., et al. (1956). Toward a theory of schizophrenia. *Behavioural Sciences, 1*, 251–264.

Berlo, D.K. (1960). *The process of communication.* San Francisco: Reinhart Press.

Coatsworth-Puspoky, R.R., Forchuk, C.C., & Ward-Griffin, C.C. (2006). Nurse–client processes in mental health: Recipients' perspectives. *Journal of Psychiatric & Mental Health Nursing, 13*(3), 347–355. doi:10.1111/j.1365-2850.2006.00968.x.

Collins, M. (1983). *Communication in health care: The human connection in the life cycle* (2nd ed.). St. Louis, MO: Mosby.

Egan, G. (2005). *Essentials of skilled helping: Managing problems, developing opportunities.* Belmont, CA: Thomson Higher Education.

Egan, G. (2009). *The skilled helper: A problem-management and opportunity development approach to helping.* Toronto: Nelson Education.

Ellis, R.B., Gates, B., & Kenworthy, N. (2003). *Interpersonal communicating in nursing* (2nd ed.). London, UK: Churchill Livingstone.

Farkas-Cameron, M.M. (1995). Clinical supervision in psychiatric nursing. *Journal of Psychosocial Nursing and Mental Health Services, 33*(2), 40–47.

Fontes, L.A. (2008). *Interviewing clients across cultures: A practitioner's guide.* New York: Guilford.

Giger, J.N., & Davidhizar, R.E. (2008). *Transcultural nursing: Assessment and intervention* (5th ed.). St. Louis, MO: Mosby.

Haber, J. (2000). Hildegard E. Peplau: The psychiatric nursing legacy of a legend. *Journal of the American Psychiatric Nursing Association, 6*, 510–562. doi:10.1067/mpn.2000.104556.

Kavanaugh, K.H. (2003). Transcultural perspectives in mental health nursing. In M. Andrews & J. Boyle (Eds.), *Transcultural concepts in nursing care.* Philadelphia: Lippincott Williams & Wilkins.

Matsumoto, D. (2006). Culture and nonverbal behaviour. In V.L. Manusov & M.L. Patterson (Eds.), *The Sage handbook of nonverbal communication* (pp. 219–235). Newbury Park, CA: Sage.

Meier, S.T., & Davis, S.R. (2001). *The elements of counseling* (4th ed.). Pacific Grove, CA: Brooks/Cole.

Mohl, P.C. (2003). Psychiatry. In A. Tasman, J. Kay, & J.A. Lieberman (Eds.), *Listening to the patient* (2nd ed.). West Sussex, England: Wiley.

Moscato, B. (1988). Psychiatric nursing. In H.S. Wilson & C.S. Kneisl (Eds.), *The one-to-one relationship* (3rd ed.). Menlo Park, CA: Addison-Wesley.

Peplau, H.E. (1952). *Interpersonal relations in nursing: A conceptual frame of reference for psychodynamic nursing.* New York: Putnam.

Shea, S.C. (1998). *Psychiatric interviewing: The art of understanding* (2nd ed.). Philadelphia: Saunders.

Sommers-Flanagan, J., & Sommers-Flanagan, R. (2003). *Clinical interviewing* (3rd ed.). Hoboken, NJ: Wiley.

Wheeler, K. (2008). *Psychotherapy for the advanced practice psychiatric nurse.* St. Louis, MO: Mosby.

# 12

# Understanding Responses to Stress

*Margaret Jordan Halter, Elizabeth M. Varcarolis*
*Adapted by Sandra Mitchell*

## KEY TERMS AND CONCEPTS

Benson's relaxation technique, 192

cognitive reframing, 194

coping styles, 190

distress, 186

eustress, 186

fight-or-flight response, 185

general adaptation syndrome (GAS), 186

guided imagery, 193

journaling, 195

meditation, 192

mindfulness, 194

physical stressors, 187

progressive muscle relaxation (PMR), 190

psychological stressors, 187

psychoneuroimmunology, 187

stressors, 185

## OBJECTIVES

1. Recognize the short- and long-term physiological consequences of stress.
2. Compare and contrast Cannon's fight-or-flight response, Selye's general adaptation syndrome, and the psychoneuroimmunological models of stress.
3. Describe how responses to stress are mediated through perception, personality, social support, culture, and spirituality.
4. Assess stress level using the Recent Life Changes Questionnaire.
5. Identify and describe holistic approaches to stress management.
6. Teach a classmate or patient a behavioural technique to help lower stress and anxiety.
7. Explain how cognitive techniques can help increase a person's tolerance for stressful events.

## Evolve WEBSITE

*Visit the Evolve website for Flashcards, Case Studies, and additional testing resources related to the content in this chapter:* http://evolve.elsevier.com/Canada/Varcarolis/psychiatric/ Pre-Test interactive review

Before turning our attention to the clinical disorders presented in the chapters that follow, we will explore the subject of stress. Stress and our responses to it are central to psychiatric disorders and the provision of mental health care. The interplay among stress, the development of psychiatric disorders, and the exacerbation (worsening) of psychiatric symptoms has been widely researched. The old adage "What doesn't kill you will make you stronger" does not hold true with the development of mental illness; early exposure to stressful events actually sensitizes people to stress in later life. In other words, we know that people who are exposed to high levels of stress as children—especially during stress-sensitive developmental periods—have a greater incidence of all mental illnesses as adults (Weber, Rockstroh, Borgelt, et al., 2008). However, we do not know if severe stress causes a vulnerability to mental illness or if vulnerability to mental illness influences the likelihood of adverse stress responses. It is most important to recognize that severe stress is unhealthy and can weaken biological resistance to psychiatric pathology in any individual; however, stress is especially harmful for those who have a genetic predisposition to these disorders.

While an understanding of the connection between stress and mental illness is essential in the psychiatric setting, it is also

**THE STRESS RESPONSE**

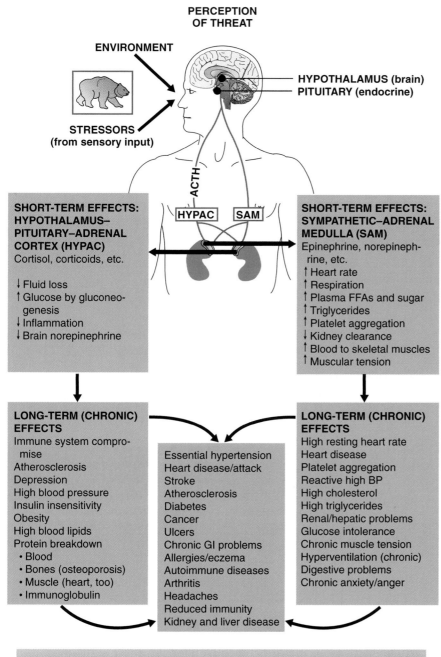

**FIGURE 12-1** The stress response. **Source:** From Brigham, D.D. (1994). Imagery for getting well: Clinical applications of behavioural medicine. New York: W.W. Norton.

*ACTH*-adrenocorticotropic hormone; *BP*-blood pressure; *FFAs*-free fatty acids; *GI*-gastrointestinal.

important when developing a plan of care for any patient, in any setting, with any diagnosis. Imagine having an appendectomy and being served with an eviction notice on the same day. How well could you cope with either situation, let alone both simultaneously? The nurse's role is to intervene to reduce stress by promoting a healing environment, facilitating successful coping, and developing future coping strategies. In this chapter, we will explore how we are equipped to respond to stress, what can go wrong with the stress response, and how to care for our patients and even ourselves during times of stress.

## RESPONSES TO AND EFFECTS OF STRESS

### Early Stress Response Theories

The earliest research into the stress response (Figure 12-1) began as a result of observations that stressors brought about physical disorders or made existing conditions worse. Stressors are psychological or physical stimuli that are incompatible with current functioning and require adaptation. Walter Cannon (1871–1945) methodically investigated the sympathetic nervous system as a pathway of the response to stress, known more commonly as fight (aggression) or flight (withdrawal). The well-known fight-or-flight response is the body's way of preparing for a situation perceived as a threat to survival. This response results in increased blood pressure, heart rate, and cardiac output.

While groundbreaking, Cannon's theory has been criticized for being simplistic since not all animals or people respond by fighting or fleeing. In the face of danger, some animals become still (e.g., a deer) to avoid being noticed or to observe the environment in a state of heightened awareness. Also, Cannon's theory was developed primarily based on the responses of animals and men. Men and women, however, have different neural responses to stress. While men experience altered prefrontal blood flow and increased salivary cortisol in response to stress, women experience increased limbic (emotional) activity and, less significantly, altered salivary cortisol (Wang, Korczykowski, Rao, et al., 2007).

Hans Selye (1907–1982), another pioneer in stress research, introduced the concept of stress into both the scientific and popular literature. Selye (1974) expanded Cannon's 1956 theory of stress in his formulation of the general adaptation syndrome (GAS). The GAS occurs in three stages:

1. The *alarm* (or *acute stress*) stage is the initial, brief, and adaptive response (fight or flight) to the stressor. During the alarm stage, three principal *stress mediators* are involved:
   - The brain's cortex and hypothalamus signal the adrenal glands to release the catecholamine adrenalin. This release, in turn, increases sympathetic system activity (e.g., increased heart rate, respirations, and blood pressure) to enhance strength and speed. Pupils dilate for a broad view of the environment, and blood is shunted away from the digestive tract (resulting in dry mouth) and kidneys to more essential organs.
   - The hypothalamus also sends messages to the adrenal cortex. The adrenal cortex produces corticosteroids to help increase muscle endurance and stamina, whereas other nonessential functions (e.g., digestion) are decreased. Unfortunately, the corticosteroids also inhibit functions such as reproduction, growth, and immunity (Sadock & Sadock, 2008).
   - Endorphins are released that reduce sensitivity to pain and injury. The alarm stage is extremely intense, and no organism can sustain this level of reactivity and excitement for long. If the organism survives, the resistance stage follows.
2. The *resistance* stage could also be called the *adaptation stage*, because it is during this time that sustained and optimal resistance to the stressor occurs. Usually, stressors are successfully overcome; however, when they are not, the organism may experience the final stage: exhaustion.
3. The *exhaustion* stage occurs when attempts to resist the stressor prove futile. At this point, resources are depleted, and the stress may become chronic, producing a wide array of psychological and physiological responses and even death.

The body responds the same physiologically regardless of whether the stress is real or only perceived as a threat and whether the threat is physical, psychological, or social. Additionally, the body cannot differentiate between the energy generated by positive and negative stimuli. Lazarus and Folkman (1984) described these reactions as distress and eustress:

- Distress is a negative, draining energy that results in anxiety, depression, confusion, helplessness, hopelessness, and fatigue. Distress may be caused by such stressors as a death in the family, financial overload, or school or work demands.
- Eustress is a positive, beneficial energy that motivates and results in feelings of happiness, hopefulness, and purposeful movement. Eustress may be the result of a much-needed vacation, being called in for an interview, the birth of a baby, or buying a new car. Eustress could lead to a depletion of physiological resources if sustained, but, fortunately or unfortunately, one does not typically become chronically happy and motivated.

Currently, Selye's GAS remains a popular theory, but it has been expanded and reinterpreted since the 1950s (McKewan, 2005). Some researchers question the notion of "nonspecific responses" and believe that different types of stressors bring about different patterns of responses. Furthermore, the GAS is most accurate in the description of how males respond when threatened. Females do not typically respond to stress by fighting or fleeing but rather by tending and befriending, a survival strategy that emphasizes the protection of young and a reliance on the social network for support.

Increased understanding of the exhaustion stage of the GAS has revealed that illness results from not only the depletion of reserves but also the stress mediators themselves. This finding is discussed in Immune Stress Responses on page 187. Table 12-1 describes some reactions to acute and prolonged (chronic) stress.

| TABLE 12-1 | SOME REACTIONS TO ACUTE AND PROLONGED (CHRONIC) STRESS |
|---|---|
| **ACUTE STRESS CAN CAUSE** | **PROLONGED (CHRONIC) STRESS CAN CAUSE** |
| Uneasiness and concern | Anxiety and panic attacks |
| Sadness | Depression or melancholia |
| Loss of appetite | Anorexia or overeating |
| Suppression of the immune system | Lowered resistance to infections, leading to increase in opportunistic viral and bacterial infections |
| Increased metabolism and use of body fats | Insulin-resistant diabetes Hypertension |
| Infertility | Amenorrhea or loss of sex drive Impotence, anovulation |
| Increased energy mobilization and use | Increased fatigue and irritability Decreased memory and learning |
| Increased cardiovascular tone | Increased risk for cardiac events (e.g., heart attack, angina, and sudden heart-related death) Increased risk of blood clots and stroke |
| Increased cardiopulmonary tone | Increased respiratory problems |

## Neurotransmitter Stress Responses

Serotonin is a brain catecholamine that plays an important role in mood, sleep, sexuality, appetite, and metabolism. It is one of the main neurotransmitters implicated in depression, and many medications used to treat depression do so by increasing the availability of serotonin (see Chapter 4). During times of stress, serotonin synthesis becomes more active. This stress-activated turnover of serotonin is at least partially mediated by the corticosteroids, and researchers believe this activation may dysregulate (impair) serotonin receptor sights and the brain's ability to use serotonin (Sadock & Sadock, 2008). The influence of stressful life events on the development of depression is well documented, but researchers still do not fully understand the relationship. This neurotransmitter stress response research sheds some new light on the process.

## Immune Stress Responses

Cannon and Selye focused on the physical and mental responses of the nervous and endocrine systems to acute and chronic stress. Later work revealed that there is also an interaction between the nervous system and the immune system during the alarm phase of the GAS. In one study, rats were given a mixture of saccharine and a drug that reduces the immune system (Ader & Cohen, 1975). Afterward, when given only the saccharine, the rats continued to have decreased immune responses, which indicated that stress itself negatively impacts the body's ability to produce a protective structure.

Studies in psychoneuroimmunology (study of the relationship between the mind, the nervous system, and the immune system) continue to provide evidence that stress, through the hypothalamic–pituitary–adrenal and sympathetic–adrenal medullary axes, can induce changes in the immune system. This model helps explain what many researchers and clinicians have believed and witnessed for centuries: there are links among stress (biopsychosocial), the immune system, and disease—a clear mind–body connection that may alter health outcomes. Stress may result in malfunctions in the immune system that are implicated in autoimmune disorders, immunodeficiency, and hypersensitivities.

Stress influences the immune system in several complex ways. As discussed earlier, corticosteroids are released in response to stress and inhibit the immune system, which increases susceptibility to illness (Sadock & Sadock, 2008). Conversely, stress can enhance the immune system and prepare the body to respond to injury. Cytokines, which are proteins and glycoproteins used for communication between cells, are normally released by immune cells when a pathogen is detected; they serve to activate and recruit other immune cells. During times of stress, these cytokines are released, and immunity is profoundly activated. But the activation is limited since the cytokines stimulate further release of corticosteroids, which inhibit the immune system.

The immune response and the resulting cytokine activity in the brain raise questions regarding their connection with psychological and cognitive states such as depression (Anisman & Merali, 2005). Some cancers are treated with a type of cytokine molecules known as interleukins. These chemotherapy drugs tend to cause or increase depression. Furthermore, elevated

## RESEARCH HIGHLIGHT
### The Immune System and Happiness

**Source:** Borak, Y. (2006). The immune system and happiness. *Autoimmunity Reviews*, 5(8), 523–537.

**Problem**
The effects of positive human emotions, especially happiness, on physiological parameters and immunity have received very little attention.

**Purpose of Study**
To determine how psychosocial factors, such as optimism and social support, moderate the stress response.

**Methods**
They are mapping the biological and cellular mechanisms by which stress affects the immune system and testing new theories (Borak, 2006).

**Key Findings**
The data support the hypothesis that individuals characterized by a more negative affective style poorly recruit their immune response and may be at risk for illness more so than those with a positive affective style.

**Implications for Nursing Practice**
Emotions are intimately involved in the initiation or progression of cancer, human immunodeficiency virus (HIV), cardiovascular disease, and autoimmune disorders. It is important for nurses to assess patients' emotions and reactions to their illness as individual responses can positively or negatively impact the healing process.

cytokines and immune activation are often seen during episodes of severe depression.

## MEDIATORS OF THE STRESS RESPONSE

### Stressors

A variety of dissimilar situations (e.g., emotional arousal, fatigue, fear, loss, humiliation, loss of blood, extreme happiness, unexpected success) all are capable of producing stress and triggering the stress response (Selye, 1993). No individual factor can be singled out as the cause of the stress response; however, stressors can be divided into two categories: physical and psychological. Physical stressors include changes to environmental conditions (e.g., trauma, excessive cold or heat), as well as physical conditions (e.g., infection, hemorrhage, hunger, pain). Psychological stressors include cognitive- or emotion-based changes, such as divorce, loss of a job, unmanageable debt, the death of a loved one, retirement, and fear of a terrorist attack, as well as changes we might consider positive, such as marriage, the arrival of a new baby, or unexpected success.

### Perception

Researchers have looked at the degree to which various life events upset a specific individual and have found that the perception of a stressor determines the person's emotional and psychological reactions to it (Rahe, 1995). Responses to stress and anxiety are affected by factors such as age, gender, culture, life experience, and lifestyle, all of which may work to either lessen or increase the degree of emotional or physical influence and the sequel of stress. For example, a man in his 40s who has a new baby, has just purchased a home, and is laid off with six months' severance pay may feel the stress of the job loss more intensely than a man in his 60s who is financially secure and is asked to take an early retirement.

## Personality

As mentioned above, part of our response to stressors is based on our own individual perceptions, which are coloured by a variety of factors, including genetic structure and vulnerability, childhood experiences, coping strategies, and personal outlook on life and the world. All these factors combine to form a unique personality with specific strengths and vulnerabilities.

## Social Support

Social support is a mediating factor with significant implications for nurses and other health care providers. Strong social support from significant others can enhance mental and physical health and act as a significant buffer against distress. A shared identity—whether with a family, social network, or colleagues—helps people overcome stressors more adaptively (Haslam & Reicher, 2006). Numerous studies have found a strong correlation between lower mortality rates and intact support systems (Koenig, McCullough, & Larson, 2001).

### Self-Help Groups

The proliferation of self-help groups attests to the need for social supports, and the explosive growth of a great variety of support groups reflects their effectiveness for many people. Many of the support groups currently available are for people going through similar stressful life events: Alcoholics Anonymous (a prototype for 12-step programs), Gamblers Anonymous, Cancer Connection, and Parents Without Partners, to note but a few.

### Low- and High-Quality Support

It is important to differentiate between social support relationships of low quality and those of high quality. Low-quality support relationships (e.g., living in an abusive home situation or with a controlling and demeaning person) often negatively affect a person's coping effectiveness in a crisis. On the other hand, high-quality relationships have been linked to less loneliness, more supportive behaviour, and greater life satisfaction (Hobfall & Vaux, 1993). High-quality emotional support is a critical factor in enhancing a person's sense of control and in rebuilding feelings of self-esteem and competency after a stressful event. Supportive, high-quality relationships are relatively free from conflict and negative interactions and are close, confiding, and reciprocal (Hobfall & Vaux, 1993).

## Culture

Each culture not only emphasizes certain problems more than others but also interprets emotional problems differently from other cultures. For example, the specific characteristics of the dysphoria of depression vary cross-culturally (Kim, 2002; Neighbors, 2003). The Hopi of North America express depressive states through feelings of guilt, shame, and sinfulness. On the other hand, First Nations people deal with stress by withdrawing and reducing their activity levels (Blue & Blue, 1981).

Although Western European and North American cultures subscribe to a psychophysiological view of stress and somatic distress, this view does not dominate in other cultures. The overwhelming majority of Asians, Africans, and Central Americans "not only express subjective distress in somatic terms, but actually experience this distress somatically, such that psychological interpretations of suffering may not be much use cross-culturally" (Gonzalez, Griffith, & Ruiz, 1995). The following vignette illustrates this point.

> **VIGNETTE**
>
> A 62-year-old woman was referred for evaluation of incapacitating abdominal pain after a medical diagnostic evaluation gave negative results. The pain began nine months earlier, approximately one month after her son was jailed for killing his girlfriend, whom the patient loved "like a daughter." The patient expected that the psychiatrist would prescribe medication that would take her pain away, and she was initially distressed to learn that she was expected to talk about her life. Although not ruling out the use of medication, the therapist explained to the patient that her pain might be related to the wrenching emotional ordeal of the past year. The therapist made it a point to validate the patient's pain and took great care not to imply that the pain was "merely" the expression of unacknowledged emotion. In particular, the therapist told the patient that he understood her pain to be real and that he did not expect her pain to be gone overnight. This approach allowed the patient to engage in a course of brief psychotherapy, during which her conflicted feelings about her son were examined, although these feelings were never specifically identified as the cause of her pain. Eventually, the patient felt strong enough to make drastic changes in her role as enabler of her children, at which point she reported that her pain was much improved (Gonzalez, Griffith, & Ruiz, 1995, p. 60).

## Spirituality and Religious Beliefs

Many spiritual and religious beliefs help people cope with stress, and these deserve closer scientific investigation. Studies have demonstrated that spiritual practices can enhance the immune system and sense of well-being (Koenig, McCullough, & Larson, 2001). Some scholars propose that spiritual well-being helps people deal with health issues, primarily because spiritual beliefs help people cope with issues of living. Thus, people with spiritual beliefs have established coping mechanisms they employ in normal life and can use when faced with illness. People who include spiritual solutions to physical or mental distress often gain a sense of comfort and support that can aid in healing and lowering stress. Even prayer, in and of itself, can elicit the relaxation response (discussed later in this chapter),

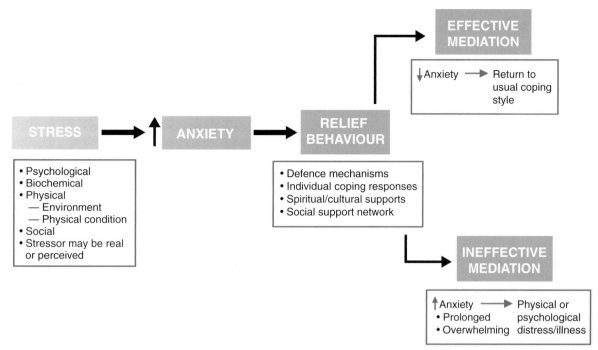

**FIGURE 12-2** Stress and anxiety operationally defined.

which is known to reduce stress physically and emotionally and to reduce stress on the immune system.

Figure 12-2 operationally defines the process of stress and the positive or negative results of attempts to relieve stress, and Box 12-1 identifies several stress busters that can be incorporated into our lives with little effort.

## NURSING MANAGEMENT OF STRESS RESPONSES

### Measuring Stress

Health indicators are a range of measures that can facilitate comparisons across time and place at national, provincial, territorial, and regional levels. Since 1999, Statistics Canada and the Canadian Institute for Health Information have collaborated on developing and providing a broad range of indicators for health regions across Canada.

Celebrating the 10th anniversary of the Health Indicators project, the *Healthy People, Healthy Places* report examined the health of the Canadian population using a selection of health indicators that focus on demography, health status, health behaviours, and the environment. In this report, the degree of stress experienced was measured by the percentage of the population aged 15 or older who reported most days to be "quite a bit stressful" or "extremely stressful" versus "not at all stressful." Highlights of the report include the following (Statistics Canada, 2010):

- Canadians who were physically active in their leisure time reported lower levels of stress.
- Seniors who perceived low levels of stress were about twice as likely to be in good health as were those with high stress levels.
- Working women were more likely than working men to report high levels of perceived life stress.

- In 2008, 21.2% of males (2.8 million) and 23.4% of females (3.2 million) aged 15 or older reported that most days were quite a bit or extremely stressful.
- Males and females aged 35 to 54 and men aged 25 to 34 years were more likely than Canadians overall to report high levels of stress. These are the ages at which people are most likely to be managing the multiple roles associated with career and family responsibilities.
- Both male and female seniors were less likely to report daily stress than were Canadians overall.
- Overall, females were more likely than males to report that most days were quite a bit or extremely stressful, particularly at ages 15 to 24 and 35 to 44.
- Although relatively few people aged 15 to 24 reported high levels of stress, the difference between the sexes was greatest in this age range; females were 1.5 times more likely than males to report that most days were quite a bit or extremely stressful.

Take a few minutes to assess your stress level for the past 6 to 12 months using the Recent Life Changes Questionnaire (Table 12-2). Keep in mind that when you administer the questionnaire, you must take into account the following:

- Not all events are perceived to have the same degree of intensity or disruptiveness.
- Culture may dictate whether or not an event is stressful or how stressful it is.
- Different people may have different thresholds beyond which disruptions occur.
- The questionnaire equates change with stress.

Other stress scales that may be useful to nursing students have been developed. You might like to try the Perceived Stress Scale (Figure 12-3). Although there are no absolute scores, this scale measures how relatively uncontrollable, unpredictable,

## BOX 12-1  EFFECTIVE STRESS BUSTERS

**Sleep**
- Chronically stressed people are often fatigued, so go to sleep 30 to 60 minutes early each night for a few weeks.
- If you are still fatigued, try going to bed another 30 minutes earlier.
- Sleeping later in the morning is not helpful and can disrupt body rhythms.

**Exercise (Aerobic)**
- Exercise:
  - Can dissipate chronic and acute stress
  - May decrease levels of anxiety, depression, and sensitivity to stress
  - Can decrease muscle tension and increase endorphin levels
- It is recommended you exercise for at least 30 minutes three or more times a week.
- It is best to exercise at least three hours before bedtime.

**Reduction or Cessation of Caffeine Intake**
- Lowering or stopping caffeine intake can lead to more energy and fewer muscle aches and help you feel more relaxed.
- Slowly wean off coffee, tea, colas, and chocolate drinks.

**Music (Classical or Soft Melodies of Choice)**
- Listening to music increases your sense of relaxation.
- Increased healing effects may result.
- Therapeutically, music can:
  - Decrease agitation and confusion in older adults
  - Increase quality of life in hospice settings

**Pets**
- Pets can bring joy and reduce stress.
- They can be an important social support.
- Pets can alleviate medical problems aggravated by stress.

**Massage**
- Massage can slow the heart rate and relax the body.
- Alertness may actually increase.

and overloaded you find your life. Try this scale in a clinical postconference for comparison and discussion.

### Assessing Coping Styles

People cope with life stressors in a variety of ways, and a number of factors can act as effective mediators to decrease stress in our lives. Rahe (1995) identified four discrete personal attributes (coping styles) people can develop to help manage stress:

1. Health-sustaining habits (e.g., medical compliance, proper diet, relaxation, adequate rest and sleep, pacing one's energy)
2. Life satisfactions (e.g., occasional escapism, reading, movie watching, work, family, hobbies, humour, spiritual solace, arts, nature)
3. Social supports (e.g., talk with trusted friends, family, counsellors, or support groups)
4. Effective and healthy responses to stress (e.g., work off anger through physical activity, go for a walk, dig in the garden, do yoga)

Examining these four coping categories can help nurses identify areas to target for improving their patients' responses to stress. Table 12-3 presents positive and negative responses to stress.

### Managing Stress Through Relaxation Techniques

Poor management of stress has been correlated with an increased incidence of a number of physical and emotional conditions, such as heart disease, poor diabetes control, chronic pain, and significant emotional distress (Slater, Steptoe, Weickgenant, et al., 2003). Psychoneuroimmunology provides the foundation for several integrative therapies, also referred to as mind–body therapies. There is now considerable evidence that many mind–body therapies can be used as effective adjuncts to conventional medical treatment for a number of common clinical conditions (Astin, Shapiro, Eisenberg, et al., 2003). Chapter 37 offers a more detailed discussion of holistic, mind–body, and integrative therapies.

Nurses should be aware of a variety of stress and anxiety reduction techniques they can teach their patients. The following are some of the known benefits of stress reduction:

- Alters the course of certain medical conditions, such as high blood pressure, arrhythmias, arthritis, cancer, and peptic ulcers
- Decreases the need for medications such as insulin, analgesics, and antihypertensives
- Diminishes or eliminates the urge for unhealthy and destructive behaviours, such as smoking, addiction to drugs, insomnia, and overeating
- Increases cognitive functions such as learning and concentration and improves study habits
- Breaks up static patterns of thinking and allows fresh and creative ways of perceiving life events
- Increases the sense of well-being through endorphin release
- Reduces anxiety, increases comfort, and helps decrease sleep disturbances

Because no single stress-management technique is right for everyone, employing a mixture of techniques brings the best results. All are useful in a variety of situations for specific individuals. Essentially, there are stress-reducing techniques for every personality type, situation, and level of stress. Give them a try. Practising relaxation techniques will help you not only help your patients reduce their stress levels but also manage your own physical responses to stressors. These techniques result in reduced heart and breathing rates, decreased blood pressure, improved oxygenation to major muscles, and reduced muscle tension. They also help manage subjective anxiety and improve appraisals of reality.

### Relaxation Exercises

In 1938, Edmund Jacobson developed a rather simple procedure that elicits a relaxation response, which he coined progressive muscle relaxation (PMR) (Sadock & Sadock, 2008). This technique can be done without any external gauges or feedback and can be practised almost anywhere. The premise behind PMR is that since anxiety results in tense muscles, one way to decrease anxiety is to nearly eliminate muscle

## TABLE 12-2   RECENT LIFE CHANGES QUESTIONNAIRE

| LIFE-CHANGING EVENT | LIFE CHANGE UNIT* | LIFE-CHANGING EVENT | LIFE CHANGE UNIT* |
|---|---|---|---|
| **Health** | | Child leaving home: | |
| An injury or illness that: | | To attend college | 41 |
| Kept you in bed a week or more or sent you to the hospital | 74 | Due to marriage | 41 |
| Was less serious than above | 44 | For other reasons | 45 |
| Major dental work | 26 | Change in arguments with spouse | 50 |
| Major change in eating habits | 27 | In-law problems | 38 |
| Major change in sleeping habits | 26 | Change in the marital status of your parents: | |
| Major change in your usual type and/or amount of recreation | 28 | Divorce | 59 |
| | | Remarriage | 50 |
| **Work** | | Separation from spouse: | |
| Change to a new type of work | 51 | Due to work | 53 |
| Change in your work hours or conditions | 35 | Due to marital problems | 76 |
| Change in your responsibilities at work: | | Divorce | 96 |
| More responsibilities | 29 | Birth of grandchild | 43 |
| Fewer responsibilities | 21 | Death of spouse | 119 |
| Promotion | 31 | Death of other family member: | |
| Demotion | 42 | Child | 123 |
| Transfer | 32 | Brother or sister | 102 |
| Troubles at work: | | Parent | 100 |
| With your boss | 29 | | |
| With co-workers | 35 | **Personal and Social** | |
| With persons under your supervision | 35 | Change in personal habits | 26 |
| Other work troubles | 28 | Beginning or ending of school or college | 38 |
| Major business adjustment | 60 | Change of school or college | 35 |
| Retirement | 52 | Change in political beliefs | 24 |
| Loss of job: | | Change in religious beliefs | 29 |
| Laid off from work | 68 | Change in social activities | 27 |
| Fired from work | 79 | Vacation | 24 |
| Correspondence course to help you in your work | 18 | New close personal relationship | 37 |
| | | Engagement to marry | 45 |
| **Home and Family** | | Girlfriend or boyfriend problems | 39 |
| Major change in living conditions | 42 | Sexual differences | 44 |
| Change in residence: | | "Falling out" of a close personal relationship | 47 |
| Move within the same town or city | 25 | An accident | 48 |
| Move to a different town, city, or state | 47 | Minor violation of the law | 20 |
| Change in family get-togethers | 25 | Being held in jail | 75 |
| Major change in health or behavior of family member | 55 | Death of a close friend | 70 |
| Marriage | 50 | Major decision regarding your immediate future | 51 |
| Pregnancy | 67 | Major personal achievement | 36 |
| Miscarriage or abortion | 65 | | |
| Gain of a new family member: | | **Financial** | |
| Birth of a child | 66 | Major change in finances: | |
| Adoption of a child | 65 | Increase in income | 38 |
| A relative moving in with you | 59 | Decrease in income | 60 |
| Spouse beginning or ending work | 46 | Investment and/or credit difficulties | 56 |
| | | Loss or damage of personal property | 43 |
| | | Moderate purchase | 20 |
| | | Major purchase | 37 |
| | | Foreclosure on a mortgage or loan | 58 |

*One-year totals ≥ 500 life change units are considered indications of high recent life stress.
**Source:** Miller, M.A., & Rahe, R.H. (1997). Life changes scaling for the 1990s. *Journal of Psychosomatic Research, 43*(3), 279–292, Copyright 1997, with permission from Elsevier. doi:10.1016/S0022-3999(97)00118-9.

**Instructions:** The questions in this scale ask you about your feelings and thoughts during the last month. In each case, please indicate with a check how often you felt or thought a certain way.

1. In the last month, how often have you been upset because of something that happened unexpectedly?
   ___0 never  ___1 almost never  ___2 sometimes  ___3 fairly often  ___4 very often

2. In the last month, how often have you felt that you were unable to control the important things in your life?
   ___0 never  ___1 almost never  ___2 sometimes  ___3 fairly often  ___4 very often

3. In the last month, how often have you felt nervous and "stressed"?
   ___0 never  ___1 almost never  ___2 sometimes  ___3 fairly often  ___4 very often

4. In the last month, how often have you felt confident about your ability to handle your personal problems?
   ___0 never  ___1 almost never  ___2 sometimes  ___3 fairly often  ___4 very often

5. In the last month, how often have you felt that things were going your way?
   ___0 never  ___1 almost never  ___2 sometimes  ___3 fairly often  ___4 very often

6. In the last month, how often have you found that you could not cope with all the things that you had to do?
   ___0 never  ___1 almost never  ___2 sometimes  ___3 fairly often  ___4 very often

7. In the last month, how often have you been able to control irritations in your life?
   ___0 never  ___1 almost never  ___2 sometimes  ___3 fairly often  ___4 very often

8. In the last month, how often have you felt that you were on top of things?
   ___0 never  ___1 almost never  ___2 sometimes  ___3 fairly often  ___4 very often

9. In the last month, how often have you been angered because of things that were outside of your control?
   ___0 never  ___1 almost never  ___2 sometimes  ___3 fairly often  ___4 very often

10. In the last month, how often have you felt difficulties were piling up so high that you could not overcome them?
   ___0 never  ___1 almost never  ___2 sometimes  ___3 fairly often  ___4 very often

**Perceived stress scale scoring**
Items 4, 5, 7, and 8 are the positively stated items. PSS-10 scores are obtained by reversing the scores on the positive items—e.g., 0 = 4, 1 = 3, 2 = 2, etc.—and then adding all 10 items.

**FIGURE 12-3** Perceived Stress Scale—10 Item (PSS-10). **Source:** Cohen, S., Kamarck, T., & Mermelstein, R. "A Global Measure of Perceived Stress." Journal of Health and Social Behavior, Vol. 24, No. 4 (Dec., 1983), Appendix A.

| TABLE 12-3 | POSITIVE AND NEGATIVE RESPONSES TO STRESS | |
| --- | --- | --- |
| **POSITIVE STRESS RESPONSES** | **NEGATIVE STRESS RESPONSES** | |
| Problem solving—figuring out how to deal with the situation | Avoidance—choosing not to deal with the situation, letting negative feelings and situations fester and continue to become chronic | |
| Using social support—calling in others who are caring and may be helpful | Self-blame—faulting oneself, which keeps the focus on minimizing one's self-esteem and prevents positive action toward resolution or working through of the feelings related to the event | |
| Reframing—redefining the situation to see both positive and negative sides, as well as the way to use the situation to one's advantage | Wishful thinking—believing that things will resolve themselves and that "everything will be fine" (a form of denial) | |

**Source:** Adapted from Lazarus, R.S., & Folkman, S. (1984). *Stress, appraisal, and coping.* New York: Springer.

contraction. This muscle relaxation is accomplished by tensing groups of muscles (beginning with the feet and ending with the face) as tightly as possible for eight seconds and suddenly releasing them. Considerable research supports the use of PMR as helpful for a number of medical conditions, such as "tension headaches" and psychiatric disorders, especially those with anxiety components (Conrad & Roth, 2006). Many good PMR scripts are available online.

Herbert Benson (1975, 1996) expanded on Jacobson's work by incorporating a state of mind that is conducive to relaxation. His technique, influenced by Eastern practices, is achieved by adopting a calm and passive attitude and focusing on a pleasant mental image in a calm and peaceful environment. **Benson's relaxation technique** allows the patient to switch from the sympathetic mode of the autonomic nervous system (fight-or-flight response) to the parasympathetic mode (a state of relaxation). Follow the steps in Box 12-2 to practise the relaxation response. Benson's relaxation technique has been combined successfully with meditation and visual imagery to treat numerous disorders, such as diabetes, high blood pressure, migraine headaches, cancer, and peptic ulcers.

### Meditation

**Meditation** follows the basic guidelines described for the relaxation response. It is a discipline for training the mind to develop

## BOX 12-2   BENSON'S RELAXATION TECHNIQUE

- Choose any word or brief phrase that reflects your belief system, such as *love, unity in faith and love, joy, shalom, one God, peace.*
- Sit in a comfortable position.
- Close your eyes.
- Deeply relax all your muscles, beginning at your feet and progressing up to your face. Keep them relaxed.
- Breathe through your nose. Become aware of your breathing. As you breathe out, say your word or phrase silently to yourself. For example, breathe IN … OUT (phrase), IN … OUT (phrase), and so forth. Breathe easily and naturally.
- Continue for 10 to 20 minutes. You may open your eyes and check the time, but do not use an alarm. When you finish, sit quietly for several minutes, at first with your eyes closed and then with your eyes open. Do not stand up for a few minutes.
- Do not worry about whether you are successful in achieving a deep level of relaxation. Maintain a passive attitude, and permit relaxation to occur at its own pace. When distracting thoughts occur, try to ignore them by not dwelling on them, and return to repeating your word or phrase. With practice, the response should come with little effort. Practise the technique once or twice daily, but not within two hours after any meal, because the digestive process seems to interfere with the elicitation of the relaxation response.

**Source:** Benson, H. (1975). *The relaxation response.* New York: William Morrow & Company, Inc.

## BOX 12-3   SCRIPT FOR GUIDED IMAGERY

- Imagine releasing all the tension in your body … letting it go.
- Now, with every breath you take, feel your body drifting down deeper and deeper into relaxation … floating down … deeper and deeper.
- Imagine a peaceful scene. You are sitting beside a clear, blue mountain stream. You are barefoot, and you feel the sun-warmed rock under your feet. You hear the sound of the stream tumbling over the rocks. The sound is hypnotic, and you relax more and more. You see the tall pine trees on the opposite shore bending in the gentle breeze. Breathe the clean, scented air, with each breath moving you deeper and deeper into relaxation. The sun warms your face.
- You are very comfortable. There is nothing to disturb you. You experience a feeling of well-being.
- You can return to this peaceful scene by taking time to relax. The positive feelings can grow stronger and stronger each time you choose to relax.
- You can return to your activities now, feeling relaxed and refreshed.

greater calm and then using that calm to bring penetrative insight into one's experience. Meditation can be used to help people reach their deep inner resources for healing, to calm the mind, and to operate more efficiently in the world. It can help people develop strategies to cope with stress, make sensible adaptive choices under pressure, and feel more engaged in life (Miller, 2000).

Meditation elicits a relaxation response by creating a hypometabolic state of quieting the sympathetic nervous system. Some people meditate using a visual object or a sound to help them focus. Others may find it useful to concentrate on their breathing while meditating. There are many meditation techniques, some with a spiritual base, such as Siddha meditation or prayer. Meditation is easy to practise anywhere. Some students find that meditating the morning of a test helps them focus and lessens anxiety. Keep in mind that meditation, like most other skills, must be practised to produce the relaxation response.

### Guided Imagery

Guided imagery is a process whereby a person is led to envision images that are both calming and health enhancing. It can be used in conjunction with Benson's relaxation technique. The content of the imagery exercises is shaped by the person helping with the imagery process. A person who has dysfunctional images can be helped to generate more effective and functional

coping images to replace the depression- or anxiety-producing ones (Miller, 2000). For example, athletes have discovered that the use of images of positive coping and success can lead to improvement in performance (Aetna InteliHealth, 2008) (Box 12-3).

Imagery techniques are a useful tool in the management of many medical conditions and are an effective means of relieving pain for many people. Pain is reduced by inducing muscle relaxation and focusing the mind away from the pain. For some, imagery techniques are healing exercises in that they not only relieve the pain but also, in some cases, diminish the source of the pain (Koenig, McCullough, & Larson, 2001). Guided imagery is used by cancer patients to help reduce chronic high levels of cortisol, epinephrine, and catecholamines, which prevent the immune system from functioning effectively, and to produce β-endorphins, which increase pain thresholds and enhance lymphocyte proliferation (Koenig, McCullough, & Larson, 2001).

Often, audio recordings are made specifically for patients and their particular situations. However, many generic guided-imagery CDs and MP3s are available to patients and health care workers.

### Breathing Exercises

Respiratory retraining, usually in the form of learning abdominal (diaphragmatic) breathing, has some definite merits in the modification of stress and anxiety reactions (Miller, 2000). One breathing exercise that has proved helpful for many patients with anxiety disorders has two parts: the first part focuses on abdominal breathing, while the second part helps patients interrupt trains of thought, thereby quieting mental noise (Box 12-4). With increasing skill, breathing becomes a tool for dampening the cognitive processes likely to induce stress and anxiety reactions.

## BOX 12-4 DEEP-BREATHING EXERCISE

- Find a comfortable position.
- Relax your shoulders and chest; let your body relax.
- Shift to relaxed, abdominal breathing. Take a deep breath through your mouth, expanding the abdomen. Hold it for three seconds and then exhale slowly through the nose; exhale completely, telling yourself to relax.
- With every breath, turn attention to the muscular sensations that accompany the expansion of the belly.
- As you concentrate on your breathing, you will start to feel focused.
- Repeat this exercise for two to five minutes.

### Physical Exercise

Physical exercise can lead to protection from the harmful effects of stress on both physical and mental states. Regular physical activity was associated with lower incidence of all psychiatric disorders except bipolar disorder and lower incidence of co-morbid conditions in subjects ages 14 to 24 in a study by Strohle, Hofler, Pfister, and colleagues (2007). Researchers have been particularly interested in the influence exercise has over depression. Blumenthal, Babyak, Doraiswamy, and colleagues (2007) found that patients who had four months of treatment either with a selective serotonin reuptake inhibitor antidepressant or with aerobic exercise had similar relief of depression. Yoga, an ancient form of exercise, has been found to be helpful for depression when used in conjunction with medication (Shapiro, Cook, Davydov, et al., 2007). Other popular forms of exercise that can decrease stress and improve well-being are walking, tai chi, dancing, cycling, aerobics, and water exercise.

### Biofeedback

Through the use of sensitive instrumentation, biofeedback provides immediate and exact information regarding muscle activity, brain waves, skin temperature, heart rate, blood pressure, and other bodily functions. Indicators of the particular internal physiological process are detected and amplified by a sensitive recording device. An individual can achieve greater voluntary control over phenomena once considered to be exclusively involuntary if he or she knows instantaneously, through an auditory or visual signal, whether a somatic activity is increasing or decreasing.

Using biofeedback requires special training, and the technique is thought to be most effective for people with low to moderate hypnotic ability. For people with higher hypnotic ability, meditation, PMR, and other cognitive-behavioural therapy techniques produce the most rapid reduction in clinical symptoms.

With increasing recognition of the role of stress in a variety of medical illnesses, including diseases affected by immune dysfunction, biofeedback has emerged as an effective strategy for stress management. The necessity of using the complex instrumentation required to detect minute levels of muscle tension or certain patterns of electroencephalographic activity is uncertain, but it has been confirmed that teaching people to relax deeply and apply these skills in response to real-life stressors can be helpful in lowering stress levels.

### Cognitive Reframing

Cognitive reframing has been found to be positively correlated with greater positive affect and higher self-esteem (Billingsley, Collins, & Miller, 2007). The goal of cognitive reframing is for an individual to change his or her perceptions of stress by reassessing a situation and replacing irrational beliefs ("I can't pass this course") with more positive self-statements ("If I choose to study for this course, I will increase my chances of success"). We can learn from most situations by asking ourselves:

- What positive things came out of this situation or experience?
- What did I learn in this situation?
- What would I have done differently?

The desired result is to reframe a disturbing event or experience as less disturbing and to give the patient a sense of control over the situation. When the perception of the disturbing event is changed, there is less stimulation to the sympathetic nervous system, which, in turn, reduces the secretion of cortisol and catecholamines that destroy the balance of the immune system (Miller, 2000).

Cognitive distortions occur when our mind convinces us of something that is not really true. These incorrect thoughts help to reinforce negative thinking or emotions. These thoughts sound rational and accurate but really only reinforce the bad feeling we have about ourselves (Beck, 1976). They often include overgeneralizations ("He always ..." or "I'll never ...") and "should" statements ("I should have done better" or "He shouldn't have said that").

Table 12-4 shows some examples of cognitive reframing of anxiety-producing thoughts. Often, cognitive reframing is used along with progressive muscle relaxation and guided imagery to reduce stress.

### Mindfulness

Mindfulness, a centuries-old form of meditation that has been dated back to Buddhist treatises, has received increased attention among health care providers. It is based on the premise that we are not aware of ourselves moment-to-moment but operate on a sort of mental autopilot (Grossman, Niemann, Schmidt, et al., 2004). Mental activity often occurs unchecked; thoughts can become negative, untrue, and unrealistic and result in anxiety, depression, and lack of focus. Happiness or lack of happiness is not caused by outside forces but by our own perceptions and interpretations of reality.

Practitioners suggest that, to become mindful, we observe and monitor the content of our consciousness and recognize that thoughts are just thoughts. Negative interpretations ("Mowing the lawn is a hot, dirty, and exhausting job") can become positive ("Mowing the lawn is fantastic exercise") when mindfulness is practised.

This moment-to-moment awareness also extends to the outer world. Being mindful includes being in the moment by paying attention to what is going on around you—what you are seeing, feeling, hearing. Imagine how much you miss during an ordinary walk to class if you spend it staring straight ahead as your mind wanders from one concern to the next. You miss the pattern of sunlight filtered through the leaves, the warmth of the sunshine on your skin, and the sounds of birds calling

| TABLE 12-4 | COGNITIVE REFRAMING OF IRRATIONAL THOUGHTS |
|---|---|
| **IRRATIONAL THOUGHT** | **POSITIVE STATEMENTS** |
| "I'll never be happy until I am loved by someone I really care about." | "If I do not get love from one person, I can still get it from others and find happiness that way."<br>"If someone I deeply care for rejects me, that will seem unfortunate, but I will hardly die."<br>"If the only person I truly care for does not return my love, I can devote more time and energy to winning someone else's love and probably find someone better for me."<br>"If no one I care for ever cares for me, I can still find enjoyment in friendships, in work, in books, and in other things." |
| "He should treat me better after all I do for him." | "I would like him to do certain things to show that he cares. If he chooses to continue to do things that hurt me after he understands what those things are, I am free to make choices about leaving or staying in this hurtful relationship." |

**Source:** Adapted from Ellis, A., & Harper, R.A. (1975). *A new guide to rational living.* North Hollywood, CA: Wilshire.

out to one another. By focusing on the here and now, rather than past and future, you are meditating and practising mindfulness.

### Journaling

Journaling is an extremely useful yet simple method of identifying stressors. It is a technique that can ease worry and obsession, help identify hopes and fears, increase energy levels and confidence, and facilitate the grieving process (Cullen, 2004). Keeping an informal diary of daily events and activities can reveal surprising information on sources of daily stress. Simply noting which activities put a strain on energy and time, which trigger anger or anxiety, and which precipitate a negative physical experience (e.g., headache, backache, fatigue) can be an important first step in stress reduction. Writing down thoughts and feelings is helpful not only in dealing with stress and stressful events but also in healing both physically and emotionally (Cullen, 2004). According to Cullen (2004), writing can strengthen the immune system, decrease reliance on pain medication, improve lung function in people with asthma, and reduce symptoms in people with rheumatoid arthritis.

### Humour

The use of humour as a cognitive approach is a good example of how a stressful situation can be "turned upside down." The intensity attached to a stressful thought or situation can be dissipated when it is made to appear absurd or comical. Essentially, the bee loses its sting.

## ▌KEY POINTS TO REMEMBER

- Stress is a universal experience and an important concept when caring for any patient in any setting.
- The body responds similarly whether stressors are real or perceived and whether the stressor is negative or positive.
- Physiologically, the body reacts to anxiety and fear by arousal of the sympathetic nervous system. Specific symptoms include rapid heart rate, increased blood pressure, diaphoresis, peripheral vasoconstriction, restlessness, repetitive questioning, feelings of frustration, and difficulty concentrating.
- Cannon introduced the fight-or-flight model of stress, and Selye, a Canadian endocrinologist, introduced the widely known general adaptation syndrome (GAS).
- The psychoneuroimmunology model describes the immune system's response to stress and its effect on neural pathways in the brain.
- Prolonged stress can lead to chronic psychological and physiological responses when not mitigated at an early stage (see Table 12-1).
- There are basically two categories of stressors: physical (e.g., heat, hunger, cold, noise, trauma) and psychological (e.g., death of a loved one, loss of job, schoolwork, humiliation).

- Age, gender, culture, life experience, and lifestyle all are important in identifying the degree of stress a person is experiencing.
- Lowering the effects of chronic stress can alter the course of many physical conditions; decrease the need for some medications; diminish or eliminate the urge for unhealthy and destructive behaviours such as smoking, insomnia, and drug addiction; and increase a person's cognitive functioning.
- Perhaps the most important factor for a nurse to assess is a person's support system. Studies have shown that high-quality social and intimate supports can go a long way toward minimizing the long-term effects of stress.
- Cultural differences exist in the extent to which people perceive an event as stressful and in the behaviours they consider appropriate to deal with a stressful event.
- Spiritual practices have been found to lead to an enhanced immune system and a sense of well-being.
- A variety of relaxation techniques are available to reduce the stress response and elicit the relaxation response, which results in improved physical and psychological functioning.

# CRITICAL THINKING

1. Assess your level of stress using the Recent Life Changes Questionnaire found in Table 12-2, and evaluate your potential for illness in the coming year. Identify stress-reduction techniques you think would be useful to learn.

2. Teach a classmate the deep-breathing exercise identified in this chapter (see Box 12-4).

3. Assess a classmate's coping styles, and have the same classmate assess yours. Discuss the relevance of your findings.

4. Using Figure 12-1, explain to a classmate the short-term effects of stress on the sympathetic–adrenal medulla system, and identify three long-term effects if the stress is not relieved. How would you use this information to provide patient teaching? If your classmate were the patient, how would his or her response indicate that effective learning had taken place?

5. Using Figure 12-1, have a classmate explain to you the short-term effects of stress on the hypothalamus–pituitary–adrenal cortex and the eventual long-term effects if the stress becomes chronic. Summarize to your classmate your understanding of what was presented. Using your knowledge of the short-term effects of stress on the hypothalamus–pituitary–adrenal cortex and the long-term effects of stress, develop and present to your clinical group a patient education model related to stress.

6. In clinical postconference, discuss a patient you have cared for who had one of the stress-related effects identified in Figure 12-1. See if you can identify some stressors in the patient's life and possible ways to lower chronic stress levels.

7. Assess the number of positive emotions, especially happiness, that you have experienced over the past week. Note the activities you were engaged in at the time. How might you increase the number of positive emotions in order to reduce your potential for illness in the coming year?

# CHAPTER REVIEW

1. The nurse is caring for a patient who is experiencing a crisis. Which symptoms would indicate that the patient is in the stage of alarm?
   1. Constricted pupils
   2. Dry mouth
   3. Decrease in heart rate
   4. Sudden drop in blood pressure

2. If it is determined that a patient will benefit from guided imagery, what teaching should the nurse provide?
   1. Focus on a visual object or sound.
   2. Become acutely aware of your breathing pattern.
   3. Envision an image of a place that is peaceful.
   4. Develop deep abdominal breathing.

3. A patient is going to undergo biofeedback. Which patient statement requires further teaching by the nurse?
   1. "This will measure my muscle activity, heart rate, and blood pressure."
   2. "It will help me recognize how my body responds to stress."
   3. "I will feel a small shock of electricity if I tell a lie."
   4. "The instruments will know if my skin temperature changes."

4. A patient has told the nurse that she knows she is going to lose her job, which scares her because she needs to work to pay her bills. Which nursing response reflects the positive stress response of problem solving?
   1. "What are your plans to find a new job?"
   2. "Can you call your parents to support you during this time?"
   3. "Is it possible that this job loss is an opportunity to find a better paying job?"
   4. "I'm sure everything will turn out just fine."

5. The nurse is caring for four patients. Which patient would be at highest risk for psychosocial compromise? The patient who has experienced:
   1. The death of a friend
   2. A divorce
   3. A recent job layoff
   4. The death of a spouse

*Visit the Evolve Web site for Chapter Review Answers and Rationales, Critical Thinking Answer Guidelines, and additional resources related to the content in this chapter:* http://evolve.elsevier.com/Canada/Varcarolis/psychiatric/

# REFERENCES

Ader, R., & Cohen, N. (1975). Behaviourally conditioned immunosuppression. *Psychosomatic Medicine, 37*(4), 333–340.

Aetna InteliHealth. (2008). Guided imagery. Retrieved from http://www.intelihealth.com/IH/ihtIH/WSIHW000/8513/34968/358820.html?d=dmtContent.

Anisman, H., & Merali, Z. (2005). Cytokines, stress, and depressive illness: Brain-immune interactions. *Annals of Medicine, 35*, 2–11. doi:10.1080/07853890310004075.

Astin, J.A., Shapiro, S.L., Eisenberg, D.M., et al. (2003). Mind–body medicine: State of science, implications for practice. *Journal of the American Board of Family Practice, 16*(2), 131–147.

Beck, A.T. (1976). *Cognitive therapies and emotional disorders.* New York: New American Library.

Benson, H. (1975). *The relaxation response* (2nd ed.). New York: William Morrow & Company, Inc.

Benson, H., & Stark, M. (1996). *Timeless healing.* New York: Scribner.

Billingsley, S.K., Collins, A.M., & Miller, M. (2007). Healthy student, healthy nurse: A stress management workshop. *Nurse Educator, 32*, 49–51. doi:10.1097/01.NNE.0000264333.42577.c6.

Blue, A.W., & Blue, M.A. (1981). The trail of stress. *The Canadian Journal of Native Studies, 1*(2), 311–330.

Blumenthal, J.A., Babyak, M.A., Doraiswamy, P.M., et al. (2007). Exercise and pharmacotherapy in the treatment of major depressive disorder. *Psychosomatic Medicine, 69*, 587–596. doi:10.1097/PSY.0b013e318148c19a.

Conrad, A., & Roth, W.T. (2006). Muscle relaxation therapy for anxiety disorders: It works but how? *Journal of Anxiety Disorders, 21*, 243–264. doi:10.1016/j.janxdis.2006.08.001.

Cullen, D. (2004, February 10). The power of the pen. *The Age.* Retrieved from http://www.theage.com.au/articles/2004/02/09/1076175101614.html.

Gonzalez, C.A., Griffith, E.E.H., & Ruiz, P. (1995). Cross-cultural issues in psychiatric treatment. In G.O. Gabbard (Ed.), *Treatment of psychiatric disorders, Vol. I* (2nd ed., pp. 55–74). Washington, DC: American Psychiatric Press.

Grossman, P., Niemann, L., Schmidt, S., et al. (2004). Mindfulness-based stress reduction and health benefits: A meta-analysis. *Journal of Psychosomatic Research, 57*, 35–43. doi:10.1016/S0022-3999(03)00573-7.

Haslam, S.A., & Reicher, S. (2006). Stressing the group: Social identity and the unfolding dynamics of responses to stress. *Journal of Applied Psychology, 91*, 1037–1052. doi:10.1037/0021-9010.91.5.1037.

Hobfall, S.E., & Vaux, A. (1993). Social support: Social resources and social context. In L. Goldberger & S. Breznitz (Eds.), *Handbook of stress: Theoretical and clinical aspects* (2nd ed., pp. 685–705). New York: Free Press.

Kim, M. (2002). Measuring depression in Korean Americans: Development of the Kim Depression Scale for Korean Americans. *Journal of Transcultural Nursing, 13*, 109–117. doi:10.1177/104365960201300203.

Koenig, H.G., McCullough, M.E., & Larson, D.B. (2001). *Handbook of religion and health.* New York: Oxford University Press.

Lazarus, R., & Folkman, S. (1984). *Stress, appraisal, and coping.* New York: Springer.

McKewan, B.S. (2005). Stressed or stressed out: What is the difference? *Journal of Psychiatry Neuroscience, 30*(5), 315–318.

Miller, W.R. (2000). *Integrating spirituality into treatment.* Washington, DC: American Psychological Association.

Neighbors, H. (2003, January). The (mis)diagnosis of African Americans: Implementing DSM criteria in the hospital and community. In *MLK Grand Rounds.* Symposium conducted at the meeting of the University of Michigan, Department of Psychiatry, Ann Harbor, MI. Retrieved from http://www.psych.med.umich.edu/.

Rahe, R.H. (1995). Stress and psychiatry. In H.I. Kaplan & B.J. Sadock (Eds.), *Comprehensive textbook of psychiatry/VI, Vol. 2* (6th ed., pp. 1545–1559). Baltimore, MD: Williams & Wilkins.

Sadock, V.A., & Sadock, B.J. (2008). *Kaplan and Sadock's concise textbook of clinical psychiatry* (3rd ed.). Philadelphia: Wolters Kluwer Health/Lippincott Williams & Wilkins.

Selye, H. (1974). *Stress without distress.* Philadelphia, PA: Lippincott.

Selye, H. (1993). History of the stress concept. In L. Goldberger & S. Breznitz (Eds.), *Handbook of stress: Theoretical and clinical aspects* (2nd ed., pp. 7–17). New York: Free Press.

Shapiro, D., Cook, I.A., Davydov, D.M., et al. (2007). Yoga as a complementary treatment of depression: Effects of traits and moods on treatment outcome. *Evidenced-Based Complementary and Alternative Medicine, 4*(4), 493–502. doi:10.1093/ecam/nel114.

Slater, M.A., Steptoe, A., Weickgenant, A., et al. (2003). Psychiatry. In A. Tasman, J. Kay, & J.A. Lieberman (Eds.), *Behavioural medicine* (2nd ed.). West Sussex, UK: Wiley.

Statistics Canada. (2010). Perceived life stress. Retrieved from http://www.statcan.gc.ca/pub/82-229-x/2009001/status/pls-eng.htm.

Strohle, A., Hofler, M., Pfister, H., et al. (2007). Physical activity and prevalence and incidence of mental disorders in adolescents and young adults. *Psychological Medicine, 37*, 1657–1666. doi:10.1017/S003329170700089X.

Wang, J., Korczykowski, M., Rao, H., et al. (2007). Gender difference in neural response to psychological stress. *Social Cognitive and Affective Neuroscience Advance Access, 2*, 227–239. doi:10.1093/scan/nsm018.

Weber, K., Rockstroh, B., Borgelt, J., et al. (2008). Stress load during childhood affects psychopathology in psychiatric patients. *BioMedCentral Psychiatry, 8*, 1–10. doi:10.1186/1471-244X-8-63.

# UNIT 4

# Psychobiological Disorders

# Anxiety, Obsessive-Compulsive, and Related Disorders

*Margaret Jordan Halter, Elizabeth M. Varcarolis,*
*Nancy Christine Shoemaker*
*Adapted by Mary Haase and Susan L. Ray*

## KEY TERMS AND CONCEPTS

## OBJECTIVES

1. Compare and contrast the four levels of anxiety in relation to perceptual field, ability to learn, and physical and other defining characteristics.
2. Identify defence mechanisms and consider one adaptive and one maladaptive use of each.
3. Identify genetic, biological, psychological, and cultural factors that may contribute to anxiety disorders.
4. Describe clinical manifestations of each anxiety disorder.
5. Formulate four appropriate nursing diagnoses that can be used in providing care to a person with an anxiety disorder.
6. Identify three defence mechanisms commonly found in patients with anxiety disorders.
7. Describe feelings that may be experienced by nurses caring for patients with anxiety disorders.
8. Propose realistic outcome criteria for a patient with (a) generalized anxiety disorder, (b) panic disorder, and (c) post-traumatic stress disorder.
9. Describe five basic nursing interventions used for patients with anxiety disorders.
10. Discuss three classes of medications appropriate for the treatment of anxiety disorders.
11. Describe advanced-practice and basic-level interventions for anxiety disorders.

## ⊖volve WEBSITE

*Visit the Evolve website for Flashcards, Case Studies, and additional testing resources related to the content in this chapter:* *http://evolve.elsevier.com/Canada/Varcarolis/psychiatric/* ( Pre-Test | interactive review )

For most people, anxiety is an everyday part of life: "I was really anxious when I couldn't find a parking space just before my final exam. I think I would have done better without that worry." For some people, however, anxiety-related symptoms become severely debilitating and interfere with normal functioning:

"Today I was so worried that I wouldn't find a parking space before the final exam, I stayed home." Or imagine being so incapacitated by anxiety, you live in dread of germs to the point that handwashing has become the focal point of your day. Consider repeatedly feeling the immediate terror of emotionally

## HOW A NURSE HELPED ME
### I Am Not the Only One

I am in my mid-fifties now, but when I was a young girl I lived a secret life. I was always a quiet girl, preferring to play dolls by myself or with Judy, my best and only friend, rather than with a group of girls. I was especially uncomfortable with the boys. I don't know what it was; I just didn't feel comfortable with them. I often felt as though others were judging me and making comments about me. I never told anyone how being around a group of people made me feel: I felt embarrassed and stupid. My parents called me "the quiet one" of the family, and I lived up to that label. I struggled through school, constantly feeling on edge and worrying that a teacher would ask me a question.

I know it seems silly, but one of my greatest fears was having to introduce myself in a group. I would start sweating, my heart pounded, I felt like I was going to die, and I was petrified that I might stutter. I became good at managing this situation by always volunteering to go first. You see, if I introduced myself first, then I could relax. I was very pleased with myself when I made this discovery. But other situations that caused even greater anxiety began to crop up. When I had to do a presentation in front of the class, I would pretend that I was ill, and my mother would let me stay home. I found that when I was extremely anxious, I would have difficulty breathing. This led to another strategy for getting out of embarrassing situations: I was diagnosed with childhood asthma, and I very quickly learned how to bring on an asthma attack and get out of going to school. My fear of being found out was always present, and I hated lying to my parents, but I was too ashamed to tell them that I was afraid of sweating, dying, or stuttering in public.

When I went on to university, I would force myself to step out of my comfort zone. I always had a sense of doom and a fear that I was going to die of embarrassment. It was not so much the situation that caused me anxiety; it was more the fear of doing something to embarrass myself that caused me anxiety. It was as if I feared the fear.

My adult years have been lonely. I wanted to talk with people and have fun, but I couldn't get over my anxiety. Then, five years ago, I met a nurse who works in psychiatry. He asked me how long I had been struggling with social anxiety disorder (social phobia). "You mean the way I feel is a disorder? I am not the only one?" He arranged for me to see a psychiatrist, who ordered a low dose of medication and enrolled me in 20 cognitive-behavioural therapy classes (in a group, of course). The change in me has been remarkable. I still get anxious in some situations, but I am able to reframe my thoughts and move on. I no longer feel as if I am going to die of embarrassment.

A therapist could be many things, but the following points describe the nurse who was able to help me with my anxiety disorder:

1. Was kind, compassionate, and easy to talk to
2. Conversed with me to get a feel for how strong or resilient my character is
3. Was able to "walk a mile in my shoes," so to speak
4. Was willing to research the problem on the Internet and in books, as needed
5. Considered my feelings and offered constructive yet gentle criticism
6. Suggested tangible ways that I could try to advance my position and rectify my problem one step at a time
7. Offered positive self-esteem-enhancing comments during the process as, more than likely, these were lacking in my life
8. Encouraged me to be proud of myself for my accomplishments
9. Challenged me occasionally so that I could continue to move forward
10. Realized when I was emotionally and physically well or exhausted or overwhelmed and in need of rest
11. Helped me recognize coping strategies for relapse prevention or maintenance of my current level of coping
12. Helped me better understand my illness and the types of evidence-informed treatments available
13. Helped to educate me about my medication and to monitor for adverse effects
14. Unmasked the real problem in my core before attempting to rectify the manifestation of my condition, which is probably very obvious
15. Took time during appointments to "read between the lines" of what I say
16. Was available if I really needed to speak with him
17. Asked questions, especially if he was unsure of what I meant
18. Gave me some homework
19. Kept the therapy on point for both of us
20. Engaged in a truly well-rounded therapeutic relationship with me
21. Learned from me as I learned from him

Being positive and being interested—it is a tall order!

**Source:** Holly, a client with an anxiety disorder.

reliving a horrific event in your life, such as hydroplaning on the highway and finding yourself facing oncoming traffic in the wrong lane. You would likely refuse to drive when it rains. This chapter will examine the concept of anxiety and defences against anxiety while providing an overview of anxiety disorders and their treatment.

## ANXIETY

Anxiety is a universal human experience and is the most basic of emotions. It can be defined as a feeling of apprehension, uneasiness, uncertainty, or dread resulting from a real or perceived threat. Whereas anxiety is a vague sense of dread related to an unspecified or unknown danger, fear is a reaction to a specific danger. Another important distinction between anxiety and fear is that anxiety affects us at a deeper level: it invades the central core of the personality and erodes feelings of self-esteem and personal worth. Physiologically, however, the body reacts to anxiety and fear in similar ways.

Normal anxiety is a healthy reaction necessary for survival. It provides us energy to carry out everyday tasks and strive toward goals; motivates us to make and survive change; and prompts constructive behaviours, such as studying for an examination, being on time for a job interview, preparing for a presentation, and working toward a promotion.

An understanding of the levels of anxiety and of the defensive patterns used in response to anxiety is fundamental to psychiatric mental health nursing care. With this understanding and practice, you will become skilled at identifying levels of anxiety, recognizing the defences used to alleviate anxiety, evaluating the possible stressors that contribute to increased anxiety, and planning interventions to lower anxiety levels (including one's own) effectively.

## LEVELS OF ANXIETY

As discussed in Chapter 3, Hildegard Peplau had a profound role in shaping the specialty of psychiatric mental health nursing. She identified anxiety as one of the most important concepts and developed an anxiety model that consists of four levels: mild, moderate, severe, and panic (Peplau, 1968). The boundaries between these levels are not distinct, and the behaviours and characteristics of individuals experiencing anxiety can and often do overlap. Identification of a patient's specific level of anxiety is essential because interventions are based on the degree of the anxiety.

### Mild Anxiety

Mild anxiety, which occurs in the normal experience of everyday living, allows an individual to perceive reality in sharp focus. A person experiencing a mild level of anxiety sees, hears, and grasps more information, and problem solving becomes more effective. Physical symptoms may include slight discomfort, restlessness, irritability, or mild tension-relieving behaviours (e.g., nail biting, foot or finger tapping, fidgeting, wringing of hands).

### Moderate Anxiety

As anxiety increases, the perceptual field narrows, and some details are excluded from observation. The person experiencing moderate anxiety sees, hears, and grasps less information and may demonstrate selective inattention, in which only certain things in the environment are seen or heard unless they are pointed out. While the person's ability to think clearly is hampered, learning and problem solving can still take place, although not at an optimal level. Physical symptoms of moderate anxiety include tension, pounding heart, increased pulse and respiratory rate, perspiration, and mild somatic symptoms (gastric discomfort, headache, urinary urgency). Voice tremors and shaking may be noticed. Mild or moderate anxiety levels can be constructive because anxiety may signal that something in the person's life needs attention or is dangerous.

### Severe Anxiety

The perceptual field of a person experiencing severe anxiety is greatly reduced. A person with severe anxiety may focus on one particular detail or many scattered details and have difficulty noticing his or her environment, even when it is pointed out by another. Learning and problem solving are not possible at this level, and the person may be dazed and confused. Behaviour becomes automatic (e.g., wringing hands, pacing) and is aimed at reducing or relieving anxiety. Somatic symptoms such as headache, nausea, dizziness, and insomnia often increase; trembling and a pounding heart are common; and the person may hyperventilate and experience a sense of impending doom or dread (see Case Study and Nursing Care Plan 13-1 on pages 224–225).

### Panic

Panic, the most extreme level of anxiety, results in noticeably disturbed behaviour. Someone in a state of panic is unable to process what is going on in the environment and may lose touch with reality, even experiencing hallucinations, or false sensory perceptions (e.g., seeing people or objects not really there). Physical manifestations may include pacing, running, shouting, screaming, or withdrawal, and actions may become erratic, uncoordinated, and impulsive. These sorts of automatic behaviours are used to reduce or relieve anxiety, although such efforts may be ineffective. Acute panic may lead to exhaustion.

Table 13-1 distinguishes among the levels of anxiety in regard to their (1) effects on perceptual field, (2) effects on the ability to learn, and (3) physical and other defining characteristics.

## DEFENCES AGAINST ANXIETY

Dysfunctional behaviour (e.g., compulsions) is a result of *defence mechanisms* (automatic coping styles that protect people from anxiety and maintain self-image by blocking feelings, conflicts, and memories). When behaviour is recognized as dysfunctional, nurses can initiate interventions to reduce anxiety. As anxiety decreases, dysfunctional behaviour will frequently decrease, although initially, as dysfunctional behaviour

## TABLE 13-1    LEVELS OF ANXIETY

| MILD | MODERATE | SEVERE | PANIC |
|---|---|---|---|
| **Perceptual Field** | | | |
| May have heightened perceptual field | Has narrow perceptual field Grasps less of what is going on | Has greatly reduced perceptual field Focuses on details or one specific detail Attention is scattered | Is unable to focus on the environment |
| Is alert and can see, hear, and grasp what is happening in the environment | Can attend to more if pointed out by another (selective inattention) | May not be able to attend to events in environment even when pointed out by another | Experiences the utmost state of terror and emotional paralysis Feels he or she "ceases to exist" |
| Can identify things that are disturbing and are producing anxiety | | Completely absorbed with self | May have hallucinations or delusions that take the place of reality |
| | | *In severe to panic levels of anxiety, the environment is blocked out. It is as if these events are not occurring.* | |
| **Ability to Learn** | | | |
| Able to work effectively toward a goal and examine alternatives | Able to solve problems but not at optimal ability | Unable to see connections between events or details | May be mute or have extreme psychomotor agitation, leading to exhaustion |
| | Benefits from guidance of others | Has distorted perceptions | Shows disorganized or irrational reasoning |
| *Mild and moderate levels of anxiety can alert the person that something is wrong and can stimulate appropriate action.* | | *Severe and panic levels prevent problem solving and discovery of effective solutions. Unproductive relief behaviours are called into play, thus perpetuating a vicious cycle.* | |
| **Physical or Other Characteristics** | | | |
| Slight discomfort Attention-seeking behaviours Restlessness, irritability, or impatience Mild tension-relieving behaviour (e.g., foot or finger tapping, lip chewing, fidgeting) | Voice tremors Change in voice pitch Difficulty concentrating Shakiness Repetitive questioning Somatic complaints, (e.g., urinary frequency and urgency, headache, backache, insomnia) Increased respiration rate Increased pulse rate Increased muscle tension More extreme tension-relieving behaviour (e.g., pacing, banging of hands on table) | Feelings of dread Ineffective functioning Confusion Purposeless activity Sense of impending doom More intense somatic complaints (e.g., dizziness, nausea, headache, sleeplessness) Hyperventilation Tachycardia Withdrawal Loud and rapid speech Threats and demands | Feeling of terror Immobility or severe hyperactivity, fight-or-flight or freeze Dilated pupils Unintelligible communication or inability to speak Severe shakiness Sleeplessness Severe withdrawal Hallucinations or delusions— likely out of touch with reality |

decreases, anxiety may actually increase until the individual learns to restructure thoughts cognitively and so on.

Sigmund Freud and his daughter, Anna Freud, outlined most of the defence mechanisms we recognize today. Although they operate all the time, defence mechanisms are not always apparent to the individual using them. The *adaptive use* of defence mechanisms helps people lower their anxiety to achieve goals in acceptable ways. The excessive application of defence mechanisms, however, results in their *maladaptive use* and is particularly problematic when immature defences are called upon. Figure 13-1 operationally defines anxiety and illustrates how defences come into play.

With the exception of sublimation and altruism, which are always healthy coping mechanisms, all defence mechanisms can be used in both healthy and unhealthy ways. Most people use a variety of defence mechanisms but not always at the same level. Keep in mind that evaluating whether the use of defence mechanisms is adaptive or maladaptive is determined, for the most

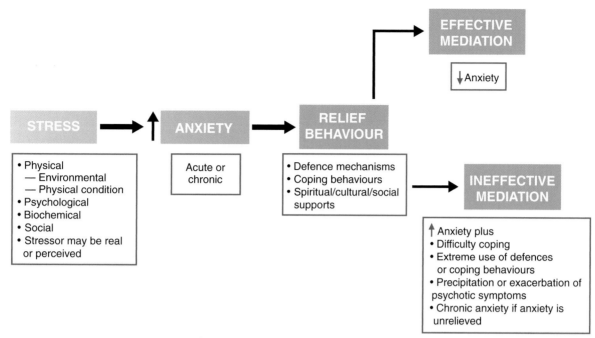

**FIGURE 13-1**   Anxiety operationally defined.

part, by their frequency, intensity, and duration of use. Table 13-2 describes defence mechanisms and their adaptive and maladaptive uses.

## ANXIETY DISORDERS

People with anxiety disorders use rigid and ineffective behaviours repetitively to try to control their anxiety. The common element of such disorders is that those affected experience a degree of anxiety so high that it interferes with personal, occupational, or social functioning. Recent studies also suggest that the presence of chronic anxiety disorders may increase the number of cardiovascular system–related deaths (Martens, de Jonge, Na, et al., 2010; Fleet, Lesperance, Arsenault, et al., 2005). Anxiety disorders tend to be persistent and are often disabling. Chapter 12 offers a more complete description of the debilitating effects of chronic stress and resultant anxiety.

## CLINICAL PICTURE

The term *anxiety disorder* refers to a number of disorders, including:

- Panic disorders
- Phobias
- Obsessive-compulsive disorder and related disorders
- Generalized anxiety disorder
- Post-traumatic stress disorder
- Acute stress disorder
- Substance-induced anxiety disorder
- Anxiety due to medical conditions
- Anxiety disorder not otherwise specified
- Attention deficit hyperactivity disorder (ADHD)

## Panic Disorders

Panic disorder (PD) is an anxiety disorder characterized by recurring severe panic attacks. It may also effect significant behavioural changes lasting at least a month and ongoing worry about having other attacks. A panic attack is the sudden onset of extreme apprehension or fear, usually associated with feelings of impending doom. The feelings of terror present during a panic attack are so severe that normal function is suspended, the perceptual field is extremely limited, severe personality disorganization is evident, and misinterpretation of reality may occur. The following vignette gives an example of a patient with signs and symptoms of a panic attack.

> **VIGNETTE**
>
> Sophia, a 30-year-old pharmacist, began to experience tension, irritability, and sleep disturbances after her mother's death from heart disease. On several occasions, Sophia has awakened gasping for breath. Her heart pounds and she feels a tight sensation like a band around her chest. Her pulse typically increases to more than 110 beats per minute, and she experiences dizziness. She fears that she is going to die. The symptoms come on within ten minutes (sudden onset) and then dissipate. On these occasions, Sophia telephones a friend to come over. The friend typically finds Sophia wringing her hands, moaning, and appearing totally disorganized. In each instance, the friend takes Sophia to the emergency department, where Sophia remains overnight for observation and tests. All diagnostic test results are normal. Because the physician finds no apparent organic basis for the episodes, she suggests they are likely panic attacks.

| TABLE 13-2 | ADAPTIVE AND MALADAPTIVE USES OF DEFENCE MECHANISMS | | |
|---|---|---|
| **DEFENCE MECHANISM** | **ADAPTIVE USE** | **MALADAPTIVE USE** |
| *Compensation* is used to make up for perceived deficiencies and to cover up shortcomings related to these deficiencies to protect the conscious mind from recognizing them. | A shorter-than-average man becomes assertively verbal and excels in business. | An individual drinks alcohol when self-esteem is low to temporarily diffuse discomfort. |
| *Conversion* is the unconscious transformation of anxiety into a physical symptom with no organic cause. Often, the symptom functions to gain attention or to provide an excuse. | A student is unable to take a final examination because of a terrible headache. | A man becomes blind after seeing his wife flirt with other men. |
| *Denial* involves escaping unpleasant, anxiety-causing thoughts, feelings, wishes, or needs by ignoring their existence. | A man reacts to news of the death of a loved one by saying, "No, I don't believe you. The doctor said he was fine." | A woman whose husband died three years earlier still keeps his clothes in the closet and talks about him in the present tense. |
| *Displacement* is the transference of emotions associated with a particular person, object, or situation to another nonthreatening person, object, or situation. | A patient criticizes a nurse after his family fails to visit. | A child who is unable to acknowledge fear of his father becomes fearful of animals. |
| *Dissociation* is a disruption in the usually integrated functions of consciousness, memory, identity, or perception of the environment. It may result in a separation between feeling and thought. Dissociation can also be manifested by compartmentalizing uncomfortable or unpleasant aspects of oneself. | An art student is able to mentally separate herself from the noisy environment as she becomes absorbed in her work. | As the result of an abusive childhood and the need to separate from its realities, a woman finds herself perpetually in a world where she feels disconnected from reality. |
| *Identification* is attributing to oneself the characteristics of another person or group, which may be done consciously or unconsciously. | An 8-year-old girl dresses up like her teacher and puts together a pretend classroom for her friends. | A young boy thinks a neighbourhood gang leader with money and drugs is someone to look up to. |
| *Intellectualization* is the process of analyzing events based on remote, cold facts (i.e., without passion), rather than incorporating feeling into the processing. | Despite the fact that a man has lost his farm to a tornado, he analyzes his options and leads his child to safety. | A man responds to the death of his wife by focusing on the details of day care and operating the household, rather than processing the grief with his children. |
| *Introjection* is the process by which the outside world is incorporated or absorbed into a person's view of the self. | After his wife's death, a man has transient complaints of chest pains and difficulty breathing—the symptoms his wife had before she died. | A woman whose parents overcriticized and belittled her as a child grows up thinking that she is no good. She has taken on her parents' evaluation of her as part of her self-image. |
| *Projection* refers to the unconscious rejection of emotionally unacceptable features and the transfer of them onto other people, objects, or situations. You can remember this defence through the childhood retort of "What you say is what you are." | A man who is unconsciously attracted to other women teases his wife about being attracted to other men. | A woman who has repressed an attraction toward other women refuses to socialize. She fears another woman will make homosexual advances toward her. |
| *Rationalization* consists of justifying illogical or unreasonable ideas, actions, or feelings by developing acceptable explanations that satisfy the teller as well as the listener. | An employee says, "I didn't get the raise because the boss doesn't like me." | A man who thinks his son was fathered by another man excuses his malicious treatment of the boy by saying, "He is lazy and disobedient" when that is not the case. |

*Continued*

| TABLE 13-2 | ADAPTIVE AND MALADAPTIVE USES OF DEFENCE MECHANISMS—cont'd | |
|---|---|---|
| **DEFENCE MECHANISM** | **ADAPTIVE USE** | **MALADAPTIVE USE** |
| *Reaction formation* occurs when unacceptable feelings or behaviours are controlled and kept outside of awareness by developing the opposite behaviour or emotion. | A recovering alcoholic constantly preaches about the evils of drink. | A woman who has an unconscious hostility toward her daughter is overprotective and hovers over her to protect her from harm, interfering with her normal growth and development. |
| *Regression* is the reversion to an earlier, more primitive, and childlike pattern of behaviour that may or may not have been previously exhibited. | A 4-year-old boy with a new baby brother starts sucking his thumb and wanting a bottle. | A man who loses a promotion starts complaining to others, hands in sloppy work, misses appointments, and comes in late for meetings. |
| *Repression* is a first-line psychological defence against anxiety. It is the unconscious temporary or long-term exclusion of unpleasant or unwanted experiences, emotions, or ideas from conscious awareness. | A man forgets his wife's birthday after a marital fight. | A woman is unable to enjoy sex after having pushed out of awareness a traumatic sexual incident from childhood. |
| *Splitting* is the inability to integrate the positive and negative qualities of oneself or others into a cohesive image. Aspects of the self and of others tend to alternate between opposite poles—for example, either good, loving, worthy, and nurturing, or bad, hateful, destructive, rejecting, and worthless. | A toddler views her parents as superhuman and wants to be like them. | A 26-year-old woman has difficulty maintaining close relationships. Although she can initially find many positive qualities about new acquaintances, eventually she becomes disillusioned when they turn out to be flawed. |
| *Sublimation* is an unconscious process of substituting mature, constructive, and socially acceptable activity for immature, destructive, and unacceptable impulses. Often, these impulses are sexual or aggressive. | A woman who is angry with her boss writes a short story about a heroic woman. | *The use of sublimation is always constructive.* |
| *Suppression* is the conscious denial of a disturbing situation or feeling. | A businessman who is preparing to make an important speech later in the day is told by his wife that morning that she wants a divorce. Although visibly upset, he puts the incident aside until after his speech, when he can give the matter his total concentration. | A woman who feels a lump in her breast shortly before leaving for a three-week vacation puts the information in the back of her mind until after returning from her vacation. |
| *Undoing*, most commonly seen in children, is atoning for an act or communication. | After flirting with her male assistant, a woman brings her husband tickets to a concert he wants to see. | A man with rigid, moralistic beliefs and repressed sexuality is driven to wash his hands to gain composure when around attractive women. |

People experiencing panic attacks may believe they are losing their minds or having a heart attack since the attacks are often accompanied by highly uncomfortable physical symptoms such as palpitations, chest pain, breathing difficulties, nausea, a choking feeling, chills, and hot flashes. Typically, panic attacks occur within ten minutes "out of the blue" (i.e., suddenly and not necessarily in response to stress), are extremely intense, last a matter of minutes, and then subside. Table 13-3 outlines a generic nursing care plan for PD.

## Panic Disorder With Agoraphobia

Panic disorder with agoraphobia is a combination of panic-attack symptoms and agoraphobia. Agoraphobia is intense, excessive anxiety or fear about being in places or situations from which escape might be difficult or embarrassing or in which help might not be available if a panic attack were to occur. Feared places are avoided in an effort to control anxiety. Situations that are commonly avoided by people with agoraphobia include being alone outside; being alone at home;

## TABLE 13-3   GENERIC CARE PLAN FOR PANIC DISORDER

**Nursing diagnosis:** *Anxiety* as evidenced by sudden onset of fear or sense of impending doom, increased pulse and respirations, shortness of breath, possible chest pain, dizziness, abdominal distress, and panic attacks

**Outcome:** Panic attacks will become less intense, and time between episodes will lengthen so that patient can function comfortably at the usual level

| SHORT-TERM GOAL | INTERVENTION | RATIONALE |
|---|---|---|
| 1. Patient's anxiety will decrease to moderate by (date). | 1a. If hyperventilation occurs, encourage patient to take slow, deep breaths. Breathing with the patient may be helpful. | 1a. Focus is shifted away from distressing symptoms. Slow, deep breathing triggers a relaxation response. |
| | 1b. Keep expectations minimal and simple. | 1b. Anxiety limits ability to attend to complex tasks. |
| 2. Patient will gain mastery over panic episodes by (date). | 2a. Help patient connect feelings before attack with onset of attack: "What were you thinking about just before the attack?" "Can you identify what you were feeling just before the attack?" | 2a. Physiological symptoms of anxiety usually appear first as the result of a stressor. They are immediately followed by automatic thoughts, such as "I'm dying" or "I'm going crazy," which are distorted assessments. |
| | 2b. Help patient recognize symptoms as resulting from anxiety, not from a catastrophic physical problem. Examples: Explain physical symptoms of anxiety. Discuss the fact that anxiety causes sensations similar to those of physical events, such as a heart attack. | 2b. Factual information and alternative interpretations can help patient recognize distortions in thought. |
| | 2c. Identify effective therapies for panic episodes. | 2c. Cognitive-behavioural treatment is highly effective. Antianxiety medication is appropriate. |
| | 2d. Teach patient abdominal breathing. | 2d. Breathing breaks the cycle of escalating symptoms of anxiety. |
| | 2e. Teach patient to reframe anxiety by using positive self-talk, such as "I can control my anxiety." | 2e. Cognitive restructuring is an effective way to replace negative self-talk. |
| | 2f. Teach patient and family about any medication ordered for patient's panic attacks. | 2f. Patient and family need to know what the medication can do, the adverse effects and toxic effects, and when to offer medication to the patient. |

travelling in a car, bus, or airplane; being on a bridge; and riding in an elevator. Avoidance behaviours, however, can be debilitating and life constricting. Consider the effect on a father whose agoraphobia renders him unable to leave home and prevents him from seeing his child's high school graduation, or the businesswoman whose avoidance of flying prevents her from attending distant business conferences.

**VIGNETTE**

Dmitri is a 28-year-old man who suffers from panic attacks with agoraphobia. He once lived a very active life, often participating in thrill-seeking activities like bungee jumping and skydiving. Dmitri's father, who had severe cardiovascular disease, died two years previously on his way to work one day. Since then, Dmitri has become increasingly fearful of the outdoors. He has gradually stopped leaving the family home because he experiences panic attacks, fearing he will die if he goes out.

### Simple Agoraphobia

Agoraphobia without a history of PD (i.e., unaccompanied by panic attacks) occurs only rarely and early in the patient's history. Over time, panic attacks usually develop as well.

### Phobias

A *phobia* is a persistent, irrational fear of a specific object, activity, or situation that leads to a desire for avoidance or to actual avoidance of the object, activity, or situation despite the awareness and reassurance that it is not dangerous. Specific phobias, which are more intense, cause impaired daily functioning and last at least half a year. They are characterized by the experience of high levels of anxiety or fear in response to specific objects or situations, such as dogs, spiders, heights, storms, water, blood, closed spaces, tunnels, and bridges. Specific phobias are common and usually do not cause sufferers much difficulty because they can contrive to avoid the feared object. See Table 13-4 for clinical names for common phobias.

| TABLE 13-4 | CLINICAL NAMES FOR COMMON PHOBIAS |
|---|---|
| **CLINICAL NAME** | **FEARED OBJECT OR SITUATION** |
| Acrophobia | Heights |
| Agoraphobia | Open spaces |
| Apiphobia | Bees |
| Astraphobia | Electrical storms |
| Claustrophobia | Closed spaces |
| Glossophobia | Talking |
| Hematophobia | Blood |
| Hydrophobia | Water |
| Monophobia | Being alone |
| Mysophobia | Germs or dirt |
| Nyctophobia | Darkness |
| Pyrophobia | Fire |
| Social phobia | Fear of a social or performance situation |
| Triskaidekaphobia | Fear of the number 13 |
| Zoophobia | Animals |

**VIGNETTE**

Abdi developed a morbid fear of elevators after being trapped in one for three hours during a power outage. As his fear and anxiety intensified, it became necessary for him to use only stairs or escalators. Abdi even became anxious if he had to enter closets or small storage rooms. He had developed claustrophobia, a fear of closed spaces.

Social phobia, also called *social anxiety disorder (SAD)*, is characterized by severe anxiety or fear provoked by exposure to a social or performance situation (e.g., fear of being scrutinized, saying something that sounds foolish in public, not being able to answer questions in a classroom, eating in public, performing on stage). Fear of public speaking is the most common social phobia.

Characteristically, phobic individuals experience overwhelming and crippling anxiety when faced with the object or situation provoking the phobia. Phobic people go to great lengths to avoid the feared object or situation. A phobic person may not be able to think about or visualize the object or situation without becoming severely anxious. The life of a phobic person becomes increasingly restricted as activities are given up in order to avoid the phobic object. All too frequently, complications ensue when people try to decrease anxiety through self-medication with alcohol or drugs.

**VIGNETTE**

David, a 22-year-old musical theatre major, has developed a fear of performing on stage. He suffers severe anxiety attacks whenever he is scheduled to appear in a student production. Recently, he has become severely anxious when faced with giving classroom readings or singing solo in music class. He is thinking about changing his major.

## Obsessive-Compulsive Disorder (OCD) and Related Disorders

Obsessions are defined as thoughts, impulses, or images that persist and recur and cannot be dismissed from the mind. Obsessions often seem senseless to the individual who experiences them (*ego-dystonic*), and their presence causes severe anxiety.

Compulsions are ritualistic behaviours or thoughts an individual feels compelled to perform in an attempt to reduce anxiety. Performing the compulsive act temporarily reduces high levels of anxiety. Primary gain is achieved by compulsive rituals, but because the relief is only temporary, the compulsive act must be repeated again and again until it feels "just right" (Haase, 2002).

Although obsessions and compulsions can exist independently of each other, they most often occur together (see Table 13-5). Obsessive-compulsive behaviour exists along a continuum. "Normal" individuals may experience mildly obsessive-compulsive behaviour. For example, nearly everyone has had the experience of having a tune run persistently through the mind despite attempts to push it away. Many people have had nagging doubts as to whether a door is locked or not. These doubts may require the person to go back to check the door once, but then they can carry on with their day. Compulsive superstitions such as touching a lucky charm or avoiding a black cat are not harmful, and mild compulsions about timeliness, orderliness, and reliability are, in fact, valued traits in Canadian society.

At the pathological end of the continuum are obsessive-compulsive symptoms that typically involve issues of contamination, fear of losing control, need for symmetry, unwanted thoughts of a sexual nature, and recurrent feelings of doubt. Pathological obsessions or compulsions cause marked distress to individuals, who often feel humiliation and shame for these behaviours. The rituals are time consuming and interfere with normal routines, social activities, and relationships with others. Severe OCD consumes so much of the individual's mental processes that the performance of cognitive tasks may be impaired.

The fifth edition of the *Diagnostic and Statistical Manual of Mental Disorders (DSM-5)* includes a new chapter on obsessive-compulsive and related disorders to reflect the increasing evidence of these disorders' relatedness to one another and distinction from other anxiety disorders, as well as to help clinicians better identify and treat individuals suffering from these disorders. Disorders in this chapter of *DSM-5* include obsessive-compulsive disorder, body dysmorphic disorder and trichotillomania (hair-pulling disorder), as well as two new disorders:

## TABLE 13-5 COMMON OBSESSIONS AND COMPULSIONS

| TYPE OF OBSESSION | EXAMPLE | ACCOMPANYING COMPULSION |
|---|---|---|
| Harm to self or others | A person thinks, *If I do not bow then harm will come to my family.* | Is repeatedly bowing and constantly seeks reassurance from family that they are safe |
| Moral or religious thoughts | A person thinks, *I will offend God if I am not doing what is right.* | Praying or confessing to parents or others |
| Feelings of doubt | *Did I turn off the stove?* repeatedly intrudes into the thoughts of a young man who has recently moved out of his family home. | Checks over and over even though he can see that the burners are off, as if seeing is not believing |
| Unwanted thoughts of a sexual nature | A young man has the recurrent thought *Am I gay?* when in the presence of a man. | Avoids the presence of men if possible; if with men, excuses self to wash hands every 10–15 minutes |
| Need for symmetry | *Everything must be in its place* is the recurrent thought in Jane's mind. | Arranges and rearranges items until she feels that the items have been arranged "just right" |
| Fear of losing control | A man repeatedly has the thought *I should hit her* when he sees a blond woman. | Abruptly turns head away and squints eyes to try to avoid seeing blondes |
| Fear of contamination | A woman ruminates, "Everything is covered in germs." | Avoids touching all objects; scrubs hands if she touches any object |

hoarding disorder and excoriation (skin-picking) disorder. For further information, visit http://www.dsm5.org.

## Generalized Anxiety Disorder

Generalized anxiety disorder (GAD) is an anxiety reaction characterized by persistent and exaggerated apprehension and tension. GAD is diagnosed when a person worries excessively about a variety of everyday problems for at least six months (Kendler, Neale, Kessler, et al., 1992). The individual with GAD also displays many of the following symptoms:

- Restlessness
- Fatigue
- Poor concentration
- Irritability
- Tension
- Sleep disturbance

The individual's anxiety is out of proportion to the true impact of the event or situation about which he or she worries. Examples of concerns typical of GAD include inadequacy in interpersonal relationships, job responsibilities, finances, the health of family members, household chores, and lateness for appointments. Sleep disturbance is common because the individual pores over the day's events and real or imagined mistakes, reviews past problems, and anticipates future difficulties. Decision making becomes difficult, owing to poor concentration and dread of making a mistake. Refer to Table 13-6 for a generic care plan for GAD.

## Post-Traumatic Stress Disorder

Post-traumatic stress disorder (PTSD) is included in a new chapter in the *DSM-5* on trauma- and stressor-related disorders. Post-traumatic stress disorder (PTSD) is an acute emotional response to a traumatic event or situation

> **VIGNETTE**
>
> Jane is a 49-year-old legal secretary. She comes to the clinic complaining of feeling "so anxious I could jump out of my skin." She is shaky and diaphoretic; she has dilated pupils, an elevated pulse, and a quivering voice. She tells the nurse, "It was probably foolish to come here. Nobody understands me." Jane's only daughter is expecting her first child. Although the pregnancy is going well, Jane worries that something is wrong with the baby. "What if it's premature? What if it's deformed?"
>
> Jane describes herself as tense and irritable. She has difficulty initiating sleep and cannot concentrate at her job. She worries about making mistakes at work, about being fired from her position, and about the financial problems that could result. She often says, "I just can't cope." Her daughter has begun calling several times a day to reassure her that all is well with the pregnancy and to try to decrease Jane's worry over other matters. The daughter has also begun shopping and housecleaning for Jane "to help her get some rest."

involving severe environmental stress (*Mosby's Dictionary of Medicine*, 2012).

The individual with PTSD persistently re-experiences a traumatic event that involved threatened or actual death or serious injury to self or others, and to which the person responded with intense fear, helplessness, or horror. PTSD may present after any traumatic event that is outside the range of usual experience, such as military combat, detention as a prisoner of war, natural disasters (e.g., floods, tornadoes, earthquakes), human disasters (e.g., plane and train accidents), crime-related events (e.g., bombing, assault, mugging, rape, being taken hostage), or diagnosis of a life-threatening illness.

| TABLE 13-6 | GENERIC CARE PLAN FOR GENERALIZED ANXIETY DISORDER |
|---|---|

**Nursing diagnosis:** *Ineffective coping* related to persistent anxiety, fatigue, and difficulty concentrating
**Outcome:** Patient will maintain role performance.

| SHORT-TERM GOAL | INTERVENTION | RATIONALE |
|---|---|---|
| 1. Patient will state that immediate distress is decreased by end of session. | 1a. Stay with patient. | 1a. Conveys acceptance and ability to give help |
| | 1b. Speak slowly and calmly. | 1b. Conveys calm and promotes security |
| | 1c. Use short, simple sentences. | 1c. Promotes comprehension |
| | 1d. Assure patient that you are in control and can assist him or her. | 1d. Counters feeling of loss of control that accompanies severe anxiety |
| | 1e. Give brief directions. | 1e. Reduces indecision; conveys belief that patient can respond in a healthy manner |
| | 1f. Decrease excessive stimuli; provide quiet environment. | 1f. Reduces need to focus on diverse stimuli; promotes ability to concentrate |
| | 1g. After assessing level of anxiety, administer appropriate dose of anxiolytic agent if warranted. | 1g. Reduces anxiety and allows patient to use coping skills |
| | 1h. Monitor and control own feelings. | 1h. Avoids transmission of anxiety (which is transmissible); displays of negative emotion can cause patient anxiety |
| 2. Patient will be able to identify source of anxiety by (date). | 2a. Encourage patient to discuss preceding events. | 2a. Promotes future change through identification of stressors |
| | 2b. Link patient's behaviour to feelings. | 2b. Promotes self-awareness |
| | 2c. Teach cognitive therapy principles:<br>• Anxiety is the result of a dysfunctional appraisal of a situation.<br>• Anxiety is the result of automatic thinking. | 2c. Provides a basis for behavioural change |
| | 2d. Ask questions that clarify and dispute illogical thinking:<br>• "What evidence do you have?"<br>• "Explain the logic in that."<br>• "Are you basing that conclusion on fact or feeling?"<br>• "What's the worst thing that could happen?" | 2d. Helps promote accurate cognition |
| | 2e. Have patient give an alternative interpretation. | 2e. Broadens perspective; helps patient think in a new way about problem or symptom |
| 3. Patient will identify strengths and coping skills by (date). | 3a. Have patient identify what has provided relief in the past. | 3a. Provides awareness of self as individual with some ability to cope |
| | 3b. Have patient write assessment of strengths. | 3b. Increases self-acceptance |
| | 3c. Reframe situation in ways that are positive. | 3c. Provides a new perspective and converts distorted thinking |

According to Ray (2009), recent changes from peacekeeping to peacemaking deployments of the Canadian military have led to an increase in trauma issues. Thus, it has been estimated that 30% of Canadian Forces veterans transitioning to civilian life have an operational stress injury (OSI) such as post-traumatic stress disorder (PTSD), addiction, or another mental health problem (Statistics Canada, 2003). PTSD symptoms often begin within three months of the trauma, but a delay of several months or years is not uncommon.

The major features of PTSD are:
• Persistent re-experiencing of the trauma through recurrent intrusive recollections of the event, dreams about the event, and flashbacks—dissociative experiences during which the event is relived (i.e., the person behaves as though he or she is experiencing the event in the present)
• Persistent avoidance of stimuli associated with the trauma, causing the individual to avoid talking about the trauma or avoid activities, people, or places that rouse memories of the trauma

- Persistent numbing of general responsiveness, as evidenced by the individual's feeling empty inside or feeling disconnected from others
- Persistent symptoms of increased arousal, as evidenced by irritability, difficulty sleeping, difficulty concentrating, hypervigilance, or exaggerated startle response

Difficulty with interpersonal, social, or occupational relationships nearly always accompanies PTSD, and trust is a common issue of concern. Child and spousal abuse may be associated with hypervigilance and irritability, and chemical abuse may begin as an attempt to self-medicate to relieve anxiety (see Case Study and Nursing Care Plan 13-2 on pages 226–227).

## Acute Stress Disorder

Acute stress disorder occurs within one month of a highly traumatic event, such as those that precipitate PTSD. To be diagnosed with acute stress disorder, the individual must display at least three dissociative symptoms either during or after the traumatic event, including a subjective sense of numbing, detachment, or absence of emotional responsiveness; a reduction in awareness of surroundings; derealization (a sense of unreality related to the environment); depersonalization (a sense of unreality or self-estrangement); or dissociative amnesia (loss of memory) (Canadian Network for Mood and Anxiety Treatments, 2013b). By definition, acute stress disorder resolves within four weeks.

---

**VIGNETTE**

Olivia, a 22-year-old college student, is sexually assaulted by a family friend. In the emergency department, she describes feeling detached from her body and being unaware of her surroundings during the assault, "as though it took place in a vacuum." She displays virtually no affect (i.e., she does not cry or appear anxious, angry, or sad). Olivia finds it difficult to concentrate on the examiner's questions. Three days later, Olivia still feels as though her mind is detached from her body; she reports having difficulty sleeping, not being able to concentrate, and startling whenever anyone touches her. When she sees the nurse four weeks after the event, Olivia expresses feelings of anger and sadness over the assault, displays the ability to concentrate, and states that she no longer feels as though her mind and body are detached. She reports being able to sleep better and not being so jittery and easily startled.

---

## Substance-Induced Anxiety Disorder

Substance-induced anxiety disorder is characterized by symptoms of anxiety, panic attacks, obsessions, and compulsions that develop with the use of a substance or within a month of discontinuing use of the substance. For a diagnosis of substance-induced anxiety disorder, the patient's history, physical examination, or laboratory findings must reveal evidence of the use of a psychoactive substance (e.g., alcohol, cocaine, heroin, hallucinogens) (Canadian Network for Mood and Anxiety Treatments, 2013a).

## Anxiety Due to Medical Conditions

In anxiety due to a medical condition, the individual's symptoms of anxiety are a direct physiological result of a medical condition, such as hyperthyroidism, pulmonary embolism, or cardiac dysrhythmias. Determining such a source of anxiety symptoms requires a careful and comprehensive assessment of multiple factors. Once again, evidence must be present in the history, physical examination, or laboratory findings for a diagnosis of anxiety due to a medical condition. Table 13-7 lists medical disorders that may contribute to anxiety symptoms.

## Anxiety Disorder Not Otherwise Specified

Anxiety disorder not otherwise specified is a diagnosis used for disorders in which anxiety or phobic avoidance predominates but the symptoms do not meet full diagnostic criteria for a specific anxiety disorder.

## Attention Deficit Hyperactivity Disorder (ADHD)

Attention deficit hyperactivity disorder (ADHD) in adults is now well established as a recognized disorder (Castellanos & Tannock, 2002), with a prevalence of 4.4% (Canadian Attention Deficit Hyperactivity Disorder Resource Alliance [CADDRA],

| TABLE 13-7 | COMMON MEDICAL CAUSES OF ANXIETY |
|---|---|
| **SYSTEM** | **DISORDERS** |
| Respiratory | Chronic obstructive pulmonary disease |
| | Pulmonary embolism |
| | Asthma |
| | Hypoxia |
| | Pulmonary edema |
| Cardiovascular | Angina pectoris |
| | Arrhythmias |
| | Congestive heart failure |
| | Hypertension |
| | Hypotension |
| | Mitral valve prolapse |
| Endocrine | Hyperthyroidism |
| | Hypoglycemia |
| | Pheochromocytoma |
| | Carcinoid syndrome |
| | Hypercortisolism |
| Neurological | Delirium |
| | Essential tremor |
| | Complex partial seizures |
| | Parkinson's disease |
| | Akathisia |
| | Otoneurological disorders |
| | Postconcussion syndrome |
| Metabolic | Hypercalcemia |
| | Hyperkalemia |
| | Hyponatremia |
| | Porphyria |

2011). Most adults who seek out a referral for assessment do so upon the diagnosis of their own child or someone they know well (CADDRA, 2011). Adults with ADHD may present with a primary complaint that is an associated symptom, such as procrastination, disorganization, lack of motivation, insomnia, rage attacks, or labile moods (CADDRA, 2011). Currently, treatment of ADHD in adults is either not available or not adequate. Adult ADHD represents a significant health care need requiring physician and nursing education, the establishment of services within the health care system, and appropriate research on treatment and service delivery. The latest practice guidelines published by the Canadian Attention Deficit Hyperactivity Disorder Resource Alliance (CADDRA) are available online at http://www.caddra.ca.

## EPIDEMIOLOGY

Anxiety disorders are the most common form of psychiatric disorders in Canada. In 2002, Statistics Canada's Canadian Community Health Survey reported that 4.7% of Canadians over the age of 15 years reported symptoms of anxiety in the previous 12 months. Of these, 1.6% met the criteria for panic disorder, 0.7% for agoraphobia, and 3.0% for social anxiety disorder. A full 11.5% of Canadian adults (more than 1 in 10) reported symptoms that indicated an anxiety disorder during their lifetime: 3.7% reported they had experienced panic disorder; 1.5%, agoraphobia; and 8.1%, social anxiety disorder. Social anxiety disorder is clearly the most common anxiety disorder in this country.

## CO-MORBIDITY

Clinicians and researchers have clearly shown that anxiety disorders frequently co-occur with other psychiatric problems. Several studies suggest that other psychiatric disorders coexist about 90% of the time in people with generalized anxiety or panic disorder, 84% in those with agoraphobia, and about 70% in those with PTSD (Sadock & Sadock, 2008). Anxiety disorders are co-morbid with major depression at a rate of 60%; in this type of co-morbidity, anxiety symptoms tend to present before depressive symptoms. In fact, treatments for both disorders are similar, leading to speculation that, genetically, anxiety and depression may be two sides of the same coin and not distinct disorders (Kendler, Gardner, Gatz, et al., 2007).

## ETIOLOGY

There is no longer any doubt that biological factors predispose some individuals to pathological anxiety states (e.g., phobias, panic attacks). However, traumatic life events, psychological factors, and sociocultural factors are also etiologically significant.

### Biological Factors
#### Genetic
Numerous studies substantiate that anxiety disorders tend to cluster in families. Twin studies demonstrate the existence of a genetic component to both panic disorder and obsessive-compulsive disorder (Pauls, 2010). First-degree biological relatives of those with OCD or phobias have a higher frequency of these disorders than exists in the general population. Nearly half of people with panic disorders have a relative who is also affected (Sadock & Sadock, 2008). Even in the case of post-traumatic stress disorder and generalized anxiety disorder, there is evidence of inherited components (Su, Wu, Zhang, et al., 2008).

### Neurobiological
Certain anatomic pathways (the limbic system) provide the transmission structure for the electrical impulses that occur when anxiety-related responses are sent or received. Neurons release chemicals (neurotransmitters) that convey these messages. The neurochemicals that regulate anxiety include epinephrine, norepinephrine, dopamine, serotonin, and gamma-aminobutyric acid (GABA).

There are various theories regarding the causes of anxiety disorders. One is the GABA–benzodiazepine theory. It is known that benzodiazepine receptors are linked to a receptor that inhibits the activity of the neurotransmitter GABA. The release of GABA slows neural transmission, inducing a calming effect. Benzodiazepine medications bind to benzodiazepine receptors, facilitating the action of GABA (Sadock & Sadock, 2008). The GABA–benzodiazepine theory proposes that abnormalities of the benzodiazepine receptors lead to unregulated anxiety levels.

Studies suggest that the stress response of the hypothalamus–pituitary–adrenal system is abnormal in patients with PTSD. Repeated trauma or stress not only alters the release of neurotransmitters but also changes the anatomy of the brain. Neuroimaging has demonstrated that the size of the right hippocampus is significantly reduced in combat veterans who suffer from PTSD (Pavić, Gregurek, Rados, et al., 2007).

### Traumatic Life Events
Erwin, Heimberg, Marx, et al. (2006) examined the frequency of the re-experience, avoidance, and hyperarousal symptoms most often associated with post-traumatic stress disorder (PTSD) among 45 persons with social anxiety disorder and 30 nonanxious controls in response to a traumatic life event. One third of the participants commonly responded to reminders of socially stressful traumatic events with avoidance and hyperarousal, suggesting a traumatic life event may predispose individuals to social anxiety disorder.

### Psychological Factors
Psychodynamic theories about the development of anxiety disorders centre on the idea that unconscious childhood conflicts are the basis for symptom development. Sigmund Freud suggested that anxiety results from the threatened breakthrough of repressed ideas or emotions from the unconscious into consciousness. Freud also suggested that the individual uses ego defence mechanisms to keep anxiety at manageable levels (see Chapter 3). The use of defence mechanisms results in behaviour that is not wholly adaptive because of its rigidity and repetitive nature.

Harry Stack Sullivan (1953) believed that anxiety is linked to the emotional distress caused when early needs go unmet or disapproval is experienced (interpersonal theory). He also suggested that anxiety is "contagious," being transmitted to the infant from the mother or caregiver. Thus, the anxiety experienced early in life becomes the prototype for anxiety experienced when unpleasant events occur later in life.

Behavioural theories suggest that anxiety is a learned response to specific environmental stimuli (*classical conditioning*). An example of classical conditioning is a boy who experiences anxiety when his abusive mother enters the room and then generalizes this anxiety as a response to all women (Sadock & Sadock, 2008). Anxiety may also be learned through the modelling of parents or peers. For example, a mother who is fearful of thunder and lightning and hides in closets during storms may transmit her anxiety to her children, who adopt her behaviour into adulthood. Such individuals can unlearn this behaviour by observing others who react normally to a storm, perhaps by lighting candles and telling stories.

Cognitive theorists believe that anxiety disorders are caused by distortions in an individual's thoughts and perceptions. Because individuals with such distortions may believe that any mistake will have catastrophic results, they experience acute anxiety.

## Sociocultural Factors

Reliable data on the incidence of anxiety disorders are sparse, but sociocultural variation in symptoms of anxiety disorders has been noted. In some cultures, most individuals express anxiety through somatic symptoms, whereas in other cultures, cognitive symptoms predominate. Panic attacks in Latin Americans and Northern Europeans often involve sensations of choking, smothering, numbness, or tingling, as well as fear of dying. In some other cultural groups, panic attacks involve fear of magic or witchcraft. Social anxiety in Japanese and Korean cultures may relate to one's beliefs that his or her blushing, eye contact, or body odour is offensive to others.

## Culture-Bound Syndromes

Up to 175 culture-bound syndromes have been identified. Culture-bound syndromes express distress about a range of personal and social problems in a culture and do not necessarily indicate psychopathology (e.g., heat in the head, heart-squeezed, bored). Some, such as trance, possession states, and fainting or seizurelike episodes, may in Western thinking be assessed as pathological (e.g., delusions or hallucinations) but are accepted expressions of distress in a particular culture. In addition, cultural idioms of distress encompass explanatory mechanisms for

 **RESEARCH HIGHLIGHT**

### Diagnosis of Asthma and the Link to an Anxiety Disorder

**Source:** Ross, C.J.M., Davis, T.M.A., & Hogg, D.Y. (2007). Screening and assessing adolescent asthmatics for anxiety disorders. *Clinical Nursing Research, 16*(1), 5–24.

**Problem**

Asthma is the most common chronic disease in the adolescent population of Canada and the United States. A possible correlation between asthma and anxiety disorders has been noted; in fact, 33% to 43% of adolescents with asthma also have at least one anxiety disorder (Katon, Lazano, Russo, et al., 2007). The high percentage of adolescents with both asthma and anxiety disorder diagnoses gives rise to concerns that having asthma may lead to development of an anxiety disorder. Research also suggests that adolescents with asthma and an anxiety disorder experience more respiratory symptoms than adolescents with just asthma. Asthma plus an anxiety disorder can result in increased mental, physical, and emotional turmoil, leading to increased use of health care resources. It is important to recognize and treat anxiety in an adolescent with asthma to avoid not only health care problems but also absences from school, development of low self-esteem, and loneliness as a result of isolation from peers.

**Purpose of Study**

The purpose of this study was to evaluate a two-stage case identification strategy designed to screen and diagnose adolescents with asthma for anxiety disorders. The specific research objectives were to compare the utility of two self-report measures as screening instruments for anxiety disorders, determine the accuracy of anxiety disorder diagnoses formulated by trained

nurses using a structured clinical interview, and determine the prevalence of *DSM-5*–defined anxiety disorders in a sample of adolescents with asthma.

**Methods**

The study included 53 adolescents (26 girls and 27 boys) aged 12 to 18 years with a diagnosis of asthma who had received medical treatment in an emergency department in the preceding year. Once participants were identified and parental permission obtained, each adolescent was evaluated by means of a two-stage assessment procedure using two self-report screening tools: the State Trait Anxiety Inventory for Children (STAI-C [Trait]) and the Multidimensional Anxiety Scale for Children (MASC).

**Key Findings**

Twenty-one participants (40%—6 boys and 15 girls) received an anxiety diagnosis. Of the 21 participants, 14 (67%) were diagnosed with two or more coexisting anxiety disorders. Five were diagnosed with two anxiety disorders; five, with three anxiety disorders; and four, with four or more anxiety disorders. The STAI-C (Trait) was found to be more effective than the MASC.

**Implications for Nursing Practice**

It is suggested that the STAI-C (Trait) be used by nurses and other health care providers to screen adolescents with asthma for anxiety disorders. Early intervention for the treatment of the diagnosed anxiety disorder and asthma may result in decreased absenteeism from school, increased self-esteem, and decreased loneliness.

behaviours or symptoms (e.g., evil eye, witchcraft, extreme emotion that upsets hot–cold balance) (Flaskerud, 2009). An online set of glossaries and indexes plus extensive information on the culture-bound syndromes and idioms of distress can be found at http://faculty.valpo.edu/jnelson/CCWebPage/Notes/CBPPPP/index.htm. Nurses need to show acceptance and respect in regard to culture-bound syndromes. However, showing acceptance and respect does not mean that the patient is not offered antipsychotics or other medications. Depending on the results of a thorough assessment, medication may be necessary.

The Considering Culture box discusses factors relevant to one anxiety disorder (ataque de nervios) primarily experienced by people from Hispanic cultures. Review Chapter 7 for more discussion of cultural issues.

## CONSIDERING CULTURE

### Ataque de Nervios

It goes without saying that technology and the commonplace nature of travel have resulted in a "smaller" world. Psychiatric mental health nurses in Canada, therefore, will be exposed to culture-bound syndromes with which they are unfamiliar. Ataque de nervios—or, in English, "attack of the nerves"—is a disorder primarily of Hispanic populations in response to stressful events (e.g., a death, acute family discord, witnessing an accident). Symptoms are dramatic, and people afflicted by ataque de nervios exhibit sudden trembling, faintness, palpitations, out-of-control shouting, heat that moves from the chest to the head, and seizurelike activities. After the episode, the affected individual often has little memory of it. This disorder is more common in socially disadvantaged females with less than a high school education.

What do these symptoms sound like to you? Some clinicians and researchers believe that ataque de nervios is closely related to an anxiety disorder and could even be a form of panic attack. However, unlike people who have panic attacks, people with this disorder are responding to a precipitating event, and they do not typically experience fear or apprehension prior to the attack.

**Sources:** Razzouk, D., Nogueira, B., & de Jesus Mari, J. (2011). The contribution of Latin American and Caribbean studies on culture-bound syndromes for the revision of the *ICD-10*: Key findings from a work in progress. *Revista Brasileira de Psiquiatria, 33*(1); and Stern, T.A., Fricchione, G.L., Cassem, N.H., et al. (2010). *Handbook of general hospital psychiatry* (6th ed.). Philadelphia: Saunders.

## APPLICATION OF THE NURSING PROCESS

## ASSESSMENT

### General Assessment

People with anxiety disorders rarely need hospitalization unless they are suicidal or have compulsions that cause injury (e.g., cutting self, banging a body part). Most patients prone to anxiety disorders are encountered incidentally in a variety of community settings. A common example is someone taken to an emergency department to rule out a heart attack when, in fact, the individual is experiencing a panic attack. It is essential for clinicians to determine whether the anxiety is secondary to another source (medical condition or substance) or is the primary problem, as in an anxiety disorder.

As previously described, the main symptoms of anxiety disorders are panic attacks, excessive anxiety, severe reactions to stress or trauma, phobias, obsessions, and compulsions.

The Hamilton Rating Scale for Anxiety is a popular tool for measuring anxiety (Table 13-8). High scores may indicate GAD or PD, although it is important to note that high anxiety scores may also be a symptom of major depressive disorder. See how you rate on this tool. Keep in mind that although the Hamilton Rating Scale highlights important areas in the assessment of anxiety, it is intended for use by experienced clinicians as a guide for planning care and not as a method of self-diagnosis.

### Other Rating Scales for Specific Anxiety Disorders

Goodman, Price, and Rasmussen (1989) developed the Yale-Brown Obsessive Compulsive Scale (YBOCS). The YBOCS has become the preferred measurement tool for OCD. It is important to note that the YBOCS is not a diagnostic tool. Rather, it is a scale used to gauge the severity and nature of OCD symptoms. Foa, Kozak, Salkovskis, et al. (1998) developed the Obsessive Compulsive Inventory (OCI) with the following subscales: washing, checking, doubting, ordering, obsessions, hoarding, and neutralizing. The Panic Disorder Severity Scale (PDSS) is a clinician-administered questionnaire developed for measuring the severity of panic disorder and for monitoring treatment outcome (Shear, Brown, Barlow, et al., 1997). The PDSS consists of seven items: panic frequency, distress during panic, panic-focused anticipatory anxiety, phobic avoidance of situations, phobic avoidance of physical sensations, impairment in work functioning, and impairment in social functioning.

### Self-Assessment

As a nurse working with an individual with an anxiety disorder, you may experience uncomfortable personal reactions. You may have feelings of frustration or anger while working with a patient with an anxiety disorder, especially if the symptoms seem to be a matter of choice or under personal control. For example, the rituals of the patient with OCD may hinder your ability to accomplish certain nursing tasks within the usual time. Communicating with such patients can be difficult since patients with OCD often correct and clarify repeatedly, as though they cannot let go of any topic. Using therapeutic communication techniques such as reflecting and paraphrasing (see Chapter 11) often prove ineffective with these patients; the patient may repeat the material and angrily imply that you have not understood. As another example, a person with a phobia may acknowledge that the fear is exaggerated and unrealistic yet continue to practise avoidant behaviour, which may bewilder the nurse.

The process of recovery for patients with anxiety is very different from that seen in a patient with an infection, who might be given antibiotics and demonstrate improvement in 24 to 72 hours.

## TABLE 13-8 HAMILTON RATING SCALE FOR ANXIETY

The symptom inventory provides scaled information that classifies anxiety behaviours and assists the clinician in targeting behaviours and achieving outcome measures. Provide a rating for each indicator based on the following scale: 0 = none; 1 = mild; 2 = moderate; 3 = disabling; 4 = severe, grossly disabling.

| ITEM | SYMPTOMS | RATING |
|---|---|---|
| 1. Anxious mood | Worry, anticipation of the worst, fearful anticipation, irritability | _____ |
| 2. Tension | Feelings of tension, fatigability, startle response, moved to tears easily, trembling, feelings of restlessness, inability to relax | _____ |
| 3. Fear | Fearful of dark, strangers, being left alone, animals, traffic, crowds | _____ |
| 4. Insomnia | Difficulty in falling asleep, broken sleep, unsatisfying sleep and fatigue on waking, dreams, nightmares, night terrors | _____ |
| 5. Intellectual (cognitive) manifestations | Difficulty in concentrating, poor memory | _____ |
| 6. Depressed mood swings | Loss of interest, lack of pleasure in hobbies, depression, early waking, diurnal | _____ |
| 7. Somatic (sensory) symptoms | Tinnitus, blurring of vision, hot and cold flushes, feelings of weakness, picking sensation | _____ |
| 8. Somatic (muscular) symptoms | Pains and aches, twitching, stiffness, myoclonic jerks, grinding of teeth, unsteady voice, increased muscular tone | _____ |
| 9. Cardiovascular symptoms | Tachycardia, palpitations, skipped beats, pain in chest, throbbing of vessels, fainting feelings | _____ |
| 10. Respiratory symptoms | Pressure of constriction in chest, choking feelings, sighing, dyspnea | _____ |
| 11. Gastrointestinal symptoms | Difficulty in swallowing, flatulence, abdominal pain, burning sensations, abdominal fullness, nausea, vomiting, borborygmi, looseness of bowels, loss of weight, constipation | _____ |
| 12. Genitourinary symptoms | Frequency of urination, urgency of urination, amenorrhea, menorrhagia, development of frigidity, premature ejaculation, loss of libido, impotence | _____ |
| 13. Autonomic symptoms | Dry mouth, flushing, pallor, tendency to sweat, giddiness, tension headache, raising of hair | _____ |
| 14. Behaviour at interview | Fidgeting, restlessness or pacing, tremor of hands, furrowed brow, strained face, sighing or rapid respiration, facial pallor, swallowing, belching, brisk tendon jerks, dilated pupils, exophthalmos | _____ |

Scoring:

14–17 = mild anxiety

18–24 = moderate anxiety

25–30 = severe anxiety

**Source:** Adapted from Hamilton, M. (1959). The assessment of anxiety states by rating. *British Journal of Medical Psychology, 32,* 50–55. doi:10.1111/j.2044-8341.1959.tb00467.x. Copyright © 2011, John Wiley and Sons.

Unlike the patient who just needs a dressing changed several times a week, the patient with anxiety requires "emotional bandaging" much more often, and behavioural change is often accomplished slowly.

When rapid progress is not made, nurses can become impatient. At the very least, they are likely to experience increased tension and fatigue from mental strain. They may also feel anger or frustration and, as a consequence, may withdraw from the patient emotionally and physically. Such negative feelings are easily transmitted to the patient, who then feels increasingly anxious and may also withdraw.

Therefore, patience, the ability to provide clear structure, and empathy are important assets when working with patients with anxiety disorders. Staging outcomes in small, attainable steps can help prevent the nurse from feeling overwhelmed by the patient's slow progress and help the patient gain a sense of control.

By having a clear understanding of the emotional pitfalls of working with patients who have anxiety disorders, a nurse is better prepared to minimize and avoid the guilt associated with strong negative feelings. It is important, then, to examine your personal feelings so you can better understand their origin and respond objectively and constructively.

## ASSESSMENT GUIDELINES
### Anxiety Disorders

1. Ensure that a sound physical and neurological examination is performed to help determine whether the anxiety is primary or secondary to another psychiatric disorder, medical condition, or substance use.
2. Assess for substance use (i.e., prescription and non-prescription medication, alcohol consumption, nicotine and caffeine consumption).
3. Determine current level of anxiety (mild, moderate, severe, or panic).
4. Assess for potential for self-harm and suicide; people suffering from high levels of intractable anxiety may become desperate and attempt suicide.
5. Perform a psychosocial assessment. Always ask the person, "What is going on in your life that may be contributing to your anxiety?" The patient may identify a problem that should be addressed by counselling (e.g., stressful marriage, recent loss, stressful job or school situation).
6. Remember that culture can affect how anxiety is manifested.

## DIAGNOSIS

The North American Nursing Diagnosis Association International (NANDA-I) provides many nursing diagnoses that can be considered for patients experiencing anxiety and anxiety disorders. The "related to" component will vary with the individual patient. Table 13-9 identifies potential nursing diagnoses for the patient experiencing anxiety. Signs and symptoms that might be found upon assessment to support the diagnosis are included.

## OUTCOMES IDENTIFICATION

The *Nursing Outcomes Classification (NOC)* identifies desired outcomes for patients with anxiety or anxiety-related disorders (Moorhead, Johnson, Maas, et al., 2008). Each outcome contains a definition and rating scale to measure the severity of the symptom or the frequency of the desired response. This rating scale enables you to evaluate outcomes in the nursing care plan. Some of the *NOC*-recommended outcomes related to anxiety include *Anxiety self-control, Anxiety level, Stress level, Coping, Social interaction skills,* and *Symptom control.* Refer to Table 13-10 for examples of intermediate and short-term indicators related to *NOC* outcomes.

## PLANNING

Anxiety disorders are encountered in all health care settings. Nurses care for people with coexisting anxiety disorders in medical-surgical units, as well as in homes, day programs, and clinics. Patients with anxiety disorders usually do not require admission to inpatient psychiatric units, so planning for their care may involve selecting interventions that can be implemented in a community setting.

Whenever possible, the patient should be encouraged to participate actively in planning. By including the patient in decision making, you increase the likelihood of positive outcomes. Shared planning is especially appropriate for someone with mild or moderate anxiety. When experiencing severe levels of anxiety, a patient may be unable to participate in planning, and the nurse may be required to take a more directive role.

## IMPLEMENTATION

### Determining Levels of Anxiety

When working with patients with anxiety disorders, you must first determine what level of anxiety they are experiencing. A general framework for anxiety interventions can then be built on a solid foundation of understanding.

### Mild to Moderate Levels of Anxiety

A person experiencing a mild to moderate level of anxiety is still able to solve problems; however, the ability to concentrate decreases as anxiety increases. A patient can be helped to focus and solve problems when you use specific nursing communication techniques, such as asking open-ended questions, giving broad openings, and exploring and seeking clarification. Closing off topics of communication and bringing up irrelevant topics can increase a person's anxiety, making the nurse, but not the patient, feel better.

Reducing the patient's anxiety level and preventing escalation to more distressing levels can be aided by providing a calm presence, recognizing the anxious person's distress, and being willing to listen. Evaluation of effective past coping mechanisms is also useful. Often, you can help the patient consider alternatives to problematic situations and offer activities that may temporarily relieve feelings of inner tension. Table 13-11 identifies interventions useful in assisting people experiencing mild to moderate levels of anxiety.

### Severe to Panic Levels of Anxiety

A person experiencing a severe to panic level of anxiety is unable to solve problems and may have a poor grasp of what is happening in the environment. Unproductive relief behaviours may take over, and the person may not be in control of his or her actions. Extreme regression and aimless running about are behavioural manifestations of a person's intense psychic pain.

Appropriate nursing interventions are to provide for the safety of the patient and others and to meet physical needs (e.g., fluids, rest) to prevent exhaustion. Anxiety reduction measures may take the form of removing the person to a quiet environment (seclusion room) with minimal stimulation and providing gross motor activities to drain some of the tension. The use of medications may have to be considered, but both medications and a seclusion room should be used only after other more personal and less restrictive interventions have failed to decrease anxiety to safer levels. Although a patient's communication may be scattered and disjointed, feeling understood can reduce anxiety and decrease the overwhelming sense of isolation.

## TABLE 13-9 POTENTIAL DIAGNOSES FOR ANXIETY DISORDERS

| SIGNS AND SYMPTOMS | NURSING DIAGNOSES |
|---|---|
| Concern that a panic attack will occur<br>Exposure to phobic object or situation<br>Presence of obsessive thoughts<br>Recurrent memories of traumatic event<br>Fear of panic attacks | Anxiety (moderate, severe, panic)<br>Fear |
| High levels of anxiety that interfere with the ability to work, disrupt relationships, and change ability to interact with others<br>Avoidance behaviours (phobia, agoraphobia)<br>Hypervigilance after a traumatic event<br>Inordinate time taken for obsession and compulsions | Ineffective coping<br>Deficient diversional activity<br>Social isolation<br>Ineffective role performance |
| Difficulty with concentration<br>Preoccupation with obsessive thoughts<br>Disorganization associated with exposure to phobic object | Ineffective health maintenance |
| Intrusive thoughts and memories of traumatic event | Post-trauma syndrome |
| Excessive use of reason and logic associated with overcautiousness and fear of making a mistake | Decisional conflict |
| Disruption in sleep related to intrusive thoughts, worrying, replaying of a traumatic event, hypervigilance, fear | Insomnia<br>Sleep deprivation<br>Fatigue |
| Feelings of hopelessness, inability to control one's life, low self-esteem related to inability to have some control in one's life | Hopelessness<br>Chronic low self-esteem<br>Spiritual distress |
| Inability to perform self-care related to rituals | Self-care deficit |
| Skin excoriation related to rituals of excessive washing or excessive picking at the skin | Impaired skin integrity |
| Inability to eat because of constant ritual performance<br>Feeling of anxiety or excessive worrying that overrides appetite and need to eat | Imbalanced nutrition: less than body requirements |
| Excessive overeating to appease intense worrying or high anxiety levels | Imbalanced nutrition: more than body requirements |

## TABLE 13-10 NOC OUTCOMES FOR ANXIETY DISORDERS

| NURSING OUTCOME AND DEFINITION | INTERMEDIATE INDICATORS | SHORT-TERM INDICATORS |
|---|---|---|
| Anxiety self-control: Personal actions to eliminate or reduce feelings of apprehension, tension, or uneasiness from an unidentifiable source | Controls anxiety response<br>Maintains role performance | Monitors intensity of anxiety<br>Uses relaxation techniques to decrease anxiety<br>Decreases environmental stimuli when anxious<br>Maintains adequate sleep |
| Coping: Personal actions to manage stressors that tax an individual's resources | Identifies multiple coping strategies<br>Modifies lifestyle as needed | Reports decrease in physical symptoms of stress<br>Identifies ineffective coping patterns<br>Verbalizes need for assistance<br>Seeks information concerning illness and treatment |
| Self-esteem: Personal judgement of self-worth | Describes pride in self<br>Describes success in social groups | Maintains eye contact<br>Maintains grooming and hygiene<br>Accepts self-limitations<br>Accepts compliments from others |
| Knowledge: Disease process: Extent of understanding conveyed about a specific disease process | Describes usual disease course | Describes signs and symptoms<br>Describes cause or contributing factors<br>Describes signs and symptoms of complications<br>Describes precautions to prevent complications |

**Source:** Moorhead, S., Johnson, M., Maas, M., et al. (2008). *Nursing outcomes classification (NOC)* (4th ed.). St. Louis, MO: Mosby.

| TABLE 13-11 | INTERVENTIONS FOR MILD TO MODERATE LEVELS OF ANXIETY |
|---|---|

**Nursing diagnosis:** *Anxiety (moderate)* related to situational event or psychological stress, as evidenced by increase in vital signs, moderate discomfort, narrowing of perceptual field, and selective inattention

| INTERVENTION | RATIONALE |
|---|---|
| Help the patient identify anxiety: "Are you comfortable right now?" | It is important to validate observations with the patient, name the anxiety, and start to work with the patient to lower anxiety. |
| Anticipate anxiety-provoking situations. | Escalation of anxiety to a more disorganizing level is prevented. |
| Use nonverbal language to demonstrate interest (e.g., lean forward, maintain eye contact, nod your head). | Verbal and nonverbal messages should be consistent. The presence of an interested person provides a stabilizing focus. |
| Encourage the patient to talk about his or her feelings and concerns. | When concerns are stated aloud, problems can be discussed and feelings of isolation decreased. |
| Avoid closing off avenues of communication that are important for the patient. Focus on the patient's concerns. | When staff anxiety increases, changing the topic or offering advice is a common temptation, but this action isolates the patient. |
| Ask questions to clarify what is being said: "I'm not sure what you mean. Give me an example." | Increased anxiety results in scattering of thoughts. Clarifying helps the patient identify thoughts and feelings. |
| Help the patient identify thoughts or feelings before the onset of anxiety. "What were you thinking right before you started to feel anxious?" | The patient is assisted in identifying thoughts and feelings, and problem solving is facilitated. |
| Encourage problem solving with the patient.* | Encouraging patients to explore alternatives increases sense of control and decreases anxiety. |
| Assist in developing alternative solutions to a problem through role play or modelling behaviours. | The patient is encouraged to try out alternative behaviours and solutions. |
| Explore behaviours that have worked to relieve anxiety in the past. | The patient is encouraged to mobilize successful coping mechanisms and strengths. |
| Provide outlets for working off excess energy (e.g., walking, playing Ping-Pong, dancing, exercising). | Physical activity can provide relief of built-up tension, increase muscle tone, and increase endorphin levels. |

*Patients experiencing mild to moderate anxiety levels can problem-solve.

Because individuals experiencing severe to panic levels of anxiety are unable to solve problems, the techniques suggested for communicating with people with mild to moderate levels of anxiety may not be effective at more severe levels. These patients are out of control, so they need to know they are safe from their own impulses. Firm, short, and simple statements are useful. Reinforcing what is observable in the environment (e.g., the door, the painting) and pointing out reality when there are distortions can also be useful interventions for severely anxious people. Table 13-12 suggests some basic nursing interventions for patients with severe to panic levels of anxiety.

Anxiety management and reduction are primary concerns when working with patients who have anxiety disorders, but they may have a variety of other needs as well. When developing a plan of care, psychiatric mental health nurses can refer to the appropriate standards of practice for their governing body. The *Nursing Interventions Classification (NIC)* offers pertinent interventions in the behavioural and safety domains (Bulechek, Butcher, & Dochterman, 2008) (see Box 13-1).

The following are basic nursing interventions:
1. Identify community resources that can offer the patient specialized, effective treatment.

2. Identify community support groups for people with specific anxiety disorders and their families.
3. Use counselling, milieu therapy, promotion of self-care activities, and psychobiological and health teaching interventions as appropriate.

### Counselling

Psychiatric mental health nurses use counselling to reduce anxiety, enhance coping and communication skills, and intervene in crises. When patients request or prefer to use integrative therapies, the nurse performs assessment and teaching as appropriate.

### Milieu Therapy

As mentioned earlier, most patients with anxiety disorders can be treated successfully as outpatients. Hospital admission is necessary only if severe anxiety or symptoms interfere with the individual's health or if the individual is suicidal. When hospitalization is necessary, the following features of the therapeutic milieu can be especially helpful to the patient:
- Structuring the daily routine to offer physical safety and predictability, thus reducing anxiety over the unknown

## TABLE 13-12  INTERVENTIONS FOR SEVERE TO PANIC LEVELS OF ANXIETY

**Nursing diagnosis:** *Anxiety (severe, panic)* related to severe threat (biochemical, environmental, psychosocial), as evidenced by verbal or physical acting out, extreme immobility, sense of impending doom, inability to differentiate reality (possible hallucinations or delusions), and inability to problem-solve

| INTERVENTION | RATIONALE |
|---|---|
| Maintain a calm manner. | Anxiety is communicated interpersonally. The quiet calm of the nurse can serve to calm the patient. The presence of anxiety can escalate anxiety in the patient. |
| Always remain with the person experiencing an acute severe to panic level of anxiety. | Alone with immense anxiety, a person feels abandoned. A caring face may be the patient's only contact with reality when confusion becomes overwhelming. |
| Minimize environmental stimuli. Move to a quieter setting and stay with the patient. | A quieter setting helps minimize further escalation of anxiety. |
| Use clear and simple statements and repetition. | A person experiencing a severe to panic level of anxiety has difficulty concentrating and processing information. |
| Use a low-pitched voice; speak slowly. | A high-pitched voice can convey anxiety. A low pitch can decrease anxiety. |
| Reinforce reality if distortions occur (e.g., seeing objects that are not there or hearing voices when no one is present). | Anxiety can be reduced by focusing on and validating what is going on in the environment. |
| Listen for themes in communication. | In severe to panic levels of anxiety, verbal communication themes may be the only indication of the patient's thoughts or feelings. |
| Attend to physical and safety needs (e.g., warmth, fluids, elimination, pain relief, family contact) when necessary. | High levels of anxiety may obscure the patient's awareness of physical needs. |
| Because safety is an overall goal, physical limits may need to be set. Speak in a firm, authoritative voice: "You may not hit anyone here. If you can't control yourself, we will help you." | A person who is out of control is often terrorized. Staff must offer the patient and others protection from destructive and self-destructive impulses. |
| Provide opportunities for exercise (e.g., walk with nurse, punching bag, Ping-Pong game). | Physical activity helps channel and dissipate tension and may temporarily lower anxiety. |
| When a person is constantly moving or pacing, offer high-calorie fluids. | Dehydration and exhaustion must be prevented. |
| Assess need for medication or seclusion after other interventions have been tried but not been successful. | Exhaustion and physical harm to self and others must be prevented. |

- Providing daily activities to promote sharing and cooperation
- Providing therapeutic interactions, including one-on-one nursing care and behaviour contracts
- Including the patient in decisions about his or her own care

### Promotion of Self-Care Activities

Patients with anxiety disorders are usually able to meet their own basic physical needs. Self-care activities that are most likely to be affected are discussed in the following sections.

### Nutrition and Fluid Intake

Patients who engage in ritualistic behaviours may be too involved with their rituals to take time to eat and drink. Some phobic patients may be so afraid of germs, they cannot eat. In general, nutritious diets with snacks should be provided. Adequate intake should be firmly encouraged, but a power struggle

should be avoided. Weighing patients frequently (e.g., three times a week) is useful in assessing whether nutrition needs are being met.

### Personal Hygiene and Grooming

Some patients, especially those with OCD and phobias, may be excessively neat and engage in time-consuming rituals associated with bathing and dressing. Hygiene, dressing, and grooming may take several hours. Maintenance of skin integrity may become a problem when the rituals involve excessive washing and skin becomes excoriated and infected.

Some patients are indecisive about bathing or about what clothing should be worn. For the latter, limiting choices to two outfits is helpful. In the event of severe indecisiveness, simply presenting the patient with the clothing to be worn may be necessary. You may also need to remain with the patient to give simple directions: "Put on your shirt. Now put on your slacks."

## BOX 13-1 *NIC* INTERVENTIONS FOR ANXIETY DISORDERS

### Coping Enhancement
*Definition of* coping enhancement: Assistance provided to a patient in adapting to perceived stressors, changes, or threats that interfere with meeting life demands and roles.

*Activities\*:*
- Provide an atmosphere of acceptance.
- Encourage verbalization of feelings, perceptions, and fears.
- Acknowledge the patient's spiritual or cultural background.
- Discourage decision making when the patient is under severe stress.

### Hope Inspiration
*Definition of* hope inspiration: Enhancement of the belief in one's capacity to initiate and sustain actions.

*Activities\*:*
- Assist the patient to identify areas of hope in life.
- Demonstrate hope by recognizing the patient's intrinsic worth and viewing the patient's illness as only one facet of the individual.
- Avoid masking the truth.
- Help the patient expand the spiritual self.

### Self-Esteem Enhancement
*Definition of* self-esteem enhancement: Assistance provided to a patient in increasing his or her personal judgement of self-worth.

*Activities\*:*
- Make positive statements about the patient.
- Monitor frequency of self-negating verbalizations.
- Explore previous achievements.
- Explore reasons for self-criticism or guilt.

### Relaxation Therapy
*Definition of* relaxation therapy: The use of techniques to encourage and elicit relaxation for the purpose of decreasing undesirable signs and symptoms such as pain, muscle tension, or anxiety.

*Activities\*:*
- Demonstrate and practise the relaxation technique with the patient.
- Provide written information about preparing and engaging in relaxation techniques.
- Anticipate the need for the use of relaxation.
- Evaluate and document the response to relaxation therapy.

*\*Partial list.*
**Source:** Bulechek, G.M., Butcher, H.K., & Dochterman, J.M. (2008). *Nursing interventions classification (NIC)* (5th ed.). St. Louis, MO: Mosby.

Matter-of-fact support is effective in assisting patients to perform as much of a task as possible independently. Encourage patients to express thoughts and feelings about self-care. This communication can provide a basis for later health teaching or for ongoing dialogue about the patient's abilities.

### Elimination
Patients with OCD may be so involved with the performance of rituals that they may suppress the urge to void and defecate, sometimes resulting in constipation or urinary tract infections. Interventions may include creating a regular schedule for taking the patient to the bathroom.

### Sleep
Patients experiencing anxiety frequently have difficulty sleeping. They may perform rituals to the exclusion of resting and sleeping, causing physical exhaustion. Those with GAD, PTSD, and acute stress disorder often experience sleep disturbance from nightmares. Teaching patients ways to promote sleep (e.g., warm bath, warm milk, relaxing music) and monitoring sleep through a sleep record are useful interventions. Chapter 21 offers an in-depth discussion of sleep disturbances.

### Pharmacological Interventions
Several classes of medications have been found to be effective in the treatment of anxiety disorders. The Drug Treatment box identifies medications approved by Health Canada for the treatment of anxiety, as well as medications that do not have specific approval but are commonly used "off-label" for anxiety disorders. Review Chapter 4 for more detailed explanations of the actions of psychotropic medications.

### Antidepressants
Antidepressants prescribed for anxiety have the secondary benefit of treating co-morbid depressive disorders. Selective serotonin reuptake inhibitors (SSRIs) are the first-line treatment for acute stress disorders and PTSD (Sadock & Sadock, 2008). Some of the SSRIs, however, exert more of an "activating" effect than others and, therefore, may increase anxiety. Sertraline (Zoloft) and paroxetine (Paxil) seem to have a more calming effect than do other SSRIs. SSRIs are preferable to the tricyclic antidepressants (TCAs) because they have a more rapid onset of action and fewer problematic adverse effects.

Monoamine oxidase inhibitors (MAOIs) are reserved for treatment-resistant conditions because of the risk for life-threatening hypertensive crisis in patients who do not follow dietary restrictions (e.g., eat foods containing tyramine). The risk for hypertensive crisis also makes the use of MAOIs contraindicated in patients with co-morbid substance abuse.

### Antianxiety Drugs
Antianxiety drugs (also called anxiolytics) are often used to treat the somatic and psychological symptoms of anxiety disorders (Pollock, Kinrys, Delong, et al., 2008). When moderate or severe anxiety is reduced, patients are better able to participate in treatment of any underlying problems. Benzodiazepines are most commonly used because they have a quick onset of action. However, due to the potential for dependence, these medications ideally should be used for short periods, only until other medications or treatments reduce symptoms. An important nursing intervention is to monitor for adverse effects of the benzodiazepines, including sedation, ataxia, and decreased

## DRUG TREATMENT OF PATIENTS WITH ANXIETY DISORDERS

| GENERIC (TRADE) | HEALTH CANADA–APPROVED USES | OFF-LABEL USES |
|---|---|---|
| **Antidepressants** | | |
| **Selective Serotonin Reuptake Inhibitors** | | |
| Citalopram hydrobromide (Celexa) | | Panic disorder<br>Social anxiety disorder<br>Obsessive-compulsive disorder<br>Generalized anxiety disorder<br>Post-traumatic stress disorder |
| Escitalopram oxalate (Cipralex) | Generalized anxiety disorder | Panic disorder<br>Social anxiety disorder<br>Obsessive-compulsive disorder<br>Post-traumatic stress disorder |
| Fluoxetine hydrochloride (Prozac) | Obsessive-compulsive disorder | Social anxiety disorder<br>Generalized anxiety disorder<br>Panic disorder<br>Post-traumatic stress disorder |
| Fluvoxamine maleate (Luvox) | Obsessive-compulsive disorder<br>Social anxiety disorder | Panic disorder<br>Generalized anxiety disorder<br>Post-traumatic stress disorder |
| Paroxetine hydrochloride (Paxil) | Panic disorder<br>Social anxiety disorder<br>Obsessive-compulsive disorder<br>Generalized anxiety disorder<br>Post-traumatic stress disorder | |
| Sertraline hydrochloride (Zoloft) | Panic disorder<br>Social anxiety disorder<br>Obsessive-compulsive disorder<br>Post-traumatic stress disorder | Generalized anxiety disorder |
| **Selective Serotonin-Norepinephrine Reuptake Inhibitors** | | |
| Duloxetine hydrochloride (Cymbalta) | Panic disorder<br>Generalized anxiety disorder | Obsessive-compulsive disorder<br>Post-traumatic stress disorder |
| Venlafaxine hydrochloride (Effexor XR) | Generalized anxiety disorder<br>Social anxiety disorder<br>Panic disorder | Obsessive-compulsive disorder<br>Post-traumatic stress disorder |
| **Tricyclics** | | |
| Amitriptyline hydrochloride (Elavil) | | Panic disorder<br>Generalized anxiety disorder<br>Post-traumatic stress disorder |
| Clomipramine hydrochloride (Anafranil) | Obsessive-compulsive disorder | Panic disorder<br>Generalized anxiety disorder<br>Post-traumatic stress disorder |
| Desipramine hydrochloride (Norpramin) | | Panic disorder<br>Generalized anxiety disorder<br>Post-traumatic stress disorder |
| Doxepin hydrochloride (Adapin, Sinequan) | | Panic disorder<br>Generalized anxiety disorder<br>Post-traumatic stress disorder |
| Imipramine hydrochloride (Tofranil) | | Panic disorder<br>Generalized anxiety disorder<br>Post-traumatic stress disorder |
| Nortriptyline hydrochloride (Aventyl, Norventyl) | | Panic disorder<br>Generalized anxiety disorder<br>Post-traumatic stress disorder |

*Continued*

## DRUG TREATMENT OF PATIENTS WITH ANXIETY DISORDERS—cont'd

| GENERIC (TRADE) | HEALTH CANADA–APPROVED USES | OFF-LABEL USES |
| --- | --- | --- |
| **Monoamine Oxidase Inhibitors** | | |
| Phenelzine sulfate (Nardil) | | Panic disorder<br>Social anxiety disorder<br>Generalized anxiety disorder<br>Post-traumatic stress disorder |
| Tranylcypromine sulfate (Parnate) | | Panic disorder<br>Social anxiety disorder<br>Generalized anxiety disorder<br>Post-traumatic stress disorder |
| **Antianxiety Agents** | | |
| **Benzodiazepines** | | |
| Alprazolam (Xanax) | Panic disorder<br>Generalized anxiety disorder | Social anxiety disorder |
| Chlordiazepoxide hydrochloride (Librax) | | Panic disorder<br>Social anxiety disorder<br>Generalized anxiety disorder |
| Clonazepam (Rivotril) | Panic disorder | Generalized anxiety disorder<br>Social anxiety disorder |
| Diazepam (Valium) | Generalized anxiety disorder | Panic disorder<br>Social anxiety disorder |
| Lorazepam (Ativan) | | Panic disorder<br>Social anxiety disorder<br>Generalized anxiety disorder |
| Oxazepam (Serax) | | Panic disorder<br>Social anxiety disorder<br>Generalized anxiety disorder |
| **Nonbenzodiazepines** | | |
| Buspirone hydrochloride (Bustab) | Generalized anxiety disorder | Social anxiety disorder<br>Obsessive-compulsive disorder |
| **Other Classes** | | |
| **Antihistamines** | | |
| Hydroxyzine hydrochloride (Atarax) | | Generalized anxiety disorder |
| Hydroxyzine pamoate (Vistaril) | | Generalized anxiety disorder |
| **β-Blockers** | | |
| Atenolol (Tenormin) | | Social anxiety disorder |
| Propranolol (Inderal) | | Social anxiety disorder |
| **Anticonvulsants** | | |
| Carbamazepine (Tegretol) | | Post-traumatic stress disorder<br>Panic disorder |
| Gabapentin (Neurontin) | | Panic disorder<br>Social anxiety disorder<br>Generalized anxiety disorder<br>Post-traumatic stress disorder |
| Valproic acid (Depakote) | | Panic disorder<br>Social anxiety disorder<br>Generalized anxiety disorder<br>Post-traumatic stress disorder |

**Sources:** Clip & save: Drug chart. (2008). *Journal of Psychosocial and Mental Health Services, 46*(5), 9; Health Canada. (2010). Drug product database (DPD). Retrieved from http://www.hc-sc.gc.ca/dhp-mps/prodpharma/databasdon/index-eng.php.; Pollack, M.H., Kinrys, G., Delong, H., et al. (2008). The pharmacotherapy of anxiety disorders. In T.A. Stern, J.F. Rosenbaum, M. Fava, et al. (Eds.), *Massachusetts General Hospital comprehensive clinical psychiatry: Expert consult.* Philadelphia: Mosby; and Stahl, S.M. (2006). *Essential psychopharmacology: The prescriber's guide* (Revised and updated ed.). New York: Cambridge.

## PATIENT AND FAMILY TEACHING
### Antianxiety Medications

1. Caution the patient:
   - Not to increase dose or frequency of ingestion without prior approval of doctor
   - That these medications reduce the ability to handle mechanical equipment (e.g., cars, machinery)
   - Not to drink alcoholic beverages or take other antianxiety drugs, because depressant effects of both would be potentiated
   - To avoid drinking beverages containing caffeine, because they decrease the desired effects of the drug
2. Recommend that the patient taking benzodiazepines avoid becoming pregnant, because these drugs increase the risk of congenital anomalies.
3. Advise the patient not to breastfeed while taking benzodiazepines, because these drugs are excreted in the milk and would have adverse effects on the infant.
4. Teach a patient who is taking monoamine oxidase inhibitors the details of a tyramine-restricted diet.
5. Teach the patient that:
   - Cessation of benzodiazepines after three to four months of daily use may cause withdrawal symptoms such as insomnia, irritability, nervousness, dry mouth, tremors, convulsions, and confusion
   - Medications should be taken with or shortly after meals or snacks to reduce gastrointestinal discomfort
   - Drug interactions can occur: antacids may delay absorption; cimetidine interferes with metabolism of benzodiazepines, causing increased sedation; central nervous system depressants, such as alcohol and barbiturates, cause increased sedation; serum phenytoin concentration may build up because of decreased metabolism

cognitive function. Benzodiazepines are not recommended for patients with a known substance abuse problem and should not be given to women during pregnancy or breastfeeding. Other important information for patients and their families is outlined in the Patient and Family Teaching box.

Buspirone (BuSpar) is an alternative antianxiety medication that does not cause dependence, but two to four weeks are required for it to reach full effect. The drug may be used for long-term treatment and should be taken regularly.

### Other Classes of Medications

Other classes of medications sometimes used to treat anxiety disorders include beta blockers, antihistamines, and anticonvulsants. These agents are often added if the first course of treatment is ineffective. Beta blockers block the nerves that stimulate the heart to beat faster and have been used to treat SAD. Anticonvulsants have shown some benefit in the management of GAD, PD, PTSD, and SAD (Sadock & Sadock, 2008). Antihistamines are a safe, nonaddictive alternative to benzodiazepines to lower anxiety levels, and again are helpful in treating patients with substance abuse problems.

Another therapeutic strategy may come in a most unusual form: D-cycloserine, an antibiotic used to treat tuberculosis, has also been demonstrated to enhance learning. D-cycloserine binds with N-methyl-D-aspartate (NMDA) receptors in the amygdala, the area of the brain that mediates fears and phobic responses, and may help patients unlearn fear responses more quickly (Stahl, 2008). Administering this drug to a patient undergoing cognitive-behavioural therapy actually promotes fear extinction, not just fear conditioning, in phobic individuals. It has also been useful when combined with extinction-based exposure therapy in the treatment of obsessive-compulsive disorder and social anxiety disorder (Hofmann, Meuret, Smits, et al., 2006; Kushner, Kim, Donahue, et al., 2007).

### Integrative Therapy

Chapter 37 identifies a number of complementary practices or integrative therapies that people use to cope with stress in their lives. Herbal and complementary therapy is popular in Canada; however, herbs and dietary supplements are not subject to the same rigorous testing as prescription medications. Also, herbs and dietary supplements are not required to be uniform, and there is no guaranteed bioequivalence of the active compound among preparations.

Problems that can occur with the use of psychotropic herbs include toxic adverse effects and herb–drug interactions. Nurses and other health care providers do well to improve their knowledge of these products so that discussions with their patients provide informed and reliable information. The Integrative Therapy box discusses kava kava, an herb often used for its sedative and antianxiety effects.

## INTEGRATIVE THERAPY
### Kava Kava

Kava kava is prepared from a South Pacific plant (Piper methysticum) and is marketed as an herbal sedative with antianxiety effects. Prior to seeking psychiatric treatment, patients with anxiety disorders may try kava kava in the belief that herbs are safer than medications, but it may have a darker side.

Kava kava is known to dramatically inhibit a liver enzyme (P450) necessary for the metabolism of many medications. This inhibition could result in liver failure, especially when taken along with alcohol or other medications such as central nervous system depressants (antianxiety agents fall into this category). This potentially dangerous interaction highlights the need for the nurse to ask about all medications the patient is taking—both prescribed and over-the-counter—before administering medications to those with anxiety disorders. Several countries have actually taken kava kava off the market, but some researchers believe that the benefits of this drug may outweigh the risks, compared to other medications used to treat anxiety.

The bottom line is that kava kava is considered to be beneficial for short-term use for mild to moderate anxiety. But as with any drug, it should be used carefully.

**Source:** Saeed, S.A., Bloch, R.M., & Antonacci, D.J. (2007). Herbal and dietary supplements for treatment of anxiety disorders. *Complementary and Alternative Medicine, 76*(4), 549–556.

## Health Teaching

Health teaching is a significant nursing intervention for patients with anxiety disorders. Patients may conceal symptoms for years before seeking treatment and often come to the attention of health care providers because of a co-occurring problem. People with PD and GAD seem more motivated than those with other anxiety disorders to get treatment; most seek help during the first year of symptoms (Wang, Berglund, Olfson, et al., 2005). Three out of every five individuals with an anxiety disorder do not consult a health care provider about their disorder (Statistics Canada, 2002). And those who do often wait years before getting medical attention.

Teaching about the specific disorder and available effective treatments is a major step toward improving the quality of life for those with anxiety disorders. Whether in a community or hospital setting, nurses can teach patients about signs and symptoms of anxiety disorders, presumed causes or risk factors (especially substance abuse), medications, the use of relaxation techniques, and the benefits of psychotherapy.

## Advanced Interventions

Nurses use several cognitive and behavioural treatment approaches, including relaxation training, modelling, systematic desensitization, flooding, response prevention, and thought stopping.

### Cognitive Therapy

Cognitive therapy is based on the belief that patients make errors in thinking that lead to mistaken negative beliefs about the self and others. For example, "I have to be perfect or my boyfriend will not love me." Through a process called *cognitive restructuring*, the therapist helps the patient (1) identify automatic negative beliefs that cause anxiety, (2) explore the basis for these thoughts, (3) re-evaluate the situation realistically, and (4) replace negative self-talk with supportive ideas.

### Behavioural Therapy

The several forms of behavioural therapy currently used involve the teaching and physical practice of activities to decrease anxious or avoidant behaviour:

- **Relaxation training**—Relaxation exercises aim to relax the breathing or muscle groups. The relaxation response is the opposite of the stress response and results in a reduced heart rate, slower breathing, and relaxed muscles. Refer to Chapter 12 for a description of different approaches to relaxation training.
- **Modelling**—The therapist or significant other acts as a role model to demonstrate appropriate behaviour in a feared situation, and then the patient imitates it. For example, the role model rides in an elevator with a claustrophobic patient.
- **Systematic desensitization**—The patient is gradually introduced to a feared object or experience through a series of steps, from the least frightening to the most frightening (graduated exposure). The patient is taught to use a relaxation technique at each step when anxiety becomes

overwhelming. For example, a patient with agoraphobia would start with opening the door to the house to go out on the steps and advance to attending a movie in a theatre. The therapist may start with imagined situations in the office before moving on to in vivo (real life) exposures.

- **Flooding**—Unlike systematic desensitization, flooding exposes the patient to a large amount of an undesirable stimulus in an effort to extinguish the anxiety response. The patient learns through prolonged exposure that survival is possible and that anxiety diminishes spontaneously. For example, an obsessive patient who usually touches objects with a paper towel may be forced to touch objects with a bare hand for one hour. By the end of that period, the anxiety level is lower.
- **Response prevention**—Patients with compulsive behaviour are not allowed to perform the compulsive ritual (e.g., hand-washing), and the patient learns that anxiety subsides even when the ritual is not completed. After trying this activity in the office, the patient learns to set time limits at home to gradually lengthen the time between rituals until the urge fades away.
- **Thought stopping**—With this technique, a negative thought or obsession is interrupted. The patient may be instructed to say "Stop!" out loud when the idea comes to mind or to snap a rubber band worn on the wrist. This distraction briefly blocks the automatic undesirable thought and cues the patient to select an alternative, more positive idea. (After learning the exercise, the patient gives the command silently.)

### Cognitive-Behavioural Therapy

Cognitive-behavioural therapy combines cognitive therapy with specific behavioural therapies to reduce the anxiety response. Cognitive-behavioural therapy includes cognitive restructuring, psychoeducation, breathing restraining and muscle relaxation, teaching of self-monitoring for panic and other symptoms, and in vivo (real life) exposure to feared objects or situations.

## EVALUATION

Identified outcomes serve as the basis for evaluation. Each *NOC* outcome has a built-in rating scale that helps the nurse measure improvement. In general, evaluation of outcomes for patients with anxiety disorders deals with questions such as the following:

- Is the patient experiencing a reduced level of anxiety?
- Does the patient recognize symptoms as anxiety related?
- Does the patient continue to display obsessions, compulsions, phobias, worrying, or other symptoms of anxiety disorders? If still present, are they more or less frequent? More or less intense?
- Is the patient able to use newly learned behaviours to manage anxiety?
- Can the patient adequately perform self-care activities?
- Can the patient maintain satisfying interpersonal relations?
- Can the patient assume usual roles?

## CASE STUDY AND NURSING CARE PLAN 13-1

### *Severe Level of Anxiety*

The following case study describes a man experiencing a severe level of acute anxiety. See if you can match his signs and symptoms with those in Table 13-1.

Ted Silvestri, a 63-year-old man, comes into the emergency department (ED) with his wife, Julie, who has taken an overdose of sleeping pills and antidepressant medications. Ten years earlier, Julie's mother died, and since that time, Julie has suffered several episodes of severe depression with suicide attempts. She has needed hospitalization during these episodes. Julie had been released from the hospital two weeks earlier after treatment for depression and threatened suicide.

Ted has a long-established routine of giving his wife her antidepressant medications in the morning and her sleeping medication at night and keeping the bottles hidden when he is not at home. Today he had forgotten to hide the medications before he went to work. His wife had taken the remaining pills from both bottles with large quantities of alcohol. When Ted returned home for lunch, Julie was comatose. In the ED, Julie suffers cardiac arrest and is taken to the intensive care unit (ICU).

Ted appears very jittery. He moves about the room aimlessly. He drops his hat, a medication card, and his keys. His hands are trembling, and he looks around the room, bewildered. He appears unable to focus on any one thing. He says over and over, in a loud, high-pitched voice, "Why didn't I hide the bottles?" He is wringing his hands and begins stomping his feet, saying, "It's all my fault. Everything is falling apart."

Other people in the waiting room appear distracted and alarmed by his behaviour. Ted seems to be oblivious to his surroundings.

### ASSESSMENT

Jean Gautier, the psychiatric nurse working in the ED, comes into the waiting room and assesses Ted's behaviour as indicative of a severe anxiety level. After talking with Ted briefly, Jean believes nursing intervention is indicated, based on the following assessment of the patient:

| Objective Data | Subjective Data |
|---|---|
| Unable to focus on anything | "Everything is falling apart." |
| Engaging in purposeless activity (walking around aimlessly) | "Why didn't I hide the bottles?" |
| Oblivious to his surroundings | "It's all my fault." |
| Showing unproductive relief behaviour (stomping, wringing hands, dropping things) | |

### DIAGNOSIS

Anxiety (severe) related to the patient's perception of responsibility for his wife's coma and possible death

**Supporting Data**
- Inability to focus
- Confusion
- The feeling that "everything is falling apart"

### OUTCOMES IDENTIFICATION

Patient will demonstrate effective coping strategies.

### PLANNING

Jean thinks that if he can lower Ted's anxiety to a moderate level, he can work with Ted to get a clear picture of his situation and place the events in a more realistic perspective. He also thinks Ted needs to talk to someone and share some of his pain and confusion to help sort out his feelings. Jean identifies two short-term goals:
1. Patient's anxiety will decrease from severe to moderate by 1600 hrs.
2. Patient will verbalize his feelings and a need for assistance by 1600 hrs.

### IMPLEMENTATION

Jean takes Ted to a quiet room in the back of the ED. He introduces himself and comments that he notices that Ted is upset. He says, "I will stay with you." At first, Ted finds it difficult to sit down and continues pacing around the room. Jean sits quietly and calmly while listening to Ted's self-recriminations. He attends carefully to what Ted is saying—and what he is not saying—to identify themes.

After a while, Ted becomes calmer and is able to sit next to Jean. Jean offers him orange juice, which he accepts and holds tightly.

Jean speaks calmly, using simple, clear statements. He uses communication tools that are helpful to Ted in sorting out his feelings and naming them.

*Continued*

**CASE STUDY AND NURSING CARE PLAN 13-1—cont'd**

*Severe Level of Anxiety*

| Dialogue | Therapeutic Tool or Comment |
|---|---|
| **Ted:** "Yes … yes … I forgot to hide the bottles. She usually tells me when she feels bad. Why didn't she tell me?" | |
| **Nurse:** "You think that if she had told you she wanted to kill herself, you would have hidden the pills?" | Jean asks for clarification of Ted's thinking. |
| **Ted:** "Yes, if I had only known, this wouldn't have happened." | |
| **Nurse:** "It sounds as if you believe you should have known what your wife was thinking without her telling you." | Here, Jean clarifies Ted's expectations that he should be able to read his wife's mind. |
| **Ted:** "Well, yes … when you put it that way … I just don't know what I'll do if she dies." | |

When Jean thinks that Ted has discussed his feelings of guilt sufficiently, he asks Ted to clarify his thinking about his wife's behaviour. Ted is able to place his feelings of guilt in a more realistic perspective. Next, Jean brings up another issue—the question of whether Ted's wife will live or die.

| Dialogue | Therapeutic Tool or Comment |
|---|---|
| **Nurse:** "You said that if your wife dies, you don't know what you will do." | Jean reflects Ted's feelings back to him. |
| **Ted:** "Oh, God" (he begins to cry) "I can't live without her. She's all I have in the world." | |
| *Silence* | |
| **Nurse:** "She means a great deal to you." | Jean reflects Ted's feelings back to him. |
| **Ted:** "Everything. Since her mother died, we are each other's only family." | |
| **Nurse:** "What would it mean to you if your wife died?" | Jean asks Ted to evaluate his feelings about his wife. |
| **Ted:** "I couldn't live by myself, alone. I couldn't stand it." (Starts to cry again.) | |
| **Nurse:** "It sounds as if being alone is very frightening to you." | Jean restates in clear terms Ted's experience and feelings. |
| **Ted:** "Yes, I don't know how I'd manage by myself." | |
| **Nurse:** "A change like that could take time to adjust to." | Jean validates that Ted's wife dying would be very painful for Ted. At the same time, he implies hope that Ted could work through the death in time. |

**Ted:** "Yes … it would be very hard."

Again, Jean gives Ted a chance to sort out his feelings and fears. Jean helps him focus on the reality that his wife may die and encourages him to express fears related to her possible death. After a while, Jean offers to go up to the ICU with Ted to see how his wife is doing. When they arrive they learn that, although Julie is still comatose, her condition has stabilized and she is breathing on her own.

After his arrival at the ICU, Ted starts to worry about whether he remembered to lock the door at home. Jean suggests that he call neighbours and ask them to check the door. Ted is now able to focus on everyday things. Jean makes arrangements to see Ted the next day when he comes in to visit his wife.

The next day, Julie has regained consciousness. She is discharged one week later. At the time of her discharge, Ted and Julie Silvestri are considering family therapy once a week with a nurse in the outpatient psychiatry department.

## EVALUATION

The first short-term goal is to lower Ted's anxiety level from severe to moderate. Jean can see that Ted has become more visibly calm: his trembling, wringing of hands, and stomping of feet have ceased, and he is able to focus on his thoughts and feelings with Jean's help.

The second short-term goal established for Ted is that he will verbalize his feelings and his need for assistance. Ted is able to identify and discuss with Jean his feelings of guilt and fear of being left alone in the world if his wife should die. Both of these feelings are overwhelming him. He is also able to state that he needs assistance in coping with these feelings in order to make tentative plans for the future.

## CASE STUDY AND NURSING CARE PLAN 13-2
### Post-Traumatic Stress Disorder

Mr. Charbonneau, 46, is brought to the emergency department by his very distraught wife after she finds him writing a suicide note and planning to shoot himself in the woods with a handgun. He had written: "I don't deserve to live. I should have died with the others." Mr. Charbonneau is subdued, shows minimal affect, and his breath has the distinct odour of alcohol. When asked about suicidal thoughts, he states that he is worthless and that his wife and family would be better off if he were dead. He refuses to contract for safety. The decision is made to hospitalize him to protect him from danger to himself.

Mr. Charbonneau's wife gives further history. Her husband is a construction contractor who served in the Canadian Armed Forces during the Afghanistan War. He lost half his squad from a roadside bombing. He walks with a permanent limp due to a

leg injury acquired during the attack. Upon returning home, he showed no signs of anxiety and refused offers of crisis treatment, stating, "I was in a war—I can handle stress." But six months later, Mrs. Charbonneau noticed that her husband had trouble sleeping, his mood was irritable or withdrawn, he avoided news reports on television, and he started drinking daily. He complained of nightmares but would not talk to her about his fears. He agreed to go to the psychiatrist only to request sleeping medication.

Mr. Charbonneau was admitted to the psychiatric unit and his care assigned to Ms. Dawson, a dually educated nurse. She observes that, as he is oriented to the unit, Mr. Charbonneau is quiet and passive but that he looks around vigilantly and is easily startled by sounds on the unit.

## ASSESSMENT

### Self-Assessment
Ms. Dawson initially feels sympathy for Mr. Charbonneau, and he reminds her of her uncle James, who served in World War II. She is concerned because his suicide plan was lethal and he is guarded in his speech, not revealing his thoughts or feelings. She realizes that as she implements suicide precautions, she must demonstrate an attitude of hope and acceptance to encourage him to develop trust. Also, she must stay neutral and not convey any pity or sympathy.

| Objective Data | Subjective Data |
|---|---|
| Sleep difficulty, nightmares | "I don't deserve to live. I should have died with the others." |
| Hypervigilance | |
| Alcohol use | |
| Irritability | |
| Withdrawn mood | |
| Constricted range of affect | |
| Feels estranged from wife and children | |
| Avoidance of news coverage with potential for emergency reports | |
| Refusal of treatment and safety contract | |
| Plan for suicide | |

## DIAGNOSIS

*Risk for suicide* related to anger and hopelessness due to severe trauma, as evidenced by suicidal plan and verbalization of intent

### Supporting Data
- Lethal plan with weapon
- Refusal to agree to a safety plan—that is, to speak to staff when experiencing suicidal ideation
- Emotional withdrawal from wife, as evidenced by his refusal to talk to her about his fears

## OUTCOMES IDENTIFICATION

Patient will consistently refrain from attempting suicide.

## PLANNING

The initial plan is to maintain safety for Mr. Charbonneau while encouraging him to express feelings and recognize that his situation is not hopeless.

*Continued*

## CASE STUDY AND NURSING CARE PLAN 13-2—cont'd

### Post-Traumatic Stress Disorder

## IMPLEMENTATION

Mr. Charbonneau's plan of care is personalized as follows:

| Short-Term Goal | Intervention | Rationale | Evaluation |
|---|---|---|---|
| 1. Patient will speak to staff whenever experiencing self-destructive thoughts. | 1a. Administer medications with mouth checks.<br>1b. Provide ongoing surveillance of patient and environment.<br>1c. Agrees to safety plan, to talk with staff when experiencing suicidal ideation<br>1d. Use direct, nonjudgemental approach in discussing suicide.<br>1e. Provide teaching about PTSD. | 1a. Addresses risk of hiding medications<br>1b. Provides one-to-one monitoring for safety<br>1c. Encourages increased self-control<br>1d. Shows acceptance of patient's situation with respect<br>1e. Offers reality of treatment | **GOAL MET**<br>After eight hours, patient agrees to safety plan every shift and starts to discuss feelings of self-harm. |
| 2. Patient will express feelings by the third day of hospitalization. | 2a. Interact with patient at regular intervals to convey caring and openness and to provide an opportunity to talk.<br>2b. Use silence and listening to encourage expression of feelings.<br>2c. Be open to expressions of loneliness and powerlessness.<br>2d. Share observations or thoughts about patient's behaviour or response. | 2a. Encourages development of trust<br><br>2b. Shows positive expectation that patient will respond<br>2c. Allows patient to voice these uncomfortable feelings<br>2d. Directs attention to here-and-now treatment situation | **GOAL MET**<br>By second day, patient occasionally answers questions about feelings and admits to anger and grief. |
| 3. Patient will express will to live by discharge from unit. | 3a. Listen to expressions of grief.<br><br>3b. Encourage patient to identify own strengths and abilities.<br>3c. Explore with patient previous methods of dealing with life problems.<br>3d. Assist in identifying available support systems.<br><br><br>3e. Refer patient to spiritual advisor of his choice. | 3a. Supports patient and communicates that such feelings are natural<br>3b. Affirms patient's worth and potential to survive<br>3c. Reinforces patient's past coping skills and ability to problem-solve now<br>3d. Addresses fact that anxiety has narrowed patient's perspective, distorting reality about loved ones.<br>3e. Allows patient opportunity to explore spiritual values and self-worth | **GOAL MET**<br>By fifth day, patient becomes tearful and states that he does not want to hurt his wife and daughter. |

## EVALUATION

See individual outcomes and evaluation within the care plan.

# KEY POINTS TO REMEMBER

- Anxiety has an unknown or unrecognized source, whereas fear is a reaction to a specific threat.
- Peplau operationally defined four levels of anxiety: mild, moderate, severe, and panic. The patient's perceptual field, ability to learn, and physical and other characteristics are different at each level (see Table 13-1).
- Defences against anxiety can be adaptive or maladaptive. Table 13-2 provides adaptive and maladaptive examples of the more common defence mechanisms.
- Anxiety disorders are the most common psychiatric disorders in Canada and frequently co-occur with depression or substance abuse.
- Research has identified genetic and biological factors in the etiology of anxiety disorders.

- Psychological theories and cultural influences are also pertinent to the understanding of anxiety disorders.
- People with anxiety disorders suffer from panic attacks, irrational fears, excessive worrying, uncontrollable rituals, or severe reactions to stress.
- People with anxiety disorders are often too embarrassed or ashamed to seek psychiatric help. Instead, they may go to primary care providers with multiple somatic complaints.
- Psychiatric treatment is effective for anxiety disorders.
- Nursing interventions include counselling, milieu therapy, promotion of self-care activities, psychobiological intervention, health teaching, and behavioural and cognitive-behavioural therapies.

# CRITICAL THINKING

1. Ethan is in his final year at college and is taking his examinations for an engineering course. The professor catches him copying from the examination of his willing partner, Jessica, and takes his exam away. Ethan's heart immediately begins to pound, his pulse and respiration rates increase, and he has to wipe perspiration from his hands and face several times. He feels as if he needs to vomit and has a throbbing in his head. When talking with the professor after the examination, he initially has difficulty focusing; when he starts to speak, his voice trembles. Ethan says that Jessica convinced him that cheating was done all the time—in fact, it was her idea. Ethan goes on to say that this "silly little exam" does not mean anything anyway, that he already passed the important courses. He tells the professor, "I thought you were the greatest, and now I see that you're a fool." The professor remains calm and explains that regardless of Ethan's thoughts on this matter, Ethan was caught cheating, he will have to take responsibility for his actions, and the choice to cheat was his. The professor will have Ethan go before the disciplinary board, which is the well-known procedure when one is caught cheating. When Ethan realizes that this incident could affect his graduating on time, he begins to yell at the professor and call him offensive names. Another professor walking past the classroom witnesses this encounter.
   a. Identify the level of anxiety Ethan was experiencing once he was caught cheating, and describe the signs and symptoms that helped you determine this level.
   b. Identify and define five defence mechanisms Ethan used to lessen his anxiety.
   c. Given the circumstances, once Ethan was caught, how could he have reacted using healthier coping defences in a manner that would have reflected more self-responsibility?

2. Ms. Halevy, a patient with OCD, washes her hands until they are cracked and bleeding. Your nursing goal is to promote healing of her hands. What interventions will you plan?

3. Mr. Olivetti is in the emergency department for the third time in a week. He is experiencing severe anxiety accompanied by many physical symptoms. He clings to you, desperately crying, "Help me! Help me! Don't let me die!" Diagnostic tests have ruled out a physical disorder. The patient outcome has been identified as "Patient anxiety level will be reduced to moderate to mild within one hour."
   a. What interventions should you use? Be comprehensive in your approach.
   b. Mr. Olivetti is given an appointment at the anxiety disorders clinic. How will you explain the importance of keeping the clinic appointment? Are there any factors you would have to consider while providing patient education?

4. Mrs. Bettencourt is a patient with GAD. She has a history of substance abuse and is now a recovering alcoholic. During a clinic visit, she tells you she plans to ask the psychiatrist to prescribe diazepam (Valium) to use when she feels anxious. She asks whether you think this is a good idea. How would you respond? What action could you take?

5. How would you assess for anxiety in an adolescent who has repeated attacks of asthma prior to examinations at school?

## CHAPTER REVIEW

1. Since learning that he will have a trial pass to a new group home tomorrow, Bill's behaviour has changed. He has started to pace rapidly, has become very distracted, and is breathing rapidly. He has trouble focusing on anything other than the group home issue and complains that he suddenly feels very nauseated. Which initial nursing response is most appropriate for Bill's level of anxiety?
   1. "You seem anxious. Would you like to talk about how you are feeling?"
   2. "If you do not calm down, I will have to give you medicine to calm you."
   3. "Bill, slow down. Listen to me. You are safe. Take a nice, deep breath. …"
   4. "We can delay the visit to the group home if that would help you calm down."

2. A patient who seems to be angry when his family again fails to visit as promised tells the nurse that he is fine and that the visit was not important to him anyway. When the nurse suggests that perhaps he might be disappointed or even a little angry that the family has again let him down, the patient responds that it is his family who is angry, not him, or else they would have visited. Which of the following defence mechanisms is this patient using to deal with his feelings?
   1. Rationalization
   2. Introjection
   3. Regression
   4. Dissociation

3. John, a construction worker, is on duty when a wall under construction suddenly falls, crushing a number of co-workers. Shaken initially, he seems to be coping well with the tragedy but later begins to experience tremors, nightmares, and periods during which he feels numb or detached from his environment. He finds himself frequently thinking about the tragedy and feeling guilty that he was spared while many others died. Which statement about this situation is most accurate?
   1. John is experiencing post-traumatic stress disorder (PTSD) and requires therapy.
   2. John has acute stress disorder and should be treated with antianxiety medications.
   3. John is experiencing anxiety and grief and should be monitored for PTSD symptoms.
   4. John is experiencing mild anxiety and a normal grief reaction; no intervention is needed.

4. Various medications are used in the treatment of severe anxiety disorders. Which class of medication used to treat anxiety is potentially addictive?
   1. Benzodiazepines
   2. Selective serotonin reuptake inhibitors (SSRIs)
   3. Beta blockers
   4. Antihistamines
   5. Nonbenzodiazepine anxiolytics

5. An older adult in the outpatient internal medicine clinic complains of feeling a sense of dread and fearfulness without apparent cause. It has been growing steadily worse and is to the point that it is interfering with the patient's sleep and volunteer work. After a brief interview and cursory physical exam, the nurse diagnoses the patient with generalized anxiety disorder and suggests a referral to the mental health clinic. Which response(s) by the medical clinic nurse would be the priority response?
   1. Complete the referral to the mental health clinic.
   2. Meet with the patient's family to discuss treatment options for generalized anxiety disorder.
   3. Instruct the client in deep-breathing and basic cognitive-behavioural techniques for coping with worry.
   4. Suggest that a battery of blood tests, including a CBC, be ordered and reviewed.

## ℮volve WEBSITE

Post-Test interactive review

*Visit the Evolve Web site for Chapter Review Answers and Rationales, Critical Thinking Answer Guidelines, and additional resources related to the content in this chapter:* http://evolve.elsevier.com/Canada/Varcarolis/psychiatric/

## REFERENCES

Bulechek, G.M., Butcher, H.K., & Dochterman, J.M. (2008). *Nursing interventions classification (NIC)* (5th ed.). St. Louis, MO: Mosby.

Canadian Attention Deficit Hyperactivity Disorder Resource Alliance (CADDRA). (2011). *Canadian ADHD practice guidelines* (3rd ed.). Toronto: Author.

Canadian Network for Mood and Anxiety Treatments. (2013a). *Anxiety: Diagnosing substance-induced anxiety disorder.* Retrieved from http://www.canmat.org/cme-anxiety-substance-induced-anxiety-disorder.php.

Canadian Network for Mood and Anxiety Treatments. (2013b). *Disorder information: Acute stress disorder.* Retrieved from: http://www.canmat.org/di-anxiety-acute-stress-disorder.php.

Castellanos, F.X., & Tannock, R. (2002). Neuroscience of attention-deficit/hyperactivity disorder: The search for endophenotypes. *National Review Neuroscience, 3*(8), 617–628.

Erwin, B.A., Heimberg, R.G., Marx, B.P., et al. (2006). Traumatic and socially stressful life events among persons with social anxiety disorder. *Anxiety Disorders, 20,* 896–914.

Flaskerud, J.H. (2009). What do we need to know about culture-bound syndromes? *Issues in Mental Health Nursing, 30,* 406–407. doi:10.1080/01612840902812947.

Fleet, R., Lesperance, F., Arsenault, A., et al. (2005). Myocardial perfusion study of panic attacks in patients with coronary artery disease. *American Journal of Cardiology, 96*(8), 1064–1068. doi:10.1016/j.amjcard.2005.06.035.

Foa, E.B., Kozak, M.J., Salkovskis, P.M., et al. (1998). The validation of a new obsessive compulsive disorder scale: The Obsessive Compulsive Inventory (OCI). *Psychological Assessment, 10,* 206–214.

Goodman, W.K., Price, L.H., & Rasmussen, S.A. (1989). The Yale-Brown Obsessive Compulsive Scale. *Archives of General Psychiatry, 46,* 1006–1011.

Haase, M. (2002). Uncommon experiences: Living with obsessive compulsive disorder. In M. van Manen (Ed.), *Writing in the dark: Phenomenological studies in interpretive inquiry* (pp. 62–83). London, ON: Althouse Press.

Hofmann, S.G., Meuret, A.E., Smits, J.A.J., et al. (2006). Augmentation of exposure therapy with d-cycloserine for social anxiety disorder. *Archives of General Psychiatry, 63*(3), 298–304.

Kendler, K.S., Gardner, C.O., Gatz, M., et al. (2007). The sources of co-morbidity between major depression and generalized anxiety disorder in a Swedish national twin sample. *Psychological Medicine, 37,* 453–462. doi:10.1017/S0033291706009135.

Kendler, K.S., Neale, M.C., Kessler, R.C., et al. (1992). Generalized anxiety disorder in women. A population-based twin study. *Archives of General Psychiatry, 49*(4), 267–272.

Kushner, M.G., Kim, S.W., Donahue, C., et al. (2007). D-cycloserine augmented exposure therapy for obsessive-compulsive disorder. *Biological Psychiatry, 62,* 835–838. doi:10.1016/j.biopsych.2006.12.020.

Martens, E.J., de Jonge, P., Na, B., et al. (2010). Scared to death? Generalized anxiety disorder and cardiovascular events in patients with stable coronary heart disease. *Archives of General Psychiatry, 67*(7), 750–758.

Moorhead, S., Johnson, M., Maas, M., et al. (2008). *Nursing outcomes classification (NOC)* (4th ed.). St. Louis, MO: Mosby.

*Mosby's Dictionary of Medicine, Nursing & Health Professions* (9th ed.) (2012). St. Louis, MO: Mosby.

Pauls, D.L. (2010). The genetics of obsessive-compulsive disorder: A review. *Dialogues in Clinical Neuroscience, 12*(2), 149–163.

Pavić, L., Gregurek, R., Rados, M., et al. (2007). Smaller right hippocampus in war veterans with posttraumatic stress disorder. *Psychiatry Research: Neuroimaging, 154,* 191–198. doi:10.1016/j.pscychresns.2006.08.005.

Peplau, H.E. (1968). A working definition of anxiety. In S.F. Burd & M.A. Marshall (Eds.), *Some clinical approaches to psychiatric nursing.* New York: Macmillan.

Pollock, M.H., Kinrys, G., Delong, H., et al. (2008). The pharmacotherapy of anxiety disorders. In T.A. Stern, J.F. Rosenbaum, M. Fava, et al. (Eds.), *Massachusetts General Hospital comprehensive clinical psychiatry: Expert consult* (pp. 565–575). Philadelphia: Mosby.

Ray, S.L. (2009). The experience of contemporary peacekeepers healing from trauma. *Nursing Inquiry, 16*(1), 53–63.

Sadock, B.J., & Sadock, V.A. (2008). *Kaplan and Sadock's concise textbook of clinical psychiatry* (3rd ed.). Philadelphia: Lippincott.

Shear, M.K., Brown, T.A., Barlow, D.H., et al. (1997). Multicenter collaborative panic disorder severity scale. *American Journal of Psychiatry, 154*(11), 1571–1575. Retrieved from http://www.ncbi.nlm.nih.gov/entrez/eutils/elink.fcgi?dbfrom=pubmed&tool=sumsearch.org/cite&retmode=ref&cmd=prlinks&id=9356566.

Stahl, S.M. (2008). *Stahl's essential psychopharmacology* (3rd ed.). Cambridge, MA: Cambridge University Press.

Statistics Canada. (2002). *Canadian community health survey: Mental health and well-being, Cycle 1.2.* Ottawa: Canada.

Statistics Canada. (2003). *Canadian Forces CCHS supplement: Briefing document.* Ottawa: Author.

Su, Y.A., Wu, J., Zhang, L., et al. (2008). Dysregulated mitochondrial genes and networks with drug targets in postmortem brain of patients with posttraumatic stress disorder (PTSD) revealed by human mitochondria-focused cDNA microarrays. *International Journal of Biological Science, 4*(4), 223–235.

Sullivan, H.S. (1953). *The interpersonal theory of psychiatry.* New York: W.W. Norton.

Wang, P.S., Berglund, P., Olfson, M., et al. (2005). Failure and delay in initial treatment contact after first onset of mental disorders in the national comorbidity survey replication. *Archives of General Psychiatry, 62*(6), 603–613.

# Depressive Disorders

*Mallie Kozy, Elizabeth M. Varcarolis*
*Adapted by Ann-Marie Urban*

## KEY TERMS AND CONCEPTS

affect, 238
anergia, 232
anger, 238
anhedonia, 238
Beck's cognitive triad, 236
diathesis–stress model of depression, 235
dysthymic disorder (DD), 233
electroconvulsive therapy (ECT), 250
hypersomnia, 232
learned helplessness, 236
light therapy, 253

major depressive disorder (MDD), 232
mood disorders, 232
norepinephrine, 235
psychomotor agitation, 238
psychomotor retardation, 238
serotonin, 235
serotonin syndrome, 246
transcranial magnetic stimulation (TMS), 251
vagus nerve stimulation (VNS), 251
vegetative signs of depression, 238

## OBJECTIVES

1. Compare and contrast major depressive disorder and dysthymic disorder.
2. Discuss the links between the diathesis-stress model of depression and the biological model of depression.
3. Assess behaviours in a patient with depression in regard to each of the following areas: (a) affect, (b) thought processes, (c) feelings, (d) physical behaviour, and (e) communication.
4. Formulate five nursing diagnoses for a patient with depression, and include outcome criteria.
5. Name unrealistic expectations a nurse may have while working with a patient with depression, and compare them to your own personal thoughts.
6. Role-play six principles of communication useful in working with patients with depression.

7. Evaluate the advantages of the selective serotonin reuptake inhibitors (SSRIs) over the tricyclic antidepressants (TCAs).
8. Compare and contrast the unique attributes of two of the atypical antidepressants.
9. Write a medication teaching plan for a patient taking a tricyclic antidepressant, including adverse effects, toxic reactions, and other drugs that can trigger an adverse reaction.
10. Write a medication teaching plan for a patient taking a monoamine oxidase inhibitor (MOA), including foods and drugs that are contraindicated.
11. Write a nursing care plan incorporating the recovery model of mental health.
12. Describe the types of depression for which electroconvulsive therapy (ECT) is most helpful.

## ⊖volve WEBSITE

*Visit the Evolve website for Flashcards, Case Studies, and additional testing resources related to the content in this chapter: http://evolve.elsevier.com/Canada/Varcarolis/psychiatric/* Pre-Test interactive review

No textbook chapter can adequately convey the personal pain and suffering experienced by the individual with depression, not to mention the pain, helplessness, and frustration felt by the affected individual's friends and loved ones. However, it is essential for nursing students to gain a fundamental understanding of this group of disorders. People of all ethnicities, cultures, ages, socioeconomic groups, education levels, and geographic areas are susceptible to depressive episodes, but some individuals are more susceptible than others. Virtually all nurses will come into contact with patients with depression or whose primary condition is complicated by depression. This chapter includes basic information and therapeutic tools that will facilitate the care of patients with depression.

## HOW A NURSE HELPED ME
### Diagnosed but Not Forgotten

*After months of my not having any interest in doing anything and withdrawing from friends and family, my husband took me to the hospital emergency room where I was admitted to the hospital's mental health unit and diagnosed with major depressive disorder (MDD). While major depression is common, I believed that this diagnosis would change my life. During my two weeks in hospital, psychiatric nurses helped me to understand the distorted beliefs I had about myself and others. Outside of the one-on-one time with the nurses, they taught me how to incorporate yoga and exercise in my treatment plan. Initially, because of my fear of gaining weight, I wanted to stop taking my venlafaxine (Effexor XR), but the nurses taught me about the importance of taking my medications even once I was feeling better. The nurses also helped me to identify a support system. My husband and girlfriend help me along when I want to give up. I also attend a monthly depression group, and if I feel as though I am slipping back into a depression, I know I can call the mental health clinic or speak to the psychiatric nurse in the emergency department. It has been ten years since I was diagnosed with major depression, and there are still times when I need help; however, I know that my life has changed and is not over.*

## CLINICAL PICTURE

This chapter describes several subtypes of major depressive disorder, as well as other proposed depressive types currently being researched as potential mood disorders. Mood disorders (also called *affective disorders*) are a group of psychiatric disorders, including depression and bipolar disorder, characterized by a pervasive disturbance of mood that is not caused by an organic abnormality (American Heritage Medical Dictionary, 2007).

### Major Depressive Disorder

Patients with a major depressive disorder (MDD) experience substantial pain and suffering, as well as psychological, social,

and occupational disability. A patient with MDD presents with a history of one or more major depressive episodes and no history of manic or hypomanic episodes. The symptoms of MDD interfere with the person's social or occupational functioning and, in some cases, may include psychotic features. Delusional or psychotic major depression is a severe form of mood disorder characterized by delusions or hallucinations. For example, patients might have delusional thoughts that interfere with their nutritional status (e.g., "God put snakes in my stomach and told me not to eat.").

The emotional, cognitive, physical, and behavioural symptoms experienced during a major depressive episode represent a change in the person's usual functioning. The course of MDD is variable. While 56% of people will experience one episode, approximately 29% will experience two episodes and 15.4% will experience three or more episodes during their life (Patten, Kennedy, Lam, et al., 2009).

### Subtypes
The diagnosis for MDD may include one of the following specifiers to describe the most recent episode of depression:
- **Psychotic features.** Indicates the presence of disorganized thinking, delusions (e.g., delusions of guilt or of being punished for sins, somatic delusions of horrible disease or body rotting, delusions of poverty or going bankrupt), or hallucinations (usually auditory, voices berating person for sins).
- **Melancholic features.** This outdated term indicates a severe form of endogenous depression (not attributable to environmental stressors) characterized by severe apathy, weight loss, profound guilt, symptoms that are worse in the morning, early morning awakening, and often, suicidal ideation.
- **Atypical features.** Refers to dominant vegetative symptoms (e.g., overeating, oversleeping). Onset is younger, psychomotor activities are slow, and anxiety is often an accompanying problem, which may cause misdiagnosis.
- **Catatonic features.** Marked by nonresponsiveness, extreme psychomotor retardation (may seem paralyzed), withdrawal, and negativity.
- **Postpartum onset.** Indicates onset within four weeks after childbirth. It is common for psychotic features to accompany this depression. Severe ruminations or delusional thoughts about the infant signify increased risk of harm to the infant.
- **Seasonal features (seasonal affective disorder [SAD]).** Indicates that episodes mostly begin in fall or winter and remit in spring. These patients have reduced cerebral metabolic activity. SAD is characterized by anergia (lack of energy or passivity), hypersomnia (excessive daytime sleep), overeating, weight gain, and a craving for carbohydrates; it responds to light therapy.

### Premenstrual Dysphoric Disorder
Patients with premenstrual dysphoric disorder have more severe symptoms than premenstrual syndrome. Symptoms begin toward the last week of the luteal phase, are absent in the

**CONSIDERING CULTURE**

*Postpartum Depression in Immigrant Women*

Women who deliver a baby in a country different from the one in which they were born may be at higher risk for postpartum depression (PPD). Various studies have shown that among immigrant populations, postpartum depression rates are around 37% compared to 7% among nonimmigrants (Zelkowitz, Saucier, Wang, et al., 2008). Research shows that risk factors for PPD are the same for immigrants as nonimmigrants, specifically prenatal depression, anxiety, somatic symptoms, and stressful marital relationship. So why is there a higher rate in immigrant women?

One reason is lack of support. Immigrant women report support networks as strong and as large as nonimmigrant women; however, a larger portion of the social network is located in a different country. This distance can put a strain on a marital relationship because immigrant women may expect and need more support from their spouses. Husbands may not be prepared to take on the kind of supportive role required by their wives.

It may be hard to detect PPD in immigrant women because of language barriers and because PPD may manifest itself in somatic complaints. Zelkowitz and colleagues (2008) found that immigrant women with PPD had more somatic complaints than women who did not have depression.

Immigrant women have special needs because of language barriers, geographically distant support networks, increased somatic symptoms, and paternal role strain (Ozeki, 2008). Nurses can develop interventions geared toward increasing support and alleviating physical complaints of female immigrants who have recently delivered.

**Sources:** Ozeki, N. (2008). Transcultural stress factors of Japanese mothers living in the United Kingdom. *Journal of Transcultural Nursing, 19*, 47–54. doi:10.1177/1043659607309137; Zelkowitz, P., Saucier, J.F., Wang, T., et al. (2008). Stability and change in depressive symptoms from pregnancy to two months postpartum in childbearing immigrant women. *Archives of Women's Mental Health, 11*, 1–11. doi:10.1007/s00737-008-0219-y.

week following menses, and include depressed mood, anxiety, affective lability, or persistent and marked anger or irritability. Other symptoms include anergia, overeating, difficulty concentrating, and feeling out of control or overwhelmed, among others.

### Other Specified Depressive Disorders

Other Specified Depressive Disorders included as diagnoses in the fifth edition of the *Diagnostic and Statistical Manual of Mental Disorders (DSM-5)*:

- **Short-duration depressive episode.** Depressive affect with at least four of the eight symptoms of MDD that persists more than four days but less than fourteen days.
- **Recurrent brief depression.** Meets criteria for MDD, but episodes last one day to one week. Depressive episode must

recur at least once per month over 12 months or more. Carries a high risk for suicide.
- **Depressive episode with insufficient symptoms.** Characterized by depressed affect and at least one of the other eight symptoms of MDD that persists at least two weeks.

### Dysthymic Disorder

Dysthymic disorder (DD) is defined as a mood disorder with chronic (long-term) depressive symptoms that are present most of the day, more days than not, for a period of at least two years (Gulli & Hesson, 2003). Individuals who suffer from dysthymic disorder have had their depressive symptoms for years and often cannot pinpoint exactly when they started to feel depressed (Gulli & Hesson, 2003). Although people with dysthymia suffer from social and occupational distress, it is not usually severe enough to warrant hospitalization unless the person becomes suicidal. The usual age of onset ranges from early childhood and teenage years to early adulthood. Patients with DD are at risk for developing major depressive episodes and other psychiatric disorders.

Differentiating MDD from DD can be difficult because the disorders have similar symptoms. The main differences are in the duration and severity of the symptoms (Patten, Kennedy, Lam, et al., 2009).

## EPIDEMIOLOGY

Depression is the leading cause of disability in the world. The lifetime prevalence of a major depressive episode or the total number of adults in Canada who will experience the disorder within their lifetime is 10.8% (Patten, Kennedy, Lam, et al., 2009). The average age of MDD onset is between 15 and 45 years of age (Patten, Kennedy, Lam, et al., 2009). Studies find that MDD is more common in women and in younger age groups; however, its prevalence decreases with age (Patten, Kennedy, Lam, et al., 2009). Several Canadian studies found that MDD tends to have higher prevalence rates in lower-income or unemployed populations and in unmarried or divorced people.

### Children and Adolescents

Children as young as 3 years of age have been diagnosed with depression. MDD is said to occur in as many as 18% of preadolescents, which is perhaps a low estimate because depression in this age group is often underdiagnosed or misdiagnosed as schizophrenia, a personality disorder, or disruptive behaviour disorder (Thorpe, Whitney, Kutcher, et al., 2001). Children and adolescents between 9 and 17 years of age have a 5% to 10% prevalence of depression (Thorpe, Whitney, Kutcher, et al., 2001). Girls 15 years and older are twice as likely as boys of the same age to experience a major depressive episode. The dominant symptom of depression in children and adolescents tends to be irritability (Joska & Stein, 2008).

### Older Adults

Although depression in older adults is common, it is not a normal result of aging. It is estimated that of the 35 million people in Canada over age 65, 2 million (almost 6%) suffer from severe depression, and another 5 million (around 14%) suffer from less severe forms of depression (National Institute of Mental Health, 2007). However, residents in long-term care, inpatients, and patients with dementia are at particular risk for MDD (Thorpe, Whitney, Kutcher, et al., 2001). Many older adults suffer from subsyndromal depression, in which they experience many, but not all, of the symptoms of a major depressive episode. These individuals have an increased risk of developing major depression (National Institute of Mental Health, 2007), and a disproportionate number of older adults with depression are likely to die by suicide. Unfortunately, the symptoms of depression often go unrecognized in this population, although older adults generally make frequent medical visits. Thus, older individuals suffering from depression are at risk for being untreated.

## CO-MORBIDITY

A depressive syndrome frequently accompanies other psychiatric disorders, such as anxiety disorders, schizophrenia, substance abuse, eating disorders, and schizoaffective disorder. People with anxiety disorders (e.g., panic disorder, generalized anxiety disorder, obsessive-compulsive disorder) commonly present with depression, as do people with personality disorders (particularly borderline personality disorder), adjustment disorder, and brief depressive reactions.

Mixed anxiety–depression is perhaps one of the most common psychiatric presentations; however, care needs to be taken since anxiety may be over-recognized and depression under-recognized (Enns, Swenson, McIntyre, et al., 2001). Symptoms of anxiety occur in an average of 60% to 90% of cases of major depression.

The presence of co-morbid anxiety disorder and depression has a negative impact on the disease course. Co-morbidity has been shown to result in a higher rate of suicide, an overlap with eating disorders and attention deficit hyperactivity disorder, greater severity of depression, greater impairment in social and occupational functioning, and poorer response to treatment (Simon & Rosenbaum, 2003; Lam, Kennedy, Grigoriadis, et al., 2009). These effects are especially true in older adults with depression who have coexisting symptoms of anxiety or an anxiety disorder (Lenze, 2003).

The incidence of major depression greatly increases with the occurrence of a medical disorder, and people with chronic medical problems are at a higher risk for depression than those in the general population. Depression is often secondary to a medical condition and may also be secondary to use of substances such as alcohol, cocaine, marijuana, heroin, and even anxiolytics and other prescription medications (Table 14-1). Depression can also be a sequela, or consequence, of bereavement and grief (Chapter 33 has an in-depth discussion of end-of-life issues and bereavement). Depression in young women has also been associated with eating disorders such as anorexia nervosa and bulimia nervosa. Adolescents may also experience anxiety and exhibit antisocial behaviour (Cunningham, Gunn, Alladin, et al., 2008).

**TABLE 14-1   DEPRESSION SECONDARY TO MEDICAL CONDITIONS AND SUBSTANCES OR MEDICATIONS**

| Medical Conditions | |
|---|---|
| Neurological | Epilepsies, Parkinson's disease, multiple sclerosis, Alzheimer's disease |
| Infectious or inflammatory | Neurosyphilis, AIDS |
| Cardiac disorders | Ischemic heart disease, cardiac failure, cardiomyopathies |
| Endocrine | Hypothyroidism, diabetes mellitus, vitamin deficiencies, parathyroid disorders |
| Inflammatory disorders | Collagen-vascular diseases, irritable bowel syndrome, chronic liver disorders |
| Neoplastic disorders | Central nervous system tumours, paraneoplastic syndromes |

| Substances or Medications | |
|---|---|
| Central nervous system depressants | Alcohol, barbiturates, benzodiazepines, clonidine |
| Central nervous system medications | Amantadine, bromocriptine, levodopa, phenothiazines, phenytoin |
| Psychostimulants | Amphetamines, cocaine |
| Systemic medications | Corticosteroids, digoxin, diltiazem, enalapril, ethionamide, isotretinoin, mefloquine, methyldopa, metoclopramide, quinolones, reserpine, statins, thiazides, vincristine |

**Source:** Joska, J.A., & Stein, D.J. (2008). Mood disorders. In R.E. Hales, S.C. Yudofsky, & G.O. Gabbard (Eds.), *Textbook of psychiatry* (5th ed., p. 464). Washington, DC: American Psychiatric Publishing.

## ETIOLOGY

Although many theories attempt to explain the cause of depression, many psychological, biological, and cultural variables make identification of any one cause difficult; furthermore, it is unlikely that there is a single cause for depression. The high variability in symptoms, response to treatment, and course of the illness support the supposition that depression results from a complex interaction of causes. For example, genetic predisposition to the illness combined with childhood stress may lead to significant changes in the central nervous system (CNS) that result in depression (Sadock & Sadock, 2008). However, there seem to be several common risk factors for depression, listed in Box 14-1.

## Biological Factors

### Genetic

Twin studies consistently show that genetic factors play a role in the development of depressive disorders. Various studies reveal that the average concordance rate for mood disorders among monozygotic twins (twins sharing the same genetic material) is about 37%. That is, if one twin is affected, the second has a 37% chance of being affected as well (Joska & Stein, 2008). Increased heritability of mood disorders is associated with an earlier age of onset, greater rate of co-morbidity, and increased risk of recurrent illness. For depression to develop, however, a genetic predisposition must also be affected by environmental factors (Sadock & Sadock, 2008).

### Biochemical

The brain is a highly complex organ that contains billions of neurons. There is much evidence to support the concept that many CNS neurotransmitter abnormalities may cause clinical depression. These neurotransmitter abnormalities may be the result of genetic or environmental factors or even of other medical conditions, such as cerebral infarction, hypothyroidism, acquired immunodeficiency syndrome (AIDS), or drug use.

Specific neurotransmitters in the brain are believed to be related to altered mood states. Two of the main neurotransmitters involved are serotonin (5-hydroxytryptamine [5-HT]) and norepinephrine. Serotonin is an important regulator of sleep, appetite, and libido; therefore, serotonin-circuit dysfunction can result in sleep disturbances, decreased appetite, low sex drive, poor impulse control, and irritability (Joska & Stein, 2008). Norepinephrine modulates attention and behaviour. It is stimulated by stressful situations, which may result in overuse and, subsequently, a deficiency of norepinephrine. A deficiency, an imbalance as compared to other neurotransmitters, or an impaired ability to use available norepinephrine can result in apathy, reduced responsiveness, and slowed psychomotor activity.

At present, research suggests that depression results from the dysregulation of a number of neurotransmitter systems in addition to serotonin and norepinephrine. The dopamine, acetylcholine, and gamma-aminobutyric acid (GABA) systems are also believed to be involved in the pathophysiology of a major depressive episode (Sadock & Sadock, 2008).

Stressful life events, especially losses, seem to be a significant factor in the development of depression. Norepinephrine, serotonin, and acetylcholine play a role in stress regulation. When these neurotransmitters become overtaxed through repeated stressful events, neurotransmitter depletion or kindling may occur.

At this time, no single mechanism of depressant action has been found. The relationships among the serotonin, norepinephrine, dopamine, acetylcholine, and GABA systems are complex and need further assessment and study. However, treatment with medication that helps regulate these neurotransmitters has proved empirically successful in the treatment of many patients. Figure 14-1 shows a positron emission tomographic (PET) scan of the brain of a woman with depression before and after taking medication. Refer to Figure 4-7 for PET scans comparing brain activity in an individual with depression and an individual without depression.

### Alterations in Hormonal Regulation

Although neuroendocrine findings are as yet inconclusive, the neuroendocrine characteristic most widely studied in relation to depression has been hyperactivity of the hypothalamic–pituitary–adrenal cortical axis. People with major depression have increased urine cortisol levels and elevated corticotropin-releasing hormone (Joska & Stein, 2008). Dexamethasone, an exogenous steroid that suppresses cortisol, is used in the dexamethasone suppression test for depression. Results of this test are abnormal in about 50% of people with depression, indicating hyperactivity of the hypothalamic–pituitary–adrenal cortical axis. However, the findings may also be abnormal in people with obsessive-compulsive disorder (OCD) and other medical conditions. Significantly, patients with MDD with psychotic features are among those with the highest rates of nonsuppression of cortisol on the dexamethasone suppression test.

### Diathesis–Stress Model

The diathesis–stress model of depression takes into account the interplay of biology and life events in the development of depressive disorders. It is believed that psychosocial stressors and interpersonal events trigger neurophysical and neurochemical changes in the brain. Early life trauma may result in long-term hyperactivity of the CNS corticotropin-releasing factor (CRF), which releases the cortisol hormone, and norepinephrine systems, with a consequent neurotoxic effect on the hippocampus, which leads to overall neuronal loss. These changes could cause sensitization of the CRF circuits to even mild stress in adulthood, leading to an exaggerated stress response (Gillespie & Nemeroff, 2007).

**FIGURE 14-1** Positron emission tomographic (PET) scans of a 45-year-old woman with recurrent depression. The scan on the left was taken when the patient was on no medication and very depressed. The scan on the right was taken several months later, when the patient was well, after she had been treated with medication for her depression. Note that her entire brain, particularly the left prefrontal cortex, is more active when she is well. **Source:** Courtesy Mark George, MD, Biological Psychiatry Branch, National Institute of Mental Health.

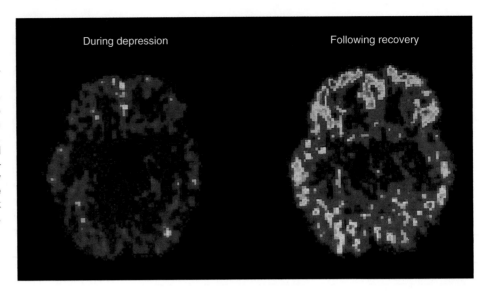

During depression          Following recovery

Some people may be born with a predisposition toward depression, which is then triggered by a stressful life event. The experience of depression further alters the neurological connections in the brain, further increasing the predisposition toward depression. The result is a vicious cycle of recurrent depressive disorder. Early, effective treatment is needed to break the cycle.

### Psychological Factors
#### Cognitive Theory
In cognitive theory, the underlying assumption is that a person's thoughts will result in emotions. If a person looks at his or her life in a positive way, the person will experience positive emotions, but negative interpretation of life events can result in sorrow, anger, and hopelessness. Cognitive theorists believe that people may acquire a psychological predisposition to depression due to early life experiences. These experiences contribute to negative, illogical, and irrational thought processes that may remain dormant until they are activated during times of stress (Beck & Rush, 1995). Beck and Rush (1995) found that people with depression process information in negative ways, even in the midst of positive factors. He believed that automatic, negative, repetitive, unintended, and not readily controllable thoughts perpetuate depression. Three thoughts constitute Beck's cognitive triad:

1. A negative, self-deprecating view of self
2. A pessimistic view of the world
3. The belief that negative reinforcement (or no validation for the self) will continue in the future

Realizing that one has an ability to interpret life events in positive ways provides an element of control over emotions and, therefore, over depression.

#### Learned Helplessness
An older but still plausible theory of depression is that of learned helplessness. Seligman (1973) stated that although anxiety is the initial response to a stressful situation, it is replaced by depression if the person feels no control over the outcome of a situation. A person who believes that an undesired event is his or her fault and that nothing can be done to change it is prone to depression. The theory of learned helplessness has been used to explain the development of depression in certain social groups, such as older adults, people living in impoverished areas, and women.

## APPLICATION OF THE NURSING PROCESS

### ASSESSMENT

Undiagnosed and untreated depression is often associated with more severe presentation of symptoms, greater risk of suicide, somatic problems, and severe anxiety or anxiety disorders. A study by Bijl, van Marwijk, de Haan, and associates (2004) concluded that individuals with depression who manifested psychological symptoms were recognized as having depression 90% of the time, in contrast to those who showed somatic symptoms (e.g., chronic pain, insomnia), who were recognized as having depression 50% of the time, and to those who had a medical disorder, in whom depression was identified 20% of the time.

#### General Assessment
##### Assessment Tools
Numerous standardized depression screening tools that help assess the type of depression are available, including the Beck Depression Inventory, the Hamilton Depression Scale, the Zung Depression Scale, and the Geriatric Depression Scale. Dr. Bagby's Depression Scale, however, is considered the leader in assessing depression. It is particularly useful for assessing depression among East Asians who manifest symptoms of depression as more physical symptoms, valuable given Canada's large East Asian population.

The Patient Health Questionnaire-9 (PHQ-9), a short inventory that highlights predominant symptoms of depression, is presented here because of its ease of use (see Figure 14-2).

The website http://heretohelp.bc.ca/screening/online/, sponsored by the BC Partners for Mental Health and Addictions Information, enables people to take an online confidential screening test for depression and anxiety and find reliable information on the illness.

## PATIENT HEALTH QUESTIONNAIRE-9 (PHQ-9)

| Over the last 2 weeks, how often have you been bothered by any of the following problems? | Not at all | Several days | More than half the days | Nearly every day |
|---|---|---|---|---|
| 1. Little interest or pleasure in doing things | 0 | 1 | 2 | 3 |
| 2. Feeling down, depressed, or hopeless | 0 | 1 | 2 | 3 |
| 3. Trouble falling or staying asleep, or sleeping too much | 0 | 1 | 2 | 3 |
| 4. Feeling tired or having little energy | 0 | 1 | 2 | 3 |
| 5. Poor appetite or overeating | 0 | 1 | 2 | 3 |
| 6. Feeling bad about yourself — or that you are a failure or have let yourself or your family down | 0 | 1 | 2 | 3 |
| 7. Trouble concentrating on things, such as reading the newspaper or watching television | 0 | 1 | 2 | 3 |
| 8. Moving or speaking so slowly that other people could have noticed? Or the opposite — being so fidgety or restless that you have been moving around a lot more than usual | 0 | 1 | 2 | 3 |
| 9. Thoughts that you would be better off dead or of hurting yourself in some way | 0 | 1 | 2 | 3 |

_____0_____ + _____ + _____ + _____

= Total score: _____

If you checked off any problems, how difficult have these problems made it for you to do your work, take care of things at home, or get along with other people?

| Not difficult at all | Somewhat difficult | Very difficult | Extremely difficult |
| ☐ | ☐ | ☐ | ☐ |

**I confirm this information is accurate.** | Patient's/Subject's initials: | Date:

A

### PHQ-9 SCORING CARD FOR SEVERITY DETERMINATION

_for healthcare professional use only_

Scoring—add up all checked boxes on PHQ-9

| Total Score | Depression Severity |
|---|---|
| 0-4 | None |
| 5-9 | Mild |
| 10-14 | Moderate |
| 15-19 | Moderately severe |
| 20-27 | Severe |

B

FIGURE 14-2 **A,** Patient Health Questionnaire-9 (PHQ-9). **B,** Scoring the PHQ-9. **Source:** © 2005 Pfizer, Inc. Developed by Drs. Robert L. Spitzer, Janet B. Williams, Kurt Kroenke, and colleagues.

## Assessment of Suicide Potential

The patient should always be evaluated for suicidal or homicidal ideation. About 15% of people with clinical depression commit suicide (Brendel, Lagomasino, Perlis, et al., 2008). Initial suicide assessment might include the following statements or questions:

- You have said you are depressed. Tell me what that is like for you.
- When you feel depressed, what thoughts go through your mind?
- Have you gone so far as to think about taking your own life?
- Do you have a suicide plan?
- Do you have the means to carry out your plan?

- Is there anything that would prevent you from carrying out your plan?

Refer to Chapter 25 for a detailed discussion of suicide, critical risk factors, warning signs, and strategies for suicide prevention. Also see Case Study and Nursing Care Plan 14-1 on pages 254–256.

## Key Assessment Findings

A depressed mood and anhedonia (loss of ability to experience joy or pleasure in living) are the key symptoms of depression. Almost 97% of people with depression have anhedonia. Anxiety, a common symptom in depression, is seen in about 60% to 90% of patients with depression. Psychomotor agitation may be evidenced by constant pacing and wringing of hands. The slowed movements of psychomotor retardation, however, are more common. Somatic complaints (e.g., headaches, malaise, backaches) are also common. Vegetative signs of depression—alterations in those activities necessary to support physical life and growth (e.g., change in bowel movements and eating habits, sleep disturbances, lack of interest in sex)—are universally present. In primary care, people with MDD experience chronic pain at a rate of 66% and disabling pain at a rate of 41%, compared to 43% and 10%, respectively, of patients who do not have depression (Arnow, Hunkeler, Blasey, et al., 2006).

## Areas to Assess
### Affect

Affect, an objective finding based on the nurse's assessment, is the outward representation of a person's internal state of being. A person who has depression sees the world through grey-coloured glasses. Posture is poor, and the patient may look older than his or her stated age. Facial expressions convey sadness and dejection, and the patient may have frequent bouts of weeping. Conversely, the patient may say that he or she is unable to cry. Feelings of worthlessness, guilt, anger, helplessness, hopelessness, and despair are readily reflected in the person's affect. For example, the patient may not make eye contact, may speak in a monotone, may show little or no facial expression (flat affect), and may make only "yes" or "no" responses. Some individuals can be very depressed yet present as the "smiling depressed."

### Thought Processes

During a depressive episode, the person's ability to solve problems and think clearly is negatively affected. Judgement is poor, and indecisiveness is common, largely because thinking is slow, and memory and concentration are poor. Depressed people also dwell on and exaggerate their perceived faults and failures and are unable to focus on their strengths and successes. They may experience delusions of being punished for doing bad deeds or being a terrible person. Common statements of delusional thinking are "I have committed unpardonable sins," "God wants me dead," and "I am wicked and should die."

### Mood

Mood is the patient's subjective experience of sustained emotions or feelings. Feelings frequently reported by people with depression include anxiety, worthlessness, guilt, helplessness, hopelessness, and anger. Feelings of worthlessness range from feeling inadequate to having an unrealistically negative evaluation of self-worth. These feelings reflect the low self-esteem that is a painful partner to depression. Statements such as "I am no good" and "I'll never amount to anything" are common.

### Feelings

Guilt is a common accompaniment to depression. A person may ruminate over present or past failings. Extreme guilt can assume psychotic proportions (e.g., "I have committed terrible sins, and God is punishing me for my evil ways.").

Helplessness is evidenced by the inability to carry out the simplest tasks (e.g., grooming, doing housework, working, caring for children), because they seem too difficult to accomplish. With feelings of helplessness come feelings of hopelessness, which are particularly correlated with suicidal feelings (Beck, Brown, Berchick, et al., 2006). Even though most depressive episodes are time limited, people experiencing them believe things will never change. This feeling of utter hopelessness can lead people to view suicide as a way out of constant mental pain. Hopelessness, one of the core characteristics of depression and risk factors for suicide, is a combined cognitive and emotional state that includes the following attributes:

- Negative expectations for the future
- Loss of control over future outcomes
- Passive acceptance of the futility of planning to achieve goals
- Emotional negativism, as expressed in despair, despondency, or depression

Anger is a strong feeling of displeasure or hostility. It is a natural outcome of profound feelings of helplessness. Anger in depression is often expressed inappropriately through destruction of property, hurtful verbal attacks, or physical aggression toward others. However, anger may be directed toward the self in the form of suicidal or subsuicidal behaviours (e.g., alcohol abuse, substance abuse, overeating, smoking, etc.). These behaviours often result in feelings of low self-esteem and worthlessness.

### Physical Behaviour

Lethargy and fatigue may result in psychomotor retardation, in which movements are extremely slow, facial expressions are decreased, and the gaze is fixed. The continuum of psychomotor retardation may range from slowed and difficult movements to complete inactivity and incontinence. Psychomotor agitation, in which patients constantly pace, bite their nails, smoke, tap their fingers, or engage in some other tension-relieving activity, may also be observed. At these times, patients commonly feel fidgety and unable to relax.

Grooming, dress, and personal hygiene are markedly neglected. People who usually take pride in their appearance and dress may be poorly groomed and allow themselves to look shabby and unkempt.

Vegetative signs of depression, including changes in eating patterns, sleep patterns, bowel habits, and libido, are universal. About 60% to 70% of people with depression report having anorexia; overeating occurs more often in DD. Many people experience insomnia, wake frequently, and have a total reduction in sleep, especially deep-stage sleep (Sadock & Sadock, 2008). One of the hallmark symptoms of depression is waking at 0300 hrs or 0400 hrs and then staying awake or sleeping for only short periods. The light sleep of a person with depression tends to prolong the agony of depression over a 24-hour period. For some, sleep is increased (hypersomnia) and provides an escape from painful feelings. In any event, sleep is rarely restful or refreshing. Changes in bowel habits depend on other physical symptoms: patients with psychomotor retardation often experience constipation; diarrhea, occurring less frequently, often presents in conjunction with psychomotor agitation. As well, interest in sex often declines during depression, which can further complicate marital and social relationships. Some men experience impotence.

## Communication

A person with depression may speak and comprehend very slowly. The lack of an immediate response by the patient to a remark does not necessarily mean the patient has not heard or chooses not to reply; the patient may need more time to comprehend what was said and then compose a reply. In extreme depression, however, a person may become mute.

## Religious Beliefs and Spirituality

The role of religious beliefs and spirituality in depression is just beginning to be understood. Arehart-Treichel (2006) found that people with depression concerned themselves with spiritual questions, such as "What is the meaning of life?" The author concluded that people with depression and anxiety, like people with other serious illnesses, seek the greater meaning of their experience and look beyond themselves for answers. Doolittle and Farrell (2004) found that certain aspects of faith and religious beliefs, such as belief in a higher power, belief in prayer, and the ability to find meaning in suffering were associated with lower rates of depression. Nurses must assess patients' spiritual health by asking how their depression has affected their faith. Encouraging a connection with religious or spiritual practices that have brought them comfort in the past may be therapeutic.

## Age Considerations

### Assessment of Children and Adolescents

Depression often is overlooked in children and adolescents because mood changes in children are frequently seen as behavioural problems and in adolescents as a part of normal development. Although children with depression may display irritability and disruptive behaviour, sadness and hopelessness are often the core issues (Grayson, 2004). Although it is normal for teens to experience a degree of mood lability, adolescents with depression will have a sustained change in mood, thinking, and motivation; they may become sexually promiscuous or engage in alcohol or substance abuse. Both age groups may withdraw from friends and become preoccupied with death.

### Assessment of Older Adults

It can be easy to overlook depression in older adults because they are more likely to complain of aches and pains than acknowledge feelings of sadness or grief. Depression may exist alongside other illnesses or occur as the result of vascular changes in the brain (National Institute of Mental Health, 2007). Patients and health care professionals may falsely believe that depression is a normal part of aging, but the nurse must assess older adults to see if the level of functioning represents a change from normal patterns.

 **RESEARCH HIGHLIGHT**

### Depression, Spirituality, and Symptom Burden

**Source:** Gusick, G. (2008). The contribution of depression and spirituality to symptom burden in chronic heart failure. *Archives of Psychiatric Nursing, 22,* 53–55. doi:10.1016/j.apnu.2007.10.004.

**Problem**

Heart failure (HF) adds greatly to disease burden in Canada. While the role of psychological factors and symptom burden in chronic illness has been explored, the role of spirituality is less well understood.

**Purpose of Study**

The purpose of the study was to see if spirituality had any relationship to depression and symptom burden in patients with HF.

**Methods**

Adults with HF attending an outpatient clinic were recruited to participate in this exploratory correlational study. The 102 participants completed questionnaires to measure depression, spiritual beliefs, and symptom burden.

**Key Findings**

- There was a positive correlation between depression scores and the frequency and intensity of HF symptoms.
- There was not a significant relationship between spirituality and symptom burden; however, the interaction between depression and spirituality accounted for a greater variance in symptom burden than depression alone. In other words, if a person had a higher depression score, spiritual beliefs appeared to have a positive influence on symptom burden.

**Implications for Nursing Practice**

When symptoms of heart failure worsen, it is usually assumed that the underlying pathology is physical, but this study underscores the fact that heart failure patients need to be screened and treated for depression. Nurses can assess for symptoms of depression and for spiritual beliefs in patients with HF, thus contributing to appropriate reduction in symptom burden.

## Self-Assessment

Patients with depression often reject the advice, encouragement, and understanding of the nurse and others, and they often appear not to respond to nursing interventions and seem resistant to change. Nurses witnessing such behaviours may feel frustrated, hopeless, and annoyed. These problematic responses can be altered by the following:

- Recognizing any unrealistic expectations for yourself or the patient

- Identifying feelings that originate with the patient
- Understanding the roles biology and genetics play in the precipitation and maintenance of a depressed mood

### Unrealistic Expectations of Self

Nursing students and others new to caring for individuals with depression may have unrealistic expectations of themselves and their patients, and problems result when these expectations are not met. Unmet expectations usually result in a nurse's feeling anxious, hurt, angry, helpless, or incompetent. Unrealistic expectations of self and others may be held even by experienced health care workers, a phenomenon contributing to staff burnout. Many of your nursing expectations may not be conscious, but when these expectations are made conscious and are worked through with peers and more experienced clinicians (supervisors), more realistic expectations can be formed and attainable outcomes identified. Realistic expectations of self and the patient can decrease feelings of helplessness and increase a nurse's self-esteem and therapeutic potential.

### Feeling What the Patient Is Feeling

It is not uncommon for nurses and other health care providers to experience intense anxiety, frustration, annoyance, hopelessness, and helplessness while caring for individuals with depression; nurses empathically sense what the patient is feeling. Novice nurses may interpret these emotions as personal reactions toward the patient with whom they are working. However, these feelings can be important diagnostic clues to the patient's experience. You can discuss feelings of annoyance, hopelessness, and helplessness with peers and supervisors to separate personal feelings from those originating with the patient. If personal feelings are not recognized, named, and examined, the nurse is likely to withdraw.

---

**VIGNETTE**

Velma is working with Aleks, a patient with depression who is living at a homeless shelter after losing his job and being evicted from his apartment. Aleks expresses a lot of hopelessness about his future and believes he will never get another job or be able to live on his own. During clinical conference, Velma states that she is feeling threatened and frustrated because Aleks rejects her suggestions and her attempts to help. She confesses that she thinks Aleks is not trying to feel better or improve his situation. Velma spends time reviewing the illness of depression, common behaviours, and patient needs. She also reviews the recovery model of mental illness. In subsequent visits, she refocuses on Aleks and stops giving him suggestions. After four weeks, Aleks has worked out a plan to live with relatives while he undergoes vocational training. He thanks Velma for listening and not making him "feel like a failure."

---

People instinctively avoid situations and other people that arouse feelings of frustration, annoyance, or intimidation. If the nurse also has unresolved feelings of anger and depression, the complexity of the situation is compounded. There is no substitute for competent and supportive supervision to facilitate growth, both professionally and personally. Being supervised by a more experienced clinician and sharing with peers help minimize feelings of confusion, frustration, and isolation and can increase your therapeutic potential and self-esteem while you care for individuals with depression.

---

**📋 ASSESSMENT GUIDELINES**

**Depression**

1. Always evaluate the patient's risk for harm to self or others. Overt hostility is highly correlated with suicide (see Chapter 25).
2. Depression is a mood disorder that can be secondary to a host of medical or other psychiatric disorders, as well as medications. A thorough medical and neurological examination helps determine if the depression is primary or secondary to another disorder. Essentially, evaluate whether:
   - The patient is psychotic
   - The patient has taken drugs or alcohol
   - Medical conditions are present
   - The patient has a history of a co-morbid psychiatric syndrome (eating disorder, borderline or anxiety disorder)
3. Assess the patient's past history of depression, what past treatments worked and did not work, and any events that may have triggered this episode of depression.
4. Assess support systems, family, significant others, and the need for information and referrals.

---

## DIAGNOSIS

Depression is a complex disorder, and individuals with depression have a variety of needs; therefore, nursing diagnoses are many. However, a high priority for the nurse is determining the risk for suicide, and the nursing diagnosis of *Risk for suicide* is always considered. Refer to Chapter 25 for assessment guidelines and interventions for suicidal individuals. Other key targets for nursing interventions are represented by the diagnoses of *Hopelessness, Ineffective coping, Social isolation, Spiritual distress,* and *Self-care deficit* (bathing, dressing, feeding, toileting). Table 14-2 identifies signs and symptoms commonly experienced in depression and offers potential nursing diagnoses.

## OUTCOMES IDENTIFICATION

### The Recovery Model

In 1993, Dr. William Anthony changed the focus of mental health to a focus on recovery from mental illness rather than treatment of it. The recovery model emphasizes that individuals with mental illnesses, including depression, can learn to live with them (Summerville, 2009). Recovery is attained through partnership with health care providers who focus on the patient's strengths. Treatment goals are mutually developed based on the patient's personal needs and values, and interventions are evidenced-informed (Summerville, 2009).

## TABLE 14-2  POTENTIAL NURSING DIAGNOSES FOR DEPRESSION

| SIGNS AND SYMPTOMS | POTENTIAL NURSING DIAGNOSES |
|---|---|
| Previous suicide attempts, putting affairs in order, giving away prized possessions, suicidal ideation (has plan, ability to carry it out), overt or covert statements regarding killing self, feelings of worthlessness, hopelessness, helplessness | Risk for suicide<br>Risk for self-mutilation<br>Risk for self-harm |
| Lack of judgement, memory difficulty, poor concentration, inaccurate interpretation of environment, negative ruminations, cognitive distortions | Altered thought processes |
| Difficulty with simple tasks, inability to function at previous level, poor problem solving, poor cognitive functioning, verbalizations of inability to cope | Ineffective coping<br>Interrupted family processes<br>Risk for impaired attachment<br>Ineffective role performance |
| Difficulty making decisions, poor concentration, inability to take action | Decisional conflict |
| Feelings of helplessness, hopelessness, powerlessness | Hopelessness<br>Powerlessness |
| Questioning of meaning of life and own existence, inability to participate in usual religious practices, conflict over spiritual beliefs, anger toward spiritual deity or religious representatives | Spiritual distress<br>Impaired religiosity<br>Risk for impaired religiosity |
| Feelings of worthlessness, poor self-image, negative sense of self, self-negating verbalizations, feeling of being a failure, expressions of shame or guilt, hypersensitivity to slights or criticism | Chronic low self-esteem<br>Situational low self-esteem |
| Withdrawal, noncommunicativeness, monosyllabic speech, avoidance of contact with others | Impaired social interaction<br>Social isolation<br>Risk for loneliness |
| Vegetative signs of depression: changes in sleeping, eating, grooming and hygiene, elimination, sexual patterns | Self-care deficit (bathing, dressing, feeding, toileting)<br>Imbalanced nutrition: less than body requirements<br>Disturbed sleep pattern<br>Constipation<br>Sexual dysfunction |

## TABLE 14-3  NOC OUTCOMES RELATED TO DEPRESSION

| NURSING OUTCOME AND DEFINITION | INTERMEDIATE INDICATORS | SHORT-TERM INDICATORS |
|---|---|---|
| Depression self-control: Personal actions to minimize melancholy and maintain interest in life events | Reports improved mood<br>Adheres to therapy schedule<br>Takes medication as prescribed<br>Follows treatment plan | Monitors intensity of depression<br>Identifies precursors of depression<br>Plans strategies to reduce effects of precursors<br>Reports changes in symptoms to health care provider |

**Source:** Data from Moorhead, S., Johnson, M., Maas, M., et al. (2008). *Nursing outcomes classification* (4th ed.). St. Louis, MO: Mosby.

Remember that MDD can be a recurrent and chronic illness. Care should be directed not only at resolution of the acute phase but also at long-term management. The nurse and the patient identify realistic outcome criteria and formulate concrete, measurable short-term and intermediate indicators. Each patient is a unique individual, and indicators should be selected according to individual needs.

Table 14-3 presents some outcome criteria from the *Nursing Outcomes Classification (NOC)* (Moorhead, Johnson, Maas, et al., 2008). Indicators for the outcomes of the vegetative or physical signs of depression (e.g., reports adequate sleep) are formulated to show, for example, evidence of weight gain, return to normal bowel activity, sleep duration of six to eight hours per night, or return of sexual desire.

## PLANNING

The planning of care for patients with depression is geared toward the patient's phase of depression, particular symptoms, and personal goals. At all times during the care of a person with depression, nurses and members of the health care team must be cognizant of the potential for suicide; therefore, assessment of risk for self-harm (or harm to others) is ongoing. A combination of therapy (cognitive, behavioural, and interpersonal) and psychopharmacology is an effective approach to the treatment of depression across all age groups.

Be aware that the vegetative signs of depression (e.g., changes in eating, sleeping, sexual satisfaction), as well as changes in concentration, activity level, social interaction, care for personal appearance, and so on, often need targeting. The planning of care for a patient with depression is based on the individual's symptoms and goals, and it attempts to encompass a variety of areas in the person's life. Safety is always the highest priority.

## IMPLEMENTATION

There are three phases in treatment and recovery from major depression:

1. The *acute phase* (six to twelve weeks) is directed at reduction of depressive symptoms and restoration of psychosocial and work function. Hospitalization may be required.
2. The *continuation phase* (four to nine months) is directed at prevention of relapse through pharmacotherapy, education, and depression-specific psychotherapy.
3. The *maintenance phase* (one year or more) of treatment is directed at prevention of reoccurrences of depression.

It is important to keep in mind that the primary goal of both the continuation and maintenance phases is keeping the patient a functional and contributing member of the community after recovery from the acute phase.

### Counselling and Communication Techniques

Some patients with depression may be so withdrawn that they are unwilling or unable to speak. Nurses often experience some difficulty communicating with patients without talking; just sitting with them in silence may seem like a waste of time or be uncomfortable. As anxiety increases, the nurse may start daydreaming, feel bored, remember something that "must be done now," and so on. It is important to be aware, however, that this time can be meaningful, especially for the nurse who has a genuine interest in learning about the patient with depression.

Determining when a withdrawn patient will be able to respond is difficult. However, certain techniques are known to be useful in guiding effective nursing interventions. Some communication techniques to use with a severely withdrawn patient are listed in the Guidelines for Communication: Communication With Severely Withdrawn People box. Counselling guidelines for use with patients with depression are offered in the Guidelines for Communication: Counselling People With Depression box.

### Health Teaching and Health Promotion

One basic premise of the recovery model of mental illness is that each person controls his or her treatment based on individual goals. Within this model, health teaching is especially important because it allows patients to make informed choices.

 **GUIDELINES FOR COMMUNICATION**

*Communicating With Severely Withdrawn People*

| INTERVENTION | RATIONALE |
|---|---|
| When a patient is mute, use the technique of making observations: "There are many new pictures on your wall." "You are wearing your new shoes." "You ate some of your breakfast." | When a patient is not ready to talk, direct questions can raise the patient's anxiety level and frustrate the nurse. Pointing to commonalities in the environment draws the patient into and reinforces reality. |
| Use simple, concrete words. | Slowed thinking and difficulty concentrating impair comprehension. |
| Allow time for the patient to respond. | Slowed thinking necessitates time to formulate a response. |
| Listen for covert messages and ask about suicide plans. | People often experience relief and a decrease in feelings of isolation when they share thoughts of suicide. |
| Avoid platitudes such as "Things will look up," "Everyone gets down once in a while," or "Tomorrow will be better." | Platitudes tend to minimize the patient's feelings and can increase feelings of guilt and worthlessness, because the patient cannot "look up" or "snap out of it." |

Health teaching is also an avenue for providing hope to the patient and should include the following information:

- Depression is an illness that is beyond a person's voluntary control.
- Although it is beyond voluntary control, depression can be managed through medication and lifestyle.
- Illness management depends in large part on understanding personal signs and symptoms of relapse.
- Illness management depends on understanding the role of medication and possible adverse effects of medication.
- Long-term management is best assured if the patient undergoes psychotherapy along with taking medication.
- Identifying and coping with the stress of interpersonal relationships—whether they are familial, social, or occupational—is key to illness management.
- Including the family in discharge planning is also important and helps the patient in the following ways:
  - Increases the family's understanding and acceptance of the family member and helps family recognize the importance of medication adherence during the aftercare period.
  - Increases the patient's use of aftercare facilities in the community.
  - Contributes to higher overall adjustment in the patient after discharge.

## GUIDELINES FOR COMMUNICATION
### *Counselling People With Depression*

| INTERVENTION | RATIONALE |
|---|---|
| Help the patient question underlying assumptions and beliefs and consider alternative explanations for problems. | Reconstructing a healthier and more hopeful attitude about the future can alter depressed mood. |
| Work with the patient to identify cognitive distortions that encourage negative self-appraisal. For example:<br>a. Overgeneralizations<br><br>b. Self-blame<br><br>c. Mind reading<br><br>d. Discounting of positive attributes | Cognitive distortions reinforce a negative, inaccurate perception of self and world.<br>a. The patient takes one fact or event and makes a general rule out of it ("He always …"; "I never …").<br>b. The patient consistently blames self for everything perceived as negative.<br>c. The patient assumes others do not like him or her without any real evidence that assumptions are correct.<br>d. The patient focuses on the negative. |
| Encourage activities that can raise self-esteem. Identify need for (a) problem-solving skills, (b) coping skills, and (c) assertiveness skills. | Many people with depression, especially women, are not taught a range of problem-solving and coping skills. Increasing social, family, and job skills can change negative self-assessment. |
| Encourage exercise, such as running or weight lifting. | Exercise can improve self-concept and potentially shift neurochemical balance. |
| Encourage formation of supportive relationships, such as through support groups, therapy, and peer support. | Such relationships reduce social isolation and enable the patient to work on personal goals and relationship needs. |
| Provide information referrals, when needed, for religious or spiritual information (e.g., readings, programs, tapes, community resources). | Spiritual and existential issues may be heightened during depressive episodes; many people find strength and comfort in spirituality or religion. |

## Promotion of Self-Care Activities

In addition to feelings of hopelessness, despair, and physical discomfort, signs of physical neglect may be apparent, in which case, nursing measures for improving physical well-being and promoting adequate self-care are initiated. Some effective interventions targeting physical needs are listed in Table 14-4. Nurses in the community can work with family members to encourage a family member with depression to perform and maintain his or her self-care activities.

## Milieu Management

When a person has acute and severe depression, admission to an inpatient setting may be indicated. The patient with depression needs protection from suicidal acts and a supervised environment for regulating treatments. Often, being removed from a stressful interpersonal situation increases therapeutic value. Hospitals have protocols regarding the care and protection of the suicidal patient (see Chapter 25).

## Pharmacological Interventions

Because mood disorders are caused by problems with neurotransmitters, it follows that medications that alter brain chemistry are an important component in the treatment of them. In most clinical trials, patients showed a response to antidepressant therapy with reduced depression rate scale scores (Lam, Kennedy, Grigoriadis, et al., 2009). It should be noted, however, that the combination of specific psychotherapies (e.g., CBT, IPT, behavioural) and antidepressant therapy is superior

to either psychotherapy or psychopharmacological treatment alone (Reynolds, Dew, Pollock, et al., 2006).

### Antidepressant Drugs

Antidepressant drugs can positively alter poor self-concept, degree of withdrawal, vegetative signs of depression, and activity level. Target symptoms include the following:
- Sleep disturbance
- Appetite disturbance (decreased or increased)
- Fatigue
- Decreased sex drive
- Psychomotor retardation or agitation
- Diurnal variations in mood (often worse in the morning)
- Impaired concentration or forgetfulness
- Anhedonia

A drawback of antidepressant drugs is that improvement in mood may take one to three weeks or longer. If a patient is acutely suicidal, electroconvulsive therapy (discussed in detail later in this chapter) can be a reliable and effective alternative.

The goal of antidepressant therapy is the complete remission of symptoms (Stahl, 2008). Often, the first antidepressant prescribed is not the one that will ultimately bring about remission; aggressive treatment helps in finding the proper treatment. An adequate trial for the treatment of depression is three months. Individuals experiencing their first depressive episode are maintained on antidepressants for six to nine months after symptoms of depression remit. Some people may have multiple episodes of depression or may have a chronic form (similar to

## TABLE 14-4  INTERVENTIONS TARGETING THE VEGETATIVE SIGNS OF DEPRESSION

| INTERVENTION | RATIONALE |
|---|---|
| **Nutrition—Anorexia** | |
| Offer small, high-calorie and high-protein snacks frequently throughout the day and evening. | Low weight and poor nutrition render the patient susceptible to illness. Small, frequent snacks are more easily tolerated than large plates of food when the patient is anorexic. |
| Offer high-protein and high-calorie fluids frequently throughout the day and evening. | These fluids prevent dehydration and can minimize constipation. |
| When possible, encourage family or friends to remain with the patient during meals. | This strategy reinforces the idea that someone cares, can raise the patient's self-esteem, and can serve as an incentive to eat. |
| Ask the patient which foods or drinks he or she likes. Offer choices. Involve the dietitian. | The patient is more likely to eat the foods provided. |
| Weigh the patient weekly and observe the patient's eating patterns. | Monitoring the patient's status gives the information needed for revision of the intervention. |
| **Sleep—Insomnia** | |
| Provide periods of rest after activities. | Fatigue can intensify feelings of depression. |
| Encourage the patient to get up and dress and to stay out of bed during the day. | Minimizing sleep during the day increases the likelihood of sleep at night. |
| Encourage the use of relaxation measures in the evening (e.g., tepid bath, warm milk). | These measures induce relaxation and sleep. |
| Reduce environmental and physical stimulants in the evening—provide decaffeinated coffee, soft lights, soft music, and quiet activities. | Decreasing caffeine and epinephrine levels increases the possibility of sleep. |
| **Self-Care Deficits** | |
| Encourage the use of toothbrush, washcloth, soap, makeup, shaving equipment, and so forth. | Being clean and well groomed can temporarily increase self-esteem. |
| When appropriate, give step-by-step reminders such as "Wash the right side of your face; now the left." | Slowed thinking and difficulty concentrating make organizing simple tasks difficult. |
| **Elimination—Constipation** | |
| Monitor intake and output, especially bowel movements. | Many patients with depression are constipated. If the condition is not checked, fecal impaction can occur. |
| Offer foods high in fibre, and provide periods of exercise. | Roughage and exercise stimulate peristalsis and help evacuation of fecal material. |
| Encourage the intake of fluids. | Fluids help prevent constipation. |
| Evaluate the need for laxatives and enemas. | These measures prevent fecal impaction. |

the chronicity of diabetes) and benefit from indefinite antidepressant therapy.

Antidepressants may precipitate a psychotic episode in a person with schizophrenia or a manic episode in a patient with bipolar disorder. Patients with bipolar disorder often receive a mood stabilizing drug along with an antidepressant.

***Choosing an antidepressant.*** All antidepressants work to increase the availability of one or more of the neurotransmitters, serotonin, norepinephrine, or dopamine. All antidepressants work equally well; however, a variety of antidepressants or a combination of antidepressants may need to be tried before the most effective regimen is found for an individual patient. Each of the antidepressants has different adverse effects, costs,

safety issues, and maintenance considerations. Selection of the appropriate antidepressant is based on the following considerations (Suehs, Argo, Bendele, et al., 2008):

- Adverse-effect profile (e.g., sexual dysfunction, weight gain)
- Ease of administration
- History of past response
- Safety and medical considerations

The Drug Treatment box provides an overview of antidepressants used in Canada.

***Selective serotonin reuptake inhibitors.*** The selective serotonin reuptake inhibitors (SSRIs) are recommended as first-line therapy for most types of depression. Essentially, the SSRIs selectively block the neuronal uptake of serotonin (e.g., 5-HT,

## DRUG TREATMENT OF PATIENTS WITH MAJOR DEPRESSION

| GENERIC (TRADE) | ACTION | NOTES | ADVERSE EFFECTS | WARNINGS |
|---|---|---|---|---|
| **Selective Serotonin Reuptake Inhibitors (SSRIs)** | | | | |
| Citalopram (Celexa) Fluoxetine (Prozac) Fluvoxamine (Luvox) Paroxetine (Paxil) Sertraline (Zoloft) Escitalopram (Cipralex) | Blocks the reuptake of serotonin | First line of treatment for major depression Some SSRIs activate and others sedate; choice depends on patient symptoms Risk of lethal overdose minimized with SSRIs | Agitation, insomnia, headache, nausea and vomiting, sexual dysfunction, and hyponatremia | Discontinuation syndrome— dizziness, insomnia, nervousness, irritability, nausea, and agitation— may occur with abrupt withdrawal (depending on half-life); taper slowly Contraindicated in people taking MAOIs |
| **Serotonin Norepinephrine Reuptake Inhibitors (SNRIs)** | | | | |
| Venlafaxine (Effexor) Duloxetine (Cymbalta) | Blocks the reuptake of serotonin and norepinephrine | Effexor is a popular next-step strategy after trying SSRIs Cymbalta has the advantage of decreasing neuropathic pain | Hypertension (venlafaxine), nausea, insomnia, dry mouth, sweating, agitation, headache, sexual dysfunction | Monitor blood pressure with Effexor, especially at higher doses and with a history of hypertension Hypertension may be particularly noted in the diastolic measurement Discontinuation syndrome (see SSRIs above) Contraindicated in people taking MAOIs |
| **Norepinephrine Reuptake Inhibitors (NRIs)** | | | | |
| | Blocks the reuptake of norepinephrine and enhances its transmission | Antidepressant effects similar to SSRIs and TCAs Useful with severe depression and impaired social functioning | Insomnia, sweating, dizziness, dry mouth, constipation, urinary hesitancy, tachycardia, decreased libido | Contraindicated in people taking MAOIs |
| **Norepinephrine Dopamine Reuptake Inhibitors (NDRIs)** | | | | |
| Bupropion (Wellbutrin) | Blocks the reuptake of norepinephrine and dopamine Not indicated for patients under 18 years of age | Stimulant action may reduce appetite May increase sexual desire Used as an aid to quit smoking | Agitation, insomnia, headache, nausea and vomiting, seizures (0.4%) | Contraindicated in people taking MAOIs High doses increase seizure risk, especially in people who are predisposed to seizures |
| **Serotonin Norepinephrine Disinhibitors (SNDIs)** | | | | |
| Mirtazapine (Remeron) | Blocks $\alpha_1$-adrenergic receptors that normally inhibit norepinephrine and serotonin | Antidepressant effects equal SSRIs and may occur faster | Weight gain, sedation, dizziness, headache; sexual dysfunction is rare | Drug-induced somnolence exaggerated by alcohol, benzodiazepines, and other CNS depressants Contraindicated in people taking MAOIs |
| **Tricyclic Antidepressants (TCAs)** | | | | |
| Amitriptyline (Elavil) Clomipramine (Anafranil) Nortriptyline (Aventyl) | Inhibits the reuptake of serotonin and norepinephrine Antagonizes adrenergic, histaminergic, and muscarinic receptors | Therapeutic effects similar to SSRIs, but adverse effects are more prominent May work better in melancholic depression TCAs can worsen many cardiac and other medical conditions | Dry mouth, constipation, urinary retention, blurred vision, orthostatic hypotension, cardiac toxicity, sedation | Lethal in overdose Use cautiously in older adults and those with cardiac disorders, elevated intraocular pressure, urinary retention, hyperthyroidism, seizure disorders, and liver or kidney dysfunction Contraindicated in people taking MAOIs |

*Continued*

## DRUG TREATMENT OF PATIENTS WITH MAJOR DEPRESSION—cont'd

| GENERIC (TRADE) | ACTION | NOTES | ADVERSE EFFECTS | WARNINGS |
|---|---|---|---|---|
| **Monoamine Oxidase Inhibitors (MAOIs)** | | | | |
| Phenelzine (Nardil) Tranylcypromine (Parnate) | Inhibits the enzyme monoamine oxidase, which normally breaks down neurotransmitters, including serotonin and norepinephrine | Efficacy similar to other antidepressants, but dietary restrictions and potential drug interactions make this drug type less desirable | Insomnia, nausea, agitation, and confusion Potential for hypertensive crisis or serotonin syndrome with concurrent use of other antidepressants | Contraindicated in people taking other antidepressants Tyramine-rich food could bring about a hypertensive crisis Many other drug interactions |
| Moclobemide (Aurorix, Manerix) | Acts on serotonin, norepinephrine and dopamine | MDD and social anxiety | Nausea and dizziness | Contraindicated if known hypersensitivity to moclobemide |

**Sources:** Canadian Pharmacists Association & Canadian Pharmaceutical Association. (2011). *Compendium of pharmaceuticals and specialties.* Toronto: Canadian Pharmaceutical Association; Lehne, R.A. (2010). *Pharmacology for nursing care* (7th ed.). St. Louis, MO: Saunders; Martinez, M., Marangell, L.B., & Martinez, J.M. (2008). *Psychopharmacology.* In R.E. Hales, S.C. Yudofsky, & G.O. Gabbard (Eds.), *Textbook of psychiatry.* Arlington, VA: American Psychiatric Publishing.

5-HT1 receptors), which increases the availability of serotonin in the synaptic cleft. Refer to Chapter 4 for a more detailed discussion of how the SSRIs work.

SSRI antidepressant drugs have a relatively low adverse-effect profile compared with the older antidepressants (tricyclics—discussed later in this chapter); they do not create dry mouth, blurred vision, or urinary retention, making it easier for patients to take these medications as prescribed. Adherence to the medication regimen is a crucial step toward recovery or remission of symptoms. The SSRIs are effective in depression with anxiety features and depression with psychomotor agitation.

Because the SSRIs cause relatively few adverse effects and have low cardiotoxicity, they are less dangerous than older antidepressants when taken in overdose. The SSRIs, selective serotonin–norepinephrine reuptake inhibitors (SNRIs), and atypical antidepressants have a low lethality risk in suicide attempts, whereas the tricyclic antidepressants have a very high potential for lethality with overdose.

**Indications.** The SSRIs have a broad base of clinical use. In addition to their use in treating depressive disorders, the SSRIs have been prescribed with success to treat some of the anxiety disorders—in particular, obsessive-compulsive disorder and panic disorder (see Chapter 13). Fluoxetine has been found to be effective in treating some women who suffer from late-luteal-phase dysphoric disorder and bulimia nervosa.

**Common adverse reactions.** Agents that selectively enhance synaptic serotonin within the CNS may induce agitation, anxiety, sleep disturbance, tremor, sexual dysfunction (primarily anorgasmia), or tension headache. The effect of the SSRIs on sexual performance may be the most significant undesirable outcome reported by patients. Autonomic reactions (e.g., dry mouth, sweating, weight change, mild nausea, loose bowel movements) may also be experienced with the SSRIs.

**Potential toxic effects.** One rare and life-threatening event associated with SSRIs is serotonin syndrome. This syndrome is

thought to be related to overactivation of the central serotonin receptors, caused by either too high a dose or interaction with other drugs. Symptoms include abdominal pain, diarrhea, sweating, fever, tachycardia, elevated blood pressure, altered mental state (delirium), myoclonus (muscle spasms), increased motor activity, irritability, hostility, and mood change. Severe manifestations can induce hyperpyrexia (excessively high fever), cardiovascular shock, or death. The risk of this syndrome seems to be greatest when an SSRI is administered in combination with a second serotonin-enhancing agent, such as a monoamine oxidase inhibitor (MAOI). A patient should discontinue all SSRIs for two to five weeks before starting an MAOI. Box 14-2 lists the signs and symptoms of serotonin syndrome and gives emergency treatment guidelines. The following Patient and Family Teaching box is a useful tool for teaching patient and family about the SSRIs.

*Tricyclic antidepressants.* The tricyclic antidepressants (TCAs) inhibit the reuptake of norepinephrine and serotonin by the presynaptic neurons in the CNS, increasing the amount of time norepinephrine and serotonin are available to the post-synaptic receptors. This increase in norepinephrine and serotonin in the brain is believed to be responsible for mood elevations.

**Indications.** The sedative effects of the TCAs are attributed to the blockage of histamine receptors (Lehne, 2010). Patients must take therapeutic doses of TCAs for 10 to 14 days or longer before they begin to work; full effects may not be seen for four to eight weeks, but an effect on some symptoms of depression, such as insomnia and anorexia, may be noted earlier. Choosing a TCA for a patient is based on what has worked for the patient or a family member in the past and the drug's adverse effects for that patient.

A stimulating TCA, such as desipramine (Norpramin) may be best for a patient who is lethargic and fatigued. If a more sedating effect is needed for agitation or restlessness, drugs such as amitriptyline (Elavil) and doxepin (Sinequan) may be more

| BOX 14-2 | SEROTONIN SYNDROME: SYMPTOMS AND INTERVENTIONS |
|---|---|

**Symptoms**

- Hyperactivity or restlessness
- Tachycardia → cardiovascular shock
- Fever → hyperpyrexia
- Elevated blood pressure
- Altered mental states (delirium)
- Irrationality, mood swings, hostility
- Seizures → status epilepticus
- Myoclonus, incoordination, tonic rigidity
- Abdominal pain, diarrhea, bloating
- Apnea → death

**Interventions**

- Remove offending agent(s)
- Initiate symptomatic treatment:
  - Serotonin-receptor blockade with cyproheptadine, methysergide, propranolol
  - Cooling blankets, chlorpromazine for hyperthermia
  - Dantrolene, diazepam for muscle rigidity or rigours
  - Anticonvulsants
  - Artificial ventilation
  - Paralysis

| BOX 14-3 | DRUGS TO BE USED WITH CAUTION WITH TRICYCLIC ANTIDEPRESSANTS (TCAS) |
|---|---|

- Monoamine oxidase inhibitors
- Phenothiazines
- Barbiturates
- Oral contraceptives (or other estrogen preparations)
- Anticoagulants
- Some antihypertensives (clonidine, guanethidine, reserpine)
- Benzodiazepines
- Alcohol
- Nicotine

### PATIENT AND FAMILY TEACHING

#### Selective Serotonin Reuptake Inhibitors (SSRIs)

- May cause sexual dysfunction or lack of sex drive. Inform nurse or primary care provider if this occurs.
- May cause insomnia, anxiety, and nervousness. Inform nurse or primary care provider if this occurs.
- May interact with other medications. Tell primary care provider about other medications patient is taking (digoxin, warfarin). SSRIs should not be taken within 14 days of the last dose of a monoamine oxidase inhibitor.
- No over-the-counter drug should be taken without first notifying primary care provider.
- Common adverse effects include fatigue, nausea, diarrhea, dry mouth, dizziness, tremor, and sexual dysfunction or lack of sex drive.
- Because of the potential for drowsiness and dizziness, patient should not drive or operate machinery until these adverse effects are ruled out.
- Alcohol should be avoided.
- Liver and renal function tests should be performed and blood counts checked periodically.
- Medication should not be discontinued abruptly. If adverse effects become bothersome, patient should ask primary care provider about changing to a different drug. Abrupt cessation can lead to serotonin withdrawal.
- Any of the following symptoms should be reported to the primary care provider immediately:
  - Increase in depression or suicidal thoughts
  - Rash or hives
  - Rapid heartbeat
  - Sore throat
  - Difficulty urinating
  - Fever, malaise
  - Anorexia and weight loss
  - Unusual bleeding
  - Initiation of hyperactive behaviour
  - Severe headache

appropriate choices. Regardless of which TCA is given, the initial dose should always be low and increased gradually.

**Common adverse reactions.** The chemical structure of the TCAs closely resembles that of antipsychotic medications, and the anticholinergic actions are similar (e.g., dry mouth, blurred vision, tachycardia, constipation, urinary retention, esophageal reflux). These adverse effects are more common and more severe in patients taking antidepressants than in patients taking antipsychotic medications. They usually are not serious and are often transitory, but urinary retention and severe constipation warrant immediate medical attention. Weight gain is also a common complaint among people taking TCAs.

The α-adrenergic blockade of the TCAs can produce postural-orthostatic hypotension and tachycardia. Postural hypotension can lead to dizziness and increase the risk of falls.

Administering the total daily dose of TCA at night is beneficial for two reasons: (1) most TCAs have sedative effects and thereby aid sleep, and (2) the minor adverse effects occur while the individual is sleeping, which increases adherence to drug therapy.

**Potential toxic effects.** The most serious effects of the TCAs are cardiovascular: dysrhythmias, tachycardia, myocardial infarction, and heart block have been reported. Because the cardiac adverse effects are so serious, TCA use is considered a risk in older adults and patients with cardiac disease. Patients should have a thorough cardiac workup before beginning TCA therapy.

**Adverse drug interactions.** Use of an MAOI along with a TCA is contraindicated. A few of the more common medications usually not given while TCAs are being used are listed in Box 14-3. A patient who is taking any of these medications along with a TCA should have medical clearance, because some of the reactions can be fatal.

**Contraindications.** People who have recently had a myocardial infarction (or other cardiovascular problems), those with narrow-angle glaucoma or a history of seizures, and

- The patient and family should be told that mood elevation may take from 7 to 28 days. Up to six to eight weeks may be required for the full effect to be reached and for major depressive symptoms to subside.
- The family should reinforce this information frequently to the family member with depression, who may have trouble remembering and may respond to ongoing reassurance.
- The patient should be reassured that drowsiness, dizziness, and hypotension usually subside after the first few weeks.
- The patient should be cautioned to be careful working around machines, driving cars, and crossing streets because of possible altered reflexes, drowsiness, or dizziness.
- Alcohol can block the effects of antidepressants. The patient should be told to refrain from drinking.
- If possible, the patient should take the full dose at bedtime to reduce the experience of adverse effects during the day.
- If the bedtime dose (or the once-a-day dose) is missed, the patient should take the dose within three hours; otherwise, the patient should wait until the usual medication time the next day. The patient should not double the dose.
- Suddenly stopping TCAs can cause nausea, altered heartbeat, nightmares, and cold sweats within two to four days. The patient should call the primary care provider or take one dose of the TCA until the primary care provider can be contacted.

women who are pregnant should not be treated with TCAs, except with extreme caution and careful monitoring.

**Patient and family teaching.** Topics for the nurse to discuss when teaching patients and their families about TCA therapy are presented in the above Patient and Family Teaching box.

*Monoamine oxidase inhibitors.* The enzyme monoamine oxidase is responsible for inactivating, or breaking down, certain monoamine neurotransmitters in the brain, such as norepinephrine, serotonin, dopamine, and tyramine. When a person ingests an MAOI, these amines do not get inactivated, and there is an increase of neurotransmitters available for synaptic release in the brain. The increase in norepinephrine, serotonin, and dopamine is the desired effect because it results in mood elevation. The increase in tyramine, on the other hand, poses a problem. When the level of tyramine increases, and it is not inactivated by monoamine oxidase, high blood pressure, hypertensive crisis, and eventually cerebrovascular accident can occur. Therefore, people taking these drugs must reduce or eliminate their intake of foods and drugs that contain high amounts of tyramine (Box 14-4 and Table 14-5).

Because people with depression are often lethargic, confused, and apathetic, adherence to strict dietary limitations may not be realistic. That is why MAOIs, although highly effective, are not often given as a first-line treatment.

**Indications.** MAOIs are particularly effective for people with atypical depression (characterized by mood reactivity, oversleeping, and overeating), along with panic disorder, social phobia, generalized anxiety disorder, obsessive-compulsive disorder, post-traumatic stress disorder, and bulimia. The MAOIs

**BOX 14-4   DRUGS THAT CAN INTERACT WITH MONOAMINE OXIDASE INHIBITORS (MAOIS)**

- Over-the-counter medications for colds, allergies, or congestion (any product containing ephedrine or phenylpropanolamine)
- Tricyclic antidepressants (imipramine, amitriptyline)
- Narcotics
- Antihypertensives (methyldopa, spironolactone)
- Amine precursors (levodopa, l-tryptophan)
- Sedatives (alcohol, barbiturates, benzodiazepines)
- General anesthetics
- Stimulants (amphetamines, cocaine)

commonly used in Canada at present are phenelzine (Nardil) and tranylcypromine sulfate (Parnate).

**Common adverse reactions.** Some common and troublesome long-term adverse effects of the MAOIs are orthostatic hypotension, weight gain, edema, change in cardiac rate and rhythm, constipation, urinary hesitancy, sexual dysfunction, vertigo, overactivity, muscle twitching, hypomanic and manic behaviour, insomnia, weakness, and fatigue.

**Potential toxic effects.** The most serious reaction to the MAOIs is an increase in blood pressure, with the possible development of intracranial hemorrhage, hyperpyrexia, convulsions, coma, and death. Therefore, routine monitoring of blood pressure, especially during the first six weeks of treatment, is necessary.

Because many drugs, foods, and beverages can cause an increase in blood pressure in patients taking MAOIs, hypertensive crisis is a constant concern. The beginning of a hypertensive crisis usually occurs within a few hours of ingestion of the contraindicated substance. The crisis may begin with headaches, stiff or sore neck, palpitations, increase or decrease in heart rate (often associated with chest pain), nausea, vomiting, or increase in temperature (pyrexia). When a hypertensive crisis is suspected, immediate medical attention is crucial. Antihypertensive medications such as the calcium channel blocker nifedipine or an α-adrenergic blocker such as phentolamine may be given (Martinez, Marangell, & Martinez, 2008). Pyrexia is treated with hypothermic blankets or ice packs.

Table 14-6 identifies common adverse effects and toxic effects of the MAOIs, and the following Patient and Family Teaching box can be used as an MAOI teaching guide for patients and their families.

**Contraindications.** The use of MAOIs may be contraindicated with each of the following:

- Cerebrovascular disease
- Hypertension and congestive heart failure
- Liver disease
- Consumption of foods containing tyramine, tryptophan, and dopamine (see Table 14-5)
- Use of certain medications (see Box 14-4)
- Recurrent or severe headaches
- Surgery in the previous 10 to 14 days
- Age younger than 16 years

## TABLE 14-5 FOODS THAT CAN INTERACT WITH MONOAMINE OXIDASE INHIBITORS (MAOIS)

### FOODS THAT CONTAIN TYRAMINE

| CATEGORY | UNSAFE FOODS (HIGH TYRAMINE CONTENT) | SAFE FOODS (LITTLE OR NO TYRAMINE) |
|---|---|---|
| Vegetables | Avocados, especially if overripe; fermented bean curd; fermented soybean; soybean paste | Most vegetables |
| Fruits | Figs, especially if overripe; bananas, in large amounts | Most fruits |
| Meats | Meats that are fermented, smoked, or otherwise aged; spoiled meats; liver, unless very fresh | Meats that are known to be fresh (exercise caution in restaurants; meats may not be fresh) |
| Sausages | Fermented varieties; bologna, pepperoni, salami, others | Nonfermented varieties |
| Fish | Dried or cured fish; fish that is fermented, smoked, or otherwise aged; spoiled fish | Fish that is known to be fresh; vacuum-packed fish, if eaten promptly or refrigerated only briefly after opening |
| Milk, milk products | Practically all cheeses | Milk, yogurt, cottage cheese, cream cheese |
| Foods with yeast | Yeast extract (e.g., Marmite, Bovril) | Baked goods that contain yeast |
| Beer, wine | Some imported beers, Chianti wines | Major domestic brands of beer; most wines |
| Other foods | Protein dietary supplements; soups (may contain protein extract); shrimp paste; soy sauce | |

### FOODS THAT CONTAIN OTHER VASOPRESSORS

| FOOD | COMMENTS |
|---|---|
| Chocolate | Contains phenylethylamine, a pressor agent; large amounts can cause a reaction. |
| Fava beans | Contain dopamine, a pressor agent; reactions are most likely with overripe beans. |
| Ginseng | Headache, tremulousness, and mania-like reactions have occurred. |
| Caffeinated beverages | Caffeine is a weak pressor agent; large amounts may cause a reaction. |

**Source:** Lehne, R.A. (2010). *Pharmacology for nursing* (7th ed., p. 351). Philadelphia: Saunders.

## TABLE 14-6 ADVERSE REACTIONS TO AND TOXIC EFFECTS OF MONOAMINE OXIDASE INHIBITORS (MAOIS)

| ADVERSE REACTIONS | COMMENTS |
|---|---|
| Hypotension<br>Insomnia<br>Changes in cardiac rhythm<br>Anorgasmia or sexual impotence<br>Urinary hesitancy or constipation<br>Weight gain | Hypotension is a normal adverse effect of MAOIs.<br>Orthostatic blood pressures should be taken—first lying down, then sitting or standing after one to two minutes. Hypotension may be a dangerous adverse effect, especially in older adults who may fall and sustain injuries as a result of dizziness from the blood pressure drop. |

| TOXIC EFFECTS | COMMENTS |
|---|---|
| Hypertensive crisis:<br>• Severe headache<br>• Tachycardia, palpitations<br>• Hypertension<br>• Nausea and vomiting | Patient should go to local emergency department immediately—blood pressure should be checked.<br>One of the following may be given to lower blood pressure:<br>• 5 mg intravenous phentolamine (Rogitine)<br>• Sublingual nifedipine to promote vasodilation<br>Patients may be prescribed a 10 mg nifedipine capsule to carry in case of emergency. |

**Source:** Data from Canadian Pharmacists Association & Canadian Pharmaceutical Association. (2011). *Compendium of pharmaceuticals and specialties.* Toronto: Canadian Pharmaceutical Association; Fava, M., & Papakostas, G.I. (2008). Antidepressants. In T.A. Stern, J.F. Rosenbaum, M. Fava, et al. (Eds.), *Comprehensive clinical psychiatry* (pp. 595–619). Philadelphia: Mosby; Lehne, R.A. (2010). *Pharmacology for nursing* (7th ed.). Philadelphia: Saunders.

## PATIENT AND FAMILY TEACHING
### Monoamine Oxidase Inhibitors (MAOIs)

- Educate and provide details to the patient and family to avoid certain foods and all medications (especially cold remedies) unless prescribed by and discussed with the patient's primary care provider (see Table 14-5 and Box 14-4 for specific food and drug restrictions).
- Give the patient a wallet card describing the MAOI regimen.
- Instruct the patient to avoid Chinese restaurants (sherry, brewer's yeast, and other contraindicated products may be used).
- Advise the patient to go to the emergency department immediately if he or she has a severe headache.
- Ideally, blood pressure should be monitored during the first six weeks of treatment (for both hypotensive and hypertensive effects).
- After the MAOI is stopped, instruct the patient that dietary and drug restrictions should be maintained for 14 days.

***Use of antidepressants by pregnant women.*** Within the past few years, concerns about the safety of taking antidepressants during pregnancy have increased. Early studies demonstrated an association between TCAs and congenital malformations of the heart and limbs, and MAOI use has been associated with severe hypertension and stroke (Mayo Foundation for Medical Education and Research, 2007). In 2005, Health Canada issued a warning for possible increased risk for birth defects with the use of SSRIs. One study indicated that women who took either SSRIs or TCAs had an increased risk of preterm birth (Iasist, 2008). Another study demonstrated a higher risk for spontaneous abortion with use of antidepressants (Hemels, Einarson, Koren, et al., 2005). Information about the effects of medications during pregnancy can be found through the Motherisk Program (http://www.motherisk.org).

Although these problems have been documented, the overall risk remains small (Mayo Foundation, 2007), and untreated depression presents its own problems. Pregnant women with depression have a higher risk of preterm birth, low-birth-weight infants, substance abuse, and nicotine use (Doskoch, 2001). The decision to take antidepressants while pregnant is one that must be made by carefully weighing the risks and benefits.

***Use of antidepressants by children and adolescents.*** In 2005, Health Canada issued a black-box warning for all antidepressants, alerting the public to the increased risk of suicidal thinking or attempts in children or adolescents under the age of 18 taking antidepressants. Following the black-box warning, the number of prescriptions written for SSRIs for children and young adults decreased, but suicides in those age groups actually increased (Dudley, Hadzi-Pavlovic, Andrews, et al., 2008). Dudley and colleagues concluded that the risk for suicide is greater in children and adolescents with depression who do not take antidepressants. To minimize the risk of suicide in people taking antidepressants, close monitoring by health care providers and patient and caregiver education are essential. Chapter 25 has a more detailed discussion of suicide risk factors and warning signs.

***Use of antidepressants by older adults.*** Polypharmacy and the normal process of aging contribute to concerns about prescribing antidepressants for older adults. SSRIs are a first-line treatment for older adults, but they have the potential for aggravated adverse effects. Starting doses are recommended to be half the lowest adult dose, with dose adjustments occurring no more frequently than every seven days. TCAs and MAOIs have adverse-effect profiles that are more dangerous for older adults, specifically cardiotoxicity with TCAs and hypotension with both classes. Any medication with an adverse effect of hypotension or sedation in older adults increases the risk of falls. Older adults should be cautioned against abrupt discontinuation of antidepressants because of the possibility of discontinuation syndrome, which causes anxiety, dysphoria, flulike symptoms, dizziness, excessive sweating, and insomnia (Akpafflong, Wilson-Lawson, & Kunik, 2008).

### Electroconvulsive Therapy

Electroconvulsive therapy (ECT) is a procedure in which electrical currents are passed through the brain, intentionally triggering a brief seizure. ECT seems to cause changes in brain chemistry that can quickly reverse symptoms of certain mental illnesses. It often works when other treatments are unsuccessful. However, despite being a highly effective somatic (physical) treatment for psychiatric disorders, ECT has a bad reputation. This may be due to media portrayals of patients being restrained on a gurney while having a full-blown seizure induced. Given the current sophistication of anesthetic and paralytic agents, ECT is actually not dramatic at all. Another possible reason for ECT's stigmatized status is that how it works remains a mystery (Stahl, 2008), although researchers have speculated about its mechanism of action. It is likely that the seizure that is induced results in mobilization and activity of neurotransmitters.

### Indications

ECT is used most commonly for depression. While as many as 50% of people taking antidepressants fail to achieve full remission, response rates as high as 80% to 90% have been reported with ECT (Kennedy, Lam, Parikh, et al., 2009), and suicidal thoughts respond to ECT in 80% of cases. Psychotic illnesses are the second most common indication for ECT. For drug-resistant patients, a combination of ECT and antipsychotic medication has resulted in sustained improvement about 80% of the time.

While medication is generally the first line of treatment, according to Sadock and Sadock (2008), ECT may be a primary treatment in the following cases:
- When a patient is suicidal, and there is a need for a rapid, definitive response
- If previous medication trials have failed
- If the patient chooses
- When there is marked agitation, marked vegetative symptoms, or catatonia
- For major depression with psychotic features
- In pregnant women

ECT is useful in treating patients with major depression, especially when psychotic symptoms are present. Patients who have depression with marked psychomotor retardation and

## RESEARCH HIGHLIGHT

### Electroconvulsive Therapy (ECT) and Older Adults

**Source:** Amazon, J., McNeely, E., Lehr, S., et al. (2008). The decision-making process of older adults who elect to receive ECT. *Journal of Psychosocial Nursing, 46*(5), 45–52.

#### Problem

Electroconvulsive therapy (ECT) remains an effective treatment option for people experiencing late-life depression; however, the decision-making process of older adults opting for ECT remains largely misunderstood. Nurses must have a better understanding of this process in order to assist older adults as they make decisions about whether or not to have ECT.

#### Purpose of Study

The purpose of the study was to explore the decision-making process of older adults electing to receive ECT.

#### Methods

Seven older adults between the ages of 60 and 90 who had received ECT participated in this exploratory phenomenological study. Each participant engaged in a one-hour, in-depth interview in which they were asked to describe the process of deciding to receive ECT. The participants' responses were analyzed for common themes.

#### Key Findings

- Four key themes that emerged were:
  - Trust in family, their physician, and God
  - Support from family, friends, and significant others
  - Past experience with positive results from ECT, either for themselves or a friend or acquaintance
  - A sense of desperation to get well
- The overriding substantive theme involved the negative impact of the stigma of both mental illness and ECT. Participants feared what other people would think if their experience of ECT was made known.

#### Implications for Nursing Practice

In addition to providing education and information to older adults considering ECT, psychiatric mental health nurses must also work to break through the stigma and discrimination these patients face.

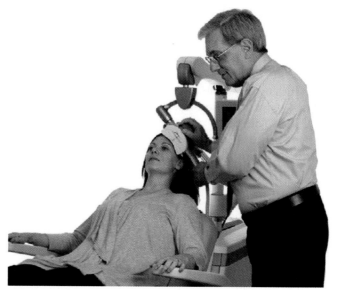

**FIGURE 14-3** Transcranial magnetic stimulation. **Source:** Photo courtesy of Neuronetics.

management. Since the heart can be stressed at the onset of the seizure and for up to ten minutes after, careful assessment and management in patients with hypertension, congestive heart failure, cardiac arrhythmias, and other cardiac conditions are warranted (Welch, 2008). ECT also stresses the brain as a result of increased cerebral oxygen, blood flow, and intracranial pressure. Conditions such as brain tumours and subdural hematomas may increase the risk of using ECT. Providers of care and patients need to weigh the risk of continued disability or potential suicide from depression against ECT treatment risks.

## Transcranial Magnetic Stimulation

Transcranial magnetic stimulation (TMS) is a noninvasive treatment modality that uses MRI-strength magnetic pulses to stimulate focal areas of the cerebral cortex (Figure 14-3). Mitchell and Loo (2006) analyzed 25 studies involving the use of TMS for patients with depression and concluded that benefits were statistically significant and treatment was safe. Ongoing research is needed to determine optimum treatment guidelines (frequency, intensity, and duration) and who would benefit most from this type of procedure.

### Indications

In 2002, Canada approved the use of TMS for patients who have been unresponsive to at least one antidepressant (Kennedy, Milev, Giacobbe, et al., 2009). A large-scale, multisite, randomized controlled trial reported that TMS is an effective stand-alone (without antidepressants) treatment (O'Reardon, Solvason, Janicak, et al., 2007). Studies have been conducted and are underway to research the safety and efficacy of TMS in the treatment of schizophrenia, anxiety disorders, and pain (George, Nahas, Borckardt, et al., 2008).

## Nerve Stimulation

The use of vagus nerve stimulation (VNS) originated as a treatment for epilepsy. VNS is approved in Canada for

stupor also respond well. ECT is also indicated for manic patients whose conditions are resistant to treatment with lithium and antipsychotic drugs and for rapid cyclers. A rapid cycler is a patient with bipolar disorder who has many episodes of mood swings close together (four or more in one year). People with schizophrenia (especially catatonic), those with schizoaffective syndromes, psychotic patients who are pregnant, and patients with Parkinson's disease can also benefit from ECT.

ECT is not necessarily effective, however, in patients with DD, atypical depression, personality disorders, drug dependence, or depression secondary to situational or social difficulties.

The usual course of ECT for a patient with depression is two or three treatments per week to a total of six to twelve treatments. Although no absolute contraindications to ECT exist, several conditions pose risks and require careful workup and

treatment-resistant depression (TRD). Clinicians noted that while VNS decreased seizures, it also appeared to improve mood in a population that normally experiences increased rates of depression (Dougherty & Rauch, 2008). The theory behind VNS relates to the action of the vagus nerve, the longest cranial nerve, which extends from the brain stem to organs in the neck, chest, and abdomen. Researchers believe that electrical stimulation of the vagus nerve results in boosting the level of neurotransmitters, thereby improving mood and also improving the action of antidepressants (Stahl, 2008).

### Indications

Nearly a decade after VNS was approved for use in Europe, the Food and Drug Administration granted approval for VNS use in the United States in 2001 for treatment-resistant depression (Kennedy, Milev, Giacobbe, et al., 2009) (Figure 14-4). The efficacy of VNS in treating depression is still being established. Other potential applications of VNS include anxiety, obesity, and pain (George, Nahas, Borckardt, et al., 2008).

### Advanced-Practice Interventions

Nurses and nurse practitioners are qualified to provide counselling, social skills training, and group therapy (Canadian Nurses Association, 2011; Registered Psychiatric Nurses of Canada, 2011). In some provinces, nurse practitioners who have met appropriate educational standards may also be certified to prescribe medication to treat depression.

### Psychotherapy

Cognitive-behavioural therapy (CBT), interpersonal therapy (IPT), time-limited focused psychotherapy, and behavioural therapy all are considered especially effective in the treatment of mild to moderate depression. However, only CBT and IPT were shown to demonstrate superiority in the maintenance phase. CBT helps people change their negative thought patterns and behaviours, whereas IPT focuses on working through personal relationships that may contribute to depression (Parikh, Segal, Grigoriadis, et al., 2009).

### Group Therapy

Group therapy is a widespread modality for the treatment of depression; it increases the number of people who can receive treatment at a decreased cost per individual. Another advantage is that groups offer patients an opportunity to socialize and share common feelings and concerns, which decreases feelings of isolation, hopelessness, helplessness, and alienation.

### Future of Treatment

There is a great need for earlier detection, earlier intervention, prevention of progression, achievement of remission, and integration of neuroscience and behavioural science in the treatment of depression (Greden, 2004). Goals include the following:
- Improved screening for high-risk ages and groups, including:
  - Individuals in late adolescence and early adulthood
  - Women in reproductive years
  - Adults and older adults with medical problems (e.g., pain)
  - People with a family history of depression
- Increased education, particularly about the linkage between physical symptoms and depression
- Psychopharmacological treatment augmented with cognitive-behavioural therapies
- Inclusion of more supplementary strategies, such as:
  - Promotion of sleep hygiene
  - Increase in exercise
  - Better overall health care

## EVALUATION

Short-term indicators and outcome criteria are frequently evaluated during the course of treatment for depression. For example, if the patient with depression came into the unit with suicidal thoughts, the nurse evaluates whether suicidal thoughts are still present, the patient is able to state alternatives to suicidal impulses in the future, the patient is able to explore thoughts and feelings that precede suicidal impulses, and so forth. Outcomes relating to thought processes, self-esteem, and social interactions are frequently formulated, because these areas are often problematic in people with depression.

Physical needs warrant nursing or medical attention. If a patient has lost weight because of anorexia, is the appetite returning? If the patient was constipated, are the bowels now functioning normally? If the patient was suffering from insomnia, is he or she now sleeping six to eight hours per night? If indicators have not been met, an analysis of the data, nursing diagnoses, goals, and planned nursing interventions is made. The care plan is reassessed and reformulated as necessary.

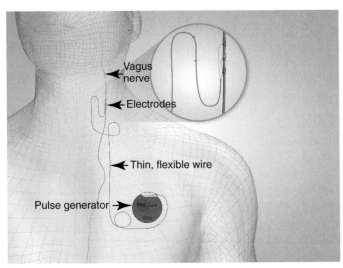

**FIGURE 14-4** Vagus nerve stimulation. **Source:** Image courtesy of Cyberonics, Inc.

## INTEGRATIVE THERAPY

### Complementary, Alternative, and Integrative Approaches

Pilkington, Rampes, and Richardson (2006) highlight an array of complementary, alternative, and integrative approaches in the treatment of depression, including the use of dietary supplements, acupuncture, aromatherapy, meditation, light therapy, homeopathy, and yoga. Herbal products and supplements for depression have become a multimillion-dollar industry; however, the long-term effects of these products have just begun to be studied. Pilkington and colleagues warn that because many of these methods are not well supported by research, they should be used with caution. The approaches briefly discussed here are light therapy, use of St. John's wort, and exercise.

#### Light Therapy

Light therapy has been researched for nearly 20 years and is accepted as a first-line treatment for seasonal affective disorder (SAD). It is estimated that 1% to 3% of Canadians suffer from symptoms of SAD (Lam, Levitt, Levitan, et al., 2006, p. 86). People with SAD often live in regions in which there are marked seasonal differences in the amount of daylight, which is thought to disrupt melatonin production, circadian rhythms, or the ability to process dopamine and norepinephrine. Whatever the cause, the effect is a seasonal depression that can impair the person's ability to cope with life stressors. Light therapy may also be useful as an adjunct in treating chronic MDD or DD with seasonal exacerbations (Ravindran, Lam, Filteau, et al., 2009).

Light therapy is thought to be effective because of the influence of light on melatonin. Melatonin is secreted by the pineal gland and is necessary for maintaining and shifting biological rhythms. Exposure to light suppresses the nocturnal secretion of melatonin, and this suppression seems to have a therapeutic effect on people with SAD (Harvard Medical School, 2008). Ideal treatment consists of 30 to 45 minutes of exposure daily to a 10,000-lux light source. Morning exposure is best; however, success has been reported when exposure occurs at other times of the day or in divided doses. Anecdotal reports suggest that increasing the available light by adding additional light sources may also help to elevate mood. For those affected by SAD, light therapy has been found to be as effective in reducing depressive symptoms as

medications. Adverse effects include headache, eyestrain, and (rarely) hypomania and will subside with decreased exposure. Concerns about eye damage from light exposure have not been validated (Harvard Medical School, 2008).

#### St. John's Wort

St. John's wort (*Hypericum perforatum*) is a flower that can be processed into tea or tablets. It is thought to increase the amount of serotonin, norepinephrine, and dopamine in the brain, resulting in antidepressant effects. Studies of St. John's wort used in the treatment of depression offer mixed results. It has generally been found to be as effective as antidepressants in the treatment of mild to moderate depression (Linde, Berner, & Kriston, 2008; Ravindran, Lam, Filteau, et al., 2009), but usefulness in severe depression has not been established (Ravindran, Lam, Filteau, et al., 2009). Because St. John's wort is not regulated in Canada, concentrations of the active ingredients may vary from preparation to preparation, an inconsistency that may account for some variation in research results. St. John's wort has the potential for adverse reactions when taken with other medications, and safety has not been established for use during pregnancy or use in children.

#### Exercise

Substantial evidence suggests that exercise can enhance mood and counteract symptoms of depression (Harris, Cronkite, & Moos, 2006). Cripps (2008) reports that the effects of exercise on symptoms of depression are biological, social, and psychological. Research shows that exercise increases available serotonin, typically low in depression. It has also been demonstrated to dampen the activity of the hypothalamic–pituitary–adrenocorticoid (HPA) axis, which is believed to be overly active in depression. People with depression who exercise regularly report an elevated mood, a greater feeling of happiness, and more social involvement. Additional benefits of exercise are its easier accessibility, lower expense, and fewer adverse effects as compared with antidepressants.

**Sources:** Cripps, F. (2008). Exercise your mind: Physical activity as a therapeutic technique for depression. *International Journal of Therapy and Rehabilitation, 15*(10), 460–464; Harris, A.H., Cronkite, R., & Moos, R. (2006). Physical activity, exercise coping, and depression in a 10-year cohort study of depressed patients. *Journal of Affective Disorders, 93*, 79–85. doi:10.1016/j.jad.2006.02.013; Harvard Medical School. (2008, January). A SAD story: Light therapy and antidepressants help people who get depressed during the winter. *Harvard Health Letter.* Retrieved from http://www.health.harvard.edu/fhg/updates/Seasonal-affective-disorder.shtml; Linde, K., Berner, M.M., & Kriston, L. (2008). St John's wort for major depression. Cochrane Database System Review, 10(4). doi:10.1002/14651858.CD000448.pub3; Pilkington, K., Rampes, H., & Richardson, J. (2006). Complementary medicine for depression. *Expert Review of Neurotherapeutics, 6*, 1741–1751; Ravindran, A.V., Lam, R.W., Filteau, M.J., et al. (2009). Canadian Network for Mood and Anxiety Treatments (CANMAT) clinical guidelines for the management of major depressive disorder in adults: V. Complementary and alternative medicine treatments. *Journal of Affective Disorders, 117*, S54–S64. Retrieved from http://www.canmat.org/resources/CANMAT%20Depression%20Guidelines%202009.pdf.

## CASE STUDY AND NURSING CARE PLAN 14-1

### *Depression*

Ms. Glessner is a 35-year-old executive secretary. She has been divorced for three years and has two sons, 11 and 13 years of age. She is brought into the emergency department (ED) by her neighbour. She has some slashes on her wrists and is bleeding. The neighbour states that both of Ms. Glessner's sons are visiting their father for the summer. Ms. Glessner has become more and more despondent since terminating a two-year relationship with a married man four weeks previously. According to the neighbour, for three years after her divorce, Ms. Glessner talked constantly about not being pretty or good enough and doubted that anyone could really love her. The neighbour states that Ms. Glessner has been withdrawn for at least three years. After the relationship with her boyfriend ended, she became even more withdrawn and sullen. Ms. Glessner is about 20 pounds overweight, and her neighbour states that Ms. Glessner often stays awake late into the night, drinking by herself and watching television. She sleeps through most of the day on the weekends.

After receiving treatment in the ED, Ms. Glessner is seen by a psychiatrist. The initial diagnosis is dysthymic disorder with suicidal ideation. A decision is made to hospitalize her briefly for suicide observation and evaluation for appropriate treatment.

The nurse, Ms. Ward, admits Ms. Glessner to the unit from the ED.

**Nurse:** "Hello, Ms. Glessner. I'm Marcia Ward. I'll be your primary nurse."

**Ms. Glessner:** "Yeah, I don't need a nurse, a doctor, or anyone else. I just want to get away from this pain."

**Nurse:** "You want to get away from your pain?"

**Ms. Glessner:** "I just said that, didn't I? Oh, what's the use? No one understands."

**Nurse:** "I would like to understand, Ms. Glessner."

**Ms. Glessner:** "Look at me. I'm fat ... ugly ... and no good to anyone. No one wants me."

**Nurse:** "Who doesn't want you?"

**Ms. Glessner:** "My husband didn't want me, and now Jerry has left me to go back to his wife."

**Nurse:** "You think because Jerry went back to his wife that no one else could care for you?"

**Ms. Glessner:** "Well, he doesn't anyway."

**Nurse:** "Because he doesn't care, you believe that no one else cares about you?"

**Ms. Glessner:** "Yes ..."

**Nurse:** "Who do you care about?"

**Ms. Glessner:** "No one ... except my sons. I do love my sons, even though I don't often show it."

**Nurse:** "Tell me more about your sons."

Ms. Ward continues to speak with Ms. Glessner. Ms. Glessner talks about her sons with some affect and apparent affection; however, she continues to state that she does not think of herself as worthwhile.

## ASSESSMENT

### Self-Assessment

Ms. Ward is aware that when patients have depression, they can be negative, think life is hopeless, and be hostile toward those who want to help. When Ms. Ward was new to the unit, she withdrew from patients with depression and sought out patients who appeared more hopeful and appreciative of her efforts. The unit coordinator was very supportive of Ms. Ward when she was first on the unit. Ms. Ward, along with other staff, was sent to clinical education sessions on working with patients with depression and was encouraged to speak up in staff meetings about the feelings many of these patients evoked in her. As a primary nurse, she was assigned a variety of patients. She found that as time went on, with the support of her peers and the opportunity to speak up at staff meetings, she was able to take what patients said less personally and not feel so responsible when patients did not respond as fast as she would like.

After two years, she had had the experience of seeing many patients who seemed hopeless and despondent on admission respond well to nursing and medical interventions and go on to lead full and satisfying lives. This also made it easier for Ms. Ward to understand that even though the patient with depression may think life is hopeless and may believe there is nothing in life to live for, change is always possible.

| Objective Data | Subjective Data |
|---|---|
| Slashed her wrists | "No one wants me." |
| Recently broke up with boyfriend | "I just want to get rid of this pain." |
| Has thought poorly of herself for three years, since divorce | "I'm fat ... ugly ... and no good to anyone." |
| Has two sons she cares about | "I do love my sons, even though I don't often show it." |
| Is 20 pounds overweight | |
| Stays awake late at night, drinking by herself | |
| Has been withdrawn since divorce | |

## DIAGNOSIS

The nurse evaluates Ms. Glessner's strengths and weaknesses and decides to concentrate on two initial nursing diagnoses that seem to have the highest priority:

1. *Risk for suicide* related to separation from two-year relationship, as evidenced by actual suicide attempt

*Continued*

## CASE STUDY AND NURSING CARE PLAN 14-1—cont'd

### *Depression*

**Supporting Data**
- Slashed her wrists
- Recently broke off with boyfriend
- Drinks at night by herself
- Withdrawn for three years since divorce

2. *Situational low self-esteem* related to divorce and recent termination of love relationship, as evidenced by derogatory statements about self

**Supporting Data**
- "No one wants me."
- "I'm fat ... ugly ... and no good to anyone."
- "I do love my sons, even though I don't often show it."

## OUTCOMES IDENTIFICATION

Patient refrains from attempting suicide.

## PLANNING

Because Ms. Glessner is discharged after 48 hours, the issue of disturbance in self-esteem continues to be addressed in her therapy after discharge. Ms. Ward later reviews the goals for her work with Ms. Glessner in the community.

## IMPLEMENTATION

Ms. Glessner's plan of care is personalized as follows:

| Short-Term Goal | Intervention | Rationale | Evaluation |
|---|---|---|---|
| 1. Patient expresses at least one reason to live, apparent by the second day of hospitalization. | 1a. Observe patient every 15 minutes while she is suicidal. <br> 1b. Remove all dangerous objects from patient. <br> 1c. Obtain a "no self-harm" contract with patient for a specific period of time, to be renegotiated (note: some provinces no longer use contracting). <br> 1d. Spend regularly scheduled periods of time with patient throughout the day. <br> 1e. Assist patient in evaluating both positive and negative aspects of her life. <br> 1f. Encourage appropriate expression of angry feelings. <br> 1g. Accept patient's negativism. | 1a, b. Patient safety is ensured. The risk for impulsive self-harmful behaviour is minimized. <br><br> 1c. Contract may help patient gain a sense of control and a feeling of responsibility. <br><br> 1d. This interaction reinforces that the patient is worthwhile and builds her experience in relating better to the nurse on a one-to-one basis. <br> 1e. A person with depression is often unable to acknowledge any positive aspects of life unless they are pointed out by others. <br> 1f. Providing for expression of pent-up hostility in a safe environment can reinforce more adaptive methods of releasing tension and may minimize need to act out self-directed anger. <br> 1g. Acceptance enhances feelings of self-worth. | **GOAL MET** <br> By the end of the second day, Ms. Glessner states she really did not want to die; she just couldn't stand the loneliness in her life. She states that she loves her sons and would never want to hurt them. |

*Continued*

## CASE STUDY AND NURSING CARE PLAN 14-1—cont'd

### Depression

| Short-Term Goal | Intervention | Rationale | Evaluation |
|---|---|---|---|
| 2. Patient will identify two outside supports she can call upon if she feels suicidal in the future. | 2a. Explore usual coping behaviours.<br><br>2b. Assist patient in identifying members of her support system.<br><br>2c. Suggest a number of community-based support groups she might wish to discuss or visit (e.g., hotlines, support groups, women's groups).<br><br>2d. Assist patient in identifying realistic alternatives she is willing to use. | 2a. Behaviours that need reinforcing and new coping skills that need to be introduced can be identified.<br><br>2b. Strengths and weaknesses in her available support can be evaluated.<br><br>2c. Patient needs to be aware of community supports to use them.<br><br>2d. Unless patient agrees with any plan, she will be unable or unwilling to follow through in a crisis. | **GOAL MET**<br>By discharge, Ms. Glessner states that she is definitely going to try cognitive-behavioural therapy. She also discusses joining a women's support group that meets once a week in a neighbouring town. |

### EVALUATION

During the course of her work with Ms. Ward, Ms. Glessner decides to go to some meetings of Parents Without Partners. She states that she is looking forward to getting back to work and feels much more hopeful about her life. She has also lost three pounds while attending Weight Watchers. She states, "I need to get back into the world." Although Ms. Glessner still has negative thoughts about herself, she admits to feeling more hopeful and better about herself, and she has learned important tools to deal with her negative thoughts.

## ■ KEY POINTS TO REMEMBER

- Anxiety is the most common psychiatric disorder.
- There are a number of subtypes of depression and depressive clinical phenomena. The two primary depressive disorders are major depressive disorder (MDD) and dysthymic disorder (DD).
- The symptoms of major depression are usually severe enough to interfere with a person's social or occupational functioning. A person with MDD may or may not have psychotic symptoms, and the symptoms usually exhibited during an episode of major depression are different from the characteristics of the normal personality prior to the onset of MDD.
- The symptoms of DD are often chronic (lasting at least two years) and are considered mild to moderate. Usually a person's social or occupational functioning is not greatly impaired. The symptoms in DD are often congruent with the person's usual pattern of functioning.
- Many theories exist about the cause of depression. The most accepted is biological (genetic and biochemical) factors; however, cognitive theory, learned helplessness theory, and the diathesis–stress theory help explain triggers to depression and maintenance of depressive thoughts and feelings.
- Nursing assessment includes the evaluation of affect, thought processes (especially suicidal thoughts), mood, feelings, physical behaviour, communication, and religious beliefs and spirituality. The nurse also must be aware of the symptoms that may mask depression.
- Nursing diagnoses can be numerous. Individuals with depression are always evaluated for risk for suicide. Some other common nursing diagnoses are *Disturbed thought processes, Chronic low self-esteem, Imbalanced nutrition, Constipation, Disturbed sleep pattern, Ineffective coping,* and *Interrupted family processes.*
- Working with people who have depression can evoke intense feelings of hopelessness and frustration in health care workers. Nurses must clarify expectations of themselves and their patients and sort personal feelings from those communicated by the patient via empathy. Peer supervision and individual supervision by an experienced nurse clinician, psychiatric social worker, or psychologist are useful in increasing therapeutic potential.
- Interventions for patients who have depression involve several approaches. Basic-level interventions include using specific principles of communication, planning activities of daily living, administering or participating in psychopharmacological therapy, maintaining a therapeutic environment, and teaching patients about the biochemical aspects of depression.
- Advanced-practice interventions may include several short-term psychotherapies that are effective in the treatment of

depression, including IPT, CBT, skills training (assertiveness and social skills), and some forms of group therapy.

- Depression is often overlooked in children, adolescents, and older adults because symptoms of depression are often mistaken for signs of normal development.
- Planning and interventions for patients with depression are based on the recovery model, which involves a therapeutic

alliance with health care providers in order to achieve outcomes based on individual patient needs and values.

- Evaluation is ongoing throughout the nursing process, and patients' outcomes are compared with the stated outcome criteria and short-term and intermediate indicators. The care plan is revised when indicators are not being met.

# CRITICAL THINKING

1. You are spending time with Mr. Plotsky, who is undergoing a workup for depression. He hardly makes eye contact, slouches in his seat, and wears a blank but sad expression. Mr. Plotsky has had numerous bouts of major depression in the past and says to you, "This will be my last depression. I will never go through this again."
   a. Since safety is the first concern, what are the appropriate questions to ask Mr. Plotsky at this time?
   b. In terms of behaviours, thought processes, activities of daily living, and ability to function at work and home, give examples of the kinds of signs and symptoms you might find when assessing a patient with depression.
   c. Mr. Plotsky tells you that he has been on every medication there is, but none have worked. He asks you about the herb St. John's wort. What should you tell him about its effectiveness for severe depression, interactions with other antidepressants, and regulatory status?
   d. What might be some somatic options for a person who is resistant to antidepressant medications?
   e. Mr. Plotsky asks what causes depression. In simple terms, how might you respond to his query?

   f. Mr. Plotsky tells you that he has never tried therapy because he thinks it is for weaklings. What information could you give him about various therapeutic modalities that have proven effective for other patients with depression?

2. You are working with Ms. Fok, a 28-year-old with MDD on long-term antidepressant therapy. She asks you about the possibility of pregnancy while taking her SSRIs.
   a. What are some of the things Ms. Fok might want to consider about taking antidepressants if she plans to get pregnant?
   b. If she decides to stop taking her antidepressants, what are some things she might do to help manage her depression?

3. You are working with Mrs. Burton, who has recently been diagnosed with chronic heart failure. In caring for Mrs. Burton, what are two key areas of assessment?

4. What are some of the key areas to consider when working with an older person considering ECT for depression?

# CHAPTER REVIEW

1. The nurse is caring for a patient who exhibits disorganized thinking and delusions. The patient repeatedly states, "I hear voices of aliens trying to contact me." The nurse should recognize this presentation as which type of major depressive disorder (MDD)?
   1. Catatonic
   2. Atypical
   3. Melancholic
   4. Psychotic

2. Which patient statement indicates learned helplessness?
   1. "I am a horrible person."
   2. "Everyone in the world is just out to get me."
   3. "It's all my fault that my husband left me for another woman."
   4. "I hate myself."

3. The nurse is planning care for a patient with depression who will be discharged to home soon. What aspect of teaching should be the priority on the nurse's discharge plan of care?

   1. Pharmacological teaching
   2. Safety risk
   3. Awareness of symptoms of increasing depression
   4. The need for interpersonal contact

4. The nurse is reviewing orders given for a patient with depression. Which order should the nurse question?
   1. A low starting dose of a tricyclic antidepressant
   2. An SSRI given initially with an MAOI
   3. Electroconvulsive therapy to treat suicidal thoughts
   4. Elavil to address the patient's agitation

5. Which of the following are considered vegetative signs of depression?
   1. Hallucinations and delusions
   2. Expressions of guilt and worthlessness
   3. Feelings of helplessness and hopelessness
   4. Changes in physiological functioning such as appetite and sleep disturbances

Ⓔvolve WEBSITE

**Post-Test** interactive review

*Visit the Evolve Web site for Chapter Review Answers and Rationales, Critical Thinking Answer Guidelines, and additional resources related to the content in this chapter: http://evolve.elsevier.com/Canada/Varcarolis/psychiatric/*

## REFERENCES

Akpafflong, M.J., Wilson-Lawson, M., & Kunik, M.E. (2008). Antidepressant-associated side effects in older adult depressed patients. *Geriatrics, 63*(4), 18–23.

*American Heritage Medical Dictionary* (2007). Boston: Houghton Mifflin Company.

Arehart-Treichel, J. (2006). Spirituality tied to higher depression, anxiety rates. *Psychiatric News, 41*(21), 26–28.

Arnow, B.A., Hunkeler, E.M., Blasey, C.M., et al. (2006). Comorbid depression, chronic pain, and disability in primary care. *Psychosomatic Medicine, 68*, 262–268. doi:10.1097/01.psy.0000204851.15499.fc.

Beck, A.T., Brown, G., Berchick, R.J., et al. (2006). Relationship between hopelessness and ultimate suicide: A replication with psychiatric outpatients. *Focus, 4*(2), 291–296.

Beck, A.T., & Rush, A.J. (1995). Cognitive therapy. In H.I. Kaplan & B.J. Sadock (Eds.), *Comprehensive textbook of psychiatry/VI: Vol. 2* (6th ed., pp. 1847–1856). Baltimore, MD: Williams & Wilkins.

Bijl, D., van Marwijk, H.W., de Haan, M., et al. (2004). Effectiveness of disease management programmes for recognition, diagnosis and treatment of depression in primary care. *European Journal of General Practice, 10*, 6–12. doi:10.3109/13814780409094220.

Brendel, R.W., Lagomasino, I.T., Perlis, R.H., et al. (2008). The suicidal patient. In T.A. Stern, J.F. Rosenbaum, M. Fava, et al. (Eds.), *Comprehensive clinical psychiatry* (pp. 733–745). St. Louis, MO: Mosby.

Canadian Nurses Association. (2011). *Advanced nursing practice: A national framework*. Retreived from http://www.cna-aiic.ca/en/search/?q=Advanced%20Practice%20Nurses.

Cunningham, S., Gunn, T., Alladin, A., et al. (2008). Anxiety, depression and hopelessness in adolescents: A structural equation model. *Journal of the Canadian Academy of Child and Adolescent Psychiatry, 17*(3), 137–144.

Doolittle, B., & Farrell, M. (2004). The association between spirituality and depression in an urban clinic. *Primary Care Companion Journal of Clinical Psychiatry, 6*(4), 114–118.

Doskoch, P. (2001). Which is more toxic to a fetus—antidepressants or maternal depression? *Neuropsychiatry Reviews, 2*(5), 1.

Dougherty, D.D., & Rauch, S.L. (2008). Neurotherapeutics. In T.A. Stern, J.F. Rosenbaum, M. Fava, et al. (Eds.), *Comprehensive clinical psychiatry* (pp. 645–650). St. Louis, MO: Mosby.

Dudley, M., Hadzi-Pavlovic, D., Andrews, D., et al. (2008). New-generation antidepressants, suicide and depressed adolescents: How should clinicians respond to changing evidence? *The Australian and New Zealand Journal of Psychiatry, 42*, 456–466. doi:10.1080/00048670802050538.

Enns, M.W., Swenson, R.J., McIntyre, R.S., et al. (2001). Clinical guidelines for the treatment of depressive disorders: VII. Comorbidity. *The Canadian Journal of Psychiatry, 46*(Suppl. 1), 77S–90S. Retrieved from http://ww1.cpa-apc.org:8080/publications/Clinical_Guidelines/depression/clinicalGuidelinesDepression.asp.

George, M.S., Nahas, Z.H., Borckardt, J.J., et al. (2008). Nonpharmacological somatic treatments. In R.E. Hales, S.C. Yudofsky, & G.O. Gabbard (Eds.), *Textbook of psychiatry* (5th ed., pp. 1133–1153). Washington, DC: American Psychiatric Publishing.

Gillespie, C.F., & Nemeroff, C.B. (2007). Corticotropin-releasing factor and the psychobiology of early-life stress. *Current Directions in Psychological Science, 16*, 85–89. doi:10.1111/j.1467-8721.2007.00481.x.

Grayson, C.E. (2004). *Depression in children*. Retrieved from http://www.medicinenet.com/depression_in_children/article.htm#suffer.

Greden, J.F. (2004). *Best practices for achieving remission in depression with physical symptoms: Current and future trends* [Paper presented in

Symposium 10E]. New York: American Psychiatric Association Annual Meeting.

Gulli, L.F., & Hesson, L. (2003). *Dysthymic disorder*. Gale Encyclopedia of Mental Disorders. New York: Gale Publishers.

Hemels, M.E.H., Einarson, A., Koren, G., et al. (2005). Antidepressant use during pregnancy and the rates of spontaneous abortions: A meta-analysis. *The Annals of Pharmacotherapy, 39*, 803–809. doi:10.1345/aph.1E547.

Iasist. (2008). *Agency for Healthcare Research and Quality*. Retrieved from http://www.iasist.com/en/resources/glossary/agency-healthcare-research-and-quality.

Joska, J.A., & Stein, D.J. (2008). Mood disorders. In R.E. Hales, S.C. Yudofsky, & G.O. Gabbard (Eds.), *Textbook of psychiatry* (5th ed., pp. 457–504). Washington, DC: American Psychiatric Publishing.

Kennedy, S.H., Lam, R.W., Parikh, S.V., et al. (2009). Canadian Network for Mood and Anxiety Treatments (CANMAT) clinical guidelines for the management of major depressive disorder in adults. *Journal of Affective Disorders, 117*, S1–S2. Retrieved from http://www.canmat.org/resources/CANMAT%20Depression%20Guidelines%202009.pdf.

Kennedy, S.H., Milev, R., Giacobbe, P., et al. (2009). Canadian Network for Mood and Anxiety Treatments (CANMAT) clinical guidelines for the management of major depressive disorder in adults: IV. Neurostimulation therapies. S44–S53. Retrieved from http://www.canmat.org/resources/CANMAT%20Depression%20Guidelines%202009.pdf.

Lam, R.W., Kennedy, S.H., Grigoriadis, S., et al. (2009). Canadian Network for Mood and Anxiety Treatments (CANMAT). Clinical guidelines for the management of major depressive disorder in adults: III. Pharmacotherapy. *Journal of Affective Disorders*, S26–S43. Retrieved from http://www.canmat.org/resources/CANMAT%20Depression%20Guidelines%202009.pdf.

Lehne, R.A. (2010). *Pharmacology for nursing care* (7th ed.). St. Louis, MO: Saunders.

Lenze, E.J. (2003). Comorbidity of depression and anxiety in the elderly. *Current Psychiatric Reports, 5*, 62–67. doi:10.1007/s11920-003-0011-7.

Martinez, M., Marangell, L.B., & Martinez, J.M. (2008). Psychopharmacology. In R.E. Hales, S.C. Yudofsky, & G.O. Gabbard (Eds.), *Textbook of psychiatry* (5th ed., pp. 1050–1073). Arlington, VA: American Psychiatric Publishing.

Mayo Foundation for Medical Education and Research. (2007). *Antidepressants: Safe during pregnancy?* Retrieved from http://www.mayoclinic.com/health/antidepressants/DN00007.

Mitchell, P.B., & Loo, C.K. (2006). Transcranial magnetic stimulation for depression. *Australian and New Zealand Journal of Psychiatry, 40*(5), 406–413.

Moorhead, S., Johnson, M., Maas, M.L. et al. (2008). *Nursing outcomes classification (NOC)* (4th ed.). St. Louis, MO: Mosby.

National Institute of Mental Health. (2007). *Older adults: Depression and suicide facts* (NIH publication No. 03–4593). Bethesda, MD: National Institutes of Health. Retrieved from http://www.nimh.nih.gov/health/publications/older-adults-depression-and-suicide-facts-fact-sheet/index.shtml.

O'Reardon, J.P., Solvason, H.B., Janicak, P.G., et al. (2007). Efficacy and safety of transcranial magnetic stimulation in the acute treatment of major depression: A multisite randomized controlled trial. *Biological Psychiatry, 62*, 1208–1216. doi:10.1016/j.biopsych.2007.01.018.

Parikh, S.V., Segal, Z.V., Grigoriadis, S., et al. (2009). Canadian Network of Mood and Anxiety Treatments (CANMAT) clinical guidelines for the management of major depressive disorder in adults: II. Psychotherapy alone or in combination with antidepressant medication. *Journal of Affective Disorders*, S15–S25. Retrieved from http://www.canmat.org/resources/CANMAT%20Depression%20Guidelines%202009.pdf.

Patten, S.B., Kennedy, S.H., Lam, R.W., et al. (2009). Canadian Network for Mood and Anxiety Treatments (CANMAT) clinical guidelines for the management of major depressive disorder in adults: I. Classification, burden and principles of management. *Journal of Affective Disorders*, S5–S14. Retrieved from http://www.canmat.org/resources/CANMAT%20Depression%20Guidelines%202009.pdf.

Registered Psychiatric Nurses of Canada. (2011). *Guidelines for registered psychiatric nurses in independent practice*. Retrieved from http://www.rpnc.ca/publications-and-resources.

Reynolds, C.F., III, Dew, M.A., Pollock, B.G., et al. (2006). Maintenance treatment of major depression in old age. *New England Journal of Medicine, 354*(11), 1130–1138.

Sadock, B.J., & Sadock, V.A. (2008). *Concise textbook of clinical psychiatry* (3rd ed.). Philadelphia: Lippincott, Williams, & Wilkins.

Seligman, M.E. (1973). Fall into hopelessness. *Psychology Today, 7*(1), 43–48.

Simon, N.M., & Rosenbaum, J.F. (2003). *Anxiety and depression comorbidity: Implications and intervention*. Retrieved from http://www.medscape.com/viewarticle/451325.

Stahl, S.M. (2008). *Stahl's essential pharmacology*. New York: Cambridge.

Suehs, B.T., Argo, T.R., Bendele, S.D., et al. (2008). *Texas Medication Algorithm Project procedural manual: Major depressive disorder algorithms*. Retrieved from http://www.dshs.state.tx.us/.

Summerville, C. (2009, January). *Recovery: More than "symptom reduction."* Toronto, ON: Paper presented at the Mental Health Commission of Canada. Retrieved from http://channal.ca/wp-content/uploads/2011/03/Presentation_-_Recovery_notes.pdf.

Thorpe, L., Whitney, D.K., Kutcher, S.P., et al. (2001). Clinical guidelines for the treatment of depressive disorders: VI. Special populations. *The Canadian Journal of Psychiatry, 46*(Suppl. 1), 63S–76S. Retrieved from http://ww1.cpa-apc.org:8080/publications/Clinical_Guidelines/depression/clinicalGuidelinesDepression.asp.

Welch, C.A. (2008). Electroconvulsive therapy. In T.A. Stern, J.F. Rosenbaum, M. Fava, et al. (Eds.), *Comprehensive clinical psychiatry* (pp. 635–644). St. Louis, MO: Mosby.

*Margaret Jordan Halter*
*Adapted by Melissa Watkins and Susan L. Ray*

## KEY TERMS AND CONCEPTS

acute phase, 268
anticonvulsant drugs, 272
bipolar I disorder, 262
bipolar II disorder, 262
clang associations, 266
continuation phase, 268
cyclothymia, 262
euphoric mood, 264

flight of ideas, 266
grandiosity, 267
hypomania, 264
maintenance phase, 269
mania, 261
rapid cycling, 262
seclusion protocol, 276

## OBJECTIVES

1. Assess a person experiencing mania for (a) mood, (b) behaviour, and (c) thought processes, and be alert to possible dysfunction.
2. Formulate three nursing diagnoses appropriate for a person with mania, and include supporting data.
3. Explain the rationales behind five methods of communication that may be used with a person experiencing mania.
4. Teach a nursing student at least four expected adverse effects of lithium carbonate therapy.
5. Distinguish between signs of early and severe lithium carbonate toxicity.
6. Write a medication care plan specifying five areas of teaching regarding lithium carbonate.

7. Compare and contrast clinical conditions that may respond better to anticonvulsant therapy with those that may respond better to lithium carbonate therapy.
8. Evaluate specific indications for the use of seclusion for a person experiencing mania.
9. Review at least three of the items presented in the patient and family teaching plan (see Patient and Family Teaching: Bipolar Disorder) with a person with bipolar disorder.
10. Distinguish the focus of treatment for a person in the acute manic phase from the focus of treatment for a person in the continuation or maintenance phase.

## Ⓔvolve WEBSITE

*Visit the Evolve website for Flashcards, Case Studies, and additional testing resources related to the content in this chapter:* *http://evolve.elsevier.com/Canada/Varcarolis/psychiatric/*    Pre-Test   interactive review

Once commonly known as *manic depression*, bipolar disorder is a chronic, recurrent illness that must be carefully managed throughout a person's life. Bipolar disorder frequently goes unrecognized, and people suffer for an average of six years before receiving a proper diagnosis and treatment (Wang, Berglund, Olfson, et al., 2005). Bipolar disorder is marked by shifts in mood, energy, and ability to function. The course of the illness is variable, and symptoms range from severe mania— an exaggerated euphoria or irritability—to severe depression (Figure 15-1). Periods of normal functioning may alternate with periods of illness (highs, lows, or a combination of both). However, many individuals continue to experience chronic interpersonal or occupational difficulties even during remission. According to the Canadian Mental Health Association's *Fast Facts About Mental Illness* (2011), approximately 1% of Canadians will experience bipolar disorder. The mortality rate among individuals with bipolar disorder is two to three times greater than that of the general population and includes higher rates of suicide (Health Canada, 2002).

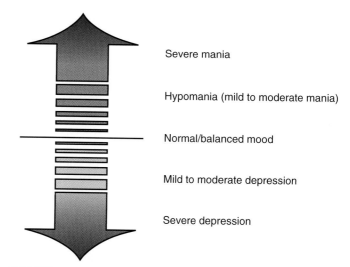

Severe mania

Hypomania (mild to moderate mania)

Normal/balanced mood

Mild to moderate depression

Severe depression

**FIGURE 15-1** Spectrum of symptoms in bipolar disorders. **Source:** Redrawn from U.S. Department of Health and Human Services, National Institute of Mental Health. (2009). *Bipolar disorder* (p. 5). Retrieved from http://www.nimh.nih.gov/health/publications/bipolar-disorder/.

## ✹ HOW A NURSE HELPED ME

### *Support and Care for My Brother and Me*

*Life was always different in our house; there were good days and bad days, but there really wasn't a dull day in our house. To my brother and me, Mom was normal—we knew no differently. But to my friends, Mom was strange and "crazy" sometimes. My brother and I often moved around, from relative to relative and from place to place. When I was 17, my mom had another episode and was in hospital once again, and I was left to raise my little brother. Mom was discharged from hospital after two months of care—a little longer than usual—but I thought nothing of this as Mom had been in and out of hospital throughout my childhood. Everything was settled for the next couple of months, but I noticed Mom giving away household items as well as buying lots of new things for the house, this time really quickly. This was a sign, I had learned over the years, that Mom was becoming unwell again. She had bought a new mobile home and airline tickets for an overseas holiday, something we never actually used. Mom had been admitted to hospital again to stabilize, as the nurses always explained to me. This hospital stay was different, as she stayed in for only two weeks and was provided a case manager to follow up with her at home. The case manager was a nurse who was invaluable to Mom's care, but the nurse was also a wealth of help and care to my brother and me. Mom's case manager came over regularly, talked to Mom about her medications and about her signs and symptoms of becoming unwell but, more importantly,*

*about her ongoing care. The nurse also helped my brother and me understand and watch for signs and symptoms of Mom's bipolar disorder. Mom was stable for a little while, and although she had no money left after the extravagant holiday she'd booked and the new mobile home in our yard, life was more stable, until Mom asked me to join her and the nurse case manager for a chat. I was to find out that Mom had cancer. She'd had it for a while, and the future was not positive. Mom died two months after that chat, and life was yet again upside down for my brother and me. It was the nurse who helped us move forward. We all thought that, since Mom had died, there would be no reason for the nurse to visit, but this was not the case. Not only did she make Mom's last days with us comfortable and some of the most stable times we'd had with Mom, but she continued to visit my brother and me, provide support for us both, and help link us with various community supports. The nurse supported my mom but also my brother and me, and, without this caring nurse and the continued support after Mom died, my brother and I would not have had the happy memories we have of Mom today. It is the nurse we thank not only for teaching us about bipolar disorder but also for bringing us to an understanding and appreciation of what a good mom we had, even during the rough times, and to the realization that there is support for people who are in the same position as my mom.*

## CLINICAL PICTURE

The three types of bipolar disorder currently identified include the following (listed from most to least severe):

- Bipolar I disorder: At least one episode of mania alternates with major depression. Psychosis may accompany the manic episode.
- Bipolar II disorder: Hypomanic episode(s) alternate with major depression. Psychosis is not present in bipolar II. The hypomania of bipolar II disorder tends to be euphoric (an exaggerated feeling of physical and mental well-being, especially when not justified by external reality) and often increases functioning (Benazzi, 2007), and the depression tends to put people at particular risk for suicide.
- Cyclothymia: Hypomanic episodes alternate with minor depressive episodes (at least two years in duration). Individuals with cyclothymia tend to have irritable hypomanic episodes.

The specifier rapid cycling (four or more mood episodes in a 12-month period) is used to indicate more severe symptoms, such as poorer global functioning, high recurrence risk, and resistance to conventional somatic treatments. Rapid cycling is seen in 5% to 15% of people with bipolar disorder (Mood Disorders Society of Canada, 2009). It is estimated to be present in 12% to 24% of patients who go to specialized clinics for mood disorders (Bauer, Beaulieu, Dunner, et al., 2008).

## EPIDEMIOLOGY

Canadian studies looking at lifetime incidence of major depression found that 7.9% to 8.6% of adults over 18 years of age and living in the community met the criteria for a diagnosis of major depression at some time in their lives (Health Canada, 2002). Other studies have reported that between 3% and 6% of adults will experience dysthymia (a serious state of chronic depression that persists for at least two years but is less acute and severe than major depressive disorder) during their lifetime and that between 0.6% and 1% of adults will have a manic episode during their lifetime (Health Canada, 2002).

The median age of onset for bipolar I is 18 years; for bipolar II, the median age of onset is 20 years (Merikangas, Akiskal, Angst, et al., 2007). Bipolar I tends to begin with a depressive episode—in women, 75% of the time; in men, 67% of the time (Sadock & Sadock, 2008). The episodes tend to increase in number and severity during the course of the illness.

Bipolar I disorder seems to be somewhat more common among males, but bipolar II disorder (characterized by the milder form of mania—hypomania—and increased depression) is more common among females (Baldassano, Marangell, Gyulai, et al., 2005). Women with bipolar disorder are more likely to abuse alcohol, commit suicide, and develop thyroid disease; men with bipolar disorder are more likely to have legal problems and commit acts of violence.

According to Vieta and Suppes (2008), bipolar II disorder is underdiagnosed and often mistaken for major depression or personality disorders, when it actually may be the most common form of bipolar disorder. Clinicians may downplay bipolar II and consider it to simply be the milder version of bipolar disorders. However, it is a source of significant morbidity and mortality, particularly due to the occurrence of severe depression. According to Benazzi (2007), one out of two people with depression may have bipolar II.

Cyclothymia usually begins in adolescence or early adulthood. There is a 15% to 50% risk that an individual with cyclothymia will subsequently develop bipolar I or bipolar II disorder.

## CO-MORBIDITY

One large-scale study, with 9282 participants, revealed that more than half of people with bipolar disorder have another Axis I psychiatric disorder (Merikangas, Akiskal, Angst, et al., 2007). Within a lifetime, the most commonly co-occurring disorders for all bipolar disorders were panic attacks (62%), alcohol abuse (39%), social phobia (38%), oppositional defiant disorder (37%), specific phobia (35%), and seasonal affective disorder (35%). Substance use disorders were much higher in bipolar I than in bipolar II disorders. Treatment for substance abuse and bipolar disorder should proceed concurrently whenever possible (Ostacher, 2011).

The incidence of borderline personality disorder occurring along with bipolar disorder is high. Patients who have borderline personality disorder have a 19.4% higher rate of bipolar disorder than do people with other personality disorders (Gunderson, Weinberg, Daversa, et al., 2006).

With advances in a global scientific database, trends are emerging that were previously unknown. One such trend is the relationship between psychiatric illnesses and physically based illnesses. In a study of nearly 37 000 people, several physical disorders were found to be associated with bipolar I (McIntyre, Konarski, Soczynska, et al., 2006). The rates of the following disorders were significantly higher: chronic fatigue syndrome, asthma, migraine, chemical sensitivity, hypertension, bronchitis, and gastric ulcers. The presence of these diseases further complicates the lives of people with bipolar I by impairing their ability to work, increasing their dependence on others, and increasing their need for health care.

## ETIOLOGY

Bipolar disorders are thought to be distinctly different from one another; for example, bipolar I disorder, bipolar II disorder, and cyclothymia have different characteristics. Other variants of bipolar disorder, including a number of other diseases whose end result is bipolar symptomatology, are currently being evaluated (Baum, Akula, Cabanero, et al., 2008; Sklar, Smoller, Fan, et al., 2008; Wellcome Trust Case Council Consortium, 2007).

Episodes of depression in bipolar disorders are different from unipolar depression (i.e., depression without episodes of mania—see Chapter 14). Depressive episodes in bipolar disorder affect younger people, produce more episodes of illness, and require more frequent hospitalization. They are also characterized by higher rates of divorce and marital conflict.

Theories of the development of bipolar disorders focus on biological, psychological, and environmental factors. Most likely, multiple independent variables contribute to the occurrence of bipolar disorder. For this reason, a biopsychosocial approach will likely be the most successful approach to treatment.

## Biological Factors
### Genetic
The bipolar disorders have a strong heritability (i.e., the influence of genetic factors is much greater than the influence of external factors). Bipolar disorders are 80% to greater than 90% heritable, whereas Parkinson's disease, for example, is only 13% to 30% heritable (Burmeister, McInnis, & Zollner, 2008). The rate of bipolar disorders may be as much as five to ten times higher for people who have a relative with bipolar disorder than the rates found in the general population.

It is likely that bipolar disorder is a polygenic disease, which means that a number of genes contribute to its expression. In a landmark study at the National Institute of Mental Health (NIMH), researchers found a connection between bipolar disorder and a genome that encodes an enzyme called *diacylglycerol kinase eta* (DGKH). Lithium carbonate is the first-line therapy for bipolar disorder, and DGKH is a crucial part of a lithium carbonate–sensitive pathway (Baum, Akula, Cabanero, et al., 2008). Other research has focused on abnormal circadian genes that may result in a superfast biological clock, which manifests itself in extreme insomnia (McClung, 2007).

The scientific community has been increasingly drawn to the concept of bipolar disorders and schizophrenia having similar genetic origins and pathology (Owen, Craddock, & Jablensky, 2007). Both disorders exhibit irregularities on chromosomes 13 and 15. It may be that the genotype has more to do with the specific expression of psychoses (altered thought, delusions, and hallucinations) than are reflected in traditional classification systems. Current psychiatric diagnostic systems will undoubtedly be modified as advances are made in molecular genetics, which will revolutionize our understanding and treatment of many psychotic disorders.

### Neurobiological
Neurotransmitters (norepinephrine, dopamine, and serotonin) have been studied since the 1960s as causal factors in mania and depression. One simple explanation is that having too few of these chemical messengers will result in depression, and having an oversupply will cause mania. However, proportions of neurotransmitters in relation to one another may be more important. Receptor site insensitivity could also be at the root of the problem—even if there is enough of a certain neurotransmitter, it is not going where it needs to go.

Additional research has found that the interrelationships in the neurotransmitter system are complex, and more elaborate theories have been developed since the amine hypotheses were originally proposed. Mood disorders are most likely a result of interactions among various chemicals, including neurotransmitters and hormones.

Brain pathways implicated in the pathophysiology of bipolar disorder are located in subregions of the prefrontal cortex (PFC) and medial temporal lobe (MTL). Dysregulation in the neurocircuits surrounding these areas has been viewed through functional imaging (e.g., positron emission tomography [PET] scans, magnetic resonance imaging [MRI]) (Pollock & Kuo, 2004). Neuroimaging studies reveal structural and functional brain changes in people with bipolar disorder. Some structural changes seem to cause the disorder, and some seem to be caused by the disorder. For example, prefrontal cortical changes are evident in the early stages of the illness, whereas lateral ventricle abnormalities develop with repeated episodes of mania or depression (or both) (Strakowski, DelBello, & Adler, 2005). Functional imaging also reveals differences in the anterior limbic regions of the brain, which are associated with emotion, motivation, memory, and fear—the areas most deeply affected by bipolar disorder.

### Neuroendocrine
The hypothalamic–pituitary–thyroid–adrenal (HPTA) axis has been closely scrutinized in people with mood disorders. Hypothyroidism is known to be associated with depressed moods, and it is seen in some patients experiencing rapid cycling. High-dose thyroid hormone administration has been suggested as a method to improve outcomes in treatment-resistant bipolar disorder (Gitlin, 2007).

### Gender
Rates of bipolar disorder among men and women are roughly equal (Mood Disorders Society of Canada, 2009). In 1999, in all except the 5- to 9-year age group, women were hospitalized for bipolar disorder at significantly higher rates than men. This statistic contrasts with the generally accepted equal ratio of prevalence of the disorder among men and women. Further research is needed to explain this distribution. Women were hospitalized for bipolar disorder most frequently between the ages of 40 and 44 years (Health Canada, 2002).

## Psychological Factors
Although there is increasing evidence for genetic and biological vulnerabilities in the etiology of the mood disorders, psychological factors may play a role in precipitating manic episodes for many individuals. In the absence of severe stressful events, it is possible that a person with a genetic predisposition and a neurochemical imbalance may never experience symptoms of bipolar disorder. However, once the disease has been triggered by an event that is perceived as stressful—for example, loss of a relationship, financial difficulties, failing an exam, being accepted to a highly desirable graduate school—it no longer requires environmental stress to continue.

## Environmental Factors
Bipolar disorder is a worldwide problem that generally affects all races and ethnic groups equally, but some evidence suggests that bipolar disorders may be more prevalent in upper socioeconomic classes. The exact reason for this finding is unclear; however, people with bipolar disorders appear to achieve higher

## CONSIDERING CULTURE

### *Cultural Conceptions and Expression of Mental Illness*

After the death of her husband, Mrs. Wong emigrated from China to live with her married daughter. During her first year in Canada, Mrs. Wong had many somatic complaints, such as headache, backache, and chest pain. These physical complaints surfaced in part because, for many, physical pain is socially much more accepted than psychological health problems and also because of the deeply entrenched holistic view of health and illness in Chinese culture. The development of mental illness is commonly attributed to the imbalance of *yin* and *yang*, disturbed flow of *chi* (energy), divine punishment due to failure to comply with ancestor worship rituals, *karma*, genetic vulnerability, physical or emotional strain, organic disorders, and character weakness. Family-shared shame and different cultural perceptions of mental illness and its causes delay treatment among many members of minority groups. Because of her reluctance to seek out a Western medicine practitioner, Mrs. Wong agreed to meet with a traditional Chinese medicine practitioner. The Chinese medicine practitioner helped her to integrate the beliefs of her original culture with resources from her newly adopted country.

**Source:** Wang, M., McCart, A., & Turnbull, A.P. (2007). Implementing positive behavior support with Chinese American families: Enhancing cultural competence. *Journal of Positive Behavior Interventions, 9*, 38–51. Copyright © 2007 by SAGE. Reprinted by Permission of SAGE Publications.

levels of education and higher occupational status than individuals with unipolar depression. The educational levels of individuals with unipolar depressive disorders, on the other hand, appear to be no different from those of individuals with no symptoms of depression within the same socioeconomic class. Also, the proportion of patients with bipolar disorders among creative writers, artists, highly educated men and women, and professional people is higher than in the general population.

## APPLICATION OF THE NURSING PROCESS

### ASSESSMENT

Individuals with bipolar disorder are often misdiagnosed or underdiagnosed. Early diagnosis and proper treatment can help people avoid:

- Suicide attempts
- Alcohol or substance abuse
- Marital or work problems
- Development of medical co-morbidity

Figure 15-2 presents the Mood Disorder Questionnaire (MDQ). This diagnostic test, while not definitive, is a helpful initial screening device.

### General Assessment

The characteristics of mania discussed in the following sections are (1) mood, (2) behaviour, (3) thought processes and speech patterns, and (4) cognitive function.

### Mood

The euphoric mood associated with mania is unstable. During euphoria, patients may state that they are experiencing an intense feeling of well-being, is "cheerful in a beautiful world," or is becoming "one with God." The overly joyous mood may seem out of proportion to what is going on, and cheerfulness may be inappropriate for the circumstances, considering they are full of energy with little or no sleep. Their mood may change quickly to irritation and anger when they are thwarted. The irritability and belligerence may be short-lived, or it may become the prominent feature of the manic phase of bipolar disorder.

People experiencing a manic state may laugh, joke, and talk in a continuous stream, with uninhibited familiarity. They often demonstrate boundless enthusiasm, treat others with confidential friendliness, and incorporate everyone into their plans and activities. They know no strangers, and energy and self-confidence seem boundless.

To people experiencing mania, no aspirations are too high, and no distances are too far—no boundaries exist to curtail them. Often during impulsive, intrusive, and demanding behaviours, they can become easily angered and show a shift in mood at anyone attempting to stop them or set limits.

As the clinical course progresses from hypomania to mania, sociability and euphoria are replaced by a stage of hostility, irritability, and paranoia. The following is a patient's description of the painful transition from hypomania to mania:

> At first when I'm high, it's tremendous ... ideas are fast ... like shooting stars you follow until brighter ones appear ... all shyness disappears, the right words and gestures are suddenly there ... uninteresting people, things become intensely interesting. Sensuality is pervasive; the desire to seduce and be seduced is irresistible. Your marrow is infused with unbelievable feelings of ease, power, well-being, omnipotence, euphoria ... you can do anything ... but somewhere this changes. ... The fast ideas become too fast and there are far too many ... overwhelming confusion replaces clarity ... you stop keeping up with it—memory goes. Infectious humour ceases to amuse—your friends become frightened ... everything now is against the grain ... you are irritable, angry, frightened, uncontrollable, and trapped in the blackest caves of the mind—caves you never knew were there. It will never end. Madness carves its own reality. (Jamison, 1995, p. 70)

### Behaviour

When people experience hypomania, they have voracious appetites for social engagement, spending, and activity, even indiscriminate sex. Constant activity and a reduced need for sleep prevent proper rest. Although short periods of sleep are possible, some patients may not sleep for several days in a row. This nonstop physical activity and the lack of sleep and food can lead to physical exhaustion and even death if not treated; it therefore constitutes an emergency.

When in full-blown mania, a person constantly goes from one activity, place, or project to another. Many projects may be started, but few if any are completed. Inactivity is impossible, even for the shortest period of time. Hyperactivity may range

## MOOD DISORDER QUESTIONNAIRE

*Instructions:* Please answer each question as best you can.

| | Yes | No |
|---|:---:|:---:|
| 1. **Has there ever been a period of time when you were not your usual self and....** | | |
| you felt so good or so hyper that other people thought you were not your normal self or you were so hyper that you got into trouble? | ○ | ○ |
| you were so irritable that you shouted at people or started fights or arguments? | ○ | ○ |
| you felt much more self-confident than usual? | ○ | ○ |
| you got much less sleep than usual and found you didn't really miss it? | ○ | ○ |
| you were much more talkative or spoke much faster than usual? | ○ | ○ |
| thoughts raced through your head or you couldn't slow down your mind? | ○ | ○ |
| you were so easily distracted by things around you that you had trouble concentrating or staying on track? | ○ | ○ |
| you had much more energy than usual? | ○ | ○ |
| you were much more active or did many more things than usual? | ○ | ○ |
| you were much more social or outgoing than usual; for example, you telephoned friends in the middle of the night? | ○ | ○ |
| you were much more interested in sex than usual? | ○ | ○ |
| you did things that were unusual for you or that other people might have thought were excessive, foolish, or risky? | ○ | ○ |
| spending money got you or your family into trouble? | ○ | ○ |
| 2. **If you answered "Yes" to more than one of the above, have several of these ever happened during the same period of time?** | ○ | ○ |

3. **How much of a problem did any of these cause you — like being unable to work; having family, money, or legal troubles; or getting into arguments or fights? Please select one response only.**

   ○ No problem    ○ Minor problem    ○ Moderate problem    ○ Serious problem

| | Yes | No |
|---|:---:|:---:|
| 4. **Have any of your blood relatives (children, siblings, parents, grandparents, aunts, uncles) had manic-depressive illness or bipolar disorder?** | ○ | ○ |
| 5. **Has a health care professional ever told you that you have manic-depressive illness or bipolar disorder?** | ○ | ○ |

*Criteria for Results:* Answering "Yes" to 7 or more of the events in question 1, answering "Yes" to question 2, and answering "Moderate problem" or "Serious problem" to question 3 is considered a positive screen result for bipolar disorder.

**FIGURE 15-2** The Mood Disorder Questionnaire (MDQ). **Source:** Hirschfeld, R., Williams, J., Spitzer, R., et al. (2000). Development and validation of a screening instrument for bipolar spectrum disorder: The Mood Disorder Questionnaire. *American Journal of Psychiatry, 157*(11), 1873–1875. © 2004 Eli Lilly and Company.

from mild, constant motion to frenetic, wild activity. Flowery and lengthy letters are written, and excessive phone calls are made. Individuals become involved in pleasurable activities that can have painful consequences. For example, spending large sums of money on frivolous items, giving money away indiscriminately, or making foolish business investments can leave an individual or family penniless. Sexual indiscretion can dissolve relationships and marriages and lead to sexually transmitted infections. Religious preoccupation is a common symptom of mania.

## RESEARCH HIGHLIGHT

### *Sleep Disruption in the Manic Phase of Bipolar Disorder*

**Source:** Roybal, K., Theobold, D., Graham, A., et al. (2007). Mania-like behaviour induced by disruption of CLOCK. *Proceedings of the National Academy of Sciences of the United States of America, 104,* 6406–6411. doi:10.1073/pnas.0609625104.

#### Problem

One of the most dramatic symptoms of bipolar disorder in the manic phase is sleep disruption. If you have ever stayed awake all night and tried to function the next day, you may have a partial appreciation for the thought impairment, decreased judgement, and emotional dysregulation experienced by people who have been awake for three nights. Researchers believe that a faulty circadian rhythm, the natural 24- to 25-hour sleep–wake cycle monitored by a body clock in the hypothalamus, may be to blame. This connection is strengthened by our knowledge that normal sleep–wake cycles are essential to mood stabilization and that sleep disruptions can trigger mania.

#### Purpose of Study

The purpose of this study was to examine the role of a specific gene in the disruption of circadian rhythms. This gene is the central transcriptional activator of molecular rhythms, or the *Clock gene.*

#### Methods

Researchers mutated the *Clock* gene in mice that served in the study. Next, the researchers implanted electrodes in the medial forebrain bundle of the mice's brains, the area that allows mice to give themselves pleasurable sensations. The researchers then measured the degree of current, or reward, that the mice gave themselves.

#### Key Findings

- *Clock*-mutant mice are similar to bipolar patients in a manic state, in their increased preference for rewarding stimuli, including brain stimulation and cocaine.
- The experimental mice displayed other behaviours associated with mania, including less depressive behaviour and decreased anxiety.
- Lithium carbonate treatment reverses manic-like behaviour in *Clock*-mutant mice.
- Once *Clock*-mutant mice had their functional *Clock* restored, their abnormal behaviour ceased.

#### Implications for Nursing Practice

The study of molecular genetics holds great promise for how people are diagnosed and treated. At a personal level, understanding the mechanics of mania may lessen professional stigma (negative attitudes of health care workers) and even our own attitudes toward people experiencing mania. When you are dealing with someone who is hypertalkative, hypersexual, and constantly making requests, it is fairly easy to become irritated and even resentful. An increased understanding of the physiology behind the disorder can go a long way.

At a hands-on level, the importance of promoting an adaptive sleep–wake cycle in people with mood disorders, particularly people with mania, is highlighted by this study. Teaching aimed at understanding the importance of not "burning the midnight oil" (staying awake all night) is important for everyone but is imperative for people with bipolar disorder. Furthermore, recognizing disturbed sleep patterns may help people to recognize symptoms of impending mania.

---

Individuals experiencing mania may be manipulative, profane, fault finding, and adept at exploiting others' vulnerabilities. They constantly push limits. These behaviours often alienate family, friends, employers, health care providers, and others.

Modes of dress often reflect the person's grandiose yet tenuous grasp of reality. Dress may be described as outlandish, bizarre, colourful, and noticeably inappropriate. Makeup may be garish and overdone. People with mania are highly distractible. Concentration is poor, and individuals with mania go from one activity to another without completing anything. Judgement is poor. Impulsive marriages and divorces can take place.

People often emerge from a manic state startled and confused by the shambles of their lives. The following description conveys one patient's experience:

> Now there are only others' recollections of your behaviour—your bizarre, frenetic, aimless behaviour—at least mania has the grace to dim memories of itself … now it's over, but is it? … Incredible feelings to sort through … Who is being too polite? Who knows what? What did I do? Why? And most hauntingly, will it—when will it—happen again? Medication to take—to resist, to resent, to forget, but always to take. Credit cards revoked … explanations at work … bad cheques and apologies overdue … memory flashes of vague men (what did I do?) … friendships gone, a marriage ruined. (Jamison, 1995, p. 86)

### Thought Processes and Speech Patterns

Flight of ideas is a nearly continuous flow of accelerated speech with abrupt changes from topic to topic that are usually based on understandable associations or plays on words. At times, the attentive listener can keep up with the flow of words, even though the direction changes from moment to moment. Speech is rapid, verbose, and circumstantial (including minute and unnecessary details). When the condition is severe, speech may be disorganized and incoherent. The incessant talking often includes joking, puns, and teasing: "How are you doing, kid? No kidding around, I'm going home … home sweet home … home is where the heart is, the heart of the matter is I want out, and that ain't hay … hey, Doc … get me out of this place."

The content of speech is often sexually explicit and ranges from grossly inappropriate to vulgar. Themes in the communication of the individual with mania may revolve around extraordinary sexual prowess, brilliant business ability, or unparalleled artistic talents (e.g., writing, painting, dancing). The person may actually have only average ability in these areas.

Speech is not only profuse but also loud, bellowing, or even screaming. One can hear the force and energy behind the rapid words. As mania escalates, flight of ideas may give way to clang associations. Clang associations are the stringing together of words because of their rhyming sounds, without regard to their meaning: "Cinema I and II, last row. Row, row, row your boat. Don't be a cutthroat. Cut your throat. Get your goat. Go out and vote. And so I wrote."

Grandiosity (inflated self-regard) is apparent in both the ideas expressed and the person's behaviour. People with mania may exaggerate their achievements or importance, state that they know famous people, or believe they have great powers. They boast of exceptional powers, and status can take delusional proportions during mania. Grandiose persecutory delusions are common. For example, people may think that God is speaking to them or that authorities are out to stop them from saving the world. Sensory perceptions may become altered as the mania escalates, and hallucinations may occur. However, no evidence of delusions or hallucinations is present during hypomania.

### Cognitive Function

The onset of bipolar disorder is often preceded by comparatively high cognitive function. However, there is growing evidence that about one third of patients with bipolar disorder display significant and persistent cognitive problems and difficulties in psychosocial areas. Cognitive deficits in bipolar disorder are milder but similar to those in patients with schizophrenia (Schretlen, Cascella, Meyer, et al., 2007). Cognitive impairments exist in both bipolar I and bipolar II but are more pronounced in bipolar I (Torrent, Sanchez-Moreno, Comes, et al., 2006).

The potential cognitive dysfunction among many people with bipolar disorder has specific clinical implications (Robinson, Thompson, Gallagher, et al., 2006):

- Cognitive function greatly affects overall function.
- Cognitive deficits correlate with a greater number of manic episodes, history of psychosis, chronicity of illness, and poor functional outcome.
- Early diagnosis and treatment are crucial to prevent illness progression, cognitive deficits, and poor outcome.
- Medication selection should consider not only the efficacy of the drug in reducing mood symptoms but also the cognitive impact of the drug on the patient.

### Self-Assessment

The person experiencing mania (who is often out of control and resists being controlled) can elicit numerous intense emotions in a nurse. The person may use humour, manipulation, power struggles, or demanding behaviour to prevent or minimize the staff's ability to set limits on and control dangerous behaviour. People with mania have the ability to "staff split," or divide the staff into the good guys and the bad guys: "The nurse on the day shift is always late with my medication and never talks with me. You are the only one who seems to care." This divisive tactic may pit one staff member or group against another, undermining a unified front and consistent plan of care. Frequent team meetings to deal with the behaviours of the person and the nurses' responses to these behaviours can help minimize staff splitting and feelings of anger and isolation. Limit setting (e.g., lights out after 2300 hrs) is the main theme in treating a person

with mania. Consistency among staff is imperative if the limit setting is to be carried out effectively.

The person can become aggressively demanding, which often triggers frustration, worry, and exasperation in health care providers. The behaviour of a person experiencing mania is often aimed at decreasing the effectiveness of staff control, which could be accomplished by staff members' getting involved in power plays. For example, the person might taunt the staff by pointing out faults or oversights and drawing negative attention to one or more staff members. Usually, this taunting is done in a loud and disruptive manner, which provokes staff to become defensive and thereby escalates the environmental tension and the person's degree of mania.

If you are working with a person experiencing mania, you may find yourself feeling helplessness, confusion, or even anger. Understanding, acknowledging, and sharing these responses and counter-transference reactions will enhance your professional ability to care for the person and perhaps promote your personal development as well. Collaborating with the interprofessional team, accessing the supervision (as a nursing student) of your nursing faculty member, and sharing your

### ⬛ ASSESSMENT GUIDELINES
#### Bipolar Disorder

1. Assess whether the person is a danger to self or others:
   - People experiencing mania can exhaust themselves to the point of death.
   - People experiencing mania may not eat or sleep, often for days at a time.
   - Poor impulse control may result in harm to others or self.
   - Uncontrolled spending may occur.
2. Assess the need for protection from uninhibited behaviours. External control may be needed to protect the person from such things as bankruptcy because people experiencing mania may give away all of their money or possessions.
3. Assess the need for hospitalization to safeguard and stabilize the person.
4. Assess medical status. A thorough medical examination helps to determine whether mania is primary (a mood disorder—bipolar disorder or cyclothymia) or secondary to another condition.
   - Mania may be secondary to a general medical condition.
   - Mania may be substance-induced (caused by use or abuse of a drug or substance or by toxin exposure).
5. Assess for any coexisting medical condition or other situation that warrants special intervention (e.g., substance abuse, anxiety disorder, legal or financial crises).
6. Assess the person's and family's understanding of bipolar disorder, knowledge of medications, and knowledge of support groups and organizations that provide information on bipolar disorder.

experience with peers in postconference may be helpful, perhaps essential.

## NURSING DIAGNOSIS

Nursing diagnoses vary among people experiencing mania. A primary consideration for a person in acute mania is the prevention of exhaustion and death from cardiac collapse. Because of the person's poor judgement, excessive and constant motor activity, probable dehydration, and difficulty evaluating reality, *Risk for injury* is a likely and appropriate diagnosis. Table 15-1 lists potential nursing diagnoses for bipolar disorders.

## OUTCOMES IDENTIFICATION

Outcome criteria will be based on which of the three phases of the illness the patient is experiencing. The *Nursing Outcomes Classification (NOC)* (Moorhead, Johnson, Maas, et al., 2008) provides useful outcomes for each phase.

### Acute Phase

The overall outcome of the acute phase is injury prevention. Outcomes in the acute phase reflect both physiological and psychiatric issues. For example, the patient will:

- Be well hydrated
- Maintain stable cardiac status
- Maintain and obtain tissue integrity
- Get sufficient sleep and rest
- Demonstrate thought self-control
- Make no attempt at self-harm

Relevant *NOC* outcomes for this phase include *Hydration, Cardiac pump effectiveness, Tissue integrity: Skin and mucous membranes, Sleep, Distorted thought self-control,* and *Suicide self-restraint.*

### Continuation Phase

The continuation phase lasts for four to nine months. Although the overall outcome of this phase is relapse prevention, many

| TABLE 15-1 | POTENTIAL NURSING DIAGNOSES FOR BIPOLAR DISORDERS | |
|---|---|
| **SIGNS AND SYMPTOMS** | **NURSING DIAGNOSES** |
| Excessive and constant motor activity<br>Poor judgement<br>Lack of rest and sleep<br>Poor nutritional intake (excessive or relentless mix of above behaviours can lead to cardiac collapse) | *Risk for injury*<br>*Risk for self-neglect* |
| Loud, profane, hostile, combative, aggressive, demanding behaviours | *Risk for other-directed violence*<br>*Risk for self-directed violence*<br>*Risk for suicide* |
| Intrusive and taunting behaviours<br>Inability to control behaviour<br>Rage reaction | *Ineffective coping*<br>*Self-neglect* |
| Manipulative, angry, or hostile verbal and physical behaviours<br>Impulsive speech and actions<br>Property destruction or lashing out at others in a rage reaction | *Defensive coping*<br>*Ineffective coping*<br>*Ineffective impulse control* |
| Racing thoughts, grandiosity, poor judgement | *Ineffective coping*<br>*Ineffective impulse control* |
| Giving away of valuables, neglect of family, impulsive major life changes (divorce, career changes) | *Interrupted family processes*<br>*Caregiver role strain* |
| Continuous pressured speech, jumping from topic to topic (flight of ideas) | *Impaired verbal communication* |
| Constant motor activity, going from one person or event to another<br>Annoyance or taunting of others, loud and crass speech<br>Provocative behaviours | *Impaired social interaction*<br>*Risk for ineffective relationships* |
| Failure to eat, groom, bathe, or dress self because person is too distracted, agitated, and disorganized | *Imbalanced nutrition: less than body requirements*<br>*Deficient fluid volume*<br>*Self-care deficit (bathing, dressing, feeding, toileting)* |
| Inability to sleep because patient is too frantic and hyperactive (sleep deprivation can lead to exhaustion and death) | *Disturbed sleep pattern* |

other outcomes must be accomplished to achieve relapse prevention. These outcomes include:

- Psychoeducational classes for the patient and family related to:
  - Knowledge of disease process
  - Knowledge of medication
  - Consequences of substance addictions for predicting future relapse
  - Knowledge of early signs and symptoms of relapse
- Support groups or therapy (cognitive-behavioural, interpersonal)
- Communication and problem-solving skills training

Relevant *NOC* outcomes for this phase include *Compliance behaviour, Knowledge: Disease process, Social support, and Substance addiction consequences.*

### Maintenance Phase

The overall outcomes for the maintenance phase continue to focus on prevention of relapse and limitation of the severity and duration of future episodes. Relevant *NOC* outcomes include *Knowledge: Disease process, Compliance behaviour, and Family support during treatment.* Additional outcomes include:

- Participation in learning interpersonal strategies related to work, interpersonal, and family problems
- Participation in psychotherapy, group, or other ongoing supportive therapy modality

## PLANNING

Planning care for an individual with bipolar disorder is usually geared toward the particular phase of mania the person is in (acute, continuation, or maintenance), as well as any other co-occurring issues identified in the assessment (e.g., risk for suicide, risk for violence to person or property, family crisis, legal crises, substance abuse, risk-taking behaviours).

### Acute Phase

During the acute phase, planning focuses on medically stabilizing the person while maintaining safety. Therefore, the hospital is usually the safest environment for accomplishing this stabilization (see Case Study and Nursing Care Plan 15-1 on pages 278–280). Nursing care is geared toward managing medications, decreasing physical activity, increasing food and fluid intake, ensuring at least four to six hours of sleep per night, alleviating any bowel or bladder problems, and intervening to see that self-care needs are met. Some patients may require seclusion or even electroconvulsive therapy (ECT) to assist with stabilization.

### Continuation Phase

During the continuation phase, planning focuses on maintaining adherence to the medication regimen and prevention of relapse. Interventions are planned in accordance with the assessment data regarding the person's interpersonal and stress-reduction skills, cognitive functioning, employment status, substance-related problems, and social support systems. During this time, psychoeducational teaching is necessary for the patient and family. The need for referrals to community

programs, groups, and support for any co-occurring disorders or problems (e.g., substance abuse, family problems, legal issues, financial crises) is evaluated.

Evaluation of the need for communication skills training and problem-solving skills training is also an important consideration. People with bipolar disorders often have interpersonal and emotional problems that affect their work, family, and social lives. Residual problems resulting from reckless, violent, withdrawn, or bizarre behaviour that may have occurred during a manic episode often leave lives shattered and family and friends hurt and distant. For some patients, cognitive-behavioural therapy (in addition to medication management) is useful to address these issues, although the focus of psychotherapeutic treatment will vary over time for each individual.

### Maintenance Phase

During the maintenance phase, planning focuses on preventing relapse and limiting the severity and duration of future episodes. Patients with bipolar disorders require medications over long periods of time or even an entire lifetime. Psychotherapy, support groups, psychoeducational groups, and periodic evaluations help patients maintain their family, social, and occupational lives.

## IMPLEMENTATION

Patients with bipolar disorders are often ambivalent about treatment. Only 39% of people experiencing symptoms of bipolar disorder seek treatment within the first year, and the median delay of treatment is six years (Wang, Berglund, Olfson, et al., 2005). Patients may minimize the destructive consequences of their behaviours or deny the seriousness of the disease, and some are reluctant to give up the increased energy, euphoria, and heightened sense of self-esteem of hypomania (Hirschfeld, Williams, Spitzer, et al., 2000). Unfortunately, nonadherence to the regimen of mood-stabilizing medication is a major cause of relapse, so establishing a therapeutic alliance with the individual with bipolar disorder is crucial.

### Acute Phase
#### Depressive Episodes

Depressive episodes of bipolar disorder have the same symptoms and risks as major depression (see Chapter 14), although they are often more intense. Hospitalization may be required if suicidal ideation, psychosis, or catatonia is present. Lithium carbonate and lamotrigine (Lamictal) are the first line of treatment for a person with bipolar disorder experiencing an acute depressive episode according to the Canadian Network for Mood and Anxiety Treatments (CANMAT) (2009). Treatment with antidepressants is not recommended (particularly for bipolar I disorder) since the patient's central nervous system (CNS) may become overactive, which results in hypomania or mania. Patients who experience depression while taking maintenance levels of medications may benefit from increased doses of the original drugs. When depressive episodes have psychotic features, an atypical antipsychotic may be added to the medication regimen.

## Manic Episodes

Hospitalization provides safety for a person experiencing acute mania (bipolar I disorder), imposes external controls on destructive behaviours, and provides for medication stabilization. There are unique approaches to communicating with and maintaining the safety of the person during the hospitalization period (Table 15-2). Staff members continuously set limits in a firm, nonthreatening, and neutral manner to prevent further escalation of mania and provide safe boundaries for the person and others.

## Continuation Phase

The continuation phase is crucial for patients and their families. The outcome for this phase is prevention of relapse, and community resources are chosen based on the needs of the person, the appropriateness of the referral, and the availability of resources. Frequently, a case manager evaluates appropriate follow-up care for patients and their families.

Medication adherence during this phase is perhaps the most important treatment outcome. Often, this follow-up is handled in a community mental health clinic. However, adherence to the medication regimen is also addressed in outpatient clinics and psychiatric home-care visits. Patients who are not too excitable and are able to tolerate a certain level of stimuli may attend an outpatient clinic. In addition to medication management, community mental health clinics offer structure, decrease social isolation, and help patients channel their time and energy. If a person is homebound, community psychiatric home care is the appropriate modality for follow-up care.

## Maintenance Phase

The goal of the maintenance phase is to prevent recurrence of an episode of bipolar disorder. The community resources cited earlier are helpful, and patients and their families often greatly benefit from mutual support and self-help groups, which will be discussed later in this chapter.

## Pharmacological Interventions

The recommendations for the management of acute mania remain mostly unchanged for the continuation and maintenance phases. Lithium carbonate, valproic acid (Depakene), and several atypical antipsychotics continue to be first-line treatments for acute mania. Tamoxifen is now suggested as a third-line augmentation option. Combining olanzapine (Zyprexa) and carbamazepine (Tegretol) is not recommended. For the management of bipolar depression, lithium, lamotrigine (Lamictal), and quetiapine (Seroquel) monotherapy; olanzapine plus a selective serotonin reuptake inhibitor (SSRI); and lithium or valproic acid plus SSRI or bupropion (Wellbutrin) remain first-line options. New data support the use of adjunctive modafinil (Alertec) as a second-line option but also indicate that aripiprazole (Abilify) should not be used as monotherapy for bipolar depression. Lithium, lamotrigine, valproic acid, and olanzapine continue to be first-line options for maintenance treatment of bipolar disorder. New data support the use of quetiapine monotherapy and adjunctive therapy for the prevention of manic and depressive episodes; aripiprazole monotherapy for the prevention of manic episodes; and risperidone (Risperdal) long-acting injection monotherapy and adjunctive therapy and adjunctive ziprasidone (Zeldox) for the prevention of mood episodes (CANMAT, 2009).

## Lithium Carbonate

Lithium carbonate ($LiCO_3$ or $Li+$) is effective in the treatment of bipolar I acute and recurrent manic and depressive episodes. Lithium inhibits about 80% of acute manic and hypomanic episodes within 10 to 21 days (Sadock & Sadock, 2008).

*Indications.* Lithium is particularly effective in reducing:
- Elation, grandiosity, and expansiveness
- Flight of ideas
- Irritability and manipulation
- Anxiety

To a lesser extent, lithium controls:
- Insomnia
- Psychomotor agitation
- Threatening or assaultive behaviour
- Distractibility
- Hypersexuality
- Paranoia

Lithium must reach therapeutic levels in the patient's blood to be effective. Reaching this level usually takes 7 to 14 days, or longer for some patients. An antipsychotic or a benzodiazepine can be used to prevent exhaustion, coronary collapse, and death until lithium reaches therapeutic levels. Antipsychotics act promptly to slow speech, inhibit aggression, and decrease psychomotor activity.

As lithium becomes effective in reducing manic behaviour, the antipsychotic drugs are usually discontinued. Although lithium is an effective intervention for treating the acute manic phase of bipolar disorder, it is not a cure (Repchinsky, 2006). Elderly patients appear to be more susceptible to adverse effects and may experience a higher incidence of neurotoxicity at lithium concentrations considered therapeutic for younger adults (Repchinsky, 2006). Many patients receive lithium for maintenance indefinitely and experience manic and depressive episodes if the drug is discontinued.

Margaret Trudeau (former wife of the late prime minister Pierre Trudeau) struggled with undiagnosed bipolar disorder for more than 30 years. In 2001, after overcoming the stigma and admitting herself into the Royal Ottawa Hospital, she was finally diagnosed with bipolar depression. Dr. Pierre Blier, chairman of Mood Disorders Research at the University of Ottawa's Institute of Mental Health Research, stated in an article, "The pivotal key for treating the illness is medication. Generally, more than one type of mood stabilizer, such as lithium, is required for treatment in conjunction with therapy to help establish patterns for those suffering the illness. It has to be tailored for the individual patient." Added Margaret, "I have my life back and I'm here to champion the cause. ... There is no shame in coming forward for help. ... I felt like I was broken for a long time, and now I feel whole again" (*Ottawa Citizen*, 2006).

*Therapeutic and toxic levels.* Lithium therapy requires reaching plasma levels of lithium that are relatively close to toxic

## TABLE 15-2 INTERVENTIONS FOR THE PATIENT EXPERIENCING ACUTE MANIA

| INTERVENTION | RATIONALE |
|---|---|
| **Communication** | |
| Use firm and calm approach: "John, come with me. Please eat this sandwich." | Structure and control are provided for the person who is out of control. Feelings of security can result: "Someone is in control." |
| Use short and concise explanations or statements. | Short attention span limits comprehension to small bits of information. |
| Remain neutral; avoid power struggles and value judgements. | Person can use inconsistencies and value judgements as justification for arguing and escalating mania. |
| Be consistent in approach and expectations. | Consistent limits and expectations minimize potential for person's manipulation of staff. |
| Have frequent staff meetings to plan consistent approaches and set agreed-on limits. | Consistency of all staff is needed to maintain controls and minimize manipulation by patient. |
| With other staff, decide on limits, tell person in simple, concrete terms with consequences. Example: "John, do not yell at or hit Peter. If you cannot control yourself, we will help you." Or "The seclusion room will help you feel less out of control and prevent harm to yourself and others." | Clear expectations help the person experience outside controls, as well as understand reasons for medication, seclusion, or restraints (if he or she is not able to control behaviours). |
| Hear and act on legitimate complaints. | Underlying feelings of helplessness are reduced, and acting-out behaviours are minimized. |
| Firmly redirect energy into more appropriate and constructive channels. | Distractibility is the nurse's most effective tool with the person experiencing mania. |
| **Structure in a Safe Milieu** | |
| Maintain low level of stimuli in patient's environment (e.g., away from bright lights, loud noises, people). | Escalation of anxiety can be decreased. |
| Provide structured solitary activities with nurse or aide. | Structure provides security and focus. |
| Provide frequent high-calorie fluids. | Serious dehydration is prevented. |
| Provide frequent rest periods. | Exhaustion is prevented. |
| Redirect violent behaviour. | Physical exercise can decrease tension and provide focus. |
| When warranted in acute mania, use phenothiazines and seclusion to minimize physical harm. | Exhaustion and death can result from dehydration, lack of sleep, and constant physical activity. |
| Observe for signs of lithium toxicity. | There is a small margin of safety between therapeutic and toxic doses. |
| Prevent person from giving away money and possessions. Hold valuables in hospital safe until rational judgement returns. | Person's "generosity" is a manic defence that is consistent with irrational, grandiose thinking. |
| **Physiological Safety: Self-Care Needs** | |
| *Nutrition* | |
| Monitor intake, output, and vital signs. | Adequate fluid and caloric intake are ensured; development of dehydration and cardiac collapse is minimized. |
| Offer frequent, high-calorie, protein drinks and finger foods (e.g., sandwiches, fruit, milkshakes). | Constant fluid and calorie replacement are needed. Person may be too active to sit at meals. Finger foods allow "eating on the run." |
| Frequently remind person to eat. "Tom, finish your milkshake." "Sally, eat this banana." | The person experiencing mania is unaware of bodily needs and is easily distracted. Needs supervision to eat. |

*Continued*

| TABLE 15-2 | INTERVENTIONS FOR THE PATIENT EXPERIENCING ACUTE MANIA—cont'd | |
| --- | --- | --- |
| **INTERVENTION** | **RATIONALE** | |
| *Sleep* | | |
| Encourage frequent rest periods during the day. | Lack of sleep can lead to exhaustion and death. | |
| Keep person in areas of low stimulation. | Relaxation is promoted, and manic behaviour is minimized. | |
| At night, provide warm baths, soothing music, and medication when indicated. Avoid giving person caffeine. | Relaxation, rest, and sleep are promoted. | |
| *Hygiene* | | |
| Supervise choice of clothes; minimize flamboyant and bizarre dress (e.g., garish stripes or plaids and loud, unmatching colours). | The potential is decreased for ridicule, which lowers self-esteem and increases the need for manic defence. The person is helped to maintain dignity. | |
| Give simple, step-by-step reminders for hygiene and dress. "Here is your razor. Here are your toothbrush and toothpaste." | Distractibility and poor concentration are countered through simple, concrete instructions. | |
| *Elimination* | | |
| Monitor bowel habits; offer fluids and foods that are high in fibre. Evaluate need for laxative. Monitor input and output. | Fecal impaction resulting from dehydration and decreased peristalsis is prevented. | |

levels. Since lithium is excreted primarily by the kidney, adequate renal function and adequate salt and fluid intake (2500 to 3000 mL) are essential for avoiding lithium accumulation and intoxication; thus, a decision to initiate lithium therapy should be preceded by a thorough clinical examination and evaluation of the patient. If lithium levels exceed 1.5 to 2 mmol/L, the drug should be discontinued and, if appropriate, administration resumed at a lower level after 24 hours (Repchinsky, 2006). A small increment exists between therapeutic and toxic levels of lithium. Lithium serum levels should usually be monitored three times weekly during the initial period of administration and periodically as required thereafter. Blood should be drawn in the morning, 8 to 12 hours after the last dose of lithium is taken. Table 15-3 details expected adverse effects of lithium, signs of lithium toxicity, and interventions for both.

***Maintenance therapy.*** Some clinicians suggest that patients with bipolar disorder need to be given lithium for 9 to 12 months, and some patients may need lifelong lithium maintenance to prevent further relapses. Many patients respond well to lower dosages during maintenance or prophylactic lithium therapy.

Lithium is unquestionably effective in preventing both manic and depressive episodes in patients with bipolar disorder. However, complete suppression occurs in only 50% of patients or fewer, even with adherence to the maintenance therapy regimen. Therefore, the patient and family should be given careful instructions about (1) the purpose and requirements of lithium therapy, (2) its adverse effects, (3) its toxic effects and complications, and (4) situations in which the physician should be contacted. The patient and family should also be advised that suddenly stopping lithium can lead to relapse and recurrence of mania. Health care providers must stress to patients and their families the importance of discontinuing maintenance therapy gradually. The following Patient and Family Teaching box outlines teaching regarding lithium therapy for the patient and family.

People taking lithium need to know that two major long-term risks of lithium therapy are hypothyroidism and impairment of the kidneys' ability to concentrate urine. Therefore, a person receiving lithium therapy must have periodic follow-ups to assess thyroid and renal function.

***Contraindications.*** Before lithium is administered, a medical evaluation is performed to assess the person's ability to tolerate the drug. In particular, baseline physical and laboratory examinations should include assessment of renal function; determination of thyroid status, including levels of thyroxine and thyroid-stimulating hormone; and evaluation for dementia or neurological disorders, which presage a poor response to lithium. Other clinical and laboratory assessments, including an electrocardiogram, are performed as needed, depending on the individual's physical condition.

Lithium therapy is generally contraindicated in patients with cardiovascular disease, brain damage, renal disease, thyroid disease, or myasthenia gravis. Whenever possible, lithium is not given to women who are pregnant because it may harm the fetus. The fear of becoming pregnant and the wish to become pregnant are both major concerns for many women taking lithium. Lithium use is also contraindicated in mothers who are breastfeeding and in children younger than 12 years of age.

### Anticonvulsant Drugs

In the 1980s, researchers hypothesized that mood instability could be viewed much the same as epilepsy and that a chain reaction of sensitivity, or *kindling*, was responsible for the worsening of bipolar symptoms over time (Ostacher & Tilley, 2008). This hypothesis led to the use of anticonvulsant drugs, such as carbamazepine (Tegretol), valproic acid (Depakene), and lamotrigine (Lamictal), as a treatment for mania that has been

## TABLE 15-3  LITHIUM ADVERSE EFFECTS AND SIGNS OF LITHIUM TOXICITY

| LEVEL | SIGNS AND SYMPTOMS | INTERVENTIONS |
|---|---|---|
| **Expected Adverse Effects** <br> <0.4–1.0 mEq/L (therapeutic level) | Fine hand tremor, polyuria, mild thirst, mild nausea and general discomfort, weight gain | Symptoms may persist throughout therapy. Symptoms often subside during treatment. Weight gain may be helped with diet, exercise, and nutritional management. |
| **Early Signs of Toxicity** <br> <1.5 mEq/L | Nausea, vomiting, diarrhea, thirst, polyuria, lethargy, slurred speech, muscle weakness, and fine hand tremor | Medication should be withheld, blood lithium levels measured, and dosage re-evaluated. Dehydration, if present, should be addressed. |
| **Advanced Signs of Toxicity** <br> 1.5–2.0 mEq/L | Coarse hand tremor, persistent gastrointestinal upset, mental confusion, muscle hyperirritability, electroencephalographic changes, incoordination, sedation | Interventions outlined above or below should be used, depending on severity of circumstances. |
| **Severe Toxicity** <br> 2.0–2.5 mEq/L | Ataxia, confusion, large output of dilute urine, serious electroencephalographic changes, blurred vision, clonic movements, seizures, stupor, severe hypotension, coma; death is usually secondary to pulmonary complications | Hospitalization is indicated. The drug is stopped, and excretion is hastened. If patient is alert, an emetic is administered. |
| >2.5 mEq/L | Convulsions, oliguria; death can occur | In addition to the interventions above, hemodialysis may be used in severe cases. |

**Source:** Data from Lehne, R.A. (2010). *Pharmacology for nursing care* (7th ed., p. 357). Philadelphia: Saunders; and Sadock, B.J., & Sadock, V.A. (2008). *Concise textbook of clinical psychiatry* (3rd ed.). Philadelphia: Lippincott, Williams & Wilkins.

## PATIENT AND FAMILY TEACHING

### Lithium Therapy

The patient and the patient's family should be given the following information, be encouraged to ask questions, and be given the material in written form as well.

1. Lithium treats your current emotional problem and also helps prevent relapse. Therefore, it is important to continue taking the drug after the current episode is over.
2. Because therapeutic and toxic dosage ranges are so close, it is important to monitor lithium blood levels very closely—more frequently at first, and then once every several months after that.
3. Lithium is not addictive.
4. It is important to eat a normal diet, with normal salt and fluid intake (1500–3000 mL/d or six 350-mL glasses of fluid). Lithium decreases sodium reabsorption in the kidneys, which could lead to a deficiency of sodium. A low sodium intake leads to a relative increase in lithium retention, which could produce toxicity.
5. You should stop taking lithium if you have excessive diarrhea, vomiting, or sweating. All of these symptoms can lead to dehydration. Dehydration can raise lithium levels in the blood to toxic levels. Inform your physician if you have any of these problems.
6. Do not take diuretics (water pills) while you are taking lithium.
7. Lithium is irritating to the lining of your stomach. Take lithium with meals.
8. It is important to have your kidneys and thyroid checked periodically, especially if you are taking lithium over a long period. Talk to your doctor about this follow-up.
9. Do not take any over-the-counter medicines without checking first with your doctor.
10. If you find that you are gaining a lot of weight, you may need to talk this change over with your doctor or dietitian.
11. Many self-help groups are available to provide support for people with bipolar disorder and their families. The local self-help group is (give name and telephone number).
12. You can find out more information by calling (give name and telephone number).
13. Keep a list of adverse effects and toxic effects handy, along with the name and number of a person to contact if these effects occur (see Table 15-3).
14. If lithium is to be discontinued, your dosage will be tapered gradually to minimize the risk of relapse.

refractory to lithium therapy. They also proved useful in treating people who need rapid de-escalation and who do not respond to other treatment approaches. Subsequent research did not support the kindling theory, however, suggesting that symptom improvement for bipolar disorder is based on another mechanism of action of these anticonvulsant drugs and not on their seizure prevention mechanism.

Anticonvulsant drugs are thought to be:

- Superior for continuously cycling patients
- More effective when there is no family history of bipolar disorder
- Effective at dampening affective swings in schizoaffective patients
- Effective at diminishing impulsive and aggressive behaviour in some nonpsychotic patients
- Helpful in cases of alcohol and benzodiazepine withdrawal
- Beneficial in controlling mania (within two weeks) and depression (within three weeks or longer)

***Divalproex sodium (Epival).*** Chemically related to valproic acid (Depakene), divalproex sodium is useful in treating lithium nonresponders who are in acute mania, experience rapid cycles, are in dysphoric mania, or have not responded to carbamazepine. It is also helpful in preventing future manic episodes. It is important to monitor liver function and platelet count periodically, although serious complications are rare. Divalproex doses can cause drowsiness and dizziness and increase thoughts of suicide; therefore, mood, ideations, and behaviour should be monitored on a regular basis. Therapeutic serum levels that range from 50 to 100 mcg/m and 50 to 125 mcg/m for mania should be monitored to prevent toxicity and overdose (Vallerand, Sanoski, & Deglin, 2013).

***Carbamazepine.*** Some patients with treatment-resistant bipolar disorder improve after taking carbamazepine (Tegretol) and lithium or carbamazepine and an antipsychotic. Carbamazepine seems to work better in patients with rapid cycling and in severely paranoid, angry patients experiencing manias than in euphoric, overactive, overfriendly patients experiencing manias. It is thought to also be more effective in dysphoric patients experiencing manias.

As with valproic acid, liver function and platelet count should be monitored periodically. Blood levels of carbamazepine should be monitored at least weekly for the first eight weeks of treatment because the drug can increase levels of liver enzymes that can speed its own metabolism. In some instances, this increase can cause bone-marrow suppression and liver inflammation.

***Lamotrigine.*** Lamotrigine (Lamictal) is a first-line treatment for bipolar depression and is approved for acute and maintenance therapy. Lamotrigine is generally well tolerated but has one serious though rare dermatological reaction: a potentially life-threatening rash. Patients should be instructed to seek immediate medical attention if a rash appears, although most are likely benign (Preston, O'Neal, & Talaga, 2005).

Adverse drug reactions (ADRs), as indicated by CANMAT, that require patient safety monitoring are:

- Both valproic acid and carbamazepine may cause blood dyscrasias, hepatotoxicity, and teratogenicity.

- Carbamazepine has also been linked to hyponatremia and serious dermatological adverse effects.
- Valproic acid has been associated with polycystic ovary syndrome, weight gain, acute pancreatitis, and hyperammonemic encephalopathy.
- The severe ADRs associated with lamotrigine are dermatological, namely Stevens-Johnson syndrome.
- Drug interactions such as lamotrigine–valproic acid and carbamazepine–hormonal contraceptives are also important to be aware of.

## Antianxiety Drugs

***Clonazepam and lorazepam.*** Diazepam (Valium), clonazepam (Rivotril), and lorazepam (Ativan) are antianxiety (anxiolytic) drugs useful in the treatment of acute mania in some patients who are resistant to other treatments. These drugs are also effective in managing the psychomotor agitation seen in mania. They should be avoided, however, in patients with a history of substance abuse.

## Atypical Antipsychotics

In addition to showing sedative properties during the early phase of treatment (help with insomnia, anxiety, agitation), the atypical antipsychotics seem to have mood-stabilizing properties. CANMAT (2009) guidelines support the use of olanzapine (Zyprexa), risperidone (Risperdal), aripiprazole (Abilify), quetiapine (Seroquel), and ziprasidone (Zeldox). For example, an initial study showed that olanzapine is better tolerated and prevents mania relapse more effectively than lithium (Tohen, 2003). Ziprasidone (Zeldox), recently approved in Canada for bipolar disorder, and quetiapine (Seroquel), both original formula and Seroquel XR (extended release), are the only medications currently approved for use in both the manic and depressive phases of bipolar disorder (Mood Disorders Society of Canada, 2009).

The Drug Treatment box provides an overview of drugs used to treat bipolar disorder that are approved by Health Canada and the *Canadian Food and Drugs Act*.

## Electroconvulsive Therapy

Electroconvulsive therapy (ECT) is used to subdue severe manic behaviour, especially in patients with treatment-resistant mania and those with rapid cycling (i.e., those who experience four or more episodes of illness a year). Depressive episodes—particularly those with severe, catatonic, or treatment-resistant depression—are an indication for this treatment and may be helpful for mania during pregnancy (Baghai, 2008). Electroconvulsive therapy may be considered as an alternative during pregnancy in cases of psychotic decompensation or suicidal ideation (CANMAT, 2009, p. 34). ECT is effective for patients with bipolar disorder who have rapid cycling, for those with paranoid-destructive features (who often respond poorly to lithium therapy), and in acutely suicidal patients. Chapter 14 offers a more detailed discussion of ECT.

## Milieu Management

Control of hyperactive behaviour during the acute phase almost always includes immediate treatment with an antipsychotic

# 💊 DRUG TREATMENT OF PATIENTS WITH BIPOLAR DISORDER

| GENERIC (TRADE) | HEALTH CANADA–APPROVED | OFF-LABEL USES | CANMAT RECOMMENDATIONS |
|---|---|---|---|
| Lithium carbonate | Acute mania Maintenance Mood Stabilizer | Depression | A first line for bipolar depression Recommended for acute mania Treatment and prevention of manic episodes |
| **Anticonvulsants** | | | |
| Valproic acid (Depakene) | Acute mania | Depression | Recommended for acute mania |
| Divalproex sodium (Epival) | | Maintenance | A first line of maintenance treatment of bipolar disorder |
| Carbamazepine (Tegretol) | Acute mania | Depression Maintenance | Recommended for maintenance treatment of bipolar disorder, mood stabilizing effect |
| Lamotrigine (Lamictal) | Maintenance | Depression (can worsen mania) | A first line for bipolar depression Recommended for maintenance treatment of bipolar disorder |
| Gabapentin (Neurontin) and topiramate (Topamax) | | Acute mania Maintenance | Recommended for maintenance treatment of bipolar disorder |
| **Atypical Antipsychotics** | | | |
| Aripiprazole (Abilify) | Mania Maintenance | Depression | |
| Olanzapine (Zyprexa) | Mania Maintenance | Depression | Recommended for acute mania |
| Quetiapine fumarate (Seroquel) | Depression Mania Maintenance | | |
| Risperidone (Risperdal) | Mania | Depression Maintenance | First line treatment for severe mania |
| Ziprasidone (Zeldox) | Acute mania Mixed features | | Acute mania |

**Source:** Data from Canadian Network for Mood and Anxiety Treatments (CANMAT). (2009). Canadian Network for Mood and Anxiety Treatments (CANMAT) and International Society for Bipolar Disorders (ISBD) collaborative update of CANMAT guidelines for the management of patients with bipolar disorder: Update 2009. Retrieved from http://www.canmat.org/resources/CANMAT%20Bipolar%20Disorder%20Guidelines%20-2009%20Update.pdf; and Health Canada. (2013). Drugs and health products. Retrieved from http://www.hc-sc.gc.ca/dhp-mps/index-eng.php.

# ⚙ INTEGRATIVE THERAPY

### Omega-3 Fatty Acids as a Treatment for Bipolar Disorder

A few generations ago, youngsters actively resisted a nightly dose of cod liver oil that mothers swore by as a method to prevent constipation. The foul-tasting, rancid-smelling liquid undoubtedly helped win the battle against constipation, but it may have had other benefits as well. Cod liver oil is rich in omega-3 fatty acids, which have drawn increasing attention as being important in mood regulation. Fish oil is the target of this attention. It contains two omega-3 fatty acids—eicosapentaenoic acid (EPA) and docosahexaenoic acid (DHA)—which are important in CNS functioning. EPA seems to be particularly important for behaviour and mood.

The interest in these particular fatty acids developed as research began to suggest that people who live in areas with low seafood consumption (especially cold-water seafood) exhibited higher rates of depression and bipolar disorder. This finding led researchers to explore the influence of omega-3 fatty acids as protection for bipolar disorder (Parker, Gibson, Brotchie, et al., 2006). Alternative treatments are especially attractive for the depressive phase of the disorder since drugs that are normally used to treat depression can catapult a person into a dangerous manic episode.

The jury is still out on the absolute benefits of either eating more fish or taking fish oil supplements (delivered in pleasant-tasting gel capsules). In a review of published trials, one group of researchers was unable to come up with clear support for increasing dietary intake of omega-3 fatty acids (Appleton, Hayward, Gunnell, et al., 2006). But Kidd (2007) conducted another large-scale analysis of current research and concluded just the opposite: that multiple studies support the benefits of fish oil for the mood swings of bipolar disorder. Given the array of health benefits some researchers have identified, adding this dietary recommendation to patients with bipolar disorder may be helpful.

**Sources:** Appleton, K.M., Hayward, R.C., Gunnell, T.J., et al. (2006). Effects of n-3 long-chain polyunsaturated fatty acids on depressed mood: Systematic review of published trials. *American Journal of Clinical Nutrition, 84*(6), 1308–1316; Kidd, P.M. (2007). Omega-3 DHA and EPA for cognition, behaviour, and mood: Clinical findings and structural-functional synergies with cell membrane phospholipids. *Alternative Medicine Review, 12*(3), 207–227; and Parker, G., Gibson, N.A., Brotchie, H., et al. (2006). Omega-3 fatty acids and mood disorders. *American Journal of Psychiatry, 163*, 969–978. doi:10.1176/appi.ajp.163.6.969.

drug. However, when a person is dangerously out of control, use of a seclusion room or restraints may also be required. A seclusion room provides comfort and relief to many patients who are unable to control their own behaviour. Seclusion serves the following purposes:

- Reduces overwhelming environmental stimuli
- Protects a person from injuring himself or herself or others, including staff
- Prevents destruction of personal property or property of others

Seclusion is warranted when documented data collected by the nursing and medical staff reflect the following points:

- Substantial risk of harm to others or self is clear.
- The person is unable to control his or her actions.
- Problematic behaviour has been sustained (continues or escalates despite other measures).
- Other measures have failed (e.g., setting limits beginning with verbal de-escalation or using chemical restraints).

The use of seclusion or restraints is associated with complex therapeutic, ethical, and legal issues. Most provincial and territorial laws prohibit the use of unnecessary physical restraint or isolation. Barring an emergency, the use of seclusion and restraints requires consent. Therefore, most hospitals have well-defined protocols for treatment with seclusion. Seclusion protocol includes a proper reporting procedure, through the appropriate channels, when a person is to be secluded. For example, the use of seclusion and restraint is permitted only on the written order of a physician and must be reviewed and rewritten every 24 hours. The order must include the type of restraint to be used. Seclusion and observation levels and care protocols must be carefully adhered to as per individual hospital or agency policy.

Seclusion protocols also identify specific nursing responsibilities, such as how often the patient's behaviour is to be observed and documented (e.g., every 15 minutes), how often the patient is to be offered food and fluids (e.g., every 30 to 60 minutes), and how often the patient is to be toileted (e.g., every one to two hours). Medication is often administered to patients in seclusion; therefore, vital signs should be measured frequently, as per hospital policy.

Careful and precise documentation is a legal necessity. The nurse documents the following:

- The behaviour leading up to the seclusion or restraint
- The actions taken to provide the least restrictive alternative
- The time the patient was placed in seclusion
- Every 15 minutes, the patient's behaviour, needs, nursing care, and vital signs
- The time and type of medications given and their effects on the patient

When a patient requires seclusion to prevent self-harm or violence toward others, it is ideal for one nurse on each shift to work with the patient on a continuous basis. Communication with a patient in seclusion is concrete and direct but also empathic and limited to brief instructions. Patients need reassurance that seclusion is only a temporary measure and that they will be returned to the unit when their behaviour is more controlled and they demonstrate the ability to safely be around others.

Frequent staff meetings regarding personal feelings are necessary to prevent using seclusion as a form of punishment or leaving a patient in seclusion for long periods of time without proper supervision. Restraints and seclusion are never to be used as punishment or for the convenience of the staff. Refer to Chapter 8 for a more detailed discussion of the legal implications of seclusion and restraints and Chapter 26 for further discussion and guidelines.

## Support Groups

Patients with bipolar disorder, as well as their friends and families, benefit from forming mutual support groups. Often, these are coordinated by organizations such as the Mood Disorders Society of Canada and the Canadian Mental Health Association.

## Health Teaching and Health Promotion

Patients and families need information about bipolar disorder, with particular emphasis on its chronic and highly recurrent nature. In addition, patients and families need to be taught the warning signs and symptoms of impending episodes. For example, changes in sleep patterns are especially important because they usually precede, accompany, or precipitate mania. Even a single night of unexplainable sleep loss can be taken as an early warning of impending mania. Health teaching stresses the importance of establishing regularity in sleep patterns, meals, exercise, and other activities. The following Patient and Family Teaching box lists health-teaching guidelines for patients with bipolar disorder and their families.

Mood stabilizers may cause weight gain and other metabolic disturbances such as altered metabolism of lipids and glucose (Fagiolini, Chengappa, Soreca, et al., 2008). These alterations increase the risk for diabetes, high blood pressure, dyslipidemia, cardiac problems, or all of these in combination (metabolic syndrome). Not only do these disturbances impair quality of life and lifespan, they are also a major reason for nonadherence. Teaching aimed at weight reduction and management is essential to keep patients physically healthy and emotionally stable.

Recovery concepts are particularly important for patients with bipolar disorder, who often have issues with adherence to treatment. The best method of addressing this problem is to follow a collaborative-care model, in which responsibilities for treatment adherence are shared (Sajatovic, Davies, Bauer, et al., 2005). In this model, patients are responsible for making it to appointments and openly communicating information, and the health care provider is responsible for keeping current on treatment methods and listening carefully as patients share perceptions. Through this sharing, treatment adherence becomes a self-managed responsibility.

## Psychotherapy

Pharmacotherapy and psychiatric mental health care and management are essential in the treatment of acute manic attacks and during the continuation and maintenance phases of bipolar disorder. Individuals with bipolar disorder must deal with the psychosocial consequences of their past episodes and their vulnerability to experiencing future episodes. They also have to face the burden of long-term treatments that may involve

## PATIENT AND FAMILY TEACHING
### Bipolar Disorder

1. Patients with bipolar disorder and their families need to know:
   - The chronic and episodic nature of bipolar disorder
   - The fact that bipolar disorder is long term and that maintenance treatment therefore will require that one or more mood-stabilizing agents be taken for a long time
   - The expected adverse effects and toxic effects of the prescribed medication, as well as whom to call and where to go in case of a toxic reaction
   - The signs and symptoms of relapse that may "come out of the blue"
   - The role of family members and others in preventing a full relapse
   - The phone numbers of emergency contact people, which should be kept in an easily accessed place
2. The use of alcohol, drugs of abuse, even small amounts of caffeine, and over-the-counter medications can produce a relapse.
3. Good sleep hygiene is critical to stability. Frequently, the early symptom of a manic episode is lack of sleep. In some cases, mania may be averted by the use of sleep medications (e.g., temazepam [Restoril]).
4. Psychosocial strategies are important for dealing with work, interpersonal, and family problems; lowering stress; enhancing a sense of personal control; and increasing community functioning.
5. Group and individual psychotherapy are invaluable for gaining insight and skills in relapse prevention, providing social support, increasing coping skills in interpersonal relations, improving adherence to the medication regimen, reducing functional morbidity, and decreasing rehospitalizations.
   Health care workers need to remember the following:
   - Minimization and denial are common defences that require gradual introduction of facts.
   - Anger and abusive remarks, although aimed at the health care provider, are symptoms of the disease and are not personal.

**Source:** Adapted from Milkowitz, D.J. (2003). Bipolar disorder. In D.H. Barlow (Ed.), *Clinical handbook of psychological disorders* (pp. 523–560). New York: Guilford Press; and Zerbe, K.J. (1999). *Women's mental health in primary care.* Philadelphia: Saunders.

unpleasant adverse effects. Many patients have strained interpersonal relationships, marital and family problems, academic and occupational problems, and legal or other social difficulties. Psychotherapy can help them work through these difficulties, decrease some of the psychic distress, and increase self-esteem. Psychotherapeutic treatments can also help patients improve their functioning between episodes and attempt to decrease the frequency of future episodes.

Cognitive-behavioural therapy (CBT) is typically used as an adjunct to pharmacotherapy and involves identifying maladaptive cognitions and behaviours that may be barriers to a person's recovery and ongoing mood stability. It is also used for bipolar disorder in children and adolescents (Feeny, Danielson, Schwartz, et al., 2006). CBT focuses on adherence to the medication regimen, early detection and intervention for manic or depressive episodes, stress and lifestyle management, and the treatment of depression and co-morbid conditions (Jones, Mulligan, Law, et al., 2012; Otto, Reilly-Harrington, & Sachs, 2003). Patients treated with cognitive therapy are more likely to take their medications as prescribed than are patients who do not participate in therapy, and psychotherapy results in greater adherence to the regimen (Jones, Mulligan, Law, et al., 2012). A formalized psychotherapy called *interpersonal and social rhythm therapy* has been tested in combination with pharmacotherapy in randomized clinical trials as treatment for patients during the maintenance phase of bipolar disorder. This therapy addresses the variables that relate to recurrence of symptoms, especially nonadherence to medication, stress management, and maintenance of social supports (Frank, 2007).

Often the patients receiving medication and therapy place more value on psychotherapy than clinicians do. Kay Redfield Jamison is an American clinical psychologist and mood disorder researcher who has suffered from bipolar disorder since her early adulthood. She describes her feelings about drug therapy and psychotherapy as follows:

> I cannot imagine leading a normal life without lithium. From startings and stoppings of it, I now know it is an essential part of my sanity. Lithium prevents my seductive but disastrous highs, diminishes my depressions, clears out the weaving of my disordered thinking, slows me, gentles me out, keeps me in my relationships, in my career, out of a hospital, and in psychotherapy. It keeps me alive, too. But psychotherapy heals, it makes some sense of the confusion, it reins in the terrifying thoughts and feelings, it brings back hope and the possibility of learning from it all. Pills cannot, do not, ease one back into reality. They bring you back headlong, careening, and faster than can be endured at times. Psychotherapy is a sanctuary, it is a battleground, and it is where I have come to believe that someday I may be able to contend with all of this. No pill can help me deal with the problem of not wanting to take pills, but no amount of therapy alone can prevent my manias and depressions. I need both. (Jamison, 1995, p. 139)

## EVALUATION

Outcome criteria often dictate the frequency of evaluation of short-term and intermediate indicators. Are the person's vital signs stable? Is he or she well hydrated? Is the person able to control personal behaviour or respond to external controls? Is the person able to sleep for four or five hours a night or take frequent, short rest periods during the day? Does the family have a clear understanding of the patient's disorder and need for medication? Do the patient and family know which community agencies might help them?

If outcomes or related indicators are not achieved satisfactorily, the preventing factors are analyzed. Were the data incorrect or insufficient? Were nursing diagnoses inappropriate or outcomes unrealistic? Was intervention poorly planned? After the outcomes and care plan are reassessed, the plan is revised, if indicated. Longer-term outcomes include adherence to the medication regimen; resumption of functioning in the community; achievement of stability in family, work, and social relationships and in mood; and improved coping skills for reducing stress.

## CASE STUDY AND NURSING CARE PLAN 15-1
### *Mania*

Hannah is brought to the emergency department after being found on the highway shortly after her car broke down. She is dressed in a long red dress, a blue and orange scarf, many long chains, and a pair of yellow shoes. The police report that when they came to her aid, she told them she was "driving to fame and fortune." She appeared overly cheerful and was constantly talking, laughing, and making jokes. At the same time, she paced up and down beside the car, sometimes tweaking the cheek of one of the policemen. She was coy and flirtatious with the police officers, saying at one point, "Boys in blue are fun to do."

When she reached into the car and started drinking from an open bottle of vodka, the police decided that her behaviour and general condition might result in harm to herself or others. When they explained to Hannah that they wanted to take her to the hospital for a general checkup, her jovial mood turned to anger and rage, yet two minutes after getting into the police car, she was singing "Jailhouse Rock."

On admission to the emergency department, Hannah is seen by a psychiatrist, and her sister is called. The sister states that Hannah stopped taking her lithium about five weeks ago and has been becoming more and more agitated and out of control. She reports that Hannah has not eaten in two days, has stayed up all night calling friends and strangers all over the province, and finally fled the house when the sister called an ambulance to take her to the hospital. The psychiatrist contacts Hannah's regular physician, and her previous history and medical management are discussed. It is decided that she should be hospitalized during the acute manic phase and restarted on lithium therapy. It is hoped that medications and a controlled environment will prevent further escalation of the manic state and prevent possible exhaustion and cardiac collapse.

## ASSESSMENT

### Self-Assessment

Jake has worked as a nurse on the psychiatric unit for two years. He has learned to deal with many of the challenging behaviours associated with the manic defence. For example, he no longer takes most of the verbal insults personally, even when the remarks are cutting and hit close to home. He is also better able to recognize and set limits on some of the tactics used by the person experiencing mania to split the staff. The staff on this unit work closely with one another, making the atmosphere positive and supportive; therefore, communication is good among staff. Frequent and effective communication is needed to prevent staff splitting, maximize external controls, and maintain consistency in nursing care.

The only aspects of Hannah's behaviour Jake thinks he may have difficulty with are the sexual advances and loud sexual comments she makes toward him. He knows that these behaviours could make him anxious, and his concern is that Hannah might pick up on his anxiety. When he discusses this concern with the senior nurse, they decide that two nurses should provide care for Hannah. A female nurse will spend time with her in her room, and Jake will spend time with her in quiet areas on the unit. It is decided that neither Jake nor any male staff member will be alone with Hannah in her room at any time. Jake will ask for relief if Hannah's sexual remarks and acting-out behaviours make him anxious.

| Objective Data | Subjective Data |
| --- | --- |
| Little if anything to eat for days | "Driving to fame and fortune." |
| Little if any sleep for days | "Boys in blue are fun to do." |
| History of mania | |
| History of lithium maintenance | |
| Very loud and distracting to others | |
| Anger when wishes are denied | |
| Flight of ideas | |
| Loud and inappropriate dress | |
| Sexually suggestive remarks and actions | |
| Remarks that suggest grandiose thinking | |
| Poor judgement | |

## DIAGNOSIS

1. *Risk for injury* related to dehydration and faulty judgement, as evidenced by inability to meet own physiological needs and set limits on own behaviour

**Supporting Data**
- Has not slept for days
- Has not consumed food or fluids for days

*Continued*

*Mania*

2. *Defensive coping* related to biochemical changes, as evidenced by change in usual communication patterns
**Supporting Data**
* Remarks suggest sexual themes
* Remarks suggesting grandiose thinking
* Flight of ideas
* Constantly talking, laughing, and making jokes

## OUTCOMES IDENTIFICATION

Physical status will remain stable during manic phase.

## PLANNING

The nurse plans interventions that will help de-escalate Hannah's activity to minimize potential physical injury (dehydration, cardiac instability) through the use of medication and provision of a nonstimulating environment.

## IMPLEMENTATION

Jake makes the following nursing care plan:

| Short-Term Goal | Intervention | Rationale | Evaluation |
|---|---|---|---|
| 1. Person will be well hydrated, as evidenced by good skin turgor and normal urinary output and specific gravity, within 24 hours. | 1a. Give olanzapine (Zyprexa) intramuscularly immediately and as ordered. | 1a. Continuous physical activity and lack of fluids can eventually lead to cardiac collapse and death. | **GOAL MET** After 3 hours, person takes small amounts of fluid (60–120 mL per hour). |
| | 1b. Check vital signs frequently (every 1–2 hours). | 1b. Cardiac status is monitored. | After 5 hours, patient starts taking 250 mL per hour with a lot of reminding and encouragement. |
| | 1c. Place person in private or quiet room (whenever possible). | 1c. Environmental stimuli are reduced—escalation of mania and distractibility are minimized. | After 24 hours, urine specific gravity is within normal limits. |
| | 1d. Stay with person and divert person away from stimulating situations. | 1d. Nurse's presence provides support. Ability to interact with others is temporarily impaired. | |
| | 1e. Offer high-calorie, high-protein drink (250 mL) every hour in quiet area. | 1e. Proper hydration is mandatory for maintenance of cardiac status. | |
| | 1f. Frequently remind person to drink: "Take 2 more sips." | 1f. Person's concentration is poor; she is easily distracted. | |
| | 1g. Offer finger food frequently, in quiet area. | 1g. Person is unable to sit; snacks she can eat while pacing are more likely to be consumed. | |
| | 1h. Maintain record of intake and output. | 1h. Such a record allows staff to make accurate nutritional assessment for person's safety. | |
| | 1i. Weigh person daily. | 1i. Monitoring of nutritional status is necessary. | |

*Continued*

## CASE STUDY AND NURSING CARE PLAN 15-1—cont'd

*Mania*

| Short-Term Goal | Intervention | Rationale | Evaluation |
|---|---|---|---|
| 2. Person will sleep or rest 3 hours during the first night in the hospital with aid of medication and nursing interventions. | 2a. Continue to direct person to areas of minimal activity.<br><br>2b. When possible, try to direct energy into productive and calming activities (e.g., pacing to slow, soft music; slow exercise; drawing alone; or writing in quiet area).<br><br>2c. Encourage short rest periods throughout the day (e.g., 3–5 minutes every hour) when possible.<br><br>2d. Drinks such as coffee, tea, and colas should be decaffeinated only.<br><br>2e. Provide nursing measures at bedtime that promote sleep— for example, warm milk, soft music. | 2a. Lower levels of stimulation can decrease excitability.<br><br>2b. Directing patient to paced, nonstimulating activities can help minimize excitability.<br><br>2c. Person may be unaware of feelings of fatigue. Can collapse from exhaustion if hyperactivity continues without periods of rest.<br><br>2d. Caffeine is a central nervous system stimulant that inhibits needed rest or sleep.<br><br>2e. Such measures promote nonstimulating and relaxing mood. | Person is awake most of the first night. Sleeps for 2 hours from 0400 to 0600 hours.<br><br>Person is able to rest on the second day for short periods and engage in quiet activities for short periods (5–10 minutes). |
| 3. Person's blood pressure (BP) and pulse (P) will be within normal limits within 24 hours, with the aid of medication and nursing interventions. | 3a. Continue to monitor BP and P frequently throughout the day (every 30 minutes).<br><br>3b. Keep staff informed, by verbal and written reports, of baseline vital signs and patient progress. | 3a. Physical condition is presently a great strain on patient's heart.<br><br>3b. Alerting all staff regarding person's status can increase medical intervention if a change in status occurs. | **GOAL MET**<br>Baseline measures on unit are not obtained because of hyperactive behaviour. Information from family physician states that baseline BP is 130/90 mm Hg and baseline P is 88 beats per minute.<br>BP at end of 24 hours is 130/70 mm Hg; P is 80 beats per minute. |

## EVALUATION

After two days, the medical staff feel that Hannah's physical status is stable. Her vital signs are within normal limits, she is consuming sufficient fluids, and her urinary output is normal. Although her hyperactivity persists, it does so to a lesser degree; she is able to get periods of rest during the day and is sleeping three to four hours during the night.

Hannah's hyperactivity continues to be a challenge to the nurses; however, she is able to participate in some activities that require gross motor movement. These activities are useful in channelling some of her aggressive energy. Shortly after her arrival on the unit, Hannah starts a fight with another patient, but seclusion is avoided because she is able to refrain from further violent episodes as a result of medication and nursing interventions. She can be directed toward solitary activities, which channel some of her energies, at least for short periods.

As the effect of the drugs progresses, Hannah's activity level decreases, and by discharge, she is able to discuss issues of concern with the nurse and make some useful decisions about her future. She is to come for follow-up at the community centre and agrees to join a family psychoeducational group for patients with bipolar disorder and their families, which she will attend with her sister.

# KEY POINTS TO REMEMBER

- Biological factors appear to play a role in the etiology of the bipolar disorders. Strong genetic correlates have been revealed, especially through twin studies. In addition, little doubt exists that neurotransmitter (norepinephrine, dopamine, serotonin) excess and imbalance are also related to bipolar mood swings, supporting the existence of neurobiological influences. Neuroendocrine and neuroanatomical findings provide strong evidence for biological influences.
- Early detection of bipolar disorder can help diminish co-morbid substance abuse, suicide, and decline in social and personal relationships and may help promote more positive outcomes. Unfortunately, bipolar disorder often goes unrecognized.
- The nurse assesses the person's level of mood (hypomania, acute mania), behaviour, and thought processes and is alert to cognitive dysfunction.
- Analyzing the objective and subjective data helps the nurse formulate appropriate nursing diagnoses. Some of the nursing diagnoses appropriate for patients with mania are *Risk for violence, Defensive coping, Ineffective coping, Disturbed thought processes*, and *Situational low self-esteem.*
- During the acute phase of mania, physical needs often take priority and demand nursing interventions. Therefore, *Deficient fluid volume, Imbalanced nutrition, Imbalanced elimination*, and *Disturbed sleep pattern* are usually addressed in the nursing plan.
- The diagnosis of *Interrupted family processes* is vital. Support groups, psychoeducation, and guidance for the family can greatly affect the person's adherence to the medication regimen.
- Planning involves identifying the specific needs of the patient and family during the three phases of mania (acute, continuation, and maintenance). Can the patient benefit from communication-skills training, improvement in coping skills, legal or financial counselling, or further psychoeducation? What community resources does the person need at this time?
- People experiencing mania can be demanding and manipulative. Examples of manipulative behaviour include pitting members of the staff against one another, loudly and persistently pointing to faults and shortcomings in staff, constantly demanding attention and favours from the staff, and provoking both patients and staff with profane and lewd remarks. The person experiencing mania constantly interrupts activities and distracts groups with continuous physical motion and incessant joking and talking. The nurse sets limits in a firm, neutral manner and tailors communication techniques and interventions to maintain the patient's safety.
- Health care workers, family, and friends often feel angry and frustrated by the person's disruptive behaviours. When these feelings are not examined and shared with others, the therapeutic potential of the staff is reduced, and feelings of confusion and helplessness remain.
- Antimanic medications are available. Lithium has a narrow therapeutic index, which necessitates thorough patient and family teaching and regular follow-up. Anticonvulsant drugs such as carbamazepine and valproic acid are useful, especially in treating people with disease that is refractory to lithium therapy. Anticonvulsant drugs are also useful in treating patients who need rapid de-escalation and do not respond to other treatment approaches.
- Antipsychotic agents may be used for their sedating and mood-stabilizing properties, especially during initial treatment.
- For some patients, ECT may be the most appropriate medical treatment.
- Individual and family teaching takes many forms and is most important in encouraging adherence to the medication regimen and reducing the risk of relapse.
- Evaluation includes examining the effectiveness of the nursing interventions, changing the outcomes as needed, and reassessing the nursing diagnoses. Evaluation is an ongoing process and is part of each of the other steps in the nursing process.

# CRITICAL THINKING

1. Jian has been diagnosed with bipolar disorder and has been taking lithium for four months. During a clinic visit, he tells you that he does not think he will be taking his lithium anymore because he feels fine and misses his old "intensity." He says he is able to function well at his job and at home with his family and that his wife agrees that he "has this thing licked."
   a. What are Jian's needs in terms of teaching?
   b. What are the needs of his family?
   c. Write a teaching plan for Jian, or use an already constructed plan that includes the following teaching topics with sound rationales:

   (1) Use of alcohol, drugs, caffeine, over-the-counter medications
   (2) Need for sleep, hygiene
   (3) Types of community resources available
   (4) Signs and symptoms of relapse

2. How would you explain the importance of a normal sleep-wake cycle to a patient with bipolar disorder?
   a. Research has shown that a faulty circadian rhythm may be to blame for sleep disruption in the mania phase of bipolar disorder. Therefore, it is important to maintain a normal sleep-wake cycle for mood stabilization because sleep disruptions can trigger mania.

# CHAPTER REVIEW

1. Which behaviour exhibited by a person with mania should the nurse choose to address first?
   1. Indiscriminate sexual relations
   2. Excessive spending of money
   3. Declaration of "being at one with the world"
   4. Demonstration of flight of ideas

2. The nurse is caring for a person experiencing mania. Which is the most appropriate nursing intervention?
   1. Provide consistency among staff members when working with the person
   2. Negotiate limits so the person has a voice in the plan of care
   3. Allow only certain staff members to interact with the person
   4. Attempt to control the person's emotions

3. The nurse is planning care for a person experiencing the acute phase of mania. Which is the priority intervention?
   1. Prevent injury
   2. Maintain stable cardiac status
   3. Get the person to demonstrate thought self-control
   4. Ensure that the person gets sufficient sleep and rest

4. What critical information should the nurse provide about the use of lithium?
   1. "You will still have hypersexual tendencies, so be certain to use protection when engaging in intercourse."
   2. "Lithium will help you to feel only the euphoria of mania but not the anxiety."
   3. "It will take one to two weeks and maybe longer for this medication to start working fully."
   4. "This medication is a cure for bipolar disorder."

5. The nurse has provided education for a person in the continuation phase, after discharge from the hospital. What indicates that the plan of care has been successful? Select all that apply.
   1. Person identifies three signs and symptoms of relapse.
   2. Person states, "My wife doesn't mind if I still drink a little."
   3. Person reports that medication has been helpful but he is ready to stop.
   4. Person states, "I no longer have a disease."

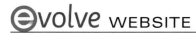 WEBSITE

Post-Test interactive review

*Visit the Evolve Web site for Chapter Review Answers and Rationales, Critical Thinking Answer Guidelines, and additional resources related to the content in this chapter:* http://evolve.elsevier.com/Canada/Varcarolis/psychiatric/

## REFERENCES

Baghai, T.C. (2008). Electroconvulsive therapy and its different indications. *Dialogues Clinical Neuroscience, 10*, 105–117.

Baldassano, C.F., Marangell, L.B., Gyulai, L., et al. (2005). Gender differences in bipolar disorder: Retrospective data from the first 500 STEP-BD participants. *Bipolar Disorder, 5*, 465–470. doi:10.1111/j.1399-5618.2005.00237.x.

Bauer, M., Beaulieu, S., Dunner, D.L., et al. (2008). Rapid cycling bipolar disorder—diagnostic concepts. *Bipolar Disorders, 10*, 153–162. doi:10.1111/j.1399-5618.2007.00560.x.

Baum, A.E., Akula, N., Cabanero, M., et al. (2008). A genome-wide association study implicates diacylglycerol kinase eta (DGKH) and several other genes in the etiology of bipolar disorder. *Molecular Psychiatry, 13*, 197–207. doi:10.1038/sj.mp.4002012.

Benazzi, F. (2007). Bipolar II disorder: Epidemiology, diagnosis, and management. *CNS Drugs, 21*(9), 727–740.

Burmeister, M., McInnis, M.G., & Zollner, S. (2008). Psychiatric genetics: Progress amid controversy. *Nature Reviews Genetics, 9*, 527–540. doi:10.1038/nrg2381.

Canadian Mental Health Association. (2011). *Fast facts about mental illness.* Retrieved from http://www.cmha.ca/bins/content_page.asp?cid=6-20-23-43.

Canadian Network for Mood and Anxiety Treatments. (2009). *Canadian Network for Mood and Anxiety Treatments (CANMAT) and International Society for Bipolar Disorders (ISBD) collaborative update of CANMAT guidelines for the management of patients with bipolar disorder: Update 2009.* Retrieved from http://www.canmat.org/resources/CANMAT%20Bipolar%20Disorder%20Guidelines%20-2009%20Update.pdf.

Fagiolini, A., Chengappa, K.N., Soreca, I., et al. (2008). Bipolar disorder and the metabolic syndrome: Causal factors, psychiatric outcomes and economic burden. *CNS Drugs, 22*(8), 655–669.

Feeny, N.C., Danielson, C.K., Schwartz, L., et al. (2006). Cognitive-behavioral therapy for bipolar disorders in adolescents: A pilot study. *Bipolar Disorder, 8*, 508–515.

Frank, E. (2007). Interpersonal and social rhythm therapy: A means of improving depression and preventing relapse in bipolar disorder. *Journal of Clinical Psychology, 63*, 463–473. doi:10.1002/jclp.20371.

Gitlin, M. (2007). Treatment-resistant bipolar disorder. *Focus, 5*(1), 49–63.

Gunderson, J.G., Weinberg, I., Daversa, M.T., et al. (2006). Descriptive and longitudinal observations on the relationship of borderline personality disorder and bipolar disorder. *American Journal of Psychiatry, 163*, 1173–1178. doi:10.1176/appi.ajp.163.7.1173.

Health Canada Editorial Board Mental Illnesses in Canada. (2002). *A report on mental illnesses in Canada (Cat. No. 0-662-32817-5).* Retrieved from http://www.phac-aspc.gc.ca/publicat/miic-mmac/.

Hirschfeld, R.M., Williams, J.B., Spitzer, R.L., et al. (2000). Development and validation of a screening instrument for bipolar spectrum disorder: The Mood Disorder Questionnaire. *American Journal of Psychiatry, 157*, 1873–1875.

Jamison, K.R. (1995). *An unquiet mind.* New York: Knopf.

Jones, S., Mulligan, L.D., Law, H., et al. (2012). A randomised controlled trial of recovery focused CBT for individuals with early bipolar disorder. *BMC Psychiatry, 12*, 204–220. doi:10.1186/1471-244X-12-204.

McClung, C.A. (2007). Circadian genes, rhythms, and the biology of mood disorders. *Pharmacology and Therapeutics, 114,* 222–232. doi:10.1016/j.pharmthera.2007.02.003.

McIntyre, R.S., Konarski, J.Z., Soczynska, J.K., et al. (2006). Medical comorbidity in bipolar disorder: Implications for functional outcomes and health service utilization. *Psychiatric Services, 57,* 1140–1144. doi:10.1176/appi.ps.57.8.1140.

Merikangas, K.R., Akiskal, H.S., Angst, J., et al. (2007). Lifetime and 12-month prevalence of bipolar spectrum disorder in the National Comorbidity Survey Replication. *Archives of General Psychiatry, 64*(5), 543–552.

Mood Disorders Society of Canada. (2009). *What is bipolar disorder?* Retrieved from http://www.mooddisorderscanada.ca/documents/Consumer%20and%20Family%20Support/Bipolar%20Brochure%20English%20FINAL%20150109.pdf.

Moorhead, S., Johnson, M., Maas, M., et al. (Eds.) (2008). *Nursing outcomes classification (NOC)* (3rd ed.). St. Louis, MO: Mosby.

Ostacher, M.J. (2011). Bipolar and substance use disorder comorbidity: Diagnostic and treatment considerations. *Focus, 9*(4), 428–434.

Ostacher, M.J., & Tilley, C.A. (2008). Anticonvulsants. In T.A. Stern, J.F. Rosenbaum, M. Fava, et al. (Eds.) *Comprehensive clinical psychiatry* (pp. 661–666). Philadelphia: Mosby Elsevier.

Ottawa Citizen (2006, May 7). *Margaret Trudeau's secret war.* Retrieved from http://www.canada.com/topics/bodyandhealth/story.html?id=8cf493ee-f0d4-421c-bfce-92adb8b2ea0b.

Otto, M.W., Reilly-Harrington, N., & Sachs, G.S. (2003). Psychoeducational and cognitive-behavioural strategies in the management of bipolar disorder [Abstract]. *Journal of Affective Disorders, 73,* 171–181. doi:10.1016/S0165-0327(01)00460-8.

Owen, M.J., Craddock, N., & Jablensky, A. (2007). The genetic deconstruction of psychosis. *Schizophrenia Bulletin, 33,* 905–911. doi:10.1093/schbul/sbm053.

Pollock, R., & Kuo, I. (2004). *Neuroimaging in bipolar disorder.* Paper presented at the 5th Invitational Congress of Biological Psychiatry, Sydney, Australia.

Preston, J.D., O'Neal, J.H., & Talaga, M.C. (2005). *Handbook of clinical psychopharmacology for therapists* (4th ed.). Oakland, CA: New Harbinger.

Repchinsky, C. (Ed.) (2006). *Compendium of pharmaceuticals and specialties (CPS): The Canadian drug reference for health professionals* (41st ed.). Ottawa: Canadian Pharmacists Association.

Robinson, L.J., Thompson, J.M., Gallagher, P., et al. (2006). A meta-analysis of cognitive deficits in euthymic patients with bipolar disorder. *Journal of Affective Disorders, 93,* 105–115. doi:10.1016/j.jad.2006.02.016.

Sadock, B.J., & Sadock, V.A. (2008). *Concise textbook of clinical psychiatry* (3rd ed.). Philadelphia: Lippincott Williams & Wilkins.

Sajatovic, M., Davies, M., Bauer, M., et al. (2005). Attitudes regarding the collaborative practice model and treatment adherence among individuals with bipolar disorder. *Comprehensive Psychiatry, 46,* 272–277. doi:10.1016/j.comppsych.2004.10.007.

Schretlen, D.J., Cascella, N.G., Meyer, S.M., et al. (2007). Neuropsychological functioning in bipolar disorder and schizophrenia. *Biological Psychiatry, 62,* 179–186. doi:10.1016/j.biopsych.2006.09.025.

Sklar, P., Smoller, J.W., Fan, J., et al. (2008). Whole-genome association study of bipolar disorder. *Molecular Psychiatry, 13,* 558–569. doi:10.1038/sj.mp.4002151.

Strakowski, S.M., DelBello, M.P., & Adler, C.M. (2005). The functional neuroanatomy of bipolar disorder: A review of neuroimaging findings. *Molecular Psychiatry, 10,* 105–116. doi:10.1038/sj.mp.4001585.

Tohen, M. (2003). *Olanzapine more effective for preventing mania relapse.* Paper presented at the 5th Invitational Congress of Bipolar Disorders, Pittsburgh, PA.

Torrent, C., Sanchez-Moreno, J., Comes, M., et al. (2006). Cognitive impairment in bipolar II disorder. *British Journal of Psychiatry, 189,* 254–259. doi:10.1192/bjp.bp.105.017269.

Vallerand, A.H., Sanoski, C.A., & Deglin, J.H. (2013). *Davis's drug guide for nurses.* Philadelphia: F.A. Davis.

Vieta, E., & Suppes, T. (2008). Bipolar II disorder: Arguments for and against a distinct diagnostic entity. *Bipolar Disorders, 10,* 163–178. doi:10.1111/j.1399-5618.2007.00561.x.

Wang, P.S., Berglund, P., Olfson, M., et al. (2005). Failure and delay in initial treatment contact after first onset of mental disorders in the National Comorbidity Survey Replication. *Archives of General Psychiatry, 62*(6), 603–613.

Wellcome Trust Case Control Consortium (2007). Genome-wide association study of 14,000 cases of seven common diseases and 3,000 shared controls. *Nature, 447,* 661–678. doi:10.1038/nature05911.

# 16

# Schizophrenia Spectrum and Other Psychotic Disorders

*Edward A. Herzog, Elizabeth M. Varcarolis*
*Adapted by Wilma Schroeder*

## KEY TERMS AND CONCEPTS

abnormal motor behaviour, 286
acute dystonia, 304
affective symptoms, 291
akathisia, 304
anosognosia, 296
anticholinergic-induced delirium, 306
associative looseness, 293
boundary impairment, 293
circumstantiality, 293
cognitive symptoms, 291
command hallucinations, 294
concrete thinking, 292
delusions, 286
depersonalization, 293
derealization, 293
disorganized thinking, 286
echolalia, 293

echopraxia, 294
extrapyramidal side effects (EPS), 304
hallucinations, 286
ideas of reference, 309
illusions, 293
negative symptoms, 286
neologisms, 293
neuroleptic malignant syndrome (NMS), 304
paranoia, 306
positive symptoms, 291
pseudoparkinsonism, 304
reality testing, 292
recovery model, 297
stereotyped behaviours, 294
tangentiality, 293
tardive dyskinesia (TD or TDK), 304
word salad, 293

## OBJECTIVES

1. Describe the progression of symptoms, focus of care, and intervention needs for the prepsychotic through maintenance phases of schizophrenia.
2. Discuss at least three of the neurobiological–anatomical–genetic findings that indicate that schizophrenia is a brain disorder.
3. Differentiate among the positive and negative symptoms of schizophrenia in terms of psychopharmacological treatment and effect on quality of life.
4. Discuss the concept of recovery for people living with schizophrenia.
5. Discuss how to deal with common reactions the nurse may experience while working with a person with schizophrenia.

6. Develop teaching plans for people taking conventional antipsychotic drugs (e.g., haloperidol [Haldol]) and atypical antipsychotic drugs (e.g., risperidone [Risperdal]).
7. Compare and contrast the conventional antipsychotic medications with atypical antipsychotics.
8. Identify nonpharmacological interventions that may be used to address symptoms of schizophrenia.
9. Create a nursing care plan that incorporates evidence-informed interventions for key areas of dysfunction in schizophrenia, including hallucinations, delusions, paranoia, cognitive disorganization, anosognosia, and impaired self-care.
10. Role-play intervening with a person who is hallucinating, delusional, and exhibiting disorganized thinking.

# ⊖volve WEBSITE

*Visit the Evolve website for Flashcards, Case Studies, and additional testing resources related to the content in this chapter:* http://evolve.elsevier.com/Canada/Varcarolis/psychiatric/     Pre-Test  interactive review

Schizophrenia spectrum and other psychotic disorders are potentially devastating brain disorders that affect a person's thinking, language, emotions, social behaviour, and ability to perceive reality accurately. The most severe disorder in this category is schizophrenia, which is the major focus of this chapter. It affects 1 in every 100 people (over 300 000 people in Canada) and is among the most disruptive and disabling of mental disorders. Unfortunately, people with this disorder are often misunderstood and stigmatized not only by the general population but even by the medical community. Negative attitudes toward people can interfere with recovery and impair their quality of life (Crowe, Deane, Oades, et al., 2006). For example, many believe that people with schizophrenia are likely to be violent, but the overall rate of violence among those with schizophrenia is no greater than that of the general public. In fact, stranger homicide by persons with psychosis is extremely rare—1 incident per 14.3 million people per year (Nielssen, Bourget, Laajasalo, et al., 2009).

- The following How a Nurse Helped Me story demonstrates the four elements of the LEAP approach (Amador, 2000), which is based on the belief that trusting relationships are key to healing partnerships:
- Listen—Both nurses listened with compassion and genuineness.
- Empathize—It is clear that both nurses were able to convey that they understood what Tammy was feeling.

## ✿ HOW A NURSE HELPED ME

### *They Helped Me to Believe in Myself*

*I live with schizoaffective disorder. I am 30 now, and I was diagnosed with a mental illness when I was 15. I experience both the psychotic symptoms often present in schizophrenia and a mood component often in the form of rapid cycling. For the first five to ten years of coping with my mental illness, the hospital was like a revolving door for me. It took me numerous years to find the right medications.*

*Through the dedication of nurses like Cheryl and Rhonda, I have been able to overcome my intense symptoms by finding balance in my chaotic moods and a decrease in my delusional symptoms and paranoia. Cheryl is a nurse who goes out of her way to be there for her patients. She uses compassion and humour to communicate with us. I have worked with Cheryl for ten years. From the very beginning, I felt a close connection with her and have felt privileged to work with her. She has had such a positive impact on my life. She believed in me even when I didn't believe in myself. She treats us each with the utmost respect. She has a gentle spirit, and she brings cheerfulness to the ward. If you are depressed or not feeling well, she is most often able to cheer you up. (That is no matter how bad you feel or how painful your day has been.) She has a fun-loving nature, and she is loved by all. Cheryl relates well to everyone. She is full of energy and*

*enthusiasm. She truly cares. She is genuine, and even if she herself is struggling that day, she is still full of kindness and empathy. Her dedication to her patients never wavers. Cheryl is definitely one of a kind.*

*Rhonda is one of the most dedicated and compassionate nurses I have ever met. She has had a tremendous influence on my life. She often works long hours to offer full support to her patients. Sometimes I have called her past 6:00 in the evening thinking I would leave a message, yet to my surprise, she is still there, and she makes time to answer my call. She is very efficient and does her job extremely well. She treats us all equally with dignity and respect. I have never felt like I have been looked down upon or judged. She has an open mind and her compassion has supported me through many rough and painful times. Rhonda has always believed in me, and this has helped me on my road to recovery. I look forward to appointments with Rhonda because she always allows me to see life situations from a positive perspective, and she provides me with ongoing encouragement. Rhonda is an awesome nurse.*

*Rhonda and Cheryl are an asset to the health care system. If all psychiatric nurses were like them, the mental health system would be amazing.*

**Source:** Story written by Tammy L. and reproduced with her permission.

- Agree—Both nurses believed in Tammy and supported her in her goals, never looking down on her or judging her but helping her on her own road to recovery.
- Partner—Clearly, both nurses respected Tammy and worked with her as partners.

LEAP is described as a technique; however, inherent in that description is the risk of seeing it only technically. The LEAP approach must be underpinned by genuineness and caring. Cheryl and Rhonda invited Tammy into a trusting and therapeutic relationship. They did not apply these components as "techniques"; instead, it appears that the LEAP principles flowed naturally out of genuine caring. Tammy's story demonstrates how empowering and healing it is to experience being truly listened to, empathized with, and collaborated with.

## CLINICAL PICTURE

Adding to observations made by Emil Kraepelin (1856–1926), Eugen Bleuler (1857–1939) coined the term *schizophrenia*. He first proposed that schizophrenia was not one illness but a heterogeneous group of illnesses with different characteristics and clinical courses. Five key features are associated with psychotic disorders:

1. Delusions: Alterations in *thought content* (what a person thinks about). Delusions are false fixed beliefs that cannot be corrected by reasoning or evidence to the contrary. "Unusual" beliefs maintained by one's culture or subculture are not delusions..
2. Hallucinations: Perception of a sensory experience for which no external stimulus exists (e.g., hearing a voice when no one is speaking).
3. Disorganized thinking: The loosening of associations, manifested as jumbled and illogical speech and impaired reasoning.
4. Abnormal motor behaviour: Alterations in behaviour, including bizarre and agitated behaviours (e.g., stilted, rigid demeanour or eccentric dress, grooming, and rituals). Grossly disorganized behaviours may include mutism, stupor, or catatonic excitement.
5. Negative symptoms: The absence of something that should be present but is not—for example, the ability to make decisions or to follow through on a plan. Negative symptoms contribute to poor social functioning and social withdrawal.

---

**VIGNETTE**

Samuel, a 25-year-old man soon to be discharged from the hospital, constantly tells the social worker he wants his own apartment. When Samuel is told that an apartment has been found for him, he asks, "But who will take care of me?" Samuel is acting out his ambivalence between his desire to be independent and his desire to be taken care of.

---

Clinicians in Canada use the criteria of the *Diagnostic and Statistical Manual of Mental Disorders*, fifth edition, for the diagnosis of schizophrenia spectrum and other psychotic disorders.

All those diagnosed with schizophrenia exhibit at least one psychotic symptom, such as delusions, hallucinations, or disorganized thinking, speech, or behaviour. The person experiences extreme difficulty with or an inability to function in family, social, or occupational realms and frequently neglects basic needs such as nutrition or hygiene. Over a period of six months, there may be times when the psychotic symptoms are absent, and in their place, the person may experience apathy or depression.

Other psychotic disorders (e.g., schizophreniform and schizoaffective disorders) are described in Box 16-1.

---

### BOX 16-1   PSYCHOTIC DISORDERS OTHER THAN SCHIZOPHRENIA

**Schizophreniform Disorder**
The features of schizophreniform disorder are similar to schizophrenia, but the total duration of the illness is less than six months. This disorder may or may not develop into schizophrenia; people who do not develop schizophrenia have a good prognosis.

**Brief Psychotic Disorder**
This disorder involves a sudden onset of psychosis or grossly disorganized or catatonic behaviour lasting less than one month. It is often precipitated by extreme stressors and is followed by a return to premorbid functioning.

**Schizoaffective Disorder**
Schizoaffective disorder is characterized by a major depressive, manic, or mixed-mood episode presenting concurrently with symptoms of schizophrenia. The symptoms are not due to any substance use or to a medical condition.

**Delusional Disorder**
Delusional disorder is characterized by nonbizarre delusions (i.e., situations that could occur in real life, such as being followed, being deceived by a spouse, or having a disease). The person's ability to function is not markedly impaired, nor is behaviour otherwise odd or psychotic. A related disorder, Capgras syndrome, involves a delusion about a significant other (e.g., family member or pet) being replaced by an imposter; this disorder may be a result of psychiatric or organic brain disease (Denes, 2007).

**Substance- or Medication-Induced Psychotic Disorder**
Psychosis may be induced by substances such as drugs of abuse, alcohol, medications, or toxins (Mauri, Volonteri, De Gaspari, et al., 2006).

**Psychosis or Catatonia Associated With Another Medical Condition or Another Mental Disorder**
Psychoses may also be caused by a medical condition (delirium, neurological or metabolic conditions, hepatic or renal diseases, and many others). Medical conditions and substance abuse must always be ruled out before a diagnosis of schizophrenia or other psychotic disorder can be made.

**Sources:** Denes, G. (2007). Capgras delusion. *Neurological Sciences, 28*, 163–164. doi:10.1007/s10072-007-0813-1; Mauri, M.C., Volonteri, L.S., De Gaspari, I.F., et al. (2006). Substance abuse in first-episode schizophrenic patients: A retrospective study. *Clinical Practice and Epidemiology in Mental Health, 2*, 1–8. doi:10.1186/1745-0179-2-4.

## EPIDEMIOLOGY

The lifetime prevalence of schizophrenia is 1% worldwide, with no differences related to race, social status, or culture. It is more common in males (1.4:1) and among persons growing up in urban areas (Tandon, Keshavan, & Nasrallah, 2008). Schizophrenia usually develops during the late teens and early twenties, although onset before the age of 10 has been reported (Masi, Mucci, & Pari, 2006). Childhood schizophrenia, although rare, does exist, occurring in 1 out of 40,000 children. Early onset (18 to 25 years) occurs more often in males and is associated with poor functioning before onset, more structural brain abnormality, and increased levels of apathy. Individuals with a later onset (25 to 35 years) are more likely to be female, have less structural brain abnormality, and have better outcomes.

## CO-MORBIDITY

Substance abuse disorders occur in nearly 50% of persons with schizophrenia (Green, Noordsy, Brunette, et al., 2008). When substance abuse occurs in people with schizophrenia, it is associated with treatment nonadherence, relapse, incarceration, homelessness, violence, suicide, and a poorer prognosis (Mauri, Volonteri, De Gaspari, et al., 2006). Nicotine dependence rates in schizophrenia range from 70% to 90% and contribute to an increased incidence of cardiovascular and respiratory disorders (Green, Noordsy, Brunette, et al., 2008).

Anxiety, depression, and suicide co-occur frequently in schizophrenia. Anxiety may be a response to symptoms (e.g., hallucinations) or circumstances (e.g., isolation, overstimulation) and may worsen schizophrenia symptoms and prognosis (Mauri, Moliterno, Rossattini, et al., 2008). Almost half of all persons with schizophrenia attempt suicide at some point in their lives, and approximately 10% succeed (Hayashi, Ishida, Miyashita, et al., 2005). Both depression and suicide attempts can occur at any point in the illness (Osborn, Levy, Nazareth, et al., 2008).

Polydipsia can lead to fatal water intoxication (indicated by hyponatremia, confusion, worsening psychotic symptoms, and ultimately coma). It is characterized by a seemingly insatiable thirst that results in a dangerous intake of water. It occurs in 7% of inpatients with schizophrenia (Gonzalez & Perez, 2008). Factors that contribute to excess water intake include taking antipsychotic medication (causes dry mouth), compulsive behaviour, and neuroendocrine abnormalities (Bralet, Ton, & Falissard, 2007).

Physical illnesses are more common among people with schizophrenia than in the general population. Even after adjusting for demographics and socioeconomic status, the death rate for people with mental illness is close to 70% higher than for the general population, and this risk of premature death is even greater for people with schizophrenia (Kisely, 2010). On average, persons with schizophrenia die 28 years prematurely due to disorders such as hypertension (22%), obesity (24%), cardiovascular disease (21%), diabetes (12%), chronic obstructive pulmonary disease (COPD) (10%), and trauma (6%) (Miller, Paschall, & Svendsen, 2007). Disturbingly, this disparity in risk has actually increased in the past 20 to 30 years (Kisely, 2010).

People with psychotic disorders may be at greater risk due to apathy, poor health habits, medications (see the discussion of metabolic syndrome later in this chapter), or failure to recognize signs of illness. Communication problems or difficulties with informed consent may also be factors (Kisely, 2010). Owing to poverty, stigma, or stereotyping (e.g., emergency department personnel assuming that because a person has a psychotic disorder, his chest pain is imaginary), they may not receive adequate health care. Despite having more contact with family physicians than the general population, persons with psychiatric disorders are less likely to be assessed and treated for conditions such as hypertension or to receive preventive care such as smoking cessation (Kisely, 2010).

Incentives and barriers to engaging people with severe mental illness in lifestyle interventions have not been extensively studied, though there is some evidence that these interventions can be effective (Roberts & Bailey, 2011). Barriers that are reported in the literature include illness symptoms, treatment effects, lack of support, and negative staff attitudes; incentives include peer and staff support, staff participation, reduction of symptoms, knowledge, and personal attributes (Roberts & Bailey, 2011).

## ETIOLOGY

Schizophrenia typically manifests in late adolescence or early adulthood. It becomes chronic or recurrent in at least 80% of those who develop it; on average, everyone has about a 0.7% chance of developing schizophrenia (Tandon, Keshavan, & Nasrallah, 2008).

Schizophrenia is a complicated disorder. In fact, what we call "schizophrenia" actually may be a group of disorders with common but varying features and multiple, overlapping etiologies. What is known is that brain chemistry, structure, and activity are different in a person with schizophrenia from those in a person who does not have the disorder.

The scientific consensus is that schizophrenia occurs when multiple inherited gene abnormalities combine with nongenetic factors (e.g., viral infections, birth injuries, prenatal malnutrition), altering the structures of the brain, affecting the brain's neurotransmitter systems, injuring the brain directly, or doing all three (Tandon, Keshavan, & Nasrallah, 2008). This effect is called the *diathesis–stress model of schizophrenia* (Walker & Tessner, 2008).

### Biological Factors
#### Genetic Factors
Schizophrenia and schizophrenia-like symptoms, such as eccentric thinking, are more prevalent in relatives of individuals with schizophrenia. According to Smoller, Finn, and Gardner-Schuster (2008):

- Compared to the usual 1% risk in the population, having a first-degree relative with schizophrenia increases the risk to 10%.

- There is variability of expression of schizophrenia, depending upon environmental factors; schizoaffective disorder and cluster-A personality disorders are more common in relatives of people with schizophrenia.
- Concordance rates in twins (how often one twin will have the disorder when the other one has it) is about 50% for identical twins and about 15% for fraternal twins.

Evidence suggests that multiple genes on different chromosomes interact with each other in complex ways to create vulnerability to schizophrenia. Genes potentially linked to schizophrenia continue to be identified, suggesting a high degree of complexity (Tandon, Keshavan, & Nasrallah, 2008).

### Neurobiological Factors

*Dopamine theory.* The dopamine theory of schizophrenia is derived from the study of the action of the first antipsychotic drugs, collectively known as *conventional* (or *first-generation*) *antipsychotics* (e.g., haloperidol [Haldol] and chlorpromazine [Largactil]). These drugs block the activity of dopamine-2 ($D_2$) receptors in the brain, limiting the activity of dopamine and reducing some of the symptoms of schizophrenia. However, because the dopamine-blocking agents do not alleviate all the symptoms of schizophrenia, it is recognized that there are other neurochemicals involved in generating the symptoms of schizophrenia. Amphetamines, cocaine, methylphenidate (Ritalin), and levodopa increase the activity of dopamine in the brain and, in biologically susceptible people, may precipitate schizophrenia's onset. If schizophrenia is already present, they may also exacerbate its symptoms.

*Other neurochemical hypotheses.* A newer class of drugs, collectively known as *atypical* (or *second-generation*) *antipsychotics,* block serotonin as well as dopamine, which suggests that serotonin may play a role in schizophrenia as well. A better understanding of how atypical agents modulate the expression and targeting of 5-hydroxytryptamine 2A (5-HT2A) and its receptors would likely lead to a better understanding of schizophrenia.

Researchers have long been aware that phenylcyclohexyl piperidine (PCP) induces a state closely resembling schizophrenia. This observation led to interest in the N-methyl-D-aspartate (NMDA) receptor complex and the possible role of glutamate in the pathophysiology of schizophrenia. Glutamate is a crucial neurotransmitter during periods of neuromaturation; abnormal maturation of the central nervous system (CNS) is considered to be a central contributing factor in schizophrenia (Goff, 2005).

### Brain Structure Abnormalities

Disruptions in communication pathways in the brain are thought to be severe in schizophrenia. Therefore, it is conceivable that structural abnormalities cause disruption of the brain's functioning. Using brain imaging techniques—computed tomography (CT), magnetic resonance imaging (MRI), and positron emission tomography (PET)—researchers have provided substantial evidence that some people with schizophrenia have structural brain abnormalities (Broome, Woolley, Tabraham, et al., 2005), including:

- Enlarged lateral cerebral ventricles, a dilated third ventricle, ventricular asymmetry, or a combination of these
- Reduced cortical, frontal lobe, hippocampal, or cerebellar volumes
- Increased size of the sulci (fissures) on the surface of the brain

In addition, MRI and CT scans demonstrate lower brain volume and more cerebrospinal fluid in people with schizophrenia. PET scans also show a lowered rate of blood flow and glucose metabolism in the frontal lobes, which govern planning, abstract thinking, social adjustment, and decision making, all of which are affected in schizophrenia. (Figure 4-5 in Chapter 4 shows a PET scan demonstrating reduced brain activity in the frontal lobe of a person with schizophrenia.) Such structural changes may worsen as the disorder continues. Postmortem studies on individuals with schizophrenia reveal a reduced volume of grey matter in the brain, especially in the temporal and frontal lobes; those with the most tissue loss had the worst symptoms (e.g., hallucinations, delusions, bizarre thoughts, depression).

### Psychological and Environmental Factors

A number of stressors, particularly those occurring during vulnerable periods of neurological development, are believed to combine with genetic vulnerabilities to produce schizophrenia. Reducing such stressors is believed to have the potential to reduce the severity of the disorder or even prevent it (Compton, 2004).

### Prenatal Stressors

A history of pregnancy or birth complications is associated with an increased risk for schizophrenia. Prenatal risk factors include viral infection, poor nutrition, hypoxia, and exposure to toxins. Psychological trauma to the mother during pregnancy (e.g., the death of a relative) can also contribute to the development of schizophrenia (Khashan, Abel, McNamee, et al., 2008). Other risk factors include a father older than 35 at the child's conception and being born during late winter or early spring (Tandon, Keshavan, & Nasrallah, 2008).

### Psychological Stressors

Although there is no evidence that stress alone causes schizophrenia, stress increases cortisol levels, impeding hypothalamic development and causing other changes that may precipitate the illness in vulnerable individuals. Schizophrenia often manifests at times of developmental and family stress, such as beginning college or moving away from one's family. Social, psychological, and physical stressors may play a significant role in both the severity and course of the disorder and the person's quality of life. Other factors increasing the risk of schizophrenia include cannabis use and exposure to psychological trauma or social defeat (Tandon, Keshavan, & Nasrallah, 2008).

### Environmental Stressors

Environmental factors are also believed to contribute to the development of schizophrenia in vulnerable people. These include exposure to social adversity (e.g., living in chronic

## CULTURAL CONSIDERATIONS

### The Stigma of Schizophrenia

Mrs. Chou, a 25-year-old woman, left China for North America six months ago to join her husband. In China, she lived with her parents and had learned English. She was shy and looked to her parents, and later to her husband, for guidance and support. Shortly after arrival in her new country, her mother developed pneumonia and died. Mrs. Chou later told her husband that if she had stayed in China, her mother would not have become ill and that evil would now come to their 1-year-old child because Mrs. Chou had not taken proper care of her mother.

Mrs. Chou became increasingly lethargic, staring into space and mumbling to herself. When Mr. Chou asked who she was talking to, she answered, "My mother."

Mr. Chou realized that something was terribly wrong with his wife, yet he was reluctant to ask either relatives or professionals for assistance since mental illness is strongly stigmatized in the Chinese culture. In fact, mental illness may be believed to be a punishment for personal failings.

Mrs. Chou was finally admitted to a psychiatric unit when Mr. Chou noticed she had quit eating and taking care of herself and was certainly unable to care for their child. During her admission assessment, she sat motionless and mute. Mr. Nolan, her primary nurse, noticed that after he checked her pulse, her arm remained in midair until he lowered it for her. Mrs. Chou was unkempt and pale, and her skin turgor was poor.

Mr. Nolan also spoke with Mr. Chou, who was visibly distressed by his wife's condition. He discovered that Mr. Chou blamed himself for his wife's illness because his relocation prevented her from caring for her ailing mother. He agreed with his wife that their mutual failings placed their child at risk of retribution. He conceded that coming to the hospital had been very difficult, owing to embarrassment both about his wife's mental illness and his own belief that he should not burden others with the care of himself and his wife. Mr. Nolan helped Mr. Chou recognize that in North American culture, family members shared caregiving burdens, professional help was more available, and stigmatization was less intense.

Gradually, Mr. Chou's distress lessened as he came to appreciate that he would not have to carry the level of burden he had anticipated. As Mrs. Chou's psychosis abated, both she and Mr. Chou came to ascribe more culpability for the illness to fate, reducing their burden of self-blame. They agreed to meet with a healer who helped them integrate the beliefs and resources of their original and adopted cultures, further reducing their guilt and distress.

**Source:** Wong, D.F.K., Tsui, H.K.P., Pearson, V., et al. (2004). Family burdens, Chinese health beliefs, and the mental health of Chinese caregivers in Hong Kong. *Transcultural Psychiatry, 4,* 497–513.

to be aware of social and economic diversity among immigrant groups, as they may face challenges different from those of the dominant cultural group. Although this was a small study, its results deserve consideration.

### Course of the Disorder

The onset of symptoms or forewarning (prodromal) symptoms may appear a month to a year before the first psychotic break or full-blown manifestations of the illness; such symptoms represent a clear deterioration in previous functioning. The course thereafter typically includes recurrent exacerbations separated by periods of reduced or dormant symptoms. Some people will have a single episode of schizophrenia without recurrences or have several episodes and none thereafter. A recent study of over 2000 persons found four patterns of the course of the illness. Although the course of schizophrenia varied, all showed an initial deterioration followed by improvement (Levine, Lurie, Kohn, et al., 2011). Remission and recovery are increasingly common outcomes with early detection, appropriate treatment, and social support. For many people, however, schizophrenia is a chronic or recurring disorder that, like diabetes or heart disease, is managed but rarely cured.

Frequently, the history of a person with schizophrenia reveals that, prior to the illness, the person was socially awkward, lonely, and perhaps depressed and expressed himself or herself in vague, odd, or unrealistic ways. In this prodromal phase, complaints about anxiety, phobias, obsessions, dissociative features, and compulsions may be noted. As anxiety mounts, indications of a thought disorder become evident. Concentration, memory, and completion of school- or job-related work deteriorate. Intrusive thoughts, "mind wandering," and the need to devote more time to maintaining one's thoughts are reported.

The person may feel that something "strange" or "wrong" is happening. Events are misinterpreted, and mystical or symbolic meanings may be given to ordinary events. For example, the person may think that certain colours have special powers or that a song on the radio is a message from God. Discerning others' emotions becomes more difficult, and other people's actions or words may be mistaken for signs of hostility or evidence of harmful intent (Chung, Kang, Shin, et al., 2008).

### Prognosis

Studies have shown that most of the deterioration occurs within the first two to five years after onset of psychosis, followed by a plateau in impairment and symptoms (Srihari, Shah, & Keshavan, 2012). For the majority of people, most symptoms can be at least somewhat controlled through medications and psychosocial interventions. With support and effective treatments, many people with schizophrenia experience a good quality of life and success within their families, occupations, and other roles. Associates may not even realize the person has schizophrenia.

In other cases, schizophrenia does not respond fully to available treatments, leaving residual symptoms and causing varying degrees of disability. Some cases require repeated or lengthy inpatient care or institutionalization. An abrupt onset of symptoms is usually a favourable prognostic sign, and those with

poverty or high-crime environments) and migration to or growing up in a foreign culture (Tandon, Keshavan, & Nasrallah, 2008; Broome, Woolley, Tabraham, et al., 2005). O'Mahony and Donnelly (2007) found that immigrant women face many difficulties accessing mental health services. These authors suggest that although knowledge and cultural practices have an influence on such access, it is necessary for health care providers

good premorbid social, sexual, and occupational functioning have a greater chance for a good remission or a complete recovery. A slow, insidious onset over two to three years is more ominous, and the younger one is at the onset of schizophrenia, the more discouraging the prognosis. A childhood history of withdrawn, reclusive, eccentric, and tense behaviour is also an unfavourable diagnostic sign, as is a preponderance of negative symptoms (Möller, 2007).

## Phases of Schizophrenia

Schizophrenia usually progresses through predictable phases, although the presenting symptoms during a given phase and the length of the phase can vary widely. The phases of schizophrenia are as follows (Chung, Kang, Shin, et al., 2008):

- **Phase I—Acute:** Onset or exacerbation of florid, disruptive symptoms (e.g., hallucinations, delusions, apathy, withdrawal) with resultant loss of functional abilities; increased care or hospitalization may be required.
- **Phase II—Stabilization:** Symptoms are diminishing, and there is movement toward one's previous level of functioning (baseline); day hospitalization or care in a residential crisis centre or a supervised group home may be needed.
- **Phase III—Maintenance:** The person is at or nearing baseline (or premorbid) functioning; symptoms are absent or diminished; level of functioning allows the person to live in the community. Ideally, recovery with few or no residual symptoms has occurred. Most people in this phase live in their own residences. Although this phase has been termed *maintenance*, current literature shows a trend toward reframing it with a greater emphasis on recovery. Some clinicians and people with schizophrenia contend that maintenance and recovery are opposing concepts, "maintenance" being a pessimistic view, and "recovery" being more optimistic. In a maintenance model, the goal of treatment is stability, while in a recovery model, the goal is to extend improvement beyond stability (Manschreck, Duckworth, Halpern, et al., 2008). This new way of looking at this final phase requires recognition that progress is not a linear process and that recovery-focused therapy may be at odds with stability-focused therapy; that is, the health care providers must be able to tolerate instability such as setbacks and struggles in the recovery process (Lysecker & Buck, 2006).

Some clinicians also designate an earlier prodromal (or prepsychotic) phase, in which subtle symptoms or deficits associated with schizophrenia are present; such symptoms may or may not herald the onset of schizophrenia. Detection and treatment programs in most major Canadian cities aim to detect psychosis in the prodromal phase and prevent acute episodes of schizophrenia. Strategies of early intervention include reducing the duration of untreated psychosis (DUP), reducing delay in treatment, and providing interventions adapted for younger people and their families in the early course of the illness (Srihari, Shah, & Keshavan, 2012). A list of Canadian programs can be found on the website of the International Early Psychosis Association at www.iepa.org.au.

There is controversy as to whether the benefits of early intervention can be maintained over time. However, a study at the Prevention and Early Intervention Program for Psychosis (PEPP) in London, Ontario, found symptom improvement was not only maintained at the five-year follow-up but increased for an additional two to five years (Norman, Manchanda, Malla, et al., 2011). This program provides continuity of care for five years, with more intense intervention in the initial two years and a gradual, individualized transfer to usual services. When compared to programs that provide only two years of treatment, the PEPP approach demonstrates better durability of benefit (Srihari, Shah, & Keshavan, 2012).

## APPLICATION OF THE NURSING PROCESS

### ASSESSMENT

Nursing assessment of people who have or may have a psychotic disorder focuses largely on symptoms, coping, functioning, and safety. Assessment involves interviewing the person and observing behaviour and other outward manifestations of the disorder. It also should include mental status and spiritual, cultural, biological, psychological, social, and environmental elements. Sound therapeutic communication skills, an understanding of the disorder and the ways the person may be experiencing the world, and the establishment of trustworthiness and a therapeutic nurse–patient relationship all strengthen the assessment. Indeed, the therapeutic relationship is of critical importance. A helping partnership between the nurse and the person with schizophrenia facilitates recovery (Anthony, 2008). Early engagement between the nurse and a person with schizophrenia is an important factor in predicting recovery and continued disease remission (Bertolote & McGorry, 2005). For example, a small study of health care providers working with immigrant women found that the care provider–patient relationship had a great influence on how these women sought mental health care (O'Mahony & Donnelly, 2007).

One effective approach to developing this trusting relationship is the LEAP approach described by Amador (2000) and referenced at the beginning of this chapter. It consists of four steps: (1) listen—try to put yourself in the other person's shoes to gain a clear idea of his or her experience; (2) empathize—seriously consider and empathize with the other person's point of view; (3) agree—find common ground and identify facts you can both agree upon; (4) partner—collaborate on accomplishing the agreed-upon goals (Amador, 2000, pp. 56–58). In this way, trust can be gained and an alliance formed.

### During the Prepsychotic Phase

Experts believe that detection and treatment of symptoms that may warn of schizophrenia's onset lessen the risk of developing the disorder or decrease the severity of the disorder if it does develop. A delay in diagnosis and treatment allows the psychotic process to become more entrenched; it can also result in relational, work, housing, and school problems (Riecher-Rössler, Gschwandtner, Borgwardt, et al., 2006).

Therefore, early assessment plays a key role in improving the prognosis for persons with schizophrenia (Chung, Kang, Shin, et al., 2008). This form of primary prevention involves

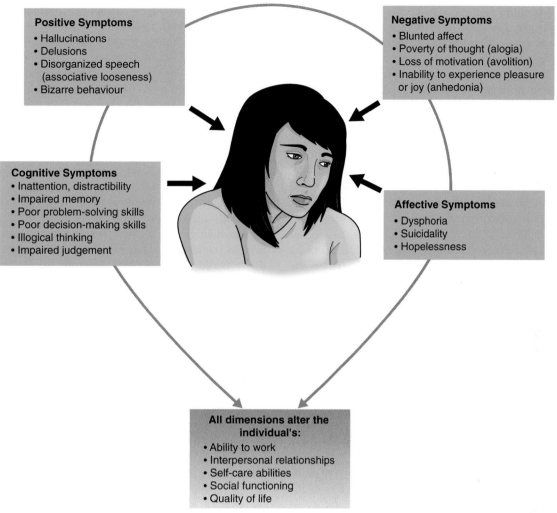

**Positive Symptoms**
- Hallucinations
- Delusions
- Disorganized speech (associative looseness)
- Bizarre behaviour

**Negative Symptoms**
- Blunted affect
- Poverty of thought (alogia)
- Loss of motivation (avolition)
- Inability to experience pleasure or joy (anhedonia)

**Cognitive Symptoms**
- Inattention, distractibility
- Impaired memory
- Poor problem-solving skills
- Poor decision-making skills
- Illogical thinking
- Impaired judgement

**Affective Symptoms**
- Dysphoria
- Suicidality
- Hopelessness

**All dimensions alter the individual's:**
- Ability to work
- Interpersonal relationships
- Self-care abilities
- Social functioning
- Quality of life

**FIGURE 16-1** Four main symptom groups of schizophrenia.

monitoring those at high risk (e.g., children of parents with schizophrenia) for symptoms such as abnormal social development and cognitive dysfunction. Intervening to reduce stressors (i.e., reduce or avoid exposure to triggers), enhancing social and coping skills (e.g., build resiliency), and administering prophylactic antipsychotic medication may also be of benefit (Bechdolf, Phillips, Francey, et al., 2006).

Similarly, in people who have already developed the disorder, minimizing the onset and duration of relapses is believed to improve the prognosis. Research suggests that with each relapse of psychosis, there is an increase in residual dysfunction and deterioration. Recognition of the early warning signs of relapse, such as reduced sleep and concentration, followed by close monitoring and intensification of treatment is essential (van Meijel, van der Gaag, Sylvain, et al., 2004). For this reason, adherence to a drug regimen of antipsychotics can be more important than the risk of adverse effects because most adverse effects are reversible, whereas the consequences of relapse may not be.

## General Assessment

Not all people with schizophrenia have the same symptoms, and some of the symptoms of schizophrenia are also found in other

disorders. Figure 16-1 describes the four main symptom groups of schizophrenia:

1. Positive symptoms: the presence of something that is not normally present
2. Negative symptoms: the absence of something that should be present but is not
3. Cognitive symptoms: abnormalities in how a person thinks
4. Affective symptoms: symptoms involving emotions and their expression

## Positive Symptoms

The positive symptoms usually appear early in the illness, and their dramatic nature captures our attention and often precipitates hospitalization. They are also the symptoms most laypeople associate with insanity, making schizophrenia the disorder most associated with being "crazy." However, positive psychotic symptoms are perhaps less important prognostically and usually respond to antipsychotic medication. Positive symptoms are associated with:

- Acute onset
- Normal premorbid functioning
- Normal social functioning during remissions

- Normal CT findings
- Normal neuropsychological test results
- Favourable response to antipsychotic medication

The positive symptoms presented here are categorized as alterations in thinking, speech, perception, and behaviour.

***Alterations in thinking.*** All people experience occasional and momentary errors in thinking (e.g., "Why are all these lights turning red when I'm already late? Someone must be trying to slow me down!"), but most can catch and correct the error by using intact reality testing—the ability to determine accurately whether or not an experience is based in reality. People with impaired reality testing, however, maintain the error, which contributes to delusions, or alterations in *thought* content. A person experiencing delusions is convinced that what he or she believes to be real *is* real. Student nurses sometimes try unsuccessfully to argue a person out of delusions by offering evidence of reality; this approach may irritate the person and slow the development of a therapeutic relationship. Table 16-1 provides definitions and examples of frequent types of delusions.

About 75% of people with schizophrenia experience delusions at some time. The most common delusions are persecutory or grandiose or those involving religious or hypochondriacal ideas. A delusion may be a response to anxiety or may reflect areas of concern for a person; for example, someone with poor self-esteem may believe he is Beethoven or an emissary of God, allowing him to feel more powerful or important. Looking for and addressing such underlying themes or needs can be a key nursing intervention. At times, delusions hold a kernel of truth. One person repeatedly told the staff that the Mafia was out to kill him. Later, staff learned that he had been selling drugs, had not paid his contacts, and gang members *were* trying to find him to hurt or even kill him.

Concrete thinking refers to an impaired ability to think abstractly. The person interprets statements literally. For example, the nurse might ask what brought the person to the hospital, and the person might answer, concretely, "a cab" (rather than explaining that he had attempted suicide). Traditionally, concreteness has been assessed through the patient's interpretation of proverbs. However, this assessment is not accurate if the person is from another culture or is otherwise unfamiliar with the proverb (Haynes & Resnick, 1993). It is preferable to use the *similarities test*, which involves asking the person to explain how two things are similar, such as an orange and an apple, a chair and a table, or a child and an adult. A description of physical characteristics ("apples and oranges are

| TABLE 16-1 | SUMMARY OF DELUSIONS | |
|---|---|---|
| **DELUSION** | **DEFINITION** | **EXAMPLE** |
| Thought insertion | Believing that another person, group of people, or external force controls thoughts | Bruce always wears a hat so that aliens don't insert thoughts into his brain. |
| Thought withdrawal | Believing that others are taking thoughts out of a person's mind | Bernadette covers her windows with foil so the police can't empty her mind. |
| Thought broadcasting | Believing that one's thoughts are being involuntarily broadcasted to others | Marcel was convinced that everyone could hear what he was thinking at all times. |
| Ideas of reference | Giving personal significance to trivial events; perceiving events as relating to you when they do not | When Maria saw staff talking, she believed they were plotting against her. |
| Ideas of influence | Believing that you have somehow influenced events that are, in fact, out of your control | Jean Pierre is convinced that he caused the flooding in Manitoba. |
| Persecution | Believing that one is being singled out for harm by others; this belief often takes the form of a plot by people in power | Saed believed that the RCMP was planning to kill him by poisoning his food. Therefore, he would eat only food he bought from machines. |
| Grandeur | Believing that one is a very powerful or important person | Sam believed he was a famous playwright and tennis pro. |
| Somatic | Believing that the body is changing in an unusual way (e.g., rotting inside) | David told the doctor that his heart had stopped and his insides were rotting away. |
| Erotomanic | Believing that another person desires you romantically | Although he barely knew her, Mary insisted that Mr. Johansen would marry her if only his current wife would stop interfering. |
| Jealousy | Believing that one's mate is unfaithful | Harry wrongly accused his girlfriend of going out with other men. His proof was that she came home from work late twice that week, even though the girlfriend's boss explained that everyone had worked late. |

both round") would be a concrete answer, while an abstract answer recognizes ideas such as classifications ("apples and oranges are fruit"). Concreteness reduces one's ability to understand and address abstract concepts such as love or the passage of time or to reality-test delusions or other symptoms. Educational strategies need to take into account a person's ability to think abstractly.

***Alterations in speech.*** Alterations in speech demonstrate difficulties with *thought process* (how a person thinks). *Associations* are the threads that tie one thought logically to another. In associative looseness, these threads are interrupted or illogically connected; thinking becomes haphazard, illogical, and difficult to follow:

> *Nurse:* "Are you going to the picnic today?"
>
> *Patient:* "I'm not an elephant hunter; no tiger teeth for me."

At times, the nurse may be able to decipher or decode the patient's messages and begin to understand the patient's feelings and needs. Any exchange in which a person feels understood is useful. Therefore, the nurse might respond to the patient in this way:

> *Nurse:* "Are you saying that you're afraid to go out with the others today?"
>
> *Patient:* "Yeah, no tiger getting me today."

Sometimes it is not possible to understand the person's meaning because his or her speech is too fragmented. For example:

> *Patient:* "I sang out for my mother … for this to hell I went. These little hills hop aboard, share the Christmas mice spread … the devil will be washed away."

If the nurse does not understand what the patient is saying, it is important that he or she let the patient know. Clear messages and honesty are a vital part of working effectively in psychiatric mental health nursing. An honest response lets the person know that the nurse does not understand, would like to understand, and can be trusted to be honest.

Other alterations in speech that can make communication challenging are *circumstantiality, tangentiality, neologisms, echolalia, clang association,* and *word salad*:

- Circumstantiality refers to the inclusion of unnecessary and often tedious details in one's conversation (e.g., describing your breakfast when asked how your day is going).
- Tangentiality is a departure from the main topic to talk about less important information; the patient goes off on tangents in a way that takes the conversation off-topic.
- Neologisms are made-up words (or idiosyncratic uses of existing words) that have meaning for the person but a different or nonexistent meaning to others (e.g., "I was going to tell him the *mannerologies* of his hospitality won't do"). This eccentric use of words represents disorganized thinking and interferes with communication.
- Echolalia is the pathological repeating of another's words and is often seen in catatonia.
- *Nurse:* "Mary, come get your medication."
- *Mary:* "Come get your medication."
- *Clang association* is the choosing of words based on their sound rather than their meaning, often rhyming and sometimes having a similar beginning sound (e.g., "On the track, have a Big Mac," "Click, clack, clutch, close"). Clanging may also be seen in neurological disorders.
- Word salad is a jumble of words that is meaningless to the listener—and perhaps to the speaker as well—because of an extreme level of disorganization.

***Alterations in perception.*** Alterations in perception are errors in one's view of reality. The most common form of altered perception in psychosis is hallucination, but depersonalization, derealization, and boundary impairment are sometimes experienced as well:

- Depersonalization is a nonspecific feeling that a person has lost his or her identity and that the self is different or unreal. People may feel that body parts do not belong to them or may sense that their body has drastically changed. For example, a person may see her fingers as snakes or her arms as rotting wood.
- Derealization is the false perception that the environment has changed. For example, everything seems bigger or smaller, or familiar surroundings have become somehow strange and unfamiliar. Both depersonalization and derealization can be interpreted as *loss of ego boundaries* (sometimes called *loose ego boundaries*).
- Boundary impairment is an impaired ability to sense where one's self ends and others' selves begin. For example, a person might drink another's beverage, believing that because it is in his vicinity, it is his.
- Hallucinations result from perceiving a sensory experience for which no external stimulus exists (e.g., hearing a voice when no one is speaking). Hallucinations differ from illusions in that illusions are misperceptions or misinterpretations of a real experience; for example, a man sees his coat on a coat rack and believes it is a bear about to attack. He does see something real but misinterprets what it is.

Causes of hallucinations include psychiatric disorders, drug abuse, medications, organic disorders, hyperthermia, toxicity (e.g., digitalis), and other conditions. Hallucinations can involve any of the five bodily senses. Table 16-2 provides definitions and examples of these types of hallucinations.

Auditory hallucinations are experienced by up to 15% of people without psychotic disorders and 60% of people with schizophrenia at some time during their lives (Hubl, Koenig, Strik, et al., 2004). Voices typically seem to come from outside the person's head, and auditory processing areas of the brain are activated during auditory hallucinations just as they are when a genuine external sound is heard (Hubl, Koenig, Strik, et al., 2004). This abnormal activation may cause hallucinations, but another leading theory is that "voices" are a misperception of one's internally generated conversation (Hoffman & Varanko, 2006). John Nash (n.d.), the world-renowned mathematician portrayed in the 2001 film *A Beautiful Mind*, described the voices he heard during the acute phase of his illness: "I thought of the voices as … something a little different from aliens. I thought of them more like angels. … It's really my subconscious talking, it was really that. … I know that now."

Voices may be of people familiar or unknown, single or multiple. They may be perceived as supportive and pleasant or

| TABLE 16-2 | SUMMARY OF HALLUCINATIONS | |
|---|---|---|
| **HALLUCINATION** | **DEFINITION** | **EXAMPLE** |
| Auditory | Hearing voices or sounds that do not exist in the environment but are misperceptions of inner thoughts or feelings | Juan hit the ambulance attendant when a voice told him the attendant was taking him to a concentration camp. |
| Visual | Seeing a person, object, animal, colours, or visual patterns that do not exist in the environment | Antoine became very frightened and screamed, "There are rats coming at me!" |
| Olfactory | Smelling odours that do not exist | Theresa "smells" her insides rotting. |
| Gustatory | Tasting sensations that do not exist | Simon will not eat his food because he "tastes" the poison they are putting in it. |
| Tactile | Feeling strange sensations on the skin where no external objects stimulate such feelings; common in delirium tremens | Jack "feels" electrical impulses tingling as they control his mind, and he covers his walls in tinfoil to block them out. |

derogatory and frightening. Voices commenting on the person's behaviour or conversing with the person are most common. A person who hears voices when no one is present often struggles to understand the experience, sometimes developing related delusions to explain the voices (e.g., the person may believe the voices are from God, the devil, or deceased relatives). People with chronic hallucinations may attempt to cope by drowning them out with loud music or competing with them by talking loudly (Farhall, Greenwood, & Jackson, 2007).

Command hallucinations are "voices" that direct the person to take an action. All hallucinations must be assessed and monitored carefully, because the voices may command the person to hurt self or others. For example, voices might command a person to "jump out the window" or "take a knife and kill my child." Command hallucinations are often terrifying and may herald a psychiatric emergency. In all cases, it is essential to assess what the person hears, the person's ability to recognize the hallucination as real or not real, and the person's ability to resist any commands. A person may falsely deny hallucinations, requiring behavioural assessment to support (validate) or refute the person's report. Outward indications of possible hallucinations include turning or tilting the head as if to listen to someone, suddenly stopping current activity as if interrupted, and moving the lips silently.

Visual hallucinations occur less frequently in schizophrenia and are more likely to occur in organic disorders such as acute alcohol withdrawal or dementia. Olfactory, tactile, or gustatory hallucinations are unusual; when present, other physical causes should be investigated (Sadock & Sadock, 2008).

*Alterations in behaviour.* Alterations in behaviour include bizarre and agitated behaviours involving such things as stilted, rigid demeanour or eccentric dress, grooming, and rituals. Other behavioural changes seen in schizophrenia include the following:

- Catatonia, a pronounced increase or decrease in the rate and amount of movement. The most common form is stuporous behaviour, in which the person moves little or not at all.

- Psychomotor retardation, a pronounced slowing of movement. It is important to differentiate the slowed movements secondary to schizophrenia from those seen in depression; careful assessment of thought content and thought processes is essential for making this determination.
- Psychomotor agitation, excited behaviour such as running or pacing rapidly, often in response to internal or external stimuli. Psychomotor agitation can pose a risk to others and to the person, who is at risk for exhaustion, collapse, and even death.
- Stereotyped behaviours, repeated motor behaviours that do not presently serve a logical purpose.
- Automatic obedience, the performance by a catatonic person of all simple commands in a robotlike fashion.
- Waxy flexibility, the extended maintenance of posture usually seen in catatonia. For example, the nurse raises the person's arm, and the person retains this position in a statuelike manner.
- Negativism, akin to resistance but may not be intentional. In *active negativism*, the person does the opposite of what he or she is told to do; *passive negativism* is a failure to do what is requested.
- Impaired impulse control, a reduced ability to resist one's impulses. Examples include performing socially inappropriate behaviours such as grabbing another's cigarette, throwing food on the floor, pushing others around, and changing TV channels while others are watching.
- Echopraxia, the mimicking of the movements of another. It is also seen in catatonia.

Behaviours such as agitation and impaired impulse control are likely to bring the person into contact with the police and justice system. One consequence of deinstitutionalization is that behaviours previously managed in psychiatric settings are increasingly brought to the attention of police, resulting in criminal charges rather than hospitalization (Jansman-Hart, Seto, Crocker, et al., 2011). As a result, the criminal justice system is becoming the entry point to mental health services for increasing numbers of people (Jansman-Hart et al., 2011).

Unfortunately, though, the prison system is not designed for mental health treatment, and the conditions there are neither therapeutic nor rehabilitative for people with mental health concerns (Zinger, 2012).

### Negative Symptoms

Negative symptoms develop slowly and are those that most interfere with a person's adjustment and ability to cope. They tend to be persistent and crippling because they render the person inert and unmotivated. Negative symptoms impede one's ability to:

- Initiate and maintain conversations and relationships
- Obtain and maintain a job
- Make decisions and follow through on plans
- Maintain adequate hygiene and grooming

Negative symptoms contribute to poor social functioning and social withdrawal. During the acute phase, they are difficult to assess because positive symptoms (such as delusions and hallucinations) dominate. Selected negative symptoms are outlined in Table 16-3.

In schizophrenia, affect—the external manifestation of feeling or emotion that is manifested in facial expression, tone of voice, and body language—may not always coincide with inner emotions. Affect in schizophrenia can usually be categorized in one of four ways:

- Flat—immobile or blank facial expression
- Blunted—reduced or minimal emotional response
- Inappropriate—emotional response incongruent with the tone or circumstances of the situation (e.g., a man laughs when told that his father has died)
- Bizarre—odd, illogical, emotional state that is grossly inappropriate or unfounded; especially prominent in disorganized schizophrenia and includes grimacing and giggling

### Cognitive Symptoms

Cognitive symptoms represent the third symptom group and are evident in most people with schizophrenia. They include difficulty with attention, memory, information processing, cognitive flexibility, and executive functions (e.g., decision making, judgement, planning, and problem solving) (Braw, Bloch, Mendelovich, et al., 2008). These impairments can leave the person unable to manage personal health care, hold a job, initiate or maintain a support system, or live alone.

### Affective Symptoms

Affective symptoms, the fourth symptom group, are common and increase a person's suffering. Assessment for depression is crucial because depression:

- May herald an impending relapse
- Increases substance abuse
- Increases suicide risk
- Further impairs functioning

This assessment can be done by inquiring into mood and the presence of depressive thoughts or suicidal ideation.

### Self-Assessment

Working with individuals with schizophrenia produces strong emotional reactions in most health care workers. The acutely ill person's intensely anxious, lonely, dependent, and distrustful presentation evokes similarly intense, uncomfortable, and frightening emotions in others. The chronicity, repeated exacerbations, and slow response to treatment that many people experience can lead to feelings of helplessness and powerlessness in staff. Some behaviour (especially violent behaviour) can produce strong emotional responses (called *counter-transference*) such as fear or anger (see Chapter 10).

Ironically, knowledge that schizophrenia is a brain disease may contribute to stigmatizing attitudes and feelings of hopelessness. Early research suggests that when public education focuses on illness without including personal contact or information about recovery, stigma actually increases or becomes entrenched (Martin & Johnson, 2008). Nurses who do not see recovering people or learn about recovery may be subject to this effect. Inpatient nurses, in particular, tend to see only the most ill people, and so it is important for them to avoid a skewed and hopeless view by staying aware of the growing numbers of people who are living well with schizophrenia. The importance of hope in the nursing of people with schizophrenia and their families is well documented, and being hopeful is an essential characteristic of mental health providers in this field (Koehn & Cutliffe, 2007).

At the same time, it is necessary to be realistic about the length of time that it may take for a patient to recover from an acute episode. It can be helpful to remember that the person

| TABLE 16-3 | SELECTED NEGATIVE SYMPTOMS OF SCHIZOPHRENIA |
|---|---|
| **NEGATIVE SYMPTOM** | **DESCRIPTION** |
| Affective blunting | A reduction in the expression, range, and intensity of affect (in *flat affect*, no facial expression is present) |
| Anergia | Lack of energy; passivity, lack of persistence at work or school; may also be a symptom of depression, so needs careful evaluation |
| Anhedonia | Inability to experience pleasure in activities that usually produce it; result of profound emotional barrenness |
| Avolition | Reduced motivation; inability to initiate tasks such as social contacts, grooming, and other activities of daily living (ADLs) |
| Poverty of content of speech | While adequate in amount, speech conveys little information because of vagueness or superficiality |
| Poverty of speech (alogia) | Reduced amount of speech—responses range from brief to one-word answers |

has essentially had a brain injury, to set realistic, achievable goals, and to acknowledge small steps. Negative symptoms, in particular, can be very slow to resolve. It may also take a long time to gain trust, so the nurse can expect the orientation phase of the helping relationship to be prolonged.

Without support and the opportunity and willingness to explore feelings with more experienced staff, the nurse may adopt nontherapeutic behaviours—denial, withdrawal, avoidance, and anger most commonly. These behaviours thwart the patient's progress and undermine the nurse's self-esteem. Comments such as "These patients are hopeless," and "All you can do is babysit these people" are indications of unrecognized or unresolved counter-transference that, if left uncorrected, interfere with both treatment and work satisfaction. Canadian nurse Jan Landeen, cited by Koehn and Cutliffe

(2007), found that strategies for increasing hope include getting to know the patient as a person, sharing patient successes, learning about treatments and research, and keeping expectations realistic.

People living with schizophrenia may experience fear, self-stigma, or shame related to their mental illness, leading them to conceal some aspects of their experience. Negativism and alogia (reduced verbalization) can also limit the person's responses. Many people with schizophrenia experience anosognosia, an inability to realize they are ill, which is caused by the illness itself. The resulting lack of insight can make assessment (and treatment) challenging, delaying completion of a full assessment and requiring additional skills on the part of the nurse. Selected techniques that may help you overcome these challenges can be found in Table 16-4.

## TABLE 16-4  INTERVENTIONS FOR OVERCOMING OBSTACLES TO ASSESSMENT

| INTERVENTION | RATIONALE | EXAMPLE |
|---|---|---|
| Use empathic comments and observations to prompt the patient to provide information. | Empathy conveys understanding and builds trust and rapport. | *Nurse:* "It must be difficult to find yourself in a psychiatric hospital." <br> *Patient:* "Yes...I'm frightened." |
| Minimize questioning, especially closed-ended questioning. <br> Seek data conversationally, using prompts and open-ended questions. | Extended questioning can increase suspiciousness, and closed questions elicit minimal information. Both become wearying and off-putting. | "Could you please tell me more about ...?" <br> "Tell me what life has been like for you lately." |
| Use short, simple sentences and introduce only one idea at a time. <br> Allow time for responses to questions. | Long sentences or rambling questions can confuse a person who has difficulty processing auditory information or is actively hallucinating. Also, a person with alogia requires more time to respond to questions. | *Therapeutic:* "Would you like to join us for a basketball game?" <br> *Nontherapeutic:* "Would you like to join us for a basketball game? Sports can be very good for you, you know, and you seem very lonely, so it would help you a lot. I really hope you will come play a game" |
| Directly but supportively seek the needed information, explaining the reasons for the assessment. | Being direct but supportive conveys genuineness, builds rapport, and helps reduce anxiety. | "You seem very sad. Sometimes sad people think about hurting themselves. Have you ever thought about hurting yourself?" |
| Judiciously use indirect, supportive (therapeutic) confrontation. <br> Seek other data to support (validate) the person's report (obtain further history from third parties, past medical records, and other treatment providers when possible), preferably with the person's permission. | Blunt contradiction or premature confrontation increases resistance. Patients may be unable or unwilling to provide information fully and reliably. Validating their reports assures the validity of the assessment. | "I realize admitting to hearing voices might be difficult to do. I notice you talking as if to others when no one is there." <br> "Your brother reports he works at a factory. Is that your understanding?" |
| Prioritize the data you seek, and avoid seeking nonessential data. | Patients may have limited tolerance for the assessment interview and answer only a limited number of inquiries. Seeking nonessential information does not benefit the person or assessment. | *Patient:* "I hate school! I wish they'd all die!" <br> *Nurse:* (less therapeutic) "Which school do you go to?" <br> *Nurse:* (more therapeutic) "Things would be better if they were dead. ..." (Paraphrasing prompts elaboration and confirmation or refutation of the comment.) |

---

### 📋 ASSESSMENT GUIDELINES

#### Schizophrenia and Other Psychotic Disorders

1. Determine if the patient has had a medical workup. Are there any indications of physical medical problems that might mimic psychosis (e.g., digitalis or anticholinergic toxicity, brain trauma, drug intoxication, delirium, fever)?
2. Assess whether the person abuses or is dependent on alcohol or drugs.
3. Assess for risk to self or others.
4. Assess for command hallucinations (e.g., voices telling the patient to harm self or another). If present, ask the person:
   - Do you recognize the voices?
   - Do you believe the voices are real?
   - Do you plan to follow the command? (A positive response to any of these questions suggests an increased risk that the person will act on the commands.)
5. Assess the patient's belief system. Is it fragmented or poorly organized? Is it systematized? Are the beliefs delusional? If yes, then ask:
   - Do you feel that you or loved ones are being threatened or are in danger?
   - Do you feel the need to act against a person or organization to protect or avenge yourself or loved ones? (A positive response to either of these questions suggests an increased risk of danger to others.)
6. Assess for suicide risk (see Chapter 25).
7. Assess for ability to ensure self safety, addressing:
   - Adequacy of food and fluid intake
   - Hygiene and self-care
   - Handling of potentially hazardous activities, such as smoking and cooking
   - Ability to transport self safely
   - Impulse control and judgement
   - Appropriate dress for weather conditions
8. Assess for coexisting disorders:
   - Depression
   - Anxiety
   - Substance abuse or dependency
   - Medical disorders (especially brain trauma, toxicity, delirium, cardiovascular disease, obesity, and diabetes)
9. Assess medications the patient has been prescribed, whether and how the patient is taking the medications, and what factors (e.g., costs, mistrust of staff, adverse effects) are affecting adherence.
10. Assess for the presence and severity of positive and negative symptoms. Complete a mental status examination, noting which symptoms are present, how they affect functioning, and how the patient is managing them.
11. Assess the patient's insight, knowledge of the illness, relationships and support systems, other coping resources, and strengths.
12. Assess the family's knowledge of and response to the patient's illness and its symptoms. Are family members overprotective? Hostile? Anxious? Are they familiar with family support groups and respite resources?

---

The Unpleasant Voices Scale has been designed for assessment of the risk of harm related to command hallucinations and can be used in conjunction with the Harm Command Safety Protocol (Gerlock, Buccheri, Buffum, et al., 2010). The Inventory of Voice Experiences, a nursing tool developed in Canada, offers increased accuracy of assessment of voices (England, 2007).

## DIAGNOSIS

People with schizophrenia have multiple disturbing and disabling symptoms that require a multifaceted approach to care and treatment of both the patient and the family. Table 16-5 lists potential nursing diagnoses for a person with schizophrenia.

## OUTCOMES IDENTIFICATION

Desired outcomes vary with the phase of the illness. *Nursing Outcomes Classification (NOC)* (Moorhead, Johnson, Maas, et al., 2008) is a useful guide. Ideally, outcomes should focus on enhancing strengths and minimizing the effects of the patient's deficits and symptoms. Outcomes should be consistent with the recovery model (see Chapter 31), which stresses hope, living a full and productive life, and eventual recovery rather than focusing on controlling symptoms and adapting to disability.

### Phase I—Acute

During the acute phase, the overall goal is the person's safety and medical stabilization. Therefore, if the person is at risk for violence to self or others, initial outcome criteria address safety issues (e.g., *Person refrains from self harm*). Another outcome is *Person consistently labels hallucinations as "not real—a symptom of an illness."* Table 16-6 gives selected short-term and intermediate indicators for the outcome *Distorted thought self-control.*

### Phase II—Stabilization

Outcome criteria during phase II focus on helping the patient adhere to treatment, become stabilized on medications, and control or cope with symptoms. The outcomes target the negative symptoms and may include ability to succeed in social, vocational, or self-care activities.

### Phase III—Maintenance

Outcome criteria for phase III focus on maintaining achievement, preventing relapse, and achieving independence and a satisfactory quality of life.

## TABLE 16-5    POTENTIAL NURSING DIAGNOSES FOR SCHIZOPHRENIA

| SYMPTOM | NURSING DIAGNOSES |
|---|---|
| **Positive Symptoms** | |
| Hears voices that others do not (*auditory hallucinations*) | *Disturbed sensory perception: auditory** |
| Hears voices telling him or her to hurt self or others (*command hallucinations*) | *Risk for self-directed violence* <br> *Risk for other-directed violence* |
| Delusions[†] | *Disturbed thought processes*[‡] |
| Shows loose association of ideas (*associative looseness*) | *Disturbed thought processes*[‡] |
| Conversation is derailed by unnecessary and tedious details (*circumstantiality*) | *Impaired verbal communication* |
| **Negative Symptoms** | |
| Uncommunicative, withdrawn | *Social isolation* |
| Expresses feelings of rejection or aloneness (lies in bed all day, positions back to door) | *Impaired social interaction* <br> *Risk for loneliness* |
| Talks about self as "bad" or "no good" | *Chronic low self-esteem* |
| Feels guilty because of "bad thoughts"; extremely sensitive to real or perceived slights | *Risk for self-directed violence* |
| Shows lack of energy (*anergia*) | *Ineffective coping* |
| Shows lack of motivation (*avolition*), unable to initiate tasks (social contact, grooming, and other aspects of daily living) | *Self-care deficit (bathing, dressing, feeding, toileting)* <br> *Constipation* |
| **Other** | |
| Families and significant others become confused or overwhelmed, lack knowledge about disorder or treatment, feel powerless in coping with the patient | *Compromised family coping* <br> *Caregiver role strain* <br> *Deficient knowledge* |
| Stops taking medication (because of anosognosia, adverse effects, drugs costs, mistrust of staff), stops going to therapy, is not supported in treatment by significant others | *Nonadherence* |

*Diagnosis retired from Herdman, T.H. (Ed.). (2012). *NANDA International nursing diagnoses: Definitions & classification, 2012–2014*. Oxford, UK: Wiley-Blackwell.
[†]Although NANDA has always classified these as "disturbed thought process," in fact, delusions are a problem of thought *content* and are classified as such in the standard mental status examination.
[‡]Diagnosis retired from Herdman, T.H. (Ed.). (2012). *NANDA International nursing diagnoses: Definitions & classification, 2012–2014*. Oxford, UK: Wiley-Blackwell.

## TABLE 16-6    *NOC* OUTCOMES RELATED TO DISTORTED THOUGHT SELF-CONTROL

| NURSING OUTCOME AND DEFINITION | INTERMEDIATE INDICATORS | SHORT-TERM INDICATORS |
|---|---|---|
| Distorted thought self-control: Self-restraint of disruptions in perception, thought processes, and thought content | Maintains affect consistent with mood <br> Interacts appropriately <br> Perceives environment and the ideas of others accurately <br> Exhibits logical thought flow patterns <br> Exhibits reality-based thinking <br> Exhibits appropriate thought content | Recognizes that hallucinations or delusions are occurring <br> Refrains from attending to and responding to hallucinations or delusions <br> Describes content of hallucinations or delusions <br> Reports decrease in hallucinations or delusions <br> Asks for validation of reality |

**Source:** Moorhead, S., Johnson, H., Maas, M., et al. (2008). *Nursing outcomes classification (NOC)* (4th ed.). St. Louis, MO: Mosby.

# PLANNING

The planning of appropriate interventions is guided by the phase of the illness and the strengths and needs of the patient. It is influenced by cultural considerations, available resources, and the patient's preferences.

## Phase I—Acute

Hospitalization is indicated if the patient is considered a danger to self or others, refuses to eat or drink, or is too disorganized or otherwise impaired to function safely in the community without supervision. The planning process focuses on the best strategies to ensure the person's safety and provide symptom stabilization. Additionally, during the patient's hospitalization, this process also includes discharge planning.

In discharge planning, the patient and interprofessional treatment team identify aftercare needs for follow-up and support. Discharge planning considers not only external factors, such as the person's living arrangements, economic resources, social supports, and family relationships, but also internal factors, such as resilience and repertoire of coping skills. Because relapse can be devastating to the person's circumstances (resulting in loss of employment, housing, and relationships) and worsen the long-term prognosis, vigorous efforts are made to connect the person and family with (and not simply refer them to) community resources that provide therapeutic programming and social, financial, and other needed support.

### Phase II—Stabilization/Phase III—Maintenance

Planning during the stabilization and maintenance phases includes providing individual and family education and skills training (psychosocial education). Relapse prevention skills are vital. Planning identifies interpersonal, coping, health care, and vocational needs and addresses how and where these needs can best be met within the community.

## IMPLEMENTATION

Interventions are geared toward the phase of schizophrenia the person is experiencing. For example, during the acute phase, the clinical focus is on crisis intervention, medication for symptom stabilization, and safety. Interventions are often hospital-based; however, people in the acute stage are increasingly being treated in the community.

### Phase I—Acute

#### Settings

A number of factors that affect the choice of treatment setting include the following:

- Level of care and restrictiveness needed to protect the person from harm to self or others
- Person's needs for external structure and support
- Person's ability to cooperate with treatment
- Need for a particular treatment available only in particular settings
- Need for treatment of a coexisting medical condition
- Availability of supportive others who can provide critical information and treatment history to staff and permit stabilization in less restrictive settings

The use of less restrictive and more cost-effective alternatives to hospitalization that work for many people include:

- Partial hospitalization: Patients sleep at home and attend treatment sessions (similar to what they would receive if admitted) during the day or evening.
- Residential crisis centres: Patients who are unable to remain in the community but do not require full in-person services can be admitted (usually for 1 to 14 days) to receive increased supervision, guidance, and medication stabilization.
- Group homes: Patients live in the community with a group of other people, sharing expenses and responsibilities. Staff

are present in the house 24 hours a day, 7 days a week to provide supervision and therapeutic activities.
- Day treatment programs: Patients reside in the community and attend structured programming during the day.

These programs may include group and individual therapy, supervised activities, and specialized skill training. It is vital that staff be aware of these and other community resources and make this information available to discharged people and their families, ideally by directly connecting them with these resources. Patients and family members should be given telephone numbers and addresses of local support groups such as their provincial Schizophrenia Society. Northern and rural communities, however, may not have local support groups.

Other community resources include community mental health centres (usually providing medication services, day treatment, access to 24-hour emergency services, psychotherapy, psychoeducation, and case management); home health services; supported employment programs, offering services from job training to on-site coaches, who help people to learn to succeed in the work environment, often via peer-led services (e.g., drop-in centres, sometimes called "clubhouses," that offer social contact, constructive activities, and sometimes employment opportunities); family educational and skills groups (e.g., the Schizophrenia Society of Canada's "Strengthening Families Together" program); and respite care for caregivers.

### Interventions

Acute phase interventions include the following:
- Psychiatric, medical, and neurological evaluation
- Psychopharmacological treatment
- Support, psychoeducation, and guidance
- Supervision and limit setting in the milieu

Due to a shortage of inpatient beds, there is pressure to keep the length of hospitalization short. This situation may create an ethical dilemma for treatment teams, as short initial hospital stays have been found to be related to high rates of readmission and shorter intervals between hospitalizations (Canadian Institute for Health Information, 2008). Typically, as soon as the acute symptoms are adequately stabilized, the patient is discharged to the community, where appropriate treatment can be continued during the stabilization and maintenance phases. However, in some cases, discharge may be delayed while appropriate housing and supports are sought.

### Phase II——Stabilization/Phase III—Maintenance

Effective long-term care of an individual with schizophrenia relies on a three-pronged approach: medication administration and adherence, nursing intervention, and community support. Family psychoeducation, a key role of the nurse, is an essential intervention. All interventions and strategies are geared to the patient's strengths, culture, personal preferences, and needs.

### Milieu Management

Effective hospital care provides (1) protection from stressful or disruptive environments and (2) structure. People in the acute phase of schizophrenia show greater improvement in a structured milieu than on an open unit that allows more freedom. A therapeutic milieu is consciously designed to maximize safety, opportunities for learning skills, therapeutic activities, and access to resources. The milieu also provides guidance, supportive peer contact, and opportunities for practising conflict resolution, stress reduction techniques, and dealing with symptoms.

## Activities and Groups

Participation in activities and groups appropriate to the patient's level of functioning may decrease withdrawal, enhance motivation, modify unacceptable behaviours, develop friendships, and increase social competence. Activities such as drawing, reading poetry, and listening to music may be used to focus conversation and promote the recognition and expression of feelings. Self-esteem is enhanced as patients experience successful task completion. Recreational activities such as picnics and outings to stores and restaurants are not simply diversions; they teach constructive leisure skills, increase social comfort, facilitate growth in social concern and interactional skills, and enhance the ability to develop boundaries and set limits on self and others. After discharge, group therapy can provide necessary structure within the patient's community milieu.

## Safety

A small percentage of people with schizophrenia, especially during the acute phase, may exhibit a risk for physical violence, typically in response to hallucinations, delusions, paranoia, impaired judgement or impulse control, or self-referentiality (believing neutral, everyday occurrences carry special personal meaning). Concurrent substance use disorders are a greater risk factor for violence than is schizophrenia alone (Fazel, Gulati, Linsell, et al., 2009). When the potential for violence exists, measures to protect the patient and others become the priority. Interventions include increasing staff supervision, reducing stimulation (e.g., noise, crowds), addressing paranoia and other contributing symptoms, providing constructive diversion and outlets for physical energy, teaching and practising coping skills, implementing cognitive-behavioural approaches (to correct unrealistic expectations or selectively extinguish aggression), de-escalating tension verbally, and, when necessary, using seclusion, chemical (i.e., medication) or physical restraints. The Harm Command Safety Protocol provides guidelines for how to respond when a person indicates intent to harm someone else (Gerlock, Buccheri, Buffum, et al., 2010). Refer to Chapter 26 for more detailed discussions of caring for the aggressive person, seclusion, and restraints.

## Counselling and Communication Techniques

Therapeutic communication techniques for patients with schizophrenia aim to lower the person's anxiety, build trust, encourage clear communication, decrease defensiveness, encourage interaction, enhance self-esteem, and reinforce skills such as reality testing and assertiveness. It is important to remember that people with schizophrenia may have memory impairment and require repetition. They may also have limited tolerance for interaction, owing to the stimulation it creates. Therefore, shorter (<30 minutes) but more frequent interactions may be more therapeutic. Interventions for paranoia and other selected presentations are discussed later in this chapter.

## Hallucinations

When a patient is having a hallucination, the nursing focus is on understanding the person's experiences and responses. Suicidal or homicidal themes or commands necessitate appropriate safety measures. For example, "voices" that tell a patient a particular individual plans to harm him or her may lead to aggressive actions against that person; one-to-one supervision of the patient or transfer of the potential victim to another unit is often essential.

Hallucinations are real to the patient who is experiencing them and may be distracting during nurse–patient interactions. Call the person by name, speak simply but in a louder voice than usual, approach the person in a nonthreatening and nonjudgemental manner, maintain eye contact, and redirect the person's focus to the conversation as needed (Farhall, Greenwood, & Jackson, 2007). The following Guidelines for Communication box lists other techniques for communicating with patients experiencing hallucinations.

### 📖 GUIDELINES FOR COMMUNICATION
#### *With People Experiencing Hallucinations*

- Ask the person directly about the hallucinations (e.g., "Are you hearing voices?" followed by "What are you hearing?").
- Watch the person for cues that he or she is hallucinating, such as darting the eyes to one side, muttering, appearing distracted, or watching a vacant area of the room.
- Avoid reacting to hallucinations as if they are real. Do not address the voices.
- Do not negate the person's experience, but offer your own perceptions (e.g., "I don't see the devil standing over you, but I understand how upsetting that must be for you").
- Focus on reality-based, "here-and-now" diversions such as conversations or simple projects. Tell the person, "The voice you hear is part of your illness; it cannot hurt you. Try to listen to me and the others you can see around you."
- Be alert to signs of anxiety in the person, which may indicate that hallucinations are increasing.

**Source:** Farhall, J., Greenwood, K.M., & Jackson, H.J. (2007). Coping with hallucinated voices in schizophrenia: A review of self-initiated strategies and therapeutic interventions. *Clinical Psychology Review, 27,* 476–493. doi:10.1016/j.cpr.2006.12.002.

## Delusions

Delusions may be the patient's attempts to understand confusion and distorted experiences. They reflect the misperception of one's circumstances, which go uncorrected in schizophrenia due to impaired reality testing. When, as a nurse, you attempt to see the world through the eyes of the patient, it is easier to understand his or her delusional experience. For example:

> ***Patient:*** "You people are all alike ... all in on the RCMP plot to destroy me."
>
> ***Nurse:*** "I don't want to hurt you, Tom. Thinking that people are out to destroy you must be very frightening."

In this example, the nurse acknowledges the patient's experience, conveys empathy about the patient's fearfulness, and avoids focusing on the content of the delusion (RCMP and plot to destroy) but labels the patient's feelings so they can be explored, as tolerated. Note that talking about the feelings is helpful, but extended focus on delusional material is not.

It is *never* useful to debate or attempt to dissuade the patient regarding the delusion. Doing so can intensify the patient's retention of irrational beliefs and cause him or her to view you as rejecting or oppositional. However, it *is* helpful to clarify misinterpretations of the environment and gently suggest, as tolerated, a more reality-based perspective. For example:

*Patient:* "I see the doctor is here; he is out to destroy me."

*Nurse:* "It is true the doctor wants to see you, but he just wants to talk to you about your treatment. Would you feel more comfortable talking to him in the day room?"

Focusing on specific reality-based activities and events in the environment helps to minimize the focus on delusional thoughts. The more time the patient spends engaged in activities or with people, the more opportunities there are to receive feedback about and become comfortable with reality.

Work with the patient to find out which coping strategies succeed and how the patient can make the best use of them. The following Guidelines for Communication box lists techniques for communicating with people experiencing delusions, and the subsequent Patient and Family Teaching box presents patient and family teaching topics for coping with hallucinations and delusions.

---

### Associative Looseness

Associative looseness often mirrors the person's abnormal thoughts and reflects poorly organized thinking. An increase in associative looseness often indicates that the person is feeling increased anxiety or is overwhelmed by internal and external stimuli. The person's ramblings may also produce confusion and frustration in the nurse. The following guidelines are useful for intervention with a patient whose speech is confused and disorganized:

- Do *not* pretend you understand the patient's words or meaning when you do not; tell the person you are having difficulty understanding.

---

### 🖐 PATIENT AND FAMILY TEACHING
#### Coping With Auditory Hallucinations or Delusions

**Distraction**
- Listening to music
- Reading (aloud may help more)
- Counting backwards from 100
- Watching television

**Interaction**
- Looking at others—if they do not seem to be hearing or fearing what you are, ignore the voices or thoughts
- Talking with another person

**Activity**
- Walking
- Cleaning the house
- Having a relaxing bath
- Playing the guitar or singing
- Going to the gym (or anyplace you enjoy being, where others will be present)

**Talking to Yourself**
- Telling the voices or thoughts to go away
- Telling yourself that the voices and thoughts are a symptom and not real
- Telling yourself that no matter what you hear, voices can be safely ignored

**Social Action**
- Talking to a trusted friend or member of the family
- Calling a help line or going to a drop-in centre
- Visiting a favourite place or a comfortable public place

**Physical Action**
- Taking extra medication when ordered (call your prescriber)
- Going for a walk or doing other exercise
- Using breathing exercises and other relaxation methods

**Sources:** Farhall, J., Greenwood, K.M., & Jackson, H.J. (2007). Coping with hallucinated voices in schizophrenia: A review of self-initiated strategies and therapeutic interventions. *Clinical Psychology Review, 27*, 476–493. doi:10.1016/j.cpr.2006.12.002.; Jenner, J.A., Neinhuis, F.J., van de Willige, G., et al. (2006). "Hitting" voices of schizophrenia patients may lastingly reduce persistent auditory hallucinations and their burden: 18-month outcome of a randomized controlled trial. *Canadian Journal of Psychiatry, 51*(3), 169–177.

---

### 📖 GUIDELINES FOR COMMUNICATION
#### With People Experiencing Delusions

- To build trust, be open, honest, and reliable.
- Respond to suspicions in a matter-of-fact, empathic, supportive, and calm manner.
- Ask the person to describe the delusions. Example: "Tell me more about someone trying to hurt you."
- Avoid debating the delusional content, but interject doubt where appropriate. Example: "It seems as though it would be hard for that petite girl to hurt you."
- Focus on the feelings that underlie or flow from the delusions. Example: "You seem to wish you could be more powerful" or "It must feel frightening to think others want to hurt you."
- Once it is understood and addressed, do not dwell further on the delusion. Instead, focus on more reality-based topics. If the person obsesses about delusions, set firm limits on the amount of time you will talk about them, and explain your reason.
- Observe for events that trigger delusions. If possible, help the person find ways to reduce or manage them.
- Validate a part of the delusion that is real. Example: "Yes, there was a man at the nurse's station, but I did not hear him talk about you."

**Source:** Data from Farhall, J., Greenwood, K.M., & Jackson, H.J. (2007). Coping with hallucinated voices in schizophrenia: A review of self-initiated strategies and therapeutic interventions. *Clinical Psychology Review, 27*, 476–493. doi:10.1016/j.cpr.2006.12.002.

- Place the difficulty in understanding on yourself, *not* on the patient. Example: "I'm having trouble following what you are saying," *not* "You're not making any sense."
- Look for recurring topics and themes in the patient's communications, and tie these to events and timelines. Example: "You've mentioned trouble with your brother several times, usually after your family has visited. Tell me about your brother and your visits with him."
- Summarize or paraphrase the patient's communications to role-model more effective ways of making his or her point and to give the person a chance to correct anything you may have misunderstood.
- Reduce stimuli in the vicinity, and speak concisely, clearly, and concretely.
- Tell the person what you *do* understand, and reinforce clear communication and accurate expression of needs, feelings, and thoughts.

## Health Teaching and Health Promotion

Education is an essential strategy and includes teaching the patient and family about the illness, including possible causes, medications and medication adverse effects, coping strategies, what to expect, and prevention of relapse. Understanding these things helps the patient and family to recognize the impact of stress, enhances their understanding of the importance of treatment to a good outcome, encourages involvement in (and support of) therapeutic activities, and identifies resources for consultation and ongoing support in dealing with the illness.

Including family members in any strategies aimed at reducing psychotic symptoms reduces family anxiety and distress and enables the family to reinforce the staff's efforts. The family plays an important role in the stability of the patient. The patient who returns to a warm, concerned, and supportive environment is less likely to experience relapse. An environment in which people are critical or their involvement in the patient's life is intrusive is associated with relapse and poorer outcomes.

Lack of understanding of the disease and its symptoms can lead others to misinterpret the patient's apathy and lack of drive as laziness, fostering a hostile response by family members, caregivers, or community. Thus, public education about the symptoms of schizophrenia can reduce tensions in families, as well as communities. The most effective education occurs over time and is available when the family is most receptive (Weisman, Duarte, Koneru, et al., 2006). The following Patient and Family Teaching box offers guidelines for patient and family teaching about schizophrenia.

## Pharmacological Interventions

Drugs used to treat psychotic disorders, antipsychotics, first became available in the 1950s. Before that time, the available medications provided only sedation, not treatment of the disorder itself. Until the 1960s, people who had even one episode of schizophrenia usually spent months or years in provincial mental health hospitals. Psychotic episodes resulted in great emotional burdens to families and people with schizophrenia. The advent of antipsychotic drugs at last provided symptom control and allowed people to live in the community.

---

### 🧑‍🤝‍🧑 PATIENT AND FAMILY TEACHING

#### *Schizophrenia*

1. Learn all you can about the illness.
   - Attend psychoeducational and support groups.
   - Join the National Network for Mental Health.
   - Contact your provincial Schizophrenia Society.
2. Develop a relapse prevention plan.
   - Know the early warning signs of relapse (e.g., avoiding others, trouble sleeping, troubling thoughts).
   - Know whom to call, what to do, and where to go when early signs of relapse appear. Make a list and keep it with you.
   - Relapse is part of the illness, not a sign of failure.
3. Take advantage of all psychoeducational tools.
   - Participate in family, group, and individual therapy.
   - Learn new ways to act and coping skills to help handle family, work, and social stress. Get information from your nurse, case manager, doctor, self-help group, community mental health group, or hospital.
   - Have a plan, on paper, of what to do to cope with stressful times.
   - Recognize that everyone needs a place to address their fears and losses and to learn new ways of coping.
4. Adhere to treatment.
   - People who adhere to treatment that works for them do the best in coping with the disorder.
   - Engaging in struggles over adherence does not help, but tying adherence to the patient's own goals does. ("Staying in treatment will help you keep your job and avoid trouble with the police.")
   - Share concerns about troubling adverse effects or concerns (e.g., sexual problems, weight gain, "feeling funny") with your nurse, case manager, doctor, or social worker; most adverse effects can be helped.
   - Keeping adverse effects a secret or stopping medication can prevent you from having the life you want.
5. Avoid alcohol and drugs; they can act on the brain and cause a relapse.
6. Keep in touch with supportive people.
7. Keep healthy—stay in balance.
   - Taking care of one's diet, health, and hygiene helps prevent medical illnesses.
   - Maintain a regular sleep pattern.
   - Keep active (hobbies, friends, groups, sports, job, special interests).
   - Nurture yourself, and practise stress-reduction activities daily.

**Source:** Data from Tandon, R., Harvey, P.D., & Nasrallah, H.A. (2003, October). *Beyond symptom control: Moving towards positive patient outcomes.* Paper presented at the American Psychiatric Association 55th Institute on Psychiatric Services Boston. Retrieved from http://www.medscape.com/viewprogram/2835_pnt.
Further information can be found in the pamphlet *For Consumers: Schizophrenia and Substance Abuse,* available at http://www.schizophrenia.ca/SSC_for_Consumers.pdf. or via the Your Recovery Journey Web site (Schizophrenia Society of Canada), http://www.your-recovery-journey.ca/.

## ⚙ INTEGRATIVE THERAPY

### Yoga as an Adjunctive Treatment for Schizophrenia

Social and occupational functioning is a problem for people with schizophrenia. Studies indicate that yoga, in conjunction with conventional medical treatment, may improve symptoms of schizophrenia, social and occupational functioning, and quality of life. Yoga is based on an ancient Indian spiritual practice that has been reported to improve the connection among the mind, body, and spirit.

In a randomized controlled study by Duraiswamy and colleagues (2007), 61 people with a diagnosis of schizophrenia participated in a trial that compared the efficacy of physical exercise (stretching and aerobic) and yoga. Participants were supervised as they performed one or the other and also practised independently for one hour each day. After four months, both groups experienced symptom reduction, but subjects who had practised yoga showed greater improvement of both negative symptoms of schizophrenia and psychological quality of life.

Machleidt and Ziegenbein (2008) found that yoga together with traditional medical treatment improved not only quality of life but also occupational and social functioning. Yoga, therefore, is a promising adjunctive treatment for schizophrenia that provides participants with an essential experience of grounding, especially in distinguishing themselves from the outside world. It may be the centring quality of the breathing work, in particular, that improves the interrelationship of mind, body, and spirit.

A subsequent systematic review and meta-analysis by Cramer, Lauche, Klose, et al. (2013) found moderate evidence of short-term benefits of yoga on quality of life. However, these researchers caution that yoga should be considered on an individual patient basis and not prescribed as a routine intervention.

**Sources:** Cramer, H., Lauche, R., Klose, P., et al. (2013). Yoga and schizophrenia: A systematic review and meta-analysis. *BioMed Central, 13*(1), 1–12. doi: 10.1186/1471-244X-13-32.; Duraiswamy, G., Thirhalli, J., Nagendra, H.R., et al. (2007). Yoga therapy as an add-on treatment in the management of patients with schizophrenia—A randomized controlled trial. *Acta Psychiatrica Scandinavica, 3*, 226–232. doi:10.1111/j.1600-0447.2007.01032.x.; Machleidt, W., & Ziegenbein, M. (2008). An appreciation of yoga-therapy in the treatment of schizophrenia. *Acta Psychiatrica Scandinavica, 117*, 397–398. doi:10.1111/j.1600-0447.2008.01159.x.

Two groups of antipsychotic drugs exist: conventional antipsychotics (traditional dopamine antagonists [$D_2$ dopamine receptor antagonists]), also known as *typical* or *first-generation antipsychotics*, and atypical antipsychotics (serotonin–dopamine antagonists [$5-HT_{2A}$ receptor antagonists]), also known as *second-generation antipsychotics*. Newer "third-generation" drugs (aripiprazole [now available] and bifeprunox [pending]) give hope for enhanced effectiveness and adverse-effect reduction (Wadenberg, 2007). Other drugs, such as anticonvulsants and antiparkinsonian drugs, are used to augment antipsychotics for patients who do not respond fully. For example, D-serine—an amino acid that enhances NMDA activity—has been shown to increase the effectiveness of selected antipsychotics (Heresco-Levy, Javitt, Ebstein, et al., 2005).

All antipsychotics are effective for most exacerbations of schizophrenia and for reduction or mitigation of relapse. The conventional antipsychotics affect primarily the positive symptoms of schizophrenia (e.g., hallucinations, delusions, disordered thinking). The atypical antipsychotics can improve negative symptoms (e.g., asociality, blunted affect, lack of motivation) as well.

Antipsychotic agents usually take effect two to six weeks after the regimen is started. Only about 10% of people with schizophrenia fail to respond to antipsychotic drug therapy; these patients should not continue to take medication that holds only risks and no benefit for them.

Polypharmacy is an issue for patients with severe and persistent symptoms that do not respond easily to a single medication. It is not unusual to find patients being prescribed a combination of antipsychotic medications, sometimes both oral and depot or both typical and atypical. These individuals may also be taking antiparkinsonian agents and other medications to combat adverse effects. It is important in these cases to have the medication regime carefully and regularly reviewed by both the physician and a pharmacist and to monitor closely for adverse effects. These patients would be at high risk of anticholinergic toxicity, a potentially life-threatening situation (see Table 16-9).

### Atypical Antipsychotics

Atypical antipsychotics first emerged in the early 1990s with clozapine (Clozaril). Unfortunately, clozapine produces agranulocytosis in 0.8% to 1% of those who take it and also increases the risk for seizures. Clozapine produced dramatic improvement in some patients whose disorder had been resistant to the earlier antipsychotics. Due to the risk for agranulocytosis, however, people taking clozapine must have weekly white blood cell counts for the first six months, then frequent monitoring thereafter, to obtain the medication. As a result, clozapine use is declining.

Atypicals are often chosen as first-line antipsychotics because they treat both the positive and negative symptoms of schizophrenia. Furthermore, they produce minimal to no extrapyramidal side effects (EPSs) or tardive dyskinesia in most people, although these effects may still occur for some patients. Adverse effects tend to be significantly less, resulting in greater adherence to treatment.

Atypical antipsychotics include risperidone (Risperdal), lurasidone (Latuda), olanzapine (Zyprexa), quetiapine (Seroquel), ziprasidone (Zeldox), and aripiprazole (Abilify), the last of which is technically a third-generation drug. These atypicals are free of the potential hematological adverse effects of clozapine and are all first-line agents because of their lower adverse-effect profile.

One significant disadvantage of the atypicals, with the exception of ziprasidone and aripiprazole, is that they have a tendency to cause significant weight gain. Metabolic syndrome—which includes weight gain, dyslipidemia, and altered glucose metabolism—is a significant concern with the administration of most atypicals and increases the risk of diabetes, hypertension, and atherosclerotic heart disease (Tschoner, Engl, Laimer, et al., 2007). An additional disadvantage of atypicals is cost: they are more expensive than conventional antipsychotics. Table 16-7 lists the classification, route, and adverse-effect profile of the antipsychotic drugs.

## Conventional Antipsychotics

Conventional antipsychotics are antagonists at the $D_2$ dopamine receptor site in both the limbic and motor centres. This blockage of $D_2$ dopamine receptor sites in the motor areas causes extrapyramidal side effects (EPS), which include akathisia, acute dystonias, pseudoparkinsonism, and tardive dyskinesia. Other adverse reactions include anticholinergic effects, orthostasis, photosensitivity, and lowered seizure threshold.

Specific drugs are often chosen for their adverse-effect profiles. For example, chlorpromazine is the most sedating agent and has fewer EPSs than do other antipsychotic agents, but it causes significant hypotension. Haloperidol (Haldol) is less sedating and induces less hypotension but has a high incidence of EPSs. As a result, haloperidol has value for treating hallucinations because of its effectiveness in controlling positive symptoms with minimal hypotension and sedation. People taking these medications may prefer less sedating drugs, but those who are agitated or excitable may do better with a more sedating medication.

Conventional antipsychotics are becoming less common in the treatment of schizophrenia because of their minimal impact on negative symptoms and their adverse effects. However, conventional antipsychotics are effective against positive symptoms, are much less expensive than atypicals, and come in a depot (long-acting injectable) form, which is given once or twice a month. (*Note*: Risperidone, an atypical antipsychotic, is also available in a depot form [Risperdal Consta].) For people who respond to them and can tolerate their adverse effects, conventional antipsychotics remain an appropriate choice (Swartz, Perkins, Stroup, et al., 2007), especially when metabolic syndrome or cost are concerns.

The conventional antipsychotics are often divided into low-potency and high-potency drugs on the basis of their anticholinergic (ACh) adverse effects, EPSs, and sedative profiles:

Low potency = high sedation + high ACh + low EPSs
High potency = low sedation + low ACh + high EPSs

Conventional antipsychotics must be used cautiously in people with seizure disorders; they can lower the seizure threshold. Three of the more common EPSs are acute dystonia (acute sustained contraction of muscles, usually of the head and neck), akathisia (psychomotor restlessness evident as pacing or fidgeting, sometimes pronounced and very distressing to patients), and pseudoparkinsonism (a medication-induced, temporary constellation of symptoms associated with Parkinson's disease: tremor, reduced accessory movements, impaired gait, and stiffening of muscles). Most patients develop tolerance to these EPSs after a few months.

EPSs can usually be minimized by lowering dosages or adding antiparkinsonian drugs, especially centrally acting anticholinergic drugs such as trihexyphenidyl and benztropine

mesylate (Cogentin). Diphenhydramine hydrochloride (Benadryl) is also useful. Lorazepam, a benzodiazepine, may be helpful in reducing akathisia. Table 16-8 identifies some of the drugs most commonly used to treat EPSs.

Unfortunately, antiparkinsonian drugs can cause significant anticholinergic adverse effects and worsen the anticholinergic adverse effects of conventional antipsychotics and other anticholinergic medications. These adverse effects include anticholinergic syndrome, which is seen in the peripheral nervous system (tachycardia, hyperthermia, hypertension, dry skin, urinary retention, functional ileus) and central nervous system (mydriasis, hallucinations, delirium, seizures, and, in some cases, coma) (Ramjan, Williams, Isbister, et al., 2007). Other troubling adverse effects of conventional antipsychotics include weight gain, sexual dysfunction, endocrine disturbances (e.g., galactorrhea), drooling, and tardive dyskinesia, discussed in the following section. Weight gain, frequently a problem for women, can be more than 45 kilograms; therefore, changing the antipsychotic may be necessary. Impotence and sexual dysfunction are occasionally reported (but frequently experienced) by men and may also necessitate a medication change.

Table 16-9 identifies common adverse effects of the conventional antipsychotic medications, their usual times of onset, and related nursing and medical interventions.

Tardive dyskinesia (TD or TDK) is a persistent EPS that usually appears after prolonged treatment and persists even after the medication has been discontinued. TD is evidenced by involuntary tonic muscular contractions that typically involve the tongue, fingers, toes, neck, trunk, or pelvis. This potentially serious EPS is most frequently seen in women and older persons and affects up to 50% of individuals receiving long-term, high-dose therapy. TD varies from mild to moderate and can be disfiguring or incapacitating; a common presentation is a guppylike mouth movement sometimes accompanied by tongue protrusion. Its appearance can contribute to the stigmatization of people with mental illness.

Early symptoms of tardive dyskinesia are fasciculations of the tongue (described as looking like a bag of worms) or constant smacking of the lips. These symptoms can progress into uncontrollable biting, chewing, or sucking motions; an open mouth; and lateral movements of the jaw. No reliable treatment exists for tardive dyskinesia. The National Institute of Mental Health (NIMH) developed the Abnormal Involuntary Movement Scale (AIMS), a brief test for the detection of tardive dyskinesia and other involuntary movements (Figure 16-2 on pp. 309–310). It examines facial, oral, extremity, and trunk movement. Regularly administering the AIMS exam to detect TD as early as possible is a key nursing role.

## Potentially Dangerous Responses to Antipsychotics

Nurses need to know about some rare—but serious and potentially fatal—effects of antipsychotic drugs, including neuroleptic malignant syndrome, agranulocytosis, liver impairment, and anticholinergic-induced delirium.

Neuroleptic malignant syndrome (NMS) occurs in about 0.2% to 1% of people who have taken conventional antipsychotics, although it can occur with atypicals as well. Acute

| TABLE 16-7 | ANTIPSYCHOTIC DRUGS: CLASSIFICATION, ROUTE, AND ADVERSE-EFFECT PROFILE |

| GENERIC (BRAND) | ROUTE | EPSS | SEDATION | ORTHOSTATIC HYPOTENSION | ANTICHOLINERGIC | WEIGHT GAIN | DIABETES |
| --- | --- | --- | --- | --- | --- | --- | --- |
| **Atypical Antipsychotics—Treat Positive and Negative Symptoms** | | | | | | | |
| Aripiprazole (Abilify) | PO | Very low | Low | Low | None | Low | Low |
| Clozapine (Clozaril) | PO | Very low | High | Moderate | High | High | High |
| Olanzapine (Zyprexa) | PO, IM | Very low | High | Moderate | High | High | High |
| Paliperidone (Invega) | PO | Moderate | Low | Low | None | Moderate | * |
| Quetiapine (Seroquel) | PO | Very low | Moderate | Moderate | None | Moderate | Moderate |
| Risperidone (Risperdal) | PO, IM | Very low | Low | Low | None | Moderate | Moderate |
| Ziprasidone (Zeldox) | PO, IM | Moderate | Moderate | Moderate | None | Low | Low |
| **Conventional Antipsychotics—Treat Positive Symptoms** | | | | | | | |
| **Low Potency** | | | | | | | |
| Chlorpromazine (generic only) | PO, IM, IV, R | Moderate | High | High | Moderate | Moderate | — |
| **Medium Potency** | | | | | | | |
| Loxapine (Loxapac) | PO | Moderate | Moderate | Low | Low | Low | — |
| Perphenazine (generic only) | PO | Moderate | Moderate | Low | Low | — | — |
| **High Potency** | | | | | | | |
| Thiothixene (Navane) | PO | High | Low | Moderate | Low | Moderate | — |
| Fluphenazine (Modecate) | PO, IM | High | Low | Low | Low | — | — |
| Haloperidol (Haldol) | PO, IM | High | Low | Low | Low | Moderate | — |
| Pimozide (Orap) | PO | High | Moderate | Low | Moderate | — | — |
| **Conventional Antipsychotics for Which Limited Data Is Available** | | | | | | | |
| Flupentixol (Fluanxol, Fluanxol Depot) | PO, IM | High | Low | Moderate | Low | — | — |
| Zuclopenthixol (Clopixol, Clopixol Depot, Clopixol Acuphase) | PO IM | — | — | — | May potentiate ACh effects of other drugs | — | — |

*Data unavailable.
*ACh* = Anticholinergic adverse effects; *EPSs* = extrapyramidal side effects.
**Sources:** Canadian Pharmacists Association. (2011). *Electronic compendium of pharmaceuticals and specialties (eCPS)*. Retrieved from https://www.e-therapeutics.ca/; Centre for Addiction and Mental Health. (2009). *Types of antipsychotics*. Retrieved from http://www.camh.net/Care_Treatment/Resources_clients_families_friends/psych_meds/antipsychotics/upm_antipsychotics_types%20.html; Lehne, R.A. (2010). *Pharmacology for nursing care* (7th ed.). St. Louis, MO: Saunders; Martinez, M., Marangell, L.B., & Martinez, J.M. (2008). Psychopharmacology. In R.E. Hales, S.C. Yudofsky, & G.O. Gabbard (Eds.), *Textbook of psychiatry*. Arlington, VA: American Psychiatric Publishing.

**TABLE 16-8  ANTIPARKINSONIAN AND ANTICHOLINERGIC AGENTS FOR TREATMENT OF EXTRAPYRAMIDAL SIDE EFFECTS**

*Note:* All anticholinergic agents (ACAs) can contribute to the risk of anticholinergic toxicity. Practise caution when using multiple ACA agents. After one to six months of long-term maintenance antipsychotic therapy, most ACAs can be withdrawn.

| GENERIC (TRADE) NAME | CHEMICAL TYPE |
| --- | --- |
| Trihexyphenidyl (Apo-Trihex, Artane)* | ACA |
| Benztropine mesylate (Cogentin)* | ACA |
| Diphenhydramine hydrochloride (Benadryl) | Antihistamine (used for its anticholinergic properties) |

*Antiparkinsonian agent.
**Source:** Tirgobov, E., Wilson, B.A., Shannon, M.T., et al. (2005). *Psychiatric drug guide.* Upper Saddle River, NJ: Pearson/Prentice Hall.

reduction in brain dopamine activity plays a role in its development. NMS is a life-threatening medical emergency and is fatal in about 10% of cases. It usually occurs early in therapy but has been reported in people after 20 years of treatment.

NMS is characterized by reduced consciousness, increased muscle tone (muscular rigidity), and autonomic dysfunction—including hyperpyrexia, labile hypertension, tachycardia, tachypnea, diaphoresis, and drooling. Treatment consists of early detection, discontinuation of the antipsychotic, management of fluid balance, temperature reduction, and monitoring for complications. Mild cases of neuroleptic malignant syndrome may be treated with benzodiazepines, vitamins E and B6, or bromocriptine. More severe cases may even be treated with electroconvulsive therapy (ECT) (Agar, 2010; Haddad & Dursun, 2007). Dantrolene, recommended in much of the literature, carries a black box warning (the most serious medication warning required by the Food and Drug Administration) for hepatotoxicity in the United States (Agar, 2010) and is not available in Canada.

Agranulocytosis is a serious, potentially fatal, adverse effect. Liver impairment may also occur. Nurses need to be aware of the prodromal signs and symptoms of these adverse effects and teach them to patients and their families (see Table 16-9).

Anticholinergic-induced delirium is a potentially life-threatening adverse effect usually seen in older adults, although it can occur in younger people as well. It is also seen in patients taking multiple antipsychotic drugs. See Table 16-9 for symptoms and treatment of this serious adverse effect.

### Adjuncts to Antipsychotic Drug Therapy

Antidepressants are recommended along with antipsychotic agents for the treatment of depression, which is common in schizophrenia. Refer to Chapter 14 for a more detailed discussion of depression and antidepressant drugs.

Antimanic (mood-stabilizing) agents have been helpful in enhancing the effectiveness of antipsychotics. Valproic acid (Epival, Valproate) is used during acute exacerbations of psychosis to hasten response to antipsychotics (Freudenreich, Weiss, & Goff, 2008). Lamotrigine may be given along with clozapine to improve therapeutic effects.

Augmentation with benzodiazepines (e.g., clonazepam) can reduce anxiety and agitation and contribute to improvement in positive and negative symptoms (Tirgobov, Wilson, Shannon, et al., 2005).

### When to Change an Antipsychotic Regimen

The following circumstances suggest a need to adjust or change the antipsychotic agent or add supplemental medications (e.g., lithium, carbamazepine, valproate):
- Inadequate improvement in target symptoms despite an adequate trial of the drug
- Persistence of dangerous or intolerable adverse effects

### Specific Interventions for Paranoia, Catatonia, and Disorganization

The following sections discuss paranoia, catatonia, and disorganization in psychoses and identify pertinent communication guidelines, self-care needs, and milieu needs.

### Paranoia

Any intense and strongly defended irrational suspicion can be regarded as paranoia. Paranoia is evident, at least intermittently, in many people without psychotic disorders but is verified as irrational and discarded by the reality-testing process. This process fails in people experiencing paranoia concomitant with psychotic disorders. For them, paranoid ideas cannot be corrected by experiences or modified by facts or reality. *Projection* is the most common defence mechanism used in paranoia: when individuals with paranoia feel angry (or self-critical), they project the feeling onto others and believe others are angry with (or harshly critical toward) them—as if to say, "I'm not angry—you are!"

Schizophrenia with predominantly paranoid symptoms usually has a later age of onset (late 20s to 30s), develops rapidly in individuals with good premorbid functioning, tends to be intermittent during the first five years of the illness, and, in some cases, is associated with a good outcome or complete recovery. People with paranoia are usually frightened and may behave defensively (e.g., a delusion that another person is planning to kill the patient can result in the patient attacking or killing that person first). The paranoia is often a defence against painful feelings of loneliness, despair, helplessness, and fear of abandonment. Useful nursing strategies are outlined in the following sections.

*Communication guidelines.* Because people with paranoia have difficulty trusting those around them, they are usually guarded, tense, and reserved. To ensure interpersonal distance, they may adopt a superior, aloof, hostile, or sarcastic attitude, disparaging and dwelling on the shortcomings of others to maintain their self-esteem. Although they may shun interpersonal contact, functional impairment other than paranoia may

| TABLE 16-9 | ADVERSE EFFECTS OF CONVENTIONAL ANTIPSYCHOTICS AND RELATED NURSING INTERVENTIONS |
|---|---|
| **ADVERSE EFFECT** | **NURSING INTERVENTIONS** |
| Dry mouth | Provide frequent sips of water, ice chips, and sugarless candy or gum; if severe, provide moisture spray |
| Urinary retention and hesitancy | Check voiding<br>Try warm towel on abdomen, and consider catheterization if no result |
| Constipation | Usually short term<br>May use stool softener<br>Ensure adequate fluid intake<br>Increase fibre intake<br>Use dietary laxatives (e.g., prune juice) |
| Blurred vision | Usually abates in 1 to 2 weeks<br>May require use of reading or magnifying glasses<br>If intolerable, consider consult regarding change in medication |
| Photosensitivity | Encourage person to wear sunglasses, sunscreen, and sun-blocking clothing<br>Limit exposure to sunlight |
| Dry eyes | Use artificial tears |
| Inhibition of ejaculation or impotence in men | Consult prescriber: person may need alternative medication |
| Anticholinergic-induced delirium: dry mucous membranes; reduced or absent peristalsis; mydriasis; nonreactive pupils; hot, dry, red skin; hyperpyrexia without diaphoresis; tachycardia; agitation; unstable vital signs; worsening of psychotic symptoms; delirium; urinary retention; seizure; repetitive motor movements | ***Potentially life-threatening medical emergency***<br>Consult prescriber immediately<br>Hold all medications<br>Implement emergency cooling measures as ordered (cooling blanket, alcohol, or ice bath)<br>Implement urinary catheterization as needed<br>Administer benzodiazepines or other sedation as ordered<br>Physostigmine may be ordered |
| Pseudoparkinsonism: masklike facies, stiff and stooped posture, shuffling gait, drooling, tremor, "pill-rolling" phenomenon<br>*Onset:* 5 hours–30 days | Administer prn antiparkinsonian agent (e.g., trihexyphenidyl or benztropine)<br>If intolerable, consult prescriber regarding medication change<br>Provide towel or handkerchief to wipe excess saliva |
| Acute dystonic reactions: acute contractions of tongue, face, neck, and back (usually tongue and jaw first)<br>Opisthotonos: tetanic heightening of entire body, head and belly up<br>Oculogyric crisis: eyes locked upward<br>Laryngeal dystonia: could threaten airway (rare)<br>Cogwheel rigidity: stiffness and clicking in elbow joints felt by the examiner during passive range of motion (early indicator of acute dystonia)<br>*Onset:* 1–5 days | Administer antiparkinsonian agent as above—give IM for more rapid effect and because of swallowing difficulty<br>Also consider diphenhydramine hydrochloride (Benadryl) 25–50 mg IM or IV<br>Relief usually occurs in 5–15 minutes<br>Prevent further dystonias with antiparkinsonian agent (see Table 16-8)<br>Experience can be frightening, and person may fear choking<br>Accompany to quiet area to provide comfort and support<br>Assist person to understand the event and avert distortion or mistrust of medications<br>Monitor airway |
| Akathisia: motor inner-driven restlessness (e.g., tapping foot incessantly, rocking forward and backward in chair, shifting weight from side to side)<br>*Onset:* 2 hours–60 days | Consult prescriber regarding possible medication change<br>Give antiparkinsonian agent<br>Tolerance to akathisia does not develop, but akathisia disappears when neuroleptic is discontinued<br>Propranolol (Inderal), lorazepam (Ativan), or diazepam (Valium) may be used<br>In severe cases, may cause great distress and contribute to suicidality |

*Continued*

| TABLE 16-9 | ADVERSE EFFECTS OF CONVENTIONAL ANTIPSYCHOTICS AND RELATED NURSING INTERVENTIONS—cont'd |
| --- | --- |
| **ADVERSE EFFECT** | **NURSING INTERVENTIONS** |
| Tardive dyskinesia (TD): *Face:* protruding and rolling tongue, blowing, smacking, licking, spastic facial distortion, smacking movements *Limbs:* Choreic: rapid, purposeless, and irregular movements Athetoid: slow, complex, and serpentine movements *Trunk:* neck and shoulder movements, dramatic hip jerks and rocking, twisting pelvic thrusts *Onset:* Months to years | No known treatment Discontinuing the drug rarely relieves symptoms Possibly 20% of people taking these drugs for >2 years may develop TD Nurses and doctors should encourage people to be screened for TD at least every 3 months Onset may merit reconsideration of meds Changes in appearance may contribute to stigmatizing response Teach patient actions to conceal involuntary movements (purposeful muscle contraction overrides involuntary tardive movements) |
| Hypotension and postural hypotension | Check blood pressure before giving agent: a systolic pressure of 80 mm Hg when standing is indication not to give the current dose Advise person to rise slowly to prevent dizziness and hold on to railings or furniture while rising to reduce falls Effect usually subsides when drug is stabilized in 1 to 2 weeks Elastic bandages may prevent pooling If condition is dangerous, consult prescriber regarding medication change, volume expanders, or pressure agents |
| Tachycardia | Always evaluate patients with existing cardiac problems before antipsychotic drugs are administered Haloperidol (Haldol) is usually the preferred drug because of its low ACh effects |
| Agranulocytosis (a rare occurrence, but a possibility the nurse should be aware of): symptoms include sore throat, fever, malaise, and mouth sores; any flulike symptoms should be carefully evaluated *Onset:* During the first 12 weeks of therapy, occurs suddenly | ***A potentially dangerous blood dyscrasia*** Blood work usually done every week for 6 months, then every 2 months Physician may order blood work to determine presence of leukopenia or agranulocytosis If test results are positive, the drug is discontinued, and reverse isolation may be initiated Mortality is high if the drug is not ceased and if treatment is not initiated Teach person to observe for signs of infection |
| Cholestatic jaundice: rare, reversible, and usually benign if caught in time; prodromal symptoms are fever, malaise, nausea, and abdominal pain; jaundice appears 1 week later | Consult prescriber regarding possible medication change Bed rest and high-protein, high-carbohydrate diet if ordered Liver function tests should be performed every 6 months |
| Neuroleptic malignant syndrome (NMS): rare, potentially fatal *Severe extrapyramidal:* severe muscle rigidity, oculogyric crisis, dysphasia, flexor-extensor posturing, cogwheeling *Hyperpyrexia:* elevated temperature (over 39°C or 103°F) *Autonomic dysfunction:* hypertension, tachycardia, diaphoresis, incontinence *Delirium, stupor, coma* *Onset:* Variable, progresses rapidly over 2–3 days *Risk factors:* Concomitant use of psychotropics, older age, female, presence of a mood disorder, and rapid dose titration (increase) | ***Acute, life-threatening medical emergency*** Stop neuroleptic Transfer stat to medical unit Bromocriptine can relieve muscle rigidity and reduce fever Cool body to reduce fever (cooling blankets, alcohol, cool water, or ice bath as ordered) Maintain hydration with oral and IV fluids; correct electrolyte imbalance Arrhythmias should be treated Small doses of heparin may decrease possibility of pulmonary emboli Early detection increases patient's chance of survival |

**Source:** Kemmerer, D.A. (2007). Anticholinergic syndrome. *Journal of Emergency Nursing, 33,* 76–78. doi:10.1016/j.jen.2006.10.013.

be minimal. These people frequently misinterpret the intent or actions of others, perceiving oversights as personal rejection. They also may personalize unrelated events (ideas of reference, or *referentiality*). For example, a patient might see a nurse talking to the psychiatrist and believe the two are talking about her.

During care, a patient suffering from paranoia may make offensive yet accurate criticisms of staff and of unit policies. It is important that responses focus on reducing the patient's anxiety and fear and not be defensive reactions or rejections of the patient. Staff conferences and clinical supervision help

---

### ABNORMAL INVOLUNTARY MOVEMENT SCALE (AIMS)

Public Health Service
Alcohol, Drug Abuse, and Mental Health Administration
National Institute of Mental Health

Name: _____
Date: _____
Prescribing Practitioner: _____

**Code:** 0 = None
1 = Minimal, may be extreme normal
2 = Mild
3 = Moderate
4 = Severe

*Instructions:* Complete Examination Procedure before making ratings.

| Movement ratings: Rate highest severity observed. Rate movements that occur upon activation one *less* than those observed spontaneously. Circle movement as well as code number that applies. | | Rater<br><br>Date | Rater<br><br>Date | Rater<br><br>Date | Rater<br><br>Date |
|---|---|---|---|---|---|
| **Facial and Oral Movements** | **1. Muscles of facial expression** (e.g., movements of forehead, eyebrows, periorbital area, cheeks, including frowning, blinking, smiling, grimacing) | 0 1 2 3 4 | 0 1 2 3 4 | 0 1 2 3 4 | 0 1 2 3 4 |
| | **2. Lips and perioral area** (e.g., puckering, pouting, smacking) | 0 1 2 3 4 | 0 1 2 3 4 | 0 1 2 3 4 | 0 1 2 3 4 |
| | **3. Jaw** (e.g., biting, clenching, chewing, mouth opening, lateral movement) | 0 1 2 3 4 | 0 1 2 3 4 | 0 1 2 3 4 | 0 1 2 3 4 |
| | **4. Tongue:** Rate only increases in movement both in and out of mouth — *not* inability to sustain movement. Darting in and out of mouth. | 0 1 2 3 4 | 0 1 2 3 4 | 0 1 2 3 4 | 0 1 2 3 4 |
| **Extremity Movements** | **5. Upper (arms, wrists, hands, fingers):** Include choreic movements (i.e., rapid, objectively purposeless, irregular, spontaneous) and athetoid movements (i.e., slow, irregular, complex, serpentine). *Do not include tremor* (i.e., repetitive, regular, rhythmic). | 0 1 2 3 4 | 0 1 2 3 4 | 0 1 2 3 4 | 0 1 2 3 4 |
| | **6. Lower (legs, knees, ankles, toes)** (e.g., lateral knee movement, foot tapping, heel dropping, foot squirming, inversion and eversion of foot) | 0 1 2 3 4 | 0 1 2 3 4 | 0 1 2 3 4 | 0 1 2 3 4 |
| **Trunk Movements** | **7. Neck, shoulder, hips** (e.g., rocking, twisting, squirming, pelvic gyrations) | 0 1 2 3 4 | 0 1 2 3 4 | 0 1 2 3 4 | 0 1 2 3 4 |
| **Global Judgments** | **8. Severity of abnormal movements overall** | 0 1 2 3 4 | 0 1 2 3 4 | 0 1 2 3 4 | 0 1 2 3 4 |
| | **9. Incapacitation due to abnormal movements** | 0 1 2 3 4 | 0 1 2 3 4 | 0 1 2 3 4 | 0 1 2 3 4 |
| | **10. Patient's awareness of abnormal movements:** Rate only patient's report.<br>No awareness    0<br>Aware, no distress    1<br>Aware, mild distress    2<br>Aware, moderate distress    3<br>Aware, severe distress    4 | 0<br>1<br>2<br>3<br>4 | 0<br>1<br>2<br>3<br>4 | 0<br>1<br>2<br>3<br>4 | 0<br>1<br>2<br>3<br>4 |
| **Dental Status** | **11. Current problems with teeth and/or dentures** | No   Yes | No   Yes | No   Yes | No   Yes |
| | **12. Are dentures usually worn?** | No   Yes | No   Yes | No   Yes | No   Yes |
| | **13. Edentia** | No   Yes | No   Yes | No   Yes | No   Yes |
| | **14. Do movements disappear in sleep?** | No   Yes | No   Yes | No   Yes | No   Yes |

**FIGURE 16-2** Abnormal Involuntary Movement Scale (AIMS).

*Continued*

**AIMS Examination Procedure**
Either before or after completing the Examination Procedure, observe the patient unobtrusively, at rest (e.g., in waiting room).

The chair to be used in this examination should be a hard, firm one without arms.

1. Ask patient to remove shoes and socks.
2. Ask patient whether there is anything in his or her mouth (e.g., gum, candy) and, if there is, to remove it.
3. Ask patient about the *current* condition of his or her teeth. Ask patient if he or she wears dentures. Do teeth or dentures bother the patient *now?*
4. Ask patient whether he or she notices any movements in mouth, face, hands, or feet. If yes, ask to describe and to what extent they *currently* bother patient or interfere with his or her activities.
5. Have patient sit in chair with hands on knees, legs slightly apart, and feet flat on floor. Look at entire body movements while in this position.
6. Ask patient to sit with hands hanging unsupported: if male, between legs; if female and wearing a dress, hanging over knees. Observe hands and other body areas.
7. Ask patient to open mouth. Observe tongue at rest within mouth. Do this twice.
8. Ask patient to protrude tongue. Observe abnormalities of tongue movement. Do this twice.
9. Ask patient to tap thumb, with each finger, as rapidly as possible for 10 to 15 seconds, separately with right hand, then with left hand. Observe each facial and leg movement.
10. Flex and extend patient's left and right arms (one at a time). Note any rigidity.
11. Ask patient to stand up. Observe in profile. Observe all body areas again, hips included.
12. Ask patient to extend both arms outstretched in front with palms down. Observe trunk, legs, and mouth.
13. Have patient walk a few paces, turn, and walk back to chair. Observe hands and gait. Do this twice.

**FIGURE 16-2, cont'd**

maintain objectivity and a therapeutic perspective about the patient's motivation and behaviour, increasing professional effectiveness.

*Self-care needs*. People with paranoia usually have stronger ego resources than do individuals in whom other symptoms predominate; this is particularly evident in occupational functioning and capacity for independent living. Grooming, dress, and self-care may not be problems and may, in fact, be meticulous. Nutrition, however, may be affected by a delusion, such as that the food is poisoned. Providing foods in commercially sealed packaging—for example, peanut butter and crackers or nutritional drinks in cartons—can improve nutrition. If people worry that others will harm them when they are asleep, they may be fearful of going to sleep—a problem that impairs restorative rest and warrants nursing intervention.

*Milieu needs*. A person with paranoia may become physically aggressive in response to his or her paranoid hallucinations or delusions. The person projects hostile drives onto others and then acts on these drives. Homosexual urges are projected onto others as well, and fear of sexual advances from others may stimulate aggression. An environment that provides a sense of security and safety minimizes anxiety and environmental distortions. Activities that distract the patient from ruminating on paranoid themes also decrease anxiety.

Case Study and Nursing Care Plan 16-1 on pages 313–315 discusses a person with paranoia.

### Catatonia: Withdrawn Phase

The essential feature of catatonia is abnormal levels of motor behaviour, either extreme motor agitation or extreme motor retardation. Other associated behaviours include posturing, waxy flexibility (described below), stereotyped behaviour,

muteness, extreme negativism or automatic obedience, echolalia, and echopraxia (discussed earlier in this chapter). The onset of catatonia is usually abrupt, and the prognosis favourable. With pharmacotherapy and improved individual management, severe catatonic symptoms are rarely seen today. Useful nursing strategies for intervening in catatonia are discussed in the following sections.

*Communication guidelines*. People with catatonia can be so withdrawn they appear stuporous or comatose. They can be mute and may remain so for hours, days, or even weeks or months if untreated. Although such patients may not appear to pay attention to events going on around them, they are acutely aware of the environment and may accurately remember events at a later date. Developing skill and confidence in working with withdrawn patients takes practice. The person's inability or refusal to cooperate or participate in activities challenges staff to work to remain objective and avert frustration and anger.

*Self-care needs*. In extreme withdrawal, a person may need to be hand- or tube-fed to maintain adequate nutritional status. Aspiration is a risk. Normal control over bladder and bowel functions may be interrupted, so the assessment and management of urinary or bowel retention or incontinence is essential. When physical movements are minimal or absent, range-of-motion exercises can reduce muscular atrophy, calcium depletion, and contractures. Dressing and grooming usually require direct assistance.

*Milieu needs*. The catatonic person's appearance may range from decreased spontaneous movement to complete stupor. Waxy flexibility is often seen; for example, if the patient raises arms over the head, he or she may maintain that position for hours or longer. Caution is advised because, even after holding a single posture for long periods, the patient may suddenly and without provocation show brief outbursts of gross motor activity in response to inner hallucinations, delusions, and changes in neurotransmitter levels.

### Catatonia: Excited Phase

*Communication guidelines.* During the excited stage of catatonia, the patient is in a state of greatly increased motor activity. He or she may talk or shout continually and incoherently, requiring the nurse's communication to be clear, direct, and loud (enough to focus the patient's attention on the nurse) and to reflect concern for the safety of the patient and others.

*Self-care needs.* A person who is constantly and intensely hyperactive can become completely exhausted and even die if medical attention is not available. Patients with coexisting medical conditions (e.g., congestive heart failure) are most at risk. Intramuscular administration of a sedating antipsychotic is often required to reduce psychomotor agitation to a safer level. During heightened physical activity, the patient requires stimulation reduction and additional fluids, calories, and rest. It is not unusual for the agitated person to be destructive or aggressive to others in response to hallucinations or delusions or inner distress. Many of the concerns and interventions are the same as those for mania. See Chapter 15 for more information about bipolar disorders.

### Disorganization

Disorganization represents the most regressed and socially impaired form of schizophrenia. A person with disorganization may have marked associative looseness, grossly inappropriate affect, bizarre mannerisms, and incoherence of speech and may display extreme social withdrawal. Delusions and hallucinations are fragmentary and poorly organized. Behaviour may be considered odd, and a giggling or grimacing response to internal stimuli is common.

Disorganization has an earlier age of onset (early to middle teens), often develops insidiously, is associated with poor premorbid functioning and a significant family history of psychiatric disorders, and carries a poor prognosis. Often, these people reside in long-term care facilities and can live safely in the community only in a structured, well-supervised setting or with intensive follow-up such as a PACT (Program for Assertive Community Treatment) service. Families of patients living at home need significant community support, respite care, and access to day hospital services. Unfortunately, a good portion of these people become homeless. See the Case Study and Nursing Care Plan for Disorganized Thinking on the Evolve Web site.

*Communication guidelines.* People with disorganization experience persistent and severe perceptual and communication problems. Communication should be concise, clear, and concrete. Tasks should be broken into discrete tasks that are performed one at a time. Repeated refocusing may be needed to keep the patient on topic or to allow task completion. This repetition can be frustrating to the nurse and others, requiring special effort to identify and correct counter-transference and nontherapeutic responses.

*Self-care needs.* In people with disorganization, grooming is neglected; hair is often dirty and matted, and clothes are unclean and often inappropriate for the weather (presenting a risk to self). Cognition, memory, and executive function are grossly impaired, and the person is frequently too disorganized to carry out simple activities of daily living (ADLs). Areas of nursing focus include encouraging optimal levels of functioning, preventing further regression, and offering alternatives for inappropriate behaviours whenever possible. Significant direct assistance for ADLs is also needed.

*Milieu needs.* People with disorganization need assistance to conform their behaviour to social expectations. Nurses should provide for the patient's privacy needs. Peer education about the disorder may reduce peer frustration and acting out.

---

**VIGNETTE**

Martin, a 36-year-old man, is accompanied to the mental health centre by his mother. Ms. Lam, Martin's nurse, obtains background information from his mother. According to her, he had been in a long-term care facility for treatment of schizophrenia for three months and, after his discharge, had been doing well at home until recently. His only employment history was five months as a janitor after high school graduation. His mother states that, as a teenager, Martin was an excellent athlete and received average grades. At age 17, he had his first psychotic break, when he took various street drugs. His behaviour became markedly bizarre (e.g., eating cat food and swallowing a rubber-soled heel, which precipitated an emergency laparotomy).

Ms. Lam meets with Martin. He is unshaven and dishevelled. He is wearing a headband that holds Popsicle sticks and paper scraps. He chain-smokes, paces, and frequently changes position. He reports that he is Alice from Alice in the Underground and that people from space hurt him with needles. His speech is marked by associative looseness and occasional blocking, and he often stops in the middle of a phrase and giggles to himself.

He starts to giggle, and Ms. Lam asks what he is thinking about. He states, "You interrupted me." He then begins to shake his head while repeating in a singsong voice, "Shake them tigers ... shake them tigers. ..." He denies suicidal or homicidal ideation. Ms. Lam notes that Martin has great difficulty accurately perceiving what is going on around him. He exhibits regressed social behaviours (e.g., eating with his hands and picking his nose in public). He has no apparent insight into his problems, telling Ms. Lam that his biggest problem is the people in space.

---

### Advanced-Practice Interventions

Services that may be provided by advanced-practice nurses and nurse therapists include psychotherapy, cognitive-behavioural therapy (CBT), group therapy, medication administration, social skills training, cognitive remediation, and family therapy. Family therapy is one of the most important interventions the advanced-practice nurse or nurse therapist can implement for the patient with schizophrenia.

### Family Therapy

Family therapy is a service usually delivered by health care providers with specific education in this area, including advanced-practice nurses, nurse therapists, master's-prepared social workers, and registered marriage and family therapists. The field of family therapy was actually originally developed as a treatment for schizophrenia. Families of people with schizophrenia, particularly direct caregivers, often endure considerable hardships while coping with the psychotic and residual symptoms of the illness. The patient and family may become isolated from other relatives, communities, and support systems. In fact, until the 1970s (and sometimes even today), families were often blamed for causing schizophrenia in the affected family member.

Family education and family therapy improve the quality of life for the person with schizophrenia and reduce the relapse rate for many.

The following example shows how a family came to distinguish between "Martha's problem" and "the problem caused by schizophrenia":

> It was a good idea, us all meeting in our own home to discuss my sister's illness. We were all able to say how it felt, and for the first time I realized that I knew very little about what she was suffering or how much—the word *schizophrenia* meant nothing to me before. I used to think she was just being lazy until she told me what it was really like. (Gamble & Brennan, 2000, p. 192)

Programs that provide support, education, coping skills training, and social network development are extremely effective. This psychoeducational approach brings educational and behavioural approaches into family treatment and does not blame families but, rather, recognizes them as secondary victims of a biological illness. In family therapy sessions, fears, faulty communication patterns, and distortions are identified; problem-solving skills are taught; healthier alternatives to conflict are explored; and guilt and anxiety can be lessened.

## EVALUATION

Evaluation is especially important in planning care for people who have psychotic disorders. Outcome expectations that are unrealistic discourage the patient and staff alike. It is critical for staff to remember that change is a process that occurs over time. For a person with schizophrenia, progress may occur erratically, and gains may be difficult to discern in the short term.

Chronically ill people must be reassessed regularly so that new data can be considered and treatment adjusted when needed. Questions to be asked include the following:

- Is the patient not progressing because a more important need is not being met?
- Is the staff making the best use of the patient's strengths and interests to promote treatment and achieve desired outcomes?
- Are other possible interventions being overlooked?
- Are new or better interventions available?
- How is the patient responding to existing or recently changed medications or other treatments?

 **RESEARCH HIGHLIGHT**

### *Cognitive Interventions for Auditory Hallucinations*

**Source:** England, M. (2007). Efficacy of cognitive nursing intervention for voice hearing. *Perspectives in Psychiatric Care, 43*, 69–76. doi:10.1111/j.1744-6163.2007.00114.x.

**Problem**

Medications alone do not always fully relieve hallucinations. Research has suggested that cognitive interventions can reduce distress stemming from residual hallucinations.

**Purpose of Study**

This study sought to determine whether structured cognitive nursing interventions would produce significant improvement in a population of people who hear voices.

**Methods**

Patients were divided into a usual-care control group and an experimental structured-cognitive-interventions group. Symptom reports, treatment adherence, and other parameters were measured before and after intervention. A clinical nurse specialist provided twelve 90-minute, individual cognitive sessions focusing on patients' thoughts about their hallucinations and alternative ways of thinking about their hallucinations that would be more reality-based and less distressing.

**Key Findings**

The cognitive-intervention group demonstrated significant improvement in self-esteem and reduced distress related to symptoms. This outcome is consistent with research showing that hearing voices is tied to poor self-esteem and the nature of one's relationship with the voices.

**Implications for Nursing Practice**

Existing cognitive interventions, when added to traditional psychopharmacology, can significantly enhance symptom management. Although within the scope of practice for nurses, such interventions are not consistently used at present. Training nurses in their use and providing other support to increase their use has the potential to contribute to a higher quality of life for patients with residual hallucinations.

- Is the patient becoming discouraged, anxious, or depressed?
- Is the patient participating in treatment? Are adverse effects controlled or troubling?
- Is functioning improving or regressing?
- What is the patient's quality of life, and is it improving?
- Is the family involved, supportive, and knowledgeable regarding the patient's disorder and treatment?

Active staff involvement and interest in the patient's progress communicate concern and caring, help the patient to maximize progress, promote participation in treatment, and reduce staff feelings of helplessness and burnout. Input from the patient can offer valuable information about why a certain desired outcome has not occurred.

## CASE STUDY AND NURSING CARE PLAN 16-1

### Paranoia in Schizophrenia

Tom, a 32-year-old man, is an inpatient at a Veterans Affairs Canada hospital. He has been separated from his wife and four children for three years. His records state that he has been in and out of hospitals for 13 years. Tom is a former master seaman who first "heard voices" at the age of 19 while he was serving in the Gulf War. He subsequently received a medical discharge.

The hospitalization was precipitated by an exacerbation of auditory hallucinations. "I thought people were following me. I hear voices, usually a woman's voice, and she's tormenting me. People say that it happens because I don't take my medications. The medications make me tired, and I can't have sex." Tom also uses marijuana, which he knows increases his paranoia. "It makes me feel good, and not much else does." Tom finished 11 years of school but did not graduate. He says he has no close friends. He spent five years in prison for manslaughter and was abusing alcohol and drugs when the crime occurred. Drug abuse has also been a contributing factor to Tom's psychiatric hospitalizations.

Ms. Lally is Tom's nurse. Tom is dressed in T-shirt and jeans, his hygiene is good, and he is well nourished. He reports that "the voices get worse at night, and I can't sleep." Ms. Lally notes in Tom's medical record that he has had two episodes of suicidal ideation, during which the voices were telling him to jump "off rooftops" and "in front of trains." During the first interview, Tom rarely makes eye contact and speaks in a low monotone. At times, he glances about the room as if distracted, mumbles to himself, and appears upset.

**Nurse:** "Tom, my name is Ms. Lally. I will be your nurse today and every day that I am here. If it is okay with you, we will meet every day for 30 minutes at 10 in the morning. We can talk about areas of concern to you."

**Tom:** "Well, don't believe what they say about me. I want to start. ... Are you married?"

**Nurse:** "This time is for you to talk about your concerns."

**Tom:** "Oh ..." (Looks furtively around the room, then lowers his eyes) "I think someone is trying to kill me. ..."

**Nurse:** "You seem to be focusing on something other than our conversation."

**Tom:** "The voices tell me things ... I can't say ..."

**Nurse:** "It seems like the voices are upsetting to you. I can't hear them. What kinds of things are they saying?"

**Tom:** "The voices tell me bad things."

Ms. Lally stays with Tom and encourages him to communicate with her. As Tom focuses more on the conversation, his anxiety appears to lessen. His thoughts become more connected, he is able to concentrate more, and he mumbles to himself less.

## ASSESSMENT

### Self-Assessment

On the first day of admission, Tom assaults another male patient, stating that the other person accused him of being a homosexual and touched him on the buttocks. After assessing the incident, the staff agrees that Tom's provocation came more from his own projections (Tom's sexual attraction to the other person) than from anything the other person did or said.

Tom's difficulty with impulse control frightens Ms. Lally. She has concerns regarding Tom's ability to curb his impulses and the possibility of Tom's striking out at her, especially when Tom is hallucinating and highly delusional. Ms. Lally mentions her concerns to the nursing coordinator, who suggests that Ms. Lally meet with Tom in the day room until he demonstrates more control and less suspicion of others. After five days, Tom is less excitable, and the sessions are moved to a room reserved for private interviews. Ms. Lally also speaks with a senior staff nurse regarding her fears. By talking to the senior nurse and understanding more clearly her own fear, Ms. Lally is able to manage her fear and identify interventions to help Tom regain a better sense of control.

| Objective Data | Subjective Data |
|---|---|
| Speaks in low monotone | "I hear voices." |
| Makes poor eye contact | "I think someone is trying to kill me. ..." |
| Weight appropriate for height | "I don't take my medications. [They] make me tired, and I can't |
| Clean, bathed, clothes match | have sex." |
| Impaired reality testing | "The voices get worse at night and I can't sleep." |
| Has a history of drug abuse (marijuana), which appears to | "[Marijuana] makes me feel good, and not much else does." |
| contribute to relapses | Voices have told him to jump "off rooftops" and "in front of |
| Has no close friends, separated from wife and children | trains." |
| Was first hospitalized at age 19 and has not worked since that | |
| time | |
| Has had suicidal impulses twice, both associated with command | |
| hallucinations | |
| Was imprisoned for five years for violence (manslaughter) and | |
| assaulted a peer in the hospital | |
| Thoughts scattered when anxious | |

## DIAGNOSIS

1. *Disturbed thought processes* related to alteration in neurological function, as evidenced by persecutory hallucinations and paranoia

*Continued*

## CASE STUDY AND NURSING CARE PLAN 16-1—cont'd

### Paranoia in Schizophrenia

**Supporting Data**

- Voices have told him to jump "off rooftops" and "in front of trains."
- "I think someone is trying to kill me."
- Abuses marijuana (although it increases paranoia) because "it makes me feel good."

2. *Nonadherence to medication regimen* related to adverse effects of therapy, as evidenced by verbalization of nonadherence and persistence of symptoms

**Supporting Data**

- Failure to take prescribed medications because "they make me tired, and I can't have sex."
- Chronic history of relapse of symptoms

### OUTCOMES IDENTIFICATION

1. Tom consistently refrains from acting on his "voices" and suspicions.
2. Tom consistently adheres to treatment regimen.

### PLANNING

The nurse plans intervention that will (1) help Tom deal with his disturbing thoughts and (2) minimize drug abuse and adverse effects of medication to increase adherence and decrease the potential for relapse and violence.

### IMPLEMENTATION

1. **Nursing diagnosis:** Disturbed thought processes
   *Outcome:* Tom consistently refrains from acting on his "voices" and suspicions when they occur.

| Short-Term Goal | Intervention | Rationale | Evaluation |
|---|---|---|---|
| 1. By the end of the first week, Tom will recognize the presence of hallucinations and identify one or more contributing factors, as evidenced by telling his nurse when they occur and what preceded them. | 1a. Meet with Tom each day for 30 minutes to establish trust and rapport.<br>1b. Explore those times when voices are most threatening and disturbing, noting the circumstances that precede them.<br>1c. Provide noncompetitive activities that focus on the here and now. | 1a. Short, consistent meetings help decrease anxiety and establish trust.<br>1b. Identifying events that increase anxiety and trigger "voices" and then learning to manage triggers, hallucinations can be reduced.<br>1c. Increased time spent in reality-based activities decreases focus on hallucinations. | **GOAL MET**<br>By the end of the first week, Tom tells the nurse when he is experiencing hallucinations. |
| 2. By the end of the first week, Tom will recognize hallucinations as "not real" and ascribe them to his illness. | 2a. Explore content of hallucinations with Tom.<br>2b. Educate Tom about the nature of hallucinations and ways to determine if "voices" are real. | 2a. Exploring hallucinations identifies suicidal or aggressive themes or command hallucinations.<br>2b. Education improves Tom's reality testing and helps him begin to attribute his experiences to schizophrenia. | **GOAL MET**<br>Tom identifies that the voices tell him he is a loser and he needs to be careful "because someone is after me." He identifies that the voices are worse at nighttime. He notes that others do not seem to hear what he hears and also states that smoking marijuana produces very threatening voices. |
| 3. By discharge, Tom will consistently report a decrease in hallucinations. | 3. Explore with Tom possible actions that can minimize anxiety and reduce hallucinations, such as whistling or reading aloud. | 3. Such activities offer alternatives while anxiety level is relatively low. | **GOAL MET**<br>Tom states that he is hearing voices less often, and they are less threatening to him. Tom identifies that if he whistles or sings, he stays calm and can control the voices. |

*Continued*

## CASE STUDY AND NURSING CARE PLAN 16-1—cont'd

*Paranoia in Schizophrenia*

2. **Nursing diagnosis:** Nonadherence to medication regimen
   *Outcome: Tom consistently adheres to medication regimen.*

| Short-Term Goal | Intervention | Rationale | Evaluation |
|---|---|---|---|
| 1. By the end of week 1, Tom will discuss his concerns about medication with staff. | 1a. Evaluate medication response and adverse-effect issues.<br>1b. Initiate medication change to olanzapine (Zyprexa). Administer a large dose at bedtime to increase sleep and a small dose during the day to decrease fatigue.<br>1c. Educate Tom regarding adverse effects—how long they last and what actions can be taken. | 1a. Such evaluation identifies drugs and dosages that have increased therapeutic value and decreased adverse effects.<br>1b. Olanzapine causes no known sexual difficulties.<br>1c. This knowledge can give an increased sense of control over symptoms. | **GOAL MET**<br>Tom identifies the reasons for stopping his medication. He agrees to try olanzapine because he trusts staff's assurances that the adverse effects will be reduced. Tom states that he sleeps better at night but is still tired during the day. |
| 2. By the end of week 2, Tom will describe two ways to reduce or cope with adverse effects and two ways the medications help him meet his goals (e.g., avoiding jail and reducing fear). | 2a. Connect Tom with the local Schizophrenia Society support group. | 2a. Being part of a group provides peer support and a chance to hear from others (further along in recovery) how medications can be helpful and adverse effects can be managed. The peer group can also offer suggestions for dealing with his loneliness and other problems. | **GOAL MET**<br>**Week 1:**<br>Tom attends meeting.<br>**Week 2:**<br>He speaks in the group about "not feeling good." Several group members say they understand and try to help him figure out why he is not feeling good. Peers tell him how taking medication has helped them feel better. |

### EVALUATION

By discharge, Tom expresses hope that the medications will help him feel better and avoid problems like jail. He has a better understanding of his medications and what to do for adverse effects. He knows that marijuana increases his symptoms and explains that when he gets lonely, he now has ideas of things other than drugs he can do to "feel good." Tom continues with the support group and outpatient counselling, stating that his reason for doing so is "because Ms. Lally really cared about me"; her caring made him want to get better and led him to trust what staff told him. He reports sleeping much better and says that he has more energy during the day.

## ▌ KEY POINTS TO REMEMBER

- Schizophrenia is a biological disorder of the brain. It is not one disorder but a group of disorders with overlapping symptoms and treatments.
- Recovery is increasingly possible with early identification, new treatments, and adequate social supports.
- The primary differences among subtypes involve the spectrum of symptoms that dominate their severity, the impairment in affect and cognition, and the impact on social and other areas of functioning.
- Psychotic symptoms are often more pronounced and obvious than are symptoms found in other disorders, making schizophrenia more likely to be apparent to others and increasing the risk of stigmatization.
- Neurochemical (catecholamines and serotonin), genetic, and neuroanatomical findings help explain the symptoms of schizophrenia. However, no one theory accounts fully for the complexities of schizophrenia.

- There are four categories of symptoms of schizophrenia: positive, negative, cognitive, and affective. Symptoms vary considerably among people and fluctuate over time.
- The positive symptoms of schizophrenia (e.g., hallucinations, delusions, associative looseness) are more pronounced and respond best to antipsychotic drug therapy.
- The negative symptoms of schizophrenia (e.g., social withdrawal and dysfunction, lack of motivation, reduced affect) respond less well to antipsychotic therapy and tend to be more debilitating.
- The degree of cognitive impairment (cognitive symptom) warrants careful assessment and active intervention to increase the patient's ability to adapt, function, and maximize his or her quality of life.
- Coexisting depression (affective symptom) must be identified and treated to reduce the potential for suicide, substance abuse, nonadherence, and relapse.

- Some applicable nursing diagnoses include *Disturbed sensory perception*, *Disturbed thought processes*, *Impaired communication*, *Ineffective coping*, *Risk for self-directed or other-directed violence*, and *Impaired family coping*.
- Outcomes are chosen based on the type and phase of schizophrenia and the person's individual needs, strengths, and level of functioning. Short-term and intermediate indicators are also developed to better track the incremental progress typical of schizophrenia.
- Interventions for people with schizophrenia include trust building, therapeutic communication techniques, support, assistance with self-care, promotion of independence, stress management, promotion of socialization, psychoeducation to promote understanding and adaptation, milieu management, cognitive-behavioural interventions, cognitive

enhancement or remediation techniques, and medication administration.
- Because antipsychotic medications are essential in the care of people with schizophrenia, the nurse must understand the properties, adverse and toxic effects, and dosages of conventional and atypical antipsychotics and other medications used to treat schizophrenia. The nurse helps the patient and family understand and appreciate the importance of medication to recovery.
- Schizophrenia can produce counter-transference responses in staff; clinical supervision and self-assessment help the nurse remain objective and therapeutic.
- Hope is closely tied to recovery; it is essential for nurses to hold hope for people with schizophrenia.

## CRITICAL THINKING

1. Jasmine, a 24-year-old woman, is hospitalized after an abrupt onset of psychosis and is diagnosed with paranoid schizophrenia. Jasmine is recently divorced and works as a legal secretary. Her work had become erratic, and her suspiciousness was attracting negative responses. Jasmine is being discharged in two days to her mother's care until she is able to resume her job. Jasmine's mother is overwhelmed and asks the nurse how she is going to cope: "I can hardly say anything to Jasmine without her getting upset. She is still mad at me because I called 911 and had her admitted. She says there is nothing wrong with her, and I'm worried she'll stop her medication once she is home. What am I going to do?"
   a. Explain Jasmine's behaviour and symptoms to a classmate as you would to Jasmine's mother.

   b. How would you respond to the mother's immediate concerns?
   c. What are some of the priority concerns the nurse should address before discharge?
   d. Identify interventions that are based on the concepts of the recovery model.
   e. What are some community resources that can help support this family? Describe how each could be helpful to this family.
   f. What do you think of the prognosis for Jasmine? Support your position with data regarding Jasmine's diagnosis and the treatment you have planned.

## CHAPTER REVIEW

1. A person is found in a closet with an empty two-litre bottle of cola taken from the staff refrigerator. The bottle was full but now is empty. Recently, staff have noticed an increase in this person's response to auditory hallucinations and the recent addition of confusion to his symptoms. For the past several days, the person has been seen drinking from the hallway water cooler and taking items from his peers' dinner trays. Which response is most appropriate for decreasing these behaviours?
   1. Place the person on every-15-minute checks to identify any further deterioration.
   2. Restrict his access to fluids, and evaluate for water intoxication via daily weights.
   3. Attempt to distract the person from excess fluid intake and other bizarre behaviour.
   4. Request an increase in antipsychotic medication, owing to the worsening of his psychosis.

2. Jim is sometimes seen moving his lips silently or murmuring to himself when he does not realize others are watching. Sometimes when he is conversing with others, he suddenly stops, appears distracted for a moment, and then resumes. Based on these observations, which symptom or set of symptoms is Jim most likely experiencing? Select all that apply.
   1. Illusions
   2. Paranoia
   3. Delusional thinking
   4. Auditory hallucinations
   5. Impaired reality testing
   6. Stereotyped behaviours

3. Maricel, a person diagnosed with schizophrenia, is encouraged to attend groups but stays in her room instead. Staff and peers encourage her participation, but her hygiene remains poor. She does not seem to care that others wish that she would behave differently. Which is the most likely explanation for Maricel's failure to respond to others' efforts to help her behave in a more adaptive fashion? Select all that apply.
   1. She is avolitional.
   2. She is displaying anergia.
   3. She is displaying negativism.
   4. She is exhibiting paranoid delusions.
   5. She is being resistant or oppositional.
   6. She is experiencing social withdrawal.
   7. She is apathetic due to her schizophrenia.

4. The nurse is attempting to interview Mr. Jones, a newly admitted involuntary person with schizophrenia. Mr. Jones seems evasive and uncomfortable and gives one-word responses that are minimally informative. Which response would be most useful for facilitating the interview?
   1. "Why did you come to the hospital today?"
   2. "It must be difficult to be admitted to a hospital against your will."
   3. "If you could cooperate for just a few minutes, we could get this done."
   4. "Did your schizophrenia get worse because you stopped taking your medication?"

5. A week later, Mr. Jones has begun to take the conventional antipsychotic haloperidol. You approach him with his bedtime dose and notice that he is sitting very stiffly and immobile. When you approach, you notice that he is diaphoretic, and when you ask if he is okay he seems unable to turn towards you or to respond verbally. You also notice that his eyes are aimed sharply upward and he seems frightened. How should the nurse respond to reduce the symptoms displayed by Mr. Jones? Select all that apply.

   1. Begin to wipe him with a washcloth wet with cold water or alcohol.
   2. Hold his medication, stat page his doctor, and check his temperature.
   3. Administer a medication such as benztropine IM to correct his dystonic reaction.
   4. Reassure him that although there is no treatment for his tardive dyskinesia, it will pass.
   5. Explain that he has anticholinergic toxicity, hold his meds, and give IM physostigmine.
   6. Hold his medication tonight, and consult his doctor after completing medication rounds.

6. The nurse is planning a cognitive intervention group for auditory hallucinations. According to the study by England (2007), what does the evidence show regarding this type of intervention?
   1. Improving self-esteem will reduce auditory hallucinations
   2. Cognitive intervention for hallucinations also improves attention deficits
   3. People with schizophrenia are too ill to benefit from cognitive therapy
   4. Providing alternate ways of thinking about hallucinations reduces distress

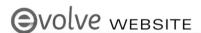 **WEBSITE**    **Post-Test** interactive review

*Visit the Evolve Web site for Chapter Review Answers and Rationales, Critical Thinking Answer Guidelines, and additional resources related to the content in this chapter: http://evolve.elsevier.com/Canada/Varcarolis/psychiatric/*

## REFERENCES

Agar, L. (2010). Recognizing neuroleptic malignant syndrome in the emergency department: A case study. *Perspectives in Psychiatric Care*, 46(2), 143–151. doi:10.1111/j.1744-6163.2010.00250.x.

Amador, X. (2000). *I'm not sick, I don't need help!* New York: Vida Press.

Anthony, K.H. (2008). Helping partnerships that facilitate recovery from severe mental illness. *Journal of Psychosocial Nursing*, 46(7), 25–33.

Bechdolf, A., Phillips, L.J., Francey, S.M., et al. (2006). Recent approaches to psychological interventions for people at risk of psychosis. *European Archive of Psychiatry and Clinical Neuroscience*, 256, 159–173. doi:10.1007/s00406-006-0623-0.

Bertolote, J., & McGorry, P. (2005). Early intervention and recovery for young people with early psychosis: Consensus statement. *British Journal of Psychiatry*, 187, S116–S119. doi:10.1192/bjp.187.48.s116.

Bralet, M., Ton, T., & Falissard, B. (2007). Schizophrenic patients with polydipsia and water intoxication more often have a form of schizophrenia first described by Kraepelin. *Psychiatry Research*, 152, 267–271. doi:10.1016/j.psychres.2006.11.009.

Braw, Y., Bloch, Y., Mendelovich, S., et al. (2008). Cognition in young schizophrenia outpatients: Comparison of first episode with multiepisode patients. *Schizophrenia Bulletin*, 34, 544–554. doi:10.1093/schbul/sbm115.

Broome, M.R., Woolley, J.B., Tabraham, P., et al. (2005). What causes the onset of psychosis? *Schizophrenia Research, 79*(1), 23–34.

Canadian Institute for Health Information (CIHI). (2008). *Hospital length of stay and readmission for individuals diagnosed with schizophrenia: Are they related?* Retrieved from https://secure.cihi.ca/estore/productSeries.htm?pc=PCC410.

Chung, Y.S., Kang, D., Shin, N.Y., et al. (2008). Deficit of theory of mind in individuals at ultra-high risk for schizophrenia. *Schizophrenia Research, 99*, 111–118.

Compton, M.T. (2004). Considering schizophrenia from a prevention perspective. *American Journal of Preventive Medicine, 26*, 178–185. Retrieved from http://www.ajpmonline.org/.

Crowe, T.P., Deane, F.P., Oades, L.G., et al. (2006). Effectiveness of a collaborative recovery training program in Australia in promoting positive views about recovery. *Psychiatric Services, 57*, 1497–1500. doi:10.1176/appi.ps.57.10.1497.

England, M. (2007). Accuracy of nurses' perceptions of voice hearing and psychiatric symptoms. *Journal of Advanced Nursing, 58*, 103–109. doi:10.1111/j.1744-6163.2007.00114.x.

Farhall, J., Greenwood, K.M., & Jackson, H.J. (2007). Coping with hallucinated voices: A review of self-initiated strategies and therapeutic interventions. *Clinical Psychology Review, 27*, 476–493. doi:10.1016/j.cpr.2006.12.002.

Fazel, S., Gulati, G., Linsell, L., et al. (2009). Schizophrenia and violence: A systematic review and meta-analysis. *PLOS Medicine, 6*(8), 1–15. doi:10.1371/journal.pmed.1000120.

Freudenreich, O., Weiss, A.P., & Goff, D.C. (2008). Psychosis and schizophrenia. In T.A. Stern, J.F. Rosenbaum, M. Fava, et al. (Eds.), *Massachusetts General Hospital comprehensive clinical psychiatry* (pp. 371–389). St. Louis, MO: Mosby.

Gamble, C., & Brennan, G. (2000). Working with families and informed careers. In C. Gamble & G. Brennan (Eds.), *Working with serious mental illness: A manual for clinical practice.* London, UK: Baillière Tindall.

Gerlock, A.A., Buccheri, R., Buffum, M.D., et al. (2010). Responding to command hallucinations to harm self and others: The Unpleasant Voices Scale and Harm Command Safety Protocol. *Journal of Psychosocial Nursing and Mental Health Services, 48*(5), 26–33. doi:10.3928/02793695-20100304-03.

Goff, D.C. (2005). Pharmacologic implications of neurobiological models of schizophrenia. *Harvard Review of Psychiatry, 13*, 352–359. doi:10.1080/10673220500433262.

Gonzalez, I., & Perez, N. (2008). High risk of polydipsia and water intoxication in schizophrenia patients. *Schizophrenia Research, 99*(1–3), 377–378.

Green, A.I., Noordsy, D.L., Brunette, M.F., et al. (2008). Substance abuse and schizophrenia: Pharmacotherapeutic intervention. *Journal of Substance Abuse Treatment, 34*, 61–71. doi:10.1016/j.jsat.2007.01.008.

Haddad, P.M., & Dursun, S.M. (2007). Neurological complications of psychiatric drugs: Clinical features and management. *Human Psychopharmacology, 23*, 15–26. doi:10.1002/hup.918.

Hayashi, T., Ishida, Y., Miyashita, T., et al. (2005). Fatal water intoxication in a schizophrenia patient—an autopsy case. *Journal of Clinical Forensic Medicine, 12*, 157–159. doi:10.1016/j.jcfm.2005.01.009.

Haynes, R.M., & Resnick, P.J. (1993). Proverb familiarity and the mental status exam. *Bulletin of the Menninger Clinic, 57*(4), 523–529.

Heresco-Levy, U., Javitt, D.C., Ebstein, R., et al. (2005). D-serine efficacy as add-on pharmacotherapy to risperidone and olanzapine for treatment-refractory schizophrenia. *Biological Psychiatry, 57*, 577–585. doi:10.1016/j.biopsych.2004.12.037.

Hoffman, R.E., & Varanko, M. (2006). Seeing voices: Fused visual/auditory verbal hallucinations reported by three persons with schizophrenia-spectrum disorder. *Acta Psychiatrica Scandinavica, 114*, 290–293.

Hubl, D., Koenig, T., Strik, W., et al. (2004). Pathways that make voices: White matter changes in auditory hallucinations. *Archives of General Psychiatry, 61*(7), 658–668.

Jansman-Hart, E.M., Seto, M.C., Crocker, A.G., et al. (2011). International trends in demand for forensic mental health services. *International Journal of Forensic Mental Health, 10*(4), 326–336. doi:10.1080/14999013.2011.625591.

Khashan, A.S., Abel, K.M., McNamee, R., et al. (2008). Higher risk of offspring schizophrenia following antenatal maternal exposure to severe adverse life events. *Archives of General Psychiatry, 65*(2), 146–152.

Kisely, S. (2010). Excess mortality from chronic physical disease in psychiatric patients: The forgotten problem. *Canadian Journal of Psychiatry, 55*(12), 749–751.

Koehn, C.V., & Cutliffe, J.R. (2007). Hope and interpersonal psychiatric/mental health nursing: A systematic review of the literature: Part one. *Journal of Psychiatric and Mental Health Nursing, 14*, 134–140. doi:10.1111/j.1365-2850.2007.01054.x.

Levine, S.Z., Lurie, I., Kohn, R., et al. (2011). Trajectories of the course of schizophrenia: From progressive deterioration to amelioration over three decades. *Schizophrenia Research, 126*, 184–191. doi:10.1016/j.schres.2010.10.026.

Lysecker, P., & Buck, K. (2006). Moving toward recovery within clients' personal narratives: Directions for a recovery-focused therapy. *Journal of Psychosocial Nursing, 44*(1), 29–35.

Manschreck, T.C., Duckworth, K.S., Halpern, L., et al. (2008). Recovery: Time for optimism? *Current Psychiatry, 7*(5), 41–58.

Martin, V., & Johnson, C. (2008). *A time for action: Tackling stigma and discrimination.* Calgary: Mental Health Commission of Canada.

Masi, G., Mucci, M., & Pari, C. (2006). Children with schizophrenia: Clinical picture and pharmacological treatment. *CNS Drugs, 20*(10), 841–866.

Mauri, M.C., Moliterno, D., Rossattini, M., et al. (2008). Depression in schizophrenia: Comparison of first- and second-generation antipsychotic drugs. *Schizophrenia Research, 99*, 7–12. doi:10.1016/j.schres.2007.10.020.

Mauri, M.C., Volonteri, L.S., De Gaspari, I.F., et al. (2006). Substance abuse in first-episode schizophrenic patients: A retrospective study. *Clinical Practice and Epidemiology in Mental Health, 2*, 1–8. doi:10.1186/1745-0179-2-4.

Miller, B.J., Paschall, C.B., & Svendsen, D.P. (2007, March). *Mortality and medical co-morbidity in patients with serious mental illness.* Poster presentation at the 8th Annual All-Ohio Institute on Community Psychiatry, Beachwood, OH.

Möller, H.J. (2007). Clinical evaluation of negative symptoms in schizophrenia. *European Psychiatry, 22*, 380–386. doi:10.1016/j.eurpsy.2007.03.010.

Moorhead, S., Johnson, M., Maas, M.L., et al. (2008). *Nursing outcomes classification (NOC)* (4th ed.). St. Louis, MO: Mosby.

Nash, J. (n.d.) *John Nash quotes.* Retrieved from http://thinkexist.com/quotes/john_nash/.

Nielssen, O., Bourget, D., Laajasalo, T., et al. (2009). Homicide of strangers by people with a psychotic illness. *Schizophrenia Bulletin, 37*, 572–579. doi:10.1093/schbul/sbp112.

Norman, R.M., Manchanda, R., Malia, A.K., et al. (2011). Symptom and functional outcomes for a 5-year early intervention program for psychoses. *Schizophrenia Research, 129*(2–3), 111–115. doi:10.1016/j.schres.2011.04.006.

O'Mahony, J.M., & Donnelly, T.T. (2007). The influence of culture on immigrant women's mental health care experiences from the perspectives of health care providers. *Issues in Mental Health Nursing, 28*, 453–471. doi:10.1080/01612840701344464.

Osborn, D., Levy, G., Nazareth, I., et al. (2008). Suicide and severe mental illnesses. *Schizophrenia Research, 99*(1–3), 134–138.

Ramjan, K.A., Williams, A.J., Isbister, G.K., et al. (2007). "Red as a beet and blind as a bat": Anticholinergic delirium in adolescents: Lessons for the paediatrician. *Journal of Paediatrics and Child Health, 43*(11), 773–780. doi:10.1111/j.1440-1754.2007.01220.x.

Riecher-Rössler, A., Gschwandtner, U., Borgwardt, S., et al. (2006). Early detection and treatment of schizophrenia: How early? *Acta Psychiatrica Scandinavica, 113*, 73–80. doi:10.1111/j.1600-0447.2005.00722.x.

Roberts, S.H., & Bailey, J.E. (2011). Incentives and barriers to lifestyle interventions for people with severe mental illness: A narrative synthesis of quantitative, qualitative, and mixed method studies. *Journal of Advanced Nursing, 67*, 690–708. doi:10.1111/j.1365-2648.2010.05546.x.

Sadock, B.J., & Sadock, V.A. (2008). *Concise textbook of clinical psychiatry* (3rd ed.). Philadelphia: Lippincott Williams & Wilkins.

Smoller, J.W., Finn, C.T., & Gardner-Schuster, E.E. (2008). Genetics and psychiatry. In T.A Stern, J.F. Rosenbaum, M. Fava, et al. (Eds.),

*Massachusetts General Hospital comprehensive clinical psychiatry* (pp. 853–883). St. Louis, MO: Mosby.

Srihari, V.H., Shah, J., & Keshavan, M.S. (2012). Is early intervention for psychosis feasible and effective? *Psychiatric Clinics of North America, 35*(3), 613–631. doi:10.1016/j.psc.2012.06.004.

Swartz, M.S., Perkins, D.O., Stroup, T.S., et al. (2007). Effects of antipsychotic medications on psychosocial functioning in patients with chronic schizophrenia: Findings from the NIMH CATIE study. *American Journal of Psychiatry, 164*, 428–436. doi:10.1176/appi.ajp.164.3.428.

Tandon, R., Keshavan, M.S., & Nasrallah, H.A. (2008). Schizophrenia, "just the facts": What we know in 2008. 2. Epidemiology and etiology. *Schizophrenia Research, 102*, 1–18. doi:10.1016/j.schres.2008.04.011.

Tirgobov, E., Wilson, B.A., Shannon, M.T., et al. (2005). *Psychiatric drug guide.* Upper Saddle River, NJ: Pearson/Prentice Hall.

Tschoner, A., Engl, J., Laimer, M., et al. (2007). Metabolic side effects of antipsychotic medication. *International Journal of Clinical Practice, 61*, 1356–1370. doi:10.1111/j.1742-1241.2007.01416.x.

van Meijel, B., van der Gaag, M., Sylvain, R.K., et al. (2004). Recognition of early warning signs in patients with schizophrenia: A review of the literature. *International Journal of Mental Health Nursing, 13*, 107–116. doi:10.1111/j.1440-0979.2004.00314.x.

Wadenberg, M.G. (2007). Bifeprunox: A novel antipsychotic agent with partial agonist properties at dopamine $D_2$ and serotonin 5-HT$_{1A}$ receptors. *Future Neurology, 2*, 153–165. doi:10.2217/14796708.2.2.153.

Walker, E., & Tessner, K. (2008). Schizophrenia. *Perspectives on Psychological Science, 3*, 30–37. doi:10.1111/j.1745-6916.2008.00059.x.

Weisman, A., Duarte, E., Koneru, V., et al. (2006). The development of a culturally informed, family-focused treatment for schizophrenia. *Family Process, 45*, 171–186. doi:10.1111/j.1545-5300.2006.00089.x.

Zinger, I. (2012). Mental health in federal corrections: Reflections and future directions. *Health Law Review, 20*(2), 22–25. Retrieved from http://www.cashra2012.ca/documents/presentation_ivan_zinger.pdf.

# 17

# Eating Disorders

*Carissa R. Enright, Kathleen Ibrahim*
*Adapted by Wendy Stanyon*

## KEY TERMS AND CONCEPTS

anorexia nervosa, 320
binge eating disorder, 320
bulimia nervosa, 320

ethnic psychopharmacology, 323
ideal body weight, 326

## OBJECTIVES

1. Discuss four theories of eating disorders.
2. Compare and contrast the signs and symptoms (clinical picture) of anorexia nervosa and bulimia nervosa.
3. Identify three life-threatening conditions, stated in terms of nursing diagnoses, for a patient with an eating disorder.
4. Identify three realistic outcome criteria for (a) a patient with anorexia nervosa and (b) a patient with bulimia nervosa.

5. Describe therapeutic interventions appropriate for anorexia nervosa and bulimia nervosa in the acute phase and long-term phase of treatment.
6. Explain the basic premise of cognitive-behavioural therapy in the treatment of eating disorders.
7. Differentiate between the long-term prognoses of anorexia nervosa, bulimia nervosa, and binge eating disorder.

## ⊖volve WEBSITE

*Visit the Evolve website for Flashcards, Case Studies, and additional testing resources related to the content in this chapter: http://evolve.elsevier.com/Canada/Varcarolis/psychiatric/*

Pre-Test  interactive review

Of all the psychiatric disorders, eating disorders may be the most perplexing. The eating and sharing of food is usually pleasurable and culturally important. It is difficult for many of us to understand how people could starve themselves or induce vomiting and seem to have little regard for how it affects them physically and socially. Cases of anorexia nervosa are documented in ancient writings; however, bulimia and binge eating necessitate an abundance of food and, therefore, may be more modern-age eating disorders. Many theories of the etiology of these disorders have been postulated, but, to date, the reasons behind the behaviour are still a mystery that drives research.

## CLINICAL PICTURE

The main types of eating disorders are anorexia nervosa, bulimia nervosa, binge eating disorder, and eating disorder not

otherwise specified (NOS). Individuals with anorexia nervosa refuse to maintain a minimally normal weight for their height and express an intense fear of gaining weight. The term *anorexia* is a misnomer because loss of appetite is rare. Some people with anorexia nervosa restrict their intake of food; others engage in binge eating and purging. Individuals with bulimia nervosa engage in repeated episodes of binge eating followed by compensatory behaviours, such as self-induced vomiting; misuse of laxatives, diuretics, or other medications; fasting; or excessive exercise. Eating disorder NOS is a category that includes disorders of eating that do not meet the criteria for either anorexia nervosa, bulimia nervosa, or binge eating disorder. All of these disorders are characterized by a significant disturbance in the perception of body shape and weight (Miyake, Okamoto, Onoda, et al., 2010).

Individuals with binge eating disorder engage in repeated episodes of binge eating, after which they experience significant distress; they do not regularly use compensatory behaviours, such as those seen in patients with bulimia nervosa.

## HOW A NURSE HELPED ME
### Patient's Challenges

*When I was 10 years old, I began overeating. It was at that time that my best friend moved away; I had other friends, but they were not the same. I am not exactly sure why, but eating helped me relax. The food demanded nothing of me—it did not judge me; it did not need me to do anything; it allowed me just to be. I knew I was smart, as I was successful at school and university.*

*Fortunately, as soon as I finished university, I had no problem finding my first teaching job. It was in a town approximately 300 kilometres away. Moving away was hard for me, but that was where the work was. I was still eating when I felt stressed, and I certainly felt stressed with the new job, in a new town, and with no friends. I was also starting to feel depressed. It was at that point that I went to the local community mental health centre for help. I met with a nurse who asked me a number of questions related to my mood, thoughts, feelings, and energy. The nurse helped me change my relationship with food by helping me understand how my thoughts and experiences impacted how much I ate. She taught me how to use a journal to record my thoughts and experiences. It helped me identify my thoughts and feelings about food, eating, and not eating. I always hated counting calories and was worried that I would have to do that; to my surprise, we talked about my daily intake of food in relationship to the nutrients my body needed. I was counting food groups and portion sizes, but not calories. Another trick she taught me to manage my stress-related food consumption was to plan ahead for the times and places where I would be eating. This really helped because, when I felt stress, I knew just when I would be eating again, so I did not panic and binge-eat. The nurse did not judge me or criticize me because I was overweight; she listened and took me seriously.*

## EPIDEMIOLOGY

Most eating disorders begin in the early teens to mid-20s, commonly following puberty, although bulimia generally occurs in later adolescence. Anorexia nervosa may start early (between ages 7 and 12), but bulimia nervosa is rarely seen in children younger than 12 years. For women, the lifetime incidence of anorexia nervosa, bulimia nervosa, and binge eating disorder are 0.9%, 1.5%, and 3.5%, respectively; and the lifetime incidence for men is 0.3%, 0.5%, and 2% (Hudson, Hiripi, Pope, et al., 2007). The rate of eating disorders among middle-aged women seems to have increased with the baby boomer

generation (those born in the mid-1900s) (Zerbe, 2003). It is extremely difficult to determine the specific number of people who have an eating disorder since fewer than half seek health care for their illness. Many people with disordered eating patterns do not meet full DSM-5 criteria and are not included in these statistics.

In a 2007 survey of the literature on the epidemiology of eating disorders, Becker (2007) highlighted the lack of research focusing on ethnicity. Keel and Klump (2003) determined women in industrialized nations are more at risk because of an abundance of food and the link between physical attractiveness and being thin. They also concluded that while anorexia can be found in all cultures, bulimia and binge eating disorder are more common in countries most influenced by Western culture. In another study published in 2002 by the Canadian Women's Health Network, Marchessault discovered more Aboriginal than non-Aboriginal girls and mothers are dissatisfied with their bodies, and Pinhas, Heinmaa, Bryden, and colleagues (2008) concluded that female Canadian Jewish adolescents are more vulnerable than their non-Jewish counterparts to developing an eating disorder and eating disorder behaviours.

There is some concern that adolescents who go on "extreme diets" that either restrict calories or prohibit certain food groups are at risk for developing an eating disorder, but it does not appear that caloric restriction as a method to reduce body weight in individuals who are overweight is in itself responsible for this risk (Williamson, Martin, Anton, et al., 2008).

Although patients with eating disorders are at risk of medical complications that may result in death, the major cause of death among those affected by eating disorders is suicide. Patients diagnosed with anorexia nervosa or bulimia nervosa may have a suicide rate that is 6.7 times greater than the norm for their age group (Pompili, Girardi, Tatarelli, et al., 2006).

## CO-MORBIDITY

Depression and anxiety are common co-morbid conditions in people with all types of eating disorders. The estimated lifetime prevalence of mood disorders in anorexia nervosa ranges from 31% to 89% and in bulimia nervosa ranges from 24% to 90%. The fact that depressive symptoms accompany any type of starvation makes determining an exact prevalence difficult (Godart, Perdereau, Rein, et al., 2007).

The incidence of obsessive-compulsive disorder (OCD) has been reported to be as high as 25% in patients with anorexia nervosa. The OCD symptoms centre on food preoccupation and may be manifested in collecting cookbooks, preparing elaborate meals for others, and hoarding food. Anxiety disorders, particularly social phobia, are also common. In addition, significant associations have been found between risk for an eating disorder and alcohol dependence, as well as the lifetime abuse of and dependence on illicit drugs (Piran & Gadalla, 2006).

People with eating disorders who are also living with depression, a substance use disorder, or difficulty with impulse control are at greater risk for relapse. There is some evidence that the younger the person is when anorexic symptoms begin, the

## RESEARCH HIGHLIGHT
### *Prevention of Eating Disorders*

**Source:** McVey, G.L., Kirsh, G., Maker, D., et al. (2010). Promoting positive body image among university students: A collaborative pilot study. *Body Image, 7*, 200–204. doi:10.1016/j.bodyim.2010.02.005.

#### Problem
Body dissatisfaction, prevalent among university students, is considered to be a risk factor for eating pathology, emphasizing the need for prevention programs.

#### Purpose of Study
To date, most research studies examining the effectiveness of interventions for eating disorders do not mention any stakeholder involvement. The purpose of this study is to pilot, in collaboration with health promotion staff and peer health educators, a prevention program designed to promote positive body image among university students.

#### Methods
A pre–post design without a control group was used to collect preliminary information about the program. Thirty-seven undergraduate students (6 males; 25 females; mean age 22.6 years) from three Canadian universities were selected from a pool of students enrolled in a peer health education program facilitated by the university-based health promotion staff. Three paper and pencil instruments were used: a survey to collect demographics, the Sociocultural Attitudes Towards Appearance Questionnaire (SATAQ) to measure the degree of internalization of sociocultural stereotypes of weight and appearance, and the Body Satisfaction Scale to assess body satisfaction. The prevention program focused on media literacy, self-esteem enhancement strategies, stress management skills, and ways to recognize healthy versus unhealthy relationships. Open-ended questions were developed to elicit participants' feedback about the program content and process.

#### Key Findings
Participants reported significant improvements in body satisfaction and reductions in the internalization of media stereotypes between the baseline and post-program period.

Participants provided positive feedback about the program and the face-to-face format.

Staff also provided positive feedback and expressed interest in incorporating strategies into their routine peer mentoring training activities.

#### Implications for Nursing Practice
Nurses are often responsible for developing health promotion resources. Knowing how to design sustainable health promotion programs capable of reaching out to students before they develop symptoms of eating disorders is invaluable.

better the chance for positive outcomes (Berkman, Lohr, & Bulik, 2007).

Personality disorders may occur in 42% to 75% of people with eating disorders. There is a high rate of avoidant personality disorders with all the eating disorders. Avoidance fits the clinical picture of being overly concerned with acceptance and approval and fearing criticism or rejection. Patients with anorexia nervosa are more likely to have a Cluster C personality disorder (avoidant, dependent, obsessive-compulsive, or passive-aggressive) (Berkman, Lohr, & Bulik, 2007). Obsessive-compulsive and dependent personality disorders are also common in patients with bulimia. Borderline personality disorder is common in patients with binge eating disorder. See Chapter 20 for more information on personality disorders.

There have been several significant conclusions in the research literature examining the relationship between trauma and eating disorders. Associated traumas now include not only childhood sexual abuse but also other forms of abuse and neglect and are more common in eating disorders involving bingeing and purging behaviours. Also, the research findings have been extended to boys and men with eating disorders (Brewerton, 2007).

## ETIOLOGY

The eating disorders—anorexia nervosa, bulimia nervosa, binge eating disorder, and eating disorder NOS—are actually entities or syndromes and are not considered to be specific diseases (Halmi, 2008). Experts tend to agree that there is no single cause of eating disorders. Eating disorders typically develop from a complex interaction of psychological risk factors, sociocultural influences, and biological or genetic predispositions (Striegel-Moore & Bulik, 2007; Mazzeo & Bulik, 2008). A number of theories attempt to explain eating disorders.

### Biological Factors
#### Genetic
There is a strong genetic link for eating disorders. In fact, data from community-based twin studies have suggested that the heritability is greater than 50% (Keel & Klump, 2003). A genetic vulnerability may lead to affect and impulse-control issues or to an underlying neurotransmitter dysfunction, but no single causative gene has been discovered to date. However, there is evidence that certain gene abnormalities may predispose a person to having symptoms of eating disorders and even confer a risk for developing full-blown eating disorders (Frieling, Römer, Wilhelm, et al., 2006).

#### Neurobiological
Research demonstrates that altered brain serotonin function contributes to dysregulation of appetite, mood, and impulse control in the eating disorders. Patients with eating disorders consistently exhibit personality traits of perfectionism, obsessive-compulsiveness, and dysphoric mood, all of which are modulated through serotonin pathways in the brain. Because these traits appear to begin in childhood—before the onset of actual eating-disorder symptoms—and persist into recovery, they are believed to contribute to a vulnerability to disordered eating (Kaye, 2007).

Tryptophan, an amino acid essential to serotonin synthesis, is available only through diet. A normal diet boosts serotonin in the brain and regulates mood. Temporary drops in dietary tryptophan may actually relieve symptoms of anxiety and dysphoria and provide a reward for caloric restriction. However, continued malnutrition will result in a physiological dysphoria. This cycle of temporary relief followed by more dysphoria sets up a positive feedback loop that reinforces the disordered eating behaviour (Kaye, 2007). The dietary need for tryptophan may account for the fact that antidepressants that boost serotonin do not improve mood symptoms until after an underweight patient has been restored to 90% of optimal weight.

Newer brain-imaging capabilities allow for more research into etiological factors of anorexia nervosa and bulimia nervosa. Overall, there is a consistent finding that patients with eating disorders who are acutely ill and those who have recovered show differences in the frontal, cingulated, temporal, or parietal regions of the brain, or a combination of these regions, in comparison to controls. More studies will be necessary before conclusions can be made about the significance of these differences (Kaye, 2007).

## Psychological Factors

Because anorexia nervosa was observed primarily in girls approaching puberty, early psychoanalytic theories linked the symptoms to an unconscious aversion to sexuality. By maintaining a childlike body, the patient avoids the anxiety associated with developing into a mature sexual being. Throughout the 1900s, many authors examined the family dynamics of these patients and concluded that a failure to separate from parents and a rebellion against the maternal bond explained the disordered eating behaviours (le Grange, Lock, Loeb, et al., 2010). Further work by Bruch (1978) explored the symptoms as a defence against an overwhelming feeling of ineffectiveness and powerlessness. Even with further insight into the intrapsychic origin of the behaviour, the process of psychoanalysis—with the goal of making unconscious processes conscious—failed to effect a cure for these syndromes (Caparrotta & Ghaffari, 2006).

Currently, cognitive-behavioural theorists suggest that eating disorders are based on learned behaviour that has positive reinforcement. For example, a mildly overweight 14-year-old has the flu and loses a little weight. She returns to school, and her friends say, "Wow, you look great," and when people say, "Wow, you look really skinny," she still hears, "Wow, you look great." Now she purposefully strives to lose weight. Her behaviour is powerfully reinforced by these comments despite the fact that her health is at risk.

Family theorists maintain that eating disorders are a problem of the whole family, and often the symptoms in the child serve to take the attention away from a distressed marriage. Families with a child who has anorexia are often described as enmeshed and perfectionistic; the child feels smothered by protectiveness and at the same time abandoned.

## Environmental Factors

The Western cultural ideal that equates feminine beauty to tall, thin models has received much attention in the media as an etiology for eating disorders. Studies have shown that culture influences the development of self-concept and satisfaction with body size. According to Statistics Canada (2011), the percentage of Canadians who are overweight or obese has risen

## CONSIDERING CULTURE
### *The Concept of Weight*

Although cultural beliefs about physical beauty do not cause eating disorders, they influence self-esteem and set the standard of beauty for men and women. An unhealthy cultural ideal, therefore, can pose health risks if not addressed.

For centuries, body weight was an indicator of wealth and the availability of food, so the ideal was to achieve a large body. Considering the more recent media focus on the effect of the Western fashion industry and its use of unnaturally thin models, it is of interest that many other cultures still have the more traditional standards that equate obesity with beauty. For example, the Saharawi of Morocco are a nomadic people who see those who are thin as ill. Young women, as they reach marriageable age, seek to rapidly increase their weight. To accomplish this, they eat large amounts of traditional foods, restrict their activity, and even take drugs such as corticosteroids to increase appetite and promote weight gain. Of the 249 women interviewed by Rguibi and Belahsen (2006), 225 were unsatisfied with their current weight. The group had a mean BMI of 29.6, with a range from 17.3 to 41.4. Only eight women wished to lose weight; the rest sought to become heavier. The authors suggest that a change in the cultural norm of beauty will be necessary to prevent the known health risks of obesity in that population.

Culturally competent care planning is made very difficult when the cultural ideal is unhealthy. In seeking to change behaviour, the nurse must acknowledge the cultural norm as important to the individual while, at the same time, providing adequate education about the risks and health consequences of the norm and helping patients find a solution that respects their culture but promotes health.

### Ethnic Psychopharmacology

**Ethnic psychopharmacology** is a field of study that examines the effects of culture, environment, genetics, biophysiology, and psychosocial factors on the prescribing and metabolism of and response to psychotherapeutic medications. Over the past several decades, researchers have identified significant differences among ethnic and racial groups related to the metabolism and clinical effectiveness of some important drugs. In addition, the field of psychiatry is showing a greater interest in the pharmacological issues related to an increasingly diverse patient population. Given their role in the health care system, nurses have a responsibility to become culturally competent in ethnic psychopharmacology.

**Source:** Campinha-Bacote, J., (2007). Becoming culturally competent in ethnic psychopharmacology. *Journal of Psychosocial Nursing, 45*(9), 27–33; Rguibi, M., & Belahsen, R. (2006). Fattening practices among Moroccan Saharawi women. *Eastern Mediterranean Health Journal, 12*(5), 619–624.

dramatically in recent years. Currently, almost a quarter of adult Canadians are obese (24.3% of men; 23.9% of women).

Record numbers of men and women are on diets to reduce body weight, but no study has been able to explain why only an estimated 0.3% to 3% of the population develops an eating disorder. Although a causal link between cultural norms of thinness and eating disorders has not been proven, all patients

## BOX 17-1 ASK MNEMONIC

*A Way to Remember the Elements of Cultural Competence in Ethnic Psychopharmacology*

**Awareness:** Am I aware of the disparities and inequalities that exist in the psychopharmacological treatment of racially and ethnically diverse populations, and do I recognize my own biases, stereotypes, and prejudices that may affect medication assessment and treatment of patients?

**Skill:** Do I know how to conduct a culturally and linguistically sensitive psychotropic medication assessment?

**Knowledge:** Do I have knowledge of factors (e.g., environment, genetics, cultural practices, generic drug substitution) involved in determining an ethnic group's response to psychotropic drugs?

## BOX 17-2 THOUGHTS AND BEHAVIOURS ASSOCIATED WITH ANOREXIA NERVOSA

- Terror of gaining weight
- Preoccupation with food
- View of self as fat even when emaciated
- Peculiar handling of food:
  - Cutting food into small bits
  - Pushing pieces of food around plate
- Possible development of rigorous exercise regimen
- Possible self-induced vomiting, use of laxatives and diuretics
- Cognition so disturbed that individual judges self-worth by his or her weight

## TABLE 17-1 POSSIBLE SIGNS AND SYMPTOMS OF ANOREXIA NERVOSA

| CLINICAL PRESENTATION | CAUSE |
| --- | --- |
| Low weight | Caloric restriction, excessive exercising |
| Amenorrhea | Low weight |
| Yellow skin | Hypercarotenemia |
| Lanugo | Starvation |
| Cold extremities | Starvation |
| Peripheral edema | Hypoalbuminemia and refeeding |
| Muscle weakening | Starvation, electrolyte imbalance |
| Constipation | Starvation |
| Abnormal laboratory values (low triiodothyronine, thyroxine levels) | Starvation |
| Abnormal computed tomographic (CT) scans, electroencephalographic (EEG) changes | Starvation |
| Cardiovascular abnormalities (hypotension, bradycardia, heart failure) | Starvation, dehydration Electrolyte imbalance |
| Impaired renal function | Dehydration |
| Hypokalemia (low potassium) | Starvation |
| Anemic pancytopenia | Starvation |
| Decreased bone density | Estrogen deficiency, low calcium intake |

with eating disorders have low self-esteem that is negatively impacted by their inability to conform to an impossible cultural standard of beauty (Vince & Walker, 2008).

Box 17-1 describes a mnemonic (ASK) that can assist nurses to remember the components of cultural competence in ethnic psychopharmacology (Campinha-Bacote, J., 2007).

# ANOREXIA NERVOSA

## APPLICATION OF THE NURSING PROCESS

## ASSESSMENT

Anorexia nervosa and bulimia nervosa are two separate syndromes that present two clinical pictures on assessment. Box 17-2 lists several thoughts and behaviours associated with anorexia nervosa, and Table 17-1 identifies clinical signs and symptoms of anorexia nervosa found on assessment, together with their causes.

Eating disorders are serious and, in extreme cases, can lead to death. Box 17-3 identifies a number of medical complications that can occur in individuals with anorexia nervosa and the laboratory findings that may result. Because the eating behaviours in these conditions are so extreme, hospitalization may become necessary. Box 17-4 identifies physical and psychiatric criteria for hospitalization of an individual with an eating disorder.

Fundamental to the care of individuals with eating disorders is establishing and maintaining a therapeutic alliance. Developing this partnership will take both time and diplomacy on the part of the nurse. In treating patients who have been sexually abused or who have otherwise been victims of boundary violations, it is critical that the nurse and other health care workers maintain and respect clear boundaries (Kluft, Bloom, & Kinzie, 2000).

### General Assessment

Individuals with the binge–purge type of anorexia nervosa may present with severe electrolyte imbalance (as a result of purging) and enter the health care system through admission to an intensive care unit. The patient with anorexia will be severely underweight and may have growth of fine, downy hair (lanugo) on the face and back. The patient will also have mottled, cool skin on the extremities and low blood pressure, pulse, and temperature readings, consistent with a malnourished, dehydrated state (see Table 17-1).

## BOX 17-3 MEDICAL COMPLICATIONS OF ANOREXIA NERVOSA

- Bradycardia
- Orthostatic changes in pulse or blood pressure
- Cardiac arrhythmias
- Prolonged QT interval and ST-T wave abnormalities
- Peripheral neuropathy
- Acrocyanosis
- Symptomatic hypotension
- Leukopenia
- Lymphocytosis
- Carotenemia (elevated carotene levels in blood), which produces skin with yellow pallor
- Hypokalemic alkalosis (with self-induced vomiting or use of laxatives and diuretics)
- Elevated serum bicarbonate levels, hypochloremia, and hypokalemia
- Electrolyte imbalances, which lead to fatigue, weakness, and lethargy
- Osteoporosis, indicated by decrease in bone density
- Fatty degeneration of liver, indicated by elevation of serum enzyme levels
- Elevated cholesterol levels
- Amenorrhea
- Abnormal thyroid functioning
- Hematuria
- Proteinuria

**Source:** Data from Halmi, K.A. (2008). Eating disorders: Anorexia nervosa, bulimia nervosa, and obesity. In R.E. Hales, S.C. Yudofsky, & G.O. Gabbard (Eds.), *Textbook of psychiatry* (5th ed., pp. 762, 769–770). Washington, DC: American Psychiatric Publishing.

## BOX 17-4 CRITERIA FOR HOSPITAL ADMISSION OF PATIENTS WITH EATING DISORDERS

**Physical Criteria**
- Weight loss, <85% below ideal
- Rapid decline in weight with food refusal even if not <85% below ideal
- Inability to gain weight with outpatient treatment
- Temperature <36°C or 97°F
- Heart rate <40 beats per minute
- Systolic blood pressure <90/60 mm Hg
- Severe dehydration
- Hypokalemia (serum potassium <3 mEq/L) or other electrolyte imbalance
- Glucose <60 mg/dL; poorly controlled diabetes
- Hepatic, renal, or cardiovascular organ compromise requiring acute treatment

**Psychiatric Criteria**
- Risk for suicide
- Failure to comply with treatment contract
- Severe depression or other psychiatric disorder that would require hospitalization
- Family crisis or dysfunction

**Source:** American Psychiatric Association (APA). (2006). Best practice guidelines for the treatment of eating disorders—Level of care guidelines. Arlington, VA: Author.

As with any comprehensive psychiatric nursing assessment, a complete evaluation of biopsychosocial function is mandatory. The areas to be covered include the patient's:
- Perception of the problem
- Eating habits
- History of dieting
- Methods used to achieve weight control (restricting, purging, exercising)
- Value attached to a specific shape and weight
- Interpersonal and social functioning
- Mental status and physiological parameters

## INTEGRATIVE THERAPY
### Ma Huang

In an attempt to lose weight and fight hunger, many patients with eating disorders turn to weight-loss products that contain herbs, such as ma huang, the Chinese name for the *Ephedra sinica* plant. Health Canada has issued several health advisories warning consumers not to use unauthorized products that contain ephedrine or ephedra in combination with caffeine or other stimulants due to the risk of serious adverse effects. Canadian retailers have also been reminded not to sell unauthorized products containing these ingredients; however, they may still be contained in natural products sold over the Internet. In a small study of patients with eating disorders, 42% of patients who actually experienced adverse effects on ephedra products decided to continue taking the herb.

**Source:** Steffen, K.J., Roerig, J.L., Mitchell, J.E., et al. (2006). A survey of herbal and alternative medication use among participants with eating-disorder symptoms. *International Journal of Eating Disorders, 39*, 741–746. doi:10.1002/eat.20233.

### Self-Assessment

When caring for the patient with anorexia, you may find it difficult to appreciate the compelling force of the illness, incorrectly believing that weight restriction, bingeing, and purging are self-imposed. If we see such self-destructive behaviours as choices, it is only natural to blame the patient for any consequent health problems. The common personality traits of these patients—perfectionism, obsessive thoughts and actions relating to food, intense feelings of shame, people pleasing, and the need to have complete control over their therapy—pose additional challenges.

In your efforts to motivate patients and take advantage of their decision to seek help and be healthier, take care not to allow encouragement to cross the line into authoritarianism and assumption of a parental role. A patient's terror at gaining weight and her or his resistance to clinical interventions may engender significant frustration in the nurse struggling to build a therapeutic relationship and be empathic. Guard against any tendency to be coercive in your approach, and be aware that one of the primary goals of treatment—weight gain—is the very thing the patient fears. When patients appear to be resistant to change, it is helpful to acknowledge the constant struggle that so characterizes the treatment.

## TABLE 17-2  *NOC* OUTCOMES RELATED TO ANOREXIA NERVOSA

| NURSING OUTCOME AND DEFINITION | SHORT-TERM INDICATORS |
| --- | --- |
| *Nutritional status: nutrient intake:* Nutrient intake to meet metabolic needs | Caloric intake<br>Protein intake<br>Fat intake<br>Carbohydrate intake |
| *Weight gain behaviour:* Personal actions to gain weight following voluntary or involuntary significant weight loss | Selects a healthy target weight<br>Commits to a healthy eating plan<br>Monitors exercise for caloric requirements<br>Sets achievable weight gain goals |
| *Anxiety self-control:* Personal action to eliminate or reduce feelings of apprehension, tension, or uneasiness from an unidentifiable source. | Monitors intensity of anxiety<br>Plans coping strategies for stressful situations<br>Uses effective coping strategies |
| *Self-esteem:* Personal judgement of self-worth | Verbalization of self-acceptance<br>Description of self<br>Acceptance of compliments from others<br>Feelings about self-worth |

**Source:** Data from Moorhead, S., Johnson, M., Maas, M.L., et al. (Eds.). (2008). *Nursing outcome classification (NOC)* (4th ed.). St. Louis, MO: Mosby.

## DIAGNOSIS

*Imbalanced nutrition: less than body requirements* is usually the most appropriate initial nursing diagnosis for individuals with anorexia (Herdman, 2012). This diagnosis generates further nursing diagnoses—for example, *Decreased cardiac output, Risk for injury* (electrolyte imbalance), and *Risk for imbalanced fluid volume* (which would take first priority when problems are addressed). Other nursing diagnoses include *Anxiety, Chronic low self-esteem, Disturbed body image, Deficient knowledge, Ineffective coping, Powerlessness,* and *Hopelessness.*

## OUTCOMES IDENTIFICATION

To evaluate the effectiveness of treatment, outcome criteria are established. Relevant categories of the *Nursing Outcomes Classification (NOC)* (Moorhead, Johnson, Maas, et al., 2008) include *Weight gain behaviour, Weight maintenance behaviour, Anxiety self-control, Nutritional status: nutrient intake, and Self-esteem.* Refer to Table 17-2 for examples of short-term *NOC* indicators for the patient with anorexia nervosa.

## PLANNING

Planning is affected by the acuity of the patient's situation. When a patient with anorexia is experiencing extreme electrolyte imbalance or weighs below 85% of his or her ideal body weight, the plan is to provide immediate medical stabilization, most likely in an inpatient unit (Wiseman, Sunday, Klapper, et al., 2001). A person's ideal body weight is based chiefly on height but is modified by factors such as gender, age, build, and degree of muscular development. With the initiation of therapeutic nutrition, malnourished patients may need treatment on a medical unit, owing to *refeeding syndrome,* a potentially catastrophic treatment complication involving a metabolic alteration in serum electrolytes, vitamin deficiencies, and sodium retention (Mehanna, Moledina, & Travis, 2008).

Once a patient is medically stable, the plan addresses the psychological issues underlying the eating disorder, usually on an outpatient basis. The nature of the treatment is determined by the intensity of the symptoms—which may vary over time—and the experienced disruption in the patient's life.

Discharge planning (living arrangements, school, work, finances, follow-up care) is a critical component in treatment. Often, family members also benefit from counselling.

## IMPLEMENTATION

### Acute Care

Typically, a patient with an eating disorder is admitted to the inpatient psychiatric facility in a crisis state. The health care team's initial focus depends on the results of a comprehensive assessment. Any acute psychiatric symptoms, such as suicidal ideation, are addressed immediately. The nurse is challenged to establish trust and monitor the patient's eating pattern.

### Psychosocial Interventions

After addressing any acute symptoms, the patient with anorexia begins a weight-restoration program that allows for incremental weight gain. Based on the patient's height, a treatment goal is set at 90% of ideal body weight, the weight at which most women are able to menstruate.

As patients begin to eat again, they ideally participate in milieu therapy, in which the cognitive distortions (errors in

## BOX 17-5   COGNITIVE DISTORTIONS

**Overgeneralization**
A single event affects unrelated situations.
- "He didn't ask me out. It must be because I'm fat."

**All-or-Nothing Thinking**
Reasoning is absolute and extreme, in mutually exclusive terms of black or white, good or bad.
- "If I allow myself to gain weight, I'll blow up like a balloon."

**Catastrophizing**
The consequences of an event are magnified.
- "If I gain weight, my weekend will be ruined."

**Personalization**
Events are overinterpreted as having personal significance.
- "I know everybody is watching me eat."

**Emotional reasoning**
Subjective emotions determine reality.
- "When I'm thin, I feel powerful."

**Source:** Adapted from Bowers, W.A. (2001). Basic principles for applying cognitive-behavioural therapy to anorexia nervosa. *Psychiatric Clinics of North America, 24,* 293–303. doi:10.1016/ S0193-953X(05)70225-2.

thinking) that perpetuate the illness are consistently addressed by all members of the interdisciplinary team. Box 17-5 identifies some types of cognitive distortions characteristic of people with eating disorders. Focus should be on the eating behaviour and underlying feelings of anxiety, dysphoria, low self-esteem, and lack of control. When possible, the distortions in body image are avoided because attempts to change this perception are often misinterpreted, as shown in the following vignette.

---

**VIGNETTE**

Alicia, a 17-year-old cheerleader, did not come to treatment for weight loss until she fainted at a football game. She insisted that she only needed to "get more energy, not get fat." When the nurse pointed out that Alicia's ribs were clearly visible and that her backbone looked like a skeleton's, Alicia grinned and said, "Thank you."

---

## Pharmacological Interventions

Research has not yet demonstrated that medications are effective as the first course of treatment of anorexia nervosa (Becker, Mickley, Derenne, et al., 2008). Further studies are needed to determine if there is a medication that is effective to treat the core symptoms of the disorder. Despite the lack of rigorous scientific studies, the selective serotonin reuptake inhibitor (SSRI) fluoxetine (Prozac) has been found clinically useful in reducing obsessive-compulsive behaviour after the patient has reached a maintenance weight. Conventional antipsychotics such as chlorpromazine (Thorazine) may be helpful for delusional or overactive patients (Halmi, 2008). Atypical antipsychotic agents such as olanzapine (Zyprexa) are helpful in improving mood and decreasing obsessional behaviours and resistance to weight gain (Attia & Walsh, 2007).

## Health Teaching and Health Promotion

Self-care activities are an important part of the treatment plan. These activities include learning more constructive coping skills, improving social skills, and developing problem-solving and decision-making skills. These skills become the focus of therapy sessions. The following vignette illustrates the need for supportive education.

---

**VIGNETTE**

A nursing assessment of a small group of three young women and one young man in a nutrition group finds that all the participants are very knowledgeable about the caloric value of common foods; as a group, they all avoid any "fatty" foods. The topic of fat-soluble vitamins and the consequences of vitamin deficiencies on the body introduced new information to all of the participants, and one of the young women started to cry, saying, "I had no idea I was doing that to my body." This show of emotion promoted a supportive interaction among the other group members as they shared their own stories of symptoms they could now identify as vitamin deficits.

---

## Milieu Management

Patients admitted to an inpatient unit designed to treat eating disorders participate in a combination of therapeutic modalities provided by a multidisciplinary team. These modalities are designed to normalize eating patterns and begin to address the medical, family, and social issues raised by the illness.

The milieu of an eating-disorder unit is purposefully organized to assist the patient in establishing more adaptive behavioural patterns, including normalization of eating. The highly structured milieu includes precise mealtimes, adherence to the selected menu, observations during and after meals, and regularly scheduled weigh-ins.

Close monitoring of patients includes monitoring all trips to the bathroom after eating to prevent self-induced vomiting. Often, patient privileges are linked to weight gain and treatment-plan adherence. The following vignette demonstrates monitoring the bathroom as a therapeutic intervention.

---

**VIGNETTE**

A 20-year-old woman who primarily restricts her eating but resorts to purging when forced to eat by her family became visibly distressed after eating all of her therapeutic meal. Although her treatment plan was to join other patients in group therapy, the patient requested permission to go to the bathroom alone because she had "embarrassing gas" she did not want overheard. The nurse negotiated to stand away from the bathroom door if the patient agreed not to flush the toilet until the nurse was able to inspect the contents. However, the patient flushed the toilet before inspection. The breaking of the contract with the nurse was discussed by the treatment team and determined to be an indication that this patient was not able to adhere to her prescribed treatment without additional structure. The treatment team established a new expectation that until the patient had gained 1 kilogram, she was to wait 30 minutes after every meal before she was allowed supervised bathroom breaks.

---

## TABLE 17-3    THE STATE OF TREATMENT FOR EATING DISORDERS, 2008

| DISORDER | EVIDENCE-INFORMED TREATMENTS AVAILABLE (ONE OR MORE LARGE-SCALE CONTROLLED TRIALS) | ONE OR MORE CONTROLLED TRIALS |
|---|---|---|
| Anorexia nervosa | None | Moderate number of controlled trials, although sample size and drop-out rates in adults present problems; family therapy for adolescents appears promising |
| Bulimia nervosa | Cognitive behavioural therapy (CBT); antidepressant medication (fluoxetine Food and Drug Administration–approved); interpersonal therapy | Brief CBT-based therapies appear promising |
| Binge eating | CBT; antidepressant medication (sibutramine, topiramate reduce both binge eating and weight); interpersonal therapy | Antidepressants appear promising with the added advantage of weight loss; brief CBT-based therapies appear promising |

**Source:** Adapted from Agras, W.S., & Robinson, A.H. (2008). Forty years of progress in the treatment of the eating disorders. *Nordic Journal of Psychiatry, 62*(47), 19–24. doi:10.1080/08039480802315632.

### Advanced-Practice Interventions

Anorexia nervosa is a chronic illness. The one-year relapse rate approaches 50%, and long-term studies show that up to 20% of patients continue to meet full criteria for anorexia nervosa after several years (Attia & Walsh, 2007). Recovery is evaluated as a stage in the process rather than a fixed event. Factors that influence the stage of recovery include percentage of ideal body weight that has been achieved, the extent to which self-worth is defined by shape and weight, and the amount of disruption existing in the patient's personal life.

The patient will require long-term treatment that might include periodic, brief hospital stays, admission to a partial hospitalization program, outpatient services, and pharmacological interventions.

Agras and Robinson (2008) reviewed the progress of treatment for eating disorders over the past 40 years. Table 17-3 outlines their findings.

### Psychotherapy

The goals of psychotherapy treatment are weight restoration with normalization of eating habits and initiation of the treatment of psychological, interpersonal, and social issues that affect each individual patient. Assisting the patient with a daily meal plan, reviewing a journal of meals and dietary intake maintained by the patient, and providing for weekly weigh-ins (ideally two to three times a week) are essential if the patient is to reach a medically stable weight.

Families frequently report feeling powerless in the face of behaviour that is mystifying. For instance, patients are often unable to experience compliments as supportive and, therefore, are unable to internalize the support. They often seek attention from others but feel shamed when they receive it. Patients express that they want their families to care for and about them but are unable to recognize expressions of care. When others do respond with love and support, patients do not perceive this as positive. The following vignette demonstrates this phenomenon.

Often family members and significant others seek ways to communicate clearly with the patient with anorexia but find that they are frequently misunderstood and that overtures of

**VIGNETTE**

In a multifamily group on an inpatient unit, Mrs. Demi (who last saw her daughter before she had gained 18 kilograms) is asked by the group leader how she regards her daughter, Lila. Mrs. Demi replies, "She looks healthy." Her daughter responds with an angry, sullen look. She ultimately verbalizes that she interprets comments about her "healthy" appearance as "You look fat." The group leader points out that it is interesting that Lila equates "healthy" with "fat." In the multifamily group, there is a commonly expressed view that the illness "is not about weight" but that thinness confers a feeling of being special and that being at a normal weight (i.e., healthy) means this special status is lost.

concern are misinterpreted. Consequently, families experience the tension of saying or doing the wrong thing and then feeling responsible if a setback occurs. Psychiatric mental health nurses have an important role in assisting families and significant others to develop strategies for improved communication and to search for ways to be comfortably supportive to the patient. Box 17-6 lists strategies for families trying to cope with a family member who has an eating disorder.

## EVALUATION

The process of evaluation is built into the outcomes specified by *NOC*. Evaluation is ongoing, and short-term indicators are revised as necessary to achieve the treatment outcomes established. The indicators provide a daily guide for evaluating success and must be continually re-evaluated for their appropriateness. Case Study and Nursing Care Plan 17-1 on pages 334–336 presents a patient with anorexia nervosa.

## BULIMIA NERVOSA

Bulimia first entered the *DSM* as a diagnosis in the third edition in 1980 but without purging or inappropriate compensatory behaviours as criteria. The diagnosis became bulimia nervosa with the addition of the preceding criteria in 1987. In the *DSM-IV-TR*, it was further subcategorized as purging or nonpurging type (Wilfley, Bishop, Wilson, et al., 2007).

| BOX 17-6 | COPING WITH A FAMILY MEMBER WHO HAS AN EATING DISORDER |
|---|---|

- Be patient. Eating disorders can be a long-term illness. Recovery takes time.
- Encourage the person to seek professional help. If the family member is truly endangering his or her life, be insistent.
- Seek outside help for yourself. Find a family or friend support group, a counsellor, or other professional who has experience in helping families.
- Recognize that when addressing the problem with the person you suspect has an eating disorder (especially if it is for the first time), the reaction may be one of denial or perhaps even hostility.
- Don't lay blame. This only reinforces the person's feelings of failure.
- Try to ensure that you don't allow the person's problems to interfere with your routine functioning.
- Let the person know that he or she is important to the family, but not more so than any other family member.
- Do not dwell on food-related discussions. Encourage the person to get involved with nonfood-related activities.
- Avoid commenting on the person's weight or appearance—your comments may not be taken in the proper context.
- People with eating disorders must feel control over their daily routine. This can be very frustrating for those around the individual, but the situation often only becomes worse when it is perceived that someone is trying to take that control away.
- Be aware that low self-esteem is often a problem for those with eating disorders. Be careful not to make comparisons to other members of the family or to others within their peer group. Recognize the person for who he or she is.
- Learn about eating disorders. Understanding is a key to coping.

**Source:** Adapted from Woodside, D.B., & Shekter-Wolfson, L. (1988/2003). *Families and eating disorders. Know the facts.* Retrieved from http://www.nedic.ca/knowthefacts/documents/Familiesandeatingdisorders.pdf.

## APPLICATION OF THE NURSING PROCESS

### ASSESSMENT

#### General Assessment

Initially, patients with bulimia nervosa do not appear to be physically or emotionally ill. They are often at or slightly above or below ideal body weight. However, as the assessment continues and the nurse makes further observations, the physical and emotional problems of the patient become apparent. On inspection, the patient demonstrates enlargement of the parotid glands, with dental erosion and caries if the patient has been inducing vomiting. Box 17-7 identifies a number of

| BOX 17-7 | MEDICAL COMPLICATIONS OF BULIMIA NERVOSA |
|---|---|

- Sinus bradycardia
- Orthostatic changes in pulse or blood pressure
- Cardiac arrhythmias
- Cardiac arrest from electrolyte disturbances or ipecac intoxication
- Cardiac murmur; mitral valve prolapse
- Electrolyte imbalances
- Elevated serum bicarbonate levels (although can be low, indicating a metabolic acidosis)
- Hypochloremia
- Hypokalemia
- Dehydration, which results in volume depletion, leading to stimulation of aldosterone production, which in turn stimulates further potassium excretion from kidneys; thus, there can be both an indirect renal loss of potassium and a direct loss through self-induced vomiting
- Severe attrition and erosion of teeth, producing irritating sensitivity and exposing the pulp of the teeth
- Loss of dental arch
- Diminished chewing ability
- Parotid gland enlargement associated with elevated serum amylase levels
- Esophageal tears caused by self-induced vomiting
- Severe abdominal pain indicative of gastric dilation
- Russell's sign (callus on knuckles from self-induced vomiting)

**Source:** Data from Halmi, K.A. (2008). Eating disorders: Anorexia nervosa, bulimia nervosa, and obesity. In R.E. Hales, S.C. Yudofsky, & G.O. Gabbard (Eds.), *Textbook of psychiatry* (5th ed., pp. 762, 769–770). Washington, DC: American Psychiatric Publishing.

medical complications that can occur and the laboratory findings that may result in individuals with bulimia nervosa. The disclosed history may reveal great difficulties with both impulsivity and compulsivity. Family relationships are frequently chaotic and reflect a lack of nurturing. Patients' lives reflect instability and troublesome interpersonal relationships as well. It is not uncommon for patients to have a history of impulsive stealing of items such as food, clothing, or jewellery (Halmi, 2008).

Box 17-8 lists several thoughts and behaviours associated with bulimia nervosa, and Table 17-4 identifies possible signs and symptoms found on assessment and their causes.

#### Self-Assessment

In working with someone with bulimia, be aware that the patient is sensitive to the perceptions of others regarding this illness and may feel significant shame and loss of control. In building a therapeutic alliance, try to empathize with the patient's feelings of low self-esteem, unworthiness, and dysphoria. If you believe the patient is not being honest (e.g., active bingeing or purging goes unreported) or is being manipulative, acknowledge such obstacles and the frustration they provoke, and construct alternative ways to view the patient's thinking and behaviour. An accepting, nonjudgemental approach, along with a comprehensive understanding of the subjective experience of the patient with bulimia, will help to build trust.

| BOX 17-8 | THOUGHTS AND BEHAVIOURS ASSOCIATED WITH BULIMIA NERVOSA |

- Binge eating behaviours
- Often, self-induced vomiting (or laxative or diuretic use) after bingeing
- History of anorexia nervosa in one fourth to one third of individuals
- Depressive signs and symptoms
- Problems with:
  - Interpersonal relationships
  - Self-concept
  - Impulsive behaviours
- Increased levels of anxiety and compulsivity
- Possible chemical dependency
- Possible impulsive stealing

| TABLE 17-4 | POSSIBLE SIGNS AND SYMPTOMS OF BULIMIA NERVOSA |

| CLINICAL PRESENTATION | CAUSE |
|---|---|
| Normal to slightly low weight | Excessive caloric intake with purging, excessive exercising |
| Dental caries, tooth erosion | Vomiting (hydrochloric acid reflux over enamel) |
| Parotid swelling | Increased serum amylase levels |
| Gastric dilation, rupture | Binge eating |
| Calluses, scars on hand (Russell's sign) | Self-induced vomiting |
| Peripheral edema | Rebound fluid, especially if diuretic used |
| Muscle weakening | Electrolyte imbalance |
| Abnormal laboratory values (electrolyte imbalance, hypokalemia, hyponatremia) | Purging: vomiting, laxative and/or diuretic use |
| Cardiovascular abnormalities (cardiomyopathy, electrocardiographic [ECG] changes) | Electrolyte imbalance—**can lead to death** |
| Cardiac failure (cardiomyopathy) | Ipecac intoxication |

## DIAGNOSIS

The assessment of the patient with bulimia nervosa yields nursing diagnoses that result from the disordered eating and weight-control behaviours. Problems resulting from purging

are a first priority because electrolyte and fluid balance and cardiac function are affected. Common nursing diagnoses include *Decreased cardiac output, Powerlessness, Chronic low self-esteem, Anxiety,* and *Ineffective coping* (substance abuse, impulsive responses to problems).

**VIGNETTE**
During the initial assessment, the nurse wonders if Brittany is actually in need of hospitalization on the eating-disorders unit. The nurse is struck by how well the patient appears, seeming healthy, well dressed, and articulate. As Brittany continues to relate her history, she tells of restricting her intake all day until early evening, when she buys her food and begins to binge as she is shopping. She arrives home and immediately induces vomiting. For the remainder of the evening and into the early morning hours, she "zones out" while watching television and binge eating. Periodically, she goes to the bathroom to vomit. She does this about 15 times during the evening. The nurse admitting Brittany to the unit reminds her of the goals of the hospitalization, including interrupting the binge–purge cycle and normalizing eating. The nurse further explains to Brittany that she has the support of the eating-disorder treatment team and the milieu of the unit to assist her toward recovery.

### ASSESSMENT GUIDELINES
**Bulimia Nervosa**
1. Medical stabilization is the first priority. Problems resulting from purging are disruptions in electrolyte and fluid balance and cardiac function. Therefore, a thorough physical examination is vital, including pertinent laboratory testing:
   - Electrolyte levels
   - Glucose level
   - Thyroid function tests
   - Complete blood count
   - ECG
2. Psychiatric evaluation is advised because treatment of psychiatric co-morbidity is important to outcome.

## OUTCOMES IDENTIFICATION

Relevant *NOC* outcomes include *Vital signs, Electrolyte and acid/base balance, Weight maintenance behaviour, Self-esteem, Hope,* and *Coping.* Table 17-5 lists selected short-term indicators for patients with bulimia nervosa.

## PLANNING

The criteria for inpatient admission of a patient with bulimia nervosa are included in Box 17-4. Like the patient with anorexia nervosa, the patient with bulimia may be treated for life-threatening complications such as gastric rupture (rare), electrolyte imbalance, and cardiac dysrhythmias. Planning will also include appropriate referrals for continuing outpatient treatment.

## RESEARCH HIGHLIGHT
### Screening Eating Disorders

**Source:** Cotton, M-A., Ball, C., & Robinson, P. (2003). Four simple questions can help screen for eating disorders. *Journal of General Internal Medicine, 18*, 53–56. doi:10.1046/j.1525-1497.2003.20374.x.

**Problem**
People with eating disorders request services from primary care providers. The best way to assess the presence of an eating disorder in a primary care setting, however, is not known.

**Purpose of Study**
This study set out to compare the performance of two short eating-disorder screening tools (the SCOFF [sick, control, one stone, fat, food] questionnaire and the Eating Disorders Screen for Primary Care [ESP]) in a primary care setting.

**Methods**
The 233 participants included primary-care-clinic patients and university students. The patients were approached in the clinic waiting room, and the university students were recruited using posters and announcements made in classes. Each participant completed both questionnaires.

**Key Findings**
It was determined that, for both the primary care patients and the university students, the ESP was a more useful tool than the SCOFF for helping clinicians determine the necessity of a more detailed assessment for a possible eating disorder. The ESP asked the following questions:
1. Are you satisfied with your eating patterns?
2. Do you ever eat in secret?
3. Does your weight affect the way you feel about yourself?
4. Have any members of your family suffered with an eating disorder?
5. Do you currently suffer with or have you ever suffered in the past with an eating disorder?

**Implications for Nursing Practice**
Using the five ESP questions can be an effective and quick method for screening people for eating disorders. If the patient identifies three or more abnormal responses, a more detailed assessment should be considered.

### VIGNETTE
Iris weighs 85% of her ideal body weight. She has a history of diuretic abuse, and she becomes very edematous when she stops their use and enters treatment. The nurse informs Iris that the edema is related to the use of diuretics and thus is transient and will resolve after Iris begins to eat normally and discontinues the diuretics. Iris cannot tolerate the weight gain and the accompanying edema that occurs when she stops taking diuretics. She restarts the diuretics, perpetuating the cycle of fluid retention and the risk of kidney damage. The nurse empathizes with Iris's inability to tolerate the feelings of anxiety and dread she experiences because of her markedly swollen extremities.

| TABLE 17-5 | *NOC* OUTCOMES RELATED TO BULIMIA NERVOSA | |
|---|---|
| **NURSING OUTCOME AND DEFINITION** | **SHORT-TERM INDICATORS** |
| *Vital signs:* Extent to which temperature, pulse, respiration, and blood pressure are within normal range | Body temperature Apical heart rate Apical heart rhythm Respiratory rate Systolic blood pressure |
| *Impulse self-control:* Self-restraint of compulsive or impulsive behaviours | Identifies harmful impulsive behaviours Identifies feelings that lead to impulsive actions Identifies consequences of impulsive actions Controls impulses |
| *Weight maintenance behaviour:* Personal actions to maintain optimum body weight | Maintains recommended eating pattern Retains ingested foods Maintains fluid balance Plans for situations that affect food and fluid intake Expresses realistic body image |
| *Hope:* Optimism that is personally satisfying and life-supporting | Expresses faith Expresses will to live Expresses optimism Sets goals |

**Source:** Data from Moorhead, S., Johnson, M., Maas, M.L., et al. (Eds.). (2008). *Nursing outcome classification (NOC)* (4th ed.). St. Louis, MO: Mosby.

## IMPLEMENTATION

### Acute Care

A patient who is medically compromised as a result of bulimia nervosa is referred to an inpatient eating-disorder unit for comprehensive treatment of the illness. The cognitive-behavioural model of treatment is highly effective and frequently serves as the cornerstone of the therapeutic approach. Inpatient units designed to treat eating disorders are specially structured to interrupt the cycle of binge eating and purging and to normalize eating habits. Therapy is begun to examine the underlying conflicts and distorted perceptions of shape and weight that sustain the illness. The patient is also evaluated for treatment of co-morbid disorders, such as major depression and substance abuse. In Canada, the addictions and mental health systems have traditionally functioned as two separate systems, each with its own range of services and particular approaches to treatment and support. The release in 2002 of the Centre for Addiction and Mental Health's best practices document, Concurrent Mental Health and Substance Use Disorders, promoted collaboration between these two sectors, resulting in the development of concurrent disorder programs in Canada.

### Milieu Management

The highly structured milieu of an inpatient eating-disorder unit has as its primary goals the interruption of the binge–purge cycle and the prevention of disordered eating behaviours. Observation during and after meals (to prevent purging), normalization of eating patterns, and maintenance of appropriate exercise are integral elements of such a unit. The multidisciplinary team uses a comprehensive treatment approach to address the emotional and behavioural problems that arise when the patient is no longer binge eating or purging. Like the interruption of other obsessive-compulsive behaviours, preventing the binge–purge pattern allows underlying anxiety to surface and be examined.

## Pharmacological Interventions

Antidepressant medication together with cognitive-behavioural psychotherapy has been shown to bring about improvement in bulimic symptoms. Limited research suggests that the SSRIs and tricyclic antidepressants helped reduce binge eating and vomiting over short terms. Fluoxetine (Prozac) treatment may help prevent relapse. Bupropion (Wellbutrin) may be effective, but due to an increased risk for seizures, it is contraindicated in patients who purge (Williams & Goodie, 2007).

## Counselling

Compared with the patient with anorexia, the patient with bulimia nervosa often more readily establishes a therapeutic alliance with the nurse, because the eating-disordered behaviours are seen as a problem. The therapeutic alliance allows the nurse, along with other members of the multidisciplinary team, to provide counselling that gives useful feedback regarding the patient's distorted beliefs.

## Health Teaching and Health Promotion

Health teaching focuses on not only the eating disorder but also meal planning, use of relaxation techniques, maintenance of a healthy diet and exercise, coping skills, the physical and emotional effects of bingeing and purging, and the impact of cognitive distortions.

Once patients reach therapeutic goals, it is recommended that they seek long-term care to solidify those goals and address the attitudes, perceptions, and psychodynamic issues that maintain the eating disorder and attend the illness.

## Advanced-Practice Interventions
### Psychotherapy

Cognitive-behavioural therapy is the most effective treatment for bulimia nervosa. Restructuring faulty perceptions and helping individuals develop accepting attitudes toward themselves and their bodies is a primary focus of therapy. When patients do not engage in bulimic behaviours, issues of self-worth and interpersonal functioning become more prominent.

Box 17-9 presents relevant *Nursing Interventions Classification (NIC)* interventions for the management of eating disorders.

## EVALUATION

Evaluation of treatment effectiveness is ongoing and built into the *NOC* categories. Outcomes are revised as necessary to reach

the desired outcomes. Case Study and Nursing Care Plan 17-2 on pages 337–338 presents a patient with bulimia nervosa.

> **VIGNETTE**
> Nadia, a 23-year-old patient with a six-year history of bulimia nervosa, struggles with issues of self-esteem. She expresses much guilt about "letting her father down" in the past by drinking alcohol excessively and binge eating and purging. She is determined that this time she is not going to fail at treatment. After her initial success in stopping the disordered behaviours, she says defiantly, "I'm doing this for me." Nadia usually experiences her behaviour as either pleasing or disappointing to others, but she begins to realize that her feeling of self-worth is very much dependent on how others see her and that she needs to develop a better sense of herself.

## BINGE EATING DISORDER

Binge eating disorder is characterized by recurring episodes of eating significantly more food than most in a relatively short period of time accompanied by feelings of guilt or distress. Overeating is frequently noted as a symptom of an affective disorder (e.g., atypical depression). Godart and colleagues (2007) conducted a critical review of the literature of studies (1985–2006) assessing the prevalence of mood disorders in individuals diagnosed with an eating disorder (anorexia nervosa and bulimia nervosa). While some research pointed to higher rates of depression among individuals with anorexia nervosa (binge–purge type) or bulimia nervosa than among individuals who do not engage in binge eating, the authors were cautious in their interpretation of the results based on the hidden biases in many of the studies and, therefore, called for further research.

Because of its efficacy with bulimia, the use of SSRIs at or near the high end of the dosage range have been studied to treat binge eating disorder and seem to help in the short term; however, patients regained significant weight after discontinuance of medication. Other medications that are under investigation include the tricyclic antidepressants, antiepileptic agents, and appetite suppressants (Williams & Goodie, 2007).

Cognitive-behavioural therapy and interpersonal therapy have been determined to be effective in eliminating binge eating; however, on average, these therapies do not produce clinically significant weight loss (Wilson, Wilfley, Agras, et al., 2010). Many advanced-practice nurses are qualified to provide these therapies.

Binge eating is one of the most common forms of eating disorders documented in individuals who are being considered for bariatric surgery. In Canada, population-adjusted rates of bariatric surgical procedures increased dramatically from 1996 to 2002 (Padwal & Lewanczuk, 2005). McAlpine, Frisch, Rome, and colleagues (2010) reviewed some of the issues related to bariatric surgery. Box 17-10 outlines the recommended preoperative and postoperative standards of care for bariatric surgery.

## BOX 17-9  *NIC* INTERVENTIONS FOR EATING-DISORDERS MANAGEMENT

*Definition:* Prevention and treatment of severe diet restriction and overexercising or bingeing and purging of food and fluids.

Activities:

- Develop a supportive relationship with patient.
- Collaborate with other members of health care team to develop treatment plan; involve patient and significant others as appropriate.
- Confer with team and patient to set a target weight if patient is not within a recommended weight range for age and body frame.
- Establish the amount of daily weight gain that is desired.
- Confer with dietitian to determine daily caloric intake necessary to attain or maintain target weight.
- Teach and reinforce concepts of good nutrition with patient (and significant others as appropriate).
- Encourage patient to discuss food preferences with dietitian.
- Monitor physiological parameters (vital signs, electrolyte levels) as needed.
- Weigh on a routine basis (e.g., at same time of day and after voiding).
- Monitor intake and output of fluids, as appropriate.
- Monitor daily caloric intake.
- Encourage patient self-monitoring of daily food intake and weight gain or maintenance as appropriate.
- Establish expectations for appropriate eating behaviours, intake of food and fluids, and amount of physical activity.
- Use behavioural contracting with patient to elicit desired weight gain or maintenance behaviours.
- Restrict food availability to scheduled, pre-served meals and snacks.
- Observe patient during and after meals and snacks to ensure that adequate intake is achieved and maintained.
- Accompany patient to bathroom during designated observation times following meals and snacks.
- Limit time spent in bathroom during periods when not under direct supervision.
- Monitor patient for behaviours related to eating, weight loss, and weight gain.
- Use behaviour modification techniques to promote behaviours that contribute to weight gain and limit weight-loss behaviours as appropriate.
- Provide reinforcement for weight gain and behaviours that promote weight gain.
- Provide support (e.g., relaxation therapy, desensitization exercises, opportunities to talk about feelings) as patient integrates new eating behaviours, changing body image, and lifestyle changes.
- Encourage patient use of daily logs to record feelings and circumstances surrounding urge to purge, vomit, or overexercise.
- Limit physical activity as needed to promote weight gain.
- Provide a supervised exercise program when appropriate.
- Allow opportunity to make limited choices about eating and exercise as weight gain progresses in desirable manner.
- Assist patient (and significant others as appropriate) to examine and resolve personal issues that may contribute to the eating disorder.
- Assist patient to develop a self-esteem that is compatible with a healthy body weight.
- Confer with the health care team on a routine basis about patient's progress.
- Initiate maintenance phase of treatment when patient has achieved target weight and has consistently shown desired eating behaviours for designated period of time.
- Monitor patient weight on a routine basis.
- Determine acceptable range of weight variation in relation to target range.
- Place responsibility for choices about eating and physical activity with patient as appropriate.
- Provide support and guidance as needed.
- Assist patient to evaluate the appropriateness and consequences of choices about eating and physical activity.
- Reinstitute weight-gain protocol if patient is unable to remain within target weight range.
- Institute a treatment program and follow-up care (medical, counselling) for home management.

**Source:** Bulechek, G.M., Butcher, H.K., & Dochterman, J.M. (2008). *Nursing interventions classification (NIC)* (5th ed., pp. 278–279). St. Louis, MO: Mosby.

## BOX 17-10  PREOPERATIVE AND POSTOPERATIVE STANDARDS OF CARE FOR BARIATRIC SURGERY

Preoperative Period—Patients:

- Should have a full understanding of the postoperative dietary requirements, necessary postsurgical supports, and the importance of stress-management strategies
- Should be screened for severe psychiatric co-morbidities
- Must have a minimum 12-month period of recovery from any eating disorder, substance abuse, manic episode, psychosis, psychiatric hospitalization, suicide attempt, or trauma-related issues before having bariatric surgery

- Should receive counselling or education to assist with lifestyle changes

Postoperative Period—Patients:

- Will receive close follow-up and support by members of a multidisciplinary team (surgery, medicine, psychiatry or psychology, nutrition and exercise science) monthly for the first six months, then every two months for the remainder of the first year postsurgery

## CASE STUDY AND NURSING CARE PLAN 17-1

### *Anorexia Nervosa*

*Cynthia, a 20-year-old woman, is brought to the inpatient eating-disorder unit of a local hospital by two older brothers, who are supporting her on either side. She is profoundly weak, holding her head up with her hands.*

## ASSESSMENT

### Self-Assessment

Nurse Mindy Jacobs is assigned to care for Cynthia. Although a young nurse, Mindy has spent the past three years working on the eating-disorders unit. When she first began, she had difficulty overidentifying with patients. Mindy has struggled with bulimia, but with treatment, she has done well. She seeks guidance from her nursing supervisor and the multidisciplinary team, which has helped her to maintain appropriate boundaries while creating a therapeutic alliance with patients.

| Objective Data | Subjective Data |
|---|---|
| Height: 157 cm<br>Weight: 26.3 kg—50% of ideal body weight<br>Blood pressure: 74/50 mm Hg<br>Pulse: 54 beats per minute<br>Anemic—hemoglobin: 90 g/L (9 g/dL)<br>Cachectic appearance, pale, with fine lanugo<br>Sad facial expression<br>Bruising on inside of each knee from sleeping on her side with knees touching | Denies being underweight: "I need treatment because I get fatigued so easily."<br>"I check my legs every night. I'm so afraid of getting fat. I hate it if my legs touch each other."<br>"I don't like to start anything until I know I can do it perfectly the first time. I wouldn't want anyone to see me make a mistake."<br>Depressed mood |

## DIAGNOSIS

1. *Imbalanced nutrition* less than body requirements related to restriction of caloric intake secondary to extreme fear of weight gain
2. *Chronic low self-esteem* related to perception that others are always judging her

## OUTCOMES IDENTIFICATION

Patient will reach 75% of ideal weight (41.7 kg) by discharge.

## PLANNING

The initial plan is to address Cynthia's unstable physiological state.

## IMPLEMENTATION

Cynthia's care plan is personalized as follows:

| Short-Term Goal | Intervention | Rationale | Evaluation |
|---|---|---|---|
| 1. Patient will gain a minimum of 1 kg and a maximum of 1.5 kg weekly through inpatient stay. | 1a. Acknowledge the emotional and physical difficulty patient is experiencing. Use patient's extreme fatigue to engage cooperation in the treatment plan.<br><br>1b. Weigh patient daily for the first week, then three times a week. Patient should be weighed in bra and panties only. There should be no oral intake, including a drink of water, before the early morning weigh-in. | 1a. A first priority is to establish a therapeutic alliance.<br><br><br><br><br>1b. These measures ensure that weight is accurate. | **Week 1:**<br>Patient increases caloric intake with liquid supplement only.<br>Patient unable to eat solid food.<br>Patient does not gain weight.<br>Patient remains hypotensive, bradycardic, anemic (hemoglobin [Hgb] = 90 g/L (9 g/dL)).<br>**Week 2:**<br>Patient gains 1 kg drinking liquid supplement—minimal solid food.<br>Patient remains hypotensive, bradycardic (Hgb = 100 g/L (10 g/dL)). |

*Continued*

## CASE STUDY AND NURSING CARE PLAN 17-1—cont'd

### Anorexia Nervosa

| Short-Term Goal | Intervention | Rationale | Evaluation |
|---|---|---|---|
| | 1c. Do not negotiate weight with patient or reweigh. Patient may choose not to look at the scale or request that she not be told the weight. | 1c. Patient may try to control and sabotage treatment. | **Week 3:** Patient gains 0.5 kg drinking liquid supplement. Patient selects meal plan but is unable to eat most solid foods. Patient's blood pressure (BP) = 84/60 mm Hg; pulse = 68 beats per minute, regular; Hgb = 110 g/L (11 g/dL). |
| | 1d. Measure vital signs tid until stable, then daily. Repeat ECG and laboratory tests until stable. | 1d. As patient begins to increase in weight, cardiovascular status improves to within normal range, and monitoring is less frequent. | **Weeks 4–6:** Patient gains an average of 1 kg/wk. Patient samples more solid foods selected from meal plan. Patient's BP = 90/60 mm Hg; pulse = 68 beats per minute, regular; Hgb = 115 g/L (11.5 g/dL). |
| | 1e. Provide a pleasant, calm atmosphere at mealtimes. Patient should be told the specific times and duration (usually a half hour) of meals. | 1e. Mealtimes become episodes of high anxiety, and knowledge of regulations decreases tension in the milieu, particularly when patient has given up so much control by entering treatment. | **Week 7:** Patient weighs 32.2 kg (almost 60% of ideal body weight); calories are mostly from liquid supplement. Patient selects balanced meals, eating more varied solid food: turkey, carrots, lettuce, fruit. Patient's Hgb = 125 g/L (12.5 g/dL); normal range of BP and pulse are maintained. Patient continues to increase participation in social aspects of eating. |
| | 1f. Administer liquid supplement as ordered. | 1f. Patient may be unable to eat solid food at first. | |
| | 1g. Observe patient during meals to prevent hiding or throwing away of food and for at least 1 hour after meals and snacks to prevent purging. | 1g, h. The compelling force of the illness is such that behaviours related to hiding or discarding food are difficult to stop. A power struggle between staff and patient may emerge, in which patient appears to comply but defies the rules (appearing to eat but throwing away food). | **Weeks 8–12:** Patient gains an average of 1 kg/wk and weighs 37.1 kg (approx. 68% of ideal body weight). Patient is eating more varied solid food, but most caloric intake is still from liquid supplement. Patient maintains normal vital signs and Hgb levels. Patient maintains social interaction during mealtimes and snacks. |
| | 1h. Encourage patient to try to eat some solid food. Preparation of patient's meals should be guided by likes and dislikes list because patient is unable to make own selections to complete menu. | | |
| | 1i. Be empathic with patient's struggle to give up control of her eating and her weight as she is expected to make minimum weight gain on a regular basis. Permit patient to verbalize feelings at these times. | 1i. Patient is expected to gain at least 0.25 kg on a specific schedule, usually three times a week (Monday, Wednesday, Friday). | **Weeks 13–16:** Patient has reached medically stable weight at the end of 16th week—41.7 kg (approx. 75% of ideal body weight). Patient continues to eat more solid food with relatively less liquid supplement. Patient is not able to participate in planned exercise program until she reaches 85% of ideal body weight. |
| | 1j. Monitor patient's weight gain. A weight gain of 1 kg/wk to 1.5 kg/wk is medically acceptable. | 1j. Weight gain of more than 2.25 kg in 1 week may result in pulmonary edema. | |
| | 1k. Provide teaching regarding healthy eating as the basis of a healthy lifestyle. | 1k. Healthy aspects of eating (e.g., increased energy, rather than gaining weight) are reinforced. | |

*Continued*

**CASE STUDY AND NURSING CARE PLAN 17-1—cont'd**

*Anorexia Nervosa*

| Short-Term Goal | Intervention | Rationale | Evaluation |
|---|---|---|---|
| | 1l. Use a cognitive-behavioural approach to address patient's expressed fears regarding weight gain. Identify and examine dysfunctional thoughts; identify and examine values and beliefs that sustain these thoughts. | 1l. Confronting irrational thoughts and beliefs is crucial to changing eating behaviours. | |
| | 1m. As patient approaches her target weight, there should be encouragement to make her own choices for menu selection. | 1m. Patient can assume more control of her meals, which is empowering for the patient with anorexia. | |
| | 1n. Emphasize social nature of eating. Encourage conversation that does not have the theme of food during mealtimes. | 1n. Eating as a social activity, shared with others and with participation in conversation, serves as both a distraction from obsessional preoccupations and a pleasurable event. | |
| | 1o. Focus on the patient's strengths, including her good work in normalizing her weight and eating habits. | 1o. Patient who is beginning to normalize weight and eating behaviours has achieved a major accomplishment, of which she should be proud. Noneating activities are explored as a source of gratification. | |
| | 1p. Provide for a planned exercise program when patient reaches target weight. | 1p. Patient experiences a strong drive to exercise; this measure accommodates this drive by planning a reasonable amount. | |
| | 1q. Encourage patient to apply all the knowledge, skills, and gains made from the various individual, family, and group therapy sessions. | 1q. Patient has been receiving intensive therapy and education, which have provided tools and techniques that are useful in maintaining healthy behaviours. | |

## EVALUATION

By the end of the sixteenth week, Cynthia has achieved a stable weight of 41.7 kilograms. This weight is approaching congruency with Cynthia's height, frame, and age. Her vital signs and hemoglobin levels are consistently normal. She is participating in therapy and consistently communicating satisfaction with her body appearance.

## CASE STUDY AND NURSING CARE PLAN 17-2

### Bulimia Nervosa

*Rima is a 30-year-old college graduate who reports that she is an aspiring actress. She is being admitted to a partial hospitalization program designed for patients with eating disorders. Rima has bulimia nervosa.*

## ASSESSMENT

### Self-Assessment

Matthew, a seasoned nurse in the area of eating disorders, is assigned to care for Rima. Matthew enjoys working with patients with bulimia because he believes he can help patients move toward health. When he first encounters Rima, he experiences an immediate negative response that surprises him. He speaks to his supervisor about these feelings and raises the question of whether or not he is the appropriate nurse to care for Rima. As he and the supervisor discuss his feelings, Matthew is able to recognize that Rima reminds him of a girlfriend he had many years earlier. The relationship ended badly. Matthew experiences an emotional release with this realization and believes that he will be able to separate his earlier negative experience from his work with Rima.

| Objective Data | Subjective Data |
|---|---|
| Height: 165 cm | "I can't stand to be fat." |
| Weight: 57.6 kg—95% of ideal body weight | "I'm ashamed that I can't control my bingeing and vomiting— |
| Blood pressure: 120/80 mm Hg sitting; 90/60 mm Hg standing | I know it's not good." |
| Pulse: 70 beats/min sitting; 96 beats/min standing | |
| Potassium level of 2.7 mmol/L (normal range, 3.3 to 5.5 mmol/L) | |
| ECG: abnormal—consistent with hypokalemia | |
| Erosion of enamel, enlarged parotid glands, consistent with a history of binge eating and purging | |

## DIAGNOSIS

1. *Risk for injury* related to low potassium and other physical changes secondary to binge eating and purging
2. *Powerlessness* related to inability to control bingeing and vomiting cycles

## OUTCOMES IDENTIFICATION

Rima will demonstrate ability to regulate eating patterns, resulting in consistently normal electrolyte balance.

## PLANNING

Rima is admitted to a partial hospitalization program designed for patients with eating disorders. She attends the program three or four days a week and participates in individual and group therapy. She will continue to work as a "temp" for a publishing house.

## IMPLEMENTATION

Rima's care plan is personalized as follows:

| Short-Term Goal | Intervention | Rationale | Evaluation |
|---|---|---|---|
| 1. Patient will identify signs and symptoms of low potassium level (K⁺), and K⁺ level will remain within normal limits throughout hospitalization. | 1a. Educate patient regarding the ill effects of self-induced vomiting, low K⁺ level, dental erosion. | 1a. Health teaching is crucial to treatment. The patient needs to be reminded of the benefits of normalization of eating behaviour. | **Week 1:**<br>Patient begins to select balanced meals.<br>Patient demonstrates knowledge of untoward effects of vomiting and K⁺ deficiency.<br>Patient begins to demonstrate understanding of repetitive nature of binge–purge cycle. |
| | 1b. Educate patient about binge–purge cycle and its self-perpetuating nature. | 1b, c. The compulsive nature of the binge–purge cycle is maintained by the sequence of intake restriction, hunger, bingeing, purging accompanied by feelings of guilt, and then repetition of the cycle over and over. | **Week 2:**<br>Patient begins to challenge irrational thoughts and beliefs.<br>Patient continues to plan nutritionally balanced meals, including dinner at home.<br>Patient begins to sample "forbidden foods" and discuss thoughts and attitudes about same. |
| | 1c. Teach patient that fasting sets one up to binge eat. | | |

*Continued*

## CASE STUDY AND NURSING CARE PLAN 17-2—cont'd

*Bulimia Nervosa*

| Short-Term Goal | Intervention | Rationale | Evaluation |
|---|---|---|---|
| | 1d. Explore ideas about trigger foods. | 1d. Patient needs to understand beliefs about trigger foods to challenge irrational thoughts. | **Week 3:**<br>Patient discusses triggers to binge and resultant behaviour.<br>Patient continues to challenge irrational thoughts and beliefs in individual and group sessions. |
| | 1e. Challenge irrational thoughts and beliefs about "forbidden" foods. | 1e. Challenge forces patient to examine own thinking and beliefs. | Patient plans meals, including "forbidden foods." |
| | 1f. Teach patient to plan and eat regularly scheduled, balanced meals. | 1f. This teaching helps to ensure success in maintaining abstinence from binge–purge activity. | **Week 4:**<br>Patient reports no binge–purge behaviours at day program or outside.<br>Patient demonstrates understanding of repetitive nature of binge–purge cycle.<br>Patient continues to challenge irrational thoughts and beliefs. |

### EVALUATION

At the end of four weeks, Rima reports no binge–purge cycles, and her potassium level remains consistently within normal limits. She is beginning to plan meals and challenge irrational thoughts and beliefs.

## KEY POINTS TO REMEMBER

- A number of theoretical models help explain the origins of eating disorders.
- Neurobiological theories identify an association among eating disorders, depression, and neuroendocrine abnormalities.
- Psychological theories explore issues of control related to eating disorders.
- Genetic theories postulate the existence of vulnerabilities that may predispose people toward eating disorders.
- Sociocultural models look at our present societal ideal of being thin.
- Men with eating disorders share many of the characteristics of women with eating disorders.
- The suicide rate of patients with eating disorders is much higher than predicted rates in similar age groups.
- Anorexia nervosa is a potentially life-threatening eating disorder that includes severe underweight; low blood pressure, pulse, and temperature; dehydration; low serum potassium level; and dysrhythmias.
- Anorexia may be treated in an inpatient treatment setting in which milieu therapy, psychotherapy (cognitive), development of self-care skills, and psychobiological interventions can be implemented.
- Long-term treatment is provided on an outpatient basis and aims to help patients maintain healthy weight. It includes treatment modalities such as individual therapy, family therapy, group therapy, psychopharmacology, and nutrition counselling.

- Patients with bulimia nervosa are typically within the normal weight range, but some may be slightly below or above ideal body weight.
- Assessment of the patient with bulimia may show enlargement of the parotid glands and dental erosion and caries if the patient has induced vomiting.
- Acute care may be necessary when life-threatening complications such as gastric rupture (rare), electrolyte imbalance, and cardiac dysrhythmias are present.
- The goal of interventions is to interrupt the binge–purge cycle.
- Psychotherapy and self-care skill training are included in the treatment plan.
- Long-term treatment focuses on therapy aimed at addressing any coexisting depression, substance abuse, or personality disorders that are causing the patient distress and interfering with the quality of life. Self-worth and interpersonal functioning eventually become issues that are useful for the patient to target.
- People with binge eating disorder report a history of major depression significantly more often than people who do not binge eat.
- Effective treatment for obese patients with binge eating disorder integrates modification of the disordered eating, improvement of depressive symptoms, and achievement of an appropriate weight.

# CRITICAL THINKING

1. Logan, a 19-year-old male model, has experienced a rapid decrease in weight over the past four months after his agent told him he would have to lose some weight or lose a coveted account. Logan is 188 centimetres tall and weighs 60 kilograms, down from his usual 80 kilograms. He is brought to the emergency department with a pulse of 40 beats per minute and severe arrhythmias. His laboratory workup reveals severe hypokalemia. He has become extremely depressed, saying, "I'm too fat! I don't want anything to eat—if I gain weight, my life will be ruined. There is nothing to live for if I can't model." Logan's parents are startled and confused, and his best friend is worried and feels powerless to help: "I tell Logan he needs to eat or he will die. I tell him he is a skeleton, but he refuses to listen to me. I don't know what to do."
   a. Which physical and psychiatric criteria suggest that Logan should be immediately hospitalized?
   b. What are five questions that could be asked to help determine if further assessment is needed regarding the possibility of an eating disorder?
   c. What are some of the questions you would eventually ask Logan when evaluating his biopsychosocial functioning?
   d. What are your feelings toward someone with anorexia? Can you make a distinction between your thoughts and feelings toward women with anorexia and toward men with anorexia?
   e. What are some things you could do for Logan's parents and friend in terms of offering them information, support, and referrals? Identify specific referrals.
   f. Explain the kinds of interventions or restrictions that may be used while Logan is hospitalized.
   g. How would you describe partial hospitalization programs when asked if Logan will have to be hospitalized for an extended period?
   h. What are some of Logan's cognitive distortions that would be a target for therapy?
   i. Identify at least five criteria that, if met, would indicate that Logan was improving.

2. You and Ambreen have been close friends since nursing school and are now working on the same surgical unit. Ambreen told you that in the past she has made several suicide attempts. Today, you come upon her bingeing off unit, and she looks embarrassed and uncomfortable when she sees you. On several occasions, you notice that she spends time in the bathroom, and you hear sounds of retching. In response to your concern, she admits that she has been binge–purging for several years but that she is now getting out of control and feels profoundly depressed.
   a. Although Ambreen does not show any physical signs of bulimia nervosa, what would you look for when assessing an individual with bulimia?
   b. What kinds of emergencies could result from bingeing and purging?
   c. What would be the most useful type of psychotherapy for Ambreen initially, and what issues would need to be addressed?
   d. What kinds of new skills does a person with bulimia need to learn to lessen the compulsion to binge and purge?
   e. What would be some signs that Ambreen is recovering?

3. The high school principal shares with you that several students (male and female) have disclosed to faculty that they have an eating disorder. The principal is concerned about the health of all the students in the school and asks you to hold a general information session.
   a. What type of health promotion material will be helpful?
   b. How could you deliver this information to the students?

# CHAPTER REVIEW

1. Which female patient should the nurse recognize as having the highest risk to have or develop bulimia nervosa? The one who:
   1. Grew up in an underserved area
   2. Lives in a society influenced by Eastern cultural beliefs
   3. Is 20 years old
   4. Is Asian Canadian

2. The nurse is caring for a 16-year-old female patient with anorexia nervosa. What should the initial nursing intervention be upon the patient's admission to the unit?
   1. Build a therapeutic relationship.
   2. Increase the patient's caloric consumption.
   3. Involve the patient in group therapy to build a support group.
   4. Self-assess to decrease tendencies toward authoritarianism.

3. The nurse is caring for a patient with bulimia. Which nursing intervention is appropriate?
   1. Monitor patient on bathroom trips after eating.
   2. Allow patient extensive private time with family members.
   3. Provide meals whenever the patient requests them.
   4. Encourage patient to select foods that she or he likes.

4. The nurse is admitting a patient who weighs 45 kilograms, is 167 centimetres tall, and is below ideal body weight. The patient's blood pressure is 130/80 mm Hg, pulse is 72 beats per minute, potassium is 2.5 mmol/L, and ECG is abnormal. Her teeth enamel is eroded, her hands are visibly shaking, and her parotid gland is enlarged. The patient states, "I am really worked up about coming to this unit." What is the priority nursing diagnosis?
   1. *Powerlessness*
   2. *Risk for injury*
   3. *Imbalanced nutrition: Less than body requirements*
   4. *Anxiety*

5. The nurse is planning care for a patient with an eating disorder. What outcomes are appropriate? Select all that apply.
   1. The patient will experience a decrease in depression.
   2. The patient will identify four methods to control anxiety.
   3. The patient will collect different kinds of cookbooks.
   4. The patient will identify two people to contact if suicidal thoughts occur.

## ⊖volve WEBSITE

Post-Test  interactive review

*Visit the Evolve Web site for Chapter Review Answers and Rationales, Critical Thinking Answer Guidelines, and additional resources related to the content in this chapter: http://evolve.elsevier.com/Canada/Varcarolis/psychiatric/*

## REFERENCES

Agras, W.S., & Robinson, A.H. (2008). Forty years of progress in the treatment of the eating disorders. *Nordic Journal of Psychiatry*, 62(47), 19–24. doi:10.1080/08039480802315632.

Attia, E., & Walsh, B.T. (2007). Anorexia nervosa. *American Journal of Psychiatry*, 164(12), 1805–1810.

Becker, A.E. (2007). Culture and eating disorders classification. *International Journal of Eating Disorders*, 40, S111–S116. doi:10.1002/eat.20435.

Becker, A.E., Mickley, D.W., Derenne, J.L., et al. (2008). Eating disorders: Evaluation and management. In T.A. Stern, J.F. Rosenbaum, M. Fava, et al. (Eds.), *Massachusetts General Hospital comprehensive clinical psychiatry* (pp. 499–518). St. Louis, MO: Mosby.

Berkman, N.D., Lohr, K.N., & Bulik, C.M. (2007). Outcomes of eating disorders: A systematic review of the literature. *International Journal of Eating Disorders*, 40, 293–309. doi:10.1002/eat.20369.

Brewerton, T.D. (2007). Eating disorders, trauma, and comorbidity: Focus on PTSD. *Eating Disorders: The Journal of Treatment & Prevention*, 15(4), 285–304. doi:10.1080/10640260701454311.

Bruch, H. (1978). *The golden cage: The enigma of anorexia nervosa.* Cambridge, MA: First Harvard University Press.

Campinha-Bacote, J. (2007). Becoming culturally competent in ethnic psychopharmacology. *Journal of Psychosocial Nursing*, 45(9), 27–33.

Caparrotta, L., & Ghaffari, K. (2006). A historical overview of the psychodynamic contributions to the understanding of eating disorders. *Psychoanalytic Psychotherapy*, 20(3), 175–196.

Centre for Addiction and Mental Health (2002). *Best practices: Concurrent mental health and substance use disorders.* Ottawa: Health Canada.

Frieling, H., Römer, K.D., Wilhelm, J., et al. (2006). Association of catecholamine-O-methyltransferase and 5-HTTLPR genotype with eating disorder–related behavior and attitudes in females with eating disorders. *Psychiatric Genetics*, 16, 205–208. doi:10.1097/01.ypg.0000218620.50386.f1.

Godart, N.T., Perdereau, F., Rein, Z., et al. (2007). Comorbidity studies of eating disorders and mood disorders. Critical review of the literature. *Journal of Affective Disorders*, 97, 37–49. doi:10.1016/j.jad.2006.06.023.

Halmi, K.A. (2008). Eating disorders: Anorexia nervosa, bulimia nervosa, and obesity. In R.E. Hales, S.C. Yudofsky, & G.O. Gabbard (Eds.), *Textbook of psychiatry* (pp. 971–998). Washington, DC: American Psychiatric Publishing.

Herdman, T.H. (Ed.), (2012). *NANDA International nursing diagnoses: Definitions & classification, 2012–2014.* Oxofrd, UK: Wiley-Blackwell.

Hudson, J.I., Hiripi, E., Pope, H.G., Jr., et al. (2007). The prevalence and correlates of eating disorders in the National Comorbidity Survey Replication. *Biological Psychiatry*, 61, 348–358. doi:10.1016/j.biopsych.2006.03.040.

Kaye, W. (2007). Neurobiology of anorexia and bulimia nervosa. *Physiology & Behavior*, 94, 112–135. doi:10.1016/j.physbeh.2007.11.037.

Keel, P.K., & Klump, K.L. (2003). Are eating disorders culture-bound syndromes? Implications for conceptualizing their etiology. *Psychological Bulletin*, 129, 747–769. doi:10.1037/0033-2909.129.5.747.

Kluft, R., Bloom, S., & Kinzie, J. (2000). Treating the traumatized patient and victims of violence. In C.C. Bell (Ed.), Psychiatric aspects of violence: Issues in prevention and treatment. New Directions in Mental Health Services, *Vol. 86* (pp. 79–102). San Francisco: Jossey-Bass.

le Grange, D., Lock, J., Loeb, K., et al. (2010). Academy for eating disorders position paper: The role of the family in eating disorders. *International Journal of Eating Disorders*, 43(1), 1–5. doi:10.1002/eat.20751.

Marchessault, G. (2002). Talking about weight with Aboriginal women. *Canadian Women's Health Network.* Retrieved from http://www.cwhn.ca/en/node/39581.

Mazzeo, S., & Bulik, C. (2008). Environmental and genetic risk factors for eating disorders: What the clinician needs to know. *Child and Adolescent Psychiatric Clinics of North America*, 18, 67–82. doi:10.1016/j.chc.2008.07.003.

McAlpine, D.E., Frisch, M.J., Rome, E.S., et al. (2010). Bariatric surgery: A primer for eating disorder professionals. *European Eating Disorders Review*, 18, 304–317. doi:10.1002/erv.1012.

Mehanna, H.M., Moledina, J., & Travis, J. (2008). Refeeding syndrome: What it is, and how to prevent and treat it. *British Medical Journal, 336,* 1495–1498. doi:10.1136/bmj.a301.

Miyake, Y., Okamoto, Y., Onoda, K., et al. (2010). Brain activation during the perception of distorted body images in eating disorders. *Psychiatry Research: Neuroimaging, 181,* 183–192. doi:10.1016/j.pscychresns.2009.09.001.

Moorhead, S., Johnson, M., Maas, M.L., et al. (2008). *Nursing outcomes classification (NOC)* (4th ed.). St. Louis, MO: Mosby.

Padwal, R.S., & Lewanczuk, R.Z. (2005). Trends in bariatric surgery in Canada, 1993–2003. *Canadian Medical Association Journal, 172,* 735. doi:10.1503/cmaj.045286.

Pinhas, L., Heinmaa, M., Bryden, P., et al. (2008). Disordered eating in Jewish adolescent girls. *Canadian Journal of Psychiatry, 53*(9), 601–608. Retrieved from http://publications.cpa-apc.org/browse/documents/25.

Piran, N., & Gadalla, T. (2006). Eating disorders and substance abuse in Canadian women: A national study. *Addiction, 102,* 105–113. doi:10.1111/j.1360-0443.2006.01633.x.

Pompili, M., Girardi, P., Tatarelli, G., et al. (2006). Suicide and attempted suicide in eating disorders, obesity and weight-image concern. *Eating Behaviors, 7,* 384–394. doi:10.1016/j.eatbeh.2005.12.004.

Statistics Canada (2011). *Canadian health measures survey: Adult obesity prevalence in Canada and the United States.* Retrieved from http://www.statscan.gc.ca.

Striegel-Moore, R.H., & Bulik, C.M. (2007). Risk factors for eating disorders. *American Psychologist, 62,* 181–198. doi:10.1037/0003-066X.62.3.181.

Vince, E.P., & Walker, I. (2008). Set of meta-analytic studies on the factors associated with disordered eating. *The Internet Journal of Mental Health, 5*(1), 2. Retrieved from http://www.ispub.com/journal/the_internet_journal_of_mental_health.html.

Wilfley, D.E., Bishop, M.E., Wilson, G.T., et al. (2007). Classification of eating disorders: Toward *DSM-V. International Journal of Eating Disorders, 40,* S123–S129. doi:10.1002/eat.20436.

Williams, P.M., & Goodie, J. (2007). Identifying and treating eating disorders. *Family Practice Recertification, 29*(8), 16–23.

Williamson, D.A., Martin, C.K., Anton, S.D., et al. (2008). Is caloric restriction associated with development of eating-disorder symptoms? Results from the CALERIE trial. *Health Psychology, 27*(1), S32–S42. doi:10.1037/0278-6133.27.1.S32.

Wilson, G.T., Wilfley, D.E., Agras, W.S., et al. (2010). Psychological treatments of binge eating disorder. *Archives of General Psychiatry, 67*(1), 94–101. doi:10.1001/archgenpsychiatry.2009.170.

Wiseman, C.V., Sunday, S.R., Klapper, F., et al. (2001). Changing patterns of hospitalization in eating disorder patients. *International Journal of Eating Disorders, 30,* 69–74. doi:10.1002/eat.1055.

Zerbe, K. (2003). Eating disorders in middle and late life: A neglected problem. *Primary Psychiatry, 10*(6), 76–78.

# 18

# Cognitive Disorders

*Jane Stein-Parbury, Charlotte Eliopoulos*
*Adapted by Cheryl L. Pollard*

## KEY TERMS AND CONCEPTS

agnosia, 353

agraphia, 355

Alzheimer's disease (AD), 348

alexia, 355

aphasia, 353

apraxia, 353

catastrophic reactions, 356

cognitive disorders, 342

confabulation, 352

delirium, 343

dementia, 348

hypermetamorphosis, 355

hyperorality, 355

perseveration, 352

primary dementia, 351

pseudodementia, 353

secondary dementia, 351

sundowning, 346

## OBJECTIVES

1. Compare and contrast the clinical picture of delirium with that of dementia and brain injury.
2. Discuss three critical needs of a person with delirium, stated in terms of nursing diagnoses.
3. Identify three outcomes for patients with delirium.
4. Summarize the essential nursing interventions for a patient with delirium.
5. Recognize the signs and symptoms occurring in the stages of Alzheimer's disease.
6. Give an example of the following symptoms assessed during the progression of Alzheimer's disease: (a) amnesia, (b) apraxia, (c) agnosia, and (d) aphasia.
7. Formulate three nursing diagnoses suitable for a patient with Alzheimer's disease, and define two outcomes for each.
8. Formulate a teaching plan for a caregiver of a patient with Alzheimer's disease, including interventions for communication, health maintenance, and a safe environment.
9. Compose a list of appropriate referrals in the community—including a support group, hotline for information, and respite services—for people with dementia and their caregivers.

## ⊖volve WEBSITE

*Visit the Evolve website for Flashcards, Case Studies, and additional testing resources related to the content in this chapter:* *http://evolve.elsevier.com/Canada/Varcarolis/psychiatric/*  Pre-Test  interactive review

The clarity and purpose of an individual's personal journey through life depend on the ability to reflect on its meaning. Cognition, therefore, is a fundamental human feature that distinguishes living from existing. This mental capacity has a distinctive, personalized impact on the individual's physical, psychological, social, and spiritual conduct of life. For example, the ability to remember the connections between related actions and how to initiate them depends on cognitive processing. Moreover, this cognitive processing has a direct relationship to activities of daily living.

Although primarily an intellectual and perceptual process, cognition is closely integrated with an individual's emotional and spiritual values. Cognitive disorders result from changes in the brain and are marked by disturbances in orientation, memory, intellect, judgement, and affect. These disorders may be described as ranging from *minor* to *major* in terms of the level of impairment.

When human beings can no longer understand facts or connect the appropriate feelings to events, they have trouble responding to the complexity of life's challenges. Emotions are overshadowed by profound disturbances in cognitive processing that either cloud or destroy the meaning of the journey.

The labyrinth of current knowledge about cognitive disorders requires compassionate understanding of the patient and family. Nursing interventions are focused on attending to needs, desires, and choices of the individual with a cognitive disorder and his or her family. The goals of the interventions are to protect welfare, preserve functional status, and promote well-being for cognitively impaired patients regardless of the reason for the impairment.

 **HOW A NURSE HELPED ME**

### What Happened to the Person I Married?

*My husband and I have been married for over 45 years. Over the past couple of years, he has become more irritable and difficult to live with. In the past, he was always very particular about his appearance and was very kind to everyone. Now, he rarely showers or bathes, almost never brushes his teeth, and wears his dirty clothes for several days. His kindness has been replaced by irritability and sarcasm. We have always had a physical relationship, but now he says sexually explicit comments that are rude and offensive. His comments are sometimes about children—he was never like that. He has also begun to masturbate in public.*

*I was very upset with these changes in behaviour. Our doctor said that he had a form of dementia that makes his impulses hard to control. Knowing this did not make it easier for me to cope, however. Fortunately, there was a mental health outreach nurse in our area. She came to see my husband and me. She helped me understand my husband's illness and provided me with information on dementia and the impulsive behaviours that are associated with different kinds of dementias. We also discussed how I could set boundaries for myself and understand that my husband's behaviours were not something I had caused. She informed me that my husband's behaviours would change as his dementia got worse. The nurse also helped me figure out what I was going to tell my daughters, who were upset that I did not want the grandchildren staying overnight anymore. We practised role-playing the discussion that I needed to have with my children. This helped build my confidence, knowing that I understood what was happening with my husband's dementia and that I was able to explain it to my kids.*

There are three main cognitive disorders: delirium, dementia, and amnestic disorder. It should be noted that the diagnosis of dementia has been retired and replaced in the fifth edition of the *Diagnostic and Statistical Manual of Mental Disorders* with *neurocognitive disorder* (which includes amnestic disorders). Many clinicians believe the term *dementia*, which literally means "without mind," was stigmatizing (Stetka & Correll, 2013) and created social barriers for people with these disorders. Cognitive disorders that do not fit the criteria for delirium or neurocognitive disorder (dementia or amnestic disorder) are referred to as *cognitive disorders not otherwise specified* and are presumed to be caused by a specific medical condition (e.g., a traumatic or an acquired brain injury), the use of a drug, or possibly both (Sadock & Sadock, 2008). Traumatic or acquired brain injuries are also associated with the onset of delirium, dementia, or both; those with such injuries experience physical and emotional symptoms that can impact their daily functioning (Becker, 2012).

This chapter addresses the broad categories of delirium and dementia, by far the most common conditions nurses encounter. It also introduces psychiatric symptoms of people with brain injuries and compares them with those of people with delirium and dementia. However, amnestic disorders are not discussed here (see Chapter 23 for that discussion). Table 18-1 offers some guidelines for distinguishing among delirium, dementia, depression, and brain injury (these last two may have similar symptoms and may co-occur in older adults).

## DELIRIUM

### CLINICAL PICTURE

Delirium is a cognitive disturbance "characterized by inattention, disorganized thinking, and a fluctuating mental status" (Gesin, Russell, Lin, et al., 2012, p. e2). It should be considered a medical emergency, and immediate attention given to prevent irreversible and serious damage (Huber, 2012). Delirium is associated with increased morbidity and mortality (Inouye, Foreman, Mion, et al., 2001). While delirium is usually short-term, it can have long-term consequences that are currently best defined through large-scale epidemiological studies (Quinlan & Rudolph, 2011; Rudolph & Marcantonio, 2011). In patients with pre-existing cognitive impairment—for example, dementia—delirium accelerates cognitive decline. While there are reports of long-term cognitive impairment (in the absence of pre-existing cognitive impairment) and functional decline following delirium, results of studies have been inconsistent. There is also an association with depression post-delirium, and evidence indicates that younger patients who have been delirious while in hospital may develop symptoms resembling those of post-traumatic stress disorder (Jones, Griffiths, Humphris, et al., 2001).

### EPIDEMIOLOGY

Delirium is the most common complication of hospitalization in older patients (Rice, Bennett, Gomez, et al., 2011). The

**TABLE 18-1   COMPARISON OF DELIRIUM, DEMENTIA, DEPRESSION, AND BRAIN INJURY**

| | DELIRIUM | DEMENTIA | DEPRESSION | BRAIN INJURY |
|---|---|---|---|---|
| **Onset** | Sudden, over hours to days | Slowly, over months | May have been gradual, with exacerbation during crisis or stress | Usually sudden; symptoms increase as damage becomes more pervasive |
| **Cause or contributing factors** | Hypoglycemia, fever, dehydration, hypotension; infection, other conditions that disrupt body's homeostasis; adverse drug reaction; head injury; change in environment (e.g., hospitalization); pain; emotional stress | Alzheimer's disease, vascular disease, human immunodeficiency virus infection, neurological disease, chronic alcoholism, head trauma | Lifelong history, losses, loneliness, crises, declining health, medical conditions | Traumatic injury (external physical force) or acquired injury (conditions other than degenerative, such as stroke, anoxia, hypoxia, tumour, toxin) |
| **Cognition** | Impaired memory, judgement, calculations, attention span; can fluctuate through the day | Impaired memory, judgement, calculations, attention span, abstract thinking; agnosia | Difficulty concentrating, forgetfulness, inattention | May have difficulty thinking and learning; poor judgement; easily distractible; disoriented, confused, or amnesic depending on injury |
| **Level of consciousness** | Altered | Not altered | Not altered | Variable alterations depending on injury |
| **Activity level** | Can be increased or reduced; restlessness, which may worsen in evening (sundowning); sleep–wake cycle may be reversed | Not altered; behaviours may worsen in evening (sundowning) | Usually decreased; lethargy, fatigue, lack of motivation; may sleep poorly and awaken in early morning | Depending on injury, may have sleep disturbances, swallowing or appetite changes, weakness or paralysis, balance or coordination difficulties |
| **Emotional state** | Rapid swings; can be fearful, anxious, suspicious, aggressive; may have hallucinations, delusions, or both | Flat; delusions | Extreme sadness, apathy, irritability, anxiety, paranoid ideation | Anxiety, depression, agitation, hyper-reactivity, disinhibition, impulsivity, labile mood depending on injury |
| **Speech and language** | Rapid, inappropriate, incoherent, rambling | Incoherent, slow (sometimes due to effort to find the right word), inappropriate, rambling, repetitious | Slow, flat, low | Depending on the injury, may experience difficulties with expressive speech, word finding, comprehension |
| **Prognosis** | Reversible with proper and timely treatment | Not reversible; progressive | Reversible with proper and timely treatment | Varies depending on the location and the extent of brain damaged |

reported incidence of delirium in hospitalized patients ranges from 3% to 56% (Michaud, Büla, Berney, et al., 2007), from 11% to 42% in medically ill older patients (Cerejeira & Mukactova-Ludinska, 2011), and from 4% to 65% in post-operative patients, depending on the type of surgery (Rudolph & Marcantonio, 2011). The high degree of variability in the reported incidence of delirium is most likely due to its under-recognition by both nurses and doctors who work in acute care settings and hospitals.

## CO-MORBIDITY AND ETIOLOGY

Delirium is always secondary to another physiological condition and is often a transient disorder. If the underlying condition is corrected, complete recovery from delirium should also occur. Delirium can be an indicator of increased frailty and vulnerability, not just an exclusively transient and fully reversible condition associated only with acute causes (Clegg, Young, & Siddiqi, 2012). The common acute causes of delirium are nervous system disease, systemic disease (such as cardiac failure), and intoxication or withdrawal from a chemical substance (see Chapter 19). Clinicians, therefore, should assume that any drug taken could result in delirium (Sadock & Sadock, 2008).

Nurses frequently encounter delirium in the general hospital setting. Although delirium is seen in children with fever and patients who are terminally ill, it occurs most frequently in older-adult patients. Surgery, the introduction of medications,

## BOX 18-1 COMMON CAUSES OF DELIRIUM

**Postoperative States, Drug Intoxications, and Withdrawals**
- Anticholinergics, benzodiazepines, alcohol, anxiolytics, opioids, and central nervous system stimulants (e.g., cocaine, crack cocaine)

**Infections**
- Systemic: pneumonia, typhoid fever, malaria, urinary tract infection, and septicemia
- Intracranial: meningitis and encephalitis

**Metabolic Disorders**
- Dehydration
- Hypoxia (pulmonary disease, heart disease, and anemia)
- Hypoglycemia
- Sodium, potassium, calcium, magnesium, and acid–base imbalances
- Hepatic encephalopathy or uremic encephalopathy
- Thiamine (vitamin B$_1$) deficiency (Wernicke's encephalopathy)
- Endocrine disorders (e.g., thyroid or parathyroid)
- Hypothermia or hyperthermia
- Diabetic acidosis

**Drugs**
- Digitalis, steroids, lithium, levodopa, anticholinergics, benzodiazepines, central nervous system depressants, tricyclic antidepressants
- Central anticholinergic syndrome due to use of multiple drugs with anticholinergic adverse effects

**Neurological Diseases**
- Seizures
- Head trauma
- Hypertensive encephalopathy

**Tumour**
- Primary cerebral

**Psychosocial Stressors**
- Relocation or other sudden changes
- Sensory deprivation or overload
- Sleep deprivation
- Immobilization
- Pain

 **RESEARCH HIGHLIGHT**

*Strategies for Preventing Delirium in Hospitalized Older Patients*

**Source:** Rice, K., Bennett, M., Gomez, M., et al. (2011). Nurses' recognition of delirium in the hospitalized older adult. *Clinical Nurse Specialist, 25*(6), 299–311. doi:10.1097/NUR.0b013e318234897b.

**Problem**
Delirium is the most frequent complication of hospitalization in older adults and is costly in relation to fiscal resources; more important, delirium is also associated with mortality and morbidity. Timely recognition is essential to offset these negative outcomes; however, delirium is often misdiagnosed or not recognized by hospital staff. Nurses are in a prime position to detect delirium.

**Purpose of Study**
The study aimed to measure staff nurses' recognition of delirium in older hospitalized patients by comparing their delirium ratings with those of expert diagnosticians, using the Confusion Assessment Method (CAM).

**Methods**
Older patients who were hospitalized in medical-surgical units and were judged to be at risk for delirium (n = 170) were assessed for delirium at least every other day until discharge. Both staff nurses and experts conducted the assessments using the CAM. The staff nurses' ratings were compared with the experts' ratings to ascertain the level of agreement.

**Key Findings**
The experts detected delirium in 7% of the patients. The staff nurses failed to recognize delirium 75% of the time, and there was poor agreement between experts and staff nurses for all observations. Predictors of staff nurses' poor recognition of delirium included older patient age, length of stay, presence of dementia, and hypoactive (quiet) delirium.

**Implications for Nursing Practice**
Nurses who work with patients at high risk for developing delirium should engage in ongoing education about its detection and management, and regular systems should be put into place to identify those patients most at risk of developing delirium. It is especially important that nurses not assess older patients who become confused as having dementia. Equally important to recognize is that some patients who become delirious will be "quietly confused."

urinary tract infections, cerebrovascular disease, and congestive heart failure are some of the most common causes (see Box 18-1). The second or third day in hospital may herald the onset of confusion and difficulty adjusting to an unfamiliar environment for many older adults.

Certain factors predispose patients to delirium, thus putting them at higher risk, including existing cognitive impairment (especially on admission to the hospital), low functional autonomy, polypharmacy (especially benzodiazepines, narcotic analgesics, and anticholinergics), and clinical severity of the primary illness (Voyer, McCuskar, Cole, et al., 2007). Consequently,

nurses should pay particular attention to those patients who are at greatest risk (see Research Highlight box).

## APPLICATION OF THE NURSING PROCESS

### ASSESSMENT

While symptoms of delirium must be managed, the goal of treatment is to determine the underlying cause and rectify it when possible (Rudolph & Marcantonio, 2011) because the underlying causes of delirium are often life threatening, and early recognition is critical to offsetting the potential consequences. Clinicians who suspect delirium and note its symptoms should undertake a thorough examination, including mental and neurological status examinations as well as a physical examination. Blood tests and a urinalysis should be done. In addition, the patient's medication regimen should be examined. A failure to quickly detect and treat delirium is associated with a significant increase in morbidity and mortality (Rice, Bennett, Gomez, et al., 2011).

### General Assessment

According to Wei, Fearing, Sternberg, and colleague (2008), there are four cardinal features of delirium that clinicians focus on in the Confusion Assessment Method (CAM):

1. Acute onset and fluctuating course
2. Inattention
3. Disorganized thinking
4. Disturbance of consciousness

Suspect the presence of delirium when a person's ability to focus, sustain, or shift attention becomes abruptly impaired and his or her awareness of the environment is reduced. Conversation is made more difficult because the person may be easily distracted by irrelevant stimuli. Questions must be repeated because the individual's attention wanders, and the person might easily get off track and need to be refocused. The person may also have difficulty with orientation—first to time, then to place, and last to person. For example, a man with delirium may think that the year is 1972, that the hospital is home, and that the nurse is his wife. Orientation to person is usually intact to the extent that the person is aware of his or her own identity.

A person with delirium may also appear withdrawn, agitated, or psychotic. Fluctuating levels of consciousness are unpredictable. Disorientation and confusion are usually markedly worse at night and during the early morning. In fact, some patients may be confused or delirious only at night and may remain lucid during the day. The phenomenon in which symptoms become more pronounced in the evening is called sundowning (also known as *sundown syndrome*). Sundowning often begins in the late afternoon as the evening approaches. This symptom-exacerbation pattern may occur in people who have either delirium or dementia.

As nurses, our frequent interaction with those in hospital places us in a prime position to prevent, detect, and treat the effects of delirium. Nursing assessment includes observation and evaluation of (1) cognitive and perceptual disturbances, (2) physical needs, and (3) moods and physical behaviours.

### Cognitive and Perceptual Disturbances

Patients experiencing delirium may be difficult to engage in conversation because they are easily distracted, display marked attention deficits, and exhibit memory impairment. In mild delirium, memory deficits are noted only on careful questioning. In more severe delirium, memory problems usually take the form of obvious difficulty in processing and remembering recent events. For example, the person might ask when a son is coming to visit, even though the son left only an hour earlier. It is critical that nurses are able to determine the presence of a delirium. In patients who also have a dementia, this task becomes more difficult. Many clinicians use the Confusion Assessment Method (CAM) (Wei, Fearing, Sternberg, et al., 2008).

Another helpful tool for clinicians to determine the presence of a component of dementia is the Montreal Cognitive Assessment (MoCA). The MoCA assesses short-term memory, visuospatial abilities, executive functioning, attention, concentration, working memory, language, and orientation to time and place (Nasreddine, Phillips, Bedirian, et al., 2005). The MoCA can be completed by an experienced clinician in approximately ten minutes.

Perceptual disturbances are also common in delirium. *Perception* is the processing of information about one's internal and external environments. Various misinterpretations of reality may take the form of illusions. For example, a person may mistake folds in the bedclothes for white rats or the cord of a window blind for a snake. Or misinterpretations may take the form of hallucinations. For example, individuals experiencing delirium may become terrified when they "see" giant spiders crawling over the bedclothes or "feel" bugs crawling on or under their skin.

The individual with delirium generally is aware that something is very wrong. Statements like "My thoughts are all jumbled" may signal cognitive problems. When perceptual disturbances are present, the emotional response is often one of fear and anxiety, which may be manifested by psychomotor agitation.

### Physical Needs

A person with delirium becomes disoriented and may try to "go home." Alternatively, a person may think that he or she *is* home and jump out of a window in an attempt to get away from "invaders." Wandering, pulling out intravenous lines and Foley catheters, and falling out of bed are common dangers that require nursing vigilance.

An individual experiencing delirium has difficulty processing stimuli in the environment, and confusion magnifies the inability to recognize reality. The physical environment should be made as simple and clear as possible. Objects such as clocks and calendars can maximize orientation to time. Glasses, hearing aids, and adequate lighting without glare can maximize the person's ability to interpret more accurately what is going on in the environment. The nurse should interact with the patient whenever the patient is awake. Short periods of social interaction help reduce anxiety and misperceptions.

Self-care deficits, injury, or hyperactivity or hypoactivity may lead to skin breakdown and possible infection. Often, this condition is compounded by poor nutrition, forced bed rest, and possible incontinence. These situations require nursing assessment and intervention.

Autonomic signs, such as tachycardia, sweating, flushed face, dilated pupils, and elevated blood pressure, are often present in delirium. These changes must be monitored and documented carefully and may require immediate medical attention as they may be an indication that the underlying physiological condition is worsening.

Changes in the sleep–wake cycle should be assessed and documented. In some cases, a complete reversal of the night–day, sleep–wake cycle can occur. The patient's level of consciousness may range from lethargy to stupor or from semi-coma to hypervigilance. In hypervigilance, patients are extraordinarily alert, and their eyes constantly scan the room; they may have difficulty falling asleep or may be actively disoriented and agitated throughout the night.

Medications should always be suspected as a potential cause of delirium (Sadock & Sadock, 2008). To recognize drug reactions or anticipate potential interactions before delirium actually occurs, health care providers must assess all medications or other substances (i.e., prescriptions, street drugs, alcohol, and over-the-counter medications, including herbal or natural therapies) the patient is taking.

### Moods and Physical Behaviours

The individual's moods and physical behaviours may change dramatically within a short period. Moods may swing back and forth among fear, anger, anxiety, euphoria, depression, and apathy. These labile moods are often accompanied by physical behaviours associated with feeling states. For example, a person may strike out from fear or anger or may cry, call for help, curse, moan, and tear off clothing one minute and become apathetic or laugh uncontrollably the next. In short, behaviour and emotions are erratic and fluctuating.

A patient's lack of concentration and disorientation complicate the health care team's interventions. The following vignette illustrates the fear and confusion a patient may experience when admitted to an intensive care unit (ICU).

### Self-Assessment

Because the behaviours exhibited by the patient with delirium can be directly attributed to temporary medical conditions, intense personal reactions in staff are less likely to arise. In fact, intense, conflicting emotions are less likely to occur in nurses working with a patient with delirium than in nurses working with a patient with dementia, which is discussed later in this chapter. Nonetheless, interacting with these patients can be frustrating for health care providers, especially given the fluctuating nature of the clinical picture.

## DIAGNOSIS

Safety needs play a substantial role in nursing care. Patients with delirium often perceive the environment in a distorted way, and objects are often misperceived (due to illusions or hallucinations). People and objects may be misinterpreted as threatening or harmful, and patients often act on these misinterpretations. For example, if feeling threatened or thinking that common medical equipment is harmful, the patient may pull off an oxygen mask, pull out an intravenous or nasogastric tube, or try to flee. In such a case, the person demonstrates a *Risk for injury* related to confusion, as evidenced by sensory deficits or perceptual deficits.

Hallucinations, distractibility, illusions, disorientation, agitation, restlessness, and misperception are major aspects of the

---

**VIGNETTE**

Peter, aged 43, survived numerous, life-threatening complications following open-heart surgery to replace his mitral valve. As a result, he spent three weeks in an intensive care unit. The night before he was to be transferred out of the unit, the nurses moved his bed to accommodate another patient who needed observation closer to the nursing unit. During the move, he heard a nurse saying, "I need to get a gas." Another nurse answered in a loud voice, "Can you get a large needle for the injection?" Peter began to get frightened, thinking the nurses were going to gas and sedate him. He became suspicious about his bed being moved and believed he was being transported, against his will, to another country to have his organs removed and donated for transplantation. His fear mounted when he realized that his wife, who had been at his bedside during his entire ICU stay, was not there. He wanted her to know that he was being taken away. His incoherent attempts to summon his wife back to his bedside confirmed what he suspected: the very people who had saved his life (although, at the time he could not appreciate this fact) were now out to get him.

Peter began to diligently watch the clock on the wall, recording every movement of the nurses to try to ascertain a pattern to their behaviour. He was planning his escape from his captors. When he was sure nobody was looking, he climbed over the bed rails and attempted to leave the unit. The nurses responded by calling security personnel to escort him back to bed. Once he was safely back in bed, the nurses applied a bed alert and then sedated him.

Peter's confusion abated the next day, at which time he was transferred from the ICU to another part of the hospital. Because he could recall the details of his confused state, both in the short and long term, he realized how distorted his thinking had been during the episode. However, the anxiety, fear, and trepidation he had experienced remained with him for months after discharge from the hospital.

What are some more helpful interventions the nurses could have used? What could the nurses have done differently? What would you have done?

---

clinical picture. When some of these symptoms are present, *Acute confusion* related to delirium is an appropriate nursing diagnosis.

If fever and dehydration are present, fluid and electrolyte balance will need to be managed. If the underlying cause of the patient's delirium results in fever, decreased skin turgor, decreased urinary output or fluid intake, and dry skin or mucous membranes, then the nursing diagnosis of *Deficient fluid volume* is appropriate. Fluid volume deficit may be related to fever, electrolyte imbalance, reduced intake, or infection.

In cases of delirium, restful sleep is not achieved, day or night; the patient may be less responsive during the day and may become disruptively wakeful during the night. *Insomnia* or *Sleep deprivation* related to impaired cerebral oxygenation or disruption in consciousness is a likely diagnosis.

Sustaining communication with a delirious patient is difficult. *Impaired verbal communication* related to cerebral hypoxia or decreased cerebral blood flow, as evidenced by confusion or clouding of consciousness, may be diagnosed.

## ASSESSMENT GUIDELINES

### Delirium

1. Assess for acute onset and fluctuating levels of consciousness, which are key in delirium.
2. Assess the person's ability to attend to the immediate environment, including responses to nursing care.
3. Establish the person's normal level of consciousness and cognition by interviewing family members or other caregivers.
4. Assess for past cognitive impairment—especially an existing dementia diagnosis—and other risk factors.
5. Identify disturbances in physiological status, especially infection, hypoxia, and pain.
6. Identify any physiological abnormalities documented in the patient's record.
7. Assess vital signs, level of consciousness, and neurological signs.
8. Assess potential for injury, especially in relation to potential for falls and wandering.
9. Maintain comfort measures, especially in relation to pain, cold, or positioning.
10. Monitor situational factors that worsen or improve symptoms.
11. Assess for availability of immediate medical interventions to help prevent irreversible brain damage.
12. Remain nonjudgemental. Confer with other staff readily when questions arise.

*Fear* is one of the most common of all nursing diagnoses and may be related to illusions, delusions, or hallucinations, as evidenced by verbal and nonverbal expressions of fearfulness. Other nursing concerns include *Self-care deficit*, *Disturbed thought processes*, and *Impaired social interaction*. Table 18-2 identifies nursing diagnoses for any confused patient with delirium or dementia.

## OUTCOMES IDENTIFICATION

The overall outcome is that the delirious patient will return to the premorbid level of functioning. Table 18-3 includes outcomes for acute confusion from the *Nursing Outcomes Classification (NOC)* (Moorhead, Johnson, Maas, et al., 2012). However, for many of the diagnoses we would use for the person experiencing delirium, *NOC* is not specific enough. Although the person can demonstrate a wide variety of needs, *Risk for injury* is always present. Appropriate outcomes are:

- During periods of lucidity, patient will be oriented to time, place, and person with the aid of nursing interventions, such as the provision of clocks, calendars, maps, and other types of orienting information.
- Patient will remain free from falls and injury while confused, with the aid of nursing safety measures while in the hospital.

Because level of consciousness can change throughout the day, the patient needs to be frequently checked for orientation.

## IMPLEMENTATION

The priorities of treatment are to keep the patient safe while attempting to identify the cause. If the underlying disorder is corrected, complete recovery is possible. If, however, the underlying disorder is not corrected and persists, irreversible neuronal damage can occur. Nursing concerns, therefore, centre on the following:

- Preventing physical harm due to confusion, aggression, or electrolyte and fluid imbalance
- Performing a comprehensive nursing assessment to aid in identifying the cause
- Assisting with proper health management to eradicate the underlying cause
- Using supportive measures to relieve distress

The *Nursing Interventions Classification (NIC)* (Bulechek, Butcher, & Dochterman, 2008) can be used as a guide to develop interventions for a person experiencing delirium (Box 18-2). Medical management of delirium involves treating the underlying organic causes. If the underlying cause of delirium is not treated, permanent brain damage may ensue. Additionally, thoughtful use of antipsychotic or antianxiety agents may also aid in controlling behavioural symptoms.

A patient in acute delirium should never be left alone. Because most hospitals and health facilities are unable to provide one-to-one supervision of the patient, family members can be encouraged to stay with the patient.

## EVALUATION

Long-term outcome criteria for a person experiencing delirium include the following:

- Patient will remain safe.
- Patient will be oriented to time, place, and person by discharge.
- Underlying cause will be treated and ameliorated.

## DEMENTIA

Dementia, a broad term, is the progressive deterioration of cognitive functioning and the global impairment of intellect with no change in consciousness. It is not a specific disease per se but, rather, a collection of symptoms that result from an underlying brain disorder. The general diagnostic label used to represent the underlying brain disorders is *neurocognitive disorder*, which may be further specified as major or mild (minor) depending on the severity of impairments. Dementia is manifested as difficulty with memory, problem solving (executive functioning), and comprehension. While the majority of dementias are irreversible, approximately 15% are due to a reversible illness (Sadock & Sadock, 2008).

## CLINICAL PICTURE

*Dementia* is the general term used to describe a decline in cognitive functioning that interferes with daily living. Alzheimer's disease (AD), the most common cause of dementia in older

## TABLE 18-2    POTENTIAL NURSING DIAGNOSES FOR THE CONFUSED PATIENT

| SYMPTOMS | NURSING DIAGNOSES |
|---|---|
| Wanders, has unsteady gait, acts out fear from hallucinations or illusions, forgets things (leaves stove on, doors open) | *Risk for injury* |
| Awake and disoriented during the night (*sundowning*), frightened at night | Disturbed sleep pattern<br>Fear<br>Acute confusion |
| Unable to take care of basic needs | Self-care deficit (bathing/hygiene, dressing, feeding, toileting)<br>Ineffective coping<br>Functional urinary incontinence<br>Imbalanced nutrition: less than body requirements<br>Risk for deficient fluid volume |
| Sees frightening things that are not there (*hallucinations*), mistakes everyday objects for something sinister and frightening (*illusions*), may become paranoid and think that others are doing things to confuse him or her (*delusions*) | Anxiety<br>Disturbed sensory perception<br>Impaired environmental interpretation syndrome<br>Disturbed thought processes |
| Does not recognize familiar people or places, has difficulty with short- or long-term memory or both, is forgetful and confused | Impaired memory<br>Impaired environmental interpretation syndrome<br>Acute or chronic confusion |
| Has difficulty with communication, cannot find words, has difficulty recognizing objects or people, is incoherent | Impaired verbal communication<br>Impaired social interaction |
| Devastated over losing place in life as known (during lucid moments), fearful and overwhelmed by what is happening to him or her | Spiritual distress<br>Hopelessness<br>Situational low self-esteem<br>Grieving |
| Family and loved ones overburdened and overwhelmed, unable to care for patient's needs | Disabled family coping<br>Interrupted family processes<br>Impaired home maintenance<br>Caregiver role strain |

## TABLE 18-3    *NOC* OUTCOMES RELATED TO ACUTE CONFUSION

*Acute confusion:* Abrupt onset of reversible disturbance of consciousness, attention, cognition, and perception that develops over a short period of time.

| NURSING OUTCOME AND DEFINITION | INTERMEDIATE INDICATORS | SHORT-TERM INDICATORS |
|---|---|---|
| *Cognitive orientation:* Ability to identify person, place, and time accurately | Identifies correct day<br>Identifies correct month<br>Identifies correct year<br>Identifies correct season<br>Identifies current place<br>Identifies significant current events | Identifies self<br>Identifies significant other |
| *Neurological status and level of consciousness:* Arousal, orientation, and attention to the environment | Oriented cognitively<br>Communicates appropriately for situation<br>Attends to environmental stimuli | Opens eyes to external stimuli<br>Obeys commands<br>Makes motor responses to noxious stimuli |

**Source:** Moorhead, S., Johnson, M., Maas, M., et al. (2012). *Nursing outcomes classification (NOC)* (5th ed.). St. Louis: Mosby.

## BOX 18-2   NIC INTERVENTIONS FOR DELIRIUM MANAGEMENT

*Definition of* delirium management: Provision of a safe and therapeutic environment for the patient who is experiencing an acute state of confusion.

Activities:
- Identify etiological factors causing delirium.
- Initiate therapies to reduce or eliminate factors causing delirium.
- Monitor neurological status on an ongoing basis.
- Provide unconditional positive regard.
- Verbally acknowledge patient's fears and feelings.
- Provide optimistic but realistic reassurance.
- Allow patient to maintain rituals that limit anxiety.
- Provide patient with information about what is happening and what can be expected to occur in the future.
- Avoid demands for abstract thinking if patient can think only in concrete terms.
- Limit need for decision making if frustrating or confusing to patient.
- Administer prn (as needed) medications for anxiety or agitation.
- Encourage visitation by significant others, as appropriate.
- Recognize and accept patient's perceptions or interpretation of reality (hallucinations or delusions).
- State your perception in a calm, reassuring, and nonargumentative manner.
- Respond to the theme or feeling tone, rather than the content, of the hallucination or delusion.
- When possible, remove stimuli that create misperception in a particular patient (e.g., pictures on the wall or television).
- Maintain a well-lit environment that reduces sharp contrasts and shadows.
- Assist with needs related to nutrition, elimination, hydration, and personal hygiene.
- Maintain a hazard-free environment.
- Place identification bracelet on patient.
- Provide appropriate level of supervision and surveillance to monitor patient and allow for therapeutic actions, as needed.
- Use physical restraints, as needed.
- Avoid frustrating patient by quizzing with orientation questions that cannot be answered.
- Reorient patient to person, place, and time, as needed.
- Provide a consistent physical environment and daily routine.
- Provide caregivers who are familiar to the patient.
- Use environmental cues (e.g., signs, pictures, clocks, calendars, colour coding of environment) to stimulate memory, reorient, and promote appropriate behaviour.
- Provide a low-stimulation environment for patients disoriented by overstimulation.
- Encourage use of aids that increase sensory input (e.g., glasses, hearing aids, dentures).
- Approach patient slowly and from the front.
- Address patient by name when initiating interaction.
- Reorient patient to health care provider with each contact.
- Communicate with simple, direct, descriptive statements.
- Prepare patient for upcoming changes in usual routine and environment before their occurrence.
- Provide new information slowly and in small doses, with frequent rest periods.
- Focus interpersonal interactions on what is familiar and meaningful to patient.

**Source:** Bulechek, G.M., Butcher, H.K., & Dochterman, J.M. (2008). *Nursing interventions classification (NIC)* (5th ed., pp. 252–257). St. Louis, MO: Mosby.

## TABLE 18-4   MEMORY DEFICIT: NORMAL AGING VERSUS DEMENTIA

| PARAMETER | NORMAL AGING | DEMENTIA |
|---|---|---|
| **Area of impairment** | Difficulty in word finding, but no aphasia, dyspraxia, agnosia | Aphasia, dyspraxia, agnosia often found |
| **Extent of impairment** | Slowing<br>Cautiousness<br>Reduced ability to solve new problems<br>Mildly impaired memory<br>Mild decline in fluid intelligence | Minor to major deceleration<br>Variable cautiousness<br>Minor to major problem-solving impairment<br>Minor to major intellectual impairment<br>Minor to major decline in fluid intelligence |
| **Rate of impairment** | Slow change over many years | More rapid though still gradual changes |

adults, is a progressive degenerative neurocognitive disorder marked by impaired memory and thinking skills (Alzheimer Society of Canada, 2009). It is a devastating disease that not only affects the person who has it but also places an enormous burden on the families and caregivers of those affected. Nurses practising in any setting will care for patients with AD and must be prepared to respond.

It is important to distinguish between normal forgetfulness and the memory deficit of AD and other dementias. Severe memory loss is *not* a normal part of growing older (Alzheimer Society of Canada, 2010a). Slight forgetfulness is a common phenomenon of the aging process (age-associated memory loss), but memory loss that interferes with one's activities of daily living is not. Table 18-4 outlines memory changes in normal aging and memory changes seen in dementia.

Many people who live to a very old age never experience significant memory loss or any other symptom of dementia. Most of us know of people in their eighties and nineties who

### Dementia and Caregiver Burden for a Chinese-Canadian Family

It has long been recognized that caregivers suffer a great deal of burden in relation to caring for a person with dementia. They are prone to emotional distress, depression, and decreased quality of life as they cope with caregiving. It also has been recognized that the experience of stress and coping varies among cultural groups, and the isolation experienced as a result of caregiving may be exacerbated by cultural differences in approaches to caregiving. For example, Asian cultures have a long tradition of respecting older adult family members and fulfilling a perceived obligation to care for them. In addition, people from Asian cultures are likely to have a collective orientation, as opposed to a Western view of individuality and autonomy. It is for these reasons that nurses must become aware of cultural meanings and understandings of caregiving for the caregiver. Many different formats of interventions have been developed to try to alleviate the caregiving burden. These formats have traditionally included individual, family, and group programs.

Recently, however, Chiu, Marziali, Colantonio, and colleagues (2009) conducted a study that explored the feasibility and usability of an online caregiver support service and evaluated the effects of that service on caregiver health outcomes. The Internet-Based Caregiver Support Service (ICSS) had intervention goals and followed therapy strategies similar to those established, utilizing individual face-to-face interventions. The primary difference was that the ICSS users accessed services via the Internet and communicated through e-mail. A caregiver information handbook was available in English and Chinese. Asynchronous e-mail communication between a client and a clinician could also occur in either English or Chinese. The researchers found evidence that tailored ethnocultural-linguistic services can impact service usability and that caregivers can benefit from asynchronous e-mail and a dedicated information Web site.

**Source:** Chiu, T., Marziali, E., Colantonio, A., et al. (2009). Internet-based caregiver support for Chinese Canadians taking care of a family member with Alzheimer disease and related dementia. *Canadian Journal on Aging, 28*(4), 323–336. doi:10.1017/S0714980809990158.

lead active lives with their intellect intact. Pablo Picasso, Duke Ellington, Ansel Adams, and George Burns are just a few examples of people who were still active in their careers when they died, and all were older than 75 years of age (Picasso was 91; George Burns was 100). The slow, minor cognitive changes associated with aging should not impede social or occupational functioning.

Although dementia often begins with a worsening of ability to remember new information, it is marked by progressive deterioration in intellectual functioning, memory, and the ability to solve problems and learn new skills; a decline in the ability to perform activities of daily living; and a progressive deterioration of personality accompanied by impairment in judgement. A person's declining intellect often leads to emotional changes such as mood lability, depression, and aggressive acting out, as well as to neurological changes that produce hallucinations and delusions.

There are several types of dementia, including dementia of the Alzheimer's type, vascular dementia, Lewy body disease, Pick's disease, alcohol-related dementias (including Korsakoff syndrome), Creutzfeldt-Jakob disease, and the dementias associated with Parkinson's disease, Huntington's disease, acquired immune deficiency syndrome (AIDS), and traumatic and acquired brain injury.

Dementias can be classified as primary or secondary. Primary dementia is irreversible, progressive, and not secondary to any other disorder. Alzheimer's disease and vascular dementias are examples of primary dementias.

Secondary dementia occurs as a result of some other pathological process (e.g., metabolic, nutritional, neurological). AIDS-related dementia is an example of a secondary dementia that is increasingly seen in health care settings. The exact prevalence of AIDS-related dementia is unknown. In a recent study involving 658 patients infected with AIDS, the researchers reported that that 11.7% were significantly cognitively impaired, 36.4% were depressed, and 19.7% had symptoms of sensory neuropathy (Wright, Brew, Arayawichanont, et al., 2008). Cognitive impairment associated with human immunodeficiency virus (HIV) is referred to as *AIDS dementia complex*. Other secondary dementias can result from viral encephalitis, pernicious anemia, folic acid deficiency, and hypothyroidism.

## EPIDEMIOLOGY

- Globally, it is estimated that 35.6 million people have dementia (a figure greater than the entire population of Canada) and that the number of people with dementia will double every 20 years to 115.4 million by 2050 (Alzheimer's Disease International, 2010).
- More than 500,000 Canadians are currently living with dementia. Of these, 71, 000 are under the age of 65.
- Among Canadians over the age of 65, 1 in 11 has dementia.
- Alzheimer's disease accounts for close to 70% of all dementias in Canada (Alzheimer Society of Canada, 2010b).
- Women comprise 72% of all Canadians living with the Alzheimer's subtype of neurocognitive disorder.
- The Alzheimer's subtype of neurocognitive disorder attacks indiscriminately, striking men and women, people of various ethnicities, rich and poor, and individuals with varying degrees of intelligence.
- Although Alzheimer's can occur at a younger age (early onset), most of those with the disease are 65 years of age or older (late onset).
- The second most common type of dementia is related to cerebrovascular disease, accounting for 20% of all dementias (Sadock & Sadock, 2008).
- Other common causes of dementia are head trauma, alcohol abuse, and movement disorders such as Parkinson's disease; these account for 1% to 5% of all cases (Sadock & Sadock, 2008).

## ETIOLOGY

Although the cause of AD is unknown, most experts agree that, like other chronic and progressive conditions, it is a result of multiple factors—genetics, lifestyle, and environment. However, the greatest risk factor is advancing age (Alzheimer's Association, 2012; Lehne, 2013).

### Biological Factors

#### Alzheimer's Tangles

The brains of people with AD reveal signs of neuronal degeneration, which begins in the hippocampus, the part of the brain responsible for recent memory, and then spreads into the cerebral cortex, the part of the brain responsible for problem solving and higher-order cognitive functioning (Lehne, 2013). Two processes contribute to cell death: (1) the accumulation of the protein β-amyloid outside the neurons, which interferes with synapses, and (2) the accumulation of the protein tau inside the neurons, which form tangles that block the flow of nutrients. The β-amyloid proteins are formed during normal metabolism and are involved in the cell communication (Casey, 2012). However, when the enzyme that is involved in breaking down these proteins, insulin-degrading enzyme, is no longer effective, protein plaques begin to accumulate; this accumulation results in synaptic dysfunction and neural cell death (Querfurth & LaFerla, 2010). As the cells die, the dysfunctional mitochondria release free radicals that trigger an inflammatory process. The increase in the concentrations of β-amyloid proteins within the neurons is believed to trigger the increase in tau protein production. Tau proteins are an important factor in the transmission of neurochemicals along the neural dendrites (Ballard, Gauthier, Corbett, et al., 2011). When the tau proteins become ineffective, through the process of phosphorylation, they adhere to one another to form neurotoxic filaments. With continued tau phosphorylation and the continued formation of neurotoxic filaments, neurofibrillary tangles form (Ballard, Gauthier, Corbett, et al., 2011). More research is needed into these mechanisms because some people who have these brain changes do not go on to develop AD (Alzheimer's Association, 2012).

### Genetic

Family history has been shown to play a role in the development of AD. For example, early-onset AD, which occurs between the ages of 30 and 60, is inherited. Three genes that lead to the devastating early-onset form of AD have been identified and probably account for half of the cases (Wright, Trinh, Blacker, et al., 2008).

A susceptibility gene has been identified for late-onset AD as well. It is a gene that makes the protein apolipoprotein E4 (APOE4), which helps carry cholesterol and is also implicated in cardiovascular disease. This gene alone does not produce Alzheimer's disease; it is the combined effect of genes and other risk factors that causes the disease to develop (Querfurth & LaFerla, 2010).

Individuals who have or have had family members with AD are understandably concerned about their own risk for developing the disease. The decision to participate in predictive genetic testing is very personal, and those considering it should weigh the psychological, legal, social, and ethical implications. Another important factor people should consider before undertaking testing is that the presence of the gene related to APOE4, which is a risk factor in developing Alzheimer's disease, cannot predict that the person will indeed develop the disease. Further information can be found on the Canadian Association of Genetic Counsellors Web site (https://cagc-accg.ca/.).

### Head Injury and Traumatic Brain Injury

Brain injury and trauma are associated with a greater risk of developing AD and other dementias. People who suffer repeated head trauma, such as boxers and football players, may be at greater risk. There is also a suggestion of a greater risk for those who suffer brain injury and carry the gene APOE4 (Alzheimer's Association, 2012).

### Cardiovascular Disease

The health of the brain is closely linked to overall heart health, and there is evidence that people with cardiovascular disease are at greater risk for AD. Likewise, lifestyle factors associated with cardiovascular disease, such as inactivity, high cholesterol, diabetes, and obesity, are considered risk factors for AD (Alzheimer's Association, 2012).

### Modifiable Factors

There is some evidence that brain health is affected by modifiable factors, such as continued mental and social activity and a healthy diet, but the research is limited by few studies and low numbers of participants (Alzheimer's Association, 2012).

## APPLICATION OF THE NURSING PROCESS

## ASSESSMENT

### General Assessment

Alzheimer's disease is commonly characterized by progressive deterioration of cognitive functioning. Initial deterioration may be so subtle and insidious that others may not notice. In the early stages of the disease, the affected person may be able to compensate for loss of memory, sometimes even hide it. This hiding is actually a form of denial, which is an unconscious protective defence against the terrifying reality of losing one's place in the world. Family members may also unconsciously deny that anything is wrong as a defence against the painful awareness that a loved one is deteriorating. As time goes on, symptoms become more obvious, and other defence mechanisms become evident, including (1) denial, (2) confabulation (the creation of stories or answers in place of actual memories, in an attempt to maintain self-esteem; it is not the same as lying because it is done unconsciously), (3) perseveration (the repetition of phrases or behaviour), and (4) avoidance of questions. The following exchange between a nurse and a patient who has remained in a hospital bed all weekend provides an example of confabulation:

*Nurse:* Good morning, Ms. Jones. How was your weekend?

*Patient:* Wonderful. I discussed politics with the prime minister, and he took me out to dinner.

*or*

*Patient:* I spent the weekend with my daughter and her family.

Symptoms observed in AD include the following:

- Amnesia or memory impairment. Initially, the person has difficulty remembering recent events. Gradually, deterioration progresses to include both recent and remote memory.
- Aphasia (loss of language ability), which progresses with the disease. Initially, the person has difficulty finding the correct word, then is reduced to a few words, and finally is reduced to babbling or mutism.
- Apraxia, which is the loss of purposeful movement in the absence of motor or sensory impairment. The person is unable to perform once-familiar and purposeful tasks. For example, in apraxia of gait, the person loses the ability to walk. In apraxia of dressing, the person is unable to put clothes on properly (may put arms in trousers or put a jacket on upside down).
- Agnosia, which is the loss of the sensory ability to recognize objects. For example, the person may lose the ability to recognize familiar sounds (auditory agnosia), such as the ring of the telephone, a car horn, or the doorbell. Loss of this ability extends to the inability to recognize familiar objects (visual or tactile agnosia), such as a glass, magazine, pencil, or toothbrush. Eventually, people are unable to recognize loved ones or even parts of their own bodies.
- Disturbances in executive functioning (planning, organizing, abstract thinking). The degeneration of neurons in the brain results in the wasting away of the brain's working components. These cells contain memories, receive sights and sounds, cause hormones to secrete, produce emotions, and command muscles into motion.

A person with AD loses a personal history, a place in the world, and the ability to recognize the environment and, eventually, loved ones. Alzheimer's robs family and friends, husbands and wives, and sons and daughters of valuable human relatedness and companionship, which results in a profound sense of grief. It robs society of productive and active participants. Because of these devastating effects, mental health care professionals and social agencies, the medical and nursing professions, and researchers are challenged to look for possible causes and treatments.

## Diagnostic Tests

A wide range of problems may be mistaken for dementia or AD. For example, in older adults, depression and dementia may have similar symptoms. It is important that nurses and other health care providers be able to assess some of the important differences among depression, dementia, and delirium (review Table 18-1).

Other disorders that often mimic dementia include drug toxicity, metabolic disorders, infections, and nutritional deficiencies. A disorder that mimics dementia is sometimes referred to as a pseudodementia. Making a diagnosis of Alzheimer's

| BOX 18-3 | BASIC MEDICAL WORKUP FOR DEMENTIA |
| --- | --- |

- Chest and skull radiographic studies
- Electroencephalography
- Electrocardiography
- Urinalysis
- Sequential multiple analyzer 12-test serum profile
- Thyroid function tests
- Folate level
- Venereal Disease Research Laboratories (VDRL), human immunodeficiency virus tests
- Serum creatinine assay
- Electrolyte assessment
- Vitamin $B_{12}$ level
- Liver function tests
- Vision and hearing evaluation
- Neuroimaging (when diagnostic issues are not clear)

disease requires ruling out all other pathophysiological conditions through careful assessment, including medical and family history, as well as through physical and laboratory tests, many of which are identified in Box 18-3.

Brain imaging with computed tomography (CT), positron emission tomography (PET), and other developing scanning technologies have diagnostic capabilities because they reveal brain atrophy and rule out other conditions such as neoplasms. The use of mental status questionnaires, such as the Mini–Mental State Examination and various other tests to identify deterioration in mental status and brain damage, is an important part of the assessment.

In addition to performing a thorough physical and neurological examination, it is important to obtain a complete medical and psychiatric history, a description of recent symptoms, a review of medications used, and a nutritional evaluation. The observations and history provided by family members are invaluable to the assessment process.

As mentioned, depression in the older adult is the disorder most frequently confused with dementia. Medical and nursing personnel should be cautioned, however, that dementia and depression or dementia and delirium can coexist. In fact, studies indicate that many people diagnosed with Alzheimer's dementia also meet the *DSM-5* criteria for a depressive disorder.

## Stages of Alzheimer's Disease

Differing classification systems exist for the stages of the Alzheimer's subtype of neurocognitive disorder. Recently, the Alzheimer's Association and the National Institute on Aging (Alzheimer's Association, 2012) have proposed revisions from the current seven-stage classification. The recommendations are that AD be identified in three stages: preclinical AD, mild cognitive impairment (MCI) due to AD, and dementia due to AD. The first stage occurs prior to any symptoms and is identified through AD biomarkers, such as β-amyloid and tau; at present, further scientific evidence about biomarkers is needed before use in the clinical setting.

## TABLE 18-5   STAGES OF ALZHEIMER'S DISEASE

| STAGE | HALLMARKS |
|---|---|
| **Stage 1**<br>*No impairment* | • No memory problems |
| **Stage 2**<br>*Very mild cognitive decline (may be age-related or due to dementia)* | • Aware of memory lapses<br>• Forgetting familiar words or the location of everyday objects<br>• No symptoms of dementia can be detected during a medical examination or by friends, family, or co-workers |
| **Stage 3**<br>*Mild cognitive decline (early-stage Alzheimer's can be diagnosed in some, but not all, individuals with these symptoms)* | • Others begin to notice difficulties.<br>• Noticeable problems coming up with the right word or name<br>• Trouble remembering names when introduced to new people<br>• Noticeable difficulty performing tasks in social or work settings<br>• Forgetting material that one has just read<br>• Losing or misplacing a valuable object<br>• Increasing trouble with planning or organizing |
| **Stage 4**<br>*Moderate cognitive decline (mild or early-stage Alzheimer's disease)* | • Forgetfulness of recent events<br>• Impaired ability to perform challenging mental arithmetic<br>• Difficulty performing complex tasks, such as planning dinner for guests, paying bills, or managing finances<br>• Becoming moody or withdrawn, especially in socially or mentally challenging situations |
| **Stage 5**<br>*Moderately severe cognitive decline (moderate or mid-stage Alzheimer's disease)* | • Gaps in memory and thinking are noticeable, and individuals begin to need help with day-to-day activities.<br>• At this stage, individuals may:<br>  • Be unable to recall their own address or telephone number or the high school or college from which they graduated<br>  • Become confused about where they are or what day it is<br>  • Have trouble with less challenging mental arithmetic<br>  • Need help choosing proper clothing for the season or the occasion<br>  • Still remember significant details about themselves and their family<br>  • Still require no assistance with eating or using the toilet |
| **Stage 6**<br>*Severe cognitive decline (moderately severe or mid-stage Alzheimer's disease)* | • Personality changes may take place and individual needs extensive help with daily activities.<br>• At this stage, individuals may:<br>  • Lose awareness of recent experiences as well as of their surroundings<br>  • Remember their own name but have difficulty with their personal history<br>  • Distinguish familiar and unfamiliar faces but have trouble remembering the name of a spouse or caregiver<br>  • Need help dressing properly and may, without supervision, make mistakes such as putting pyjamas over daytime clothes or shoes on the wrong feet<br>  • Experience major changes in sleep patterns—sleeping during the day and becoming restless at night<br>  • Need help handling details of toileting<br>  • Have increasingly frequent trouble controlling their bladder or bowels<br>  • Experience major behavioural changes, including suspiciousness and delusions or compulsive, repetitive behaviour<br>  • Tend to wander or become lost |
| **Stage 7**<br>*Very severe cognitive decline (severe or late-stage Alzheimer's disease)* | • Loss of ability to respond to the environment, to carry on a conversation, and, eventually, to control movement<br>• May still say words or phrases<br>• Needs help with daily personal care, including eating or using the toilet<br>• May also lose the ability to smile, to sit without support, and to hold the head up.<br>• Reflexes become abnormal, muscles grow rigid, and swallowing is impaired |

**Source:** Adapted from Alzheimer's Association. (n.d.). *Seven stages of Alzheimer's*. Retrieved from http://www.alz.org/alzheimers_disease_stages_of_alzheimers.asp.

The proposed second and third stages correspond to the *DSM-5* criteria for mild and major neurocognitive disorders (ND), the major differentiation of which is how much the disease is disrupting functional daily living. In relation to the seven stages outlined in Table 18-5, stage 1 relates to the pre-clinical stage, stages 3 and 4 to MCI (mild ND), while stages 5 to 7 are consistent with dementia due to AD (major ND). Table 18-5 can be used as a guide as we review the seven stages of AD and highlight the deficits associated with each stage.

## Mild Cognitive Impairment due to AD

The loss of intellectual ability is insidious. The person with mild AD loses energy, drive, and initiative and has difficulty learning new things. Because personality and social behaviour remain intact, others tend to minimize and underestimate the loss of the individual's abilities. The individual may still continue to work, but the extent of the dementia becomes evident in new or demanding situations. Depression may occur early in the disease but usually lessens as the disease progresses.

---

**VIGNETTE**

Mrs. Wakulak, 78 years old, a retired schoolteacher, has always enjoyed an active life and good health, other than an overactive thyroid, which has been successfully treated and controlled. Remarkably, her only hospitalizations were for the births of her two children, now grown and married. She is a vibrant person who takes enormous pride in her appearance and in her beautifully clean home. She is beginning to forget things that she previously has taken for granted but jokes about her failing memory as "senior moments."

During a recent visit, her daughter found Mrs. Wakulak quite distressed while in the kitchen. Mrs. Wakulak was attempting to make dinner for family guests and planned on her famous specialty, perogies. The ingredients were strewn all over the kitchen, and Mrs. Wakulak was frantically searching for a recipe. Her daughter was quite taken aback as neither of them had ever used a written recipe. Her daughter managed to settle Mrs. Wakulak and helped by giving step-by-step instructions in the construction of the perogies. Quietly, she was quite worried about her mother's failing memory, fearing that it was more than usual aging. Her daughter tried to broach the subject with her dad, a loving and loyal companion to Mrs. Wakulak. When she shared her concerns, his reply was simply, "I don't know what you are talking about." Clearly, he was not able to admit what was becoming obvious to others.

The situation reached a crisis point when her daughter discovered that Mrs. Wakulak was no longer taking her thyroid medications because she was confused between them and a calcium-sparing medication. Mrs. Wakulak had taken medication for her thyroid for 30 years, and yet she could not remember it now. This change signalled a progression in her condition.

It was painful, but her husband, too, began to realize that Mrs. Wakulak was not functioning. Her once clean house was dirty and in a state of disarray. She no longer could coordinate her clothing and often wore the same outfit for a number of days because she became overwhelmed by having to make a clothing choice, and, often, her clothes were dirty and her makeup was applied in a haphazard manner.

---

## Dementia due to AD

As AD progresses, the person often becomes unable to identify familiar objects or people, even a spouse (*agnosia*), and needs repeated instructions and directions to perform the simplest tasks (*apraxia*): "Here is the face cloth. Pick up the soap. Now, put water on the face cloth and rub the face cloth with the soap." Often, the individual cannot remember where the toilet is and becomes incontinent. Total care is necessary at this point, and the burden on the family can be emotionally, financially, and physically devastating. The world is very frightening to the person with AD because nothing makes sense any longer. Agitation, violence, paranoia, and delusions are commonly seen. Another problem that is frightening to family members and caregivers is wandering behaviour.

Late in AD, the following symptoms may occur: agraphia (inability to write), alexia (inability to read), hyperorality (the need to taste and chew, resulting in putting everything in one's mouth), blunting of emotions, visual agnosia (loss of ability to recognize familiar objects), and hypermetamorphosis (manifested by touching of everything in sight).

---

**VIGNETTE**

Mrs. Wakulak no longer was able to participate in or enjoy previous activities such as reading the newspaper and watching the morning news shows. She would stare at both the paper and television, attempting to understand but unable to retain any information. She was often restless during the day, going from one random activity to another, often rearranging her favourite knick-knacks in her curio cupboard. She would attempt to wash clothes but forget to put laundry detergent in the machine. She would empty half-filled drinking glasses into the gas range top in her kitchen. If these mistakes were pointed out, she would become defensive and angry, stating, "I have always done it this way."

Eating became difficult as she did not seem to recognize food on her plate, and she was unable to use a knife and fork to cut her food. Sometimes, she would pick up a spoon and ask what it was. Her weight began to decrease.

While Mrs. Wakulak had always slept well throughout her adult life, she began to wander around in the middle of the night, often waking her husband to ask him questions. She would go to the kitchen and empty the cupboards for no apparent reason. She would enter her wardrobe and rearrange her clothing, often leaving items lying on the floor.

When she set paper towels alight by leaving them on the gas range and then lighting it, her family and husband realized that she could no longer function safely at home. Her husband was unable to leave her alone, even for short periods of time because she would be become extremely distressed, almost to the point of panic. She and her husband moved into an assisted-living facility.

---

## Self-Assessment

Working with cognitively impaired people in any setting places a tremendous amount of responsibility on caregivers. The behavioural problems people with dementia may display can cause stress for professionals and family caregivers alike.

Nurses working in facilities designed for people who are cognitively impaired (e.g., assisted-living, supported-living, long-term care, extended care facilities) need special education and skills. Education must include information about the process of the disease and effective interventions, as well as knowledge regarding antipsychotic drugs. Support and educational opportunities should be readily available, not just to nurses but also to nursing aides, who are often directly responsible for administering basic care.

Because stress is common among those working with patients with cognitive impairments, staff need to be proactive in minimizing its effects through the use of the following strategies:

- Having a clear understanding of the disease so that expectations for the person are realistic
- Establishing realistic outcomes (perhaps as minor as *Patient feeds self with spoon*) for the person and recognizing when they are achieved, remembering that even the smallest achievement can be a significant accomplishment for the impaired individual
- Maintaining good self-care and protecting ourselves from the negative effects of stress by obtaining adequate sleep and rest, eating a nutritious diet, exercising, engaging in relaxing activities, and addressing our own emotional and spiritual needs

### 📋 ASSESSMENT GUIDELINES

**Dementia**

1. Evaluate the person's current level of cognitive and daily functioning.
2. Identify any threats to the person's safety and security and arrange their reduction.
3. Evaluate the safety of the person's home environment (e.g., with regard to wandering, eating inedible objects, falling, engaging in provocative behaviours toward others).
4. Review the medications (including herbs and complementary agents) the person is currently taking.
5. Interview family to gain a complete picture of the person's background and personality.
6. Explore how well the family is prepared for and informed about the progress of dementia, depending on cause (if known).
7. Discuss with the family members how they are coping with the requirements of caregiving and what their main issues are at this time.
8. Review the resources available to the family. Ask family members to describe the help they receive from other family members, friends, and community resources. Determine if caregivers are aware of community support groups and resources.
9. Identify the needs of the family for teaching and guidance—for example, how to manage catastrophic reactions (overreactions to a seemingly normal, non-threatening situation commonly experienced in AD), lability of mood, aggressive behaviours, and sundowning.

## DIAGNOSIS

Caring for a person with dementia requires a great deal of patience, creativity, and maturity. The needs of such a person can be enormous for nursing staff and for families who care for their loved ones in the home. As the disease progresses, so do the needs of the person and the demands on the caregivers, staff, and family.

One of the most important areas of concern identified by both staff and families is safety. Many people with AD wander and may be lost for hours or days. Wandering, along with behaviours such as rummaging, may be perceived as purposeful to the person with AD. Wandering may result from changes in the physical environment, fear caused by hallucinations or delusions, or lack of exercise.

Seizures are common in the later stages of this disease. Injuries from falls and accidents can occur during any stage as confusion and disorientation progress. The potential for burns exists if the person is a smoker or is unattended when using the stove. Prescription drugs can be taken incorrectly, or bottles of noxious fluids can be mistakenly ingested, resulting in a medical crisis. Therefore, *Risk for injury* is always present.

As the person's ability to recognize or name objects decreases, *Impaired verbal communication* becomes a problem. As memory diminishes and disorientation increases, *Impaired environmental interpretation syndrome*, *Impaired memory*, and *Confusion* occur.

Additional family issues may emerge. Perhaps some of the most crucial aspects of caregiving are support, education, and referrals for the family. The family loses an integral part of its unit, as well as the love, the function, the support, the companionship, and the warmth that this person once provided. *Caregiver role strain* is always present, and planning with the family and arranging community supports are vital parts of appropriate care. *Anticipatory grieving* is also an important phenomenon to assess and may be a significant target for intervention. Helping the family grieve can make the task ahead somewhat clearer (Gibson, 2009). Review Table 18-2 for potential nursing diagnoses for confused patients.

## OUTCOMES IDENTIFICATION

Families who have a member with dementia face an exhaustive list of issues that need to be addressed. Table 18-6 provides a checklist that may help nurses and families identify areas for intervention. Self-care needs, impaired environmental interpretation, chronic confusion, ineffective individual coping, and caregiver role strain are just a few of the areas nurses and other health care providers will need to target (Box 18-4).

## PLANNING

Planning care for a person with dementia is geared toward the person's immediate needs. Refer to Table 18-6 for help in identifying potential areas of care. The Functional Dementia Scale (Figure 18-1) can be used by nurses and families to plan

## TABLE 18-6  PROBLEMS THAT MAY AFFECT PEOPLE WITH DEMENTIA AND THEIR FAMILIES

| PROBLEM | EXAMPLES | PROBLEM | EXAMPLES |
|---|---|---|---|
| Memory impairment | Forgets appointments, visits, etc. Forgets to change clothes, wash, go to the toilet Forgets to eat, take medications Loses things | Uncontrolled behaviour | Restlessness day or night Vulgar table or toilet habits Undressing Sexual disinhibition Shoplifting |
| Disorientation | Time: mixes night and day, mixes days of appointments, wears summer clothes in winter, forgets age Place: loses way around house Person: has difficulty recognizing visitors, family, spouse | Incontinence | Urine Feces Urination or defecation in the wrong place |
| Need for physical help | Dressing Washing, bathing Toileting Eating Performing housework Maintaining mobility | Emotional reactions | Catastrophic reactions Demands for attention Depression Distress and anxiety Frustration and anger Embarrassment and withdrawal Lack of emotional control |
| Risks in the home | Falls Fire from cigarettes, cooking, heating Flooding Admission of strangers to home Wandering out | Other reactions | Suspiciousness Hoarding and hiding |
| Risks outside the home | Competence, judgement, and risks at work Driving, road sense Getting lost | Mistaken beliefs | Still at work Parents or spouse still alive Hallucinations |
| Apathy | Little conversation Lack of interest Poor self-care | Decision making | Indecisive Easily influenced Refuses help Makes unwise decisions |
| Poor communication | Aphasia | Burden on family | Disruption of social life Distress, guilt, rejection Family discord |
| Repetitiveness | Repetition of questions or stories Repetition of actions | | |

strategies for addressing immediate needs and to track progression of the dementia. The Cognitive Performance Scale, derived from the interRAI assessments, which reflect memory, decision-making skills, communication, and eating, can also be used as a tool to track the progression of dementia (Canadian Institute for Health Information, 2010).

Identifying a patient's level of functioning and assessing caregivers' needs help health care providers focus planning and identify appropriate community resources. Does the patient or family need the following?

- Transportation services
- Supervision and care when primary caregiver is out of the home
- Referrals to adult day programs
- Information on support groups within the community
- Meals on Wheels
- Information on respite and residential services
- Telephone numbers for helplines
- Home health aides
- Home care services
- Additional psychopharmaceuticals to manage distressing or harmful behaviours

## IMPLEMENTATION

The attitude of unconditional positive regard is the nurse's single most effective tool in caring for people with dementia. Positive regard induces patients to cooperate, reduces catastrophic outbreaks, and increases family members' satisfaction with the care provided. Box 18-5 lists *NIC* interventions related to the management of dementia.

A considerable number of individuals with dementia have secondary behavioural disturbances, including depression, hallucinations, delusions, agitation, insomnia, and wandering. Because these symptoms impair the person's ability to function, increase the need for supervision, and influence the need for institutionalization, the control of these symptoms is a priority in managing AD. Helping the individual achieve the highest

---

### BOX 18-4   *NOC* OUTCOMES RELATED TO DEMENTIA*

**Injury**
- Person will remain safe in the hospital or at home.
- With the aid of an identification bracelet and neighbourhood or hospital alert, the person will be returned within one hour of wandering.
- With the aid of interventions, person will remain burn free.
- With the aid of guidance and environmental manipulation, person will not hurt himself or herself if a fall occurs.
- Person will ingest only correct doses of prescribed medications and appropriate food and fluids.

**Communication**
- Person will communicate needs.
- Person will state needs in alternative modes when he or she is aphasic (e.g., will signal correct word on hearing it or will refer to picture or label).
- Person will wear prescribed glasses or hearing aid each day.

**Agitation Level**
- Person will have rest periods if pacing and restless.
- Person will cooperate with caregiving activities.
- Person will experience minimal frustrating experiences.
- Person will express frustrations in an appropriate manner.

**Caregiver Role Strain**
- Family members will have the opportunity to express "unacceptable" feelings in a supportive environment.

- Family members will have access to professional counselling.
- Family members will name two organizations within their geographical area that can offer emotional support and help with legal and financial burdens.
- Family members will participate in ill member's plan of care, with encouragement from staff.
- Family members will state that they have outside help that allows them to take personal time for themselves each week or month.

**Impaired Environmental Interpretation: Chronic Confusion**
- Person will acknowledge the reality of an object or a sound that was misinterpreted (illusion), after it is pointed out.
- Person will state that he or she feels safe after experiencing delusions or illusions.
- Person will remain nonaggressive when experiencing paranoid ideation.

**Self-Care Needs**
- Person will participate in self-care at optimal level.
- Person will be able to follow step-by-step instructions for dressing, bathing, and grooming.
- Person will put on own clothes appropriately, with aid of fastening tape (Velcro) and nursing supervision.
- Person's skin will remain intact and free from signs of pressure.

*Partial list.
**Source:** From Moorhead, S., Johnson, M., Maas, M.L., et al. (2012). *Nursing outcomes classification (NOC)* (4th ed.). St. Louis, MO: Mosby.

---

### FUNCTIONAL DEMENTIA SCALE

Circle one rating for each item:
1. None or little of the time
2. Some of the time
3. Good part of the time
4. Most or all of the time

Client: _____
Observer: _____
Position or relation to patient: _____
Facility: _____
Date: _____

| | | | | |
|---|---|---|---|---|
| 1 | 2 | 3 | 4 | 1. Has difficulty in completing simple tasks on own (e.g., dressing, bathing, doing arithmetic). |
| 1 | 2 | 3 | 4 | 2. Spends time either sitting or in apparently purposeless activity. |
| 1 | 2 | 3 | 4 | 3. Wanders at night or needs to be restrained to prevent wandering. |
| 1 | 2 | 3 | 4 | 4. Hears things that are not there. |
| 1 | 2 | 3 | 4 | 5. Requires supervision or assistance in eating. |
| 1 | 2 | 3 | 4 | 6. Loses things. |
| 1 | 2 | 3 | 4 | 7. Appearance is disorderly if left to own devices. |
| 1 | 2 | 3 | 4 | 8. Moans. |
| 1 | 2 | 3 | 4 | 9. Cannot control bowel function. |
| 1 | 2 | 3 | 4 | 10. Threatens to harm others. |
| 1 | 2 | 3 | 4 | 11. Cannot control bladder function. |
| 1 | 2 | 3 | 4 | 12. Needs to be watched so doesn't injure self (e.g., by careless smoking, leaving the stove on, falling). |
| 1 | 2 | 3 | 4 | 13. Destructive of materials around him/her (e.g., breaks furniture, throws food trays, tears up magazines). |
| 1 | 2 | 3 | 4 | 14. Shouts or yells. |
| 1 | 2 | 3 | 4 | 15. Accuses others of doing bodily harm or stealing his or her possessions — when you are sure the accusations are not true. |
| 1 | 2 | 3 | 4 | 16. Is unaware of limitations imposed by illness. |
| 1 | 2 | 3 | 4 | 17. Becomes confused and does not know where he or she is. |
| 1 | 2 | 3 | 4 | 18. Has trouble remembering. |
| 1 | 2 | 3 | 4 | 19. Has sudden changes of mood (e.g., gets upset, angered, or cries easily). |
| 1 | 2 | 3 | 4 | 20. If left alone, wanders aimlessly during the day or needs to be restrained to prevent wandering. |

**FIGURE 18-1** Functional Dementia Scale. **Source:** Moore, J.T., Bobula, J.A., Short, T.B., et al. (1983). A functional dementia scale. *Journal of Family Practice, 16*(3), 499–503.

## BOX 18-5 *NIC* INTERVENTIONS FOR DEMENTIA MANAGEMENT

Definition of *dementia management:* Provision of a modified environment for the patient who is experiencing a chronic confusional state.

Activities:

- Include family members in planning, providing, and evaluating care, to the extent desired by the patient and family.
- Identify usual patterns of behaviour for such activities as sleep, medication use, elimination, food intake, and self-care.
- Determine physical, social, and psychological history of patient, usual habits, and routines.
- Determine type and extent of cognitive deficit(s), using standardized assessment tool.
- Monitor cognitive functioning, using standardized assessment tool.
- Determine behavioural expectations appropriate for patient's cognitive status.
- Provide a low-stimulation environment (e.g., quiet, soothing music; nonvivid and simple decor with familiar patterns; performance expectations that do not exceed cognitive processing ability; dining in small groups).
- Provide adequate but nonglare lighting.
- Identify and remove potential dangers for patient in environment.
- Place identification bracelet on patient.
- Provide a consistent physical environment and daily routine.
- Prepare for interaction with eye contact and touch, as appropriate.
- Introduce self when initiating contact.
- Address patient distinctly by name when initiating interaction, and speak slowly.
- Give one simple direction at a time.
- Speak in a clear, low, warm, respectful tone of voice.
- Use distraction, rather than confrontation, to manage behaviour.
- Provide unconditional positive regard.
- Avoid touch and proximity if they cause stress or anxiety.
- Provide caregivers who are familiar to the patient (e.g., avoid frequent rotations of staff assignments).
- Avoid unfamiliar situations when possible (e.g., room changes and appointments without familiar people present).
- Provide rest periods to prevent fatigue and reduce stress.
- Monitor nutrition and weight.
- Provide space for safe pacing and wandering.
- Avoid frustrating patient by quizzing with orientation questions that cannot be answered.
- Provide cues—such as current events, seasons, location, and names—to assist orientation.
- Seat patient at a small table in groups of three to five for meals, as appropriate.
- Allow patient to eat alone if appropriate.
- Provide finger foods to maintain nutrition for patient who will not sit and eat.
- Provide patient a general orientation to the season of the year by using appropriate cues (e.g., holiday decorations; seasonal decorations and activities; access to contained, outdoor area).
- Decrease noise levels by avoiding paging systems and call lights that ring or buzz.
- Select television or radio programs based on cognitive processing abilities and interests.
- Select one-to-one and group activities geared to patient's cognitive abilities and interests.
- Label familiar photos with names of the individuals in the photos.
- Select artwork for patient's rooms featuring landscapes, scenery, or other familiar images.
- Ask family members and friends to see patient one or two at a time, if needed, to reduce stimulation.
- Discuss with family members and friends how best to interact with patient.
- Assist family to understand that it may be impossible for patient to learn new material.
- Limit number of choices patient has to make so as not to cause anxiety.
- Provide boundaries, such as red or yellow tape on the floor when low-stimulus units are not available.
- Place patient's name in large block letters in room and on clothing, as needed.
- Use symbols, rather than written signs, to assist patient in locating room, bathroom, or other area.
- Monitor carefully for physiological causes of increased confusion that may be acute and reversible.
- Remove or cover mirrors if patient is frightened or agitated by them.
- Discuss home safety issues and interventions.

**Source:** Bulechek, G.M., Butcher, H.K., Dochterman, J.M., et al. (2012). *Nursing interventions classification (NIC)* (6th ed.). St. Louis, MO: Mosby.

possible level of independence and function is the foundation of care.

But intervention with family members is also critical. The effects of losing a family member to dementia—that is, watching the deterioration of a person who has had an important role within the family unit and who is loved and is a vital part of his or her family's history—can be devastating. The following interventions are useful: counselling, health teaching, community supports, family support, and pharmacological interventions and integrative therapies.

### Counselling and Communication Techniques

How one chooses to communicate with a person with dementia affects that person's ability to maintain self-esteem and his or

her ability to participate in care. People with dementia often find it difficult to express themselves. Potential reasons for this difficulty are listed below.

- Cannot find the right words
- Invent new words to describe things
- Frequently lose their train of thought
- Rely on nonverbal gestures

The following Guidelines for Communication box provides special guidelines for nurses, family members, and other caregivers to use in communicating with a cognitively impaired person.

### Health Teaching and Health Promotion

Educating families who have a cognitively impaired member is one of the most important health-teaching duties nurses

**GUIDELINES FOR COMMUNICATION**

*With People With Dementia*

| INTERVENTION | RATIONALE |
|---|---|
| Always identify yourself and call the person by name at each meeting. | The person's short-term memory is impaired—requires frequent orientation to time and environment. |
| Speak slowly. | The person needs time to process information. |
| Use short, simple words and phrases. | The person may not be able to understand complex statements or abstract ideas. |
| Maintain face-to-face contact. | Verbal and nonverbal clues are maximized. |
| Be near the person when talking, one or two arm-lengths away. | This distance can help the person focus on the speaker while maintaining personal space. |
| Focus on one piece of information at a time. | Attention span of the person is poor, and the person is easily distracted—bite-sized information helps the person focus. Too much data can be overwhelming and can increase anxiety. |
| Talk with the person about familiar and meaningful things. | Self-expression is promoted, and reality is reinforced. |
| Encourage reminiscing about happy times in life. | Remembering accomplishments and shared joys helps distract the person from deficit and gives meaning to existence. |
| When the person is delusional, acknowledge the person's feelings and reinforce reality. Do not argue or refute delusions. | Acknowledging feelings helps the person feel understood. Pointing out realities may help the person focus on realities. Arguing can enhance adherence to false beliefs. |
| If the person gets into an argument with another person, stop the argument and temporarily separate those involved. After a short while (five minutes), explain to each person matter-of-factly why you had to intervene. | Escalation to physical acting out is prevented. The person's right to know is respected. Explaining in an adult manner helps maintain self-esteem. |
| When the person becomes verbally aggressive, acknowledge the person's feelings, and shift the topic to more familiar ground (e.g., "I know this is upsetting for you, because you always cared for others. Tell me about your children.") | Confusion and disorientation easily increase anxiety. Acknowledging feelings makes the person feel more understood and less alone. Topics the person has mastery over can remind him or her of areas of competent functioning and can increase self-esteem. |
| Have the person wear prescription glasses or hearing aid(s). | Environmental awareness, orientation, and comprehension are increased, which in turn increase awareness of personal needs and the presence of others. |
| Keep the person's room well lit. | Environmental clues are maximized. |
| Have clocks, calendars, and personal items (e.g., family pictures, meaningful books) in clear view of the person while he or she is in bed. | These objects assist in maintaining personal identity. |
| Reinforce the person's pictures, nonverbal gestures, Xs on calendars, and other methods used to anchor the person in reality. | When aphasia starts to hinder communication, alternative methods of communication need to be instituted. |

**Source:** Data from Bulechek, G.M., Butcher, H.K., Dochterman, J.M., et al. (2012). *Nursing interventions classification (NIC)* (6th ed.). St. Louis, MO: Mosby.

encounter. Families who are caring for a member in the home need to know about strategies for communicating and for structuring self-care activities (see Patient and Family Teaching: Guidelines for Self-Care in Dementia).

Most important, families need to know where to get help. Help includes professional counselling and education regarding the process and progression of the disease. Families especially need to know about and be referred to community-based groups that can help shoulder this burden (e.g., adult support programs, senior citizen groups, organizations providing home visits and respite care, family support groups). A list with definitions of some of the types of services available in the person's

community, as well as the names and telephone numbers of the providers of these services, should be given to the family.

### Referral to Community Supports

The Alzheimer Society of Canada is a national umbrella agency that provides various forms of assistance to people with the disease and their families. The society offers educational resources on Alzheimer's disease and related dementias, guidelines for providing quality care, ethical guidelines to help people address sensitive issues, and information and referrals for support programs and services, some of which may help prevent total emotional and physical fatigue in

## PATIENT AND FAMILY TEACHING

### Guidelines for Self-Care in Dementia

| INTERVENTION | RATIONALE |
| --- | --- |
| **Dressing and Bathing** | |
| Always have the person perform all tasks within his or her present capacity. | Maintains the person's self-esteem and uses muscle groups<br>Impedes staff burnout<br>Minimizes further regression |
| Always have the person wear own clothes, even if in the hospital. | Helps maintain the person's identity and dignity |
| Use clothing with elastic, and substitute fastening tape (Velcro) for buttons and zippers. | Minimizes the person's confusion<br>Eases independence of functioning |
| Label clothing items with the person's name and name of item. | Helps identify the person if he or she wanders<br>Gives the person additional clues when aphasia or agnosia occurs |
| Give step-by-step instructions whenever necessary (e.g., "Take this blouse. Put in one arm ... now the other arm. Pull it together in front. Now ...") | Uses the person's ability to focus on small pieces of information more easily<br>Allows the person to perform at optimal level |
| Make sure that water in faucets is not too hot. | Ensures safety in person who is lacking judgement or is unaware of many safety hazards |
| If the person is resistant to performing self-care, come back later and ask again. | Respects that the person's moods may be labile—the person often complies after a short interval |
| **Nutrition** | |
| Monitor food and fluid intake. | Helps to prevent anorexia or refusal to eat because of confusion |
| Offer finger food that the person can take away from the dinner table. | Increases intake throughout the day—the person may eat only small amounts at meals |
| Weigh the person regularly (once a week). | Monitors fluid and nutritional status |
| During periods of hyperorality, watch that the person does not eat nonfood items (e.g., ceramic fruit or food-shaped soaps). | Ensures safety of the person who puts everything into mouth or who is unable to differentiate inedible objects made in the shape and colour of food |
| **Bowel and Bladder Function** | |
| Begin bowel and bladder program early; start with bladder control. | Helps prevent incontinence by establishing same time of day for bowel movements and toileting—in early morning, after meals and snacks, and before bedtime |
| Evaluate use of disposable incontinence products. | Prevents embarrassment |
| Label bathroom door, as well as doors to other rooms. | Maximizes independent toileting by offering additional environmental clues |
| **Sleep** | |
| Because the person may awaken, be frightened, or cry out at night, keep area well lit. | Reinforces orientation<br>Minimizes possible illusions |
| Maintain a calm atmosphere during the day. | Encourages a calming night's sleep |
| Order nonbarbiturates (e.g., chloral hydrate) if necessary. | Avoids paradoxical reaction of agitation, often caused by barbiturates |
| If medications are indicated, consider neuroleptics with sedative properties, which may be the most helpful (e.g., haloperidol [Haldol]). | Helps clear thinking<br>Sedates |
| Avoid the use of restraints. | Avoids inciting fear in the person, who may fight against restraints until exhausted to a dangerous degree |

caregivers. In partnership with the Royal Canadian Mounted Police, the Alzheimer Society of Canada also has developed the Safely Home registry, a national registry to help find lost Alzheimer's patients and assist them in returning home (Alzheimer Society of Canada, 2011). More information about this registry can found on the Alzheimer Society of Canada's Web site: http://www.alzheimer.ca/en. The support programs and services available from the Alzheimer Society vary from community to community; examples of services it provides are found in Table 18-7.

Although many families manage the care of their loved one until death, other families eventually find that they can no

| TABLE 18-7 | **TYPES OF SERVICES THAT MAY BE AVAILABLE TO PEOPLE WITH DEMENTIA** |
|---|---|
| **TYPE OF SERVICE** | **SERVICES PROVIDED** |
| **Family/caregiver** | Caregivers have a right to:<br>Easy access to services<br>Respite care<br>Full involvement in decision making<br>Assessment of the needs of both the caregiver and the person with dementia<br>Information and referral<br>Case management: coordination of community resources and follow-up |
| **Community services** | Adult support programs: provide activities, socialization, and supervision in an outpatient setting<br>Physician services<br>Protective services: prevent, eliminate, or remedy effects of abuse or neglect<br>Recreational services<br>Transportation<br>Mental health services<br>Legal services |
| **Home care** | Meals on Wheels<br>Home health aide services<br>Homemaker services<br>Respite services<br>Occupational therapy<br>Paid companion or sitter services<br>Physiotherapy<br>Skilled nursing care<br>Personal care services: assistance in basic self-care activities<br>Social work services<br>Telephone reassurance: regular telephone calls to individuals who are isolated and homebound*<br>Personal emergency response systems: telephone-based systems to alert others that a person who is alone is in need of emergency assistance* |

*Vital for those living alone.

longer deal with the labile and aggressive behaviour, incontinence, wandering, unsafe habits, or disruptive nocturnal activity. Family members need to know where and how to place their loved one for care if such a move becomes necessary. Families need information, support, and legal and financial guidance at this time. When the nurse is unable to provide the relevant information, proper referrals by the social worker are needed. Information regarding advance directives, durable power of attorney, and guardianship should be included in the communication with the family. The following Patient and Family Teaching box provides useful guidelines for families for structuring a safe environment and planning appropriate activities.

## Pharmacological Interventions

There is currently no cure for Alzheimer's disease. There are, however, four drugs approved by Health Canada that slow the progression of the illness (Raina, Santaguida, Ismaila, et al., 2008). Since a deficiency of acetylcholine has been linked to AD, medications aimed at preventing its breakdown (cholinesterase inhibitors) have been developed, including donepezil (Aricept), rivastigmine (Exelon), and galantamine (Reminyl). Memantine (Ebixa) normalizes levels of glutamate, a neurotransmitter that may contribute to neurodegeneration (Wright, Trinh, Blacker, et al., 2008). Although these medications are used widely and have been shown to have statistically significant effects when compared to placebos, it seems that they produce only a clinically marginal effect on cognition, behaviour, or quality of life (Raina, Santaguida, Ismaila, et al., 2008). Nonetheless, they do delay the cognitive progression of dementia and assist with some of the behavioural symptoms.

Some of the troubling behaviours exhibited by people with dementia, with which their caregivers must cope, are psychotic symptoms (hallucinations, paranoia), severe mood swings (depression is very common), anxiety (agitation), and irritability and anger (verbal or physical aggression). Often, medications are useful in managing these sorts of symptoms, but such medications need to be used with extreme caution. The rule of thumb when using pharmacological measures with older adults is "start low and go slow." In addition, because people with dementia are at high risk for delirium, adding medications to their regimen should always be done with caution. Note that in 2005, Health Canada warned that the use of atypical antipsychotics is no longer indicated for dementia-related psychosis, because they are associated with increased risk of death (Health Canada, 2005).

The Drug Treatment box on page 364 presents drugs used in Canada to treat AD and its related psychological symptoms.

Of clinical relevance to nurses is evidence that suggests that personalized nursing care, in which the idiosyncratic needs of the person are recognized and met, is effective as a nonpharmacological treatment for many symptoms associated with dementia (Ayalon, Gunn, Feliciano, et al., 2006). With this evidence in mind, nurses should try to decipher patients' needs as expressed in their behaviour since people with dementia do not always communicate their needs verbally.

### An Overview of Drugs Approved for Treatment of AD

***Donepezil (Aricept).*** This drug was approved by Health Canada in 1997. It inhibits acetylcholine breakdown and also appears to slow down deterioration in cognitive functions. Donepezil is the drug of choice for AD because of its once per day dosing and fewer adverse effects (Lehne, 2013). In studies of donepezil, some individuals with AD did experience diarrhea and nausea while taking the drug.

***Rivastigmine (Exelon).*** This drug was approved by Health Canada in 2000. It is a brain-selective acetylcholinesterase inhibitor. Its most common adverse effects are nausea, vomiting, loss of appetite, and weight loss. In most cases, these effects are temporary (Apotex, 2009). Rivastigmine should always be taken with food to reduce gastrointestinal adverse effects.

## PATIENT AND FAMILY TEACHING
### Guidelines for Care at Home

| INTERVENTION | RATIONALE |
| --- | --- |
| **Safe Environment** | |
| Gradually restrict use of the car. | Ensures safety as the person's judgement becomes impaired |
| Remove throw rugs and other objects in person's path. | Minimizes tripping and falling |
| Minimize sensory stimulation. | Decreases sensory overload, which can increase anxiety and confusion |
| If the person becomes verbally upset, listen briefly, give support, and then change the topic. | Aims to prevent escalation of anger |
| | Distracts person to more productive topics and activities |
| Label all rooms and drawers. Label often-used objects (e.g., hairbrushes, toothbrushes). | May keep the person from wandering into other people's rooms |
| | Increases environmental clues to familiar objects |
| Install safety bars in bathroom. | Prevents falls |
| Supervise the person when he or she smokes. | Minimizes danger of burns |
| If the person has history of seizures, keep padded tongue blades at beside. Educate family on how to deal with seizures. | Ensures safety—seizure activity is common in advanced Alzheimer's disease |
| **Wandering** | |
| If the person wanders during the night, put his or her mattress on the floor. | Prevents falls when the person is confused. |
| Have the person wear medical alert bracelet that cannot be removed (with name, address, and telephone number). | Ensures easy identification by police, neighbours, or hospital personnel |
| Provide police department with recent pictures. | |
| Alert local police and neighbours about wanderer. | May reduce time necessary to return the person to home or hospital |
| If the person is in hospital, have him or her wear brightly coloured vest with name, unit, and phone number printed on back. | Makes the person easily identifiable |
| Put complex locks on door. | Reduces opportunity to wander |
| Place locks at top of door. | Ensures safety—in moderate and late Alzheimer's-type dementia, ability to look up and reach upward is lost |
| Encourage physical activity during the day. | May decrease wandering at night |
| Explore the feasibility of installing sensor devices. | Provides warning if the person wanders |
| **Useful Activities** | |
| Provide picture magazines and children's books when the person's reading ability diminishes. | Allows continuation of usual activities that the person can still enjoy |
| | Provides focus |
| Provide simple activities that allow exercise of large muscles. | Provides socialization (e.g., exercise groups, dance groups, walking groups) |
| | Increases circulation and maintains muscle tone |
| Encourage group activities that are familiar and simple to perform. | Increases socialization (e.g., activities such as group singing, dancing, reminiscing, working with clay and paint) |
| | Minimizes feelings of alienation |

**Galantamine (Reminyl).** This drug was approved by Health Canada in 2005. It is a reversible cholinesterase inhibitor that acts by inhibiting the protein cholinesterase, which breaks down acetylcholine, a neurochemical important for memory (Lehne, 2013). Galantamine is prescribed in the first and second stages of AD.

**Memantine (Ebixa).** This drug was approved by Health Canada in 2004 for moderate to severe stages of the disorder, but it is not approved by Health Canada for mild symptoms (Lundbeck, 2011). Memantine regulates the activity of glutamate, a chemical involved in learning and memory (Lundbeck, 2011).

### The Future of Drug Therapy

Among the most exciting developments in the treatment of AD are clinical trials of an amyloid vaccine (AN-1792), which—it is hoped—will clear the brain of amyloid plaques. Unfortunately, the latest research reports that although AN-1792 did clear the amyloid plaques of people with AD, it did not alleviate the progression of the disease (Holmes,

## DRUG TREATMENT OF PATIENTS WITH ALZHEIMER'S DISEASE

| GENERIC (TRADE) | ACTION | INDICATIONS | ADVERSE EFFECTS | WARNINGS |
|---|---|---|---|---|
| **Cholinesterase Inhibitors** | | | | |
| Donepezil* (Aricept) Rivastigmine* (Exelon) Galantamine* (Reminyl) | Prevents the breakdown of acetylcholamine and thereby increases its availability at cholinergic synapses | Modestly improves cognition, behaviour, function; slows disease progression in mild to moderate AD; no Canadian clinical guidelines for the discontinuation of these drugs | Nausea, vomiting, diarrhea, insomnia, fatigue, muscle cramps, incontinence, bradycardia, and syncope | Tacrine is no longer used extensively, owing to hepatotoxicity. Donepezil is better tolerated; dosage is only once a day and is preferred. |
| **N-Methyl-D-Aspartate (NMDA) Antagonist** | | | | |
| Memantine* (Ebixa) | Normalizes levels of glutamate, which in excessive quantities contributes to neurodegeneration | Treatment of moderate to severe Alzheimer's disease; no evidence that it modifies underlying disease | Dizziness, agitation, headache, constipation, and confusion | Clearance is reduced with renal impairment. Use cautiously with moderate renal impairment. Do not use with severe renal impairment. |
| **Selective Serotonin Reuptake Inhibitors** | | | | |
| Citalopram (Celexa) Escitalopram (Cipralex) Fluoxetine (Prozac) Paroxetine (Paxil) Sertraline (Zoloft) | Blocks the reuptake of serotonin, thereby making more available and improving mood | Useful with depression, irritability, sleep disturbances, and anxiety | Agitation, insomnia, headache, nausea and vomiting, sexual dysfunction, and hyponatremia | Discontinuation syndrome—dizziness, insomnia, nervousness, irritability, nausea, and agitation—may occur with abrupt withdrawal (depending on half-life). Taper slowly. |
| **Antianxiety Agents** | | | | |
| Lorazepam (Ativan) Oxazepam (Serax) | Facilitates the action of the inhibitory neurotransmitter GABA | Anxiety, restlessness, verbally disruptive behaviour, and resistance | Drowsiness, dizziness, headaches; restlessness, insomnia, and increased anxiety possible | Use cautiously due to risk for further memory impairment, sedation, and falls. |
| **Atypical Antipsychotics** | | | | |
| Aripiprazole (Abilify) Olanzapine (Zyprexa) Quetiapine (Seroquel) Risperidone (Risperdal) Ziprasidone (Zeldox) | Blocks serotonin and dopamine receptors | Not Health Canada–approved in elderly patients with dementia; extreme caution must be used if these drugs are prescribed with the intent of reducing paranoid thinking, hallucinations, and agitation | Many, including weight gain, increased serum glucose, and hyperlipidemia (see Chapters 4 and 16 for others) | The safety and efficacy in this population has not been established. |
| **Anticonvulsants** | | | | |
| Carbamazepine (Tegretol) Valproic acid/divalproex sodium (Epival) | Reduces the excitability of neurotransmission | Agitated and aggressive behaviour and emotional lability | Ataxia, sedation, confusion, and (rarely) bone marrow suppression | Monitor the complete blood count and liver-associated enzymes. |

*Approved by Health Canada for treatment of Alzheimer's disease.

**Sources:** Bourgeois, J.A., Seaman, J.S., & Servis, M.E. (2008). Delirium, dementia, and amnestic and other cognitive disorders. In R.E. Hales, S.C. Yudofsky, & G.O. Gabbard (Eds.), *Textbook of psychiatry* (pp. 221–250). Arlington, VA: American Psychiatric Publishing; Lehne, R.A. (2010). *Pharmacology for nursing care* (7th ed.). Philadelphia: Saunders; and Wright, C.I., Trinh, N., Blacker, D., et al. (2008). Dementia. In T.A. Stern, J.F. Rosenbaum, M. Fava, et al. (Eds.), *Massachusetts General Hospital comprehensive clinical psychiatry* (pp. 231–246). St. Louis, MO: Mosby.

Boche, Wilkinson, et al., 2008). While the news is disappointing, it should not rule out the potential for other therapies (Holtzman, 2008).

Additional research is ongoing, with focuses on:

- The development of other cholinesterase inhibitors
- The use of cholesterol-lowering agents
- The use of anti-inflammatory agents as a preventive measure
- The use of neurotrophic agents with the potential to regenerate brain cells
- The use of diabetic treatments that might decrease blood vessel inflammation in the brain

Additional information about current clinical studies can be found on the Alzheimer Society of Canada Web site: http://www.alzheimer.ca.

### Integrative Therapy

A number of herbal or all-natural drugs are currently under investigation. However, there is not yet enough scientific evidence concerning either their effectiveness or harmfulness. Keep in mind that the designation "all-natural" or "herbal" does not mean that a substance is safe. Some alternative treatments being investigated are ginkgo biloba, as discussed in the Integrative

Therapy box. According to Kidd (2008), omega-3 fatty acids, other antioxidant nutrients, and vitamins—especially folate, $B_6$, $B_{12}$, C, and E—may also be helpful in the treatment of AD.

## EVALUATION

The outcome criteria for a person with cognitive impairments need to be measurable, within the capabilities of the individual, and evaluated frequently. As the person's condition continues to deteriorate, outcomes must be altered to reflect the person's diminished functioning. Frequent evaluation and reformulation of outcome criteria and short-term indicators also help reduce staff and family frustration and minimize the person with dementia's anxiety by ensuring that tasks are not more complicated than the person can accomplish.

The overall outcomes for treatment are to promote the person's optimal level of functioning and to delay further regression whenever possible. Working closely with family members and providing them with the names of available resources and support sources may help increase the quality of life for both the family and the patient with AD (see Case Study and Nursing Care Plan 18-1, pages 365–368).

### INTEGRATIVE THERAPY

#### Ginkgo Biloba

Many people take ginkgo biloba, believing it will improve their memory and possibly prevent progression of dementia. However, the evidence is inconsistent and unconvincing (Birks & Grimley-Evans, 2008). In a recent randomized, controlled pilot study (Dodge, 2008), researchers found that ginkgo biloba neither altered the progression of dementia nor protected against a decline in memory. Nevertheless, there were some improvements on both counts when the researchers took adherence into consideration.

Further, the group taking ginkgo had a greater incidence of ischemic strokes and transient ischemic attacks. The study also found that use of ginkgo could pose risks for people who are taking warfarin, heparin, aspirin, or other anticoagulants. Those who use this herbal product, therefore, should inform their attending health care providers.

**Source:** Birks, J., & Grimley-Evans, J. (2009). Ginkgo biloba for cognitive impairment and dementia. *Cochrane Database of Systematic Reviews 2009, 1*, Art. No. CD003120. Chichester, UK: John Wiley and Sons. doi:10.1002/14651858.CD003120.pub3.; Dodge, H.H., Zitzelbergerk, T., Oken, B.S., et al. (2008). A randomized placebo-controlled trial of ginkgo biloba for the prevention of cognitive decline. *Neurology, 70*, 1809–1817. doi:10.1212/01.wnl.0000303814.13509.db.

### CASE STUDY AND NURSING CARE PLAN 18-1

#### Cognitive Impairment

During the past four years, Mr. Ludwig has demonstrated rapidly progressive memory impairment, disorientation, and deterioration in his ability to function, related to Alzheimer's disease. He is a 67-year-old man who retired at age 62 to spend some of his remaining "youth" with his wife and to travel, garden, visit family, and finally get to do the things they always wanted to do. At age 63, he was diagnosed with Alzheimer's disease.

Mr. Ludwig has been taken care of at home by his wife and his daughter, Kelly. Kelly is divorced and has returned home with her two young daughters.

The family members find themselves close to physical and mental exhaustion. Mr. Ludwig is becoming increasingly incontinent as he cannot consistently find the bathroom. He wanders

away from home, despite close supervision. The police and neighbours bring him back home an average of four times a week. Once, he was lost for five days after he had somehow boarded a bus for Vancouver, 1000 kilometres from home. He was robbed and beaten before being found by the police and returned home.

He frequently wanders into his granddaughters' rooms at night while they are sleeping and tries to get into bed with them. Too young to understand that their grandfather is lonely and confused, they fear that he is going to hurt them. Four times in the past two weeks, he has fallen while getting out of bed at night, thinking he is in a sleeping bag, camping out in the mountains. After a conflicted and painful two months, the family places him in a care facility for people with Alzheimer's disease.

*Continued*

## CASE STUDY AND NURSING CARE PLAN 18-1—cont'd

### Cognitive Impairment

Mrs. Ludwig tells the admitting nurse, Mr. Behar, that her husband wanders almost all the time and that he has difficulty finding the right words for things (aphasia) and becomes frustrated and angry when that happens. Sometimes he does not seem to recognize the family (agnosia). Once, he thought that Kelly was a thief breaking into the house and attacked her with a broom handle. The telling of this story causes Kelly to break down into heavy sobs: "What's happened to my father? He was so kind and gentle. Oh, God ... I've lost my father."

Mrs. Ludwig tells Mr. Behar that her husband can sometimes participate in dressing himself; at other times, he needs total assistance. At this point, Mrs. Ludwig begins to cry uncontrollably, saying, "I can't bear to part with him, but I can't do it anymore. I feel as if I've betrayed him."

Mr. Behar then focuses his attention on Mrs. Ludwig and her experience. He states, "This is a difficult decision for you." Mr. Behar suggests that Mrs. Ludwig talk to other families who have a cognitively impaired member. "It might help you to know that you are not alone, and having contact with others to share your grief can be healing." One of the organizations he suggests is the Alzheimer Society of Canada, a well-known group that provides support and information to caregivers.

## ASSESSMENT

### Self-Assessment

Mr. Behar has worked on his particular unit for four years. It is a unit designed especially for cognitively impaired individuals, which makes nursing care of these patients easier than on a regular unit. He applied for this position shortly after his own father died of complications secondary to Alzheimer's disease. Mr. Behar refers to the process of living and dying with this disease as horrifying; his goal is to help other people go through it with caring, dignity, and the highest level of functioning as possible.

Caring for Mr. Ludwig and his family is becoming especially personal. Mr. Behar is struck by the similarity between this family's situation and his own. Mr. Ludwig is about the same age his father had been, looks similar to him, and has many of his mannerisms. Mrs. Ludwig and her daughter Kelly seem to be responding in much the same way his family did. He finds that he is having stronger than usual counter-transference feelings with this family and even became teary when Mrs. Ludwig did.

The evening after he met the Ludwigs, Mr. Behar went home utterly exhausted and continued to think about them and his own father. He shared these feelings with his wife, and the two of them spent some time talking about his father and all they had been through together, good and bad. In the end, Mr. Behar sat back, breathed a long, deep sigh of relief, and thanked his wife for being there for him. He told her that he supposed he will never really get over the death of his father, but he is getting better every day.

When Mr. Behar returned to work, he nearly walked right into Mr. Ludwig, who was standing at the doorway wearing two shirts, a pair of pyjama bottoms, and a baseball cap. "Are you the man who's taking me to pick up my car?" he asks. Mr. Behar smiles and says, "It looks like you have quite a day planned. Let's start with a cup of coffee," and redirects him to the day hall.

| Objective Data | Subjective Data |
|---|---|
| Patient: | "I can't bear to part with him." |
| • Wanders away from home about four times a week | "I feel as if I've betrayed him." |
| • Was lost for five days and was robbed and beaten | "I've lost my father." |
| • Is often incontinent when he cannot find the bathroom | |
| • Has difficulty finding words | |
| • Has difficulty identifying members of the family at times | |
| • Has difficulty dressing himself at times | |
| • Falls out of bed at night | |
| • Has memory impairment | |
| • Is disoriented much of the time | |
| • Gets into bed with granddaughters at night when wandering | |
| Family is undergoing intense feelings of loss and guilt | |

## DIAGNOSIS

1. *Risk for injury* related to confusion, as evidenced by wandering

**Supporting Data**
• Wanders away from home about four times a week
• Wanders despite supervision
• Falls out of bed at night
• Gets into other people's beds
• Wanders at night

*Continued*

## CASE STUDY AND NURSING CARE PLAN 18-1—cont'd

### Cognitive Impairment

2. *Functional urinary incontinence* related to disturbed cognition, as evidenced by inability to find the toilet
**Supporting Data**
• Incontinent when he cannot find the bathroom

3. *Self-care deficit* (self-dressing) related to impaired cognitive functioning, as evidenced by impaired ability to put on and take off clothing
**Supporting Data**
• Sometimes he is able to dress with help of wife
• At other times he is too confused to dress self at all

4. *Anticipatory grieving* related to loss and deterioration of family member
**Supporting Data**
• "I can't bear to part with him."
• "I feel as if I've betrayed him."
• "I've lost my father."
• Family undergoing intense feelings of loss and guilt

## OUTCOMES IDENTIFICATION

Although Mr. Ludwig has many unmet needs that require nursing interventions, Mr. Behar decides to focus on the four initial nursing diagnoses. As other problems arise, they will be addressed.

| Nursing Diagnosis | Long-Term Goals | Short-Term Goals |
|---|---|---|
| 1. *Risk for injury* related to confusion, as evidenced by wandering | 1. Resident will remain safe in nursing home. | 1a. Throughout nursing home stay, resident will not fall out of bed.<br>1b. Throughout nursing home stay, resident will wander only in protected area.<br>1c. Resident will be returned within two hours if he succeeds in escaping from the unit. |
| 2. *Functional urinary incontinence* related to disturbed cognition, as evidenced by inability to find the toilet | 2. Resident will experience less incontinence (fewer episodes) by fourth week of hospitalization. | 2a. By the end of four weeks, resident will participate in unit orientation to find toilet.<br>2b. By the end of four weeks, resident will find the toilet most of the time. |
| 3. *Self-care deficit* (self-dressing) related to impaired cognitive functioning, as evidenced by impaired ability to put on and take off clothing | 3. Resident will participate in dressing himself 80% of the time. | 3a. By the end of four weeks, resident will follow step-by-step instructions for dressing most of the time.<br>3b. By the end of four weeks, resident will dress in own clothes with aid of fastening tape. |
| 4. *Anticipatory grieving* related to loss and deterioration of family member | 4. In three months' time, all family members will state that they feel they have more support and are able to talk about their grieving. | 4a. After three months, family members will state that they have opportunity to express "unacceptable" feelings in supportive environment.<br>4b. After three months, family members will state that they have found support from others who have a family member with Alzheimer's disease. |

## PLANNING

Mr. Behar plans care to ensure Mr. Ludwig's safety, provide for the maintenance of his hygiene needs and incontinence, and assist Mrs. Ludwig as she deals with her husband's deterioration.

*Continued*

**CASE STUDY AND NURSING CARE PLAN 18-1—cont'd**

*Cognitive Impairment*

## IMPLEMENTATION

Using the concepts of *NIC*, Mr. Behar's plan of care (nursing diagnosis: *Risk for injury* related to confusion, as evidenced by wandering) was personalized as follows:

| Short-Term Outcome | Intervention | Rationale | Evaluation |
|---|---|---|---|
| 1. Throughout stay in nursing home, resident will not fall out of bed. | 1a. Spend time with resident on admission. | 1a. Time spent with resident lowers anxiety and provides orientation to time and place. Resident's confusion is increased by change. | **GOAL MET** Mattress on floor prevents falls out of bed. |
| | 1b. Label resident's room in big, colourful letters. | 1b. Labels offer clues in new surroundings. | |
| | 1c. Remove mattress from bed and place on floor. | 1c. Placing the mattress on the floor prevents falls out of bed. | |
| | 1d. Keep room well lit at all times. | 1d. Lighting provides important environmental clues and helps lower possibility of illusions. | |
| | 1e. Show resident clock and calendar in room. | 1e. These items foster orientation to time. | |
| | 1f. Keep window shade up. | 1f. This visibility allows day–night variations. | |
| 2. Throughout nursing home stay, resident will wander only in protected area. | 2a. At night, take resident to large, protected, well-lit room. | 2a. Resident is able to wander safely in protected environment. | **GOAL MET** Resident continues to wander at night but, with supervision, keeps out of other residents' rooms most of the time. By fourth week, resident starts to nap on couch in large room after snacks during the night. |
| | 2b. Alert physician to check resident for cardiac decompensation. | 2b. Physical check addresses possible underlying cause of nocturnal wakefulness and wandering. | |
| | 2c. Offer snacks when resident is up—milk, decaffeinated tea, sandwich. | 2c. Snacks help replace fluid and caloric expenditure. | |
| | 2d. Allow soft music on radio. | 2d. Music helps induce relaxation. | |
| | 2e. Spend short, frequent intervals with resident. | 2e. Time with others decreases resident's feelings of isolation and increases orientation. | |
| | 2f. Take resident to bathroom after snacks. | 2f. Bathroom visits after eating help prevent incontinence. | |
| | 2g. During day, offer activities that include use of large muscle groups. | 2g. For some residents, using large muscle groups helps decrease wandering. | |
| 3. Resident will be returned within two hours if he succeeds in escaping from the unit. | 3a. Order MedicAlert bracelet for resident (with name, unit, hospital, and phone number). | 3a. If resident gets out of hospital, he can be identified. | **GOAL MET** By fourth week, resident wanders off unit only once; is found in lobby and returned by security guard within 45 minutes. |
| | 3b. Place brightly coloured vest on resident with name, unit, and phone number taped on back. | 3b. If resident wanders in hospital, he can be identified and returned. | |
| | 3c. Check resident's whereabouts periodically during the day and especially at night. | 3c. Regular checks help monitor resident's activities. | |

## EVALUATION

Although Mr. Ludwig continues to display wandering behaviours, his wandering is contained to safe areas of the unit, except for one instance when he wanders to the lobby. However, then, he is stopped by security and safely returned to the unit within 45 minutes. He has not fallen out of bed. Nursing interventions such as placing his mattress on the floor and ensuring adequate lighting increase his safety while at the same time acknowledging that he continues to exhibit wandering behaviours.

# KEY POINTS TO REMEMBER

- *Cognitive disorder* is a term that refers to disorders that result from changes in the brain and that are marked by disturbances in orientation, memory, intellect, judgement, and affect.
- Delirium and dementia are the cognitive disorders most frequently seen by health care workers.
- Delirium is marked by acute onset, disturbance in consciousness, and symptoms of disorientation and confusion that fluctuate by the minute, hour, or time of day.
- Delirium is always secondary to an underlying condition; therefore, it is transient and may last from hours to days once the underlying cause is treated. If the cause is not treated, permanent damage to neurons can result.
- Dementia usually has a more insidious onset than delirium. Global deterioration of cognitive functioning (e.g., memory, judgement, ability to think abstractly, orientation) is often progressive and irreversible, depending on the underlying cause.
- Dementia may be primary (e.g., Alzheimer's disease [AD], vascular dementia, Pick's disease, Lewy body disease). In this case, the disease is irreversible.

- Alzheimer's disease accounts for close to 70% of all cases of dementia, and vascular dementia accounts for about 20%.
- There are various theories regarding the cause of AD, but none is definitive.
- Signs and symptoms change according to the various stages of AD.
- The symptoms of AD include confabulation, perseveration, aphasia, apraxia, agnosia, and hyperorality.
- No known cause or cure exists for AD, although a number of drugs that increase the brain's supply of acetylcholine (a nerve-communication chemical) are helpful in slowing the progress of the disease.
- People with AD have many unmet needs and present numerous management challenges to both their families and health care workers.
- Specific nursing interventions for cognitively impaired individuals can increase communication, safety, and self-care and are described in the chapter. The need for family teaching and support is strong.

# CRITICAL THINKING

1. Mrs. Kendel is an 82-year-old woman who has Alzheimer's disease. She lives with her husband, who has been trying to care for her in their home. Mrs. Kendel is having trouble dressing. She has put her blouse on backwards and sometimes puts her bra on over her blouse. She often forgets where things are. She makes an effort to cook but has recently attempted to "put out" the electric burners of the stove with pitchers of water. Once in a while, she cannot find the bathroom in time, often mistaking a closet for it. At times, she cries because she is aware that she is losing her sense of place in the world. She and her husband have always been close, loving companions, and he wants to keep her at home as long as possible.
   a. Assist Mr. Kendel by writing out a list of suggestions that he can try at home that might help facilitate (a) communication, (b) activities of daily living, and (c) maintenance of a safe home environment.
   b. Identify at least three interventions that are appropriate to this situation for each of the problems Mrs. Kendel is having.
   c. Identify resources available for maintaining Mrs. Kendel in her home for as long as possible. Provide the name of a self-help group that you would urge Mr. Kendel to join.

2. Share with your class or clinical group the name and function of at least three community agencies in your area that could be an appropriate referral for a family with a member with dementia. (For one, you can contact the Alzheimer Society of Canada: http://www.alzheimer.ca).

# CHAPTER REVIEW

1. A 73-year-old woman with pneumonia becomes agitated after being admitted to the intensive care unit through the emergency department. She continually tries to leave her bed despite being too weak to walk. Her vital signs are erratic, and her thinking seems disorganized. During her first 24 hours in ICU, the patient varies from somnolent to agitated, and from laughing to angry. Her daughter reports that the patient "was never like this at home." What is the most likely explanation for the situation?

   1. Pneumonia has worsened the patient's early-stage dementia.
   2. The patient is experiencing delirium secondary to the pneumonia.
   3. The patient is sundowning due to the decreased stimulation of the intensive care unit.
   4. The patient does not want to be in the hospital and is angry that staff will not let her leave.

2. Intervention(s) appropriate for a hospitalized patient experiencing delirium include which of the following? Select all that apply.
   1. Immediately placing the patient in restraints if she begins to hallucinate or act irrationally or unsafely
   2. Assuring that a clock and a sign indicating the day and date is displayed where the patient can see it easily
   3. Being prepared for possible hostile responses to efforts to take vital signs or provide direct physical care
   4. Preventing sensory deprivation by placing the patient near the nurses' station and leaving the television and multiple lights turned on 24 hours per day
   5. Speaking with the patient frequently for short periods for reassurance, assisting the patient in remaining oriented, and ensuring the patient's safety
   6. Anticipating that the patient may try to leave if agitated and providing a secure environment with direct observation to prevent wandering
   7. Promoting normalized sleep patterns by encouraging the patient to remain awake during the day and facilitating rest at night

3. Which statement about dementia is accurate?
   1. The majority of people over age 85 are affected by dementia.
   2. Disorientation is the dominant and most disruptive symptom of dementia.
   3. People with dementia tend to be distressed by it and complain about its symptoms.
   4. Hypertension, diminished activity levels, and head injury increase the risk for dementia.

4. Mrs. Smythe dies at the age of 82. In the two months following her death, her husband, aged 84 and in good health, has begun to pay less attention to his hygiene and seems less aware of his surroundings. He complains of difficulty concentrating and sleeping and reports that he lacks energy. His family sometimes has to remind and encourage him to shower, take his medications, and eat, all of which he then does. Which response is most appropriate?
   1. Arrange for an appointment with a therapist for evaluation and treatment of suspected depression.
   2. Reorient Mr. Smythe by pointing out the day and date each time you have occasion to interact with him.
   3. Meet with family and support persons to help them accept, anticipate, and prepare for the progression of his stage 2 dementia.
   4. Avoid touch and proximity, which are likely to be uncomfortable for Mr. Smythe and may provoke aggression when he is disoriented.

5. Which of the following interventions would be beneficial for those caring for a loved one with Alzheimer's disease? Select all that apply.
   1. Guide the family to restrict the patient's driving as soon as signs of forgetfulness are exhibited.
   2. Recommend switching to hospital-type gowns to facilitate bathing, dressing, and other physical care of the patient.
   3. Discourage wandering by installing complex locks or locks placed at the tops of doors, where the patient cannot readily reach them.
   4. For situations in which the patient becomes upset, teach loved ones to listen briefly, provide support, and then change the topic.
   5. Encourage caregivers to care for themselves, as well as the patient, via use of support resources such as adult day care or respite care.
   6. If the patient is prone to wander away, encourage family to notify police and neighbours of the patient's condition, wandering behaviour, and description.

# ℮volve WEBSITE

Post-Test interactive review

*Visit the Evolve Web site for Chapter Review Answers and Rationales, Critical Thinking Answer Guidelines, and additional resources related to the content in this chapter: http://evolve.elsevier.com/Canada/Varcarolis/psychiatric/*

## REFERENCES

Alzheimer Society of Canada. (2009). *Alzheimer's disease: What is Alzheimer's disease.* Toronto: Author.

Alzheimer Society of Canada. (2010a). *Alzheimer's disease fact sheet.* Toronto: Author.

Alzheimer Society of Canada. (2010b). *Alzheimer's disease statistics.* Toronto: Author.

Alzheimer Society of Canada. (2011). *About Safely Home registry.* Retrieved from http://www.safelyhome.ca/en/safelyhome/aboutsafelyhome.asp.

Alzheimer's Association. (2012). Alzheimer's disease facts and figures. *Alzheimer's and Dementia, 8,* 131–168. Retrieved from http://www.alz.org/alzheimers_disease_facts_and_figures.asp.

Alzheimer's Disease International. (2010). *World Alzheimer report 2010: The global economic impact of dementia.* London, UK: Author.

Apotex. (2009). *Product monograph: Apo-Rivastigmine.* Weston, ON: Author.

Ayalon, L., Gunn, A.M., Feliciano, L., et al. (2006). Effectiveness of nonpharmacological interventions for the management of neuropsychiatric symptoms in patients with dementia. *Archives of Internal Medicine, 166*(20), 2182–2188.

Ballard, C., Gauthier, S., Corbett, A., et al. (2011). Alzheimer's disease. *The Lancet, 377*(9770), 1019–1031. doi:10.1016/S0140-6736(10)61349-9.

Becker, C. (2012). Nursing care of the brain injury patient on a locked neurobehavioral unit. *Rehabilitation Nursing, 37*(4), 18–33. doi:10.1002/rnj.50.

Bulechek, G.M., Butcher, H.K., & Dochterman, J.M. (2008). *Nursing interventions classification (NIC)* (5th ed.). St. Louis, MO: Mosby.

Canadian Institute for Health Information. (2010). *Caring for seniors with Alzheimer's disease and other forms of dementia.* Ottawa: Author.

Casey, G. (2012). Alzheimer's and other dementias. *Kai Tiaki Nursing New Zealand, 18*(6), 20–24. Retrieved from http://www.nzno.org.nz/services/journals_-_kai_tiaki.

Cerejeira, J., & Mukactova-Ludinska, E. (2011). A clinical update on delirium: From early recognition to effective management. *Nursing Research and Practice, 2011,* 1–12. doi:10.1155/2011/875196.

Clegg, A., Young, J., & Siddiqi, N. (2012). Delirium in cardiac patients: A clinical review. *British Journal of Cardiac Nursing, 7*(3), 111–115. Retrieved from http://www.cardiac-nursing.co.uk/.

Gesin, G., Russell, B., Lin, A., et al. (2012). Impact of a delirium screening tool and multifaceted education on nurses' knowledge of delirium and ability to evaluate it correctly. *American Journal of Critical Care, 21*(1), e1–e11. doi:10.4037/ajcc2012605.

Gibson, J. (2009). Living with loss. *Mental Health Practice, 12*(5), 22–24.

Health Canada. (2005). *Increased mortality associated with the use of atypical antipsychotic drugs in elderly patients with dementia.* Ottawa: Health Canada, Canadian Adverse Drug Reaction Monitoring Program.

Holmes, C., Boche, D., Wilkinson, D., et al. (2008). Long-term effects of Aβ$_{42}$ immunisation in Alzheimer's disease: Follow-up of a randomised, placebo-controlled phase I trial. *Lancet, 372,* 216–223. doi:10.1016/S0140-6736(08)61075-2.

Holtzman, D.M. (2008). Alzheimer's disease: Moving towards a vaccine. *Nature, 454,* 418–420. doi:10.1038/454418a.

Huber, G. (2012). Prevention and management of delirium in geriatric rehabilitation. *Topics in Geriatric Rehabilitation, 28*(3), 148–156.

Inouye, S.K., Foreman, M.D., Mion, L., et al. (2001). Nurses' recognition of delirium and its symptoms: Comparison of nurses and researcher ratings. *Archives of Internal Medicine, 161*(20), 2467–2473. doi:10.1001/archinte.161.20.2467.

Jones, C., Griffiths, R., Humphris, G., et al. (2001). Memory, delusions, and the development of acute posttraumatic stress disorder-related symptoms after intensive care. *Critical Care Medicine 29*(3), 573–580. doi:10.1097/00003246-200103000-00019.

Kidd, P.M. (2008). Alzheimer's disease, amnestic mild cognitive impairment, and age-associated memory impairment: Current understanding and progress toward integrative prevention. *Alternative Medicine Review, 13*(2), 85–115.

Lehne, R.A. (2013). *Pharmacology for nursing care* (8th ed.). St Louis, MO: Elsevier.

Lundbeck. (2011). *Product monograph: Ebixa (memantine hydrochloride).* Montreal: Author.

Michaud, L., Büla, C., Berney, A., et al. (2007). Delirium: Guidelines for general hospitals. *Journal of Psychosomatic Research, 62*(3), 371–383. Retrieved from http://www.journals.elsevier.com/journal-of-psychosomatic-research/.

Moorhead, S., Johnson, M., Maas, M., et al. (2012). *Nursing outcomes classification (NOC)* (5th ed.). St. Louis, MO: Mosby.

Nasreddine, Z., Phillips, N., Bedirian, V., et al. (2005). The Montreal Cognitive Assessment (MoCA): A brief screening tool for mild cognitive impairment. *Journal of the American Geriatrics Society, 53*(4), 695–699. Retrieved from http://onlinelibrary.wiley.com/journal/10.1111/(ISSN)1532-5415.

Querfurth, H.W., & LaFerla, F.M. (2010). Mechanisms of disease: Alzheimer's disease. *The New England Journal of Medicine, 362*(4), 329–344.

Quinlan, N., & Rudolph, J. (2011). Postoperative delirium and functional decline after noncardiac surgery. *Journal of the American Geriatrics Society 59*(S2), S301–S304. doi:10.1111/j.1532-5415.2011.03679.x.

Raina, P., Santaguida, P., Ismaila, A., et al. (2008). Effectiveness of cholinesterase inhibitors and memantine for treating dementia: Evidence review for a clinical practice guideline. *Annals of Internal Medicine, 148*(5), 379–397.

Rice, K., Bennett, M., Gomez, M., et al. (2011). Nurses' recognition of delirium in the hospitalized older adult. *Clinical Nurse Specialist, 25*(6), 299–311. doi:10.1097/NUR.0b013e318234897b.

Rudolph, J., & Marcantonio, E. (2011). Postoperative delirium: Acute change with long-term implications. *Anesthesia & Analgesia, 112*(5), 1202–1211. doi:10.1213/ANE.0b013e3182147f6d.

Sadock, B.J., & Sadock, A. (2008). *Concise textbook of clinical psychiatry* (3rd ed.). Philadelphia: Lippincott Williams & Wilkins.

Stetka, B., & Correll, C. (2012, May 21). A guide to DSM-5. *Medscape.* Retrieved from http://www.medscape.com/viewarticle/803884_13.

Voyer, P., McCuskar, J., Cole, M.G., et al. (2007). Factors associated with delirium severity among older patients. *Journal of Clinical Nursing, 16,* 819–831. doi:10.1111/j.1365-2702.2006.01808.x.

Wei, L.A., Fearing, M.A., Sternberg, E.J., et al. (2008). The confusion assessment method: A systematic review of current usage. *Journal of the American Geriatrics Society, 56,* 823–830. doi:10.1111/j.1532-5415.2008.01674.x.

Wright, C.I., Trinh, N., Blacker, D., et al. (2008). Dementia. In T.A. Stern, J.F. Rosenbaum, M. Fava, et al. (Eds.), *Massachusetts General Hospital comprehensive clinical psychiatry* (pp. 231–246). Philadelphia: Saunders.

Wright, E., Brew, B., Arayawichanont, A., et al. (2008). Neurologic disorders are prevalent in HIV-positive outpatients in the Asia-Pacific region. *Neurology, 71,* 50–56. doi:10.1212/01.wnl.0000316390.17248.65.

## KEY TERMS AND CONCEPTS

## OBJECTIVES

1. Compare and contrast the terms substance use, abuse, dependence, tolerance, and addiction.
2. Discuss four components of the assessment process, including assessment of readiness for change, to be used with a person who is experiencing substance abuse or other addictions.
3. Describe the difference between the behaviours of a person with alcoholism and a nondrinker in relation to blood alcohol level.
4. Discuss the symptoms of alcohol withdrawal and alcohol delirium and the recommended treatments for each.
5. Describe the signs of alcohol poisoning and the appropriate treatment based on the individual's presentation.
6. List the appropriate steps to take if a co-worker is impaired.
7. Recognize signs of substance abuse or impaired practice in colleagues.
8. Compare and contrast the signs and symptoms of intoxication, overdose, and withdrawal for cocaine and amphetamines.
9. Distinguish between the symptoms of opioid intoxication and those of opioid withdrawal.
10. Identify two short-term goals for a person who abuses alcohol in terms of (a) withdrawal, (b) active treatment, and (c) health maintenance.
11. Analyze the pros and cons of the following treatments for opioid addictions: methadone, therapeutic communities, and abstinence-oriented self-help programs.
12. Explore the principles and practices of motivational interviewing as an evidence-informed intervention and an approach to communication for recovery.
13. Recognize the phenomenon of relapse as it affects people who abuse substances during different phases of treatment.
14. Evaluate four indications that a person is successfully recovering from substance abuse.

# evolve WEBSITE

*Visit the Evolve website for Flashcards, Case Studies, and additional testing resources related to the content in this chapter: http://evolve.elsevier.com/Canada/Varcarolis/psychiatric/* 〔ＰＲＥ-ＴＥＳＴ〕〔interactive review〕

Canada is a society in which people use a host of substances and behaviours for various purposes: to restore health, reduce pain and anxiety, increase energy, aid weight loss or gain, create a feeling of euphoria, take part in social rituals, create community or intimacy, induce relaxation or sleep, and enhance alertness. Most of us have been personally affected by the use of, misuse of, abuse of, dependence on, tolerance of, or addiction to alcohol, other substances, or behaviours by a relative, friend, or even ourselves. The degree to which each of us has been affected can range from casual knowledge to frustration or profound family dysfunction and lasting emotional scars. This chapter explores the clinical trajectory and implications of addictive disorders, as well as the screening for addictions and the assessment of and nursing care for those experiencing addictions.

## CLINICAL PICTURE

The diagnosis of a substance-related disorder or behavioural addiction requires knowledge of the class of drug use, specific behaviours and patterns of use, and the severity of symptoms (considered mild, moderate, or severe), which may include tolerance and withdrawal. Cox and Leyton (2009) identified that the progression of addiction reflects a continuum, ranging from no use to experiences of addiction and recovery. Along the trajectory, they identify the important factors of vulnerability

## ❋ HOW A NURSE HELPED ME

### *Kari Cared Enough to Take Action*

*I was introduced to opioids years ago after an injury to my back in a work-related accident. All through my nursing education, I continued to use opioids to control the pain. Eventually, my need for more Dilaudid forced me to see doctors in different cities and towns. I didn't want my family or friends to know; but more importantly I didn't want my employer to know. When my own family doctor suggested going on methadone as a way to control my Dilaudid use and my pain, I willingly agreed. At first, the methadone seemed to be working, but my anxiety and fear about being found out caused nausea and vomiting. One day, I took an ampoule of Gravol 100 mg home from work. I was pleased with the effects; my anxiety abated [as did the nausea and vomiting]. I started carrying two or three ampoules of Gravol 100 mg in my uniform pocket (just in case I needed it at work). Each shift, I would restock my supply of Gravol. I knew how wrong this was, but the feeling of relief I got from the Gravol was profound.*

*One day, I mentioned this to the nurse at the methadone clinic. I thought by telling her, maybe they would increase my dose or the clinic doctor would prescribe something better.*

*The nurse, Kari, was kind, nonjudgemental, but very worried about my mixing of these two medications and working under the influence. The next day, Kari asked how much I had used the day before, my plan for stopping, and solutions I had tried to diminish my anxiety at work. The next day, Kari invited me into her office at the clinic, where we discussed our nursing practice standards and her responsibility for reporting me to the professional nursing association. I think I was angry at first; the clinic is supposed to be confidential; my right to privacy and confidentiality was supposed to be first and foremost!*

*Then the next day, Kari asked what I had planned to do: was I going to report my using and pilfering of Gravol from my work, or did I want her to? I didn't realize until later how much relief I felt; no more avoiding. It was time to get more help. Thanks to Kari, I booked myself into an inpatient treatment program with the help of my family doctor. I went to my union and my association and told them what was happening. The association suspended my licence, as I knew they would, but because Kari cared enough about my patients—and me—to take action, the association accepted my plan of recovery. I can't begin to imagine my life had that one nurse not taken the initiative to put professional practice into my vision of recovery. My use affected not only myself and my family but my patients and my colleagues. I used to be ashamed and angry about my personal life at work, and my work life at home. Now my recovery is having a positive effect in all aspects of my life and the lives of my patients.*

**Source:** Canadian Nurses Association. (2009). *Position statement: Problematic substance use by nurses.* Retrieved from http://www2.cna-aiic.ca/CNA/documents/pdf/publications/PS98_Problematic_Substance_Use_e.pdf.

to addiction, exposure to the conditions that contribute to addiction, and the experiences of addiction and recovery, all of which can be influenced at individual or social levels (p. 34).

Inherited genetic predispositions are often important; their effects depend on one's context and surrounding environment. In fact, it is vital to recognize that all factors can be socially, physically, and environmentally influenced, providing multiple opportunities to alter the addiction trajectory. A combination of prevention and treatment strategies, including social policies, can change individual, familial, and social experiences, altering an individual's course along this continuum. The addiction trajectory is described in more detail below.

## No Use

In this stage, the individual does not use alcohol or other substances and does not participate in addictive behaviours (e.g., gambling). Just as someone can be predisposed to substance use due to biological (genetic), psychological, or social factors, one's personal disposition or social environment may dissuade the use of certain substances or behaviours. People have their own reasons not to become involved in using a substance or engaging in a behaviour (e.g., religious beliefs, professional or legal concerns, their age, an abstinence treatment plan as part of prior recovery from addiction).

## Use

People may begin to experiment with alcohol, other drugs, or behaviours to see what it is like, to fit in with peers, or perhaps to escape from personal troubles. Some people may use a substance or behaviour to enhance an already pleasurable experience and, therefore, consider their use a social habit, such as enjoying a drink of alcohol with friends. However, some argue that the social use of a substance is not merely using in social situations; rather, it is using in a socially and culturally responsible way. There are few, if any, negative consequences of social use. The concept of social use excludes youth under the age of majority who drink alcohol and anyone who uses illegal drugs—circumstances that can result in negative legal or parental consequences.

## Misuse

The misuse of a substance or behaviour results in problems associated with its use. People who misuse alcohol, other drugs, or behaviours may experience lapses in memory, get in trouble at home or school because of impairment, spend more money than intended on gambling or shopping, or do something regrettable while under the influence of alcohol or another drug. All these problems, although they may seem small at the time, can escalate into much larger problems.

## Abuse

Identifying abuse of a substance or behaviour is possible once the problems resulting from misuse become much more regular. The person uses a substance or engages in a damaging behaviour more frequently, interfering with major areas of his or her life, such as family, parents, school, legal issues, money, friends, and leisure. The person may become obsessive about when, how, and where to get the substance or behaviour of abuse (e.g., money to gamble, access to technology to play games, new sexual partners).

## Dependency

At the dependency stage, the person has lost the ability to choose to use or not to use. Using substances or engaging in a behaviour such as gambling, gaming, shopping, or having casual sexual activity has become a way of life. The person may experience physical or psychological withdrawal, cravings for the substance of abuse, and decreased physical, mental, and emotional health. The person now has an addiction—the persistent, compulsive dependence on or use of a substance or behaviour despite its negative consequences and the increasing frequency of those consequences.

With regular use of a substance or behaviour, a person develops *tolerance*. Tolerance is a physiological experience that occurs when a person's reaction to a substance decreases with repeated administrations of the same dose. At this point, if the person attempts to stop using the substance or engaging in the behaviour, he or she may experience symptoms of withdrawal. Withdrawal causes physiological changes as the blood and tissue concentrations of a drug decrease after heavy and prolonged use of a substance.

Other phenomena frequently encountered by those who abuse substances are flashbacks, synergistic effects, and antagonistic effects. These occurrences are discussed briefly here, although they are seen in many situations, not just in substance abuse. It is important to recognize that a diagnosis of substance use disorder does not depend on the presence of tolerance or withdrawal symptoms (Erickson, 2007).

## Flashbacks

Flashbacks are transitory recurrences of perceptual disturbance that can be caused by a person's earlier hallucinogenic drug use but occur when the person is in a drug-free state (Halpern & Pope, 2003). Often, flashbacks are mild and perhaps pleasant, but at other times, individuals experience recurrences of frightening images or thoughts. Case studies have reported the typical course of experiences, which includes visual distortions, time expansion, loss of ego boundaries, and intense emotions; however, clinical research is limited (Halpern & Pope, 2003).

## Synergistic Effects

*Synergy* is the capacity of two or more drugs acting together to create a greater total effect than the sum of the effects if taken independently. For example, combinations of alcohol plus a benzodiazepine, alcohol plus an opiate, and alcohol plus a barbiturate all produce synergistic effects. Mixing alcohol with drugs can have unpleasant and sometimes fatal effects.

## Antagonistic Effects

Drugs are often combined to weaken or inhibit the effect of one of the drugs (i.e., for *antagonistic effect*). For example, those taking tranquilizers to aid sleep may use excessive caffeine or other stimulants to counteract the sedative effects of the primary prescription. Users of cocaine will often mix it with heroin (referred to as a *speedball*). The heroin, a central nervous system (CNS) depressant, may soften the intense letdown of withdrawal from cocaine, a CNS stimulant. Doctors may even prescribe drugs to counteract the effects of another. For instance, naloxone (Targin), an opioid antagonist, may be prescribed for people who have overdosed on an opioid (e.g., heroin, oxycodone) to reverse respiratory and CNS depression.

### Codependence

Codependence is a cluster of behaviours and psychological characteristics of overdependence on meeting the needs of others. These characteristics were originally identified through research involving the families of alcoholic patients. Living with an individual who abuses alcohol or other substances is a source of stress and requires adjustments to the family system. People who are codependent often exhibit over-responsible behaviour (e.g., doing for others what others could just as well do for themselves). Codependent individuals can also demonstrate overly passive behaviours, making their own needs a lower priority while being excessively preoccupied by the needs of others (e.g., attempting to control someone else's drug or alcohol use; feeling responsible or guilty for the other person's behaviour; "walking on eggshells" to avoid causing problems for the other person; assuming the duties and responsibilities of the other person). This cluster of responses and behaviours may prevent those experiencing codependence from living full and satisfying lives.

Not everyone in relationships with people who have substance use disorders will experience codependence. Navigating the difficult consequences of substance abuse, however, will almost always negatively impact relationships with family, friends, co-workers, and others.

## EPIDEMIOLOGY

In Health Canada's 2011 Canadian Alcohol and Drug Use Monitoring Survey, the prevalence of past-year alcohol use for Canadians over age 15 was 78%, a slight increase over previous years' reportings (Health Canada, 2011). In the same year, 14.4% of Canadians aged 15 years and older exceeded the quantity of alcohol consumption to be considered a chronic longer-term health risk, and 10.1% exceeded the quantity to be considered an acute health risk (e.g., alcohol poisoning). The rate of drug use by youth 15 to 24 years of age remains much higher than that reported by adults 25 years and older: three times higher for cannabis use (21.6% versus 6.7%), and nearly five times higher for other drugs (4.8% versus 1.1%). Binge drinking among Canadian men is ranked as the highest in the world (Wilsnack, Vogeltanz, Wilsnack, et al., 2000). Alcohol dependence is highest in men, young people, those self-identifying as Caucasian, those from Aboriginal communities, those with low incomes, and those who are unmarried (Health Canada, 2011).

Wesley-Esquimaux and Snowball (2010) found that alcohol abuse has been identified as a core issue in some communities across Canada. They noted that "excessive alcohol use or binging has been strongly tied to the hundreds of suicide attempts and violence in northern Aboriginal communities" (p. 392). Further,

their review identified how co-morbid substance abuse, mental illness, and violence in communities were all further complicated by the culturally and socially disconnected services available to Aboriginal people in urban centres (Wesley-Esquimaux & Snowball, 2010).

## CO-MORBIDITY

### Psychiatric Co-Morbidity

The complex combination of both substance abuse or behavioural addiction and a mental health condition known as concurrent disorder or, interchangeably, *dual diagnosis* is considered "so common, dual diagnosis should be expected rather than considered the exception" (Minkoff, 2001, p. 597). Alcohol dependence is associated with abuse of other substances, mood and anxiety disorders, and paranoid, histrionic, and antisocial personality disorders (Hasin, Stinson, Ogburn, et al., 2007). Antisocial personality disorders are associated with drug use (Compton, Thomas, Stinson, et al., 2007). Other examples of common concurrent disorders include major depression with cocaine abuse, alcoholism with generalized anxiety disorder, alcoholism and polydrug abuse with schizophrenia, and borderline personality disorder with episodic polydrug abuse (Mancini, Hardiman, & Eversman, 2008). Drug dependence is significantly associated with generalized anxiety disorders and mood disorders.

While the exact incidence and prevalence of concurrent disorders in Canada are not clear, the poor clinical and social outcomes have been described (Rush, Fogg, Nadeau, et al., 2008; Schulte, Meier, Stirling, et al., 2010). Patients with concurrent disorders often experience more severe and chronic medical, social, and emotional problems. Because they have two or more disorders, they are vulnerable to both substance abuse relapse and worsening of the psychiatric disorder. In addition, substance abuse relapse often leads to psychiatric decompensation, and the worsening of psychiatric problems often leads to substance abuse relapse, creating a vicious circle (Mancini, Hardiman, & Eversman, 2008).

Compared with patients who have a single disorder, patients with co-occurring disorders often require longer treatment, experience more crises, and progress more gradually in treatment. Among the challenges of meeting the needs of people with concurrent disorders are poorly integrated services that lack attention to cultural or community concerns (Wesley-Esquimaux & Snowball, 2010). Gradually, however, these concerns are being addressed across Canada in services reform (Canadian Centre on Substance Abuse, 2013).

### Medical Co-Morbidity

Alcohol abuse is the most prevalent of the substance abuse disorders. Therefore, alcohol-related medical problems are the co-morbidities most commonly seen in medical settings. Alcohol can affect all organ systems, in particular the CNS (resulting in disorders such as Wernicke's encephalopathy and Korsakoff syndrome) and the gastrointestinal system (resulting in disorders such as esophagitis, gastritis, pancreatitis, alcoholic hepatitis, and cirrhosis of the liver). Also commonly associated with long-term alcohol use or abuse are tuberculosis, all types of accidents, suicide, and homicide. Alcohol use during pregnancy can have negative consequences for the fetus and result in fetal alcohol spectrum disorder (FASD).

In the case of drug users, the route of drug administration influences the possible co-morbid medical complications. Those who use intravenous drugs have a higher incidence of infections and associated problems from infection, including hepatitis and human immunodeficiency virus (HIV), cellulitis, and sclerosing of veins. Those who abuse intranasal substances may be prone to sinusitis and perforated nasal septum. Smoking substances increases the likelihood of respiratory problems and saliva or airborne infections if sharing pipes or cigarettes. Table 19-1 lists physical complications associated with various classes of drugs and their routes of administration.

## ETIOLOGY

Substance use disorders and addictions are characterized by use, abuse, and even dependence and also by certain patterns of behaviour: (1) loss of control of substance consumption or of behaviour, (2) continued substance use or behaviour despite associated problems, and (3) cravings and a tendency to relapse after efforts to change behaviour. The reason one person may experience substance use disorder or behavioural addiction while another does not seems to relate to physical, developmental, psychosocial, and environmental factors, as well as genetic vulnerability (Bailey, Hill, Oesterle, et al., 2006). The difficulty in determining cause and effect is that substance use disorders are generally diagnosed many years after the onset of use, and various factors—biological, psychological, and sociocultural—coexist over the course of those years.

### Biological Factors

In recent years, scientists have discovered that alcohol and drug use affects specific neurotransmitters and areas of the brain. The main systems that seem to be involved in substance abuse are the opioid, catecholamine (especially dopamine), and gamma-aminobutyric acid (GABA) systems (Sadock & Sadock, 2008). Cocaine and amphetamines increase levels of norepinephrine, serotonin, and dopamine. Opioid drugs act on opioid receptors. Alcohol or other CNS depressants will act on GABA receptors and increase the bioavailability of glutamate, norepinephrine, and dopamine. These increases help explain the addictive and cross-tolerance effects—that is, the resistance to certain compounds of one drug due to a tolerance developed to a similar drug compound that occurs when alcohol is combined with barbiturates and benzodiazepines.

Berridge (2007) posited that dopamine is responsible for a phenomenon termed *incentive salience*, which causes the cravings experienced by those addicted to substances when they are not currently using the substance. Incentive salience explains the high rate of first-year relapse for people who abuse substances. Addictive substances that directly activate dopamine transmission or induce neural sensitization cause those addicted to become *cue-sensitive*, meaning that when presented with a stimulus previously associated with use of the addictive

drug, the person will experience an overwhelming urge to use the drug.

### Psychological Factors

While the idea of "addictive personalities" is a myth, certain psychological factors are associated with substance abuse and addiction, include the following:

- Lack of tolerance for frustration and pain
- Lack of success in life
- Lack of affectionate and meaningful relationships
- Low self-esteem, lack of self-regard
- Risk-taking propensity
- Impulsivity

Several psychological theories contribute to our understanding of substance abuse and addiction.

Psychodynamic theories view substance use as a defence against anxious impulses, a form of oral regression (dependency), or a form of self-medication for depression (Sadock & Sadock, 2008). Cognitive and behavioural responses to stressful experiences may contribute to increased initial substance intake or behaviours, ongoing use, abuse, and recurrence of substance use or relapse (Abizaid, Anisman, Matheson, et al., 2009). Cognitive or expectancy theory suggests that addictive behaviours are chosen over healthy behaviours due to one's expectations (Wiers & Hoffmann, 2010). A person may expect the benefits of an addictive behaviour to outweigh the risks. Such expectations about substance use may develop by observing others (similar to the social learning and other developmental theories of addiction). Similarly, psychological theory related to personality links personality disorders, as well as problems with impulse control, to increased substance abuse, alcohol abuse in particular (Cox & Leyton, 2009). Biological theorists suggest that cognitive and psychological change occurs as a result of the abuse of certain substances (Stavro, Pelletier & Potvin, 2013). These theories call into question the cognitive cause and patterns of substance abuse and addiction.

According to social learning theory, observing the addictive behaviours of others can lead to the development of a substance use disorder or addiction (Aaron, 2012). When applying a psychological theory of causation, such as social learning theory or cognitive theory, the nurse considers the individual environment and dynamics in psychological treatment planning and outcomes.

### Sociocultural Factors

Sociocultural factors express the social relationships, politics, and environments beyond individual psychological environments. Sociocultural theories attempt to explain differences in the incidence of substance use in various groups. Social and cultural norms influence when, what, and how a person uses substances, as well as the responses and involvement of family or community members (see Chapter 7). For example, in Asian Canadian cultures, the prevalence rate for alcohol abuse is relatively low, due in part to a deficiency in about 50% of the population of aldehyde dehydrogenase, the chemical that breaks down alcohol acetaldehyde. As the level of alcohol acetaldehyde increases in the blood, a severe flush and palpitations may occur

| TABLE 19-1 | PHYSICAL COMPLICATIONS RELATED TO SUBSTANCE ABUSE | |
|---|---|---|
| **SUBSTANCE** | **ROUTE(S)** | **PHYSICAL COMPLICATIONS** |
| Opioids (e.g., heroin)<br>Phenylcyclohexyl piperidine (PCP)<br>Cocaine or crack | Intravenous* | Acquired immune deficiency syndrome (AIDS)<br>Hepatitis<br>Bacterial endocarditis<br>Renal failure<br>Cardiac arrest<br>Coma<br>Seizures<br>Respiratory arrest<br>Dermatitis<br>Pulmonary emboli<br>Tetanus<br>Abscesses—osteomyelitis<br>Septicemia |
| Cocaine | Intravenous*<br>Intranasal<br>Smoking | Perforation of nasal septum (when taken intranasally)<br>Respiratory paralysis<br>Cardiovascular collapse<br>Hyperpyrexia |
| Caffeine | Ingestion | Gastroesophageal reflux<br>Peptic ulcer<br>Increased intraocular pressure in unregulated glaucoma<br>Tachycardia<br>Increased plasma glucose and lipid levels |
| PCP | Ingestion | Respiratory arrest |
| Marijuana | Smoking<br>Ingestion | Impaired lung structure<br>Chromosomal mutation—increased incidence of birth defects<br>Micronucleic white blood cells—increased risk of disease due to decreased resistance to infection<br>Possible long-term effects on short-term memory |
| Nicotine | Smoking<br>Chewing | Emphysema<br>Cancer of the larynx and esophagus<br>Lung cancer<br>Peripheral vascular diseases<br>Cancer of the mouth<br>Cardiovascular disease<br>Hypertension |
| Heroin | Intravenous*<br>Smoking | Constipation<br>Dermatitis<br>Malnutrition<br>Hypoglycemia<br>Dental caries<br>Amenorrhea |
| Inhalants | Sniffing<br>Snorting<br>Bagging (inhalation of fumes from a plastic bag)<br>Huffing (placement of inhalant-soaked rag in the mouth) | Respiratory arrest<br>Tachycardia<br>Arrhythmias<br>Nervous system damage |

*Complications listed can result from any drug taken intravenously.

(Linneberg, Gonzalez-Quintela, Vidal, et al., 2010), symptoms that may deter people from drinking.

Another sociocultural theory correlates substance use with the degree of socioeconomic stress. Involvement in a community that participates in an addictive behaviour may provide a sense of belonging and identity. Social factors can be considered at family, community or societal, and even political levels in terms of causation and intervention for substance abuse or addiction. For instance, a community or societal social factor may be heard in the patient who states: "I don't mean to spend my money like that, but my friends like to go to the casino. I just want to tag along and then suddenly ..." Similarly, those in certain work or social groups may find expectations around substance use to be a norm—for instance, having alcoholic drinks at fundraising events or taking clients for drinks. Other environments may have social cultures that involve drug use, and these demands can contribute to substance use disorders and addictions.

Gender differences regarding substance use and addiction are notable. Internationally, women, in general, are diagnosed with substance use at lower rates than men (Galea, Nandi, & Vlahov, 2004). One reason may be that, in many cultural groups, women who use and abuse substances are viewed much more negatively than men who do the same. These statistics may be artificially deflated since women may hide such behaviours to conform to social norms. The perceived need to hide may also prevent women from receiving necessary treatment and services.

## APPLICATION OF THE NURSING PROCESS

### ASSESSMENT

#### Assessment of Substance Use and Substance-Induced Disorders

Assessment of chemical impairment, substance use, abuse, dependence, tolerance, and withdrawal is becoming more complex because of the increase in polydrug abuse, co-occurring psychiatric disorders, and co-morbid physical illnesses, including HIV infection, acquired immune deficiency syndrome (AIDS), dementia, and encephalopathy. Also, changes in the diagnostic criteria for substance use and substance-induced disorders will lead to changes in practice. Depending on the context of the assessment (acute care, intensive care unit, community clinic, street level), different practice guidelines will be considered; the assessment of safety of the patient and others, however, will always be a priority.

Sensitivity to cultural and contextual concerns of patients and families is also important in assessing, interpreting symptoms, making diagnoses, providing clinical care, and designing prevention strategies (see Chapter 7). Steps to follow in assessment include (1) level of acute intoxication, (2) history and past substance use, (3) medical history, (4) psychiatric history, and (5) psychosocial assessment. General nursing assessment can be augmented with specific substance use assessment and addiction screening, family assessment, and the assessment of readiness for change in preparation for interventions (see Box 19-1).

---

**BOX 19-1** **GENERAL ASSESSMENT GUIDELINES FOR PATIENTS WHO USE SUBSTANCES**

**History of Patient's Past Substance Use**
- What is the date of first use, the number of substances being taken, pattern of use, amount, frequency, periods of sobriety, and time last taken?
- Was patient treated previously for substance abuse? What was the outcome?
- Is there a history of blackouts, delirium, or seizures?
- Is there a history of withdrawal symptoms, overdoses, or complications from past substance use?
- Is there a family history of drug or alcohol problems?

**Medical History**
- Does the patient have any coexisting physical conditions (e.g., HIV)?
- What medications does the patient currently take?
- What is the patient's current medical status?
- What is the patient's current mental status?

**Psychiatric History**
- Is there a history of concurrent psychiatric disorders? Depression? Personality disorder? Conduct disorder? Schizophrenia?
- Has the patient undergone treatment for a specific disorder? What medications were given, and what was the outcome?
- Is there a history of abuse (e.g., physical, sexual)? Family violence?
- Is there a history of suicidal ideation? Violence toward others?
- Is the patient currently having suicidal thoughts?

**Psychosocial Issues**
- Does the patient have a poor work record related to substance use?
- How has the patient's substance use affected his or her relationships with others?
  - Family
  - Friends
  - Professional relationships
  - Community involvement
- How has the substance use affected the patient's ability to meet usual role expectations (e.g., parent, spouse, friend, employee)?
- Is there a police or criminal record, or have there been legal problems related to substance use (e.g., vehicle accidents, driving while intoxicated, physical violence)?
- Whom does the patient identify as his or her support system? Whom does the patient trust? Who cares for the patient? Who will help the patient if the patient asks for help?
- Does the patient use coping styles that contribute to the maintenance of his or her drug or alcohol lifestyle?
- What is the patient's readiness for change?

**Source:** Center for Substance Abuse Treatment. (1999). From precontemplation to contemplation: Building readiness. In *Enhancing motivation for change in substance abuse treatment* (Treatment Improvement Protocol [TIP] Series, No. 35). Rockville, MD: Substance Abuse and Mental Health Services Administration. Retrieved from http://www.ncbi.nlm.nih.gov/books/NBK64968/.

## Assessment of Acute Intoxication and of Active and Historical Substance Use or Behavioural Addiction

Acute intoxication and history of substance use or behavioural addictions are important aspects of assessment. Although acute intoxication may or may not be obvious, it is crucial for intoxication to be ascertained to ensure an accurate clinical picture and to prevent possible drug interactions or misdiagnoses. Intracranial hematomas, subdural hematomas, and other conditions can go unnoticed if symptoms of acute alcohol intoxication and withdrawal are not distinguished from the symptoms of a brain injury. Therefore, neurological signs (pupil size, equality, and reaction to light) should be assessed, especially in comatose patients suspected of having traumatic injuries. In addition, questions about alcohol abuse should be asked as part of the assessment of any trauma. Blood alcohol level (BAL), a measurement of the percentage of alcohol in the bloodstream, tested through urinalysis and breath screening devices, can be useful for acute assessment purposes.

Assessment strategies must include collection of data pertaining to both patterns of substance use and psychiatric impairment. Unexplained exacerbations of psychiatric disorders may be due to acute substance abuse or to dependence. Substance abuse can go undetected in patients with depression, anxiety, or suicidal ideation unless a thorough history is taken. Similarly, the understanding and treatment of people with substance use disorders are enhanced by inquiries about symptoms of depression and anxiety.

Once specific data are obtained, it is helpful to know if the person is abusing or is actively dependent on the substance or behaviour and the severity of symptoms (mild to severe) as assessed by the symptoms present. In addition to an overall assessment interview, any number of more focused screening tools may also be used. One measure for assessing alcohol abuse is the Michigan Alcoholism Screening Test (MAST). The MAST, validated for use with many populations, is a 25-point questionnaire designed to provide a rapid and effective screening for lifetime alcohol-related problems and alcoholism (Selzer, 1971; Teitelbaum & Mullen, 2000). Another popular tool is the CAGE Questionnaire (Ewing, 1984), which was originally developed and tested for alcohol abuse screening and has since been adapted to identify problem use of other substances or behaviours. The four questions to be asked in the screening process are remembered by the mnemonic *CAGE*:

1. Have you felt you ought to *Cut* down on your drinking, substance use, or behaviour?
2. Have people *Annoyed* you by criticizing your drinking, substance use, or behaviour?
3. Have you felt *Guilty* about your drinking, substance use, or behaviour?
4. Have you had a drink (or used another substance or behaviour) first thing in the morning to steady your nerves or get yourself going for the day (an *Eye-opener*)?

Each question with an answer of yes scores one point, and the higher the score, the greater the problems with the substance or behaviour. A score of two or more is considered clinically significant.

If the patient is not able to respond to questions or provide a description of current or historical substance use, the nurse should assess for observable indications of substance abuse, such as dilated or constricted pupils, abnormal vital signs, needle marks, tremors, and alcohol on the breath, and obtain information from family and friends. A patient's clothing and belongings, if he or she is admitted to a health care or addictions services clinic, may also be screened or searched for drug paraphernalia, such as used syringes, crack vials, white powder, razor blades, bent spoons, and pipes.

 **ASSESSMENT GUIDELINES**

### Acute Chemical Impairment

1. Assess for a severe or major withdrawal syndrome.
2. Assess for an overdose of a drug or alcohol that warrants immediate medical attention.
3. Assess the patient for suicidal thoughts or other self-destructive behaviours.
4. Evaluate the patient for any physical complications related to drug abuse.
5. Explore the patient's interests in doing something about his or her drug or alcohol problem.
6. Assess the patient's and family's knowledge of community resources for alcohol and drug treatment.

### Signs of Intoxication and Withdrawal

Each class of drugs has its own physiological signs and symptoms of intoxication, which are summarized in the tables for each substance class. Both intoxication and withdrawal may require observation and medical attention or nursing care and can constitute psychiatric emergencies.

### Central Nervous System Depressants

CNS depressant drugs include alcohol, benzodiazepines, and barbiturates. Symptoms of intoxication, overdose, and withdrawal and possible treatments are presented in Table 19-2.

Withdrawal reactions from alcohol and other CNS depressants are associated with severe morbidity and mortality, unlike withdrawal from other drugs (McKeon, Frye, & Delanty, 2007). The syndrome for alcohol withdrawal is the same as that for the entire class of CNS depressant drugs; therefore, alcohol is used in this discussion as the prototype. Alcohol withdrawal, if uncomplicated, is typically complete within five to seven days. Symptoms of withdrawal, however, continue for a longer period and are more severe for older than younger patients. Withdrawal may be delayed, however, when another CNS depressant is the main drug of choice or when the patient is withdrawing from a combination of alcohol and other CNS depressants. Multiple drug and alcohol dependencies can result in simultaneous withdrawal syndromes that present a bizarre clinical picture and may pose problems for safe withdrawal. Further details about alcohol withdrawal and the more severe alcohol withdrawal delirium are provided below.

***Alcohol poisoning.*** Alcohol poisoning—a state of toxicity that can result when an individual has consumed large amounts

## TABLE 19-2  CENTRAL NERVOUS SYSTEM DEPRESSANTS

| DRUG | SIGNS OF INTOXICATION | EFFECTS OF OVERDOSE | POSSIBLE TREATMENTS FOR OVERDOSE | EFFECTS OF WITHDRAWAL | POSSIBLE TREATMENTS FOR WITHDRAWAL |
|---|---|---|---|---|---|
| Barbiturates Benzodiazepines Chloral hydrate Glutethimide Meprobamate Alcohol | *Physical:* Slurred speech Incoordination Unsteady gait Drowsiness Decreased blood pressure *Psychological– perceptual:* Disinhibition of sexual or aggressive drives Impaired judgement Impaired social or occupational function Impaired attention or memory Irritability | Cardiovascular or respiratory depression or arrest (mostly with barbiturates) Coma Shock Convulsions Death | Monitor vital signs every 15 minutes. Monitor for respiratory depression. Oxygen, intubation, or mechanical ventilation may be prescribed. If recent ingestion, induced vomiting, gastric lavage, or activated charcoal may be prescribed. Monitor ECG and lab values for shock. Intravenous (IV) fluids may be prescribed. Continue monitoring VS frequently for respiratory complications, cardiac arrest, and possible seizures. | *Cessation of prolonged or heavy use:* Nausea and vomiting Tachycardia Diaphoresis Anxiety or irritability Tremors in hands, fingers, eyelids Marked insomnia Grand mal seizures *After 5–15 years of heavy use:* Delirium | The physician may prescribe a carefully titrated drug in a similar classification so as to minimize symptoms of withdrawal. *Note:* Abrupt withdrawal can lead to death. |

**Source:** Rowe, B., & Lang, E.S. (2009). *Evidenced based emergency medicine.* Oxford, UK: Wiley-Blackwell.

of alcohol either quickly or over time—can cause death from aspiration of emesis or a shutdown of body systems due to severe CNS depression. Signs of alcohol poisoning include an inability to rouse the individual, severe dehydration, cool or clammy skin, respirations less than 10 per minute, cyanosis of the gums or under the fingernails, and emesis while semiconscious or unconscious. Refer to Table 19-2 for important assessment and treatment information regarding alcohol intoxication and poisoning.

**Alcohol withdrawal.** The early signs of alcohol withdrawal, a physical reaction to the cessation or reduction of alcohol (ethanol) intake, can develop within a few hours of the last intake. Symptoms peak after 24 to 48 hours and then rapidly and dramatically disappear unless the withdrawal progresses to *alcohol withdrawal delirium* (see page 381). Severity of withdrawal tends to be dose related, with heavier drinkers experiencing more severe symptoms. Withdrawal severity is also related to age, with those over 65 years experiencing more severe symptoms. During withdrawal, the patient may appear hyperalert, manifest jerky movements and irritability, startle easily, and experience subjective distress often described as "shaking inside." Grand mal seizures may appear 7 to 48 hours after cessation of alcohol intake, particularly in people with a history of seizures. Careful assessment, including this history and any other risk factors, followed by appropriate medical and nursing interventions, can prevent the more serious withdrawal reaction of delirium.

A competent, supportive manner on the part of the nurse can allay anxiety and provide a sense of security. Consistently and frequently orienting the patient to time and place may be necessary. Encouraging family or close friends (one at a time) to stay with the patient in quiet surroundings can also help increase orientation and minimize confusion and anxiety.

During withdrawal, some patients may experience illusions, which are usually terrifying. Illusions are misinterpretations, usually of a threatening nature, of objects in the environment. For example, a person may think spots on the wallpaper are blood-sucking ants. However, illusions can be clarified to reduce the patient's terror: "See, they are not ants; they are just part of the wallpaper pattern."

Some patients may be argumentative, hostile, or demanding due to the difficult physical experiences but also because of deep-seated anxiety and feelings of guilt and shame. The nurse can relieve some of these feelings by demonstrating an accepting attitude and showing strong support for efforts at recovery.

**Alcohol intoxication.** Alcohol is the only drug for which objective measures of intoxication (i.e., blood alcohol level) exist. The relationship between BAL and behaviour in a nontolerant individual is shown in Table 19-3. Assessing the patient's behaviour can assist the nurse in (1) ascertaining whether the person accurately reported recent drinking and (2) determining level of intoxication and possible tolerance, as patient behaviours may indicate greater or lesser levels of tolerance. As tolerance develops, a discrepancy is seen between the BAL and expected behaviour: a person with tolerance to alcohol may have a high BAL but minimal signs of impairment. Alternatively, a person who is highly sensitive to alcohol or

| TABLE 19-3 | RELATIONSHIP BETWEEN BLOOD ALCOHOL LEVEL AND EFFECTS IN A NONTOLERANT DRINKER | |
|---|---|---|
| BLOOD ALCOHOL LEVEL (mg%) | BLOOD ALCOHOL ACCUMULATION (NUMBER OF DRINKS) | EFFECTS |
| 0.05 | 1–2 | Changes in mood and behaviour; impaired judgement |
| 0.10 | 5–6 | Clumsiness in voluntary motor activity |
| 0.20 | 10–12 | Depressed function of entire motor area of the brain, causing staggering and ataxia; emotional lability |
| 0.30 | 15–18 | Confusion, stupor |
| 0.40 | 20–24 | Coma |
| 0.50 | 25–30 | Death due to respiratory depression |

compromised medically may have a low BAL but demonstrate a high level of intoxication.

***Alcohol withdrawal delirium.*** Alcohol withdrawal delirium is an altered level of consciousness that presents with seizures following acute alcohol withdrawal. It is considered a medical emergency and can result in death even if treated (Monte, Rabuñal, Casariego, et al., 2010). Death is usually due to cardiopathy, cirrhosis, or other co-morbidities requiring mechanical ventilation (Monte, Rabuñal, Casariego, et al., 2010). The state of delirium usually peaks 48 to 72 hours after cessation or reduction of intake (although it can peak later) and lasts two to three days. Features of alcohol withdrawal delirium include the following:

- Autonomic hyperactivity (e.g., tachycardia, diaphoresis, elevated blood pressure)
- Severe disturbance in sensorium (e.g., disorientation, clouding of consciousness)
- Perceptual disturbances (e.g., visual or tactile hallucinations)
- Fluctuating levels of consciousness (ranging from hyperexcitability to lethargy)
- Delusions
- Anxiety and agitated behaviours
- Fever (38°C to 39°C)
- Insomnia
- Anorexia

If these symptoms are observed, immediate medical attention—including ongoing assessment and supervised treatment—is warranted. The Pharmacological Interventions section later in this chapter has a full discussion of medical treatments.

### Central Nervous System Stimulants

The nursing history, physical examination, and laboratory tests are methods of gathering data about drug-related physical problems (McKeon, Frye, & Delanty, 2007). The extent of a person's impairment depends on individual susceptibility, the amount of drug used, and the route of administration.

Table 19-4 outlines the physical and psychological effects of intoxication from amphetamines and other psychostimulants, possible life-threatening results of overdose, and emergency

measures for both overdose and withdrawal. All stimulants accelerate the normal functioning of the body and affect the CNS. Common signs of stimulant abuse include dilation of the pupils, dryness of the nasal cavity, and excessive motor activity.

When someone who has ingested a stimulant experiences chest pain, has an irregular pulse, or has a history of heart trouble, the person should immediately be taken to an emergency department.

***Cocaine and crack.*** Cocaine is a naturally occurring stimulant extracted from the leaf of the coca bush, and crack is a cheap, widely available, alkalinized form of cocaine. When smoked, crack takes effect in four to six seconds, producing a fleeting high (five to seven minutes), followed by a period of deep depression that reinforces addictive behaviour patterns and nearly guarantees continued use of the drug.

Cocaine is classified as a schedule II substance with high abuse potential. It has some recognized medical uses. Cocaine exerts two main effects on the body: anaesthetic and stimulant. As an anaesthetic, it blocks the conduction of electrical impulses within the nerve cells involved in sensory transmission, primarily pain transmission. As a stimulant, it fuels sexual arousal and violent behaviour.

Cocaine blocks the reuptake of norepinephrine, dopamine, and serotonin, causing an imbalance of neurotransmitters (dopamine and norepinephrine) that may be responsible for many of the physical withdrawal symptoms reported by those who use cocaine regularly: depression, paranoia, lethargy, anxiety, insomnia, nausea and vomiting, sweating and chills, and an intense craving for the drug. These signs all result from the body's struggle to regain its normal chemical balance.

Koob and Le Moal (2006) have identified three distinct phases of withdrawal:

1. This phase, the *crash phase*, can last up to four days. Those who use cocaine report depression, anergia, and an acute onset of agitated depression. Craving for the drug peaks during this phase, as do anxiety and paranoia. Inpatient care to prevent access to further doses of the drug is helpful during the first and second phase of withdrawal.

| TABLE 19-4 | CENTRAL NERVOUS SYSTEM STIMULANTS: INTOXICATION, OVERDOSE, AND WITHDRAWAL | | | | |
|---|---|---|---|---|---|
| DRUG | EFFECTS OF INTOXICATION | EFFECTS OF OVERDOSE | POSSIBLE TREATMENTS FOR OVERDOSE | EFFECTS OF WITHDRAWAL | POSSIBLE TREATMENTS FOR WITHDRAWAL |
| Cocaine, crack (short-acting) High obtained by (method) in (time frame): snorted, 3 minutes; injected, 30 seconds; smoked (for crack), 4–6 seconds Average high lasts 15–30 minutes for cocaine; 5–7 minutes for crack | Physical: Tachycardia Dilated pupils Elevated blood pressure Nausea and vomiting Insomnia Psychological– perceptual: Agitation and aggression Grandiosity Impaired judgement Impaired social and occupational functioning Euphoria | Respiratory distress Ataxia Hyperpyrexia Convulsions Coma Stroke Myocardial infarction Death | Antipsychotics, medical and nursing management for: Fever (ambient cooling) Convulsions (diazepam) Respiratory distress or cardiovascular shock (resuscitation and medical treatment to control hypertension, tachycardia, and respirations) Acidification of urine (ammonium chloride for amphetamine) | Fatigue Depression Agitation Apathy Anxiety Sleepiness Disorientation Lethargy Craving | Supportive measures Diazepam (Valium) or lorazepam (Ativan) may be prescribed for mild to moderate withdrawal symptoms |
| Amphetamines (long-acting) Dextroamphetamine Methamphetamine Ice (synthesized for street use) | Increased energy Severe effects: State resembling paranoid schizophrenia Paranoia with delusions Psychosis Visual, auditory, and tactile hallucinations Severe to panic levels of anxiety Potential for violence Note: Paranoia and ideas of reference may persist for months afterward | Same as above | Same as above | Same as above | Same as above |

Source: Sofuoglu, M., Poling, J., Gonzalez, G., et al. (2006). Cocaine withdrawal symptoms predict medication response in cocaine users. American Journal of Drug and Alcohol Abuse, 32, 617–628. doi:10.1080/00952990600920680.

2. During the second phase, the user feels a prolonged sense of dysphoria and anhedonia, a lack of motivation, and intense cravings for the substance of abuse. This phase can last up to ten weeks. Relapse is most likely during the second phase of withdrawal.
3. The third phase is characterized by intermittent craving and can last indefinitely.

**Caffeine and nicotine.** Most people consume caffeine through coffee, tea, energy drinks, or soft drinks. People may ingest these substances as a drug (e.g., "I've got to have two cups in the morning to function" or "When I'm working a construction job, I just need a few energy drinks a day, and I'm good to go"), for social reasons (e.g., "Let's get together for coffee"), or as a reward (e.g., "After I finish this job, I'm going to take a coffee break").

While smoking rates have gone down in the past 20 years, nicotine is one of the most heavily used addictive drugs in Canada. Among people aged 15 years and older, 19% smoke cigarettes, with the highest rates seen in teenage girls (Alberta Health Services, 2009). A high proportion of psychiatric outpatients are nicotine dependent: up to 90% of patients with schizophrenia and about 70% of patients with bipolar I disorder or another substance abuse disorder (Sadock & Sadock, 2008). Champix and nicotine-replacement therapy have proven to be successful smoking-cessation treatments for many individuals.

### Opioids

The opioid drug class includes opium, morphine, heroin, codeine, fentanyl and its analogues, methadone, and meperidine. An opioid is a derivative or synthetic that affects the CNS

| TABLE 19-5 | **OPIOIDS: INTOXICATION, OVERDOSE, AND WITHDRAWAL** |

| DRUG | EFFECTS OF INTOXICATION | EFFECTS OF OVERDOSE | POSSIBLE TREATMENTS FOR OVERDOSE | EFFECTS OF WITHDRAWAL | POSSIBLE TREATMENTS FOR WITHDRAWAL |
|---|---|---|---|---|---|
| Opium (paregoric) Heroin Meperidine (Demerol) Morphine Codeine Methadone (Metadol) Hydromorphone (Dilaudid) Fentanyl (Abstral— sublingual) Fentanyl analogues | *Physical:* Constricted pupils Decreased respiration Drowsiness Decreased blood pressure Slurred speech Psychomotor retardation *Psychological– perceptual:* Initial euphoria followed by dysphoria and impairment of attention, judgement, and memory | Possible dilation of pupils due to anoxia Respiratory depression or arrest Coma Shock Convulsions Death | Opioid antagonist (e.g., naloxone [Targin]) to quickly reverse CNS depression | Yawning Insomnia Irritability Rhinorrhea Panic Diaphoresis Cramps Nausea and vomiting Muscle aches ("bone pain") Chills Fever Lacrimation Diarrhea | Methadone tapering* Clonidine– naltrexone detoxification Buprenorphine substitution** |

**Source:** Veilleux, J.C., Colvina, P.J., Andersona, J., et al. (2010). A review of opioid dependence treatment: Pharmacological and psychosocial interventions to treat opioid addiction. *Clinical Psychology Review, 30*, 155–166. doi:10.1016/j.cpr.2009.10.006.
*Methadone tapering is managed very slowly and in careful consultation with the patient with regard to their readiness.
**Buprenorphine tapering is currently under review in Ontario but is not widely used to manage withdrawal in Canada.

## RESEARCH HIGHLIGHT

### Smoking Cessation Support via Mobile Texting

**Source:** Free, C., Knight, R., Robertson, S., et al. (2011). Smoking cessation support delivered via mobile phone text messaging (txt2stop): A single-blind, randomised trial. *The Lancet, 378*, 49–55. doi:10.1016/S0140-6736(11)60701-0.

#### Problem
Most of those killed by tobacco started smoking as teenagers, and smoking contributes to the death of one of every two of those who smoke past 35 years of age. Stopping smoking at an early age conveys greater health benefits.

#### Purpose of Study
For many people, mobile phones are part of their everyday lives and are always carried with them; therefore, a text intervention can take place at any time. The purpose of this study was to assess the effectiveness of a mobile phone–based smoking intervention.

#### Methods
Participants were recruited through various media, including Web sites, primary care facilities, and pharmacies. Inclusion criteria were that participants were 16 or older, had a mobile phone, and were willing to attempt to stop smoking. In the next month, 5800 participants were randomized into two groups based on age, gender, education, and nicotine addiction score. Individuals in the treatment group received motivational and behavioural text messages while the control group received text messages related only to the importance of participation in the trial. At six months post-trial, salivary tests were used to confirm self-reported abstinence.

#### Key Findings
Text messages via mobile phones doubled smoking cessation rates in the treatment group but were similar to cessation rates in other behavioural interventions like group, one-to-one, or telephone advice programs. Mobile phones simply provide a new channel for individualized programs to be delivered inexpensively wherever the person is located.

#### Implications for Nursing Practice
Researchers suggest that the use of mobile text messages should be considered as part of existing cessation programs. The researchers also suggest that using mobile technology may be effective in changing other behavioural risk factors.

and the autonomic nervous system. Medically, it is used primarily as an analgesic (painkiller). Consistent use causes tolerance and distressing withdrawal symptoms. Table 19-5 lists signs and symptoms of intoxication, overdose, withdrawal, and possible treatments.

Heroin is one of the most widely abused opioids. Heroin intoxication can be classified into four distinct phases. The first phase is a euphoria or rush that occurs almost immediately after injection of the drug. Those who use heroin frequently characterize this euphoria in terms of sexual arousal. The euphoric phase is characterized physiologically by facial flushing and a deepening of the voice. The second phase is classified as "the high" and has been described as a sense of well-being. This phase can extend for several hours. The third phase, often termed "the nod," is an escape from reality that can range from lethargy to virtual unconsciousness. The fourth phase is the period before withdrawal occurs. During the fourth phase, those using heroin often seek more of the drug in order to avoid withdrawal.

## Marijuana

Marijuana (*Cannabis sativa*) is a hemp plant. Tetrahydrocannabinol (THC) is the active ingredient found in the resin secreted from the flowering tops and leaves of the cannabis plant. THC has mixed depressant and hallucinogenic properties. Marijuana, the leaves of the cannabis plant, is generally smoked, but it also can be ingested. Desired effects include euphoria, detachment, and relaxation. Other effects include talkativeness, slowed perception of time, inappropriate hilarity, heightened sensitivity to external stimuli, and anxiety or

paranoia. Long-term use of cannabis can result in lethargy, anhedonia, difficulty concentrating, and loss of memory.

Overdose and withdrawal symptoms (other than cravings for the substance of abuse) rarely occur. Medical indications exist for the use of THC (e.g., control of chemotherapy-induced nausea, reduction of intraocular pressure in glaucoma, appetite stimulation in AIDS wasting syndrome). Controversy over the approach to provision and prescription is unfolding in Canada. As of March 31, 2014, the federal government will no longer issue prescriptions nor allow personal production of the cannabis plant, instead favouring licensed commercial producers.

## Hallucinogens

A hallucinogen produces abnormal mental phenomena in the cognitive and perceptual spheres—for example, distortion in space and time, hallucinations, delusions (paranoid or grandiose), and synesthesia. Table 19-6 outlines the signs and symptoms of hallucinogen intoxication and overdose.

Diazepam (Valium) or lorazepam (Ativan) may be prescribed to treat PCP-induced aggressiveness, psychotic

### TABLE 19-6  HALLUCINOGENS: INTOXICATION, OVERDOSE, AND WITHDRAWAL

| DRUG | PHYSICAL EFFECTS OF INTOXICATION | PSYCHOLOGICAL-PERCEPTUAL EFFECTS OF INTOXICATION | EFFECTS OF OVERDOSE | POSSIBLE TREATMENTS FOR OVERDOSE |
|---|---|---|---|---|
| Lysergic acid diethylamide (LSD) Mescaline (peyote) Psilocybin (mushrooms) | Pupil dilation Tachycardia Diaphoresis Palpitations Tremors Incoordination Elevated temperature, pulse, respiration | Fear of going crazy Paranoid ideas Marked anxiety, depression Synesthesia (e.g., colours are heard; sounds are seen) Depersonalization Hallucinations, although sensorium is clear Grandiosity (e.g., thinking one can fly) | Psychosis Brain damage Death | Keep patient in room with low stimuli—minimal light, sound, activity. Have one person stay with patient. Provide reassurance. Speak slowly and clearly in quiet voice. Diazepam or chloral hydrate may be prescribed for extreme anxiety or tension. |
| Phencyclidine piperidine (PCP) | Vertical or horizontal nystagmus Increased blood pressure, pulse, and temperature Ataxia Muscle rigidity Seizures Blank stare Chronic jerking Agitated, repetitive movements Belligerence, assaultiveness, impulsiveness Impaired judgement, impaired social and occupational functioning | *Severe effects:* Hallucinations, paranoia Bizarre behaviour (e.g., barking like a dog, grimacing, repetitive chanting speech) Regressive behaviour Violent bizarre behaviours Very labile behaviours | Psychosis Possible hypertensive crisis or cardiovascular accident Respiratory arrest Hyperthermia Seizures | *If alert:* Put in room with minimal stimuli. Do not attempt to talk down! Speak slowly, clearly, and in a quiet voice. *Monitor and be prepared to intervene for:* Hyperthermia High blood pressure Respiratory distress Hypertension |

**Source:** Meehan Y.J., Bryant, S.M., & Aks, S.E. (2010). Drugs of abuse: The highs and lows of altered mental states in the emergency department. *Emergency Medicine Clinics of North America, 28*, 663–682. doi:10.1016/j.emc.2010.03.012.

symptoms, hypertension, and tachycardia while olanzapine (Zyprexa) or risperidone (Risperdal) may be prescribed for psychotic events (Bey & Patel, 2007).

*Lysergic acid diethylamide (LSD) and LSD-like drugs.* LSD (also known as *acid*), mescaline (peyote), and psilocybin (mushrooms) are hallucinogens. Mescaline and the mushroom *Psilocybemexicana* (from which psilocybin is isolated) have been used in religious rites by Canadian Aboriginal peoples for centuries. A hallucinogenic experience produced by LSD or other substances is commonly called a *trip*.

*Phencyclidine piperidine (PCP).* PCP is also known as *angel dust, horse tranquilizer,* and *peace pill.* When the drug is taken orally, the onset of symptoms occurs about one hour after ingestion. When it is taken intravenously or intranasally or smoked, the onset of symptoms may occur within five minutes. The signs and symptoms of PCP intoxication range from acute anxiety to acute psychosis. The drug produces a generalized anaesthesia that lessens the sensations of touch and pain. Chronic use of PCP can result in long-term effects such as dulled thinking, lethargy, loss of impulse control, poor memory, and depression.

Suicidal risk is always assessed, especially in cases of toxicity or coma. If the patient awakens and appears to be suicidal, the nurse should determine whether previous suicide attempts have occurred and whether there is a family history of suicide.

Additional history may be obtained through family and a review of medical records. Refer to Chapter 25 for more information on suicide assessment.

## Inhalants

About 2.3% to 5.3% of adolescents in Canada say they have sniffed inhalants—usually volatile solvents such as spray paint, glue, cigarette lighter fluid, and propellant gases used in aerosols—at least once in their lives (Collin, 2006). Types of inhalants, signs of intoxication, and adverse effects are outlined in Table 19-7. Inhalant use may be an early marker of substance abuse and should be the focus of increased preventive efforts and early diagnosis and treatment (Collins, Pan, Johnson, et al., 2008).

## Club Drugs

Ecstasy (3, 4-methylenedioxymethamphetamine), also called *MDMA, Adam, yaba,* and *XTC,* is a prototype of a class of substituted amphetamines that also includes MDA (methylenedioxyamphetamine, or "love") and MDE (3, 4-methylenedioxyethylamphetamine, or "Eve"). These recreational drugs produce subjective effects resembling those of stimulants and hallucinogens. MDMA causes a significant release of the neurochemicals serotonin, dopamine, and norepinephrine. The brain's saturation of these neurotransmitters

## TABLE 19-7 INHALANTS: INTOXICATION, OVERDOSE, AND TREATMENT

| DRUG | INTOXICATION | ADVERSE EFFECTS/ OVERDOSE | TREATMENT |
|---|---|---|---|
| Organic solvents (gases or liquids that vaporize at room temperature): Toluene Gasoline Lighter fluid Paint thinner Nail-polish remover Benzene Acetone Chloroform Model-airplane glue | Alcohol-like effects: euphoria, impaired judgement, slurred speech, flushing, CNS depression Visual hallucinations and disorientation | Chronic use is toxic to heart, liver, and kidneys. Toxicity may result in sudden death from anoxia, vagal stimulation, respiratory depression, and dysthymia. | Support affected systems; no antidotes |
| Volatile nitrites: Room deodorizers Products sold for recreational use | Enhancement of sexual pleasure | Venodilation causes profound systolic blood pressure drop (dizziness, lightheadedness, palpitations, pulsate headache). Toxic dose may result in methemoglobinemia. | Toxicity may be treated with oxygen. |
| Anaesthetics: Gas—especially nitrous oxide (used in dental procedures and as a propellant for whipped cream) Liquid Local | Giggling, laughter Euphoria | Numbness, weakness, sensory loss, loss of balance. May cause physical dependence. Possible polyneuropathy and myelopathy when use is chronic. | Neuropathy may be treated with $B_{12}$. |

**Source:** Data from Lehne, R.E. (2010). *Pharmacology for nursing care* (7th ed.). Philadelphia: Saunders; and Ruiz, P., Strain, E.C., & Langrod, J.G. (2007). *The substance abuse handbook.* Philadelphia: Lippincott Williams & Wilkins.

causes those who use MDMA to exhibit major empathy toward others, reduces inhibitions, elicits introspection, and results in an outpouring of good feelings about others, the current environment, and the world. The release of serotonin also intensely sharpens the senses of those using the substance.

Those using MDMA may be hyperactive and have inexhaustible energy (e.g., dancing all night long), dilated pupils with impaired reaction to light, elevated temperature, elevated pulse, elevated blood pressure, diaphoresis, dystonia, bruxism (grinding of the teeth), and other symptoms of stimulant use, such as tachycardia, mydriasis (dilation of the pupils), tremors, arrhythmias, parkinsonism, esophoria (eyes turning inward), central serotonin syndrome, and severe hyponatremia. Those using MDMA must drink a large quantity of water during use to prevent dehydration and hyperthermia.

After the effects of MDMA wear off, the person using the substance commonly goes through a period of depression. This depression is caused by a depletion of serotonin, levels of which do not return to normal within the CNS for at least three to four days. Those using MDMA describe the period after use as *blue Tuesdays*. Use of additional MDMA after serotonin stores have been depleted does not produce the same effects as the initial use, and thereafter, those using the substance tend to experience only the symptoms associated with the use of a stimulant amphetamine.

### Date Rape Drugs

The drugs most frequently used to facilitate a sexual assault (rape) are flunitrazepam (Rohypnol, or "roofies," a fast-acting benzodiazepine) and γ-hydroxybutyric acid (GHB) and its congeners (Crawford, O'Dougherty-Wright, & Bircheimer, 2008). These drugs are odourless, tasteless, and colourless; mix easily with drinks; and can render a person unconscious in a matter of minutes. Perpetrators use these drugs because they rapidly produce disinhibition and relaxation of voluntary muscles; they also cause the victim to have lasting anterograde amnesia for events that occur. Alcohol potentiates their effects. Refer to Chapter 28 for additional discussion of the use of these drugs in sexual assault.

### Psychological Changes

Certain psychological characteristics are associated with substance abuse, including denial, depression, anxiety, dependency, hopelessness, low self-esteem, and various psychiatric disorders. It is often difficult to determine which comes first: psychological changes or substance abuse. Some people self-medicate to cope with psychiatric symptoms. Some people develop psychiatric symptoms due to substance abuse.

People who abuse substances feel threatened on many levels in their interactions with nurses. First, they are concerned about being rejected because not all nurses are willing to care for people with addictions. In fact, many patients have reported experiences of rejection in past encounters with nursing personnel. Second, people who abuse substances may be anxious about giving up the substance they think they need to survive. Third, people with addictions often are concerned about failing at recovering. Addiction is a chronic, relapsing condition. In

fact, relapse is one of the criteria for diagnosing addiction. Most addicts have tried recovery at least once before and have since experienced relapse. As a result, many become discouraged about their chances of ever succeeding. Such feelings of discouragement and a high level of hopelessness can act as barriers to recovery.

Concerns about failure or potential relapse on the path of recovery can threaten the person's sense of security and sense of self, increasing anxiety levels. To protect against these feelings, the person with an addiction often establishes a predictable defensive style that includes various defence mechanisms (e.g., denial, projection, rationalization), as well as characteristic thought processes (e.g., all-or-none thinking, selective attention) and behaviours (e.g., conflict minimization and avoidance, passivity, manipulation). Typically, the person is unable to give up these maladaptive coping styles until more positive and functional skills are learned.

### Assessment of Readiness for Change

Various scales and tools have been developed to assist in the assessment process. The Rhode Island Change Assessment Scale (URICA), one such tool, is designed to measure the stages of change across diverse problem behaviours. Some interventions, such as motivational interviewing—an approach that can assist clinicians in helping patients through the fluctuations between the various phases toward change (Miller & Rollnick, 2002)—have evolved from the Transtheoretical Model of Change, which was originally explained by Prochaska and DiClemente (1984). This model describes the stages and decision making whereby people modify a problem behaviour or acquire a positive behaviour. The model serves as the basis for health care providers' development of effective interventions to promote health behaviour change and for planning treatment. It has proven useful for encouraging such positive behaviours as smoking cessation, exercise, weight control, condom use for protection against HIV, sunscreen use, stress management, medical compliance, and drug and alcohol abstinence. The model may also help to explain differences in individuals' success during treatment for addictions.

The Transtheoretical Model of Change theorizes that people pass through a series of stages toward making changes: (1) precontemplation, (2) contemplation, (3) preparation, (4) action, and (5) maintenance.

In the precontemplation phase, the individual is not currently considering change or intending to take action in the foreseeable future (usually in the next six months). Traditional health promotion or treatment programs are often not designed for such individuals and are not matched to their needs. Approaches to support the patient at this stage include the following:

- Validating the lack of readiness
- Encouraging re-evaluation of current behaviour
- Encouraging self-exploration, rather than action
- Explaining and personalizing the risk

The stage during which a person is thinking of changing is referred to as the contemplation phase. In this phase, the patient is ambivalent about change and likely not considering change within the next month. Supportive approaches might include these:

- Encouraging evaluation of the pros and cons of behaviour change
- Re-evaluating group image through group activities
- Identifying and promoting new, positive-outcome expectations

The preparation phase occurs when the patient, who may have had some experience with change, is actively making attempts at behaviour change, even if in a trial or testing process, or has plans to take action within the month (e.g., joining a health education class, consulting a counsellor, talking to a physician, buying a self-help book, or relying on a self-change approach). Supportive approaches at this phase include these:

- Encouraging the evaluation of the pros and cons of behaviour change
- Identifying and promoting new positive-outcome expectations
- Encouraging realistic, practical, and small initial steps
- Offering referrals to and support of action-oriented programs (e.g., smoking-cessation, weight-loss, or exercise programs)

In the action phase, the patient is actively working toward the desired behavioural change, including modifying his or her environment, experiences, or behaviour. At this stage, the patient will have made specific, overt modifications in lifestyle within the past six months, and measures should be taken against relapse. Supportive approaches include these:

- Helping the patient with restructuring cues and triggers and solidifying social support
- Enhancing self-efficacy for dealing with obstacles
- Helping to guard against feelings of loss and frustration

The patient in the maintenance phase focuses on actively working to maintain changes made and prevent relapse. At this stage, patients are less tempted to relapse and are becoming increasingly confident that they can continue their changed behaviour. Approaches include the following:

- Planning for follow-up support
- Reinforcing internal rewards
- Discussing strategies for coping with triggers and relapse

Relapse, not explained formally in the model, is a phase that cycles back to previous stages. It refers to reverting to an earlier stage of change, toward the old behaviours, after progressing through some of the later stages. Relapse can be an expected part of change, and supportive approaches that are particularly helpful to assist the patient and family include the following:

- Evaluating triggers for relapse
- Reassessing motivation and barriers to change
- Planning and rehearsing new and stronger coping strategies

## Self-Assessment and Self-Awareness

To offer support and motivation toward recovery, a nurse must examine his or her own attitudes, feelings, and beliefs about addiction and persons with addictions. Such reflection often means nurses must examine their own substance use and the substance use of others in their lives, a potentially difficult task. A history of substance abuse in a nurse's own family can interfere with the helping relationship and contribute to counter-transference (see Chapter 10). The negative or positive experiences a nurse has had with family members or others with addictions can influence interpersonal interactions with patients and impact treatment outcomes. Therefore, attending to personal feelings that arise when working with people experiencing addictions is vital, as are ongoing self-reflection and supervision that encourages reflection on the nurse's responses as well as the patients. Nurses who do not attend to—and work through—expected negative feelings that arise while providing care may engage in power struggles with patients, resulting in an ineffective therapeutic process (Centre for Addiction and Mental Health, 2008). These issues can also become evident when a fellow nurse has a substance abuse problem.

## Nurses and Addiction in the Workplace

"Current estimates place rates of substance misuse, abuse, and addiction rates as high as 20% among practicing nurses" (Monroe & Kenaga, 2011, p. 504). Fear of retribution or disciplinary action often prevents nurses either from seeking help for themselves or from reporting a colleague or friend. Supporting the treatment and recovery of a fellow nurse experiencing an addiction can be challenging, but the situation is not uncommon, nor is being supportive impossible. The choices for action are varied, and the only choice that is clearly wrong is doing nothing. Without intervention or treatment, the problems associated with addiction escalate, and the potential for patient harm increases.

A nurse experiencing an addiction may often volunteer to work additional shifts to be nearer to the supply of the substance of abuse. The nurse may leave the unit frequently or spend a lot of time in the bathroom. When the nurse with an addiction is on duty, more patients may complain that their pain is unrelieved by their opioid analgesic or that they are unable to sleep, despite receiving sedative medications. Increases in inaccurate drug counts and reports of vial breakage may occur.

The Canadian Nurses Association's (2008) Code of Ethics requires nurses to recognize when their own personal problems might interfere with their effectiveness and take action. The code of ethics also requires nurses to recognize signs of substance abuse or impaired practice in colleagues and to report such behaviour to the nurse manager. Intervention is the responsibility of the nurse manager and other nursing administrators. However, clear documentation by co-workers (specific dates, times, events, consequences) is crucial. The nurse manager's major concerns are with job performance and patient safety. Once the nurse manager has been informed, the legal and ethical responsibilities for in-house reporting have been met. If the nurse experiencing an addiction remains in the situation, and no action is taken by the nurse manager, then co-workers must take the information to the next level in the management structure or look to the provincial or territorial regulatory body for consultation and guidance. These measures can prevent harm to patients under the care of the nurse who is abusing substances and can save a colleague's professional career or even life.

Reporting a colleague who has a problem with misuse, abuse, or addiction is not easy, even though it is a professional responsibility. In efforts to avoid conflict or difficult emotions, nurse colleagues may deny or rationalize the problem, thus enabling the nurse who is abusing substances. The nurse then is at risk for endangering the lives of those in his or her care and for experiencing more harmful consequences of addiction. In light of the duty of professional responsibility, nurses can ask themselves the difficult questions: if they have co-signed controlled-substance "wastes" that were not actually witnessed; if they have ever corrected the narcotic count to account for a discrepancy; or if they have ever excused or rationalized behaviour that might be related to substance abuse. Box 19-2 can be used to assess whether there is a specific drug diversion or a potential misuse of drugs for personal gain in the workplace by a nurse colleague.

---

**BOX 19-2   SIGNS OF WORKPLACE DIVERSION OF DRUGS**

- Arriving early, staying late, and coming to work on scheduled days off
- Excessive wasting of drugs
- Regularly signing out large quantities of controlled drugs
- Volunteering often to give medication to other nurses' patients
- Taking frequent bathroom breaks
- Patients' reporting unrelieved pain despite adequate prescription of pain medication
- Discrepancies in the documentation of controlled substance administration
- Medications' being signed out for patients who have been discharged or transferred or who are off the unit for procedures or tests
- Minimizing the seriousness of the theft, claiming it would be wasted anyway

**Source:** Maher-Brisen, P. (2007). Addiction: An occupational hazard in nursing. *American Journal of Nursing, 107,* 78–79. doi:10.1097/01. NAJ.0000282302.49183.67.

---

Referral to a treatment program is one important treatment option for nurses with addictions. Programs for professionals experiencing addictions have been developed in most Canadian provinces. Some provincial and territorial professional nursing associations support nurses who are experiencing substance misuse or addiction and may withhold disciplinary action if treatment is sought. The aims of supportive policy and specific treatment programs for nurses are to protect patients and to keep the nurse in active practice (perhaps with limitations) or return the nurse to practice after suspension and professional help. More severe consequences—restricting or withholding the ability of the nurse to provide direct patient care—are put into place for nurses who show signs of ongoing impairment.

## Communication Techniques for Assessment and Interventions

Accurate assessment and effective intervention planning and implementation for colleagues and patients depends upon development of a therapeutic relationship (see Chapter 10) and effective communication (see Chapter 11). Communication strategies are designed to address behaviours that many people with substance abuse disorders have in common, including dysfunctional anger, manipulation, impulsiveness, and grandiosity. Communication approaches for the practice of motivational interviewing as an intervention are discussed later in this chapter, on pages 391 and 392. The nurse's ability to develop a therapeutic relationship with a patient with an addiction can help the patient feel safe enough to start looking at problems with some degree of openness and honesty. The following is a portion of an intake interview with a patient upon admission to a treatment program.

| Dialogue | Therapeutic Tool or Comment |
|---|---|
| **Nurse:** "Elyse, I get the impression that life must have been very difficult for you lately." | Validating and empathizing |
| **Elyse:** (long pause) "I don't think you would understand." | |
| **Nurse:** "I guess sometimes it feels as if no one understands, but I would like to try." | Reflecting and empathizing |
| **Elyse:** "At times I feel I can't go on anymore … so many losses." | |
| **Nurse:** "Loss is difficult. Elyse, tell me about your losses." | Encouraging the patient to share her painful feelings |
| **Elyse:** "My brother's sudden death. … We were so close. … I depended on him so much." | |
| **Nurse:** "It must have been difficult for you to lose him so suddenly." | Empathizing |
| **Elyse:** (long pause) "No one knows. … Then Joseph, he left. …" (Elyse starts to cry) | |
| **Nurse:** (sitting in silence as Elyse cries, then asking for more information about the feelings expressed) "Tell me about this experience." | Encouraging the expression of feelings while feelings are close to the surface |
| **Elyse:** "I don't know. … I just wonder, why does everyone leave me? Oh, I hate them all. … I wish I had a Valium now." | |
| **Nurse:** "And what does the Valium do to help you?" | Beginning to explore the drug dependence in a gentle, nonthreatening manner |

The next example demonstrates the use of therapeutic leverage (i.e., making abstinence and sobriety worthwhile for those abusing the substance). It is presented as a dialogue between a nurse and a 17-year-old young man whose parents are divorced and whose father abuses him when drinking. He was picked up three times during the preceding seven months for possession of cocaine.

| Dialogue | Therapeutic Tool or Comment |
|---|---|
| **Nurse:** "I understand you entered the treatment program yesterday afternoon following your court appearance." | Placing the event in time and sequence; validating the precipitating event |
| **Kang:** "Yeah—it was my dad's idea." | |
| **Nurse:** "Well, what do you think of the idea?" | Encouraging evaluation (actions first; thoughts; then feelings) |
| **Kang:** "I don't like it. I don't need this place. I'm not a junkie—I just use crack … that's all. I can handle it." | |
| **Nurse:** "From what I've heard, your involvement with crack has gotten you into trouble." | Pointing out realities |
| **Kang:** "Yeah, well, I guess I can't deny that … but I still don't think I need this place." | |
| **Nurse:** "Are you saying that you don't think you need a treatment program?" | Validating the patient's perception |
| **Kang:** "Well, I don't know. I guess maybe I am a little messed up." | |
| **Nurse:** " 'Messed up.' " | Restating |
| **Kang:** "Yeah." | |
| **Nurse:** "What is one thing about you that's messed up?" | Encouraging the patient to be specific rather than global |
| **Kang:** (silence) "I guess I feel like I don't belong anywhere." | |
| **Nurse:** "Talk more about that." | Clarifying |

## DIAGNOSIS

Formulation of appropriate nursing diagnoses depends on accurate assessment and screening. Whereas the criteria for medical diagnosis emphasize patterns of use and physical symptoms, *nursing* diagnoses identify how dependence on substances of abuse interferes with a person's ability to deal with the activities and demands of daily living.

Nursing diagnoses for patients with psychoactive substance use disorders are many and varied because of the large range of physical and psychological effects of drug abuse or dependence on people using these substances as well as on their family. Co-morbid psychiatric problems alongside addictions (referred to as *concurrent disorders*) also must be addressed. Potential nursing diagnoses for people with substance use disorders are listed in Table 19-8.

## OUTCOMES IDENTIFICATION

*Nursing Outcomes Classification (NOC)* categories (Moorhead, Johnson, Maas, et al., 2008) for outcome criteria for patients

with substance use disorders can be divided into withdrawal, initial and active drug treatment, and health maintenance. When the patient has a concurrent disorder, the nurse will also develop nursing outcomes for the psychiatric disorder. Specific *NOC* outcomes and examples of patient goals follow.

### Withdrawal

*Fluid balance:* Patient's blood pressure will not be compromised.

*Neurological status: Consciousness:* Patient will have no seizure activity.

*Distorted thought self-control:* Patient will consistently describe content of hallucinations.

### Initial and Active Substance Abuse Treatment

*Risk control: Substance use:* Patient will consistently demonstrate a commitment to substance use control strategies.

*Risk control: Substance use:* Patient will consistently acknowledge personal consequences associated with substance abuse.

*Substance addiction consequences:* Patient will demonstrate no difficulty supporting self financially.

### Health Maintenance

*Knowledge: Substance abuse control:* Patient will describe actions to prevent and manage relapses in substance use.

*Family coping:* Family will consistently demonstrate care for needs of all family members.

## PLANNING

Planning care requires attention to the patient's social status, income, ethnic background, gender, age, substance use history, and current condition. Planning must also address the patient's major psychological, social, and medical problems, as well as the substance-using behaviour. Involvement of appropriate family members is essential.

Unfortunately, a person's social status and social relations often deteriorate as a result of addiction. Job demotion or loss of job, with resultant reduced or nonexistent income, may occur. Meeting basic needs for food, shelter, and clothing is thereby hampered. Marriage and other close relationships often deteriorate, and the patient is then left alone and isolated. A lack of interpersonal and social supports is a complicating factor in treatment planning for people experiencing addiction. Case Study and Nursing Care Plan 19-1 on pages 396–398 presents a discussion of a patient with concurrent alcohol dependence and depression.

## IMPLEMENTATION

The aim of treatment is self-responsibility and motivation, not compliance with an imposed program. A major challenge is improving treatment effectiveness by matching subtypes of patients to specific types of treatment. Although those experiencing substance-related disorders and addictions may share some characteristics and dynamics, significant differences exist with regard to physiological, psychological, and sociocultural

| TABLE 19-8 | POTENTIAL NURSING DIAGNOSES FOR SUBSTANCE ABUSE OR BEHAVIOURAL ADDICTIONS |
|---|---|
| **SIGNS AND SYMPTOMS** | **NURSING DIAGNOSES** |
| Vomiting<br>Diarrhea<br>Poor nutritional and fluid intake | *Imbalanced nutrition: Less than body requirements*<br>*Deficient fluid volume* |
| Audiovisual hallucinations<br>Impaired judgement<br>Memory deficits<br>Cognitive impairments related to substance intoxication or withdrawal (e.g., deficits in problem solving, ability to attend to tasks, and grasp ideas) | *Disturbed thought processes*<br>*Disturbed sensory perception* |
| Changes in sleep–wake cycle (e.g., interference with stage 4 sleep, inability to sleep, or long periods of sleeping related to effects of or withdrawal from substance) | *Disturbed sleep pattern* |
| Lack of self-care (hygiene, grooming, failure to care for basic health needs) | *Ineffective health maintenance*<br>*Self-care deficit*<br>*Noncompliance to health care regimen* |
| Feelings of hopelessness, inability to change<br>Feelings of worthlessness<br>Feeling that life has no meaning or future | *Hopelessness*<br>*Spiritual distress*<br>*Situational low self-esteem*<br>*Chronic low self-esteem*<br>*Risk for self-directed violence*<br>*Risk for suicide* |
| Family crises and family pain<br>Ineffective parenting<br>Emotional neglect of others<br>Increased incidence of physical and sexual abuse of others<br>Increased self-hate projected to others | *Interrupted family processes*<br>*Impaired parenting*<br>*Risk for other-directed violence* |
| Excessive substance abuse affecting all areas of a person's life: loss of friends, poor job performance, increased illness rates, proneness to accidents and overdoses | *Ineffective coping*<br>*Impaired verbal communication*<br>*Social isolation*<br>*Risk for loneliness*<br>*Anxiety*<br>*Risk for suicide* |
| Increased health problems related to substance used and route of use, as well as overdose | *Activity intolerance*<br>*Ineffective airway clearance*<br>*Ineffective breathing pattern*<br>*Impaired oral mucous membrane*<br>*Risk for infection*<br>*Decreased cardiac output*<br>*Sexual dysfunction* |
| Total preoccupation with (and majority of time consumed by) taking and withdrawing from drug | *Delayed growth and development*<br>*Ineffective coping*<br>*Impaired social interaction*<br>*Dysfunctional family processes* |

processes for all individuals. These differences influence the recovery process either positively or negatively. In terms of treatment, a recent systematic review of randomized control trials for concurrent disorders showed that no one psychosocial treatment has an advantage over another. There was, however, evidence that motivational interviewing reduces substance use, suggesting that it is a crucial component in

the effectiveness of treatment for patients with concurrent disorders (Cleary, Hunt, Matheson, et al., 2008). Cumulative evidence in another systematic review supported integrating outpatient concurrent-disorder treatments into a single package and also further noted success with motivational interviewing even in short-term therapy (Drake, Mueser, Brunette, et al., 2004).

Proposing abstinence as a treatment goal is safest for those with more than one substance use disorder. Abstinence is strongly related to good work adjustment, positive health status, comfortable interpersonal relationships, and general social stability. Often, the choice of treatment or approach depends on the patient's needs, treatment goals, motivation, and personal circumstances including family needs and financial resources. Outpatient programs work best for people with substance abuse disorders who are employed and have an active social support system. People who have no support and structure in their day may do better in inpatient or residential programs when these programs are available.

Beyond personal concerns and choice of treatment, neuropsychological deficits have been associated with long-term alcohol abuse and may impact treatment choices or potential benefits. Such deficits have been found in abstract reasoning ability, ability to use feedback in learning new concepts, attention and concentration spans, cognitive flexibility, and subtle memory functions. These cognitive impairments undoubtedly have an impact on the process of treatment for alcohol or other substance abuse.

At all levels of practice, the nurse can play an important role in the intervention process by recognizing the signs of substance abuse in both the patient and the family and by being familiar with the resources available to help with the problem. Approaches to treatment implementation, including substance abuse interventions, motivational interviewing, pharmacological interventions, and advanced-practice interventions, are discussed below, as are implementation strategies at all levels of prevention.

## Substance Abuse Interventions

A useful tool for helping patients resistant to seeking help or engaging in treatment is an approach known as substance abuse intervention, commonly referred to as *an intervention*. In an intervention, significant others arrange to meet with the person experiencing an addiction to point out current problems and offer treatment alternatives. The concept behind this approach is that addiction is a progressive illness and rarely goes into remission without outside help. The steps or elements of an intervention are outlined in Box 19-3 and can be applied to abuse of not only alcohol but also other substances or behavioural addictions.

## Motivational Interviewing

Through motivational interviewing, nurses communicate with patients in a manner that can address the patient's likely indecision, ambivalence, resistance, and other such fluctuations on the path to recovery (Miller & Rollnick, 2002). The most significant predictor of treatment success, considering the ambivalence of most of these patients, is an empathic, hopeful, and consistently motivational approach (Minkoff, 2001). Miller and Rollnick (2002) established eight steps to the motivational interviewing process: establishing rapport, setting the agenda, assessing readiness to change, sharpening focus, identifying ambivalence, eliciting self-motivating statements, handling resistance, and shifting focus and transition (see Box 19-4).

### BOX 19-3  STEPS IN SUBSTANCE ABUSE INTERVENTION (FOR THOSE RESISTING TREATMENT)

1. All the people concerned about and affected by the person's substance abuse gather to present their case. The intervention must be rehearsed, usually with the support and guidance of a counsellor, before it is actually carried out. The goal is to get the substance-abusing person into treatment.
2. Each person presents specific evidence related to the substance abuse. This information should be written down in advance so as not to have to rely on memory in a tense situation.
3. Timing must be right:
   • There must be current evidence available.
   • The intervention must take place after a crisis precipitated by substance use and not when the person is under the influence of the substance or in severe withdrawal.
4. The intervention requires privacy. It must be held in a place where no interruptions can occur.
5. The person will use defences, and those in the intervention must not react to them.
6. Substance abuse is understood as a disease. Those affected by the substance use demonstrate compassion alongside genuine but firm concern.
7. Treatment alternatives are presented.
8. Those involved in the intervention prepare responses to possible outcomes.
   • If the person agrees to treatment, then he or she is taken immediately to a detoxification unit, where arrangements must have already been made.
   • If the person refuses treatment, then those who staged the intervention state that this decision forces them to make decisions of their own because they are no longer willing to live with the challenging behaviours of the person experiencing an addiction.

**Source:** Adapted from Johnson, V.E. (1986). *Intervention: How to help someone who doesn't want help.* Reprinted with permission of Hazelden Foundation, Center City, MN.

## Pharmacological Interventions

The predominant biological therapies are intended to support detoxification (management of withdrawal) or to alter drug use (e.g., methadone [Metadol], and naltrexone [ReVia]) (Sadock & Sadock, 2008).

### Detoxification or Alcohol Withdrawal Treatment

Not all people who stop drinking require biological management of withdrawal. The decision to medicate depends on the duration and extent of substance use, the prior history of withdrawal complications, and overall health status. Medication should not be given until the symptoms of withdrawal are observable. Drugs that are useful in treating patients with alcohol withdrawal delirium are listed in the Drug Treatment box on page 393.

**Naltrexone.** Naltrexone (ReVia), an agent used for opioid addiction, is sometimes used in the treatment of alcoholism, especially for those with intense cravings and somatic

## BOX 19-4   THE MOTIVATIONAL INTERVIEWING PROCESS

1. **Establish rapport.** Chapters 10 and 11 discuss establishing rapport with patients, but in the case of motivational interviewing, rapport may be fostered by simply asking permission to discuss the patient's behaviour or concern. For example:
   "Do you mind if we spend a few minutes talking about ... ?"
   "How do you feel about the behaviour (or desired behaviour change)?"

2. **Set the agenda.** Working with the patient to create an agenda helps the nurse and patient clarify the immediate concerns of interest for the patient and sets the boundaries of the helping relationship. For example:
   "What do you know about ... ?"
   "Are you interested in learning more about ... ?"
   "Are you able to come back to the clinic to discuss your plans further?"

3. **Assess readiness to change.** Motivation is not static and can change rapidly from day to day. Patients enter treatment at different levels of motivation or readiness to change, and many are ambivalent about changing—there are often aspects about the addiction that the patient is still benefiting from in some way. Assessing the patient's readiness to change prepares the nurse to tailor treatment to that stage. Such assessment can be made using a Readiness to Change Ruler, much like a pain scale. This scaling strategy conceptualizes readiness or motivation to change along a continuum and asks patients to use a ruler with a 10-point scale where 1 equals "definitely not ready to change" and 10 equals "definitely ready to change."

4. **Sharpen the focus.** The nurse can work with the patient to draw a table of costs and benefits of substance use or addiction and also identify specific facilitators of and barriers to change. For example:
   "Over the past two months, you have been talking about stopping using crack, and it seems that just recently you have started to recognize that the less good things about using are outweighing the good things. What is changing for you now that has you leaning toward stopping?"

5. **Identify ambivalence.** While identifying motivators is important, it is also important to address the fluctuation in motivation common in any behaviour change. Uncovering ambivalence and paradox can be achieved through statements that point out the contradictions in the patient's motivations for change. For example:
   "You have been continuing to engage in drinking binges, and yet you say that you want to get your driver's licence back and regain the trust of your parents."

6. **Elicit self-motivating statements.** This approach encourages the patient to state his or her own cognitive recognition of the problem, affective expression of concern, a direct intention toward change, and a sense of optimism. A *cognitive recognition of the problem* may be heard in a statement such as "I guess this is more serious than I thought." While a patient may have heard others express concern many times, self-recognition is a more powerful drive for change. An *affective expression of concern* about the perceived problem, such as "I'm really worried about what is happening to me," anchors the significance of the problem in the patient's own words. A *direct intention to change behaviour*—for example, "I've got to do something about this"—sets out a goal. Last, an expression of *optimism* about one's ability to change reinforces a sense of hope. A nurse may be able to elicit a statement of optimism by asking a patient what he or she can achieve in treatment. A patient may respond with "I know that if I try, I can really do it" or "I have maintained my sobriety for a long period of time before and know it is possible." The nurse can repeat these statements or have the patient write these statements down for future reference.

7. **Handle resistance.** There is a risk involved in recognizing the patient's resistance to change and inviting the patient to argue his or her case, but the nurse, nevertheless, should address resistance head-on. The patient may not be able to argue for ongoing change and motivation and may instead retreat to a previous phase of change. In that case, the nurse must be accepting and work with the patient to handle the resistance and the shifting phase of change. Handling resistance requires the nurse to ask questions about readiness and desire for change. The following questions provide examples of addressing the resistance honestly in the interview and reviewing motivation:
   "I know you have been coming to treatment for two months, but you are still drinking heavily. Maybe now is not the right time to change?"
   "So it sounds as though you have a lot going on with trying to balance a career and family, and these priorities are competing with your treatment at this time."

8. **Shift focus and transition.** Through all phases of change, there will be times to illuminate a shift in focus or transition to a new phase of motivation. Making a declaration about such shifts allows the patient to hear your evaluation and to argue for whatever change is developing. One example of shifting focus for motivation is provided by the following long-term outpatient treatment scenario:
   "Your goal to be able to regain visitation of your son, coupled with your girlfriend leaving you because you continued to use crack, makes it easy to understand why you are now committed to not using crack anymore."

**Source:** Adapted from Sobell, L.C., & Sobell, M.B. (2008). *Motivational interviewing strategies and techniques: Rationales and examples.* Retrieved from http://www.nova.edu/gsc/forms/mi_rationale_techniques.pdf.

symptoms. Naltrexone works by blocking opioid receptors, thereby interfering with the mechanism of reinforcement and reducing or eliminating the alcohol craving (Rösner, Hackl-Herrwerth, Leucht, et al., 2010). Long-acting injectable forms with the brand names Vivitrex or Vivitrol, Naltrel, and Depotrex are being tested and show promise as having relatively stable plasma levels, allowing for more sustained effects;

these drugs may have fewer adverse effects than naltrexone (Johnson, 2007).

***Acamprosate.*** Acamprosate (Campral) is another medication, approved by Health Canada in 2008, used to treat alcoholism. Acamprosate is prescribed for people who have quit drinking and wish to remain abstinent; however, its helpfulness for people who have not undergone detoxification is not yet

## DRUG TREATMENT OF PATIENTS WITH ALCOHOL WITHDRAWAL DELIRIUM

| DRUG CLASS | SPECIFIC DRUGS | PURPOSE |
|---|---|---|
| Benzodiazepines | Chlordiazepoxide (Librax) Diazepam (Valium) (usually not recommended due to its short half-life and frequent dosing schedule) Lorazepam (Ativan) | Decrease withdrawal symptoms, stabilize vital signs, and prevent seizures and delirium tremens |
| α-adrenergic blockers | Clonidine (Catapres) | Reduce autonomic withdrawal symptoms |

**Source:** Adapted from Lehne, R.E. (2013). *Pharmacology for nursing care* (8th ed.). Philadelphia: Saunders.

demonstrated (Sadock & Sadock, 2008). Acamprosate is believed to effect a reduction in one's intake of alcohol through suppression of excitatory neurotransmission and enhanced inhibitory transmission (Lehne, 2010).

*Topiramate.* Similar to acamprosate, topiramate (Topamax) decreases alcohol cravings by inhibiting the release of mesocorticolimbic dopamine, which has been associated with alcohol craving (Paparrigopoulos, Tzavellas, Karaiskos, et al., 2011).

### Biological Treatment of Opioid Addiction

*Methadone.* Methadone (Metadol) is a synthetic opioid that blocks the craving for and effects of opioids. It has to be taken every day, is highly addicting, and, when stopped, produces withdrawal symptoms. Therefore, for methadone to be effective, the patient must take a dose at a prescribed level that will prevent withdrawal symptoms, block drug craving, and block any effects of illicit use of short-acting opioids.

Methadone is the only medication currently approved for the treatment of pregnant women with an opioid addiction. The clinical studies available demonstrate that methadone maintenance treatment (MMT) at the appropriate dosage, when combined with prenatal care and a comprehensive program of support, can significantly improve fetal and neonatal outcome (Burns, Mattick, Lim, et al., 2007).

Methadone is not indicated as a first-line therapy for adolescents with opioid dependence. There may, however, be individual adolescents for whom methadone is a reasonable option, depending on history of use, opioid tolerance, previous attempts at stopping, and history of withdrawal symptoms. However, health care providers should discuss other treatment options with youth before initiating MMT (Health Canada, 2008).

*Naltrexone.* Naltrexone (ReVia) is a relatively pure antagonist that blocks the euphoric effects of opioids. It has low toxicity and few adverse effects and does not produce dependence. A single dose provides an effective opioid blockade for up to 72 hours. Taking naltrexone three times a week is sufficient to maintain a fairly high level of opioid blockade. For many

patients, long-term use results in gradual extinction of cravings. As previously mentioned, it has also been approved for the treatment of alcoholism because it decreases the pleasant, reinforcing effects of alcohol.

*Clonidine.* Clonidine (Catapres) was initially marketed for high blood pressure, but it is also an effective somatic treatment, combined with naltrexone, for some chemical-dependent individuals. Clonidine is a nonopioid suppresser of opioid withdrawal symptoms. It is also nonaddictive.

*Buprenorphine.* Buprenorphine (Suboxone) is a partial opioid agonist. At appropriate doses (up to 24 mg/d sublingually depending on provincial or territorial practice standards), the drug blocks signs and symptoms of opioid withdrawal. Buprenorphine has been shown to suppress opioid use in both inpatient and outpatient settings (Finch, Kamien, & Amass, 2007).

### Biological Treatment of Nicotine Addiction

Transdermal administration of nicotine doubles long-term tobacco abstinence rates. The nicotine patch is preferred over nicotine gum because compliance with the treatment regimen is better, blood levels are steadier, long-term dependence seldom occurs, and instructions are less complicated. Anti-nicotine vaccines are being developed and tested and show promise in the treatment of nicotine addiction (Hass, 2011).

### Implementation at Primary, Secondary, and Tertiary Levels of Prevention

#### Primary Prevention

Prevention models in health care are classified as primary, secondary, and tertiary. In terms of substance use and addiction prevention, primary approaches are those efforts focused on reducing the demand for a substance or behaviour, as well as stopping the occurrence of alcohol or drug use or abuse and addictive behaviours (Rassool, 2010). Examples include implementing healthy public policy; offering health education related to addiction; taxing and labelling products (e.g., cigarettes, alcohol); and promoting educational campaigns (e.g., addiction and mental health in the workplace).

#### Secondary Prevention

Secondary prevention seeks to limit further health deterioration and social harm from the use, abuse, dependence, and addiction to substances and behaviours. Examples include programs of early recognition, awareness campaigns, relapse prevention, community support, harm reduction approaches, and strategies for safe prescribing guidelines (Rassool, 2010).

*Harm-reduction approaches.* Harm reduction refers to a range of programs, policies, and interventions designed to reduce or minimize the adverse consequences associated with drug use, such as overdose, infections, and spread of communicable diseases. The family, community, and society in general are also adversely affected by drug use and abuse. Many who use these substances will not or cannot abstain from drug use; therefore, there is a need to provide options that minimize related harm (e.g., needle-exchange programs, safe injection sites, medical cannabis, safer-sex programs).

Leonard et al. (as cited in Canadian Centre on Substance Abuse, 2008) report that those using cocaine inject less when they have easier access to pipes. These types of programs can serve as a bridge to treatment or to discontinuing drug use in the long term.

Actions taken in Portugal provide a good example of how harm reduction works. In 2001, Portugal decriminalized drug use. Rather than declaring a war on drugs, the government has implemented several programs that focus on reducing the harmful effects of drug use. These programs combined have resulted in a 50% reduction of "hard drug" and intravenous drug use. More compelling is that the rate of newly reported cases of HIV, hepatitis B and C, and drug-related mortality rates have all significantly decreased (Greenwald, 2009).

***Relapse prevention.*** Relapses during recovery are common. Relapse prevention aims to help the individual learn from periods of relapse so that periods of sobriety can be lengthened over time. Lapses and relapses, therefore, are not viewed as failures. Relapse can result in a renewed and refined effort toward change.

| Dialogue | Therapeutic Tool or Comment |
|---|---|
| **Sylvain:** "I was in the emergency department Friday afternoon when you were brought in by ambulance." | Placing the event in time and sequence, validating the precipitating event |
| **Bill:** "Were you? I guess a lot of people thought it was over for me." | |
| **Sylvain:** "It certainly looked quite serious." | Emphasizing the reality—prevents minimizing the situation |
| **Bill:** "Yeah. I should never have left the program. I was doing better, and I just didn't think I needed it anymore." | |
| **Sylvain:** "You said you were doing well." | Reflecting |
| **Bill:** "Yeah. I had a job, and I was beginning to save some money. Wow! I can't believe I blew this whole thing." | |
| **Sylvain:** "I don't know that you really did. Your counsellor in the program phoned your doctor this morning to find out how you were doing." | Pointing out reality |
| **Bill:** "Do you think they'll take me back?" | |
| **Sylvain:** "Why don't we talk some more, and after we finish, I'll speak with the other staff about your situation. If you would like to get back into the program, you can call your counsellor, and we'll support your decision." | Gathering information Supporting decision making |

General strategies for relapse prevention are cognitive and behavioural: recognizing and learning how to avoid or cope with threats to recovery, changing lifestyle, learning how to

**VIGNETTE**

Bill, a 20-year-old single man, was brought to the emergency department after having been found unconscious in his room at home. He was accompanied by his mother, with whom he shares a small apartment. When his mother was not able to rouse him, she dialled 911 for an ambulance. A syringe and some white powder were found next to Bill.

On admission, Bill had laboured breathing, and his pupils were constricted. Vital signs were taken; his blood pressure was 60/40 mm Hg, and his pulse was 132 beats per minute. Bill's situation was determined to be life threatening. Although extremely distressed, Bill's mother was able to report to the staff that Bill had a substance abuse problem and had been injecting heroin for six months before recently entering a methadone maintenance program one year ago. It was decided at this point to administer an opioid antagonist, and naloxone was given intramuscularly. Bill's breathing improved, and he was able to respond to verbal stimuli. Bill's mother later told staff that Bill had been in the methadone maintenance program over the past year but that he had not attended the program or received his methadone for about one week. At the staff's urging, she called the program, and an outreach worker, Sylvain, arranged to talk to her and Bill at the hospital. Bill made an appointment to follow up with Sylvain at the methadone clinic the following Monday. Sylvain recognized that Bill's future would ultimately depend on Bill's own actions but that he could offer some motivation and guide Bill's insight.

On Monday, Sylvain spoke with Bill about his situation, what changes he wanted for himself, his drug use, some of the things that had jeopardized his recovery in the past, and what Bill thought he might need in order to get back into recovery. Bill stated, "I know I can do it if I can concentrate on health and life. If I lose that concentration, it just is old habit to use again. I can see how I slipped off track." Sylvain and Bill agreed to meet regularly, and while it took several months, Bill stopped using heroin, is holding down a good job in construction, and appears motivated. Naltrexone (ReVia) was given in conjunction with motivational interviewing and relapse-prevention training, and Bill is now regularly attending Narcotics Anonymous meetings. It has been an intensive treatment program, but Bill is the first person to say it is worth the time and concentration.

participate in activities without drugs, and securing help from other people or from social support services. Box 19-5 identifies relapse-prevention strategies.

***Self-help groups for patient and family or friends.*** Counselling and support should be encouraged for all family and friends of a person experiencing problems with alcohol, other substance use, or addictions. Al-Anon and Alateen are self-help groups that offer support and guidance for adults and teenagers, respectively. Self-help groups assist family members and friends in dealing with many common issues. Their work is based on a combination of educational and operational principles centred on acceptance of the disease model of addiction, including pragmatic methods for avoiding enabling behaviours.

***Twelve-step programs.*** One of the most effective treatment modalities for all addictions has been the 12-step program. Alcoholics Anonymous (AA) is the prototype for all the 12-step programs that were subsequently developed for many types of addiction. These programs offer the behavioural, cognitive, and

## BOX 19-5   RELAPSE-PREVENTION STRATEGIES

**Basics**

- It is important to keep the program simple at first. Remember that 40% to 50% of patients who abuse substances have mild to moderate cognitive problems while actively using substances. Providing prompts and assistance for the patient's recall may be beneficial. For example:
- Reviewing instructions from health team members.
- Encouraging use of a notebook to write down important information, appointments, schedules, and telephone numbers.

**Skills**

Patients may take advantage of cognitive-behavioural therapy to increase their coping skills. The patient can identify which important life skills are needed by inquiring about the following:

- Which situations are challenging and stress-producing?
- What situations command new skills or abilities?
- What abilities and skills are currently strong?

**Relapse-Prevention Groups**

Support membership in a relapse-prevention group. These groups help patients work on the following:

- Rehearsing stressful situations using a variety of techniques
- Finding ways to deal with current problems or ones that are likely to arise without the drugs, alcohol, or behavioural addiction
- Providing role models to support change

**Enhancement of Personal Insight**

Therapy—group, individual, or family—can help a patient gain insight and control over a variety of psychological concerns. For example:

- What triggers the use or addiction?
- What constitutes a healthy, supportive relationship?
- How can self-esteem, self-worth, and coping be strengthened?
- What does the addiction offer that would be difficult to give up? What would be the loss without the use or addiction? What could replace the loss?

**Source:** Adapted from Zerbe, K.J. (1999). *Women's mental health in primary care* (pp. 94–95). Philadelphia: Saunders.

dynamic structure needed by those in recovery from addiction. Three basic concepts are fundamental to all 12-step programs:

1. Individuals with addictive disorders are powerless over their addiction, and their lives are unmanageable.
2. Although individuals with addictive disorders are not responsible for their disease, they are responsible for their recovery.
3. Individuals can no longer blame people, places, and things for their addiction; they must face their problems and their feelings.

Using the 12 steps, often referred to as "working the steps," helps a person refrain from addictive behaviours while fostering individual change and growth. Other 12-step programs include Narcotics Anonymous (NA) and Cocaine Anonymous (CA). A

referral to the 12-step program that best fits the patient's addiction is recommended at discharge. Obtaining a sponsor prior to discharge can increase the patient's likelihood of attendance at 12-step meetings. Sponsors are individuals who are recovering from addiction and can provide addicted people with ideas and methods to deal with cravings for the substance of abuse and with coping deficits that may arise after prolonged substance use and abuse. Most programs offer assistance in facilitating sponsorship.

### Tertiary Prevention

Tertiary prevention is concerned with limiting and reducing complications and dysfunction related to the experience of substance or behavioural abuse and addiction. Effective care, treatment, and rehabilitation programs and services are characteristic of tertiary prevention approaches (Rassool, 2010). Specialized addiction detoxification programs, recovery programs, and concurrent disorder programs are examples of tertiary-level services.

*Residential treatment programs.* Residential treatment programs are best suited for individuals who have a long history of substance abuse or behavioural addiction. The goal of this intensive form of treatment is to effect a rapid change in behaviour with restricted access to the substance of abuse and with supervision and support for abstinence from the substance of abuse. Programs typically offer patients therapy for the development of skills to support awareness and treatment success and provide support to family members. Most residential programs in Canada are designed for short-stay intensive therapy, after which patients receive referrals to ongoing aftercare, or therapeutic communities, where they can choose between inpatient and outpatient support. A therapeutic community may be either a personal treatment choice or a court-mandated program.

*Intensive outpatient programs.* Most treatment for substance-abusing patients takes place in the community in the form of intensive outpatient programs. This form of program is becoming more popular because of the flexibility, diversity, cost-effectiveness, and responsiveness to the specific needs of the individual seeking treatment.

*Outpatient treatment programs and employee assistance programs.* Outpatient treatment programs and employee assistance programs may offer vocational education and placement, counselling, and individual or group psychotherapy. Employee assistance programs have been developed to deliver short-term outpatient mental health services for employees with this benefit. Many hospitals, institutions, and corporations offer their employees counselling and support as an alternative to job termination when the employee's work performance is negatively affected by a personal impairment.

### Advanced-Practice Interventions
#### Psychotherapy

Nurses with advanced training may conduct psychotherapy with substance-using patients. Psychotherapy assists patients in identifying and using alternative coping mechanisms to reduce reliance on substances. Eventually, psychotherapy can assist those recovering from addictions to become increasingly comfortable with sobriety. Evidence-informed practice and data indicate that cognitive-behavioural, motivational enhancement, behavioural, psychodynamic, interpersonal, and family therapies are all effective for selected substance use disorders. See Chapters 36 and 37 for discussions of group and family therapy.

Throughout therapy, confidentiality must be maintained *except* in circumstances that conflict with requirements for mandatory reporting (e.g., child abuse, danger to self or others).

Nurses should be aware of the following critical issues that arise during the first six months of sobriety:

- Physical changes take place as the body adapts to functioning without substances.
- Signals that previously were cues to engage in drinking and drug use continue to occur in the patient's internal and external world. Different responses to these cues need to be learned.
- Emotional responses (feelings that were formerly diluted by substance use) are now experienced fully. Because they are so unfamiliar, they can produce anxiety.
- Family's and co-workers' responses to the patient's new behaviour must be addressed. Sobriety disrupts a system, and everyone in that system needs to adjust to the change.

- New coping skills must be developed to prevent relapse and ensure prolonged sobriety.

Psychotherapy needs to be directive, open and honest, and caring. The therapeutic process involves teaching the patient to identify the physical and emotional changes that are occurring in the here and now and then assisting in the problem-solving process.

## EVALUATION

Favourable treatment outcome is judged by increased lengths of time of abstinence, decreased denial, acceptable occupational functioning, improved family relationships, and—ultimately—ability to sustain healthy relationships and habits. The ability to use existing supports and skills learned in treatment is important for ongoing recovery. For example, recovery is actively viable if, in response to cues to use the substance, the patient calls his or her sponsor or other recovering people; increases attendance at 12-step meetings, aftercare, or other group meetings; or writes feelings in a log and considers alternative actions. Continuous monitoring and evaluation increase the chances for prolonged recovery.

## CASE STUDY AND NURSING CARE PLAN 19-1

### Alcohol Dependence With Depression

*Mr. Steriovski, aged 49 years, and his wife arrive in the emergency department one evening, fearful that he has had a stroke. His right hand is limp, he is unable to hyperextend his right wrist, and sensation to the fingertips in the hand is impaired.*

*Mr. Steriovski looks much older than his stated age; in fact, he looks about 65. His complexion is ruddy and flushed. History taking is difficult. Mr. Steriovski answers only what is asked of him, volunteering no additional information. He states that he took a nap that afternoon, and when he awakened, he noticed the problems with his right arm.*

*Ms. Winkler, the admitting nurse, begins the assessment. Mr. Steriovski reveals that he has been unemployed for four years because the company he worked for went bankrupt. He has been unable to find a new job but has a job interview in ten days. His wife is now working full-time, so the family finances are okay. They have two grown children who no longer live at home. As he relates this information, his lips momentarily start to tremble and his eyes fill with tears.*

*Mr. Steriovski denies any significant medical illness except for high blood pressure, just diagnosed last year. His father has a history of depression, and his mother is a recovering alcoholic. Ms. Winkler shares with him the fact that depression and alcoholism run in families. She asks Mr. Steriovski (1) whether he knows this and (2) whether it concerns him with regard to his own drinking. He says that he knows and that he does not want to think about it.*

*Ms. Winkler speaks separately with Mr. Steriovski's wife and asks if there is anything she would like to add. Mrs. Steriovski's shoulders slump; she sighs and says, "I have spent the entire day talking to a counsellor at the local treatment centre to see if I can get him in. He won't admit that he has a problem." Mrs.*

*Steriovski recounts a six-year history of steadily increasing alcohol use. She says that she could not admit to herself that her husband was an excessive drinker. "He tried to hide it, but gradually I knew. I could tell from little changes that he was intoxicated. I couldn't believe it was happening because he had been through the same thing with his mother. I thought I knew him. Actually, I guess I did when he was working. Being unemployed and unable to find a job has really devastated him. And now he's going to job interviews intoxicated."*

*She describes her feelings, which are like an emotional roller coaster—elated and hopeful when he seems to be doing okay; dejected and desperate when he loses control. Mrs. Steriovski hates going to work for fear of what her husband might do while she is gone. She says she is terrified that one day he will get into a car wreck and kill himself, because he often drives when intoxicated. He tells her not to worry, because the life insurance policy is paid up.*

*Meanwhile, the physician in the emergency department has examined Mr. Steriovski. The diagnosis is radial nerve palsy. Mr. Steriovski most likely passed out while lying on his arm. Because he was intoxicated, he did not feel the signals that his nerves sent out to warn him to move (numbness, tingling). He was in this position for so long that the resultant cutoff of circulation was sufficient to cause some temporary nerve damage.*

*Mr. Steriovski's blood alcohol level (BAL) is 0.31 mg%—more than three times the legal limit (0.08 mg%) for intoxication in Canada. Even though he has a high BAL, Mr. Steriovski is alert and oriented, not slurring his speech or giving any other outward signs of intoxication. The difference between Mr. Steriovski's BAL and his behaviour indicates the development of tolerance, a symptom of physical dependence.*

*Continued*

## CASE STUDY AND NURSING CARE PLAN 19-1—cont'd

*Alcohol Dependence With Depression*

### ASSESSMENT

**Self-Awareness**

Ms. Winkler has developed her capacity and skills in working with people who abuse alcohol. She grew up in a home in which alcohol transformed her father from a caring and responsible parent to one who was physically and verbally abusive to his wife and children. He eventually lost his job and left home. Ms. Winkler was determined to be everything he was not and firmly resolved never to drink or use drugs.

As a new nurse, Ms. Winkler became extremely frustrated and angry with patients like Mr. Steriovski and found herself being overly protective of the family. At the end of a particular day in which she had to work with yet another intoxicated patient, she felt drained, depressed, and despondent. It became such a problem that she knew she needed to either leave her job or deal with the dynamics underlying her responses. She began to attend the support group Al-Anon. There, she was able to talk about her feelings with others who had similar backgrounds. Ms. Winkler was also provided with tools for dealing with her feelings and gained a greater understanding for the pathology behind alcohol abuse.

As Ms. Winkler approaches her work with the Steriovski family, she does so with new confidence. She feels empathy and understanding for Mrs. Steriovski, but she is able to maintain emotional boundaries and does not feel drained by their interactions. While she still feels a little frustration with Mr. Steriovski, she recognizes these feelings and focuses on him as a person with a serious disorder.

Ms. Winkler organizes her data into objective and subjective components.

| Objective Data | Subjective Data |
|---|---|
| Driving when intoxicated | Denies he has an alcohol problem |
| Covert references to death | Denies he has depression |
| Nerve damage from passing out while lying on arm | |
| Increased alcohol use since becoming unemployed | |
| Ability to find employment impaired by alcohol use | |
| Disruption in marital relationship because of alcohol use | |
| Inability to see effects of his drinking | |
| Family history of alcoholism and depression | |
| BAL three times the legal limit of intoxication; has developed tolerance | |

### DIAGNOSIS

From the data, the nurse formulates the following nursing diagnoses:

1. *Risk for suicide* related to depressed mood
**Supporting Data**
• Dangerous behaviour: driving when drinking
• Full payment of life insurance policy

2. *Ineffective coping* related to alcohol use
**Supporting Data**
• Increased alcohol use during stressful period of unemployment
• Impairment in capacity to obtain employment caused by alcohol use
• Disruption in marital relationship because of alcohol use
• Inability to see effect of his drinking on his life functioning

### OUTCOMES IDENTIFICATION

1. The patient will refrain from attempting suicide.
2. The patient will report increase in psychological comfort.

### PLANNING

The initial plan is to allow Mr. Steriovski to sober up in the emergency department before discussing goals. Once he is sober, the nurse will establish realistic outcomes with him.

### IMPLEMENTATION

Mr. Steriovski's plan of care is personalized as follows:
1. **Nursing diagnosis:** *Risk for suicide*
  **Outcome:** Patient will consistently demonstrate suicide self-restraint.

*Continued*

## CASE STUDY AND NURSING CARE PLAN 19-1—cont'd

### Alcohol Dependence With Depression

| Short-Term Goal | Intervention | Rationale | Evaluation |
|---|---|---|---|
| 1. Patient will seek treatment for depression. | 1a. Determine presence and degree of suicidal risk.<br>1b. Refer patient to mental health care provider for evaluation and treatment. | 1a. Risk for suicide is increased in substance-using patients.<br>1b. Addressing both substance use and mental health treatment needs improves outcomes. | **GOAL MET**<br>After three weeks, patient attends appointment at local clinic and has started taking an antidepressant. |

**2. Nursing diagnosis:** *Ineffective coping*
**Outcome:** Patient will demonstrate mild to no change in health status and social functioning due to substance addiction.

| Short-Term Goal | Intervention | Rationale | Evaluation |
|---|---|---|---|
| 1. Patient will consistently acknowledge personal consequences associated with alcohol misuse. | 1a. Identify with patient those factors (genetics, stress) that contribute to chemical dependence.<br>1b. Assist patient to identify negative effects of chemical dependency. | 1a. Emphasis on alcoholism as a disease can lower guilt and increase self-esteem.<br>1b. Identifying negative effects helps patient decrease denial and increase problem solving. | **GOAL MET**<br>Patient admits that he cannot find a new job when he is intoxicated. |
| 2. Patient will commit to alcohol-use-control strategies. | 2a. Determine history of alcohol use.<br>2b. Identify support groups in community for long-term substance use treatment (for wife also). | 2a. Determining history identifies high-risk situations.<br>2b. Alcohol dependence requires long-term treatment; AA is effective. | **GOAL MET**<br>After three weeks, patient states that he attends AA every day. He is learning about his triggers and new coping skills. His wife attends Al-Anon. |

### EVALUATION

See individual outcomes and evaluation in the care plan.

## KEY POINTS TO REMEMBER

- Substance use and dependence occur on a continuum, and addiction develops over a period of time.
- The cause of substance use disorders is a combination of genetic, biological, and environmental factors.
- Assessment of patients with substance use disorders needs to be comprehensive, aimed at identifying common medical and psychiatric co-morbidities.
- Patients with concurrent disorders have more severe symptoms, experience more crises, and require longer treatment for successful outcomes.
- Substance use disorders affect the family system of the patient and may lead to codependent behaviour in family members. Codependency is characterized by dependence on the needs and controls within a relationship, even to the detriment of one's own needs and self-control.
- Assessment of readiness for change is an essential part of the assessment process and can support appropriate treatment strategies.

- Relapse is an expected phase of change from addiction, and treatment includes a significant focus on teaching relapse prevention.
- Motivational interviewing, a form of intervention, can lead to appropriate treatment strategies and improved outcomes.
- Successful treatments include an integrative approach, self-help groups, psychotherapy, therapeutic communities, and psychopharmacotherapy.
- Nurses need to be aware of their own feelings about substance use so they can provide empathy and motivate change for patients.
- Nurses should be vigilant for signs of impairment and addiction in colleagues to ensure patient safety and referral to treatment for the nurse experiencing an addiction.

# CRITICAL THINKING

1. Write a paragraph describing reactions you might have to a drug-dependent patient to whom you are assigned.
   a. Would your response be different depending on the substance (e.g., alcohol versus heroin or marijuana versus cocaine)? Give reasons for your answers.
   b. Would your response be different if the substance-dependent person were a professional colleague? How?

2. Aline is a 15-year-old girl who has started using heroin.
   a. When Aline asks you why she needs to take more and more to get "high," how would you explain to her the concept of tolerance?
   b. If she had recently used heroin, what would you find on assessment of physical and psychological–perceptual signs and symptoms?
   c. If she were brought to the emergency department for overdosing on heroin, what would be the emergency care? What might be effective long-term care?

3. Robert is a 45-year-old mechanic. He has a 20-year history of heavy drinking and he says he wants to quit drinking.
   a. Role-play with a classmate an initial assessment. Identify the kinds of information you would need to have in order to plan holistic care.
   b. Robert decided to stop drinking abruptly. He is now in the emergency department with delirium tremens. What are the dangers for him? What are the appropriate medical interventions?
   c. What are some possible treatment alternatives for Robert when he is safely detoxified? How would you explain to him the usefulness and function of Alcoholics Anonymous? What are some additional treatment options that might be useful to Robert? What are available as referrals for him in your community?

# CHAPTER REVIEW

1. The nurse is caring for a patient with an addictive disorder who is currently drug-free. The patient is experiencing repeated occurrences of vivid, frightening images and thoughts. Which term would the nurse use to document this finding?
   1. Tolerance
   2. Flashbacks
   3. Withdrawal
   4. Synergistic effect

2. Which condition would the nurse be most concerned about when caring for a patient who abuses alcohol?
   1. Cirrhosis of the liver
   2. Suicidal potential
   3. Wernicke's encephalopathy
   4. Korsakoff syndrome

3. Which patient response to the question "Have you ever drunk more alcohol or used more drugs than you meant to?" should immediately cause the nurse to assess further?
   1. "No, I have never used drugs or alcohol."
   2. "I have drunk alcohol before but have never let myself get drunk."
   3. "I figured you'd ask me about that."
   4. "Yes, I did that once and will never do it again."

4. Which patient behaviours should the nurse suspect as related to alcohol withdrawal?
   1. Hyperalert state, jerky movements, easily startled
   2. Tachycardia, diaphoresis, elevated blood pressure
   3. Peripheral vascular collapse, electrolyte imbalance
   4. Paranoid delusions, fever, fluctuating levels of consciousness

5. A patient at your community mental health centre smokes up to a half a pack of cigarettes daily but has tried with limited success to cut back over the past two weeks. Today he asked the pharmacist about the various products that could aid his attempts to quit smoking in time for him to manage a long overseas flight next month and travel with friends who are allergic to smoke. What phase of change is this patient demonstrating?
   1. Precontemplation
   2. Contemplation
   3. Preparation
   4. Action

**ⓔvolve** WEBSITE

Post-Test interactive review

*Visit the Evolve Web site for Chapter Review Answers and Rationales, Critical Thinking Answer Guidelines, and additional resources related to the content in this chapter:* http://evolve.elsevier.com/Canada/Varcarolis/psychiatric/

# REFERENCES

Aaron, M. (2012). The pathways of problematic sexual behavior: A literature review of factors affecting adult sexual behavior in survivors of childhood sexual abuse. *Sexual Addiction & Compulsivity, 19*(3), 199–218. doi: 10.1080/10720162.2012.690678.

Abizaid, A., Anisman, H., Matheson, K., et al. (2009). Stress, trauma and substance use disorders. In Canadian Centre on Substance Abuse, *Substance abuse in Canada: Concurrent disorders* (pp. 12–19). Ottawa: Canadian Centre on Substance Abuse. Retrieved from http://www.ccsa.ca/2010%20CCSA%20Documents/ccsa-011811-2010.pdf.

Alberta Health Services. (2009). *Tobacco facts.* Retrieved from http://www.albertahealthservices.ca/hp/if-hp-tr-en-tobacco.pdf.

Bailey, J.A., Hill, K.G., Oesterle, S., et al. (2006). Linking substance use and problem behaviour across three generations. *Journal of Abnormal Child Psychology, 34*, 273–292. doi:10.1007/s10802-006-9033-z.

Berridge, K.C. (2007). The debate over dopamine's role in reward: The case for incentive salience. *Psychopharmacology, 191*, 391–431. doi:10.1007/s00213-006-0578-x.

Bey, T., & Patel, A. (2007). Phencyclidine intoxication and adverse effects: A clinical and pharmacological review of an illicit drug. *California Journal of Emergency Medicine, 8*(1), 9–14. Retrieved from http://www.ncbi.nlm.nih.gov/pmc/articles/PMC2859735/pdf/cjem8_1p0009.pdf.

Burns, L.A., Mattick, R.P., Lim, K., et al. (2007). Methadone in pregnancy: Treatment retention and neonatal outcomes. *Addiction, 102*(2), 264–270. doi:10.1111/j.1360-0443.2006.01651.x.

Canadian Centre on Substance Abuse. (2008). *Harm reduction: What's in a name?* Ottawa: Author. Retrieved from http://www.ccsa.ca/2008%20CCSA%20Documents2/ccsa0115302008e.pdf.

Canadian Centre on Substance Abuse. (2013). *Systems approach workbook: Integrating substance use and mental health systems.* Ottawa: Author. Retrieved from http://www.nts-snt.ca/2013%20Document%20Library/nts-systems-approach-integrating-substance-use-and-mental-health-systems-en.pdf.

Canadian Nurses Association. (2008). *Code of ethics for registered nurses.* Ottawa: Author.

Centre for Addiction and Mental Health. (2008). *Clinical supervision handbook: A guide for clinical supervisors for addiction and mental health.* Toronto: Author.

Cleary, M., Hunt, G., Matheson, S., et al. (2008). Psychosocial interventions for people with both severe mental illness and substance misuse. *Cochrane Database of Systematic Reviews, 1*.

Collin, C. (2006). *Substance abuse issues and public policy in Canada: IV. Prevalence of use and its consequences* (No. PRB 06-19E). Ottawa: Library of Parliament. Retrieved from http://www.parl.gc.ca/Content/LOP/ResearchPublications/prb0619-e.pdf.

Collins, D., Pan, Z., Johnson, K., et al. (2008). Individual and contextual predictors of inhalant use among 8th graders: A multilevel analysis. *Journal of Drug Education, 38*, 193–210. doi:10.2190/DE.38.3.a.

Compton, W.M., Thomas, Y.F., Stinson, F.S., et al. (2007). Prevalence, correlates, disability and comorbidity of *DSM-IV* drug abuse and dependence in the United States. *Archives of General Psychiatry, 64*(5), 566–576. Retrieved from http://archpsyc.ama-assn.org/content/vol64/issue5/index.dtl.

Cox, S., & Leyton, M. (2009). Impulsivity and substance use disorders. In Canadian Centre on Substance Abuse, *Substance abuse in Canada: Concurrent disorders* (pp. 30–37). Ottawa: Canadian Centre on Substance Abuse. Retrieved from http://www.ccsa.ca/2010%20CCSA%20Documents/ccsa-011811-2010.pdf.

Crawford, E., Wright, M., & Birchmeier, Z. (2008). Drug-facilitated sexual assault: College women's risk perception and behavioral choices. *Journal of American College Health, 57*(3), 261–272.

Drake, R.E., Mueser, K.T., Brunette, M.F., et al. (2004). A review of treatments for people with severe mental illnesses and co-occurring substance use disorders. *Psychiatric Rehabilitation Journal, 27*(4), 360–374.

Erickson, C.K. (2007). *The science of addiction: From neurobiology to treatment.* New York: Norton.

Ewing, J.A. (1984). Detecting alcoholism: The CAGE Questionnaire. *Journal of the American Medical Association, 252*, 1905–1907.

Finch, J.W., Kamien, J.B., & Amass, L. (2007). Two-year experience with buprenorphine-naloxone (Suboxone) for maintenance treatment of opioid dependence within a private practice setting. *Journal of Addiction Medicine, 1*, 104–110. doi:10.1097/ADM.0b013e31809b5df2.

Galea, S., Nandi, A., & Vlahov, D. (2004). The social epidemiology of substance use. *Epidemiologic Reviews, 26*(1), 36–52. doi:10.1093/epirev/mxh007.

Greenwald, G. (2009). *Drug decriminalization in Portugal: Lessons for creating fair and successful drug policies.* Washington, DC: Cato Institute. Retrieved from http://www.cato.org/pubs/wtpapers/greenwald_whitepaper.pdf.

Halpern, J.H., & Pope, H.G. (2003). Review: Hallucinogen persisting perception disorder: What do we know after 50 years? *Drug and Alcohol Dependence, 69*, 109–119.

Hasin, D.S., Stinson, F.S., Ogburn, E., et al. (2007). Prevalence, correlates, disability, and comorbidity of *DSM-IV* alcohol abuse and dependence in the United States. *Archives of General Psychiatry, 64*, 830–842. doi:10.1001/archpsyc.64.7.830.

Hass, C. (2011). A vaccine against nicotine—New hope or mere hype? [Web log post]. *Clinical Correlations.* Retrieved from http://www.clinicalcorrelations.org/?p=3935.

Health Canada. (2008). *Best practices. Methadone maintenance treatment.* Ottawa: Author.

Health Canada. (2011). *Canadian alcohol and drug use monitoring survey.* Retrieved from http://www.hc-sc.gc.ca/hc-ps/drugs-drogues/stat/_2011/summary-sommaire-eng.php.

Johnson, B.A. (2007). Naltrexone long-acting formulation in the treatment of alcohol dependence. *Therapeutics and Clinical Risk Management, 3*(5), 741–749. Retrieved from http://www.dovepress.com/naltrexone-long-acting-formulation-in-the-treatment-of-alcohol-depende-peer-reviewed-article-TCRM.

Koob, G.F., & Le Moal, M. (2006). *Neurobiology of addiction.* Oxford, UK: Elsevier.

Lehne, R.A. (2010). *Pharmacology for nursing care* (7th ed.). Philadelphia: Saunders.

Linneberg, A., Gonzalez-Quintela, A., Vidal, C., et al. (2010). Genetic determinants of both ethanol and acetaldehyde metabolism influence alcohol hypersensitivity and drinking behaviour among Scandinavians. *Clinical & Experimental Allergy, 40*, 123–130. doi:10.1111/j.1365-2222.2009.03398.x.

Mancini, M.A., Hardiman, E.R., & Eversman, M.H. (2008). A review of the compatibility of harm re-education and recovery-oriented best practices for dual disorders. *Best Practices in Mental Health, 4*(2), 99–113. Retrieved from http://wilsonweb.com.

McKeon, A., Frye, M.A., & Delanty, N. (2007). The alcohol withdrawal syndrome. *Journal of Neurology, Neurosurgery, and Psychiatry, 79*, 854–862. doi:10.1136/jnnp.2007.128322.

Miller, W.R., & Rollnick, S. (Eds.), (2002). *Motivational interviewing: Preparing people for change* (2nd ed.). New York: Guilford Press.

Minkoff, K. (2001). Developing standards of care for individuals with co-occurring psychiatric and substance use disorders. *Psychiatric Services, 52*(5), 597–599.

Monroe, T., & Kenaga, H. (2011). Don't ask, don't tell. Substance abuse and addiction among nurses. *Journal of Clinical Nursing, 20*, 504–509. doi:10.1111/j.1365-2702.2010.03518.x.

Monte, R., Rabuñal, R., Casariego, E., et al. (2010). Analysis of the factors determining survival of alcoholic withdrawal syndrome patients in a general hospital. *Alcohol & Alcoholism, 45*, 151–158. doi:10.1093/alcalc/agp087.

Moorhead, S., Johnson, M., Maas, M.L., et al. (2008). *Nursing outcomes classification (NOC)* (4th ed.). St. Louis, MO: Mosby.

Paparrigopoulos, T., Tzavellas, E., Karaiskos, D., et al. (2011). Treatment of alcohol dependence with low-dose topiramate: An open-label controlled study. *BMC Psychiatry, 11*, 1–7. doi:10.1186/1471-244X-11-41.

Prochaska, J.O., & DiClemente, C.C. (1984). *The transtheoretical approach: Towards a systematic eclectic framework.* Homewood, IL: Dow Jones Irwin.

Rassool, G.H. (2010). *Addiction for nurses.* Oxford, UK: Wiley-Blackwell.

Rösner, S., Hackl-Herrwerth, A., Leucht, S., et al. (2010). Opioid antagonists for alcohol dependence. *Cochrane Database of Systematic Reviews, 12.* doi:10.1002/14651858.CD001867.pub3.

Rush, B., Fogg, B., Nadeau, L., et al. (2008). *On the integration of mental health and substance use services and systems: Main report.* Retrieved from http://www.ccsa.ca/ceca/pdf/Main-reportFINALa.pdf.

Sadock, B.J., & Sadock, V.A. (2008). *Concise textbook of clinical psychiatry* (3rd ed.). Philadelphia: Lippincott Williams & Wilkins.

Schulte, S.J., Meier, P.S., Stirling, J., et al. (2010). Unrecognised dual diagnosis a risk factor for dropout of addiction treatment. *Mental Health and Substance Use, 3*(2), 94–109. doi.org/10.1080/17523281003705199.

Selzer, M.L. (1971). The Michigan Alcoholism Screening Test (MAST): The quest for a new diagnostic instrument. *American Journal of Psychiatry, 127*, 1653–1658.

Stavro, K., Pelletier, J., & Potvin, S. (2013). Widespread and sustained cognitive deficits in alcoholism: A meta-analysis. *Addiction Biology, 18*(2), 203–213. doi:10.1111/j.1369-1600.2011.00418.x.

Teitelbaum, L., & Mullen, B. (2000). Validity of the MAST in psychiatric settings: A META-analytic integration. *Journal of Studies on Alcohol, 61*(2), 254–261.

Wesley-Esquimaux, C.C., & Snowball, A. (2010). Viewing violence, mental illness and addiction through a wise practices lens. *International Journal of Mental Health and Addiction, 8*, 390–407. doi:10.1007/s11469-009-9265-6.

Wiers, R.W., & Hoffmann, W. (2010). Implicit cognition and health psychology: Changing perspectives and new interventions. *The European Health Psychologist, 12*(1), 4–6.

Wilsnack, R.W., Vogeltanz, N.D., Wilsnack, S.C., et al. (2000). Gender differences in alcohol consumption and adverse drinking consequences: Cross-cultural patterns. *Addiction, 95*(2), 251–265.

# 20

# Personality Disorders

*Claudia A. Cihlar*
*Adapted by Melissa Watkins and Cheryl L. Pollard*

## KEY TERMS AND CONCEPTS

antisocial personality disorder, 404

avoidant personality disorder, 406

borderline personality disorder, 405

dialectical behaviour therapy (DBT), 417

narcissistic personality disorder, 405

obsessive-compulsive personality disorder, 406

persona, 402

personality, 403

personality disorders, 403

schizotypal personality disorder, 404

splitting, 405

## OBJECTIVES

1. Analyze the interaction of biological determinants and psychosocial stress factors in the etiology of personality disorders.
2. Identify and distinguish among the three clusters of personality disorders.
3. Identify six personality disorders.
4. Describe the major characteristics of schizotypal, antisocial, borderline, narcissistic, avoidant, and obsessive-compulsive personality disorders and give an example of each.
5. Describe the emotional and clinical needs of nurses and other staff when working with patients who meet criteria for personality disorders.

6. Formulate a nursing diagnosis for each of the personality disorders.
7. Discuss two nursing outcomes for patients with borderline personality disorder.
8. Plan basic nursing care interventions for a patient with impulsive, aggressive, or manipulative behaviours.
9. Identify the role of the advanced-practice nurse when working with patients with personality disorders.

## ⊖volve WEBSITE

*Visit the Evolve website for Flashcards, Case Studies, and additional testing resources related to the content in this chapter:* *http://evolve.elsevier.com/Canada/Varcarolis/psychiatric/*    Pre-Test  interactive review

Often, we meet someone and think, "She's quite a strange person" or "What an unusual character he is." When we make evaluations such as these about other people, we are reacting to their personalities. *Personality* comes from the Latin word persona, which means "mask" and may refer to the person as other people see him or her. What is a personality? Categorizing personalities has been attempted since at least as early as the fifth century. Evidence from early Western and Eastern scholars

reveals our interest in understanding the basis for personality and its various dimensions, including the characteristics of disordered personality.

Early Chinese culture characterized personality in the language of energy balance. Western scholars spoke of disordered personality as an imbalance of the "humours" of phlegm, blood, and bile. The scientist Galen proposed that these humours produced psychological profiles of personality identified as

## HOW A NURSE HELPED ME
### My Reality Check

I was 22 and going through a bitter divorce. I was very angry and felt hopeless. Becoming more depressed, I had thoughts about harming myself and my husband (soon to be ex-husband). I was drinking to help numb my anger. One night, I was drunk and cut my wrists. As I lay bleeding in the bathtub, I phoned my parents to say goodbye. They phoned the ambulance, and I was taken to the hospital and admitted to the "psych" unit. My parents had often told me that I did not make good decisions for myself. I chose the wrong kind of man and the wrong kinds of friends, drank too much, and spent too much. Behind my back, my friends would say that I had a "personality problem." I didn't expect to hear the nurses tell me I had a personality problem, too. I hated being in hospital, but my family felt it was the best thing for me, as they were at their wits' end with me (well, that's what they told me).

I felt I was fairly bright and thought that I would be able to beat the system. I didn't feel I needed any help, and I certainly didn't need to be in hospital. Manipulation was the key: I knew how to sweet-talk to get my way—well, it worked with my family! I went with the routine; I played by the rules, and, yes, I was able to justify my behaviour to the doctor, social worker, and most of the nurses. I behaved the way I did because I had been abandoned. The divorce was my husband's fault, not mine. My parents didn't understand the emotional turmoil I was going through. I had no support. My nurse applied what I felt were strict rules: if I wanted anything, I had to go through her; I couldn't ask the other nurses. This gave me only

more reason to try to manipulate my nurse and play the "sweet card." This game, as I referred to it, went on for weeks, but I finally realized she was always one step ahead of me.

My nurse would sit down and talk to me about how I showed patterns of being overdramatic and displayed erratic behaviour. She gave me some examples of her claim, something I found hard to take, and I became quietly resistive to her "talks." But now, looking back many years later, I see that her description seems fairly close to how I acted. It took me a long time, with two more admissions to hospital (because of self-harming), to understand some of my behaviours. There were other discussions, or as my nurse called them "therapy," about my manipulative behaviours. I blamed my parents, my friends, and my ex-husband for my behaviour, and I still do to an extent. But I have learned to control my blaming and emotional behaviours to a degree.

I never said thank you to that particular nurse, who gave me a "reality check," as I didn't think the sessions were in my best interest at the time. But I now realize that the nurse was helping me take control of my life and provided me with various coping skills that I have since applied in my interactions with others. I still have good and bad days, but I know that this particular nurse helped guide me to be stronger and more controlled. I'm now a person who takes responsibility for her behaviours, something I didn't realize she was teaching me through those "therapy" sessions.

phlegmatic (calm and unemotional), sanguine (lighthearted and unemotional), melancholic (creative and depressive), and choleric (energetic and passionate) (Kagan, 2005). In the nineteenth century, Sigmund Freud proposed a construct of personality that caused a paradigm shift from a biological imbalance to a psychological perspective for both healthy and disordered personality. Freud's hypothesis that personality emerged from childhood experiences rather than from one's chemistry gave birth to the psychoanalytic movement.

Personality can be described operationally in terms of functioning. We know that personality can be protective for a person in times of difficulty but may also be a liability if one's personality results in ongoing relationship problems or leads to emotional distress on a regular basis (Clarkin & Huprich, 2011). Personality, then, determines the quality of experiences among people and serves as a guide for one-to-one interaction and in social groups. Based on this description, we can tell when a personality is unhealthy—that is, "when it interferes

with, or complicates, social and interpersonal function" (Blais, Smallwood, Groves, et al., 2008, p. 527). In contemporary society, there is a general consensus that personality disorders exist on a continuum of severity and likely represent more extreme variations in normal personality development.

## CLINICAL PICTURE

Individuals with personality disorders display significant challenges in self-identity or self-direction, and they have problems with empathy or intimacy within their relationships. Treating personality disorders is difficult and complex, as people with these disorders have difficulty recognizing or owning the fact that their difficulties are problems of their personality. They may truly believe the problems originate outside of themselves (Perry, Presniak, & Olson, 2013). People with personality disorders may injure themselves. In Canada in 2009–2010, about seven of ten adults hospitalized for self-injury had a mental illness (diagnosis on the hospital record). Of these admissions, 6% had a personality disorder (Canadian Institute for Health Information, 2011).

Judgements about an individual's personality functioning must take into account the person's ethnic, cultural, and social background (Mohanty, 2013). Patients who differ from the majority culture or the culture of the clinician may be at risk for overdiagnosis of a personality disorder. Therefore, it is important to obtain additional information from others who are knowledgeable about the particular cultural or ethnic norms before determining the presence of a personality disorder.

Six personality disorders are presented in the next section: schizotypal, antisocial, borderline, narcissistic, avoidant, and obsessive-compulsive. The discussion will focus on the prevalence of each disorder, the description of its common difficulties and main pathological traits, the neurobiological evidence for the disorder, and, lastly, a vignette to illustrate each type.

## Cluster A Personality Disorders

Cluster A personality disorders include paranoid personality disorder, schizoid personality disorder, and schizotypal personality disorder. Patients diagnosed with these disorders share characteristics of eccentric behaviours, such as social isolation and detachment. They may also display perception distortions, unusual levels of suspiciousness, magical thinking, and cognitive impairment. Schizotypal personality disorder is discussed in more detail below.

### Schizotypal Personality Disorder

Schizotypal personality disorder (STPD) is expressed in strikingly odd characteristics, including magical thinking, derealization, perceptual distortions, and rigid, peculiar ideas. People with this type of disorder firmly believe in their interpretation of events. Responding inappropriately to cultural social cues is common. Speech patterns may be distinctive and bizarre. STPD is less common than other personality disorder types; it occurs at a rate of less than 1% in the general population (Torgersen, 2009). Despite its low prevalence, STPD is so unusual and debilitating that it is one of the most studied personality disorders (Hummelen, Pedersen, & Karterud, 2012). Although this disorder shares some symptoms in common with schizophrenia, they are distinct disorders.

The main pathological traits that describe STPD are eccentricity (odd or unusual beliefs and thought processes); social detachment (a preference for social isolation); and unwarranted suspiciousness or anxiousness. STPD results in great difficulty maintaining relationships. People with STPD tend to misinterpret the motivations of others, thinking others are purposefully out to get them, so they avoid developing close and intimate relationships. The positive and negative symptoms seen in people with schizophrenia also exist with STPD; however, people with STPD are less vulnerable to psychotic episodes (Skodol, Bender, Morey, et al., 2011). They may exhibit odd beliefs (e.g., being overly superstitious) or magical thinking (e.g., thinking of themselves as psychic).

Genetics may play a role in the development of STPD. It has been found that family members of people with STPD are more likely to have a history of schizophrenia. There is rapidly growing evidence that people with STPD have structural abnormalities of the brain such as ventricular enlargement, reduction in the volume of their striatal structures, and altered dopamine transmission mechanisms (Skodol, Bender, Morey, et al., 2011).

---

**VIGNETTE**

Raymond is a 55-year-old single male who lives with his mother. He is the youngest of seven children raised in a farming community. Three of his siblings are deaf, and Raymond also has some hearing loss. Raymond started therapy with Wei, an advanced-practice registered nurse (APRN) in psychiatric mental health, after he suffered a career-ending injury, from which he is completely disabled. Wei and Raymond have been working together for several years on quality-of-life issues and depression. Raymond is frequently distressed by his unwavering belief that everyone in his hometown greets him with sexual gestures and believes he is gay. This belief extends to truck drivers who come through the town; he believes they talk about his sexuality on their CB radios. These beliefs create great distress and anxiety for him. He occasionally yells at people or gestures back. Wei has been helping Raymond to understand how his perceptions may be faulty and how his hearing loss may contribute to his perceptual difficulties and anxiety. Raymond and Wei have invited his mother into the discussion so she can support him at home.

---

## Cluster B Personality Disorders

Cluster B personality disorders include antisocial personality disorder, borderline personality disorder, histrionic personality disorder, and narcissistic personality disorder. Patients diagnosed with cluster B personality disorders show patterns of responding to life demands with dramatic, emotional, or erratic behaviour. Problems with impulse control, emotion processing and regulation, and interpersonal difficulties characterize this cluster of disorders. Insight into these issues is generally limited. To get their needs met, individuals with cluster B personality disorders may resort to behaviours that are considered desperate or entitled, including acting out, committing antisocial acts, or manipulating people and circumstances. Antisocial, borderline, and narcissistic personality disorders are discussed in more detail below.

### Antisocial Personality Disorder

The main pathological features of antisocial personality disorder (ASPD) are antagonistic behaviours such as deceit, manipulativeness for personal gain, and hostility if the person's needs are blocked. People with ASPD also display disinhibited behaviours such as high risk-taking, disregard for responsibility, and impulsivity. In the past, people with ASPD have been called *psychopaths* or *sociopaths*. ASPD is the most researched personality disorder. The prevalence of ASPD is about 1.1% in community studies (Skodol, Bender, Morey, et al., 2011). In people with ASPD, there is a clear history of conduct disorder in childhood, and individuals show no remorse for hurting others. They repeatedly neglect responsibilities, tell lies, and perform destructive or illegal acts without developing any insight into predictable consequences. Individuals with this personality disorder are concerned mostly with gaining personal power or pleasure, and, in their relationships, they focus on their own gratification to an extreme that defies conforming to ethical or community standards consistent with their culture. They have difficulty with intimacy and will exploit others if it benefits them in relationships. People with ASPD usually present for treatment for depression or for the consequences of high-risk behaviours, such as substance abuse, or they may be court-ordered to seek treatment. This disorder may be underdiagnosed in women and overdiagnosed in patients of lower socioeconomic status.

> **VIGNETTE**
> Manwell is a 27-year-old divorced cab driver who is referred to the hospital by the court for a mental health evaluation after an assault charge. He told the arresting officer that he has bipolar disorder. He has a history of substance abuse and multiple arrests for disorderly conduct or assault. During his intake interview, he is polite and even flirtatious with the female nurse. He insists that he is not responsible for his behaviour because he is manic. The only symptom he describes is irritability. He points out that he cannot tolerate any psychotropic medications because of the adverse effects. He also notes that he has dropped out of three clinics after several visits because "the staff don't understand me."

## Borderline Personality Disorder

Borderline personality disorder (BPD) is the most well-known and dramatic of the personality disorders and is characterized by severe impairments in functioning, a high mortality rate (approximately 30%), and extensive utilization of health care services (Madarasz, Manzardo, Mortensen, et al., 2012). However, with effective treatment, people with BPD experience high rates of remission and low rates of relapse (Gunderson, 2011).

BPD occurs at a rate of about 1.6% in community studies (Skodol, Bender, Morey, et al., 2011). The major features of this disorder are patterns of marked instability in emotion regulation, unstable interpersonal relationships, identity or self-image distortions, and unstable mood.

One of the pathological personality traits seen in people with BPD is negative affect. This affect is characterized by emotional lability—that is, moods that alternate rapidly from one emotional extreme to another. Other characteristics of a negative affect include responding to situations with emotions that are out of proportion to the circumstances, pathological fear of separation, and intense sensitivity to perceived personal rejection. Other disruptive traits common in people with BPD are impulsivity and antagonism. Impulsivity results in damaged relationships and even suicide attempts. Antagonism is marked by hostility, anger, and irritability in relationships.

In addition, ineffective and harmful self-soothing habits, such as cutting, promiscuous sexual behaviour, and numbing with substances, are common and may result in unintentional death. Chronic suicidal ideation is also a common feature of

this disorder and influences the likelihood of accidental death. Co-occurring mood, anxiety, or substance disorders complicate the treatment and prognosis of the condition.

Splitting, the primary defence or coping style used by people with BPD, is the inability to incorporate positive and negative aspects of oneself or others into a whole image. This kind of dichotomous thinking and coping behaviour is believed to be partly a result of the person's failed experiences with adult personality integration and is likely influenced by exposure to earlier psychological, sexual, or physical trauma. For example, the individual may tend to idealize another person (e.g., friend, lover, health care provider) at the start of a new relationship, hoping that this person will meet all of his or her needs. But at the first disappointment or frustration, the individual quickly shifts to devaluation, despising the other person.

Individuals with BPD seek out treatment for depression, anxiety, suicidal and self-harming behaviours, and other impulsive behaviours, including substance use. Repeat hospitalizations are frequently sought out by the person with BPD and are viewed as a way to decrease self-destructive risk, but they are not regarded as an effective long-term solution.

BPD has been found to run in families and is highly associated with genetic factors such as hypersensitivity, impulsivity, and emotional dysregulation (Gunderson, 2011). People with BPD may have a hyper-responsive amygdala and impairment in the prefrontal cortex that make them more vulnerable to emotionally charged words, facial expressions, and interpersonal exchanges.

> **VIGNETTE**
> Shaina is a 38-year-old married woman with one young son. She works full time as a dietitian in a primary care network. Shaina was diagnosed with fibromyalgia two years ago and is in treatment at a pain clinic. Most days, she comes home from work fatigued and goes to bed, leaving her son to play by himself after school or with friends until her husband gets home from work. Shaina also has struggled with an eating disorder since she was a teenager. When she feels guilty for ignoring her son's needs, she binges and then purges to relieve her negative emotions. Shaina recognizes that this behaviour helps only temporarily and adds to her fatigue, but she still feels helpless to stop it. When her son asks her to play with him or take him to an activity, she becomes angry with him and then feels angry at herself. Shaina has been referred by the palliative care nurse at the pain clinic to a dialectical behaviour therapy group (discussed later in this chapter) to learn skills to deal with her chronic pain and discover alternative self-soothing strategies for her bingeing and purging behaviours.

## Narcissistic Personality Disorder

Narcissistic personality disorder (NPD) is thought to be the least frequently occurring personality disorder. In the community, it exists at less than 1%, but it is seen in clinical populations more frequently (Torgersen, 2009). NPD is also less associated with impairment in individual functioning and quality of life than are other personality disorders. Narcissistic personality disorder has the primary feature of arrogance with a grandiose

## CONSIDERING CULTURE
### Gender Bias in Diagnosing Personality Disorders

There may be a culture-bound gender bias in the diagnosing of personality disorders. Borderline personality disorder (BPD) is an example of such a bias: well-respected diagnostic manuals report a 3 : 1 gender ratio of females to males for BPD (Sansone & Sansone, 2011). However, Grant, Chou, Goldstein, and colleagues (2008), in a well-executed epidemiological survey, found BPD to be equally prevalent in men and women. Thus, a subtle clinician bias has increased the predominance of female BPD diagnosis. This bias may have developed from women with BPD undertaking more self-harming behaviours, which result in an admission to treatment, versus men with BPD who have more substance abuse and antisocial features, which result in their incarceration. This difference might lead staff working in the psychiatric treatment facility to think that there are more females with BPD. Also, the emotional aspects of BPD may present differently in women and men (Verona, Sprague, & Javdani, 2012), and, as a result, it is important for health care providers to think of this disorder more broadly than as a women's issue.

**Sources:** Grant, B., Chou, S., Goldstein, R., et al. (2008). Prevalence, correlates, disability, and comorbidity of DSM-IV borderline personality disorder: Results from the wave 2 national epidemiologic survey on alcohol and related conditions. *Journal of Clinical Psychiatry, 69*(4), 533–545. Retrieved from http://www.ncbi .nlm.nih.gov/pubmed/18426259; Sansone, R., & Sansone, L. (2011). Gender patterns in borderline personality disorder. *Innovations in Clinical Neuroscience, 8*(5), 16–20. Retrieved from http://www .ncbi.nlm.nih.gov/pmc/articles/PMC3115767/; Verona, E., Sprague, J., & Javdani, S. (2012). Gender and factor-level interactions in psychopathy: Implications for self-directed violence risk and borderline personality disorder symptoms. *Personality Disorders, 3*(3), 247–262. doi:10.1037/a0025945.

view of self-importance. The individual with this disorder has a need for constant admiration, along with a lack of empathy for others, which strains most relationships. People with NPD experience a feeling of personal entitlement; when paired with their lack of social empathy, it may result in the exploitation of other people, particularly vulnerable individuals (Vater, Ritter, Schröder-Abé, et al., 2013). Underneath the surface of arrogance, people with NPD feel intense shame and fear of abandonment. They are afraid of their own mistakes, as well as the mistakes of others. Narcissistic individuals may seek help for depression or validation by therapists or family and friends for their emotional pain due to not being appreciated enough by others for their efforts or special qualities.

### Cluster C Personality Disorders

Cluster C personality disorders include avoidant personality disorder, dependent personality disorder, and obsessive-compulsive personality disorder. Patients with these types of personality disorders show patterns of anxious and fearful behaviours, rigid patterns of social shyness, hypersensitivity, need for orderliness, and relationship dependency. Avoidant and obsessive-compulsive personality disorders are discussed in more detail below.

### VIGNETTE

Dr. Abigail McLaughlin is a 40-year-old female attending psychiatrist at a university outpatient centre. She is twice divorced and has no children. Her grooming and makeup are impeccable, and she likes to chat about her expensive shopping habits. She is quite intelligent and is the only doctor on the staff trained in psychoanalysis. In clinical team meetings, she often discusses this fact, repeatedly telling others that psychoanalysis is the best treatment for mental illness. She frequently makes derogatory remarks to psychiatric residents if they suggest alternative treatment approaches for new cases. She is usually late to staff meetings, and when she is not speaking, she yawns and shifts noisily in her seat. She has a reputation for exhibiting angry outbursts at therapists in the hallway for minor mistakes, such as a scheduling error for a patient. She underwent seven years of psychoanalysis but does not consider it to have been therapy—it "was for training purposes only."

### Avoidant Personality Disorder

The central characteristics of avoidant personality disorder (AVPD) are an extreme sensitivity to rejection and robust avoidance of interpersonal situations. A timid temperament in infancy and childhood may be associated with this disorder. Individuals with AVPD demonstrate poor self-confidence and are prone to misinterpreting others' feedback because they are overly sensitive to rejection. Although they strongly desire close interpersonal relationships, they avoid them. AVPD is one of the most prevalent personality disorders (Samuels, 2011). Canadian researchers Cox, Pagura, Stein, and colleagues (2009) have estimated an AVPD lifetime prevalence rate of 2.4%. This study was conducted using epidemiological data from a sample of the United States population. Unfortunately, these researchers did not conduct a similar study using a sample of the Canadian population. Studies have found a shared association between people who have AVPD and people with social phobia (Skodol, Bender, Morey, et al., 2011).

### VIGNETTE

Annemarie is a 35-year-old single female who works as a receptionist for a computer repair company. As a child, she had few friends and never participated in extracurricular activities. Annemarie lives alone in her own apartment and has never had an intimate adult relationship. On the job, she rarely talks to co-workers and prefers to work alone. If she has any questions, she asks the supervisor and carefully follows directions. Although she has seven years of experience and a good work record, she refuses the offer of a promotion because it would require her to interact with customers.

### Obsessive-Compulsive Personality Disorder

Obsessive-compulsive personality disorder (OCPD), along with AVPD, is the most prevalent personality disorder in the general community and in clinical populations. Along with BPD, this disorder is associated with the highest burden of medical costs, and OCPD affects workplace productivity losses

(Skodol, Bender, Morey, et al., 2011). The main pathological personality traits are rigidity and inflexible standards of self and others, along with persistence to goals long after necessary and even if it is self-defeating or harmful to relationships.

People with OCPD feel genuine affection for friends and family but do not have insight about their own difficult behaviour. Internally, they are fearful of imminent catastrophe. They rehearse over and over how they will respond in social situations. They do not have full-blown obsessions or compulsions but may seek treatment for anxiety or mood disorders.

---

**VIGNETTE**

Robert is a 45-year-old single male postal worker in a small town. He lives alone and has never married. He is well groomed and wears a clean, neatly ironed uniform every day. He carefully follows all policies and procedures and is quite resistant whenever there is any update or change. He frequently challenges the supervisor about policy details and has been referred to the regional personnel office countless times for resolution of these conflicts. In staff meetings, he gives excessive circumstantial details and writes extra material on the back of any required report form. When dealing with the public, he sometimes gets into arguments with customers about postal rules or the schedule. Other staff members do not consider him to be a team player because he seldom volunteers to help others. Even if he is asked to help someone, he is quick to criticize his peer's performance. Although he has worked in the same office for ten years, he has never advanced beyond the front-line position. He is fairly content with his work and has never been in psychiatric treatment.

---

## EPIDEMIOLOGY

In the past decade, the epidemiology of personality disorders has become clearer. Personality disorders are more frequently seen in people receiving extensive medical and psychiatric services (Samuels, 2011). While narcissistic and schizotypal personality disorders are relatively rare, borderline, avoidant, and obsessive-compulsive personality disorders have been established by meta-analyses (pulling together the best and most relevant research) to be common among both community and clinical populations.

While studies vary in their estimates of prevalence depending on their methodologies, the ICD-10 criteria suggest that personality disorders affect about 10% of the world's population (Samuels, 2011). Culture has a definite influence on the rate of diagnosing personality disorders. For example, an Australian study reports substantially higher prevalence rates than North American studies do (Samuels, 2011). Differences may reflect the view of personality and behaviour as deviant rather than normal in a particular culture and within certain study methods. Or it may reflect better diagnosing practices or a system that has resources to assist people with personality disorders. It is generally agreed that there are insufficient studies to address the role of ethnicity and race on the prevalence of personality disorders (McGilloway, Hall, Lee, et al., 2010).

---

### 🌐 CONSIDERING CULTURE

#### Ageism, Culture of Aging, and Personality Disorders in Older Adults

Ageism, or the discrimination of a person based upon his or her age, has become ubiquitous in our Western culture with its emphasis on youth. This bias includes the beliefs of caregivers in health care settings designed to serve the needs of older adults. Aging stereotypes interfere with the accurate assessment of older adults, including those with personality disorders, because the changes associated with aging may further complicate the provision of their care.

In addition, aging brings with it natural changes in social relationships, most notably, more social isolation and loss. Not only is the older adult with a personality disorder impacted by these developmental relationship changes but—because personality disorders profoundly affect the ability to function effectively in relationships—there is also a greater likelihood that issues will become exacerbated and affect the person's care in later life.

**Essential Considerations**

- The incidence of personality disorders late in life is not fully known but may be overlooked by health care providers due to cultural biases about aging.
- Personality disorders do present in later life, often in conjunction with other mental health disorders such as depression or anxiety.
- A hallmark feature of personality disorders is a pervasive impairment in interpersonal relationships, and this impairment becomes a risk factor for greater social isolation as a person ages.
- For a person with reduced capacity for coping, age-related stressors such as grief and loss may strain the person's ability to tolerate these developmental changes and may strain family members as the person becomes more dependent on them.
- The health care system designed to help the older adult may tax the already reduced capacity of an individual with a more rigid personality to accept bureaucratic-style treatment conditions.
- Nurses and case managers are more successful in addressing the needs of older adults with personality disorders when they examine their own biases about aging and personality disorders. It is also helpful for professionals to use a flexible approach that supports a "goodness of fit" style that recognizes strength-based values of the patient, the family members, and the system of care involved with their patients.

**Sources:** Magoteaux, A.L., & Bonnivier, J.F. (2009). Distinguishing between personality disorders, stereotypes, and eccentricities in older adults. *Journal of Psychosocial Nursing. 47*(7), 19–24; Supiano, K.P., & Carroll, A.M. (2009). Personality disorders in older clients and their families: A challenge for geriatric case managers. *Care Management Journals, 10*(4), 146–150.

---

## CO-MORBIDITY

Normal personality traits are amplified during the experience of a crisis and any illness; therefore, it is premature and not in the best interest of the individual for a personality disorder to be diagnosed during the active phase of another illness, especially a psychiatric episode or major stressful life event such as grief and loss or trauma.

Co-morbid personality disorders influence the expression of primary mental health symptoms, often amplifying the symptoms or level of emotional dysregulation. Evidence-informed studies confirm that personality disorders also frequently co-occur with disorders of mood, anxiety, disordered eating, and substance abuse. Other studies confirm that personality disorders are more common among people who are homeless or incarcerated. Recent studies have also suggested that personality disorders are more common in older adults than originally thought and frequently become evident when accompanied by major depression or anxiety (Magoteaux & Bonnivier, 2009).

Childhood neglect and trauma have been established as risk factors for personality disorders (Samuels, 2011). This association has been linked to possible biological mechanisms involving corticotropin-releasing hormone in response to early life stress and emotional reactivity (Lee, Hempel, Tenharmsel, et al., 2012).

## ETIOLOGY

Personality disorders are the result of complex biological and psychosocial phenomena that are influenced by multifaceted variables involving genetic, neurobiological, neurochemical, and environmental factors.

### Biological Factors
#### Genetics

While genetics are thought to influence the development of personality disorders, individual genes are not believed to be associated with particular personality traits; thus, the relationship among genes and traits is a complex one (Taylor, Asmundson, & Jang, 2011).

Several possible hypotheses attempt to account for the personality differences among people in the same family. One may be that a child's temperament can elicit different responses from family members. Individual children may perceive family experiences in unique ways and therefore respond differently from other family members (Hernandez, Arntz, Gaviria, et al., 2012). Children are also affected by forces outside the family that influence personality development. It may be that personality is influenced even by the intrauterine environment, although there are less data to support this hypothesis.

### Neurobiology and Neurochemistry

Biological influences on personality expression are a promising area of research in understanding these disorders. Influences on the development of personality disorders probably incorporate a complex interaction of genetics, neurobiology, and neurochemistry. The Chemical Neurotransmitter Theory proposes that certain neurotransmitters may regulate and influence temperament. Research in brain imaging has also revealed some differences in the size and function of specific structures of the brain in people with some personality disorders (Leichsenring, Leibing, Kruse, et al., 2011).

### Psychosocial Factors
#### Psychological Factors

Several psychological theories may help to explain the development of personality disorders. Learning theory emphasizes that children develop maladaptive responses based on modelling of or reinforcement by important people in the child's life. Cognitive theories emphasize the role of beliefs and assumptions in creating emotional and behavioural responses that influence one's experiences within the family environment.

Psychoanalytic theory focuses on the use of primitive defence mechanisms by individuals with personality disorders. Defence mechanisms such as repression, suppression, regression, undoing, and splitting have been identified as dominant (Kernberg, 1985). The role of psychoanalytic theory, while historically relevant and interesting, is not confirmable through evidence-informed research methods.

### Environmental Factors

Behavioural genetics research has shown that about half of the variance accounting for personality traits emerges from the environment (Hernandez, Arntz, Gaviria, et al., 2012). These findings suggest that while the family environment is influential on development, there are other environmental factors besides upbringing that shape an individual's personality. One need only think about the individual differences among siblings raised together to illustrate this point.

### Diathesis–Stress Model

The diathesis–stress model is a general theory that explains psychopathology using a systems approach. This theory helps us understand how personality disorders emerge from the multifaceted factors of biology and environment (Paris, 2005). *Diathesis* refers to genetic and biological vulnerabilities and includes personality traits and temperament. *Temperament* is our tendency to respond to challenges in predictable ways. Examples of descriptors of temperament may be *laid back*, referring to a calm temperament, or *uptight*, referring to an anxious temperament. These characteristics remain stable throughout a person's life. In this model, *stress* refers to immediate influences on personality such as the physical, social, psychological, and emotional environment. *Stress* also includes what happened in the past, such as growing up in one's family with exposure to unique experiences and patterns of interaction. The diathesis–stress model proposes that, under conditions of stress, some people have maladaptive personality development, resulting in the emergence of a personality disorder (Paris, 2005).

There is a two-way directionality among stressors and diatheses. Genetic and biological traits are believed to influence the way an individual responds to the environment while, at the same time, the environment is thought to influence the expression of inherited traits. Many studies have suggested a strong correlation between trauma, neglect, and other dysfunctional family or social patterns of interaction and the development of personality disorders among individuals with particular personality traits and temperament.

The following is a summary of factors that are theorized to influence the development of each disorder (Skodol & Gunderson, 2008):

- Schizotypal personality disorder is a schizophrenia spectrum disorder and is genetically linked, meaning that there is a higher incidence of schizophrenia-related disorders in family members of people with STPD.
- Antisocial personality disorder is genetically linked, and twin studies indicate a predisposition to this disorder. This predisposition is set into motion by a childhood environment of inconsistent parenting, significant abuse, and extreme neglect.
- Borderline personality disorder has traditionally been thought to develop as a result of early abandonment, which results in an unstable view of self and others. This abandonment is made more intense by a biological predisposition, and twin studies identify a heritability of 69%.
- Narcissistic personality disorder may be the result of childhood neglect and criticism. The child does not learn that other people can be a source of comfort and support. As adults, they hide feelings of emptiness with an exterior of invulnerability and self-sufficiency. Little is known about inborn traits or heritability for this disorder.
- Avoidant personality disorder has been linked with parental and peer rejection and criticism. A biological predisposition to anxiety and physiological arousal in social situations has also been suggested. Genetically, this disorder may be part of a continuum of disorders related to social phobia (social anxiety disorder; see Chapter 13).
- Obsessive-compulsive personality disorder may be related to excessive parental criticism, control, and shame. The child responds to this negativity by trying to control his or her environment through perfectionism and orderliness. Heritable traits such as compulsivity, oppositionality, lack of emotional expressiveness, and perfectionism have all been implicated in this disorder.

## APPLICATION OF THE NURSING PROCESS

## ASSESSMENT

### Assessment Tools

The preferred method for determining a diagnosis of personality disorder is the semi-structured interview obtained by clinicians. These types of interviews have standard questions and a standard format for asking the questions. These interviews go beyond asking the patient to self-report on symptoms because individuals with personality disorders often lack insight into their behaviours and motivations and therefore have difficulty accurately describing themselves (Huprich, 2011). One way to elicit more objective information is to ask the person if family members and colleagues perceive them in a certain way. For example, "You said that you don't think you're emotionally distant. How would your wife describe you?" Cultural norms and expectations also need to be considered when evaluating the presence of a personality disorder. Personality disorders are often assessed through identifying pathology within one or more personality dimensions. The five main dimensions of personalities are (1) extraversion versus introversion, (2) antagonism versus compliance, (3) constraint versus impulsivity, (4) emotional dysregulation versus emotional stability, and (5) unconventionality versus closedness to experience (Simms, Goldberg, Roberts, et al., 2011). See Table 20-1.

Open-ended or subjective interviews, which do not have standard questions or a standard question format, are more likely to result in biased and culturally based decisions about diagnosis (McGilloway, Hall, Lee, et al., 2010). Self-report inventories, such as the well-known Minnesota Multiphasic Personality Inventory (MMPI), are useful because they have built-in validity and reliability scales for the clinician to refer to when interpreting test results. In general, studies have found that inventories may show higher false positive scores that result in overdiagnosing of personality disorders (Widiger & Mullins-Sweatt, 2008).

### Patient History

Taking a full medical history can help determine if the problem is a psychiatric one, a medical one, or both. Medical illness should never be ruled out as the cause for problem behaviour until the data support this conclusion. Important issues in assessing for personality disorders include a history of suicidal or aggressive ideation or actions, current use of medications and illegal substances, ability to handle money, and legal history.

Significant topics about which further details must be obtained include current or past physical, sexual, or emotional abuse and level of current risk for harm from self or others. At times, immediate interventions may be needed to ensure the safety of the person or others. Information regarding prior use of any medication, including psychopharmacological agents, is important. This information gives evidence of other contacts the person has made for help and indicates how the health care provider found the person at that time.

### Self-Assessment

Because enduring patterns of interpersonal difficulties are central to the problems faced by people diagnosed with personality disorders, it is understandable that their relationship problems with their caregivers surface in the treatment milieu. Anticipating that people with personality disorders will likely have a disrupted, intense interpersonal experience with caregivers is helpful to the caregivers as they monitor their own personal stress responses. It is important to keep in mind that these dysfunctional behaviours may really represent the person's best efforts to cope because they lack the necessary skills to be effective in their lives.

For individuals with borderline personality disorder, the therapeutic alliance often follows an initial upward curve of idealization (sometimes preceded by a brief initial rejection) by the person toward the caregivers. This reaction is then followed by a devaluation of the caregivers because the patient is disappointed by the treatment team failing to meet his or her unrealistic expectations. This process is often acted out in the treatment milieu and can interrupt the delivery of care. For example, a female patient may briefly idealize her male nurse on the inpatient unit, telling staff and patients alike that she is "the luckiest person because she has the best nurse in the hospital." The rest of the team understands that this comment is an exaggeration. After days of her constant dramatic praise for the nurse and subtle insults to the rest of the staff, some members of the team may start to feel inadequate and resentful of the nurse. They begin to make critical remarks about minor events to prove that the nurse is not perfect. A similar scenario can occur if the person constantly complains about one staff member; some colleagues are then torn between defending and criticizing the targeted staff member.

Inexperience working with this heterogeneous population, lack of appropriate education or supervision, and limited

| TABLE 20-1 | FIVE DIMENSIONS OF PERSONALITY |
|---|---|
| **PERSONALITY DIMENSIONS** | **ATTITUDES AND BEHAVIOURS** |
| Extraversion versus introversion | Activity, aloofness, assertiveness, detachment, entitlement, excitement-seeking, exhibitionism, exploratory excitability, extravagance, gregariousness, histrionic sexualization, intimacy problems, optimism, positive emotionality, restricted expression, schizoid orientation, shyness, sociability, social avoidance, social closeness, social potency, stimulus-seeking, warmth, well-being |
| Antagonism versus compliance | Aggression, agreeableness, alienation, altruism, attachment, callousness, compassion, compliance, conduct problems, dependency, diffidence, empathy, entitlement, helpfulness, insecure attachment, interpersonal disesteem, manipulativeness, mistrust, modesty, narcissism, passive oppositionality, psychopathy, pure-heartedness, rejection, sentimentality, social acceptance, social closeness, straightforwardness, submissiveness, suspiciousness, tender-mindedness, trust |
| Constraint versus impulsivity | Achievement-striving, childishness, competence, compulsivity, conscientiousness, deliberation, disorderliness, dutifulness, eagerness of effort, harm avoidance, impulsivity, irresponsibility, obsessionality, order, perfectionism, propriety, resourcefulness, responsibility, risk-taking, self-discipline, traditionalism, workaholism |
| Emotional dysregulation versus emotional stability | Affective lability, alienation, angry hostility, anticipatory worry, anxiousness, dependency, depressiveness, dysphoria, emotional dysregulation, fear of uncertainty, hostility, hypochondriasis, identity problems, inferiority, introspection, irritability, negative affect, pessimism, self-acceptance, self-consciousness, self-harm, sensitivity, stress reaction, unhappiness, vulnerability, worthlessness |
| Unconventionality versus closedness to experience | Absorption, dissociation, eccentric perceptions, eccentricity, openness to experience, perceptual cognitive distortion, rigidity, spiritual acceptance, thought disorder, transpersonal identification |

**Source:** Adapted from Simms, L., Goldberg, L., Roberts, J., et al. (2011). Computerized adaptive assessment of personality disorder: Introducing the CAT-PD project. *Journal of Personality Assessment, 93*(4), 380–389. doi:10.1080/00223891.2011.577475. Reprinted by permission of the publisher (Taylor & Francis Ltd, http://www.tandf.co.uk/journals).

 **RESEARCH HIGHLIGHT**

*Family Members' Experiences With Borderline Personality Disorder*

**Source:** Ekdahl, S., Idvall, E., Samuelsson, M., et al. (2011). A life tiptoeing: Being a significant other to persons with borderline personality disorder. *Archives of Psychiatric Nursing, 25*(6), e69–e76. doi:10.1016/j.apnu.2011.06.005.

**Problem**

Individuals with BPD characteristically struggle to create effective interpersonal relationships due to challenges with heightened emotional sensitivity, a reduced ability to be empathic to others, and a preoccupation with the fear of abandonment by others. These issues negatively affect relationships with both family and health care providers. This problem is especially important because the support of family is a major factor in recovery from a psychiatric illness episode or crisis. Research in the area of the family's lived experience with BPD is scarce. In recent years, a greater effort has been made to educate families about how to cope with a loved one who suffers from this disorder. One study found that family members with greater knowledge of BPD showed poorer health.

**Purpose of Study**

The purpose of this study was to explore how family members experience living close to a person with BPD and how they experience their encounters with health care providers.

**Methods**

The study was qualitative and used a purposeful sampling method, which means that people believed to have the best knowledge of the problem were invited to participate. Participants were recruited from a Swedish association of family members with BPD. Nineteen participants emerged from a possible population of 30 members. The majority were parents (N = 17), followed by a spouse (N = 1), and an adult child (N = 1). Most were female family members (14). Data was collected in two steps: (1) a questionnaire about the patient's health condition, strain in the family, and encounters with health care providers and (2) group interviews focused on living close to someone with BPD and the experiences of health and psychiatric care.

*Continued*

RESEARCH HIGHLIGHT—cont'd

## Family Members' Experiences With Borderline Personality Disorder

**Key Findings**

- The first major theme included four phenomena of family lived experience: tiptoeing, powerlessness, guilt, and lifelong grief:
  - *Tiptoeing* refers to the burden of 24-hour worry and duty that disrupt daily life, especially involving incidents of self-harm or suicide attempts, and living in constant crisis.
  - Feelings of powerlessness, guilt, and lifelong grief included perceived neglect of siblings, strained marital relationships, and perceived inability to ask for support from others, including health care providers, due to prejudiced beliefs about the disorder.
- A second major theme emerged in the area of family member encounters with health care providers, including psychiatric mental health care providers:
  - Families described feeling left out when the patient was hospitalized but burdened without help once the patient was discharged. They felt as though health care providers viewed them as obstacles in the treatment process. They expressed that the issue of privacy and confidentiality contributed to secrecy in treatment.

- The issue of lost trust surfaced as family members expressed their view that care often lacked a comprehensive view of the person and family in context, and although they described meeting kind and caring nurses, they felt betrayed by the inability of providers to keep their family member safe when in their care.

**Implications for Nursing Practice**

This study supports findings from other research on family involvement. Specifically, families and patients benefit from more involvement in the treatment process before they are discharged home. Nurses and other team members have both an obligation and an opportunity to consider the needs of the patient in the context of his or her family. Nurses can be leaders in facilitating two types of groups: family education groups that focus on teaching skills about interpersonal effectiveness with the person with BPD and individual family meetings to identify the needs of families around discharge planning.

clinical support contribute to the maintenance of personal defence mechanisms. Clinical supervision and additional education are helpful and supportive to staff on the front lines of care (Koivu, Saarinen, & Hyrkas, 2012). Awareness of and monitoring of one's own stress responses to people's behaviours facilitate more effective and therapeutic intervention, regardless of the specific approach to their care.

Finding an approach that works with people in the setting in which they are treated is important. Therapies such as dialectical behaviour therapy and mindfulness-based therapies offer staff evidence-informed interventions, clinical structure, and formalized support for identifying best practices.

## ASSESSMENT GUIDELINES

### Personality Disorders

1. Assess for suicidal or homicidal thoughts. If such thoughts are present, the person needs immediate attention.
2. Determine whether the person has a medical disorder or another psychiatric disorder that may be responsible for the symptoms (especially a substance use disorder).
3. View the assessment about personality functioning from within the person's ethnic, cultural, and social background.
4. Ascertain whether the person experienced a recent important loss. Personality disorders are often exacerbated after the loss of significant supporting people or in a disruptive social situation.
5. Evaluate for a change in personality, in middle adulthood or later, that signals the need for a thorough medical workup or assessment for unrecognized substance use disorder.

| TABLE 20-2 | POTENTIAL NURSING DIAGNOSES FOR PERSONALITY DISORDERS |
|---|---|
| **SIGNS AND SYMPTOMS** | **NURSING DIAGNOSES** |
| Crisis, high levels of anxiety | *Ineffective coping* <br> *Anxiety* <br> *Self-mutilation* |
| Anger and aggression; child, elder, or spouse abuse | *Risk for other-directed violence* <br> *Ineffective coping* <br> *Impaired parenting* <br> *Disabled family coping* |
| Withdrawal | *Social isolation* |
| Paranoia | *Fear* <br> *Disturbed sensory perception* <br> *Disturbed thought processes* <br> *Defensive coping* |
| Depression | *Hopelessness* <br> *Risk for suicide* <br> *Self-mutilation* <br> *Chronic low self-esteem* <br> *Spiritual distress* |
| Difficulty in relationships, manipulation | *Ineffective coping* <br> *Impaired social interaction* <br> *Defensive coping* <br> *Interrupted family processes* <br> *Risk for loneliness* |
| Failure to keep medical appointments, late arrival for appointments, failure to follow prescribed medical procedure or medication regimen | *Ineffective therapeutic regimen management* <br> *Nonadherence* |

## DIAGNOSIS

When people with personality disorders are admitted to psychiatric institutions, it is usually because of symptoms of co-morbid disorders, dangerous behaviour, or court-ordered treatment. BPD and ASPD both present a challenge for health care providers because the behaviours central to these disorders often cause disruption in psychiatric and medical-surgical settings. Emotions such as anxiety, rage, and depression and behaviours such as withdrawal, paranoia, and manipulation are among the most frequent concerns that health care workers must address. Table 20-2 lists common potential nursing diagnoses related to personality disorders.

## OUTCOMES IDENTIFICATION

Realistic outcomes are established for individuals with personality disorders based on the perspective that personality change occurs with one behavioural solution and one learned skill at a time. This change can be expected to take much time and repetition. In the acute care setting, the focus is on the presenting problem, which may be depression or severe anxiety. During the hospital stay, the chronic behaviour problems of individuals with personality disorders are not expected to be resolved but rather to be met with appropriate therapeutic feedback.

Pertinent categories of nursing outcomes based on the Nursing Outcomes Classification (NOC) include Aggression self-control, Impulse self-control, Social interaction skills, Personal resiliency, Fear level, Abusive behaviour self-restraint, and Self-mutilation restraint (Moorhead, Johnson, Maas, et al., 2008). Table 20-3 gives examples of other potential nursing outcomes for manipulative, aggressive, and impulsive behaviours.

## PLANNING

It is often difficult to create a therapeutic relationship with individuals who have antisocial or borderline personality disorders because most of them have experienced failed relationships, including therapeutic alliances. Their distrust of

| TABLE 20-3 | *NOC* OUTCOMES FOR MANIPULATIVE, AGGRESSIVE, AND IMPULSIVE BEHAVIOURS | |
| --- | --- | --- |
| **NURSING OUTCOME AND DEFINITION** | **INTERMEDIATE INDICATORS** | **SHORT-TERM INDICATORS** |
| *Social interaction skills:* Personal behaviours that promote effective relationships | Uses conflict-resolution methods | Exhibits receptiveness<br>Exhibits sensitivity to others<br>Cooperates with others<br>Uses assertive behaviours as appropriate<br>Uses confrontation as appropriate |
| *Personal resiliency:* Positive adaptation and function of an individual following significant adversity or crisis | Uses effective coping strategies | Expresses emotion<br>Seeks emotional support<br>Uses strategies to promote safety<br>Takes responsibility for own actions<br>Uses strategies to avoid violent situations<br>Identifies available community resources<br>Obtains needed support<br>Self-initiates goal-directed behaviour<br>Expresses belief in ability to perform action<br>Expresses that performance will lead to desired outcome |
| *Aggression self-control:* Self-restraint of assaultive, combative, or destructive behaviours toward others | Communicates needs appropriately | Identifies when frustrated<br>Identifies when angry<br>Identifies responsibility to maintain control<br>Identifies alternatives to aggression<br>Identifies alternatives to verbal outbursts<br>Vents negative feelings appropriately<br>Refrains from striking or harming others |
| *Impulse self-control:* Self-restraint of compulsive or impulsive behaviours | Controls impulses | Identifies harmful impulsive behaviours<br>Identifies feelings that lead to impulsive actions<br>Identifies consequences of impulsive actions to self or others<br>Avoids high-risk environments and situations<br>Seeks help when experiencing impulses |

**Source:** Data from Moorhead, S., Johnson, M., Maas, M.L, et al. (2008). *Nursing outcomes classification (NOC)* (4th ed.). St. Louis, MO: Mosby.

relationships and hostility toward others can make establishing a therapeutic relationship difficult. When they blame and attack others, the nurse needs to understand the context of their complaints; that is, these attacks spring from the feeling of being threatened. The more intense their complaints are, the greater their fear of potential harm or loss is. Lacking the ability to trust, people with personality disorders require a sense of control over what is happening to them. Giving them

realistic choices (e.g., selection of a particular group activity) may enhance adherence to treatment. It is also important to plan individual patient treatment within the context of their family. Patients, families, and health care providers can access further information on personality disorders from the Internet; two reliable Canadian sites are the Canadian Mental Health Association (www.cmha.ca) and HeretoHelp (www.heretohelp.bc.ca). Refer to Table 20-4 for guidelines for

## TABLE 20-4  NURSING AND THERAPY GUIDELINES FOR PERSONALITY DISORDERS

| PERSONALITY DISORDER | CHARACTERISTICS | NURSING GUIDELINES | SUGGESTED THERAPIES |
|---|---|---|---|
| Antisocial | Ability to seem normal<br>No anxiety or depression<br>Manipulative<br>Exploitive of others<br>Aggressive<br>Seductive<br>Callous toward others | 1. Try to prevent or reduce untoward effects of manipulation (flattery, seductiveness, instilling of guilt):<br>• Set clear and realistic limits on specific behaviour.<br>• Ensure that limits are adhered to by all staff.<br>• Carefully document signs of manipulation or aggression.<br>• Document behaviours (give times, dates, circumstances).<br>• Provide clear boundaries and consequences.<br>2. Be aware that antisocial patients can instill guilt when they are not getting what they want. Guard against being manipulated through feelings of guilt.<br>3. Substance abuse is best handled through a well-organized treatment program before counselling and other forms of therapy are started. | More responsive to psychotherapy when hospitalized than when jailed<br>Pharmacotherapy for anxiety, rage, and depression<br>Careful use of addictive agents (e.g., benzodiazepines)<br>Methylphenidate (Ritalin) may help ADHD<br>Anticonvulsants may help impulsive behaviour |
| Avoidant | Excessively anxious in social situations<br>Hypersensitive to negative evaluation<br>Desiring of social interaction | 1. A friendly, accepting, reassuring approach is the best way to treat patients.<br>2. Being pushed into social situations can cause extreme and severe anxiety. | Psychotherapy focused on trust<br>Group therapy<br>Assertiveness training<br>Antidepressants and antianxiety agents helpful; β-adrenergic receptor antagonists (e.g., atenolol) help reduce autonomic nervous system hyperactivity |
| Borderline | Separation anxiety<br>Manifestation of ideas of reference<br>Impulsive (suicide, self-mutilation)<br>Splitting (adoring then devaluing people) | 1. Set realistic goals; use clear action words.<br>2. Be aware of manipulative behaviours (flattery, seductiveness, instilling of guilt).<br>3. Provide clear and consistent boundaries and limits.<br>4. Use clear and straightforward communication.<br>5. When behavioural problems emerge, calmly review the therapeutic goals and boundaries of treatment.<br>6. Avoid rejecting or rescuing.<br>7. Assess for suicidal and self-mutilating behaviours, especially during times of stress. | Individual psychotherapy<br>Dialectical behaviour therapy<br>Group therapy<br>Antipsychotics to control anger and brief psychosis<br>Antidepressants such as SSRIs and MAOIs<br>Benzodiazepines to ease anxiety |

*Continued*

| TABLE 20-4 | NURSING AND THERAPY GUIDELINES FOR PERSONALITY DISORDERS—cont'd | | |
|---|---|---|---|
| **PERSONALITY DISORDER** | **CHARACTERISTICS** | **NURSING GUIDELINES** | **SUGGESTED THERAPIES** |
| Narcissistic | Exploitive<br>Grandiose<br>Disparaging<br>Filled with rage<br>Very sensitive to rejection, criticism<br>Inability to show empathy<br>Poor handling of aging | 1. Remain neutral; avoid engaging in power struggles or becoming defensive in response to the patient's disparaging remarks.<br>2. Convey unassuming self-confidence. | Psychotherapy only after patient acknowledges narcissism<br>Group therapy to help empathy<br>Lithium to help with mood swings; antidepressants also used |
| Obsessive-compulsive | Perfectionistic<br>Has need for control<br>Inflexible, rigid<br>Preoccupied with details<br>Highly critical of self and others | 1. Guard against power struggles with patient. Need for control is very high.<br>2. The most common defence mechanisms are intellectualization, rationalization, reaction formation, isolation, and undoing. | Supportive or insightful psychotherapy<br>Clomipramine (Anafranil) and SSRIs for obsessional thinking and depression |
| Schizotypal | Manifestation of ideas of reference<br>Cognitive and perceptual distortions<br>Social ineptness<br>Anxiety | 1. Respect patient's need for social isolation.<br>2. Be aware of patient's suspiciousness, and employ appropriate interventions.<br>3. Perform careful diagnostic assessment as needed to uncover any other medical or psychological symptoms that may need intervention (e.g., suicidal thoughts). | Supportive psychotherapy<br>Cognitive and behavioural measures<br>Group therapy to try to improve social skills<br>Low-dose antipsychotics and antidepressants |

**Source:** Sadock, B.J., & Sadock, V.A. (2008). *Concise textbook of clinical psychiatry* (3rd ed.). Philadelphia: Lippincott Williams & Wilkins.

nursing care for the major personality disorders. Case Study and Nursing Care Plan 20-1 on pages 418–420 presents a person with BPD.

## IMPLEMENTATION

People with BPD are impulsive (e.g., suicidal, self-mutilating), aggressive, manipulative, and even psychotic during periods of stress. Individuals with ASPD are often involuntarily admitted and are manipulative, aggressive, and impulsive. Refer to Boxes 20-1, 20-2, and 20-3 on pages 414–415 for interventions to address these behaviours, based on the *Nursing Interventions Classification (NIC)* (Bulechek, Butcher, Dochterman, et al., 2012).

### Safety and Teamwork

When individuals with personality disorders are admitted to the hospital, are partially hospitalized, or are in day-treatment settings, milieu management is a significant part of treatment. The primary goal is management of the person's affect in a group context. Community meetings, coping skills groups, and socializing groups are all helpful for individuals with personality disorders. Patients have the opportunity to interact with peers and staff to discuss goals and learn problem-solving skills. Dealing with emotional issues that arise in the milieu requires

| BOX 20-1 | *NIC* INTERVENTIONS FOR MANIPULATIVE BEHAVIOUR |
|---|---|

**Limit Setting**

*Definition of* limit setting: Establishing the parameters of desirable and acceptable personal behaviour
  Activities*:
- Discuss concerns about behaviour with person.
- Identify (with input when appropriate) undesirable personal behaviour.
- Discuss with person, when appropriate, what desirable behaviour is in a given situation or setting.
- Establish consequences (with person's input when appropriate) for occurrence or nonoccurrence of desired behaviours.
- Communicate established behavioural expectations and consequences to person in language that is easily understood and nonpunitive.
- Refrain from arguing or bargaining with person about established behavioural expectations and consequences.
- Monitor person for occurrence or nonoccurrence of desired behaviour.
- Modify behavioural expectations and consequences, as needed, to accommodate reasonable changes in person's situation.

*Partial list.
**Source:** Bulechek, G.M., Butcher, H.K., Dochterman, J.M., et al. (2012). *Nursing interventions classification (NIC)* (6th ed.). St. Louis, MO: Mosby.

## BOX 20-2 *NIC* INTERVENTIONS FOR AGGRESSIVE BEHAVIOUR

### Anger Control Assistance

*Definition of* anger control assistance: Facilitation of the expression of anger in an adaptive, nonviolent manner
  *Activities\*:*
  - Determine appropriate behavioural expectations for expression of anger, given person's level of cognitive and physical functioning.
  - Limit access to frustrating situations until person is able to express anger in an adaptive manner.
  - Encourage person to seek assistance from nursing staff during periods of increasing tension.
  - Monitor potential for inappropriate aggression, and intervene before its expression.
  - Prevent physical harm if anger is directed at self or others (e.g., restraint and removal of potential weapons).
  - Provide physical outlets for expression of anger or tension (e.g., punching bag, sports, clay, journal writing).
  - Provide reassurance to person that nursing staff will intervene to prevent person from losing control.
  - Assist person in identifying source of anger.
  - Identify function that anger, frustration, and rage serve for person.
  - Identify consequences of inappropriate expression of anger.

\*Partial list.
**Source:** Bulechek, G.M., Butcher, H.K., Dochterman, J.M., et al. (2012). *Nursing interventions classification (NIC)* (6th ed.). St. Louis, MO: Mosby.

## BOX 20-3 *NIC* INTERVENTIONS FOR IMPULSIVE BEHAVIOUR

### Impulse-Control Training

*Definition of* impulse-control training: Assisting the person to mediate impulsive behaviour through application of problem-solving strategies to social and interpersonal situations
  *Activities\*:*
  - Assist person to identify the problem or situation that requires thoughtful action.
  - Assist person to identify possible courses of action and their costs and benefits.
  - Teach person to cue himself or herself to "stop and think" before acting impulsively.
  - Assist person to evaluate the outcome of the chosen course of action.
  - Provide positive reinforcement (e.g., praise and rewards) for successful outcomes.
  - Encourage person to self-reward for successful outcomes.
  - Provide opportunities for person to practise problem solving (role-playing) within the therapeutic environment.
  - Encourage person to practise problem solving in social and interpersonal situations outside the therapeutic environment, followed by evaluation of outcome.

\*Partial list.
**Source:** Bulechek, G.M., Butcher, H.K., Dochterman, J.M., et al. (2012). *Nursing interventions classification (NIC)* (6th ed.). St. Louis, MO: Mosby.

a calm, united approach by the staff to maintain safety and enhance self-control.

Common problems resulting from *staff splitting* (the patient's characterization of staff members as good or bad, which can result in some staff feeling bad about themselves, about colleagues, or about the patient) can be minimized if the interprofessional teams hold weekly staff meetings in which staff members are allowed to ventilate their feelings about conflicts with their patients and other staff.

When patients are actively involved in developing their treatment plans (e.g., being included in daily staff rounds to set goals and evaluate progress), they typically take more responsibility for themselves and the success of implementing the plan. Having limits and being confronted about negative behaviour are better accepted by the person if staff members first employ empathic mirroring (i.e., reflecting back to the person an understanding of the person's distress without a value judgement). For example, the nurse can listen to a person's emotional complaints about the staff and hospital without correcting any errors but simply noting that the person truly feels hurt. Showing empathy may also decrease aggressive outbursts if the person feels that staff members are trying to understand feelings of frustration. Table 20-5 depicts a therapeutic nurse–patient interaction after an antisocial patient initiates a fight with a peer in an inpatient unit.

A final approach that is useful for people with borderline personality disorder relates to the response to superficial self-destructive behaviours. Acting in accordance with unit policies, the nurse remains neutral and dresses the cutting wound in a matter-of-fact manner. Then the person is instructed to write down the sequence of events leading up to the injury, as well as the consequences, before staff will discuss the event. This cognitive exercise encourages the person to think independently about his or her own behaviour instead of merely ventilating feelings. It facilitates the discussion with staff about alternative actions.

### Pharmacological Interventions

People with personality disorders may be helped by a broad array of psychotropic agents, all geared toward maintaining cognitive function and relieving symptoms. Depending on the chief complaint, antidepressant, anxiolytic, or antipsychotic medication may be ordered for symptom relief and improved quality of life (Ripoll, 2012; Ripoll, Triebwasser, & Siever, 2011), but the treatment efficacy of these medications remains questionable, as they do not specifically treat the underlying personality disorder (Crawford, Kakad, Rendel, et al., 2011). Recently published studies by Ripoll (2012) and Ripoll, Triebwasser, and Siever (2011) show some trends in medication efficacy for the following personality disorders:

- People with schizotypal personality disorders seem to benefit from low-dose atypical antipsychotic agents for their psychoticlike symptoms and day-to-day functioning.
- People with antisocial personality disorders respond to mood-stabilizing medications like lithium to help with aggression and impulsivity.

| TABLE 20-5 | DIALOGUE WITH A PERSON WITH MANIPULATIVE, AGGRESSIVE, AND IMPULSIVE TRAITS | |
|---|---|---|

| DIALOGUE | THERAPEUTIC TOOL/COMMENT |
|---|---|
| **Nurse:** "Borys, I would like to talk with you about what happened this morning."<br>**Borys:** "OK, shoot." | Be clear as to purpose of interview. |
| **Nurse:** "Tell me what started the incident."<br>**Borys:** "Well, as I told you before, I always had to fight to get what I wanted in life. My father and mother abandoned me emotionally when I was a child." | Use open-ended statements. Maintain a nonjudgemental attitude. |
| **Nurse:** "Yes, but tell me about this morning."<br>**Borys:** "OK. I disliked Richard from the first. He has it in for me, I just know it. He doesn't get along with anyone here. Just two days ago, he almost had a fight." | Redirect person to present problem or situation. |
| **Nurse:** "Borys, what do you mean, Richard has it in for you?"<br>**Borys:** "When I'm talking to one of the nurses, he stares and makes comments under his breath." | Explore situation. |
| **Nurse:** "What does he say?"<br>**Borys:** "How I'm 'in' with the nurses. I'm just trying to do what's expected of me here." | Encourage description. |
| **Nurse:** "You mean that Richard is envious of your relationship with the nurses?"<br>**Borys:** "Right. He really doesn't want to be here. He doesn't care about all that therapeutic junk." | Validate person's meaning. |
| **Nurse:** "You seem to know a lot about how Richard thinks. I wonder how that is."<br>**Borys:** "He reminds me of someone I knew when I was young. His name was Joe. We called him 'Bones.'" | Assist the person to recognize that he or she is assuming to know what others are thinking and that the interpretations may not be based in reality. |
| **Nurse:** "Tell me more about Bones."<br>**Borys:** "We called him Bones because he was skinny. He was into drugs and never ate. He was also called Bones because he was selfish. He never shared anything. He never even had a girl that I knew about." | Explore situation further. |
| **Nurse:** "So Richard reminds you of someone who is selfish and lonely?"<br>**Borys:** "That's right. I've had three marriages and girlfriends on the side. No one can take them away from me." (angrily) "Just let them try!" | Make interpretation of information. Note increasing anxiety. |
| **Nurse:** "What makes you so angry now?"<br>**Borys:** "Richard! I know he wants to be like me, but he can't. I'll hurt him if he makes any more comments about me." | Identify feelings and explore threat or anxiety. |
| **Nurse:** "Borys, you will not hurt anyone here on the unit."<br>**Borys:** "I'm sorry, I didn't mean that." | Set limits on, and expectations of, person's behaviour. |
| **Nurse:** "It's important that we examine your part in the incident this morning and ways to cope without threats or violence." | Focus on person's responsibility and suggest alternative methods of coping with situation. |
| **Borys:** "Listen, I know I've gotten into trouble because I can't control my temper, but that's because I won't get any respect until I can show them I don't fear them." | Person exhibits rationalization. |

*Continued*

| TABLE 20-5 | DIALOGUE WITH A PERSON WITH MANIPULATIVE, AGGRESSIVE, AND IMPULSIVE TRAITS—cont'd | |
|---|---|---|

| DIALOGUE | THERAPEUTIC TOOL/COMMENT |
|---|---|
| **Nurse:** "Who do you mean by 'them'?"<br>**Borys:** "People like Richard." | Clarify pronoun. |
| **Nurse:** "You've told me that fighting was a way of survival as a child, but as an adult, there are other ways of handling situations that make you angry." | Show understanding and suggest other means of coping. |
| **Borys:** "You're right. I've thought about this. Do you think it would help if you gave me some meds to control my anger?" | Person exhibits superficial and concrete thinking—possible manipulation. |
| **Nurse:** "I wasn't thinking of medications but of a plan for being aware of your anger and talking it out instead of fighting it out."<br>**Borys:** "I told you before, I have to fight. If I can't fight, I cut myself." | Clarify meaning toward behaviour change. Start to explore alternatives person can use when angry instead of fighting. |
| **Nurse:** "Have you thought about the consequences of your fighting or cutting?" | Identify results of impulsive behaviour. |
| **Borys:** "I feel bad afterwards. Sometimes I wish it hadn't happened." | Person continues to explore. |

- People with borderline personality disorder often respond to anticonvulsant mood-stabilizing medications, low-dose antipsychotic medications, and omega-3 supplementation for mood and emotion dysregulation symptoms. Naltrexone hydrochloride (ReVia), an opioid receptor antagonist, has been found to reduce self-injuring behaviours.
- People with avoidant personality disorder seem to respond positively to similar medications used for anxiety disorders, such as SSRIs like citalopram (Celexa) and SNRIs such as duloxetine (Cymbalta).

Pharmacological evidence is lacking for the treatment of people with narcissistic and obsessive-compulsive personality disorders.

## Case Management

Many people with personality disorders function at a high level, but a significant number need assistance to maintain their independence. Case management is helpful for individuals with personality disorders who are persistently and severely impaired. Many have had multiple hospitalizations, have been unable to maintain work or personal relationships, and are relatively alone in their attempts to care for themselves. In the acute care setting, case management focuses on three goals: to gather pertinent history from current or previous providers; to support reintegration with family or loved ones as appropriate; and to ensure appropriate referrals to outpatient care, including substance disorder treatment, if needed. In the long-term outpatient setting, case-management objectives include reducing

hospitalization by providing resources for crisis services and enhancing the social support system.

## Advanced-Practice Interventions

The mental health nurse treats individuals with personality disorders in a variety of inpatient and community settings. Research shows that treatment can be effective for many people with personality disorders, especially when a co-morbid major mental illness is targeted. See Table 20-4 for a summary of nursing and therapy guidelines for personality disorders.

Advanced-practice nurses are likely to interact with staff members regarding the treatment of individuals with personality disorders as part of their practice and clinical supervision responsibilities. They can assist staff members in a therapeutic alliance. For example, they mentor and teach additional techniques that staff members can use to develop rapport and trust with patients diagnosed with STPD when these patients are experiencing heightened anxiety from being hospitalized. Nurses should understand that the patient's ability to interpret subtle, affective cues is limited, and straightforward communication is necessary (Long, Dolley, & Hollin, 2012).

## Psychotherapy

APRNs are highly involved in and are often the clinical leaders in providing individual and group psychotherapy using dialectical behaviour therapy (DBT). DBT is an evidence-informed therapy developed by Dr. Marsha Linehan to treat chronically suicidal people with BPD (Linehan, 1993). Data on the successful use of DBT with individuals experiencing co-morbid personality disorders and other psychiatric disorders (e.g., OCPD

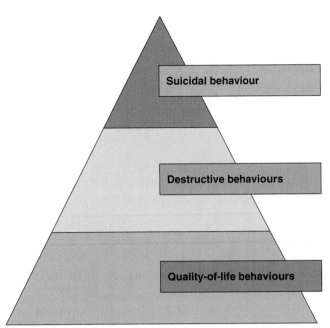

**FIGURE 20-1** Dialectical behaviour therapy treatment targets.

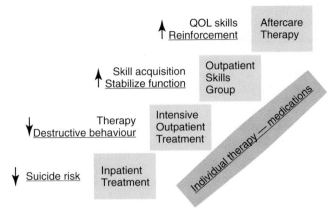

**FIGURE 20-2** Dialectical behaviour therapy treatment hierarchy. *QOL:* quality of life.

plus major depression, generalized anxiety, substance abuse, or an eating disorder) have been confirmed.

DBT combines cognitive and behavioural techniques with mindfulness, which emphasizes being aware of thoughts and actively shaping them. The goals of DBT are to increase the person's ability to manage distress and improve interpersonal effectiveness. Treatment focuses on behaviour targets, beginning with identification of and interventions for suicidal behaviours and then progressing to a focus on interrupting destructive behaviours (Figure 20-1). Finally, DBT addresses quality-of-life behaviours across a hierarchy of care (Figure 20-2). Optimally, DBT is delivered as a skills training group program combined with individual therapy with a DBT-trained therapist who may be a nurse, social worker, or psychologist.

## EVALUATION

Evaluating treatment effectiveness for individuals with personality disorders is difficult. Nurses may never know the real results of their interventions, particularly in acute care settings. Even in long-term outpatient treatment programs, many people with personality disorders find the relationship too intimate an experience to remain in long enough for successful treatment. As noted earlier, however, some motivated individuals may be able to learn to change their behaviour, especially if positive experiences are repeated.

Each therapeutic experience offers an opportunity for the person to observe himself or herself interacting with caregivers who consistently try to teach positive coping skills. Perhaps effectiveness can be measured by how successfully the nurse is able to be genuine with the person, maintain a helpful posture, offer substantial instruction, and still care for himself or herself. Specific short-term outcomes may be accomplished, and overall, the person can be given the message of hope that quality of life can always be improved.

---

### CASE STUDY AND NURSING CARE PLAN 20-1

#### *Borderline Personality Disorder*

*Ada is a 24-year-old single administrative assistant who lives alone. She has been seen in the emergency department several times for superficial suicide attempts. She is admitted because she has cut her wrists, ankles, and vagina with glass and has lost a lot of blood. This event is precipitated by her graduation from business college.*

*Upon admission, she is sweet, serene, and grateful to all the nurses, calling them "angels of mercy." Within a week, she is angry at half of the nurses and demands a new primary nurse, saying that the one she has (to whom she had grown attached) hates her. She has a history of heavy drinking and has managed*

*to sneak alcohol onto the unit. She has been found in bed with a young man. She continually breaks unit rules and then pleads to have this behaviour forgiven and forgotten. When angry, she threatens to cut herself again. When asked why she cut herself, Ada states, "I was tired." She appears restless and tense and frequently asks for antianxiety medication. When asked what she is anxious about, she says, "Uh ... I don't know ... I feel so empty inside." Ada frequently paces up and down the halls, looking both angry and bored. Her admitting diagnoses include substance abuse disorder and borderline personality disorder.*

*Continued*

## CASE STUDY AND NURSING CARE PLAN 20-1—cont'd
*Borderline Personality Disorder*

## ASSESSMENT

**Self-Assessment**

Annie is a recent nurse graduate and Ada's primary nurse. Ada's therapist impresses upon Annie the difficulty health care workers have in dealing effectively with people with BPDs. They constantly act out their feelings in self-destructive and maladaptive ways. They usually are not aware of their feelings or what triggered their actions. Most difficult for many health care workers is dealing with the intense feelings and reactions individuals with BPD can provoke in others. Annie sets up meetings twice a week with Ada's therapist to discuss the quality of the therapeutic relationship with Ada. At the next meeting, common goals and intervention strategies are discussed. This type of staff meeting, sometimes referred to as *supervision*, is a way to facilitate self-reflection for Annie and to help her work more effectively with Ada.

| Objective Data | Subjective Data |
|---|---|
| • Makes frequent, superficial suicide attempts | • Initially was attached to her primary nurse; now says her primary nurse "hates" her, and she demands another nurse |
| • Requests antianxiety medication frequently | |
| • Paces up and down the hall much of the day | • Appears restless and tense |
| • Threatens self-mutilation when anxious | • Complains of feeling empty inside |
| • Brings alcohol onto the unit | • Looks angry and bored much of the time |
| • Is found in bed with man | |

## DIAGNOSIS

Annie formulates two initial nursing diagnoses that have the highest priority during this time:

1. *Ineffective coping* related to inadequate psychological resources, as evidenced by self-destructive behaviours
**Supporting Data**
• After stating that her nurse hates her, Ada sneaks alcohol onto the unit, is found in bed with a man, and demands a new primary nurse.

2. *Self-mutilation* related to borderline personality disorder, as evidenced by suicidal gestures and poor impulse control
**Supporting Data**
• Is admitted following self-mutilation
• Threatens self-mutilation when anxious
• Threatens self-mutilation on unit

## OUTCOMES IDENTIFICATION

1. Person will consistently demonstrate the use of effective coping strategies.
2. Person will refrain from injuring self.

## PLANNING

The initial plan is to maintain personal safety and to encourage verbalization of feelings and impulses instead of action.

## IMPLEMENTATION

Annie's plan of care is personalized as follows:
**Nursing diagnosis:** *Ineffective coping*
**Outcome:** Ada will consistently demonstrate the use of effective coping strategies.

| Short-Term Goal | Intervention | Rationale | Evaluation |
|---|---|---|---|
| Ada will consistently demonstrate a decrease in stress as evidenced by talking about feelings with staff every day and an absence of acting-out behaviours. | 1. Encourage verbalization of feelings, perceptions, and fears. | 1. Discussing and understanding the dynamics of frustration help reduce the frustration by helping the person take positive action. | **GOAL MET** Ada was able to experience problems and deal with them appropriately. Acting out was minimal or absent. *Example:* Ada had an appointment for a job interview. She wanted to stay in bed and avoid the interview, but instead, she talked with the nurse about her fear of "growing up" and was able to get up and go to the interview. |
| | 2. Support the use of appropriate defence mechanisms. | 2. Discussing and understanding the meaning of defences help reduce the potential for acting out. | |

*Continued*

**CASE STUDY AND NURSING CARE PLAN 20-1—cont'd**

*Borderline Personality Disorder*

**Nursing diagnosis:** *Self-mutilation*
**Outcome:** Ada will refrain from injuring herself.

| Short-Term Goal | Intervention | Rationale | Evaluation |
|---|---|---|---|
| Ada will consistently demonstrate that she will seek help when feeling the urge to injure herself, as evidenced by the absence of self-injurious behaviours and talking to staff about her troubling feelings on a daily basis. | 1. Assist the person to identify situations and feelings that may prompt self-harm.<br><br>2. Instruct the person in coping strategies.<br><br>3. Provide ongoing surveillance of the person and environment. | 1. Observing, describing, and analyzing thoughts and feelings reduce the potential for acting them out destructively.<br><br>2. Alternative behaviours are offered that can be more satisfying and growth promoting.<br><br>3. Times of increased anxiety, frustration, or anger without external controls could increase the probability of the person using self-mutilating behaviours. | **GOAL MET**<br>Ada was able to experience troubling thoughts and feelings without self-mutilation. She stated, "I was mad at my therapist today and decided to cut my arms after the session. Instead, I told her I was angry, and together we figured out why." |

**EVALUATION**

See individual outcomes and evaluation in the care plan.

## KEY POINTS TO REMEMBER

- All personality disorders share characteristics of inflexibility and difficulties in interpersonal relationships that impair social or occupational functioning.
- Personality disorders are most likely caused by a combination of biological and psychosocial factors.
- People with personality disorders often enter psychiatric treatment because of distress from a co-morbid major mental illness.
- Nurses may experience intense emotional reactions to individuals with personality disorders and need to make use of clinical supervision to maintain objectivity.
- Despite the relatively fixed patterns of maladaptive behaviour, some individuals with personality disorders are able to change their behaviours over time as a result of treatment.

## CRITICAL THINKING

1. Vasily is undergoing surgery for a broken leg. He is suspicious of the staff and believes that the IV he is receiving for hydration and pre-anaesthesia will be used for harmful purposes. He keeps his eyes closed and refuses to answer or look at his family, who describe him as odd. He has schizotypal personality disorder.
   a. Explain how being friendly and outgoing may be threatening to Vasily.
   b. Explain how being matter-of-fact and neutral and sticking to the facts would be effective to Vasily.
   c. What could be done to give Vasily some control over his situation as a hospitalized person?
   d. How could you best handle his sarcasm and hostility so both you and he would feel most comfortable?

2. Cherie is brought to the emergency department by her brother after slashing her wrist with a razor. She has previously been in the emergency department for drug overdose and has a history of addictions. Cherie can be sarcastic, belittling, and aggressive to those who try to care for her. She has a history of difficulty with interpersonal relationships at her job. When the psychiatric triage nurse comes in to see her, Cherie is initially adoring and compliant, telling him, "You are the best nurse I've ever had, and I truly want to change." But when he refuses to support her request for diazepam (Valium) and meperidine (Demerol) for "pain," she yells at him, "You are a stupid excuse for a nurse. I want to see the doctor immediately." Cherie has borderline personality disorder.
   a. What defence mechanisms is Cherie using?
   b. How could the nurse handle this situation while setting limits and demonstrating concern?
   c. How do family members of a person with BPD typically describe their experiences?

## CHAPTER REVIEW

1. A person complains that most staff do not like her or care what happens to her, but you are special and she can tell that you are a caring person. She talks with you about being unsure of what she wants to do with her life and her "mixed-up feelings" about relationships. When you tell her that you will be on vacation next week, she becomes very angry. Two hours later, she is found using a curling iron to burn her underarms and explains that it "makes the numbness stop." Given this presentation, you would deduce that this person most likely has which personality disorder?
   1. Obsessive-compulsive
   2. Borderline
   3. Antisocial
   4. Schizotypal

2. Which statement about people with personality disorders is most accurate?
   1. Unlike those with mood or psychotic disorders, they are at very low risk of suicide.
   2. They tend not to perceive themselves as having a problem but instead believe their problems are caused by how others behave toward them.
   3. They are believed to be purely psychological disorders, that is, disorders arising from psychological rather than neurological or other physiological abnormalities.
   4. Their symptoms are not as disabling as most other mental disorders; therefore, their care tends to be less challenging and complicated for staff.

3. A person shows the nurse multiple fresh, serious (but non–life-threatening) self-inflicted cuts on her forearm. Which response would be most therapeutic?
   1. Convey empathy and explore issues that led to the self-injury as you administer first aid to the wounds.
   2. Care for the wounds; then search the person for sharp objects, and place the person on one-to-one observation or in seclusion for her own safety.
   3. Recognizing that the self-injury is, at its heart, a maladaptive attempt to obtain attention, extinguish the behaviour by minimizing the attention paid to it.
   4. Maintain a neutral demeanour while dressing the wounds, and then assign the person to write a list of circumstances that led to the injury before discussing it further.

4. A patient is flirting with a peer and is overheard asking him to intercede with staff so that she will be given privileges to leave the inpatient mental health unit. Later, she offers a back rub to a nurse if that nurse will give her the prn sedation (sedation as needed) early, although it has been ordered for 1000 hrs. Which response to such behaviours would be most therapeutic?
   1. Inform the patient that she is being manipulative.
   2. Advise the other people that this patient is being manipulative and that they should ignore her when she behaves this way.
   3. Bargain with the patient to determine a reasonable compromise regarding how much of such behaviour is acceptable before the patient crosses the line.
   4. Ignore the behaviour for the time being so the patient will find it unrewarding and in turn seek other, and hopefully more adaptive, ways to meet her needs.

5. A person becomes frustrated and angry when trying to get his MP3 player and headset to function properly and angrily throws it across the room, nearly hitting a peer with it. Which intervention would be the most therapeutic?
   1. Place the person in seclusion for one hour to allow him to de-escalate and think about his behaviour.
   2. Point out that the behaviour is unacceptable.
   3. Offer to help him learn about the operation of the MP3 player.
   4. Explore with the person his feelings as he works out how to operate his MP3 player.

## ⊖volve WEBSITE

Post-Test | interactive review

*Visit the Evolve Web site for Chapter Review Answers and Rationales, Critical Thinking Answer Guidelines, and additional resources related to the content in this chapter:* http://evolve.elsevier.com/Canada/Varcarolis/psychiatric/

# REFERENCES

Blais, M.A., Smallwood, P., Groves, J.E., et al. (2008). Personality and personality disorders. In T.A. Stern, J.F. Rosenbaum, M. Fava, et al. (Eds.), *Massachusetts General Hospital comprehensive clinical psychiatry* (pp. 527–540). Philadelphia: Saunders.

Bulechek, G.M., Butcher, H.K., Dochterman, J.M., et al. (2012). *Nursing interventions classification (NIC)* (6th ed.). St. Louis: Mosby.

Canadian Institute for Health Information, Statistics Canada. (2011). *Health Indicators 2011*. Retrieved from https://secure.cihi.ca/freeproducts/health_indicators_2011_en.pdf.

Clarkin, J., & Huprich, S. (2011). Do DSM-5 personality disorder proposals meet criteria for clinical utility? *Journal of Personality Disorders, 25*(2), 192–205. Retrieved from http://guilfordjournals.com/doi/abs/10.1521/pedi.2011.25.2.192.

Cox, B., Pagura, J., Stein, M., et al. (2009). The relationship between generalized social phobia and avoidant personality disorder in a national mental health survey. *Depression & Anxiety, 26*(4), 354–362. doi:10.1002/da.20475.

Crawford, M., Kakad, S., Rendel, C., et al. (2011). Medication prescribed to people with personality disorder: The influence of patient factors and treatment setting. *Acta Psychiatrica Scandinavica, 124*(5), 396–402. doi:10.1111/j.1600-0447.2011.01728.x.

Gunderson, J. (2011). Borderline personality disorder. *The New England Journal of Medicine, 364*, 2037–2042. doi:10.1056/NEJMcp1007358.

Hernandez, A., Arntz, A., Gaviria, A., et al. (2012). Relationships between childhood maltreatment, parenting style, and borderline personality disorder criteria. *Journal of Personality Disorders, 26*(5), 727–736. Retrieved from http://www.ncbi.nlm.nih.gov/pubmed/23013341.

Hummelen, B., Pedersen, G., & Karterud, S. (2012). Some suggestions for the DSM-5 schizotypal personality disorder construct. *Comprehensive Psychiatry, 53*(4), 341–349. doi:10.1016/j.comppsych.2011.05.009.

Huprich, S. (2011). Contributions from personality and psychodynamically orientated assessment to the development of the DSM-5 personality disorders. *Journal of Personality Assessment, 93*(4), 354–361. doi:1080/00223891.2011.577473.

Kagan, J. (2005). Personality and temperament. In M. Rosenbluth, S.H. Kennedy, & R.M. Bagby (Eds.), *Depression and personality: Conceptual and clinical challenges* (pp. 3–8). Washington, DC: American Psychiatric Publishing.

Kernberg, O. (1985). *Internal world and external reality*. London: Aronson.

Koivu, A., Saarinen, P., & Hyrkas, K. (2012). Who benefits from clinical supervision and how? The association between clinical supervision and the work-related well-being of female hospital nurses. *Journal of Clinical Nursing, 21*(17–18), 2567–2578. doi:10.1111/j.1365-2702.2011.04041.x.

Lee, R., Hempel, J., Tenharmsel, A., et al. (2012). The neuroendocrinology of childhood trauma in personality disorder. *Psychoneuroendocrinology, 37*(1), 78–86. doi:0.1016/j.psycneuen.2011.05.006.

Leichsenring, F., Leibing, E., Kruse, J., et al. (2011). Borderline personality disorder. *Lancet, 377*(9759), 74–84. doi:10.1016/S0140-6736(10)61422-5.

Linehan, M.M. (1993). *Cognitive behavioural treatment of borderline personality disorder*. New York: Guilford.

Long, C., Dolley, O., & Hollin, C. (2012). Engagement in psychosocial treatment: Its relationship to outcome and care pathway progress for women in medium-secure settings. *Criminal Behaviour & Mental Health, 22*(5), 336–349. doi:10.1002/cbm.1824.

Madarasz, W., Manzardo, A., Mortensen, E., et al. (2012). Forty-five-year mortality rate as a function of the number and type of psychiatric diagnoses found in a large Danish birth cohort. *Canadian Journal of Psychiatry, 57*(8), 505–511. Retrieved from http://www.ncbi.nlm.nih.gov/pubmed/22854033.

Magoteaux, A., & Bonnivier, J. (2009). Distinguishing between personality disorders, stereotypes, and eccentricities in older adults. *Journal of Psychosocial Nursing, 47*(7), 19–24. doi:10.3928/02793695-20090527-04.

McGilloway, A., Hall, R., Lee, T., et al. (2010). A systematic review of personality disorder, race, and ethnicity: Prevalence, aetiology and treatment. *BMC Psychiatry, 10*(33), 1–14. doi:10.1186/1471-244X-10-33.

Mohanty, J. (2013). Ethnic and racial socialization and self-esteem of Asian adoptees: The mediating role of multiple identities. *Journal of Adolescence, 36*(1), 161–170. doi:10.1016/j.adolescence.2012.10.003.

Moorhead, S., Johnson, M., Maas, M.L., et al. (2008). *Nursing outcomes classification (NOC)* (4th ed.). St. Louis, MO: Mosby.

Paris, J. (2005). A current integrative perspective on personality disorders. In J.M. Oldham, A.E. Skodol, & D.S. Bender (Eds.), *Textbook of personality disorders* (pp. 119–128). Washington, DC: American Psychiatric Publishing.

Perry, J., Presniak, M., & Olson, T. (2013). Defense mechanisms in schizotypal, borderline, antisocial, and narcissistic personality disorders. *Psychiatry: Interpersonal & Biological Processes, 76*(1), 32–52. doi:10.1521/psyc.2013.76.1.32.

Ripoll, L. (2012). Clinical psychopharmacology of borderline personality disorder: An update on the available evidence in light of the Diagnostic and Statistical Manual of Mental Disorders–5. *Current Opinion in Psychiatry, 25*(1), 52–58. doi:10.1097/YCO.0b013e32834c3f19.

Ripoll, L., Triebwasser, J., & Siever, L. (2011). Evidence-based pharmacotherapy for personality disorders. *International Journal of Neuropsychopharmacology, 14*(9), 1257–1288. doi:10.1017/S1461145711000071.

Samuels, J. (2011). Personality disorders: Epidemiology and public health issues. *International Review of Psychiatry, 23*(3), 223–233. doi:10.3109/09540261.2011.588200.

Simms, L., Goldberg, L., Roberts, J., et al. (2011). Computerized adaptive assessment of personality disorder: Introducing the CAT-PD project. *Journal of Personality Assessment, 93*(4), 380–389. doi:10.1080/00223891.2011.577475.

Skodol, A., Bender, D., Morey, L., et al. (2011). Personality disorder types proposed for DSM-5. *Journal of Personality Disorders, 25*(2), 136–169. doi:10.1521/pedi.2011.25.2.136.

Skodol, A.E., & Gunderson, J.G. (2008). Personality disorders. In R.E. Hales, S.C. Yudofsky, & G.O. Gabbard (Eds.), *Textbook of Psychiatry* (pp. 821–860). Washington, DC: American Psychiatric Publishing.

Taylor, S., Asmundson, G., & Jang, K. (2011). Etiology of obsessive-compulsive symptoms and obsessive-compulsive personality traits: Common genes, mostly different environments. *Depression & Anxiety, 28*(10), 863–869. doi:10.1002/da.20859.

Torgersen, S. (2009). Prevalence, sociodemographics and functional impairment. In J.M. Oldham, A.E. Skodol, & D.S. Bender (Eds.), *Essentials of Personality Disorders* (pp. 83–102). Washington, DC: American Psychiatric Publishing.

Vater, A., Ritter, K., Schröder-Abé, M., et al. (2013). When grandiosity and vulnerability collide: Implicit and explicit self-esteem in patients with narcissistic personality disorder. *Journal of Behavior Therapy & Experimental Psychiatry, 44*(1), 37–47. doi:10.1016/j.jbtep.2012.07.001.

Widiger, T., & Mullins-Sweatt, S. (2008). Personality disorders. In A. Tassman, J. Kay, J. Lieberman, et al. (Eds.), *Psychiatry* (3rd ed., pp. 1718–1753). London, UK: John Wiley & Sons.

# Sleep–Wake Disorders

*Margaret Trussler*
*Adapted by Holly Symonds-Brown*

## KEY TERMS AND CONCEPTS

confusional arousal disorders, 429
dyssomnias, 423
excessive sleepiness (ES), 424
hypersomnia disorders, 428
insomnia disorders, 428
sleep architecture, 426
sleep continuity, 426

sleep deprivation, 424
sleep efficiency, 427
sleep fragmentation, 426
sleep hygiene, 428
sleep latency, 425
sleep restriction, 436
stimulus control, 437

## OBJECTIVES

1. Discuss the impact of inadequate sleep on health and well-being.
2. Describe the social and economic impact of sleep disturbance and chronic sleep deprivation.
3. Identify the risks to personal and community safety imposed by sleep disturbance and chronic sleep deprivation.
4. Describe normal sleep physiology, and explain the variations in normal sleep.
5. Differentiate between insomnia and hypersomnia, and identify at least two examples of each.
6. Identify the predisposing, precipitating, and perpetuating factors for patients with insomnia.
7. Identify and describe the use of two assessment tools in the evaluation of patients experiencing sleep disturbance.
8. Develop a teaching plan for a patient with insomnia, incorporating principles of sleep restriction, stimulus control, and cognitive-behavioural therapy.
9. Formulate three nursing diagnoses for people experiencing a sleep disturbance.
10. Develop a nursing care plan for the person experiencing sleep disturbance incorporating basic sleep hygiene principles.

## ⊝volve WEBSITE

*Visit the Evolve website for Flashcards, Case Studies, and additional testing resources related to the content in this chapter:* http://evolve.elsevier.com/Canada/Varcarolis/psychiatric/  Pre-Test interactive review

---

Sleep disturbances vary in severity, duration, quality, or timing, all of which can have adverse health consequences. These disturbances are broadly referred to as dyssomnias. Understandably, energy level and cognitive focus can be impaired as a result of dyssomnias, but mood can also be affected. Disturbed sleep certainly worsens the distress and impairment caused by mental illnesses and is also a potential warning sign for additional mental or physical conditions. For instance, disturbed sleep may be a sign of medical or neurological problems such as Parkinson's disease, heart failure, or osteoarthritis, among other conditions.

Sleep and sleep–wake disorders are receiving increased attention in medical, nursing, research, and social science literature. The Canadian Sleep Society was established in 1986 to facilitate research, training, health-information dissemination, and other activities with respect to the basic understanding of sleep and sleep–wake disorders. Over the past 25 years, there has been an exponential growth in our scientific understanding of these disorders. However, despite the investment in sleep-related research and tremendous growth in our understanding of sleep physiology and pathology, application of the findings has been slow.

In this chapter, we briefly review the components of normal sleep, sleep regulation, and functions of sleep; give an overview of the most common sleep disturbances encountered in the clinical environment, with a focus on their relationship to psychiatric illness; and discuss the nurse's role in the assessment and management of a patient with a sleep disturbance.

## HOW A NURSE HELPED ME

### Worrying the Night Away

*Kelly, a 30-year-old woman, was referred to the mental health nurse by her family physician for an assessment of her insomnia. Kelly reported a three-month history of insomnia that had resulted in a progressively harder time falling asleep. Kelly reported that she would toss and turn for two to three hours before falling asleep. Due to her children's schedules, she was usually up early so was becoming more fatigued and irritable because of her lack of sleep. Kelly was adamant with her physician that she did not want to take sleeping pills.*

*The mental health nurse visited Kelly at her home and conducted a complete mental status exam, including formal depression or anxiety inventories and psychosocial, sleep history, and sleep hygiene surveys. Kelly reported no other signs of mental health problems, no acute stressors other than the ongoing challenges of parenting two young children aged 2 and 3. She reported difficulty winding down in the evening and felt that, at bedtime, she was constantly thinking of things she should be getting done. During the winter, she had decreased her exercise and was drinking four or five cups of coffee a day due to her fatigue. The mental health nurse spent the first session with Kelly educating her about sleep hygiene and some cognitive strategies for decreasing worrying at bedtime. Kelly felt she could try decreasing her caffeine intake to two to three cups of coffee before 4 p.m. and wanted to try getting out for a walk each day for 20 minutes. She agreed to try a worry list each day at 3 p.m. rather than at bedtime.*

*The second session, a week later, focused on Kelly's new bedtime routine practices, which included a warm shower and a book rather than TV and cleaning. She reported surprise at how the "worry time" strategies seemed to be working. At the final follow-up visit one month later, Kelly was reporting improved sleep and energy levels.*

## SLEEP

In a fast-paced society, people subject themselves to schedules that disrupt normal sleep physiology, so sleep is often forfeited. The National Sleep Foundation (2008) recommends that the average adult get seven to nine hours of sleep each night, yet epidemiological surveys suggest that mean sleep duration among Canadian adults has decreased during the past century (Hurst, 2008; Williams, 2001), and over three million Canadians report ongoing difficulties with sleep (Morin, LeBlanc, Belanger, et al., 2011).

Sleep has become an expendable commodity. People frequently cut back on sleep to meet other social and professional demands, with compensated work time and travel time being the most potent determinants of total sleep time (Basner, Fomberstein, Razavi, et al., 2007).

## CONSEQUENCES OF SLEEP LOSS

The major consequence of acute or chronic sleep curtailment is excessive sleepiness (ES). ES is a subjective report of difficulty staying awake that is serious enough to impact social and vocational functioning and increase the risk for accident or injury. The terms *excessive sleepiness, excessive daytime sleepiness, hypersomnia,* and *hypersomnolence* are often used interchangeably. While hypersomnia is considered a disease classification, ES is a symptom of a sleep disorder or other disease but not itself a disease per se. While self-imposed sleep restriction is a common cause of ES, disruption of the normal sleep cycle (as seen in those who do shift work), underlying sleep–wake disorders, medications, alcohol, and many medical disorders are important causes of excessive sleepiness (Ohayon, Dauvilliers, & Reynolds, 2012).

We need only look to our own experiences with acute or total sleep loss to recognize its consequences. After a poor night's sleep, we feel tired, lethargic, and irritable. The effects of chronic sleep deprivation may be less obvious but may have a greater overall impact on health and well-being. The discrepancy between hours of sleep obtained and hours of sleep required for optimal functioning creates a state of sleep deprivation, which has widespread implications for health, safety, and quality of life. Adults who sleep less than six hours a night are more likely to report fair to poor general health, frequent physical distress, frequent mental distress, limitations in activities of daily living, depressive symptoms, anxiety, and pain (Strine & Chapman, 2005). Chronic sleep deprivation has also been linked to diabetes, obesity, and heart disease (Bailes, Baltzan, Rizzo, et al., 2009; Barone & Menna-Barreto, 2011).

Sleep loss diminishes safety, resulting in the loss of lives and property. Some of the most devastating environmental and human tragedies of our time can be linked to human error due to sleep loss and fatigue. The grounding of the Exxon Valdez, the nuclear meltdown at Chernobyl, and the explosion of the Union Carbide chemical plant in India are prime examples (Canadian Centre for Occupational Health & Safety, 2007). Sleepiness while driving has become a national epidemic: in

2004, 17.8% of all fatal car collisions and 25.5% of injuries from collisions were associated with driver sleepiness (Elzohairy, 2008). The Insurance Bureau of Canada (2011) has stated that more than 400 Canadians die and even more are injured each year due to fatigue-related motor vehicle collisions. In fact, sleep deprivation can produce psychomotor impairments equivalent to those induced by alcohol consumption at or above the legal limit for drivers. Currently, a blood alcohol concentration (BAC) of 0.08%, or 80 milligrams of alcohol in 100 millilitres of blood, is the legal limit in Canada, with individual provincial and territorial acts existing to respond to those driving with lower BACs (Canada Safety Council, 2013). Interestingly, daytime wakefulness in excess of 17 to 19 hours is known to affect psychomotor ability to the same degree as a BAC of between 0.05% and 0.1% (Helis, 2009; Williamson & Feyer, 2007).

There is relatively little comprehensive data available on the economic burden of sleep disruption. However, considering its prevalence, its impact on overall health and quality of life, and the indirect costs associated with property loss and damage, the economic burden has been estimated to reach several billions of dollars in North America (Hossain & Shapiro, 2002). Chronic insomnia alone, for example, has been estimated to incur nearly $14 billion in direct expenses annually (Walsh, 2004), and sleep loss–related fatigue, $150 billion a year in absenteeism, accidents, property damage, and decreased or lost productivity ("Sleep Disorders Create," 2001).

Formal training in sleep or sleep–wake disorders within medical and nursing education is limited, and the number of trained clinicians and scientists is insufficient (Institute of Medicine, 2006). Awareness among health care providers regarding the prevalence and burden of sleep disruption and the problem of inadequate sleep is lacking, so providers do not routinely screen for sleep disturbance or inquire about overall sleep quality (Sorscher, 2008). Consequently, there is inadequate recognition, diagnosis, management, and treatment of sleep disturbance.

## NORMAL SLEEP CYCLE

Sleep is a dynamic neurological process that involves complex interaction between the central nervous system and the environment. Behaviourally, sleep is associated with low or absent motor activity, a reduced response to environmental stimuli, and closed eyes. Neurophysiologically, sleep is categorized according to specific brainwave patterns, eye movements, and general muscle tone. Sleep is measured electrophysiologically through an electroencephalogram (EEG) and consists of two distinct physiological states: non–rapid eye movement (NREM) sleep and rapid eye movement (REM) sleep. Figure 21-1 shows the EEG patterns characteristic of these sleep stages.

NREM sleep is divided into four stages characterized by progressive or deeper sleep. Stage 1 is a brief transition between wakefulness and sleep and accounts for between 2% and 5% of sleep time. The time it takes to go to sleep is referred to as sleep latency. During stage 1 sleep, body temperature declines and muscles relax. Slow, rolling eye movements are common. People lose awareness of their environment but are generally easily

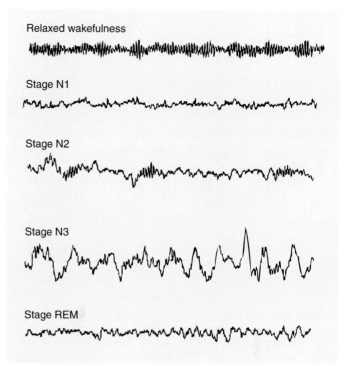

**FIGURE 21-1** Stages of sleep. **Source:** Reprinted with permission of Sleep Health Centers, Boston, MA.

aroused. Stage 2 sleep occupies 45% to 55% of total sleep time. Heart rate and respiratory rate decline. Arousal from stage 2 sleep requires more intense stimuli than does arousal from stage 1. Stages 3 and 4 are collectively known as slow wave sleep or delta sleep. Stage 3 is relatively short and constitutes only about 3% to 8% of sleep time; stage 4 is longer and represents 10% to 15% of sleep time. Slow wave sleep is characterized by further reduction in heart rate, respiratory rate, blood pressure, and response to external stimuli. The four stages of NREM sleep make up 75% to 80% of total sleep time (Carskadon & Dement, 2011).

REM sleep comprises 20% to 25% of total sleep time and is characterized by reduction and absence of skeletal muscle tone (muscle atonia), bursts of rapid eye movement, myoclonic twitches of the facial and limb muscles, reports of dreaming, and autonomic nervous system variability. The atonia in REM sleep is thought to prevent the acting out of nightmares and dreams (Carskadon & Dement, 2011).

Sleep normally begins with NREM sleep. Continuous EEG recordings of sleep demonstrate an alternating cycling between NREM and REM sleep. Typically, four to six cycles of NREM and REM sleep occur over 90- to 120-minute intervals across the sleep period. There is also a distinct organization to sleep, with NREM predominating during the first half of the sleep period and REM sleep predominating during the second half. The shortest REM period occurs 60 to 90 minutes after sleep onset and lasts only for several minutes. The longest REM period occurs at the end of the sleep period and can last up to an hour. This later REM cycle is why many people remember dreaming upon waking in the morning (Carskadon & Dement, 2011).

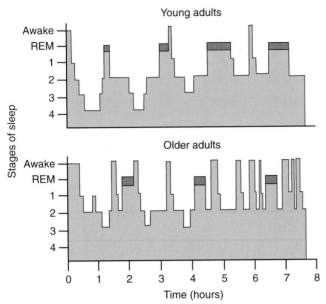

**FIGURE 21-2** Hypnogram depicting the progression of the stages of sleep in a young adult and an older adult. A comparison of the two hypnograms illustrates the typical sleep architecture differences found between older and young adults. The hypnogram for the older adult shows more awakenings (shown as the spikes in the graph), less REM sleep (purple rectangles), and delayed sleep latency (length of line on far left of graph) than that of the young adult. **Source:** Duthie, E.H., Katz, P.R., & Malone, M. (2007). *Practice of geriatrics* (4th ed.). Philadelphia: Saunders.

The structural organization of NREM and REM sleep is known as sleep architecture and is often displayed graphically as a hypnogram, as in Figure 21-2, which depicts the progression of the stages of sleep in a young adult and an older adult. The visual depiction of sleep is helpful in identifying sleep continuity (the distribution of sleep and wakefulness across the sleep period), as well as changes in sleep that may occur as a result of aging, illness, or certain medications. Disruption of sleep stages as indicated by excessive amounts of stage 1 sleep, multiple brief arousals, and frequent shifts in sleep staging is known as sleep fragmentation.

The function of alterations between NREM and REM sleep is not yet understood, but irregular cycling, absent sleep stages, and sleep fragmentation are associated with many sleep–wake disorders (Zepelin, Siegel, & Tober, 2005). For example, in people with depression, the latency to REM sleep, or period of time to go from a full, wakeful state to REM sleep, is frequently reduced. People with depression also experience a reduction in the percentage of slow wave sleep. Benzodiazepines tend to suppress slow wave sleep, whereas serotonergic drugs suppress REM sleep.

## REGULATION OF SLEEP

Although the regulation of sleep and wakefulness is not completely understood, it is believed to be a complex interaction

between two processes: one that promotes sleep, known as the *homeostatic process* or *sleep drive*, and one that promotes wakefulness, known as the *circadian process* or *circadian drive*. The homeostatic process is dependent on the number of hours a person is awake. The longer the period of wakefulness, the stronger the sleep drive. During sleep, the sleep drive gradually dissipates.

Circadian drives are near-24-hour cycles of behaviour and physiology generated and influenced by endogenous and exogenous factors. The exogenous factors are various clues from the environment known as *zeitgebers* (time-givers) that help set our internal clock to a 24-hour cycle. The strongest external cue for wakefulness is light, whereas darkness is a cue for sleep. Other environmental cues include the timing of social events, such as meals, work, or exercise (Czeisler, Buxton, & Khalsa, 2005). The endogenous component, known as the *master biological clock*, is located in the suprachiasmatic nucleus (SCN) of the hypothalamus. This clock regulates not only sleep but a host of other biological and physiological functions within the body. Information about the lighting conditions of the external environment is relayed to the SCN from the retina via the retinohypothalamic tract. The SCN also receives information from the thalamus and the midbrain. These two pathways transmit photic (light-related) and nonphotic information to the circadian clock through an expansive network. They also exert control over endocrine regulation, body temperature, sleep–wake cycles, metabolism, autonomic regulation, psychomotor and cognitive performance, attention, memory, and emotion (Czeisler, Buxton, & Khalsa, 2005).

In addition to the circadian and homeostatic processes, several neurotransmitter systems are responsible for sleep and wakefulness. The neurotransmitters responsible for wakefulness are dopamine, norepinephrine, acetylcholine, histamine, glutamate, and hypocretin. Sleep-promoting neurotransmitters include adenosine, gamma-aminobutyric acid (GABA), and serotonin (Siegel, 2004). Any medication that crosses the blood–brain barrier may affect sleep and wakefulness through the modulation of these neurotransmitters. Many of the medications used in psychiatry manipulate these neurotransmitter systems. For example, amphetamines—which promote wakefulness—increase the release of dopamine and norepinephrine. Caffeine (methylxanthine)—which promotes alertness—functions by blocking adenosine. Prescribers of medications must be aware of the effects of drugs on neurotransmitters that are involved in sleep and wakefulness.

## FUNCTIONS OF SLEEP

Despite remarkable advances in the understanding of sleep–wake disorders and the biological and physiological process of sleep, very little is known about the true function of sleep. Most of the information regarding the function of sleep comes to us from animal models of sleep deprivation and human models of partial sleep deprivation. Based on these models, several theories have been proposed and include brain tissue restoration, body restoration (NREM sleep), energy conservation, memory reinforcement and consolidation (REM sleep), regulation of immune function, metabolism and regulation of certain hormones, and thermoregulation (Banks & Dinges, 2011; Bonnet, 2011).

## SLEEP REQUIREMENTS

Sleep architecture and efficiency may change over time, but there is little change in the amount of sleep required once we reach adulthood. Sleep requirement varies considerably from individual to individual and to some degree is probably genetically mediated. While most adults require seven to eight hours of sleep for optimal functioning, a small percentage of individuals are defined as long sleepers (requiring ten or more hours per night) and short sleepers (requiring less than five hours per night) (American Academy of Sleep Medicine, 2005). The amount of sleep required is determined by the amount at which a person feels fully awake and able to sustain normal levels of performance during the period of wakefulness.

Many people have a misconception regarding sleep need and tend to allow circumstances to dictate the amount of sleep obtained. The most accurate way to determine one's sleep requirement is to establish a routine bedtime and allow oneself to sleep undisturbed without an alarm for several days. This test is usually best accomplished during an extended period of leisure time, such as during a vacation. The average of several nights' undisturbed sleep is a good estimate of total sleep requirement (Epstein, 2007).

## SLEEP PATTERNS

Sleep architecture changes over the lifespan. The percentage of each stage of sleep, as well as the overall sleep efficiency, or ratio of sleep duration to time spent in bed, varies according to age. For example, infants sleep 16 to 18 hours a day, enter sleep through REM (not NREM) sleep, and spend up to 50% of sleep time in REM sleep. By age 3, the percentage of REM sleep decreases to 20% to 25% and stays relatively constant throughout old age. The amount of slow wave sleep is maximal in young children and declines with age to almost none, particularly in men. This deficit results in a tendency for middle-of-the-night awakenings and reduced sleep efficiency with age (Bliwise, 2011).

## SLEEP–WAKE DISORDERS

The causation of sleep–wake disorders is multifactorial, with distinct and often overlapping biological (neurological or neurochemical), psychological, and social origins. Distinct aspects of causation impact specific disorders, and since different causes call for different treatment approaches, the assessment phase of the nursing process must be emphasized.

Sleep testing is often indicated for people complaining of sleep disturbance or ES that impairs social and vocational functioning. Four common diagnostic procedures are used in the evaluation of sleep–wake disorders: polysomnography (PSG),

the multiple sleep latency test (MSLT), the maintenance of wakefulness test (MWT), and actigraphy.

The PSG, the most common sleep test, is used to diagnose and evaluate people with sleep disorders related to breathing, nocturnal seizure disorders, and various parasomnias, or unusual behaviours during sleep (Kushida, Littner, Morgenthaler, et al., 2005). The MSLT is a daytime nap test used to measure sleepiness objectively in a sleep-conducive setting. One day following a PSG evaluation, the MSLT is routinely performed for patients suspected of having narcolepsy. An MWT evaluates a person's ability to remain awake in a situation conducive to sleep and is used to document adequate alertness in individuals with careers for which sleepiness would pose a risk to public safety (Littner, Kushida, Wise, et al., 2005). Actigraphy involves using a wristwatch-type device that records body movement over a period of time and is helpful in evaluating sleep patterns and sleep duration. It is used in patients with circadian rhythm disorders and insomnia (Morgenthaler, Alessi, Friedman, et al., 2007).

## CLINICAL PICTURE

In the *Diagnostic and Statistical Manual of Mental Disorders*, fifth edition (*DSM-5*), sleep–wake disorders are classified into three major categories: insomnia, hypersomnia, and confusional arousal disorders, with a variety of subtypes for each (Reynolds, Redline, & DSM-V Sleep-Wake Disorders Workgroup and Advisors, 2010). Additional clusters of sleep–wake disorders include those related to breathing and circadian rhythm. Diagnostic criteria for all include disturbed sleep causing marked distress and impaired daytime functioning. As introduced at the start of this chapter, sleep–wake disorders may be experienced independently or as co-occurring disorders and require clinical attention so as to achieve optimal outcomes for sleep, mental health, and physical health. The most common insomnia, hypersomnia, and confusional arousal disorders, as well as breathing and sensory and movement disorders affecting sleep, are described in more detail in this chapter with particular attention to diagnostic criteria, care, and interventions for insomnia disorders.

### Insomnia Disorders

Insomnia disorders are those sleep disturbances not directly attributable to another medical, psychiatric, or substance abuse disorder. Individuals who experience insomnia complain that they have difficulty with sleep initiation, sleep maintenance, early awakening, or nonrefreshing, nonrestorative sleep. People experiencing insomnia disorders will also have altered daytime functioning associated with the sleep disturbance, such as impaired social or vocational functioning, decreased concentration or memory impairment, somatic complaints, or mood disturbance. A disorder is not manifested by a few nights of poor sleep. In order to be classified as a disorder, symptoms must be present for three or more nights a week for more than three months, with an impairment in functioning.

Insomnia is best understood as a state of constant hyperarousal that involves biological, psychological, and social factors (Institute of Medicine, 2006). In addition to a thorough medical, psychiatric, and substance use history, it is helpful to use Spielman's 3P model of insomnia to comprehensively assess the causes of insomnia, suggest appropriate interventions, and provide rationales for treatment (Spielman & Glovinsky, 2004). This model suggests that three factors contribute to the insomnia complaint: predisposing, precipitating, and perpetuating factors.

*Predisposing factors* are individual factors that create a vulnerability to insomnia. These may include a prior history of poor-quality sleep, history of depression and anxiety, or a state of hyperarousal. People at risk for insomnia may describe themselves as light sleepers and "night owls." *Precipitating factors* are external events that trigger insomnia. Personal and vocational difficulties, medical and psychiatric disorders, grief, and changes in role or identity (as seen with retirement) are examples. *Perpetuating factors* are sleep practices and attributes that maintain

---

### BOX 21-1 SLEEP HYGIENE

- Maintain a regular sleep–wake schedule.
- Develop a presleep routine that signals the end of the day.
- Reserve the bedroom for sleep and a place for intimacy.
- Create an environment that is conducive to sleep (taking into consideration light, temperature, and clothing).
- Avoid clock watching.
- Limit caffeinated beverages to one or two a day and none in the evening.
- Avoid heavy meals before bedtime.
- Use alcohol cautiously, and avoid use for several hours before bed.
- Avoid daytime napping.
- Exercise daily but not right before bed.

**Source:** Epstein, L. (2007). *The Harvard Medical School guide to a good night's sleep.* New York: McGraw-Hill.

---

the sleep complaint, such as excessive caffeine or alcohol use, spending excessive amounts of time in bed or napping, and worry about the consequences of insomnia (Spielman & Glovinsky, 2004).

Successful treatment of insomnia involves an integration of the basic principles of sleep hygiene (conditions and practices that promote continuous and effective sleep) (see Box 21-1), behavioural therapies, and, in some instances, the use of hypnotic medication. Treatment is always targeted to the particular subtype, so, in some cases, lifestyle and breathing interventions are indicated (for instance, with sleep apnea disorders). Sedative and hypnotic medication is always used with caution, particularly when the patient has breathing-related insomnia, when addiction may be a concern, or when physical health or illness compromise breathing or central nervous system functioning. Both sedative or anxiolytic medications and over-the-counter sleeping aids have adverse effects; over-the-counter products also demonstrate limited effectiveness. Melatonin, a naturally occurring hormone, is a popular over-the-counter nutraceutical, but little data support its use in the management of insomnia (see the Integrative Therapy box).

### Hypersomnia Disorders
#### Hypersomnia

Hypersomnia disorders are defined as excessive sleepiness that occurs three or more times per week for three or more months despite a main sleep lasting seven hours or longer. The disorder is evidenced by either prolonged night-time sleep episodes or daytime sleep episodes that occur almost daily and cause significant distress and social and vocational impairment. Key diagnostic features of hypersomnia disorders are a report of continuous yet not refreshing nor restorative sleep and difficulty waking up, either in the morning or at the end of a nap. Some individuals with these disorders can sleep up to 20 hours a day. Diagnosis is determined by clinical evaluation and a PSG and MSLT. Treatment is through lifestyle modification and stimulant medication.

## INTEGRATIVE THERAPY
### *Melatonin for Insomnia*

Many people with insomnia turn to over-the-counter solutions. Melatonin is a hormone secreted by the pineal gland in response to information it receives from the suprachiasmatic nucleus regarding light and dark. It is available as a synthetic product at most health food stores and pharmacies. Normally, as night approaches, melatonin is secreted and blood levels rise, producing a sensation of sleepiness. Melatonin levels stay elevated throughout the night but begin to decline in the early morning hours and are essentially undetectable during the day. It would stand to reason then that melatonin supplementation would be a safe and effective soporific.

Unfortunately, research into the role of melatonin in the management of insomnia has been disappointing, with most data pointing to little to no benefit at all. It does seem, however, that melatonin may be effective in the management of circadian rhythm disorders such as jet lag, shift-work disorder, and advances and delays in the sleep cycle.

Although there have been no documented reports of toxicity or overdose of synthetic melatonin, it is important to tell patients that (1) there is no identified effective dosage range and (2) because melatonin is available over the counter and unregulated by Health Canada, there is no standardization of nutraceutical ingredients. Reported adverse effects include nausea, headache, and orthostatic blood pressure changes.

**Sources:** Passarell, S., & Duong, M. (2008). Diagnosis and treatment of insomnia. *American Journal of Health-Systems Pharmacy, 65,* 927–934. doi:10.2146/ajhp060640; and U.S. Department of Health & Human Services, Agency for Healthcare Research and Quality. (2004). *Melatonin for treatment of sleep—wake disorders* (Structured abstract [AHRQ Publication No. 05-E002-1]). Rockville, MD: Author. Retrieved from http://archive.ahrq.gov/downloads/pub/evidence/pdf/melatonin/melatonin.pdf.

## Narcolepsy

The classic tetrad of narcolepsy includes episodes of irresistible attacks of refreshing sleep, cataplexy (muscle weakness), sleep paralysis (waking in a state of temporary paralysis), and hypnagogic hallucinations (dreaming while awake). While everyone with narcolepsy reports impairing degrees of excessive sleepiness, not everyone experiences cataplexy, sleep paralysis, and hypnagogic hallucinations, making diagnosis sometimes difficult. Diagnosis focuses on narcolepsy with or without cataplexy, so all points of assessment are important. When cataplexy is present, narcolepsy is almost always caused by an immune-mediated destruction of orexin (also referred to as hypocretin) neuropeptides located in the lateral hypothalamus. This condition is not considered a hypersomnia but rather its own category of disorder, and the cataplexy is then typically managed with sodium oxybate and antidepressant drugs.

Narcolepsy is also distinguished from other hypersomnia disorders in that patients generally feel refreshed upon waking. Associated symptoms include disturbed night-time sleep with multiple middle-of-the-night awakenings and automatic behaviours characterized by memory lapses. Diagnosis is determined by clinical evaluation and a PSG and MSLT. Treatment is through lifestyle modifications and stimulant medication.

## Confusional Arousal Disorders

Confusional arousal disorders are recurrent episodes of incomplete awakening from sleep with or without terror or movement, usually occurring during the first third of the major sleep episode, and contributing to impaired night-time and day-time safety or functioning. Varying subtypes exist and include sleepwalking, sleep terrors, nightmare disorder, sleep paralysis, and rapid eye movement behaviour disorder.

## Sleepwalking

Also referred to as *somnambulism*, sleepwalking consists of a sequence of complex behaviours that begin in the first third of the night during deep NREM sleep (stages 3 and 4) and usually progress, without full consciousness or later memory, to leaving bed and walking about (activities may include dressing, going to the bathroom, screaming, and even driving). Because of the possibility of accident or injury, somnambulism in adults should be evaluated by a sleep specialist. A PSG is sometimes indicated to rule out the possibility of an underlying disorder of sleep fragmentation. Treatment consists of instructing the person and family regarding safety measures such as installing alarms or locks on windows and doors and gating stairways. Attention to sleep hygiene, limiting alcohol prior to bed, obtaining adequate amounts of sleep, and stress reduction help to prevent episodes.

## Sleep Terrors

Sleep terrors are recurrent episodes of abrupt awakening from sleep, usually occurring during the first third of the major sleep episode and beginning with a panicky scream. There is intense fear and signs of autonomic arousal, such as mydriasis, tachycardia, rapid breathing, and sweating, during each episode.

## Nightmare Disorder

Characterized by long, frightening dreams from which people awaken scared, nightmares almost always occur during REM sleep, usually after a long REM period late in the night. For some people, nightmare disorder is a lifetime condition; for others, nightmares occur only at times of stress and illness. Diagnosis is determined by clinical evaluation. Recurring nightmares can occur with post-traumatic stress disorder, so a thorough psychiatric exam and psychosocial history is necessary. Treatment is dependent on the frequency and severity of the symptoms, as well as the underlying cause. Treatment can include cognitive-behavioural strategies, pharmacotherapy, or both. Many people do well with lifestyle-modification measures, attention to sleep hygiene, and stress reduction.

## Sleep Paralysis

Sleep paralysis is the sensation of paralysis at sleep onset or upon waking. The patient describes a complete awareness of their surroundings but is unable to move. For many people, sleep paralysis causes extreme anxiety and even panic. For a number of people, sleep paralysis events are rare or isolated and do not require any long-term treatment. Reassurance that the sensation is harmless and temporary is helpful. For those individuals with more frequent or severe episodes, further evaluation and treatment by a sleep specialist are warranted. Because sleep paralysis can be seen in people with narcolepsy, screening for narcolepsy is also indicated.

### Rapid Eye Movement Behaviour Disorder

Rapid eye movement behaviour disorder (RBD) is characterized by the absence of muscle atonia during sleep. People with this disorder display elaborate motor activity associated with dream mentation. These people are actually acting out their dreams. RBD is most frequently seen in older-adult men but can be the heralding symptom of neurological pathology such as Parkinson's disease. Serotonergic medications (such as selective serotonin reuptake inhibitors [SSRIs] or selective serotonin-norepinephrine reuptake inhibitors [SNRIs]) can induce or exacerbate episodes. Diagnosis is determined by clinical evaluation and a PSG with video recording. Treatment focuses on patient and sleep partner safety. Placing the mattress on the floor is sometimes necessary to prevent injury as a result of falling out of bed. The use of intermediate-acting benzodiazepine can be helpful, especially in cases of severe disruption to the sleep partner and concerns about safety.

### Kleine–Levin Syndrome

Kleine–Levin syndrome is characterized by recurrent episodes of excessive sleep (more than 11 hrs/d). These episodes of hypersomnia occur at least once a year and are between two days and four weeks in duration. When awake, during at least one of these episodes, cognition is abnormal with a feeling of disorientation, unreality, or confusion. During episodes, patients may experience abnormal behaviour such as megaphagia or hypersexuality. Between episodes, the patient experiences normal alertness, cognitive functioning, and behaviours.

### Sleep–Wake Disorders Related to Breathing
#### Obstructive Sleep Apnea Hypopnea Syndrome

The most common disorder of breathing and sleeping is obstructive sleep apnea hypopnea syndrome, which is characterized by repeated episodes of upper airway collapse and obstruction that result in sleep fragmentation. Essentially, patients with obstructive sleep apnea hypopnea syndrome are not able to sleep and breathe at the same time. Typical symptoms include loud, disruptive snoring; witnessed apnea episodes; and excessive daytime sleepiness. Obesity is an important risk factor for obstructive sleep apnea. Diagnosis is determined by clinical evaluation and a PSG. Treatment is with continuous positive airway pressure (CPAP) therapy.

### Primary Central Sleep Apnea

Another form of sleep disorder related to breathing, primary central sleep apnea is characterized by experiences of at least one of the following: excessive daytime sleepiness, frequent arousals and awakenings during sleep or insomnia complaints,

or awakening short of breath. The PSG will show five or more central apneas per hour of sleep.

### Primary Alveolar Hypoventilation

In the case of primary alveolar hypoventilation, PSG monitoring demonstrates episodes of shallow breathing longer than ten seconds in duration associated with arterial oxygen desaturation and frequent arousals from sleep associated with the breathing disturbances or bradytachycardia. Patients often report excessive daytime sleepiness, frequent arousals and awakenings during sleep, or insomnia complaints.

### Circadian Rhythm Sleep Disorder

Circadian rhythm sleep disorder is characterized by a persistent or recurrent pattern-of-sleep disruption. It results from an altered function of the circadian timing system or from a mismatch between the individual's natural circadian sleep–wake cycle and external demands regarding the timing and duration of sleep—for example, as occurs with shift work or jet lag. Diagnosis is determined by clinical evaluation, sleep diaries, and actigraphy. Treatment is with aggressive lifestyle-management strategies aimed at adapting to or modifying the required sleep schedule.

### Restless Legs Syndrome (Willis-Ekbom Disease)

Restless legs syndrome (RLS) is a sensory and movement disorder characterized by an uncomfortable sensation in the legs (occasionally affecting the arms and trunk) accompanied by an urge to move. Symptoms begin or worsen during periods of inactivity and are relieved or reduced by physical activity such as walking, stretching, or flexing. Symptoms are worse in the evening and at bedtime and can have a significant impact on the individual's ability to fall asleep and stay asleep. Symptoms may be induced or exacerbated by serotonergic agents such as SSRIs or SNRIs (Goldstein, 2011; Pack & Pien, 2011).

---

**VIGNETTE**

Nahla is a 32-year-old woman who was referred by her primary care provider for a psychiatric evaluation for complaints of anxiety and restlessness. She reported feeling fine during the day, but in the evening, she felt nervous and anxious. The symptoms always started at the same time. As soon as she would settle down for the evening to watch some television, she would begin to have a restless sensation in her legs that would make her jump up and pace up and down. She described the sensation as having "soda pop fizzing through my veins." Sometimes she would go out for a walk at night even if it was very late in order to "calm down." These episodes began to occur almost nightly, and, as a result, she was having difficulty getting a good night's sleep. She began to dread the approach of nightfall. A full clinical evaluation suggested the diagnosis of RLS, and a course of the dopamine agonist pramipexole was initiated in the evening, resulting in dramatic improvement in her symptoms and total resolution of her sleep complaint.

Diagnosis is determined by clinical evaluation. Many people with RLS also have periodic limb movements during sleep that are observed during a PSG. Treatment is through lifestyle modification and dopamine agonist therapy, such as pramipexole (Mirapex) and ropinirole (Requip) (Reynolds, Redline, & DSM-V Sleep-Wake Disorders Workgroup and Advisors, 2010).

## EPIDEMIOLOGY

Sleep–wake problems are highly prevalent and occur across all age groups, cultures, and genders. It is estimated that three million Canadian adults suffer from a chronic disorder of sleep and wakefulness (Tjepkema, 2005). Obstructive sleep apnea hypopnea syndrome, a disorder of breathing and sleeping, affects over 3% of adult Canadians (Public Health Agency of Canada, 2009). Circadian rhythm sleep disorder, a misalignment of the normal sleep–wake pattern to accommodate vocational demands, affects up to 32% of night workers and 26% of rotating workers (Sack, Auckley, Auger, et al., 2007). Insomnia is the most common sleep disturbance and is estimated to affect 10% to 40% of the population, depending on the criteria used (Hossain & Shapiro, 2002). As many as 85% to 90% of insomnia disorders are considered co-morbid psychiatric or medical disorders, substance use, or medication effect (Ohayon, 2002).

## CO-MORBIDITY

Multiple studies suggest that sleeping less than seven hours per night may have a significant impact on cardiovascular, endocrine, immune, and neurological function (Institute of Medicine, 2006). Short sleep duration has been associated with obesity, cardiovascular disease and hypertension, and impaired glucose tolerance and diabetes (Gottlieb, Punjabi, Newman, et al., 2005; Gottlieb, Redline, Nieto, et al., 2006; Hasler, Buysse, Klaghoffer, et al., 2004). Many sleep–wake disorders increase the risk for the development of certain medical conditions. For example, obstructive sleep apnea has been associated with hypertension, diabetes, cardiovascular disease, and stroke (Tracova, Dorkova, Molcanyiova, et al., 2008). A Canadian study by Kling, McLeod, and Koehoorn (2010) showed that sleep problems were associated with increased risk for workplace injury and that women were at higher risk for work injuries related to sleep problems. Individuals with neurological disease, such as Alzheimer's and Parkinson's disease, frequently experience sleep disturbance that worsens with the progression of the illness. Sleep disturbance is a major factor contributing to long-term care facility placement for people with dementia.

Most psychiatric disorders are associated with sleep disturbance. Insomnia is the most frequent complaint, but reports of hypersomnia are also common. About 85% of people with a major mood disorder will report some type of a sleep disturbance over the course of the illness. In addition, there is evidence to demonstrate that sleep disruption itself may be a precipitating factor in triggering mood and other psychiatric disorders and increases the risk for relapse, making the

---

### RESEARCH HIGHLIGHT

#### Sleep and Sociocultural Factors

**Source:** Lauderdale, D., Knutson, K., Yan, L., et al. (2006). Objectively measured sleep characteristics among early-middle-aged adults: The CARDIA study. *American Journal of Epidemiology, 164*, 5–16. doi:10.1093/aje/kwj199.

**Problem**
Little is known about the associations among sleep and socioeconomic status, gender, ethnicity, and health.

**Purpose of Study**
The authors of this study proposed to examine whether time in bed, sleep latency, total sleep duration, and sleep efficiency vary by gender, ethnicity, demographic, socioeconomic, employment, household, and lifestyle (smoking, alcohol, physical activity) factors.

**Methods**
The authors used wrist actigraphy and sleep logs over three nights to measure time in bed, sleep latency, total sleep duration, and sleep efficiency in 669 middle-aged adults (ages 38 to 50), who were participating at one of the four Coronary Artery Risk Development in Young Adults (CARDIA) study sites. Of the participants, 30% were White women; 26%, White men; 28%, Black women; and 16%, Black men.

**Key Findings**
- Self-reported sleep duration was greater than actigraphic-determined sleep.
- Black men had significantly less total sleep time (5.1 hours a night) than White women (6.7 hours per night).
- Increased levels of income were associated with shorter sleep latency, longer sleep duration, and greater sleep efficiency.
- Not unexpectedly, alcohol and smoking were associated with longer sleep latency and less sleep efficiency.

**Implications for Nursing Practice**
Nurses play a key role in identifying individuals at increased risk for illness, accident, and injury. Self-reported sleep may be underestimated, so nurses should use available clinical tools such as sleep diaries to help patients accurately estimate total sleep time. In addition, recognition that gender, race, and socioeconomic status may play a role in sleep quality and quantity has important implications for both nursing assessment and treatment planning. Interventions aimed at identifying and intervening with vulnerable populations may improve long-term health outcomes. The need to identify people at risk for sleep disturbance secondary to alcohol and tobacco use is clear.

---

identification and management of sleep disturbance in people with affective disorders critical (Ohayon & Roth, 2003). Of special concern is that depressed people who experience a sleep disturbance demonstrate greater degrees of suicidal ideation (Chellappa & Araujo, 2007). Sleep disturbance is common in people with alcoholism, and insomnia occurs in 36% to 72% of patients in early recovery and persists for months or even years. Sleep disturbance increases the risk for relapse to alcohol abuse. Targeting sleep disturbance during recovery may support continued abstinence (Arndt, Conroy, & Bower, 2007).

## Sleep–Wake Disorders and Mental Illness

People with sleep–wake disorders tend to focus on their sleep problems and may ignore the symptoms of other mental health or physical health disorders. It is not unusual for patients to present to a sleep–wake disorders centre for a sleep evaluation and later be diagnosed with an additional sleep–wake disorder, a psychiatric disorder, or both. For example, a person may be assessed for a breathing-related sleep–wake disorder and also diagnosed with insomnia, or diagnosed with co-morbid restless legs syndrome and insomnia. People with major depressive disorder frequently experience insomnia that involves relatively normal sleep onset followed by repeated awakenings during the second half of the night and early-morning waking. They usually then are in a difficult mood in the morning. Many patients point to the sleep disruption as the cause of the mood disturbance and report that if they could just get a good night's sleep, the mood symptoms would improve.

Difficulty with sleep latency is common with all anxiety disorders, and it is not unusual for people with a previously undiagnosed anxiety disorder to present for treatment of an insomnia complaint of lifelong duration. Management of the underlying anxiety diagnosis in conjunction with the insomnia complaint results in the best clinical outcome. Finally, people with schizophrenia have prolonged sleep latencies, sleep fragmentation, and multiple middle-of-the-night awakenings. It is believed that decreased slow wave sleep plays a factor in the cognitive and negative symptoms of schizophrenia (Lee & Douglass, 2010). Poor health habits such as excessive caffeine use, smoking, and inattention to a regular sleep schedule also contribute to sleep complaints. Those who take medications used to treat schizophrenia are at increased risk for weight gain, an adverse effect, and, consequently, the development of obstructive sleep apnea and should be screened accordingly (Lee & Douglass, 2010).

Hypersomnia is seen in many patients with mental conditions, including mood disorders. Many people report excessive daytime sleepiness in the beginning stages of a mild depressive disorder. A similar complaint is characteristic of the depressed phase of bipolar I disorder. Uncomplicated grief may temporarily be associated with hypersomnia. Personality disorders, dissociative disorders, somatoform disorders, and dissociative fugue are all associated with hypersomnia. Treatment is directed at both the sleep–wake disorder and the psychiatric disorder (Reynolds, Redline, & DSM-V Sleep-Wake Disorders Workgroup and Advisors, 2010).

## Sleep and General Health

Many medical conditions are also associated with insomnia. For instance, people with conditions accompanied by pain and discomfort, such as arthritis and cardiovascular and pulmonary disease, frequently complain of insomnia. Insomnia is also associated with neoplasms, vascular lesions, infections, and

> **VIGNETTE**
>
> Margret had been living with treatment-resistant schizophrenia for many years. Despite multiple medication trials, she had poor control of her symptoms and was frequently hospitalized. Last year she was started on clozapine (Clozaril); within a few months, she had a dramatic reduction in her command hallucinations and total resolution of paranoid delusions. Her family was thrilled. She was finally working and living in a group home. Over the past few months, however, the group home staff noticed a change in Margret's sleep patterns. She frequently wakes during the night and, in the morning, complains of a headache and a sore throat. When she returns home from work in the afternoon, it is not unusual for her to take a nap for 60 minutes or longer. In addition, the group home staff members express concern that she has gained over 18 kilograms in the past year and feel she is out of shape. They have been trying to get her motivated to exercise, but she complains of feeling too tired. While Margret was home on a family visit, her mother noted loud snoring and discussed this detail with the psychiatrist. A PSG was performed and demonstrated a severe degree of obstructive sleep apnea, most likely related to her recent weight gain. Continuous positive airway pressure (CPAP) therapy was initiated, and she was able to return to her baseline level of functioning.

> **VIGNETTE**
>
> Robbie Carson is a student nurse assigned to Mrs. Ventresca in a nursing home. Robbie is in his psychiatric nursing rotation, part of which is spent in a skilled nursing facility taking care of people with dementia. When Robbie receives the report in the morning, he learns that Mrs. Ventresca has been experiencing significant sleep disturbance. She seems to have difficulty falling asleep and frequently wakes up groaning during the night. Robbie notes that Mrs. Ventresca is very confused, as well as agitated. She grimaces whenever she moves. Robbie believes Mrs. Ventresca is in pain. He checks her history to find that she has had arthritis for many years. He then checks her medication profile and discovers that Mrs. Ventresca is not on any pain medication for her arthritis. He speaks to the charge nurse, who calls the physician. Immediately, the physician orders acetaminophen at bedtime for Mrs. Ventresca. Over the next few days, not only is there a dramatic improvement in Mrs. Ventresca's sleep, but her confusion abates, and the agitation disappears.

degenerative and traumatic conditions. Chronic fatigue syndrome and hypothyroidism have been associated with hypersomnia. The relationship between chronic medical disorders and sleep disturbance highlights the importance of screening people with medical disorders for sleep complaints. Treatment is directed at both the sleep–wake disorder and the underlying medical condition (Sadock & Sadock, 2008).

A substance-induced sleep disorder can result from the use or recent discontinuance of a substance or medication. While it is quite obvious that many prescriptions and over-the-counter medications may affect sleep, there is less appreciation for the effects of commonly used substances on sleep. Alcohol, nicotine, and caffeine all have an impact on sleep quantity and quality. Alcohol—despite its great soporific effects—decreases deep sleep (stage 3 and 4) and REM sleep and is responsible for middle-of-the-night awakenings with difficulty returning to sleep. Nicotine is a central nervous system stimulant, increasing heart rate, blood pressure, and respiratory rate. As nicotine levels decline through the night, people wake in response to mild withdrawal symptoms. Caffeine blocks the neurotransmitter adenosine, promoting wakefulness. It increases sleep latency, reduces slow wave sleep, and acts as a diuretic, causing middle-of-the-night awakening for urination (Epstein, 2007).

## APPLICATION OF THE NURSING PROCESS

Regardless of the clinical environment or the presenting complaint, every patient can benefit from a sleep evaluation. Assessment of the person's sleep allows the nurse to identify short- and long-term health risks associated with sleep–wake disorders and sleep deprivation, provide health teaching and counselling regarding sleep needs, and improve clinical outcomes in those experiencing a sleep disturbance.

## ASSESSMENT

### General Assessment

#### Sleep Patterns

People frequently do not report sleep difficulties or discuss their sleep-related concerns with health care providers. They tend to minimize or adapt to the consequences of sleep disturbance. Furthermore, there is a lack of knowledge about the impact sleep disturbance and sleep deprivation have on overall functioning and health. Many people do not complain of sleep disturbance directly but, rather, complain of associated symptoms such as fatigue, decreased concentration, mood disturbance, or physical ailments.

In assessing the patient with a sleep complaint, you must recognize the 24-hour nature of the sleep disturbance. Sleep disturbance is not confined to the seven or eight hours devoted to sleep. Sleep diaries (see Figure 21-3) are helpful in identifying sleep patterns and behaviours that may be contributing to the sleep complaint. Assigning the person the homework of completing a sleep diary for two weeks will help guide the assessment and direct the plan of care. The following questions and comments provide direction for the assessment:

- When did you begin having trouble with sleep? Have you had trouble with sleep in the past?
- Describe your pre-bedtime routine. What are the activities you customarily engage in before sleep?
- Describe your sleeping environment. Are there things in your sleep environment that are hampering your sleep (such as noise, light, temperature, overall comfort)?
- Do you use your bedroom for things other than sleep or sexual activity (such as working, eating, or watching television)?
- What time do you go to bed? How long does it take to fall asleep?

- Once asleep, are you disturbed by middle-of-the-night awakening? If so, what wakes you up? Are you able to return to sleep?
- If you are unable to sleep, what do you do?
- What time do you wake up? What time do you get out of bed?
- How much time do you actually think you sleep?
- Do you sleep longer on weekends or days off?
- Do you nap? If so, for how long? Do you feel refreshed after napping?
- Can you identify any stress or problem that may have initially contributed to your sleep difficulties? Is there any particular issue or problem troubling you now?
- How have you dealt with that stress or problem?
- Tell me about your daily habits. I am interested in your diet, exercise, and medications you take. I am interested in whether or not you smoke or drink caffeinated or alcoholic beverages.
- Can you describe for me the thoughts you experience when you are lying in bed unable to get to sleep?
- What changes, if any, have you made to improve your sleep? What were the results?

#### Identifying Sleep–Wake Disorders

It is helpful to think about sleep–wake disorders according to the predominant symptoms of insomnia, hypersomnia, and arousal disorders. Box 21-2 provides pertinent screening questions for each diagnosis. An affirmative answer to any of these questions demands further investigation and evaluation.

#### Functioning and Safety

As previously described, sleep disturbance can result in increased risk for accident and injury and impose serious limitations on quality of life. Several screening tools are available to assist the clinician in evaluating sleep quality and the safety risk associated with ES. The Pittsburgh Sleep Quality Index (PSQI) is a subjective measure of sleep quality. A global sum of five or greater indicates poor quality and patterns of sleep (Buysse, Reynolds III, Monk, et al., 1989). The Epworth Sleepiness Scale (ESS) is a validated psychometric tool used to measure subject reports of sleepiness and has been validated by objective measures using the MSLT. Scores of less than 10 are considered normal, 10 to 15 is moderately sleepy, and greater than 15 is excessively sleepy. In addition to these screening tools, the following questions provide direction for further assessment:

- Have you had an accident or injury as a result of sleepiness?
- Are you sleepy when you drive a car? What do you do if you are sleepy while driving?
- What kind of work do you do? Do you operate heavy equipment or machinery? How many hours a week do you work? How long is your commute?
- How does your sleep disturbance affect your work performance?
- Do you avoid social obligations as a result of your sleep problems?

Two-week sleep diary

INSTRUCTIONS:
1 Write the date, day of the week, and type of day: Work, School, Day off, or Vacation.
2 Put the letter "C" in the box when you have coffee, cola, or tea. Put "M" when you take any medicine. Put "A" when you drink alcohol. Put "E" when you exercise.
3 Put a line (I) to show when you go to bed. Shade in the box that shows when you think you fell asleep.
4 Shade in all the boxes that show when you are asleep at night or when you take a nap during the day.
5 Leave boxes unshaded to show when you wake up at night and when you are awake during the day.

SAMPLE ENTRY BELOW: On a Monday when I worked, I jogged on my lunch break at 1 PM, had a glass of wine with dinner at 6 PM, fell asleep watching TV from 7 to 8 PM, went to bed at 10:30 PM, fell asleep around midnight, woke up and couldn't get back to sleep at about 4 AM, went back to sleep from 5 to 7 AM, and had coffee and medicine at 7:00 AM.

| Today's Date | Day of the Week | Type of Day Work, School, Off, Vacation | Noon | 1 PM | 2 | 3 | 4 | 5 | 6 PM | 7 | 8 | 9 | 10 | 11 PM | Midnight | 1 AM | 2 | 3 | 4 | 5 | 6 AM | 7 | 8 | 9 | 10 | 11 |
|---|---|---|---|---|---|---|---|---|---|---|---|---|---|---|---|---|---|---|---|---|---|---|---|---|---|---|
| sample | Mon. | Work | | E | | | | | A | | | | I | | | | | | | | C M | | | | | |

**FIGURE 21-3** Two-week sleep diary. **Source:** Adapted from American Academy of Sleep Medicine. (n.d.). *Two week sleep diary.* Retrieved from http://yoursleep.aasmnet.org/pdf/sleepdiary.pdf.

## BOX 21-2    PRIMARY SYMPTOMS OF SLEEP–WAKE DISORDERS SCREENING QUESTIONS

**Insomnia**

- Do you have difficulty falling asleep, staying asleep, or early-morning awakenings?
- Do you feel not refreshed and not restored in the morning?
- Have you noticed any problems with your energy, mood, concentration, or work quality as a result of your sleep problem?
- Is your desired sleep schedule in conflict with your social and vocational goals? What is your preferred sleep schedule? (*also for Circadian rhythm disturbance*)

**Hypersomnia**

- Have you ever been told that you snore or that it looks as though you stop breathing in your sleep? (*obstructive sleep apnea*)
- Do you have an unpleasant or uncomfortable sensation in your legs (or arms) that prevents you from sleeping or wakes you up from sleep and makes you want to move? (*RLS*)
- Do you have episodes of sleepiness you cannot control? (*narcolepsy*)
- Do you ever feel unrested even after an extended sleep period? (*hypersomnia*)

**Confusional Arousal Disorders**

- Have you ever been told that you have done anything unusual in your sleep, such as walking (*somnambulism*) or talking (*somniloquy*)?
- Have you ever been told that you act out your dreams? (*REM sleep behaviour disorder*)
- Have you ever had an unusual experience associated with sleep, such as the inability to move upon awakening or falling asleep? (*sleep paralysis*)

- Do you feel as though your sleep disturbance is affecting your physical health? How so?

### Self-Assessment

Nurses are especially vulnerable to the effects of sleep deprivation and sleep disruption. Rotating shifts and night work result in circadian rhythm disruption that can cause problems with insomnia and excessive sleepiness. Long shifts and overtime hours may lead to a decrease in total available sleep time. Inadequate sleep time and sleep quality have been shown to impair performance and judgement, both of which may affect personal safety and quality of care. In addition, nurses who work rotating or night shifts may pose an increased risk for accident or injury to self and the community as a result of excessive sleepiness while driving.

Nurses need to be able to recognize the effects of chronic partial sleep deprivation on their performance and functioning and take measures to ensure that they are well rested and able to provide safe and competent care. Self-evaluation for a possible sleep disorder and for the ability to cope with the rigours

of shift work is warranted. Consultation with a sleep professional is indicated if there is significant disruption to sleep, physical and mental health, job performance, job satisfaction, and social functioning. Paying attention to issues of sleep hygiene, limiting overtime hours, limiting shift work to eight hours, and obtaining seven to eight hours of sleep within a 24-hour period are essential for personal, individual, and community safety.

## DIAGNOSIS

There are four specific North American Nursing Diagnosis Association International (NANDA-I) nursing diagnoses for sleep disturbance (Herdman, 2012):

1. *Sleep deprivation*—prolonged periods of time without sleep (sustained natural, periodic suspension of relative consciousness)
2. *Insomnia*—a disruption in amount and quality of sleep that impairs functioning
3. *Readiness for enhanced sleep*—a pattern of natural, periodic suspension of consciousness that provides adequate rest, sustains a desired lifestyle, and can be strengthened
4. *Disturbed sleep pattern*—Time-limited interruptions of sleep amount and quality due to external factor

## OUTCOMES IDENTIFICATION

The *Nursing Outcomes Classification (NOC)* (Moorhead, Johnson, Maas, et al., 2008) identifies several appropriate outcomes for the person experiencing sleep disruption, including *Sleep, Rest, Risk control*, and *Personal well-being*. Table 21-1 provides selected intermediate and short-term indicators for these categories.

## PLANNING

The majority of people with sleep–wake disorders are treated in the community. The exceptions are cases in which the person has a primary psychiatric disorder or a medical condition that requires hospitalization. Because longstanding sleep problems are associated with a host of occupational, social, interpersonal, psychiatric, and medical conditions, the treatment is multifaceted and frequently requires a team approach under the leadership of a sleep disorder specialist. The role of the nurse is generally to conduct a full assessment, provide support to the patient and family while the appropriate interventions are determined, and teach the patient and family strategies that may improve sleep.

## IMPLEMENTATION

### Counselling

The nurse's counselling role begins with the assessment of the sleep disorder. The nurse's questions and responses to the patient and family provide support and reassurance that the sleep problems are treatable. For many people, the distress

## TABLE 21-1   *NOC* OUTCOMES FOR SLEEP DISTURBANCES

| NURSING OUTCOME AND DEFINITION | INTERMEDIATE INDICATORS | SHORT-TERM INDICATORS |
|---|---|---|
| *Sleep:* Natural periodic suspension of consciousness during which the body is restored | Sleeps through the night consistently with improvements to sleep pattern and sleep quality | Hours of sleep improve to enable restorative state<br>Sleep routine established<br>Appropriate and functional wakefulness resumes |
| *Rest:* Quantity and pattern of diminished activity for mental and physical rejuvenation | Physically rested<br>Emotionally rested<br>Mentally rested<br>Energy restored after rest | Amount of rest sufficient<br>Rest pattern supports functioning<br>Rest quality supports functioning<br>Rested appearance |
| *Risk control:* Personal actions to prevent, eliminate, or reduce modifiable health risks | Acknowledges risk factors<br>Modifies lifestyle to reduce risk factors | Develops effective risk-control strategies<br>Commits to risk-control strategies |
| *Personal well-being:* Extent of positive perception of one's health status and life circumstances | Spiritual life is satisfactory<br>Physical health is satisfactory<br>Cognitive functioning is improved | Performance of activities of daily living<br>Performance of usual roles |

**Source:** Data from Moorhead, S., Johnson, M., Maas, M., et al. (2008). *Nursing outcomes classification (NOC)* (4th ed.). St. Louis, MO: Mosby.

caused by chronic sleep difficulties sets up a conditioned barrier of hopelessness. Through the nurse's counselling approach, this hopelessness is identified and countered with encouragement, positive suggestions, and the belief that the person will be able to manage sleep difficulties.

### Health Teaching and Health Promotion

The nurse's role in health teaching cannot be overemphasized. Most individuals do not think about their sleep. This means that they also do not recognize the importance of a sleep routine or consider factors that influence good sleep. In addition, there are many myths regarding what constitutes "good sleep" and what factors contribute to sleep quality (see Box 21-1). Education about sleep testing, sleep–wake disorders, and sleep hygiene can be done verbally or with the use of educational materials such as those available through the Canadian Sleep Society or Canadian Lung Association. The nurse may also be involved in teaching relaxation techniques, such as meditation, guided imagery, progressive muscle relaxation, or controlled breathing exercises. Use of these techniques has been linked to sustained benefits for patients with primary insomnia (Sadock & Sadock, 2008).

### Pharmacological Interventions

Many people use medication to address their sleep problems. Nurses frequently provide education about the benefits of a particular drug, the adverse effects, and the fact that medications are usually prescribed for no more than two weeks, because tolerance and withdrawal may result (Sadock & Sadock, 2008). In many settings, the nurse also monitors the effectiveness of the medication.

The Drug Treatment box provides information about hypnotics approved by Health Canada for treatment of insomnia.

Generally, however, long-term use of hypnotic medication is discouraged because nonpharmacological treatments have

shown efficacy in reducing insomnia. Many antidepressants and atypical antipsychotics are also used off-label (i.e., without specific approval from Health Canada) in the treatment of sleep–wake disorders because of their sedative properties.

### Cognitive-Behavioural Therapy for Insomnia

Cognitive-behavioural therapy for insomnia (CBT-I) includes educational, behavioural, and cognitive components; it targets factors that perpetuate insomnia over time (Morin, 2004). It is the most researched nonpharmacological intervention for insomnia and is considered to be a first-line treatment option (Mitchell, Gerhman, Perlis, et al., 2012). The counsellor's first objectives are to provide education regarding sleep and sleep needs and help the person to set realistic expectations regarding sleep. Patients should be asked what they believe constitutes healthy sleep, and counsellors should then clarify any misconceptions. Eliciting information about the total number of hours spent sleeping typically has little value. Many people are stuck on a set number of sleep hours rather than on the quality of sleep obtained. Focusing on the number of hours slept rather than the quality of sleep and daytime functioning increases the insomnia experience.

The next approach involves modifying poor sleep habits and establishing a regular sleep–wake schedule. Keeping a sleep diary (see Figure 21-3) for a period of two weeks is helpful in establishing overall sleep patterns and determining overall sleep efficiency ([total sleep time divided by total time in bed] × 100). After reviewing sleep diaries, patients are sometimes surprised to discover that their sleep problems are not as bad as previously believed. Sleep restriction, or limiting the total sleep time, creates a temporary, mild state of sleep deprivation and strengthens the sleep homeostatic drive. This technique decreases sleep latency and improves sleep continuity and quality. If, for example, a person's sleep diary indicates that he or she is in bed for eight hours but sleeping only six hours, sleep is restricted to six hours, and the bedtime and wake time are adjusted

## DRUG TREATMENT OF PATIENTS WITH INSOMNIA

| GENERIC (BRAND) NAME | ONSET OF ACTION (MIN.) | DURATION OF ACTION | HEALTH CANADA– APPROVED FOR INSOMNIA | HABIT FORMING |
|---|---|---|---|---|
| **Benzodiazepines** | | | | |
| Flurazepam (Dalmane, Som Pam) | 30–60 | Long | Yes | Yes, all drugs in this class |
| Nitrazepam (Mogadon, Nitrazadon) | 30–60 | Long | Yes | are Schedule IV |
| Temazepam (Restoril) | 45–60 | Intermediate | Yes | |
| Triazolam | 15–30 | Short | Yes | |
| **Benzodiazepine-Like Drugs** | | | | |
| Zopiclone (Imovane, Rhovane) | 60 | Intermediate | Yes | Yes, all drugs in this class are Schedule IV |
| **Antidepressant** | | | | |
| Trazodone (Oleptro) | 60–120 | Long | No | No |
| **Antihistamines** | | | | |
| Diphenhydramine (Benedryl, Nytol) | 60–180 | Long | Yes | Tolerance to hypnotic effects develops in 1–2 weeks |

**Source:** Adapted from Health Canada. (2009). *Authorized sleep-aid medications in Canada.* Retrieved from http://www.hc-sc.gc.ca/ahc-asc/media/advisories-avis/_2009/2009_161-list-eng.php.

accordingly. The sleep time should not be reduced below five hours, regardless of sleep efficiency, and patients should be cautioned about the dangers of driving while undergoing a trial of sleep restriction. Once sleep efficiency is improved, total sleep time is gradually increased by 10- to 20-minute increments.

CBT-I also involves using stimulus control. Based on classical conditioning theory, stimulus control employs five basic principles that decrease the negative associations with the bed or bedroom and strengthen the stimulus for sleep. Patients should be instructed to do the following:

1. Go to bed only when sleepy.
2. Use the bed or bedroom only for sleep and intimacy (no television, reading, or other activities in the bedroom).
3. Get out of bed if unable to sleep and engage in a quiet-time activity such as reading or crossword puzzles (no television, work, or computer).
4. Maintain a regular sleep–wake schedule, with getting up at the same time each day being the most important factor.
5. Avoid daytime napping (if napping is necessary to avoid accident or injury, it should be limited to 20 to 30 minutes maximum).

Other objectives of CBT-I are aimed at identifying and correcting maladaptive attitudes and beliefs about sleep that perpetuate insomnia. For example, people frequently amplify the consequences of their insomnia and attribute most daytime experiences to their sleep complaint. They may rationalize maladaptive coping behaviours such as excessive time in bed to "catch up" on lost sleep and may exhibit unrealistic expectations about sleep. The practitioner offers alternative interpretations regarding the sleep complaint to assist the person to think about the insomnia in a different way, empowering the patient to be in control of his or her sleep (Morin, 2004). Because CBT-I approaches are not immediately effective and may take several weeks of practice before improvement is seen, success is dependent on both a high degree of motivation in the patient and a commitment on the part of the practitioner.

Other nonpharmacological methods for treating insomnia are exercise, tai chi, acupuncture, yoga, and mindfulness. All of these approaches have been researched and demonstrate some evidence of improvement in sleep quality and insomnia, but the quantity and quality of research available is limited (Cheuk, Yeung, Chung, et al., 2012).

### VIGNETTE

Josette Harris is a 52-year-old woman who complains of difficulty falling asleep and staying asleep every night. It is not unusual for Josette to take several hours to fall asleep, and once she does fall asleep, she is able to sleep for only two to three hours at a time. She tosses and turns and lies in bed "hoping to fall asleep." She estimates that she is sleeping only about four or five hours a night. Josette reports that this has been going on for at least a year but that it seems to be getting progressively worse over the past several months. Because she sleeps poorly at night, she has been staying in bed until 9:00 or 10:00 in the morning and has been late for work several times during the past three months. She feels tired during her waking hours and has difficulty focusing on the task at hand in her accounting job. To improve her work performance, she has been drinking five or six cups of coffee during the day. Even though she feels tired, she is unable to nap. Family members complain that she is irritable and short-tempered with them. Interestingly, she reports that she was able to sleep fairly well while on vacation last month. Josette completes a sleep diary for a two-week period and undergoes a complete assessment. There seems to be no underlying medical or psychiatric disorder associated with her sleep complaint. She is diagnosed with an insomnia disorder and begins a cognitive-behavioural therapy program.

**Advanced-Practice Interventions**

Although psychotherapy offers little value in the treatment of primary insomnia, there is a component of primary insomnia that involves a conditioned response. The initial episode of insomnia is frequently associated with a stressful event or crisis that produces anxiety. This anxiety becomes associated with worry about not being able to get to sleep and leads to preoccupation with getting enough sleep. The more the person tries to sleep, the more elusive sleep becomes, and the greater the person's anxiety. The advanced-practice nurse may be closely involved in the use of cognitive-behavioural therapy to manage insomnia.

# EVALUATION

Evaluation is based on whether or not the person experiences improved sleep quality as evidenced by decreased sleep latency, fewer night-time awakenings, and a shorter time to get back to sleep after waking. This evaluation is accomplished through an individual's report and maintenance of a sleep diary. Just as important as objective changes in the person's sleep pattern is the person's perception of improvement. Objectively, the improvement may be quite modest, but the person may perceive that he or she is no longer controlled by sleep (or the lack of it) but is exerting control over sleep through lifestyle changes and a better sleep routine.

# ■ KEY POINTS TO REMEMBER

- Sleep disturbance has major implications for overall health, quality of life, and personal and community safety.
- Research into the physiology of normal sleep, as well as sleep–wake disorders, is expanding.
- Most people with a mood disorder will report sleep disturbance; recognition and treatment of sleep disturbance in people with psychiatric disorders improves clinical outcomes.
- Regardless of the clinical environment or the presenting complaint, all patients can benefit from an evaluation of their sleep needs.

- It is helpful to categorize sleep disturbance according to the three major symptom categories of insomnia, hypersomnia, and confusional arousal disorders.
- Primary insomnia can be effectively treated with nonpharmacological interventions such as CBT-I, sleep restriction, stimulus control, and attention to issues of sleep hygiene. Long-term pharmacological management is generally not indicated.

# ■ CRITICAL THINKING

1. Jabar is a 46-year-old who complains of waking frequently at night. Consequently, he is tired all day and knows that he has not been functioning as well as he should. Whenever he can manage it, he goes out to his car at lunchtime to take a 60-minute nap because he has fallen asleep at his desk in the past and been given a disciplinary warning. He is drinking two to three cups of coffee in the afternoon so that he does not feel sleepy while driving home.
   a. What questions would you ask to determine whether Jabar might have a sleep disorder?
   b. What recommendations will you make for him to improve his sleep hygiene?
   c. What instructions and education should you give this person regarding personal and community safety?

2. Your patient, Vivian, has been using temazepam (Restoril) for several years to treat insomnia. She has been reading that long-term use of hypnotics is not healthy or productive and wants to quit taking them. However, she is focused on needing nine hours of sleep each night and is extremely worried about what will happen when she quits the temazepam.

   a. What instructions would you provide to Vivian regarding stimulus control, sleep restriction, and cognitive restructuring of her sleep complaint?
   b. Identify alternative pharmacological therapies.

3. Mrs. Levine is a 72-year-old woman with a history of major depression. She takes fluoxetine (Prozac) 10 mg every day and has experienced significant relief from depression. While listing her medications, she tells you she is using a variety of over-the-counter sleep aids because she has been having some difficulty sleeping recently. These over-the-counter products include diphenhydramine, melatonin, valerian, and something that her neighbour gave her to try.
   a. In light of the person's age and history of depression, what are your concerns?
   b. What further assessment is required?
   c. What specific question would you need to ask concerning her use of Prozac?
   d. What instructions and education will you provide?

4. Suzie Au, a 47-year-old business executive and single mother of two teenage sons, has presented to the urban mental health centre complaining that she is "hanging on by my fingernails," that taking care of her business and her boys is taking all of her energy, and that she has suffered from constant insomnia for several years but that it has worsened over the past few months. Her lack of sleep has forced her to give up her social life, including gym workouts. She feels stressed and worries that her ability to cope will soon disappear unless she can improve the quality of her sleep. She has begun to drink four or five cups of coffee per day to keep awake and tries to catch a nap whenever possible.

a. What strategy or tool would enable Suzie to provide an accurate self-appraisal of the characteristics of her sleep?
b. What further assessments would you need to do?
c. What immediate instructions and education will you offer Suzie in regard to her current coping strategies?
d. What short-term goals would be appropriate for Suzie?

## CHAPTER REVIEW

1. A person states that he needs only five to six hours of sleep per night to feel rested. How should the nurse interpret this statement?
   1. The person is not sleeping enough.
   2. The person is sleeping too much.
   3. The person is sleeping according to his own body's needs.
   4. The person is not getting enough REM sleep.

2. The nurse is planning care for a person with primary insomnia. What is an appropriate outcome?
   1. The person will sleep 12 hours nightly.
   2. The person will go to bed and wake up at consistent times daily.
   3. The person will take one nap daily to restore energy.
   4. The person will drink a cup of warm tea before bedtime.

3. The nurse is providing teaching for a person who has been taking a hypnotic medication to sleep. What statement by the nurse is appropriate?
   1. "You can use this medication for as long as you would like."
   2. "It would be better to take an over-the-counter medication instead."
   3. "Melatonin has been shown to be just as effective as hypnotic medications."
   4. "Be certain to follow up with your doctor regularly while you take this medication."

4. Because of the likelihood of underestimated or inaccurate self-assessment of sleep, what tool would be most appropriate for the nurse to use in obtaining an assessment from a patient suspected of having a sleep–wake disorder?
   1. A mini mental status exam
   2. An anxiety inventory
   3. A sleep diary
   4. A family history assessment

5. Which behaviour would alert the nurse to a circadian rhythm sleep disorder?
   1. Excessive sleepiness for at least one month, accompanied by prolonged sleep episodes
   2. Multiple episodes of brief daytime sleeping followed by disturbed nighttime sleep
   3. Persistent patterns of sleep disruption after travelling for business
   4. Repeated episodes of upper airway collapse and obstruction that results in sleep fragmentation

## Evolve WEBSITE

Post-Test interactive review

*Visit the Evolve Web site for Chapter Review Answers and Rationales, Critical Thinking Answer Guidelines, and additional resources related to the content in this chapter:* http://evolve.elsevier.com/Canada/Varcarolis/psychiatric/

## REFERENCES

American Academy of Sleep Medicine. (2005). *The international classification of sleep disorders (ICSD)* (2nd ed.). Westchester, IL: Author.

Arnedt, J.T., Conroy, D.A., & Bower, K.J. (2007). Treatment options for sleep disturbance during alcohol recovery. *Journal of Addictive Diseases, 26,* 41–54. doi:10.1300/J069v26n04_06.

Bailes, S., Baltzan, M., Rizzo, D., et al. (2009). Sleep disorder symptoms are common and unspoken in Canadian general practice. *Family Practice, 26,* 294–300. doi:10.1093/famprac/cmp031.

Banks, S., & Dinges, D.F. (2011). Chronic sleep deprivation. In M. Kryger, T. Roth, & W. Dement (Eds.), *Principles and practice of sleep medicine* (5th ed., pp. 67–75). Philadelphia: Saunders.

Barone, M.T., & Menna-Barreto, L. (2011). Diabetes and sleep: A complex cause-and-effect relationship. *Diabetes Research and Clinical Practice, 91,* 129–137. doi:10.1016/j.diabres.2010.07.011

Basner, M., Fomberstein, K., Razavi, F., et al. (2007). American Time Use Survey: Sleep time and its relationship to waking activities. *Sleep, 30*(9), 1085–1095.

Bliwise, D. (2011). Normal aging. In M. Kryger, T. Roth, & W. Dement (Eds.), *Principles and practice of sleep medicine* (5th ed., pp. 27–41). Philadelphia: Saunders.

Bonnet, M. (2011). Acute sleep deprivation. In M. Kryger, T. Roth, & W. Dement (Eds.), *Principles and practice of sleep medicine* (5th ed., pp. 54–66). Philadelphia: Saunders.

Buysse, D.J., Reynolds, C.F., III, Monk, T.H., et al. (1989). The Pittsburgh Sleep Quality Index: A new instrument for psychiatric practice and research. *Psychiatry Research, 28,* 193–213. doi:10.1016/0165 -1781(89)90047-4.

Canada Safety Council. (2013). *Canada's blood alcohol laws among the strictest in the Western world.* Ottawa: Author. Retrieved from https:// canadasafetycouncil.org/traffic-safety/canada-s-blood-alcohol-laws -among-strictest-western-world.

Canadian Centre for Occupational Health & Safety. (2007). Fatigue: The foe you don't want to know at work. *Health & Safety Report, 5*(11). Retrieved from http://www.ccohs.ca/newsletters/hsreport/issues/2007/11/ ezine.html#inthenews.

Carskadon, M.A., & Dement, W.C. (2011). Normal human sleep: An overview. In M. Kryger, T. Roth, & W. Dement (Eds.), *Principles and practice of sleep medicine* (5th ed., pp. 16–26). Philadelphia: Saunders.

Chellappa, S.L., & Araujo, J.F. (2007). Sleep disorders and suicidal ideation in patients with depressive disorder. *Psychiatry Research, 153,* 131–136. doi:10.1016/j.psychres.2006.05.007.

Cheuk, D.K., Yeung, W.F., Chung, K.F., et al. (2012). Acupuncture for insomnia. *Cochrane Database of Systematic Review, 12*(9). doi:10.1002/14651858.CD005472.pub3.

Czeisler, C., Buxton, O., & Khalsa, S. (2005). The human circadian system and sleep–wake regulation. In M. Kryger, T. Roth, & W. Dement (Eds.), *Principles and practice of sleep medicine* (4th ed., pp. 136–154). Philadelphia: Saunders.

Elzohairy, Y. (2008). Fatal and injury fatigue-related crashes on Ontario's roads. In M. Yakabuski, (Ed.), *Highway safety roundtable: Working together to understand driver fatigue: Report on symposium proceedings.* Symposium conducted at the meeting of the Insurance Board of Canada, Toronto, ON. Retrieved from http://www.ibc.ca/en/Car_Insurance/ documents/driver_fatigue/Understanding_Driver_Fatigue_HSR -Feb2008.pdf.

Epstein, L. (2007). *The Harvard Medical School guide to a good night's sleep.* New York: McGraw-Hill.

Goldstein, C.A. (2011). Parasomnias. In T. Freedon, J.V. Dyonzak, & C.A. Goldstein (Eds.), *Sleep medicine, part I: Insomnia, hypersomnia, and parasomnias. Disease-a-Month 57*(7), (pp. 364–388). New York: Elsevier.

Gottlieb, D.J., Punjabi, N.M., Newman, A.B., et al. (2005). Association of sleep time with diabetes mellitus and impaired glucose tolerance. *Archives of Internal Medicine, 165*(8), 863–867.

Gottlieb, D.J., Redline, S., Nieto, F.J., et al. (2006). Association of usual sleep duration with hypertension: The sleep heart health study. *Sleep, 29*(8), 1009–1014.

Hasler, G., Buysse, D.J., Klaghoffer, R., et al. (2004). The association between short sleep duration and obesity in young adults: A 13-year prospective study. *Sleep, 27*(4), 661–666.

Helis, J. (2009). *Canadian blood alcohol laws: An international perspective. Update to the 2002–2006 report.* Ottawa: Canadian Safety Council. Retrieved from http://canadasafetycouncil.org/sites/default/files/PDF_en/ bac-update-09_0.pdf.

Herdman, T.H. (Ed.). (2012). *NANDA International nursing diagnoses: Definitions & classification, 2012–2014.* Oxford, UK: Wiley-Blackwell.

Hossain, J.L., & Shapiro, C.M. (2002). The prevalence, cost implications, and management of sleep disorders: An overview. *Sleep and Breathing, 6*(2), 85–102.

Hurst, M. (2008). Who gets any sleep these days? Sleep patterns of Canadians (Statistics Canada, Catalogue no. 11-008X). *Canadian Social Trends,*

85(Spring), 39–45. Retrieved from http://www.statcan.gc.ca/pub/11 -008-x/2008001/article/10553-eng.pdf.

Institute of Medicine. (2006). *Sleep disorders and sleep deprivation: An unmet public health problem.* Washington, DC: National Academies Press.

Insurance Bureau of Canada. (2011). *Driver fatigue: Are you driving impaired?* Retrieved from http://www.ibc.ca/en/Car_Insurance/Driver_Fatigue/.

Kling, R.N., McLeod, C.B., & Koehoorn, M. (2010). Sleep problems and workplace injuries in Canada. *Sleep, 33*(5), 611–618.

Kushida, C., Littner, M., Morgenthaler, T., et al. (2005). Practice parameters for the indications for polysomnography and related procedures. *Sleep, 28*(4), 499–521.

Lee, E.K., & Douglass, A.B. (2010). Sleep in psychiatric disorders: Where are we now? *The Canadian Journal of Psychiatry, 55*(7), 403–412.

Littner, M., Kushida, C., Wise, M., et al. (2005). Practice parameters for clinical use of the multiple sleep latency test and maintenance of wakefulness test. *Sleep, 28*(1), 113–121.

Mitchell, M.D., Gerhman, P., Perlis, M., et al. (2012). Comparative effectiveness of cognitive behavioural therapy for insomnia: A systematic review. *BMC Family Practice, 13*(40). doi:10.1186/1471-2296-13-40.

Moorhead, S., Johnson, M., Maas, M., et al. (2008). *Nursing outcomes classification (NOC)* (4th ed.). St. Louis, MO: Mosby.

Morgenthaler, T., Alessi, C., Friedman, L., et al. (2007). Practice parameters for the use of actigraphy in the assessment of sleep and sleep disorders: An update for 2007. *Sleep, 30*(4), 519–529.

Morin, C. (2004). Cognitive-behavioural approaches to the treatment of insomnia. *Journal of Clinical Psychiatry, 65*(Suppl. 16), 33–40.

Morin, C.M., LeBlanc, M., Belanger, L., et al. (2011). Prevalence of insomnia and its treatment in Canada. *Canadian Journal of Psychiatry, 56*(9), 540–548.

National Sleep Foundation. (2008). *Sleep in America poll summary of findings.* Retrieved from http://www.sleepfoundation.org/article/press-release/ sleep-america-poll-summary-findings.

Ohayon, M. (2002). Epidemiology of insomnia: What we know and what we still need to learn. *Sleep Medicine Reviews, 6,* 97–111. doi:10.1177/ 0886260504268766.

Ohayon, M.M., Dauvilliers, Y., Reynolds, C.F. (2012). Operational definitions and algorithms for excessive sleepiness in the general population: Implications for DSM-5 nosology. *Archives of General Psychiatry, 69,* 71–79.

Ohayon, M., & Roth, T. (2003). Place of chronic insomnia in the course of depression and anxiety disorders. *Journal of Psychiatric Research, 37,* 9–15. doi:10.1016/S0022-3956(02)00052-3.

Pack, A.I., & Pien, G.W. (2011). Update on sleep and its disorders. *Annual Review of Medicine, 62,* 447–460. doi:10.1146/annurev-med-050409 -104056.

Public Health Agency of Canada. (2009). *What is the impact of sleep apnea on Canadians? Fast facts from the Canadian community health survey—Sleep apnea rapid response.* Retrieved from http://www.phac-aspc.gc.ca/cd-mc/ sleepapnea-apneesommeil/pdf/sleep-apnea.pdf.

Reynolds, C.F., Redline, S., & DSM-V Sleep-Wake Disorders Workgroup and Advisors. (2010). The DSM-V sleep–wake disorders nosology: An update and an invitation to the sleep community. *Journal of Clinical Sleep Medicine, 6*(1), 9–10.

Sack, R., Auckley, D., Auger, R., et al. (2007). Circadian rhythms sleep disorders, Part I: Basic principles, shift work and jet lag disorders. *Sleep, 30*(11), 1460–1524.

Sadock, B.J., & Sadock, A. (2008). *Kaplan & Sadock's concise textbook of clinical psychiatry* (3rd ed.). Philadelphia: Lippincott Williams & Wilkins.

Siegel, J. (2004). The neurotransmitters of sleep. *Journal of Clinical Psychiatry, 65*(Suppl. 16), 4–7.

Sleep disorders create growing opportunities for hospitals. (2001). *Health Care Strategic Management, 19*(2), 16–17.

Sorscher, A. (2008). How is your sleep: A neglected topic for health care screening. *Journal of the American Board of Family Medicine, 21,* 141–148. doi:10.3122/jabfm.2008.02.070167.

Spielman, A., & Glovinsky, P. (2004). A conceptual framework of insomnia for primary care providers: Predisposing, precipitating, and perpetuating factors. *Sleep Medicine Alert, 9*(1), 1–6.

Strine, T.W., & Chapman, D.P. (2005). Association of frequent sleep insufficiency with health-related quality of life and health behaviors. *Sleep Medicine, 6,* 23–27. doi:10.1016/j.sleep.2004.06.003.

Tjepkema, M. (2005). *Insomnia. Health Reports, 17*(1), 9–25.

Tracova, R., Dorkova, Z., Molcanyiova, A., et al. (2008). Cardiovascular risk and insulin resistance in patients with obstructive sleep apnea. *Medical Science Monitor, 14*(9), CR438–CR444.

Walsh, J.K. (2004). Clinical and socioeconomic correlates of insomnia. *Journal of Clinical Psychiatry, 65*(Suppl. 8), 13–29.

Williams, C. (2001). You snooze, you lose? Sleep patterns in Canada. (Statistics Canada, Catalogue no. 11-008-XIE). *Canadian Social Trends, 60*(Spring), 10–14. Retrieved from http://www.statcan.gc.ca/pub/11-008-x/2000004/article/5558-eng.pdf.

Williamson, A.M., & Feyer, A.M. (2007). Moderate sleep deprivation produces impairments in cognitive and motor performance equivalent to legally prescribed levels of alcohol intoxication. *Occupational and Environmental Medicine, 57,* 649–655. doi:10.1136/oem.57.10.649.

Zepelin, H., Siegel, J.M., & Tober, I. (2005). Mammalian sleep. In M. Kryger, T. Roth, & W. Dement (Eds.), *Principles and practice of sleep medicine* (4th ed., pp. 88–92). Philadelphia: Saunders.

# 22

# Sexual Dysfunction, Gender Dysphoria, and Paraphilias

*Margaret Jordan Halter, Verna Benner Carson*
*Adapted by Joanne Louis*

## KEY TERMS AND CONCEPTS

## OBJECTIVES

1. Describe sexuality and sexual activity.
2. Define at least three areas of sexual dysfunction, and describe the treatment for each.
3. Consider the impact of medical problems and treatments on normal sexual functioning.
4. Examine the importance of nurses' being knowledgeable about and comfortable discussing topics pertaining to sexuality.
5. Describe treatments available for sexual dysfunction.
6. Apply assessment techniques for sexual history.
7. Identify sexual preoccupations considered to be sexual disorders.
8. Discuss personal values and biases regarding sexuality and sexual behaviours.
9. Develop a plan of care for individuals diagnosed with sexual disorders.

## ⊖volve WEBSITE

*Visit the Evolve website for Flashcards, Case Studies, and additional testing resources related to the content in this chapter: http://evolve.elsevier.com/Canada/Varcarolis/psychiatric/*   Pre-Test   interactive review

Everyday professional nursing practice requires us to engage in matter-of-fact discussions with patients on topics generally considered to be private. We perform head-to-toe assessments in which we inquire about everything from headaches and sore throats to difficulties urinating and problems with constipation. The realities of providing physical care necessitate becoming comfortable with a number of skills that relate to privacy and modesty—performing breast examinations, initiating urinary catheters, and inserting rectal medications.

Health promotion and disease prevention are key responsibilities for nurses. All nurses must assess a patient's sexuality and be prepared to educate, dispel myths, assist with values clarification, refer to appropriate care providers when indicated, and share resources. These actions alleviate or decrease patient illness and suffering and reduce health care costs through prevention. As a nursing student, you are introduced to complex aspects of sexual behaviour that should help facilitate thoughtful discussion of the topic, make you aware of your personal belief systems, and help you consider the broader perspective of sexual issues as they exist in contemporary society.

This chapter addresses two general categories of concern related to sexuality. The first half of the chapter examines the

**HOW A NURSE HELPED ME**

*An Ordinary Family*

*In many ways, we were an ordinary family—a mom, a dad, an adopted daughter, and a dog. Our adopted daughter, Jasmine, was home for the holidays. At 15, she was a weekly boarder at a specialist school for high-ability dyslexics. As we chatted, Jasmine began to make hurtful comments about her father. The following evening, she burst into my bedroom and told me her father had been sexually abusing her for the past five years. "He won't leave me alone," she sobbed. "He's always feeling me up. He brushes against my breasts, so I know it's not accidental. Tonight, he touched me between my legs."*

*In a panic, I took Jasmine to the emergency department of the local hospital. At the emergency department, a sexual assault nurse examiner (SANE) explained to Jasmine and me that a SANE is a nurse who is specially trained to provide comprehensive and sensitive health care for pediatric and adult survivors of sexual assault. She provided much needed emotional support, did a physical assessment, documented injuries, collected forensic samples, provided medications, wrote a medical–legal report, and testified in court. My husband served 18 months in jail and was placed on the sex offender registry for five years. Ongoing counselling with the SANE for Jasmine and me helped me to realize that my (now ex-) husband was a pedophile. It was hard to move past the denial and to open myself up to this knowledge. In the end, the SANE helped me to reclaim my life and for my daughter to reclaim hers.*

 **CONSIDERING CULTURE**

*Sexual Orientation and Gender Identity*

When we think about culture, we often relate it to concepts such as language, ethnicity, and race. Yet culture can be an important consideration in our discussion of sexual orientation and gender identity. We live in a world where the idea of sexual relationships, marriage, and childbearing occur in the context of a monogamous male–female relationship. Having traditionally dominated the way that society is structured, these ideas have created a heterosexual culture within Canadian society. It is important, however, to move beyond these traditional notions of sexuality and recognize that sexual orientation and gender identity can be diverse. Lesbian, gay, bisexual, and transgender issues are increasingly visible in our society. As nurses, we must recognize the dominance of our heterosexual culture and its shaping of our own values and beliefs when providing care for all patients.

**Sources:** Dean, J.J. (2011). The cultural construction of heterosexual identities. *Sociology Compass, 5,* 679–687. doi:10.1111/j.1751-9020.2011.00395.x; Eliason M.J., Dibble, S., & Dejoseph, J. (2010). Nursing's silence on lesbian, gay, bisexual, and transgender issues: The need for emancipatory efforts. *Advances in Nursing Science, 33*(3), 206–218. doi:10.1097/ANS.0b013e3181e63e49; Mann, K., Gordon, J. & MacLeod, A. (2007). Reflection and reflective practice in health professions education: A systematic review. *Advances in Health Sciences Education, 14*(4), 595–621. doi: 10.1007/s10459-007-9090-2.

normal sexual response cycle, clinical disorders related to the disruption or malfunction of this cycle, and guidelines for nursing care. The second half focuses on disorders related to sexual focus and preoccupation. These disorders may be sources of discomfort and distress to the person experiencing them (e.g., as in gender dysphoria) or may be a source of pain and trauma for others whose rights are violated (e.g., as in pedophilia).

## SEXUALITY

Generally speaking, sexuality is the way that people experience and express themselves as sexual beings. Biologically, *sexual activity* includes sexual intercourse and sexual contact in all its forms. Many factors affect interest in sexual activity, including age, physical and emotional health, availability of a sexual partner, and the context of an individual's life. In fact, for many people, lack of sexual desire is not a source of distress either to the person or to his or her partner; in such situations, decreased or absent sexual desire is not viewed as an illness. However, low

sexual desire may be a source of frustration, both for those experiencing it and for their partners. It is associated with other psychiatric or medical conditions. Conversely, excessive sexual desire becomes a problem when it creates difficulties for the individual's partner or when such excessive desire drives the person to demand sexual compliance from or force it upon unwilling partners.

Testosterone (normally present in both males and females but in a much higher level in males) appears to be essential to sexual desire in both men and women. Men who have lost the ability to produce testosterone describe the change in their sexual feelings in terms such as "I still have the basic inclination for sex but do not seem to have the energy to put it into effect." Testosterone replacement therapy appears to restore sexual energy for some of these men.

Estrogen does not seem to have a similar direct effect on sexual desire in women. A secondary effect, however, may be present in the requirement of estrogen for the maintenance of normal vaginal elasticity and lubrication. If these traits are lost due to estrogen deficiency, as may occur in some postmenopausal women or in younger women who have had their ovaries removed, dyspareunia (see page 445) and vaginismus (see page 445) may result. Other causes of dyspareunia and vaginismus include vaginal infections and lesions. Physical distress during sexual activity leads to psychological distress as pain is anticipated, compounding the problem.

During sexual activity, sexual tension increases, a period called *sexual excitement*. Traditionally, penile erection and vaginal lubrication have been used as indicators of the presence of sexual excitement. If erection or lubrication does not occur in what, for the individual, is a sexually stimulating and appropriate situation, then there has been an inhibition of sexual excitement, regardless of the causative factors.

Orgasm is attained only at high levels of sexual tension in both women and men. Sexual tension (also called *sexual arousal*) is produced by a combination of mental activity—including thoughts, fantasies, and dreams—and erotic stimulation of erogenous areas, which may be specific to each individual. Most men require some penile stimulation, and most women some clitoral stimulation, either directly or indirectly, to produce the high levels of sexual tension necessary for orgasm to occur.

Most women who have experienced one orgasm may have repeated orgasms during the continuation of the same sexual activity. The occurrence of multiple orgasms depends on the maintenance of high levels of sexual tension through continued stimulation. On the other hand, once men ejaculate as a part of orgasm, they go through a refractory period. This is the time required to produce another ejaculate, which varies primarily with age. In a young man, this refractory period is measured in minutes, whereas in an older man, it may last several hours.

Once sexual stimulation has ceased, sexual tension subsides to baseline levels, and the physiological changes that had occurred dissipate. This is a period of psychological vulnerability and can be experienced in a number of ways ranging from pleasure to discomfort.

## SEXUAL DYSFUNCTION

A sexual dysfunction is a diminished or absent feeling of sexual interest or desire, absence of sexual thoughts or fantasies, and a lack of responsive desire. The motivations for attempting to become sexually aroused are scarce or absent. The lack of interest is considered to be beyond a normal lessening due to life cycle and relationship duration (Hatzimouratidis & Hatzichristou, 2007). It may prevent or reduce a person's ability to enjoy sex. In evaluating a patient with a sexual dysfunction, a physical assessment—including laboratory studies—is performed before exploring psychological factors, such as emotional issues, life situation, and experiences.

## CLINICAL PICTURE

There are seven major classes of sexual dysfunction. In women, sexual dysfunctions include persistent or recurrent disorders of sexual interest or desire, subjective sexual arousal disorders (despite stimulation or increased lubrication of the vagina, the person does not feel aroused), genital arousal disorders, orgasm disorder, and pain and difficulty with attempted or completed intercourse (Basson, Althof, Davis, et al., 2004). Erectile dysfunction, orgasm or ejaculation disorders, priapism, and Peyronie's disease are disorders of sexual function in men (Lue, Giuliano, Montorsi, et al., 2004). Sexual dysfunctions can result from physiological problems, interpersonal conflicts, a combination of physiological and interpersonal problems, a general medical condition, or substance use, or a person can experience

sexual dysfunction not otherwise specified, often as a result of stress (Sadock & Sadock, 2008).

### Sexual Desire Disorders

Sexual desire disorders are based on damage to biological sex drive, self-esteem, acceptance of personal sexuality, sexual experiences, and relationship issues (Sadock & Sadock, 2008). They are divided into two classes: (1) hypoactive sexual desire disorder, characterized by a deficiency or absence of sexual fantasies or desire for sexual activity, and (2) *sexual aversion disorder*, characterized by an aversion to and avoidance of genital sexual contact with a sexual partner or by masturbation.

Sexual difficulties affect 10% to 15% of sexually active women (Basson, 2011). A meta-analysis (summary of data) of all recent epidemiological studies ranks it as high as 24% to 34% (Segraves & Woodard, 2006). This disorder may be related to chronic stress and depression, prolonged suppression of sexual impulses, or a deteriorating relationship.

Although the incidence of sexual aversion disorder is unknown, it is thought to be common and more prevalent in men (Shafer, 2008). About 25% of the time, it is co-morbid with panic disorder.

### Sexual Arousal Disorders

*Female sexual arousal disorder* is physiologically characterized by persistent or recurrent partial or complete failure to attain or maintain the lubrication and swelling response of sexual excitement until the completion of the sexual act. To receive this diagnosis, the lack of arousal must be distressing to the woman. Sexual arousal disorder can be a lifelong problem, or it may be acquired (i.e., developed following normal functioning) (Becker & Stinson, 2008). The condition may be the result of hormonal alterations in testosterone, estrogen, prolactin, and thyroxin. Medications such as antihistamines and anticholinergics may result in decreased lubrication (Sadock & Sadock, 2008).

*Male erectile disorder* (also called *erectile dysfunction* or *impotence*) is characterized by the recurrent and persistent partial or complete failure to attain or maintain an erection to perform the sex act (Sadock & Sadock, 2008). Rarely, this problem may be a lifelong condition in which a man has never been able to obtain an erection sufficient for intercourse; more commonly, it is an acquired condition (i.e., the man has previously been able to have sexual intercourse but has lost the ability). Acquired erectile disorder affects 10% to 20% of all men and constitutes about half the complaints of sexual dysfunction in men. In young men, the disorder is uncommon, and the cause is usually psychological.

### Orgasm Disorders
### Female Orgasmic Disorder

*Female orgasmic disorder*, sometimes referred to as *inhibited female orgasm* or *anorgasmia*, is defined as the recurrent or persistent inhibition of female orgasm as manifested by the recurrent delay in, or absence of, orgasm after a normal sexual excitement phase (achieved by masturbation or coitus). It may be a lifelong disorder (i.e., never having achieved orgasm) or acquired (i.e., having had at least one orgasm and then having difficulties). The prevalence of either type of this disorder is estimated at 30% (Sadock & Sadock, 2008). Psychological factors (including fears of pregnancy, rejection, or loss of control), hostility, and cultural or societal restrictions may be causative factors. Some evidence suggests that female orgasmic disorder may be inherited.

## INTEGRATIVE THERAPY

### Nonhormonal Treatment of Menopausal Symptoms

Warnings about the risk for breast cancer and strokes have led increasing numbers of women to request nonhormonal treatments for perimenopausal and menopausal symptoms related to sexual arousal, but relatively few high-quality studies examine these treatments (Hickey, Saunders, & Stuckey, 2007).

One herbal treatment that has received attention as possibly reducing these symptoms due to its estrogenlike effects is black cohosh (*Cimicifuga racemosa*), which is sold as a dietary supplement. Concerns have been expressed, however, regarding both its minor adverse effects, such as gastrointestinal problems, and its more serious adverse effects, such as liver toxicity. Despite black cohosh's availability and marketing as a treatment for sexual dysfunction related to menopause, a search of literature reveals little data as to its efficacy. The bottom line is that women do not have enough information about any herbal therapy, including black cohosh, that may promote sexual responsiveness.

**Sources:** Cumming, G.P., Herald, J., Moncur, R., et al. (2007). Women's attitudes to hormone replacement therapy, alternative therapy, and sexual health: A web-based survey. *Menopause International, 13*, 79–83. doi:10.1258/175404507780796424; and Hickey, C., Saunders, B., & Stuckey, B. (2007). Non-hormonal treatments for menopausal symptoms. *Maturitas, 57*, 85–89. doi:10.1016/j.maturitas.2007.02.016.

### Male Orgasmic Disorder

In *male orgasmic disorder*, sometimes called *inhibited orgasm* or *retarded ejaculation*, a man achieves ejaculation during sexual activity only with great difficulty. A man with a lifelong orgasmic disorder has never been able to ejaculate during coitus; this condition may result from a rigid background in which sex is considered a sin (Rose, 2005). Lifelong orgasmic disorder is an uncommon diagnosis. Acquired orgasmic disorder, on the other hand, develops after previously normal functioning and is fairly common. Interpersonal problems may be the cause. Physical conditions, substance abuse, and prescribed medications may also precipitate this problem and should be assessed. The prevalence of male orgasmic disorder has been reported at 5% (Sadock & Sadock, 2008).

### Premature Ejaculation

In cases of premature ejaculation, a man persistently or recurrently achieves orgasm and ejaculation before he wishes to. Diagnosis is made when a man regularly ejaculates before or immediately after the penis attempts penetration. The patient's age, the newness of the relationship, and how often the man has intercourse should be considered. About 35% to 40% of men who are treated for sexual disorders complain of premature ejaculation (Lue, Giuliano, Montorsi, et al., 2004). Physical factors may be involved; for example, some men may be more tactilely sensitive and respond more intensely to stimulation. Psychological factors include fear about performance and stressful relationships in which the man feels hurried.

### Sexual Pain Disorders

#### Dyspareunia

Dyspareunia—recurrent or persistent genital pain—can occur in either men or women during or after intercourse. Dyspareunia is more common in women and is frequently associated with vaginismus (Basson, Althof, Davis, et al., 2004). Psychological factors include a history of childhood abuse or sexual assault and anxiety about sex, but the pain is real and makes sex unpleasant at the least and unbearable in extreme cases.

#### Vaginismus

Vaginismus is an involuntary constriction response of the muscles that close the vagina. This condition interferes with penetration and intercourse and may even be elicited during a normal gynecological examination with a speculum (Basson, Althof, Davis et al., 2004).

### Other Sexual Dysfunctions and Problems

*Sexual dysfunction due to a general medical condition* includes sexual desire disorders, orgasm disorders, and sexual pain disorders, but the cause of each is related to a medical condition, such as cardiovascular, neurological, or endocrine disease.

The medical diagnosis *substance-induced sexual dysfunction* is used when evidence of substance intoxication or withdrawal is apparent from the patient's history, physical examination, or laboratory findings. Distressing sexual dysfunction occurs within a month of significant substance intoxication or withdrawal. Specified substances include alcohol, amphetamines or related substances, cocaine, opioids, sedatives, hypnotics, antianxiety agents, and other known and unknown substances. The abuse of recreational substances can have a variety of effects on sexual functioning. In small doses, many substances enhance sexual performance. With continued use, however, sexual difficulties become the norm.

*Sexual dysfunction not otherwise specified* is a category that covers sexual dysfunctions that cannot be classified under one of the other categories. Examples include the experience of physiological sexual excitement and orgasm with no erotic sensation, including even when under anaesthesia. Women with a condition similar to premature ejaculation are classified as having this disorder. Disorders of excessive, rather than inhibited, sexual dysfunction (e.g., compulsive masturbation or coitus [sex addiction] or genital pain occurring during masturbation) may be classified in this category.

Sexual problems can also result from head trauma, chromosomal abnormalities, and psychosis. Patients who have experienced head trauma with damage to the frontal lobe of the brain may display symptoms of promiscuity, poor judgement, inability to recognize triggers that set off sexual desires, and poor impulse control.

Patients with schizophrenia may experience an alteration in sex drive only during the acute phase of illness or on an ongoing basis, depending partly on the severity of the illness. While schizophrenia is not necessarily associated with sexual dysfunction or deviant sexual behaviour, the symptoms of schizophrenia and even the treatment with antipsychotic medications may make the patient vulnerable to disturbances in sexual functioning and often cause the patient to be childlike and passive in relationships. In addition, patients with chronic schizophrenia have difficulty communicating their needs and concerns to others. For the patient with schizophrenia, self-concept and ego strength deteriorate over time, further decreasing the patient's ability to develop or maintain intimate relationships. The primary goal of the treatment team while the patient with schizophrenia is hospitalized is the control of acute symptoms. Sometimes the acute symptoms present as delusions, which can be sexual or be of a paranoid type that drives the patient away from meaningful relationships and produces a sexual problem due to the resulting alienation. Delusions may also be of a grandiose nature, with the patient believing himself or herself to be a great lover or someone who has a "special mission" of a sexual nature.

## EPIDEMIOLOGY

The prevalence of specific sexual dysfunctions was addressed in the previous discussion; however, some general statements may be made concerning these disorders as a category. Overall, they are more common in women than in men (Shafer, 2008) and become more prevalent with age. In later life, 20% to 30% of men and 40% to 45% of women report difficulties (Becker & Stinson, 2008).

## CO-MORBIDITY

Sexual functioning may be adversely affected any time there is a disturbance in an individual's ability to develop and maintain stable relationships—an outcome especially likely for patients with schizophrenia who are experiencing difficulty coping with stress, a decrease in reality-based orientation to the world, and defence mechanisms that lead to withdrawn behaviour. Sexual dysfunction may also be associated with depression and personality disorders (Becker & Stinson, 2008). However, several physical conditions are also related to sexual dysfunction (see Table 22-1).

## ETIOLOGY

Pioneers in the study of human sexuality included Helen Singer Kaplan (1929–1995). According to Kaplan (1974), sexual dysfunctions are the result of a combination of factors, such as:
- Misinformation or ignorance regarding sexual and social interaction
- Unconscious guilt and anxiety regarding sex
- Anxiety related to performance, especially in the case of erectile and orgasmic dysfunction
- Poor communication between partners about feelings and what they desire sexually

Additional factors related to sexual dysfunction have since been identified, including unacknowledged sexual orientation (may lead to poor performance with the opposite sex), sexual trauma, or the presence of one sexual problem that can lead to another (e.g., difficulty maintaining an erection may lead to hypoactive sexual desire [Becker & Stinson, 2008]).

## APPLICATION OF THE NURSING PROCESS
### ASSESSMENT
#### Self-Assessment

Despite a learned fearlessness when it comes to addressing other intimate issues, nurses, as well as other health care providers, often find the topic of sexuality a source of discomfort. Although most recognize that addressing sexuality is part of holistic care, many do not routinely include the topic when doing assessments (Mick, 2007). According to Dhalwani (2008), our discomfort in assessing sexual history is related to personal embarrassment, concerns about embarrassing the patient, poor training, inexperience, inadequate time, and beliefs that sexual history is not important. Indeed, you may experience discomfort exploring sexual issues with patients, fearing that this discussion will be embarrassing to both you and the patient. You may fear that you will not know what questions to ask or why the questions should be asked. Our views regarding sexuality are based on our individual beliefs about ourselves as human beings and on what is learned from older individuals such as parents. Multiple factors, including societal attitudes and traditions, parental views, cultural practices, spiritual and religious teaching, socioeconomic status, and education, affect our sexual behaviours and our attitudes toward the sexual behaviours of others, including our patients.

Nursing curricula typically have a deficiency in training nurses in the fundamentals of sexuality and nursing care (Walsh Brennan, Barnsteiner, de Leon Siantz, et al., 2012). When a nurse is interviewing patients, concerns related to age and gender differences are understandable. If the patient is approximately your age, you might worry that talking about sexuality may not be appropriate or that the patient might conclude that you are a little too interested. Discussing issues related to sexuality with people who are your parents' or grandparents' age may also create a level of discomfort, especially if you grew up in a home where such topics were avoided, and you had to rely on your friends for information (or misinformation) about sex.

Remembering your position as a professional and addressing the topics in a tone and manner appropriate to a professional will increase your comfort, along with the patient's. Patients want to know how, for example, medications or treatments will affect their relationships and ability to have satisfying sex lives. Nurses can set a comfort level for discussing such issues and fostering opportunities to address feelings and fears. Also, letting the patient know why you are asking such personal questions increases openness and cooperation. For example, "People who are depressed sometimes find that the depression affects their sexual desire. Since you have been depressed, have you noticed a change in your interest in sex?" Sometimes a more subtle approach that shifts the focus away from the patient is

## TABLE 22-1   MEDICAL CONDITIONS AND SURGICAL PROCEDURES THAT CAUSE SEXUAL DYSFUNCTION

| SYSTEM/STATE | ORGANIC DISORDERS | SEXUAL IMPAIRMENT |
|---|---|---|
| Endocrine | Hypothyroidism, adrenal dysfunction, hypogonadism, diabetes mellitus | Low libido, impotence, decreased vaginal lubrication, early impotence |
| Vascular | Hypertension, atherosclerosis, stroke, venous insufficiency, sickle-cell disorder | Impotence, but ejaculation and libido intact |
| Neurological | Spinal cord damage, diabetic neuropathy, herniated disk, alcoholic neuropathy, multiple sclerosis, temporal lobe epilepsy | Sexual disorder—early signs: low or high libido, impotence, impaired orgasm |
| Genital | *Male*—priapism, Peyronie's disease, urethritis, prostatitis, hydrocele<br>*Female*—Imperforate hymen, vaginitis, pelvic inflammatory disease, endometriosis | Low libido, impotence<br>Vaginismus, dyspareunia, low libido, decreased arousal |
| Systemic | Renal, pulmonary, hepatic, advanced malignancies, infections | Low libido, impotence, decreased arousal |
| Psychiatric | | Low libido, erectile dysfunction<br>Increased libido<br>Low libido, erectile dysfunction, reduced vaginal lubrication, anorgasmia, "anti-fantasies" focusing on partner's negative qualities (OCD only) |
| | Depression<br>Bipolar disorder (manic phase)<br>Generalized anxiety disorder, panic disorder, post-traumatic stress disorder (PTSD), obsessive-compulsive disorder (OCD)<br><br>Schizophrenia<br>Personality disorders (passive-aggressive, obsessive-compulsive, histrionic) | Low desire, bizarre sexual fantasies<br>Low libido, erectile dysfunction, premature ejaculation, anorgasmia |
| Surgical–postoperative | *Male*—Prostatectomy, abdominal–perineal bowel resection<br>*Female*—Episiotomy, vaginal prolapse repair, oophorectomy<br>*Male and female*—Leg amputation, colostomy, ileostomy | Impotence, no loss of libido, ejaculatory impairment<br>Dyspareunia, vaginismus, decreased lubrication<br>Mechanical difficulties in sex, low self-image, fear of odour |

**Source:** Data from Shafer, L.C. (2008). Sexual disorders and sexual dysfunction. In T.A. Stern, J.F. Rosenbaum, M. Fava, et al. (Eds.), *Massachusetts General Hospital comprehensive clinical psychiatry* (pp. 487–497). St. Louis, MO: Mosby.

helpful. "Since you have been depressed, has your husband felt as though you are less interested in him?"

Perhaps the most helpful consideration is recognizing that assessing sexuality is part of holistic nursing care. Your role and responsibility are to assist the patient in dealing with responses to illness or the treatment of the illness. Understanding your patient's concerns, acknowledging the patient's discomfort, and providing useful feedback will enhance your professional abilities to care for your patient and perhaps even improve self-understanding.

Patients may cue the nurse about the presence of sexual concerns without explicitly verbalizing them. Box 22-1 presents a discussion of these cues.

### General Assessment

Many psychiatric hospitals use a nursing history tool that is biologically oriented but typically has few questions about sexual functioning, but sexual assessment requires both subjective and objective data. Health history questions pertaining to the reproductive system should not be limited to menstrual history, parity, history of sexually transmitted diseases, method of contraception, and questions regarding safer-sex practices. The sexual history should include the patient's perception of physiological functioning and behavioural, emotional, and spiritual aspects of sexuality. It also should address cultural and religious beliefs with regard to sexual behaviour and sexual knowledge base.

The nurse may ask the patient about the presence of discomfort in sexual functioning. Usually, it is more comfortable for the patient if the nurse first asks questions in a general manner and then proceeds to the patient's experience. For example: "Some people who are prescribed this medication find it difficult to achieve an erection. Have you had this problem?" This technique allows the patient to feel that he or she is not alone

## BOX 22-1   PATIENT CUES THAT MAY INDICATE CONCERNS ABOUT SEXUALITY

**Nonverbal Behaviours**

- Showing discomfort by blushing, looking away, making tight fists, fidgeting, crying
- Openly engaging in overt sexual behaviours (e.g., touching own body parts, masturbating, exposing genitals, placing nurse's hand on genitals, making sexually suggestive sounds)

**Verbal Behaviours**

- Telling sexually explicit jokes
- Making sexual comments about the nurse
- Asking inappropriate questions about the nurse's sexual activity
- Discussing sexual exploits
- Expressing concern about relationship with partner:
  - "I don't feel the same about my partner."
  - "My partner doesn't feel the same about me."
  - "We're not as close."
  - "Our relationship has changed."
  - "My personal life has changed."
- Expressing concern that sexuality has been diminished (e.g., feeling less of a man, less of a woman):
  - "I've lost my manhood."
  - "I'm not as desirable as I once was."
- Expressing concern over lack of sexual desire:
  - "I'm not interested in sex anymore."
  - "My desire has changed."
  - "I'm not the man (or woman) I used to be."
  - "We don't click anymore."
- Expressing concern over sexual performance:
  - "I don't get wet."
  - "I've lost my power."
  - "Will I still be able to get hard?"
  - "What will happen to my ability to perform?"
  - "I can't perform like I used to."
- Expressing concern about one's love life:
  - "My love life has changed."
  - "The spark is gone."
- Expressing concern over the sexual impact of medications, surgery, or some other medical treatment:
  - "Will this medication interfere with my sex life?"
  - "Will I still be able to perform sexually after surgery?"

in experiencing such effects. Table 22-2 provides facilitative statements for the interviewer conducting a sexual assessment.

A comprehensive assessment of sexual dysfunction in females includes an assessment of the symptoms experienced and the current and past context of symptoms. It is important to identify the nature and duration of the patient's relationships, societal values, beliefs, traumas, and losses that impact the sexual dysfunction. Also, the role of the partner and level of distress caused by symptoms should be explored (Basson, Althof, Davis, et al., 2004). For males, a sexual function assessment should include erectile insufficiency, altered sexual desire, ejaculation, orgasm, sexually related genital pain disorders, and partner sexual function (Lue, Giuliano, Montorsi, et al., 2004).

During the assessment, both the nurse and the patient are free to ask questions and clarify information. It is reasonable to defer a lengthy sexual health assessment when acute psychiatric symptoms preclude a calm, thoughtful discussion. As symptoms subside and rapport is developed, the assessment may be resumed. With experience, the nurse is able to identify those patients who are at greater risk for difficulties in sexual functioning. This includes patients with a history of certain medical problems or surgical procedures (see Table 22-1) and patients taking some medications (see Table 22-3).

### ASSESSMENT GUIDELINES
#### Sexual Dysfunction

1. The interviewer should reflect on his or her personal biases and judgemental attitudes that could block open discussion of sexual issues.
2. A sexual assessment should be conducted in a setting that allows privacy and eliminates distractions.
3. Although note taking may be necessary for the beginner, it can be distracting to the patient and interrupt the flow of the interview. When note taking is necessary, it should be unobtrusive and kept to a minimum.
4. Good eye contact, relaxed posture, and friendly facial expressions communicate openness and receptivity on the part of the nurse and facilitate the patient's comfort.

## DIAGNOSIS

A comprehensive sexual assessment can reveal areas of sexual concern and dysfunction for the patient. These data are analyzed to determine the appropriate nursing diagnoses. Sexuality is the eighth domain of the North American Nursing Diagnosis Association International (NANDA-I), (Herdman, 2012). This domain includes sexual identity, sexual function, and reproduction. Priority nursing diagnoses, their definitions, and possible etiology follow from this NANDA domain.

The following nursing diagnoses are included under the sexuality domain:

- Sexual dysfunction
- Ineffective sexuality pattern
- Ineffective childbearing process
- Readiness for enhanced childbearing process
- Risk for ineffective childbearing process
- Risk for disturbed maternal–fetal dyad

Ineffective sexuality pattern is indicated by expressions of concern regarding one's own sexuality. Possible etiology may include the following:

- Impaired relationship with significant other
- Knowledge deficit about alternative responses to illness

## OUTCOMES IDENTIFICATION

Some sexual problems can be remedied by achieving short-term outcomes that use education as a nursing intervention. Frequently, sexual myths and misinformation can be corrected, giving the patient almost instant relief from perceived problems.

| TABLE 22-2 | FACILITATIVE STATEMENTS FOR THE INTERVIEWER CONDUCTING A SEXUAL ASSESSMENT | |
|---|---|---|

| PURPOSE | FACILITATIVE STATEMENT |
|---|---|
| To provide a rationale for a question | "As a nurse, I'm concerned about all aspects of your health. Many individuals have concern about sexual matters, especially when they are sick or having other health problems." |
| To give statements of generality or normality | "Most people are hesitant to discuss ..." "Many people worry about feeling ..." "Many people have concerns about ..." |
| To identify sexual dysfunction | "Most people have difficulties sometime during their sexual relationships. What have yours been?" |
| To obtain information | "The degree to which people have sexual outlets varies considerably. Some have sexual partners. Some obtain sexual satisfaction through masturbation. Others need no outlet at all. What has been your pattern?" |
| To identify sexual myths | "While growing up, most of us have heard some sexual myths or half-truths that continue to puzzle us. Are there any that come to mind?" |
| To determine whether sexual orientation is a source of conflict | "How do you feel about your sexual orientation?" |
| To determine whether gender identity is a source of conflict | "Do you identify as a man or a woman? Or does neither of these classifications describe your sense of self?" |
| To identify an older person's concerns about sexual function | "Many people, as they get older, believe or worry that aging signals the end of their sex life. Much misinformation continues this myth. What is your understanding about sexuality during the later years? How has the passage of time affected your sexuality (sex life)?" |
| To obtain and give information (miscellaneous areas) | "Frequently people have questions about ..." "What questions do you have about ..." "What would you like to know about ..." |
| To close the history | "Is there anything further in the area of sexuality that you would like to bring up now?" |

**Source:** Adapted from Green, R. (1975). *Human sexuality: A health practitioner's text.* Baltimore, MD: Williams & Wilkins.

The *Nursing Outcomes Classification (NOC)* (Moorhead, Johnson, Maas, et al., 2008) identifies a number of outcomes related to sexual dysfunction or ineffective sexuality patterns. Included are *Abuse recovery: Emotional/physical/sexual, Sexual functioning, Sexual identity, Role performance,* and *Self-esteem.* Table 22-4 provides selected intermediate and short-term indicators for *Sexual functioning* and *Sexual identity.*

## PLANNING

Planning nursing care for the patient with a sexual dysfunction may occur as part of care for a coexisting disorder since nurses may encounter such patients in any setting in which the patient seeks treatment for any of a variety of conditions. Once the assessment is completed, priority nursing diagnoses are developed and implemented in collaboration with the patient.

## IMPLEMENTATION

While all nurses need to be able to facilitate a discussion about sexuality with the patient, an understanding of sexual function and dysfunction is essential for nurses who work in psychiatry, as well as almost any specialty area in nursing, including

oncology, cardiology, and neurology. To be a facilitator, the nurse must be nonjudgemental, have basic knowledge of sexual functioning, and have the ability to conduct a basic sexual assessment. Once the assessment is completed, the nurse may have the knowledge, skills, and judgement to address the patient's sexual health concern. Or the nurse may need to know when and to whom to refer the patient with a sexual complaint. Depending on the nature of the problem, the patient may need a referral to a professional such as a marital counsellor, psychiatrist, gynecologist, urologist, clinical nurse specialist, or sex therapist.

Box 22-2 provides sample interventions for sexual counselling from the *Nursing Interventions Classification (NIC)* (Bulechek, Butcher, & Dochterman, 2008).

### Pharmacological Interventions

Treatments for sexual dysfunction are increasingly becoming the target of the pharmaceutical industry. Despite an increased interest in treatment for hypoactive sexual desire disorder in women, there is a deficiency of approved treatments, and treatment guidelines are negligible—partly due to vague criteria for this disorder (Segraves & Woodard, 2006). Most of the available treatments for sexual dysfunction are targeted at male

## TABLE 22-3  MEDICATIONS THAT CAN CAUSE SEXUAL DYSFUNCTION

| CATEGORY | MEDICATION | SEXUAL SIDE EFFECT |
|---|---|---|
| Cardiovascular medications | Methyldopa | Low libido, impotence, anorgasmia |
| | Thiazides (diuretics) | Low libido, impotence, decreased lubrication |
| | Clonidine (Catapres) | Impotence, anorgasmia |
| | Propranolol (Inderal) | Low libido |
| | Digoxin (Lanoxin) | Gynecomastia, low libido, impotence |
| Gastrointestinal medications | Cimetidine | Low libido, impotence |
| Hormones | Estrogen (also called *oestrogens*) | Low libido in men |
| | Progesterone (also known as *P4* [pregn-4-ene-3,20-dione]) | Low libido, impotence |
| Sedatives | Alcohol | Higher doses cause sexual problems |
| | Barbiturates (phenobarbital) | Impotence |
| Antianxiety medications | Alprazolam (Xanax) | Low libido, delayed ejaculation |
| | Diazepam (Valium) | |
| Antipsychotics | Haloperidol (Haldol) | Low libido, impotence, anorgasmia |
| Antidepressants | *MAOIs (Phenelzine [Nardil]) | Impotence, retarded ejaculation, anorgasmia |
| | Tricyclics (imipramine [Impril]) | Low libido, impotence, retarded ejaculation |
| | *SSRIs (fluoxetine [Prozac]; sertraline [Zoloft]) | Low libido, impotence, retarded ejaculation |
| | Atypical (trazodone [Trazorel]) | Priapism, retarded or retrograde ejaculation |
| Antimanic medications | Lithium | Low libido, impotence |
| Anticonvulsants | Carbamazepine (CBZ) (Tegretol) | Low libido, impotence, priapism |
| Opiates | Oxycodone (Percocet) | Low libido, orgasmic dysfunction |

*MAOIs: monoamine oxidase inhibitors; SSRIs: selective serotonin reuptake inhibitors.
**Sources:** Data from Basson, R. (2011). Female sexual dysfunction. In J. Gray (Ed.), *Therapeutic choices*. Ottawa: Canadian Pharmaceutical Society; Basson, R. (2011). Male sexual dysfunction. In J. Gray (Ed.), *Therapeutic choices*. Ottawa: Canadian Pharmaceutical Society; Shafer, L.C. (2008). Sexual disorders and sexual dysfunction. In T.A. Stern, J.F. Rosenbaum, M. Fava, et al. (Eds.), *Massachusetts General Hospital comprehensive clinical psychiatry* (pp. 487–497). St Louis, MO: Mosby.

## TABLE 22-4  *NOC* OUTCOMES FOR SEXUAL DYSFUNCTION

| NURSING OUTCOME AND DEFINITION | INTERMEDIATE INDICATORS | SHORT-TERM INDICATORS |
|---|---|---|
| *Sexual functioning:* Integration of physical, social, emotional, and intellectual aspects of sexual expression and performance | Expresses ability to perform sexually despite physical imperfections<br>Expresses comfort with sexual expression | Attains sexual arousal<br>Adapts sexual technique as needed<br>Sustains penile or clitoral erection through orgasm |
| *Sexual identity:* Acknowledgement and acceptance of own sexual identity | Challenges negative images of sexual self<br>Reports healthy sexual functioning | Affirms self as a sexual being<br>Exhibits clear sense of sexual orientation<br>Seeks social support |

**Source:** Data from Moorhead, S., Johnson, M., Maas, M., et al. (Eds.). (2008). *Nursing outcomes classification (NOC)* (4th ed.). St. Louis, MO: Mosby.

dysfunction. In fact, there are no treatments approved by Health Canada for female sexual disorders (Research Highlight box). Table 22-5 summarizes treatments for sexual dysfunction.

### Health Teaching and Health Promotion

While medication may be the treatment of choice for certain conditions, such as premature ejaculation secondary and erectile dysfunction, nurses should help patients weigh the risks and benefits of any type of pharmacotherapy. Men with

situational premature ejaculation can be treated with pharmacotherapy, behavioural therapy, or both, and those men with significant contributing psychogenic or relationship factors may benefit from concomitant pharmacotherapy and behavioural therapy. Behavioural therapy may augment pharmacotherapy to enhance relapse prevention (Lue, Giuliano, Montorsi, et al., 2004).

Helping patients to evaluate for themselves the benefits and the risks of psychopharmacotherapy empowers patients to

| BOX 22-2 | *NIC* INTERVENTIONS FOR SEXUAL COUNSELLING |
|---|---|

*Definition of* sexual counselling: Use of an interactive helping process focusing on the need to make adjustments in sexual practice or to enhance coping with a sexual event or disorder

Activities*:
- Establish a therapeutic relationship based on trust and respect.
- Provide privacy and ensure confidentiality.
- Discuss the effect of the illness or health situation on sexuality.
- Discuss the effect of medications on sexuality, as appropriate.
- Avoid displaying aversion to an altered body part.
- Provide factual information about sexual myths and misinformation that patient may verbalize.
- Provide reassurance that current and new sexual practices are healthy, as appropriate.
- Include the spouse or sexual partner in the counselling as much as possible, as appropriate.
- Refer patient to a sex therapist, as appropriate.

*Partial list.
**Source:** Data from Bulechek, G.M., Butcher, H.K., & Dochterman, J.M. (Eds.). (2008). *Nursing interventions classification (NIC)* (5th ed.). St. Louis, MO: Mosby.

choose the best course of action for them and helps them to be informed patients (Higgins, 2007).

## Advanced-Practice Interventions

Advanced-practice nurses can become qualified to treat sexual dysfunction through advanced training and certification. General therapies include psychoanalytic, couples and group therapy, and hypnotherapy. The treatment depends on the cause of the sexual dysfunction—for example, treatment of vaginismus involves psychoeducation, cognitive behavioural therapy, and the use of vaginal inserts, pelvic floor physiotherapy, and electromyography (EMG) biofeedback (Basson, Althof, Davis, et al., 2004). Some specific therapies available for sexual dysfunction include the following:

- Sensate focus: a therapeutic treatment in which patients progress from general touching and cuddling without intercourse to more intimate forms of expression
- Systematic desensitization: a combination of relaxation exercises and sexually anxiety-producing stimuli
- Masturbation training: an approach that helps women learn about their bodies and their responses in order to understand their sexual responsiveness (especially helpful in women who have never had an orgasm)

## RESEARCH HIGHLIGHT

### *Testosterone for Postmenopausal Women With Low Libido*

**Source:** Davis, S., Moreau, M., Kroll, R., et al. (2008). Testosterone for low libido in postmenopausal women not taking estrogen. *New England Journal of Medicine, 359,* 2005–2017. doi:10.1056/NEJMoa0707302.

#### Problem

Nearly one third of women in the United States may experience lack of sexual interest, and about one fourth cannot achieve orgasm. Postmenopausal women in particular can be distressed by a loss of sexual interest. When taken along with estrogen and progesterone, testosterone has been demonstrated to increase sexual interest in postmenopausal women; however, many women are (understandably) reluctant to take estrogen or progesterone due to the increased risk of breast cancer, heart attacks, and strokes.

#### Purpose of Study

The purpose of this study was to determine if testosterone, a hormone that is actually more prevalent in the bloodstreams of premenopausal women than estrogen is, would improve sexual well-being in postmenopausal women.

#### Methods

This international study included 814 naturally or surgically postmenopausal women. They were randomly selected to be in one of two groups. One group received a testosterone patch, and the other received a placebo patch. The length of the study was 52 weeks.

#### Key Findings

- Participants who received the testosterone patch reported an average increase of 2.1 satisfying sexual episodes per month versus a 0.7 increase among the placebo group.
- Of participants who reported benefits from the treatment, 85% said they would like to continue the treatment.
- A significant reduction in distress was also found in participants receiving treatment.
- Of women who had the testosterone patch, 30% reported adrenergic adverse effects such as unwanted hair growth.
- Breast cancer was diagnosed in four women in the treatment group but none in the placebo group. (One woman was diagnosed in the first four months of the study, and another had symptoms prior to the study.)

#### Implications for Nursing Practice

Testosterone is already being widely prescribed off-label (without formal Food and Drug Administration [FDA] approval) in the United States, primarily to postmenopausal women who are experiencing a decreased sex drive. The study supports this prescribing practice yet calls into question the risk to benefit ratio. The report of four cases of breast cancer in the treatment group may be coincidental, but certainly this type of therapy will be studied more.

Menopause is a mystery to many women, and its symptoms may be bewildering. Sexual interest and emotional distress are two symptoms relevant to psychiatric mental health nurses, professionals who are in a position to educate women about their options. Keeping current in research by reading studies such as these improves nurses' ability to provide the best care possible for their patients.

| TABLE 22-5 | PHARMACOLOGICAL, PSYCHOSOCIAL, AND OTHER TREATMENTS FOR SEXUAL DYSFUNCTION | | |
|---|---|---|---|
| **SEXUAL DISORDER** | **PHARMACOLOGICAL TREATMENT** | **PSYCHOSOCIAL APPROACHES** | **OTHER** |
| Hypoactive sexual desire disorder (absence of desire) | Menopausal women: low-dose testosterone gel (can be prescribed for women taking estrogen) | Counselling when the couple's emotional intimacy is insufficient or to address psychological factors that are inhibiting the effectiveness of sexual stimulation<br>Sensate focus exercises<br>Masturbation training<br>Erotic material | Screen for and treat mood disorders.<br>Address biological factors that limit the effectiveness of stimulation. |
| Sexual aversion disorder (fear and avoidance of sexual activity) | Tricyclic antidepressants<br>Antianxiety medications | Sensate focus exercises<br>Masturbation training<br>Erotic material<br>Systematic desensitization<br>Sex therapy | |
| Female sexual arousal disorder | There are no approved pharmacological treatments<br>Local estrogen used in estrogen-deficient states—conjugated estrogen vaginal cream (Premarin)<br>Vaginal lubricants (e.g., Astroglide) or moisturizers (e.g., Replens) used for intercourse | Cognitive behavioural therapy (CBT)<br>Sexual therapy<br>Mindfulness meditation | Address medications and any possible adverse effects and other biological factors such as depression.<br>Counsel or refer when the couple's emotional intimacy is insufficient.<br>Address psychological factors. |
| Male erectile disorder | Phosphodiesterase type 5 (PDE5) inhibitors: sildenafil (Viagra), vardenafil (Levitra), tadalafil (Cialis)<br>Prostaglandin E1 analogues:<br>Alprostadil intracavernosal injection (Caverject), alprostadil by urethral instillation (Muse) | Sensate focus exercises<br>Group therapy<br>Hypnotherapy<br>Systematic desensitization<br>Psychodynamic therapy<br>Couples therapy | Suggest a vacuum erection device. |
| Female orgasmic disorder | Sildenafil (Viagra) | Masturbation training<br>Couples therapy<br>Kegel vaginal exercises | |
| Male orgasmic disorder | Sildenafil (Viagra) | Masturbatory training<br>Systematic desensitization | Address sexual avoidance.<br>Address lack of subjective sexual arousal.<br>Address intra- and interpersonal psychological issues. |
| Premature ejaculation | SSRIs to slow down the ejaculatory reflex by increasing serotonergic transmission: paroxetine, clomipramine, sertraline, fluoxetine<br>Combined PDE5 inhibitors to target those patients with erectile dysfunction<br>Intracavernosal therapy for those with severe premature ejaculation (aids erectile persistence after ejaculation so as to improve partner satisfaction) | Techniques:<br>Stop/start<br>Squeeze<br>Quiet | |

**Sources:** Data from Basson, R. (2011). Female sexual dysfunction. In J. Gray (Ed.), *Therapeutic choices*. Ottawa: Canadian Pharmaceutical Society; Basson, R. (2011). Male sexual dysfunction. In J. Gray (Ed.), *Therapeutic choices*. Ottawa: Canadian Pharmaceutical Society; Becker, J.V., & Stinson, J.D. (2008). Human sexuality and sexual dysfunctions. In R.E. Hales, S.C. Yudofsky, & Gabbard, G.O. (Eds.), *Textbook of psychiatry* (5th ed., pp. 711–728). Washington, DC: American Psychiatric Publishing; and Shafer, L.C. (2008). Sexual disorders and sexual function. In T.A. Stern, J.F. Rosenbaum, M. Fava, et al. (Eds.), *Massachusetts General Hospital comprehensive clinical psychiatry* (pp. 487–497). Philadelphia: Mosby.

**VIGNETTE**

Maria is a 67-year-old woman who has been divorced for many years. She is seeing the nurse prior to having her annual checkup. She has recently started an intimate relationship with a 75-year-old widower. Maria has not been sexually active for five years, and she confides in her nurse practitioner, "I really haven't even thought about sex for so long." After discussing and eliminating the possibility of a physiological cause for her lack of interest in sex, Maria's nurse practitioner recommends that Maria begins to become comfortable with her body by practising masturbation. During the assessment, Maria and the nurse practitioner discuss healthy communication, safer-sex practices, and topical estrogen for vaginal lubrication. Maria feels comfortable and begins talking again about "how great life can be if you have the right partner."

## EVALUATION

Acceptance of sexual dysfunction (e.g., anorgasmia) is a part, but not necessarily the defining characteristic, of treatment. The degree to which the patient does not harbour negative attitudes about sex is also important. Nurses should evaluate the expected outcomes of the interventions to treat sexual dysfunction and the level of control and personal satisfaction achieved by the patient.

## SEXUAL DISORDERS

### CLINICAL PICTURE

In the first part of this chapter, we examined normal sexual functioning and sexual dysfunction. We now turn our attention to sexual disorders—psychiatric disorders in which sexual problems are considered to be socially atypical, have the potential to disrupt meaningful relationships, and may result in insult or even significant injury to other people. Two types of sexual disorders—gender dysphoria and paraphilias—will be described.

### Gender Dysphoria

When we inquire about the birth of a new infant, one of the first things we want to know is whether the baby is a boy or a girl. Actually, we are asking about the sex of the child (i.e., whether its chromosomes are XX or XY). However, biological assignment does not determine whether individuals think of themselves as male or female. Gender identity, the sense of maleness or femaleness, is not inborn but usually is established by the age of 3 years (Becker & Johnson, 2008). Although we may be predisposed to male or female gender orientation, gender identity is mainly a product of how we are raised.

When biological sex differs from gender identity, the individual experiences gender dysphoria, a sexual disorder characterized by the strong feeling of being the wrong sex or the feeling that one's body is inconsistent with the internal sense of being either male or female (Walsh Brennan, Barnsteiner, de Leon Siantz, et al., 2012). Those with gender dysphoria experience some degree of incongruity between their anatomical sex and their gender identity.

Little is known about the origins of gender dysphoria, but childhood patterns that continue into adolescence or adulthood seem to be fairly consistent. As early as 2 to 4 years of age, some children may have cross-gender interests and activities. However, only a small percentage of children who display gender dysphoria characteristics will continue to show these characteristics into adolescence or adulthood. Those with gender dysphoria continue to prefer opposite-sex behaviour into adulthood. These individuals never consider themselves to be homosexual. The biological male who falls in love with a man believes himself actually to be a woman who loves that man. He might describe himself by saying, "I am a woman trapped in a man's body." Thus, a desire for congruity in gender identity and physiology becomes important for many individuals, resulting in the most extreme case of gender dysphoria, called transsexualism, characterized by a person wishing to change his or her anatomical sexual characteristics to those of the opposite sex (Hinderliter, 2010).

### Paraphilias

People do not consciously decide what arouses them sexually. Rather, during the maturation process, they discover the nature of their own sexual orientation and interests. Individuals differ from one another in terms of the types of partners they find to be erotically appealing and the types of behaviours they find to be erotically stimulating. They also differ in the intensity of the sexual drive, in the degree of difficulty they experience in trying to resist sexual urges, and in their attitudes about whether or not such urges should be resisted.

Paraphilias are distressing and repetitive sexual fantasies, urges, or behaviours. These fantasies, urges, or behaviours occur for a significant period of time and interfere with satisfactory sexual relations or with everyday functioning, and they cause a sense of distress for these individuals. Typically, they involve nonhuman articles, nonconsenting partners, or both. (Experimenting with paraphiliac behaviour from time to time does not constitute a disorder.) Paraphilias are further classified as fetishism, pedophilia, exhibitionism, voyeurism, transvestic fetishism, sexual sadism, frotteurism, and paraphilia not otherwise specified (NOS) (Hinderliter, 2010). These terms refer to acts or sexual stimuli that are outside of what society considers normal but are necessary for some individuals to experience desire, arousal, and orgasm (Sadock & Sadock, 2008).

### Fetishism

Fetishism is characterized by intense sexually arousing fantasies, urges, or behaviours in which the individual uses a nonliving object in a sexual manner. It is characterized by a sexual focus on objects—such as shoes, gloves, or stockings—that are intimately associated with the human body. The individual requires this object in order to become sexually aroused. This interest may replace sexual partners altogether or may be included as part of a consenting relationship. Fetishes may become all-consuming and destructive. They occur in more men than women (Sadock & Sadock, 2008).

## Pedophilia

Pedophilia is, unfortunately, the most common paraphilia. It involves sexual activity with a prepubescent child (generally 13 years or younger). This behaviour is unacceptable in most cultures, including Canada's, and represents a profound violation of the boundaries of the child. Because pedophilia is illegal, its exact incidence is unknown. The Criminal Code of Canada (1985) defines a number of criminal offences (e.g., genital fondling, oral sex) perpetrated against those under the age of 16. The nature of child molestation ranges from undressing and looking at the child to genital fondling or oral sex to penetration and even to torture (Shafer, 2008).

Although most people believe that girls are more frequently molested, 60% of identified victims are boys. Pedophiles who are attracted to females tend to prefer 8- to 10-year-old children, whereas those who are attracted to males prefer older children and teens. A significant number of pedophiles have previous or current involvement in voyeurism, exhibitionism, or rape (Sadock & Sadock, 2008).

## Exhibitionism

Exhibitionism, an illegal activity, is the intentional display of the genitals in a public place. Almost 100% of cases of exhibitionism involve a man exposing himself to a woman (e.g., walking around exposed in a busy shopping mall or exposing himself on a doorstep after ringing the doorbell). Excitement results from the anticipation of the act, and the individual masturbates while exposing himself or afterward. The person with exhibitionism becomes aroused by observers' responses of shock and even disgust, and some fantasize that the person will also be aroused by the experience and actually want to be with them sexually.

On the other hand, some people with exhibitionism experience deep shame and judge themselves by the same standard that society does and consider themselves perverts. They may cover their actions and live in intense fear that they will be recognized and embarrass themselves and their families.

Although exhibitionism is illegal, it seems to be done more for shock value than as a precursor to sexual assault. Actual contact is rarely sought. Since few people are arrested for this behaviour after age 40, it has been speculated that the disorder resolves with age (Shafer, 2008).

## Voyeurism

Voyeurism is another illegal activity. It is marked by the seeking of sexual arousal through viewing, usually secretly, other people in intimate situations (e.g., naked, in the process of disrobing, engaging in sexual activity). In the language of the layperson, a person who engages in this behaviour is called a "peeping Tom." The disorder often begins in adolescence and may become a chronic condition and the only type of sexual activity for the person. Voyeurism may be driven by anger and a need to retaliate. Typically, people who engage in voyeurism also engage in other compulsive sexual behaviour and are frequently addicted to viewing pornography and going to strip clubs.

Like an exhibitionist, a person who engages in voyeurism may also be consumed by dissonance. The drive to engage in this activity does not make sense, considering the lengths to which the voyeur goes and the risks taken. As with all obsessions and compulsions, the person's shame and anxiety are temporarily relieved by engaging in the very activity that brings it about.

## Transvestic Fetishism

In transvestic fetishism, sexual satisfaction is achieved by dressing in the clothing of the opposite gender. This behaviour is related to fetishism but often goes beyond the use of one particular object. Generally, transvestic fetishism develops early in life and is associated with someone with whom the person is closely associated, whether in a loving relationship or through abuse. Unlike in gender dysphoria, there are no sexual-orientation issues, and people with transvestic fetishism do not desire a surgical sex change. People with transvestic fetishism are usually heterosexual; many cross-dress only in specific sexual situations, and they often receive the cooperation and support of their partners. This paraphilia is more common in men than in women. Over time, some men, as well as some women, with transvestic fetishism may desire to dress and live permanently as the opposite sex.

## Sexual Sadism

Sadism is a term derived from the Marquis de Sade (1740–1814), a well-known French writer who was obsessed with sexual violence. Sexual sadism is the achievement of sexual satisfaction from the physical or psychological suffering (including humiliation) of the victim. The sadist inflicts pain and suffering on (usually) nonconsenting persons. Most people with this disorder are male, and the onset usually occurs prior to age 18 (Sadock & Sadock, 2008).

Consenting partners of sadists may be sexual masochists. Sexual masochism involves the achievement of sexual satisfaction by being humiliated, beaten, bound, or otherwise made to suffer. Sexual masochistic practices are more common among men than among women (Sadock & Sadock, 2008). In any case, consenting participants tend to know the related acts constitute a "game," and actual humiliation or pain is thereby avoided.

## Frotteurism

Frotteurism is characterized by rubbing or touching a nonconsenting person. In fact, the word *frotteurism* originates from the French word *frotter*, which means to "rub or scrape." The disorder is usually seen in men and typically occurs in busy public places, particularly in subways and buses, where the individual can escape after touching the victim (Becker & Johnson, 2008). People with this disorder often have no close relationships, and this sort of aggressive contact is their only means of sexual gratification (Sadock & Sadock, 2008).

## Paraphilia Not Otherwise Specified

The diagnosis of paraphilia not otherwise specified accounts for various paraphilias that do not meet the criteria for the other categories. Included in this grouping are the following:

- Telephone and computer scatologia—obscene phone calling to an unsuspecting person or sending obscene messages or video images by email
- Necrophilia—obsession with having a sexual encounter with a cadaver

- Partialism—a concentration of sexual activity on one part of the body to the exclusion of all other parts
- Zoophilia—incorporation of animals into sexual activity
- Urophilia—sexual activity that involves urinating on one's partner or being urinated on
- Hypoxyphilia—desire to achieve an altered state of consciousness secondary to hypoxia while experiencing orgasm; a medication such as nitrous oxide may be used to produce hypoxia

Many of the people involved in nonstandard sexual practices find no need for therapy because their sexual activities are carried out with a consenting adult partner, and they are neither illegal nor physically or emotionally harmful to either partner. If, however, the person is experiencing relationship difficulties, wishes to change the sexual behaviours, becomes involved in illegal activity, or is physically or emotionally harming others or being harmed, therapy is indicated.

## EPIDEMIOLOGY

Some parents report symptoms of gender identity disturbances that were apparent before the age of 3 (Sadock & Sadock, 2008). This condition is extremely uncommon and affects three to four times as many males as females (Becker & Johnson, 2008).

Although the paraphilias are uncommon, the repetitive and consuming nature of the disorders make the occurrence highly frequent (Sadock & Sadock, 2008). The behaviours associated with the disorder tend to peak in the decade between 15 and 25 years of age and then become virtually nonexistent by age 50. Patients with paraphilias often have more than one paraphilia, which can occur simultaneously or at different points in their lives.

## CO-MORBIDITY

Personality disorders are present in about 60% of people with gender dysphoria. The most common are borderline, antisocial, and narcissistic. Substance abuse and self-destructive behaviour are also common. Attention deficit hyperactivity disorders (ADHD) in childhood, substance abuse, phobic disorders, and major depression or dysthymia are strongly associated with paraphilias (Shafer, 2008).

## ETIOLOGY

### Biological Factors

While biological factors are not thought to cause sexual disorders, they are believed to influence their development (Becker & Johnson, 2008). Hormones may play a role since it has been determined that decreased levels of testosterone in males and increased levels in women are associated with transsexualism.

Various theories attempt to identify what predisposes an individual to the development of paraphilias, but these theories are far from conclusive since they have focused primarily on violent offenders. Some people with paraphilias have diseases of the temporal lobe (Becker & Stinson, 2008), and inappropriate sexual arousal has been linked to abnormal levels of androgens.

### Psychosocial Factors

Learning theorists suggest that the absence of same-sex role models may contribute to gender dysphoria. In this scenario, caregivers provide either covert or overt approval for cross-gender identification and behaviours. Psychoanalytic theorists have posited that male children who are deprived of their mothers seek to internally meld or become one with their mothers. This melding prevents them from developing fully as a separate entity. Clinical studies indicate that boys who have gender dysphoria have overly close relationships with their mothers and are disconnected from their fathers.

Psychoanalytic theories about the origin of fetishism and transvestism suggest that castration anxiety (overwhelming fear of damage to or loss of the penis) can cause males to seek a "safer" substitute for the mother, thus resulting in these paraphilias. The need for a safe substitute may also result in extreme behaviours such as pedophilia, exhibitionism, and voyeurism (Shafer, 2008). Learning theorists explain paraphilias in terms of timing and reinforcement. During vulnerable periods, especially puberty, sexual exploration is common; if it is pleasurable and there are no negative consequences, the activity becomes reinforced and is repeated. For example, if an adolescent boy experiments sexually with a 7-year-old boy, does not get caught, and continues to fantasize, he may develop arousal to young boys. Cognitive theorists identify paraphilias as results of cognitive distortions. Errors in thought make deviant and destructive sexual behaviours seem acceptable. For example, belief that there is agreement on the part of a child makes it okay in the individual's mind to have relations with that child, or watching others engage in sexual relations is okay "as long as no one gets hurt." Perhaps the perpetrator of exhibitionistic behaviour believes that young girls get as excited as he does when he exposes himself.

## APPLICATION OF THE NURSING PROCESS

### ASSESSMENT

#### Self-Assessment

It is common for students to read descriptions of sexual disorders and respond with disgust to behaviours that seem objectionable or ridiculous. It is also common to respond with frustration, anger, and even hostility to people with disorders like sexual masochism and pedophilia. While it may be difficult, stop and consider that these deviations are not the sum total of who the patients are. There are other aspects to their temperament, and they may well have traits of character more to your liking, such as kindness over cruelty, caring over noncaring, sensitivity over insensitivity, conscientiousness over lack of conscience, and so on. Furthermore, they can legitimately suffer from the full range of mental, emotional, and spiritual distress anyone can. You may even know individuals who you care for on many levels, despite carefully guarded secret obsessions.

It may be argued that people have control over their thoughts and deviant sexual behaviours. In fact, the notion of control is the basis for placing blame or stigmatizing anyone with a psychiatric disorder. While you may not blame a person with schizophrenia for exhibiting psychotic symptoms, it is easier to conclude that any sexual deviance could be stopped if the patient really wanted to stop and simply made up his or her mind to do so. However, when it comes to appetites or drives such as hunger, thirst, pain, and the need for sleep or sex, biological regulatory systems may exert tremendous influence that overcomes willpower. A major issue in trying to understand human behaviour is determining where to draw the line between considering a person to be the product of life experiences and biological makeup and considering him or her (by virtue of having subjective consciousness) to be an active agent capable of transcending previous determinants.

Nurses may also experience some dissonance when they think about providing care for someone who engages in what they view as objectionable, or even reprehensible, acts. Some may have known someone who was the victim of a voyeur or a pedophile, or some may have personally been victimized. Exploring sexual disorders, even in an academic context, may evoke significant distress. In such a case, talking with a faculty member, a primary care provider, or someone at a mental health clinic can be helpful and important and may even result in better personal understanding and coping.

### General Assessment

Patients with gender dysphoria and paraphilias rarely are hospitalized as a direct result of their condition. People with both gender dysphoria and paraphilias may be overrepresented in psychiatric care settings, however, owing to the frequency of co-morbid psychiatric conditions that are undoubtedly exacerbated by the sexual disorder. Nurses who work in forensic settings such as prisons and jails may care for inmates who are imprisoned due to consequences of paraphilias (e.g., sexual

impulse disorders). Depression with suicidal ideation and substance abuse are common co-morbid conditions and should be assessed using principles outlined in Chapters 14 and 19.

During a thorough assessment for any psychiatric disorder (or medical condition), the nurse may discover symptoms of gender dysphoria or one of the paraphilias. For example, when the nurse asks a patient about his family, he may remark that he and his wife "aren't getting along so great lately." As this area of concern is explored further, he reveals, "My wife wants to do the same old boring things ... you know, sexually ... all the time." As the assessment continues, the nurse may learn that he is focused on sadistic sorts of activities, is obsessed with pornography, and no longer becomes aroused by his wife.

### ASSESSMENT GUIDELINES
#### Sexual Disorders

1. Assess the potential for self-harm because patients with gender dysphoria and paraphilias may become despondent and be a suicide risk.
2. Keep the main focus of the assessment on the presenting problem (e.g., depression with suicidal ideation).
3. Elicit the patient's perception of the impact of the sexual disorder upon the current illness.

## DIAGNOSIS

Nursing diagnoses for individuals with gender dysphoria or a paraphilia are suggested in Table 22-6. Other diagnoses should be considered, depending upon the co-morbid psychiatric condition that has precipitated the admission.

### TABLE 22-6　POTENTIAL NURSING DIAGNOSES FOR PEOPLE WITH SEXUAL DISORDERS

| SIGNS AND SYMPTOMS | NURSING DIAGNOSES |
| --- | --- |
| History of violating the boundaries of others | Risk for other-directed violence |
| Profound shame and worthlessness | Risk for self-directed violence |
| Uncomfortable with sexual obsessions | Ineffective sexuality pattern |
| Regret and shame related to sexual obsessions and behaviours; belief of being different and deviant; poor eye contact | Self-esteem disturbance |
| States, "I am a woman trapped in a man's body." | Disturbed personal identity |
| Responds to stress with deviant sexual behaviour. Abuses substances | Ineffective coping |
| Isolates self from others; has difficulty and disinterest in connecting in a meaningful way with others | Impaired social interaction |
| Disorganization or dysfunction in usual patterns of behaviour (e.g., absence from work, withdrawal from relationships, changes in role function) | Ineffective role performance |
| Feeling of being out of control, deviant sexual behaviours, and awareness of being different | Anxiety |
| Inability to explain actions or behaviours | Spiritual distress |

| TABLE 22-7 | *NOC* OUTCOMES FOR SEXUAL DISORDERS | |
| --- | --- | --- |
| **NURSING OUTCOME AND DEFINITION** | **INTERMEDIATE INDICATORS** | **SHORT-TERM INDICATORS** |
| *Sexual identity:* Acknowledgement and acceptance of own sexual identity | Seeks social support | Uses healthy coping behaviours to resolve sexual identity issues<br>Reports healthy sexual functioning |
| *Impulse self-control:* Self-restraint of compulsive or impulsive behaviours | Identifies harmful impulsive behaviours<br>Identifies feelings that lead to impulsive actions<br>Identifies consequences of impulsive actions | Avoids high-risk environments<br>Avoids high-risk situations<br>Upholds contract to control behaviour<br>Maintains self-control without supervision |

**Source:** Data from Moorhead, S., Johnson, M., Maas, M., et al. (Eds.). (2008). *Nursing outcomes classification (NOC)* (4th ed.). St. Louis, MO: Mosby.

## OUTCOMES IDENTIFICATION

*NOC* (Moorhead, Johnson, Maas, et al., 2008) identifies a number of outcomes for patients with either ineffective sexuality patterns or risk for other-directed violence. Included are *Sexual identity* and *Impulse self-control.* Table 22-7 provides selected intermediate and short-term indicators for these outcomes.

## PLANNING

The planning of nursing care for the patient with gender dysphoria or a paraphilia is influenced by the setting and presenting problem. The basic-level nurse may encounter such a patient during treatment for a co-morbid condition, especially when the patient is admitted to the hospital for suicidal thoughts and behaviour. Sometimes psychiatric care and treatment are mandated, such as when a voyeur or exhibitionist gets caught.

The care plan will focus on safety and crisis intervention. The patient may also be treated for co-morbid depression or anxiety disorders in the community setting. Planning will address the major complaint, along with the sexual disorder.

## IMPLEMENTATION

Interventions are aimed at offering a nonjudgemental emotional presence while exploring identity issues, self-esteem, and anxiety and encouraging an optimal level of functioning. Patients with a potential for violating the boundaries of others may require closer observation and firm limit setting. Box 22-3 lists examples of basic-level *NIC* interventions for gender dysphoria.

### Health Teaching and Health Promotion

Education for the patient with a sexual disorder is typically geared toward reducing symptoms related to the presenting problem, typically depression and anxiety. Patients with paraphilias can be taught to journal their feelings and begin to identify triggers for pathological behaviour.

| BOX 22-3 | *NIC* INTERVENTIONS FOR GENDER DYSPHORIA AND PARAPHILIAS |
| --- | --- |

**Behaviour Management: Sexual**
*Definition of* behaviour management: sexual: Delineation and prevention of socially unacceptable sexual behaviours
*Activities\*:*
- Discuss consequences of unacceptable behaviour.
- Discuss the negative impact that behaviour has on others.
- Encourage expression of feelings about past crises.
- Provide opportunities for caregivers to process their feelings about the patient.

**Self-Esteem Enhancement**
*Definition of* self-esteem enhancement: Assisting a patient to increase his or her personal judgement of self-worth
*Activities\*:*
- Encourage patient to identify strengths.
- Assist in setting realistic goals to achieve higher self-esteem.
- Assist patient to accept dependence on others, as appropriate.
- Explore previous achievements of success.
- Encourage patient to accept new challenges.

**Social Skills Behaviour Modification**
*Definition of* social skills behaviour modification: Assisting the patient to develop or improve interpersonal social skills
*Activities\*:*
- Assist in identifying problems resulting from social skill deficits.
- Encourage verbalization of feelings regarding social interaction.
- Identify a specific skill to improve. Identify steps to reach skill and role-play the steps.

\*Partial list.
**Source:** Data from Bulechek, G.M., Butcher, H.K., & Dochterman, J.M. (Eds.). (2008). *Nursing interventions classification (NIC)* (5th ed.). St. Louis, MO: Mosby.

## Milieu Management

When the patient with gender dysphoria or a paraphilia is in a crisis that requires hospitalization, providing a safe environment is fundamental. Limit setting is done consistently when needed, and all patients on a psychiatric inpatient unit should be informed upon admission about rules regarding personal contact between patients and between patients and staff.

Individuals with paraphilias tend to isolate themselves as the unit environment may be a challenge for them. Sharing meals with others may result in discomfort, and the patient might wonder what other people know about him or her. A particular challenge may be interacting in formal group settings and meeting the expectation of participation. But the group setting may actually provide patients with the greatest opportunity for growth in that they can experience others as humans with feelings, perhaps learning how much anguish and pain personal violations have caused them. The group milieu can also mean having others present who empathize with one's background and current distress.

## Pharmacological Interventions

While there is no single treatment for sexual disorders, two classes of pharmacological medications—antiandrogens and serotonergic antidepressants—are prescribed during treatment. Medications that reduce levels of testosterone may be used to treat sex offenders. The medications that are frequently used are progestin derivatives, including medroxyprogesterone acetate (MPA) (an analogue of progesterone) and cyproterone acetate (CPA) (an inhibitor of testosterone) (Garcia & Thibaut, 2011). Both of these medications act to decrease libido and break the individual's pattern of compulsive deviant sexual behaviour. They work best in patients with paraphilias and a high sex drive, such as pedophiles and exhibitionists, and less well in those with a low sex drive or an antisocial personality (Becker & Johnson, 2008). However, medication is not used independently; other interventions complement pharmacotherapy.

Current research is focusing on the use of SSRIs in the treatment of sexual disorders. Fluoxetine (Prozac) has been used successfully to treat patients with exhibitionism, voyeurism, and pedophilia and persons who have committed rape. In addition to fluoxetine, other medications, such as clomipramine (Anafranil) and fluvoxamine (Luvox) (Garcia & Thibaut, 2011), have been used in the treatment of sexual obsessions, addictions, and paraphilias. The role of the nurse in pharmacotherapy is to educate patients regarding the specific medication prescribed and to monitor the medication's effectiveness and watch for adverse effects (Becker & Johnson, 2008).

## Advanced-Practice Interventions
### Psychotherapy

Psychotherapy is recommended to address gender dysphoria and co-morbid conditions (Shafer, 2008). If the patient is considered appropriate for sex reassignment, psychotherapy is usually initiated to prepare the patient for the new gender role. The patient is then instructed to live in the new gender role—including going to work or attending school—before surgery is performed to help the individual determine whether he or she can interact successfully with members of society in the new gender mode. Legal and social arrangements are made: the name is changed on various documents, and new employment is obtained if it is necessary to leave a former job because of discrimination. Relationship issues, such as what to tell parents, children, and former spouses, must be resolved. After one or two years, if these measures have been successful and the patient still wishes reassignment, hormone treatment is begun: males take estrogen, and females take androgen. After one to two years of hormone therapy, the patient may be considered for surgical reassignment if it is still desired. In the male-to-female patient, multiple sexual reassignment surgeries may occur depending on the wishes of the patient, from a bilateral orchiectomy to the creation of an artificial vagina. Female-to-male patients may undergo bilateral mastectomy and optional hysterectomy with removal of the ovaries. Efforts to create an artificial penis have had mixed results. Psychotherapy is indicated after surgery to help the patient adjust to the surgical changes and discuss sexual functioning and satisfaction (Becker & Johnson, 2008). Box 22-4 describes a case of sexual reassignment gone wrong.

The usual treatment plan for working with patients with paraphilias is cognitive-behavioural therapy. An attempt is made to help the person learn a new sexual response pattern that will eliminate the need for the problematic activity. Techniques range from positive reinforcement for appropriate object choices to aversion techniques, in which mild electric shocks may be applied for inappropriate choices. Other treatment

---

**BOX 22-4  NATURE OR NURTURE? A CASE OF SEX REASSIGNMENT GONE WRONG**

Accidents in early infancy may result in sexual reassignment. One such fascinating case is that of David Reimer, a Canadian-born identical-twin male whose penis was destroyed as the result of a botched circumcision. Under the advice of health care providers, the child underwent surgical reassignment and later received hormonal therapy in puberty to induce the development of breasts and secondary female sex characteristics.

While the family psychologist proclaimed the reassignment from male to female a success and concluded that gender identity was primarily based on socialization, David never felt comfortable. He rejected his female designation of Brenda and began living his life as a male at age 14. Shortly after he learned of his biological sex, he had the reassignment surgically reversed, married a woman, and became stepfather to her three children.

However, David always felt uncomfortable and ultimately committed suicide. His case bolstered support for the biological influence of prenatal and early-life exposure to male hormones on gender identity. David Reimer's life is chronicled in the book *As Nature Made Him*, which raises questions about gender reassignment and the modification of a nonconsenting minor's genitals.

**Source:** From Colapinto, J. (2006). *As nature made him: The boy who was raised as a girl.* New York: Harper Collins.

modalities include psychodynamic techniques designed to help the patient understand the origin of the paraphilia.

Advanced-practice nurses may seek specialized training to enable them to work effectively with patients with gender dysphoria and paraphilias. This preparation allows the advanced-practice nurse to practise sex therapy and conduct sex research. In the United States, the American Association of Sex Educators, Counselors, and Therapists (AASECT) provides credentialing based on academic preparation, clinical supervision, experience, and skills. Credentialing is a method by which patients of mental health care services can be assured of the professional competency of the therapist treating them. Currently, however, there is no standard training offered within Canada to practise sex therapy.

## EVALUATION

Evaluation for patients with sexual disorders is partly based on determining whether the outcomes for the presenting problem were achieved, although outcomes specific to the sexual disorder are also evaluated. Long-term goals, such as *Achieves healthy sexual functioning*, can be aimed at only during an inpatient stay; realistically, however, such outcomes require continued outpatient therapy. People with sexual impulse disorders, especially those that generate victims, may be required to continue treatment, which has been demonstrated to reduce recidivism (relapse into the offending behaviour) (Becker & Johnson, 2008).

In regards to gender dysphoria, the issues may have only been touched upon during inpatient care. Long-term therapy is required. In rare cases, psychotherapy results in the reversal of this disorder (Becker & Johnson, 2008). Ultimately, the patient may opt for sexual reassignment.

## KEY POINTS TO REMEMBER

- A *sexual dysfunction* is defined as a disturbance in the normal sexual response cycle.
- There are seven different types of sexual dysfunction.
- Sexual problems are considered to be socially atypical, have the potential to disrupt meaningful relationships, and may result in insult or even significant injury to other people.
- Health care workers are often uncomfortable asking questions related to sexuality. Providing professional and holistic care requires that nurses include this vital area of assessment.
- Certain medical and surgical conditions and some medications result in a variety of sexual dysfunctions, including low libido, impotence, erectile dysfunction, anorgasmia, and priapism.
- There are distinctions between biological sex and gender identity. *Gender dysphoria* is the strong and persistent feeling of unease about one's maleness or femaleness.
- *Paraphilia* is a term used to identify repetitive or preferred sexual fantasies or behaviours that involve preference for use of a nonhuman object, repetitive sexual activity with humans involving real or simulated suffering or humiliation, or repetitive sexual activity with nonconsenting partners.
- In addition to conducting a sexual assessment, nurses are involved in milieu and behavioural therapy, counselling, education, and medication management.
- Nursing interventions for paraphilias involve administration of medications (e.g., medroxyprogesterone [Depo-Provera] and SSRIs) and therapy.
- Advanced-practice nurses may specialize in the area of sexual counselling, treatment, and therapy.

## CRITICAL THINKING

1. As a nurse on an adolescent psychiatric mental health unit, you often encounter teenagers who are misinformed about growth and development as well as sexuality. What information would you include in a series of teaching sessions that would help these adolescents acquire a greater understanding of the developmental changes they are going through?

2. In order to understand your own beliefs, answer these questions:

a. Are you comfortable with your own sexuality? Are you comfortable with those who have a sexual orientation different from your own?
b. What factors have influenced your beliefs and values regarding sexuality?
c. How could you be helpful to someone who has a sexual disorder?
d. What do you think is the impact of sexually explicit television, music videos, and movies on your sexual attitudes, values, and beliefs?

3. During a one-to-one session, Mrs. Chase, a patient who was admitted to your inpatient psychiatric unit with depression and anxiety, confides concern about her 17-year-old son, Alex. She becomes tearful and says, "I don't know what I've done wrong. Alex was arrested for exposing himself to a group of girls at school. I'm worried that he may begin doing even worse things."
   a. Provide Mrs. Chase with information regarding Alex's sexual disorder.
   b. Consider the type of feelings that you experience when you hear about Alex's behaviour. What do you need to be aware of in order to be most helpful to Mrs. Chase?

4. Mrs. Peterson, a 50-year-old postmenopausal, married woman, complains of decreased sex drive during her annual physical examination. What treatment option would you, as an advanced-practice nurse, offer Mrs. Peterson? What are the possible risks of this treatment option that you would address with Mrs. Peterson?

## CHAPTER REVIEW

1. A 27-year-old patient states that since her marriage ended two years ago, she has found herself lacking interest and motivation in sexual activity. Which response is most likely to be therapeutic?
   1. "What was your view of sex before your divorce?"
   2. "Tell me more about your life since your marriage ended."
   3. "Often, physical illness causes decreased desire in women."
   4. "This is a common problem, what with all the stress women face."

2. A young, newly married man with schizophrenia presents in the emergency department with a complaint of "demons sticking needles in my penis." Which initial response by the triage nurse would be appropriate?
   1. Arrange for the patient to be evaluated by the doctor or advanced-practice nurse on duty because the patient may be expressing real pain in a delusional manner.
   2. Request an order for lab tests to rule out a sexually transmitted infection, given that the patient has recently begun sexual relations with his new wife and may have been exposed.
   3. Complete the triage process, and refer the patient to the psychiatric nurse for a mental health evaluation since he appears to be psychotic and possibly having a relapse.
   4. Reassure the patient that it is not possible for demons to be in the emergency room and, with his permission, ask to speak with his wife to get a better understanding of his needs.

3. A young male patient tells you that somehow he feels that he should not be a man, that inside he is a woman. This is likely an example of:
   1. Fetishism
   2. Frotteurism
   3. Transsexualism
   4. Transvestic fetishism

4. Farah is the nurse assigned to work with Mr. Roberts, a transgendered male on a step-down unit. He is in counselling as part of the process of seeking sexual reassignment surgery and has female clothing in his hospital locker. Farah is anxious at the prospect of working with someone like Mr. Roberts and spends only the briefest periods of time possible responding to his needs. What are the best descriptions of what is occurring here? Select all that apply.
   1. Farah may believe that Mr. Roberts has chosen to behave in a deviant fashion, rather than that he has gender dysphoria.
   2. Farah is failing to maintain professional objectivity because of her values and beliefs about this particular patient's decisions and behaviour.
   3. Farah is experiencing a common negative response to a situation about which she has limited knowledge and little understanding.
   4. Farah may be having difficulty looking beyond Mr. Roberts's gender issues and, as a result, is failing to see or respond to him simply as a person.
   5. Nurses have a right to have personal feelings about social issues, and as long as Mr. Roberts's minimal care needs are addressed, Farah is within her rights to respond this way.
   6. Farah may be disgusted by Mr. Roberts because she is confusing his disorder with the predatory behaviour sometimes exhibited by patients with paraphilias such as pedophilia.

5. Ms. Thierry is the nurse working with Mr. Wilson, a patient in his early thirties who is in good health overall and is being evaluated for erectile dysfunction by his family physician. Mr. Wilson is very embarrassed by his condition, is distressed by the impact he feels it is having on his marriage, and reports that he "does not feel like a man" as a result of this disorder. Which of the following is a realistic short-term outcome to expect when caring for this patient? Mr. Wilson:
   1. Reports that he has begun to feel like a man
   2. Is able to maintain an erection through orgasm
   3. Reports that he has accepted his impaired erectile function
   4. Demonstrates an accurate understanding of the meaning of his disorder

# ⊘volve WEBSITE

Post-Test interactive review

*Visit the Evolve Web site for Chapter Review Answers and Rationales, Critical Thinking Answer Guidelines, and additional resources related to the content in this chapter: http://evolve.elsevier.com/Canada/Varcarolis/psychiatric/*

## REFERENCES

Basson, R. (2011). Female sexual dysfunction. In J. Gray (Ed.), *Therapeutic choices* (6th ed.) Ottawa: Canadian Pharmacists Association.

Basson, R., Althof, S., Davis, S., et al. (2004). Summary of the recommendations on sexual dysfunctions in women. *Journal of Sexual Medicine, 1*(1), 24–34.

Becker, J.V., & Johnson, B.R. (2008). Gender identity disorders and paraphilias. In R.E. Hales, S.C. Yudofsky, & G.O. Gabbard (Eds.), *Textbook of psychiatry* (5th ed., pp. 729–753). Washington, DC: American Psychiatric Publishing.

Becker, J.V., & Stinson, J.D. (2008). Human sexuality and sexual dysfunctions. In R.E. Hales, S.C. Yudofsky, & G.O. Gabbard (Eds.), *Textbook of psychiatry* (5th ed., pp. 711–728). Washington, DC: American Psychiatric Publishing.

Bulechek, G.M., Butcher, H.K., & Dochterman, J.M. (2008). *Nursing interventions classification (NIC)* (5th ed.). St. Louis, MO: Mosby.

Criminal Code, R.S.C., c. C-46. (1985). Retrieved from http://laws-lois.justice.gc.ca/eng/acts/C-46/.

Dhalwani, N.N. (2008). Barriers and facilitators in sexual history taking. From *Health care challenges in diverse populations.* Paper presented at the 19th International Nursing Research Congress Focusing on Evidence-Based Practice: Research Sessions, Singapore. Retrieved from http://stti.confex.com/stti/congrs08/techprogram/paper_39904.htm.

Garcia, F.D., & Thibaut, F. (2011). Current concepts in the pharmacotherapy of paraphilias. *Drugs, 71*(6), 771–790. doi:10.2165/11585490-000000000-00000.

Hatzimouratidis, K., & Hatzichristou, D. (2007). Sexual dysfunctions: Classifications and definitions. *Journal of Sexual Medicine, 4*(1), 241–250.

Herdman, T.H. (Ed.). (2012). *NANDA International nursing diagnoses: Definitions & classification, 2012–2014.* Oxford, UK: Wiley-Blackwell.

Higgins, A. (2007). Impact of psychotropic medication on sexuality: Literature review. *British Journal of Nursing, 16*(9), 545–550.

Hinderliter, A.C. (2010). Defining paraphilia in *DSM-5*: Do not disregard grammar. *Journal of Sex & Marital Therapy, 37*(1), 17–31.

Kaplan, H.S. (1974). *The new sex therapy: Active treatment of sexual dysfunctions.* New York: Brunner/Mazel.

Lue, T.F., Giuliano, F., Montorsi, F., et al. (2004). Summary of the recommendations on sexual dysfunctions in men. *Journal of Sexual Medicine, 1*(1), 6–23.

Mick, J.M. (2007). Sexuality assessment: 10 strategies for improvement. *Clinical Journal of Oncology Nursing, 11,* 671–675. doi:10.1188/07.CJON.671-675.

Moorhead, S., Johnson, M., Maas, M., et al. (2008). *Nursing outcomes classification (NOC)* (4th ed.). St. Louis, MO: Mosby.

Rose, S. (2005). Going too far? Sex, sin and social policy. *Social Forces, 84*(2), 1207–1232. doi:10.1353/sof.2006.0032.

Sadock, B.J., & Sadock, V.A. (2008). *Kaplan & Sadock's concise textbook of clinical psychiatry* (3rd ed.). Philadelphia: Lippincott Williams & Wilkins.

Segraves, R., & Woodard, T. (2006). Female hypoactive sexual desire disorder: History and current status. *Journal of Sexual Medicine, 3,* 408–418. doi:10.1111/j.1743-6109.2006.00246.x.

Shafer, L.C. (2008). Sexual disorders and sexual dysfunction. In T.A. Stern, J.F. Rosenbaum, M. Fava, et al. (Eds.), *Massachusetts General Hospital comprehensive clinical psychiatry* (pp. 487–497). St. Louis, MO: Mosby.

Walsh Brennan, A.M, Barnsteiner, J., de Leon Siantz, M.L., et al. (2012). Lesbian, gay, bisexual, transgendered, or intersexed content for nursing curricula. *Journal of Professional Nursing, 28*(2), 96–104.

# 23

# Somatic Symptom Disorders and Dissociative Disorders

*Cheryl L. Pollard, Mary Haase*
*With contributions from Kathleen Wheeler, Lois Angelo, and Faye J. Grund*

## KEY TERMS AND CONCEPTS

alternate personality (alter), 480
conversion disorder, 464
dissociative amnesia, 480
dissociative disorders, 479
dissociative fugue, 480
dissociative identity disorder (DID), 480
factitious disorders, 476

illness anxiety disorder, 464
*la belle indifférence*, 465
malingering, 477
Munchausen's syndrome, 477
secondary gains, 468
somatic symptom disorders, 463
subpersonality, 480

## OBJECTIVES

1. Compare and contrast essential characteristics of the somatic symptom, factitious, and dissociative disorders.
2. Identify a clinical example of what would be found in different somatic symptom disorders.
3. Describe five psychosocial interventions that would be appropriate for a patient with somatic complaints.
4. Identify concerns that both patients and health care providers have regarding somatization.

5. List three of the most common somatic complaints seen in primary care.
6. Explain the key symptoms of dissociative disorders.
7. Compare and contrast dissociative amnesia and dissociative fugue.
8. Identify nursing interventions for patients with somatic symptom and dissociative disorders.

## ⊖volve WEBSITE

*Visit the Evolve website for Flashcards, Case Studies, and additional testing resources related to the content in this chapter: http://evolve.elsevier.com/Canada/Varcarolis/psychiatric/* Pre-Test interactive review

Anxiety exerts a powerful influence on the mind and may lead to clinical conditions known as anxiety disorders. Although patients with anxiety disorders often have some somatic (physical) symptoms, the predominant complaint is mental or emotional distress. In somatic symptom and dissociative disorders, patients rarely describe themselves as having mental or emotional symptoms related to anxiety. Instead, patients' primary focus is on physical symptoms. These conditions are relatively rare in psychiatric settings, but nurses may encounter patients with such disorders in the general medical or surgical setting, in specialized units, or in primary care clinics. This chapter helps to prepare nurses to utilize a holistic approach in nursing

care so that we may address the multidimensional interplay of biological, psychological, and cultural needs and their effects on the somatization process. It is important both for psychiatric mental health nurses caring for patients with physical illnesses and for nurses working outside of psychiatric settings to be aware of the influence of environment, stress, lifestyle, and coping skills of each patient. This chapter presents an overview of somatic symptom disorders and associated nursing care; briefly discusses factitious disorders, in which symptoms of illness are intentionally induced; and concludes with a presentation of dissociative disorders and associated nursing care.

## 🌸 HOW A NURSE HELPED ME

### *My Body Hurts—But I Don't Think They Believe Me*

*My body hurt. Some days I was not able to get out of bed. I had seen many doctors, mostly specialists: an internist, two neurologists, a gastroenterologist, and my general practitioner (GP). No one could tell me what was wrong with me. Each doctor I saw would give me a different diagnosis. My GP referred me to home care as I was not able to meet my own needs. I think that he also wanted someone to check in on me since I lived alone. A home care nurse assigned a health care aide to come and help me with bathing and dressing. I appreciated this. However, there were days when I was able to get up and get dressed on my own. On these days, I asked my health care aide to help me with meal preparation. She helped me cut up carrots and potatoes. Cutting the harder foods was difficult even on my good days I always felt weak. Unfortunately, when the home care nurse found out that the health care aide was not always focusing on getting me dressed or bathed, she came to talk to me. She wondered why there were days that I could manage and days I could not. Although she never said it out loud, I thought she was frustrated and maybe even a little angry. She referred me to Mental Health. I was not happy about that—in fact, I was angry with the nurse for suggesting that I might be crazy or that I was "faking it."*

*Then, a mental health nurse came to see me at my home. She asked me questions about my physical symptoms, how I was managing, if I had worries, and if I thought about*

*suicide. We talked about my experiences with my pain, how my body functioned, and the impact my pain had on my life. We also talked about how frustrating it was not to know what was happening with my body. I felt hopeless. I knew that I hurt and that I was not able to do everything I used to be able to do—and that there was nothing I could do about it. After the mental health nurse completed her assessment, she asked if I would agree to see her again. I agreed. During her subsequent visits, she taught me about the link between my thoughts and my pain. She told me she was using cognitive behavioural therapy. I learned that not only do my thoughts impact my pain but they also have a direct relationship with my mood. I also became aware of how I was reacting to the changes in my body and in my abilities and how others reacted to me. I was still in pain, and some days I was able to do things around the house, and some days I was not. This situation had not changed, but I felt better.*

*The mental health nurse arranged a meeting with my home care nurse. The three of us discussed my illness and how my abilities seemed to vary. My mental health nurse shared information about my diagnosis and what treatment approaches we were using and really advocated for me. We all came to an agreement that I "was not faking it." Now my health care aide can help me with what I need the most help with. Some days, it is having a bath and getting dressed; other days, it is cutting carrots.*

## SOMATIC SYMPTOM DISORDERS

Somatic symptom disorders (*soma* is the Greek word for "body") are a complex spectrum of physical signs and symptoms, without any evidence of disease, that have a psychiatric foundation—that is, they are physical manifestations of emotional states. Instead of feeling anxiety, depression, or irritability, some individuals experience pain, paralysis, unexplained skin rashes, or other physical symptoms (Webb, 2010). These illnesses are often misunderstood and mislabelled. For example, in the Middle Ages, a person who exhibited physical symptoms for no known cause was said to have a "disease of the soul." It was often women who had these "diseases," and many believed they were bewitched or possessed by the devil (Soltis-Jarrett, 2010, p. 183). Freud later used the term *hysteria*, the Greek term meaning "uterus," to refer to somatic and "histrionic" behaviours—behaviours that were attention seeking, emotionally over-reactive, and often inappropriately seductive. Our understanding of the complexity of these disorders has only just begun (Hale & Reck, 2010), but generally, these disorders baffle both patients and health care providers. Patients worry that their problems are imaginary and then worry, when they do not

get a diagnosis, that they will actually die (Dickson, Hay-Smith, & Dean, 2009). Somatic symptom disorders demonstrate complex mind–body interactions, and they cause significant impairment in social and occupational functioning resulting in real distress to the patient.

*Somatization*, the expression of psychological stress through physical symptoms, can affect women, men, and children (Silber, 2011); in fact, somatic symptom disorder symptoms account for nearly 25% of primary care clinic visits (Landa, Peterson, & Fallon, 2012). Anxiety, depression, and trauma exert a powerful influence on the mind and may lead to a variety of clinical conditions—both mental and physical. When psychiatric disorders are present along with general medical conditions, increased health care costs and lengths of stay may result. They also can negatively impact outcomes and increase morbidity and mortality (Konnopka, Löbner, Luppa, et al., 2012).

## CLINICAL PICTURE

The somatic disorders include the following:
- Somatic symptom disorder (SSD)
- Illness anxiety disorder (previously *hypochondriasis*)

- Conversion disorder (also called *functional neurological disorder*)
- Psychological factors affecting medical condition
- Factitious disorder

## Somatic Symptom Disorder

Somatic symptom disorder manifests itself through thoughts, feelings, and behaviours caused by excessive worry about physical signs and symptoms. The disorder is characterized by the combination of distressing symptoms and an excessive or a maladaptive response without significant physical findings and medical diagnosis. Patients' suffering is authentic, however, and they typically experience a high level of functional impairment.

The predominance of somatization in women is significant. It has been proposed that women are more aware of their bodily sensations, have different health-seeking behaviours when faced with physical and psychological distress, and use more health care services than men (So, 2008). In particular, young women, aged 16 to 25, are more likely to receive a somatic diagnosis than men or older individuals (Huang & McCarron, 2011).

Symptoms may be initiated, exacerbated, or maintained by a combination of biological, psychological, and cultural factors. Somatic symptom disorder is difficult to distinguish from physical disorders with organic causes, and the patient's history is extremely important for an accurate diagnosis. Often, the patient has a co-morbid psychiatric disorder such as depression, anxiety, or a personality disorder.

The person with somatic symptom disorder may often seek out medical care, which rarely alleviates his or her concerns. Included in the most common symptoms for visits to primary care providers are chest pain, fatigue, dizziness, headache, swelling, back pain, shortness of breath, insomnia, abdominal pain, and numbness. These symptoms account for 40% of all visits to primary care providers; however, a biological cause for these symptoms is identified in only 26% of patients (Edwards, Stern, Clark, et al., 2010). Health-related quality of life is frequently severely impaired, and patients appraise their bodily symptoms as unduly troublesome, threatening, or harmful, often fearing the worst about their health. Some patients feel that their medical assessment and treatment have been inadequate. When the health care provider is unable to provide a clear diagnosis for discomfort, patients can feel discounted, misunderstood, devalued, and stigmatized by the suggestion that the problem is "only in their heads" (Noyes, Longley, Langbehn, et al., 2010).

Likewise, health care providers experience frustration in caring for people who are not organically ill. Providers tend to use less patient-centred communication with these patients as compared to those with straightforward symptoms, even though somatic symptom visits require more time (Huang & McCarron, 2011). Patient personality can contribute to an inadequate workup: for example, a "difficult" patient may receive a somatic diagnosis more readily than a "pleasant" patient. In fact, studies show that the strongest predictor of misdiagnosing somatic disorders is the primary care provider's dissatisfaction with the clinical encounter (Huang & McCarron, 2011).

## Illness Anxiety Disorder

Previously known as *hypochondriasis*, illness anxiety disorder results in the misinterpretation of physical sensations as evidence of a serious illness. Illness anxiety can be quite obsessive as thoughts about illness may be intrusive and hard to dismiss even when patients realize their fears are unrealistic (MacDonald, 2011). People with this disorder experience extreme worry and fear about the possibility of having a disease. Even normal body changes, such as a change in heart rate or abdominal cramps, can be seen as red flags for serious illness and imminent death. Frequent exposure to media messages reminding us to seek regular medical screenings may also contribute to fears about health (MacDonald, 2011). For example, studies show a relationship between exposure to breast cancer coverage in television programs and a heightened fear of breast cancer (Lemal & den Bulck, 2009).

In response to a patient's symptoms, primary care providers may suggest a consultation with a mental health professional, but the suggestion typically is refused. The course of the illness is chronic and relapsing, with symptoms becoming amplified during times of increased stress (Greenburg, Braun, & Cassem, 2008). Depressive symptoms may be a catalyst for the diagnosis of illness anxiety (Dols, Rhebergen, Eikelenboom, et al., 2012).

Overall, a patient with illness anxiety disorder uses 41% to 78% more health care services, excluding laboratory tests and X-rays prescribed in primary care, per year than patients with well-defined medical conditions (Fink, 2010). Because illness anxiety disorder is so prevalent, it is important that clinicians achieve basic skills in treating and identifying this disorder. Addressing patient health concerns at an early stage may prevent repeated consultations, multiple trials of medications, and medical examinations (Fink, 2010).

## Conversion Disorder

Conversion disorder (also known as *functional neurological disorder*) manifests itself as neurological symptoms in the absence of a neurological diagnosis (Feinstein, 2011). Conversion disorder is marked by the presence of deficits in voluntary motor or sensory functions, including paralysis, blindness, movement disorder, gait disorder, numbness, paresthesia (tingling or burning sensations), loss of hearing, or seizures resembling epilepsy.

Conversion disorder is a clinical problem that requires the application of multiple perspectives—biological, psychological, and social—to fully understand the symptoms of individual patients. Patients with conversion disorder symptoms may be found to have "no neurological disorder" by the neurologist and "no psychiatric disorder" by the psychiatrist, thus adding to the complexity of treatment planning (Stone, Vuilleumier, & Friedman, 2010).

Conversion disorder is attributed to the channelling of emotional conflicts or stressors into physical symptoms; however, some MRI studies suggest that patients with conversion disorder have an abnormal pattern of cerebral activation (Feinstein, 2011). While some patients become quite distressed about their symptoms, many show a lack of emotional concern about them (*la belle indifférence*). Imagine someone casually discussing sudden blindness. Care providers should assume an organic cause for the symptoms until physical pathology has been ruled out. Patients truly believe in the presence of the symptoms; they are not fabricated or under voluntary control.

Experiences of childhood physical or sexual abuse are common among patients with conversion disorder, and co-morbid psychiatric conditions include depression, anxiety, post-traumatic stress disorder, other somatic disorders, and personality disorders. There are also cases in which a co-morbid medical or neurological condition exists, and the conversion disorder is an exaggeration of the physical problem (Nicholson, Stone, & Kanaan, 2011).

The course of the disorder is related to its acuity. In cases of acute onset during stressful events, remission rate is high; in cases of a more gradual onset, the disorder is not as readily treatable. Symptoms generally remit by themselves 95% of the time (Sadock & Sadock, 2008). However, recurrence is as high as 25%, often within the first year.

---

**VIGNETTE**

Gerald is a 63-year-old, married real estate agent who was recently hospitalized for heart failure. Because of insomnia, lack of appetite, and some anger problems toward his wife, his primary care provider has referred him for a mental health consultation. During this consultation, Gerald complains of waking up at night obsessing about possibly losing his job, his lack of retirement savings, and providing for his wife in case he dies. He states, "I am very scared, and I worry about my health and being forced to retire. I don't know where I would get the money to live. I am too old to start another career." These observations were reported to the nurse practitioner. After a thorough assessment and medical workup, it is determined that Gerald is experiencing depression and severe anxiety, which precipitated increased symptoms of heart failure. Gerald has responded well to couples therapy and a men's support group. His blood pressure has decreased, and his mood is improved. Gerald has been able to return to work.

---

## EPIDEMIOLOGY

Specific prevalence rates for somatic symptom disorders in the general population are unknown. Instead, the literature describes their occurrence in the population of individuals who seek medical care but do not have an underlying physiological cause for their symptoms.

A comprehensive physical examination with appropriate diagnostic studies is necessary to rule out the following medical conditions, which can be confused with somatic symptom disorders:

- Multiple sclerosis
- Brain tumour
- Hyperthyroidism
- Hyperparathyroidism
- Lupus erythematosus
- Myasthenia gravis

A thorough psychosocial history is also required to confirm a somatic symptom disorder diagnosis, as well as any co-morbid psychiatric disorders. Table 23-1 gives further information on the age of onset, gender predilection, and co-morbidity with other psychiatric disorders.

## CO-MORBIDITY

Both the medical and mental health communities recognize the interrelationships between psychiatric and medical illnesses (Shidhaye, Mendenhall, Sumathipala, et al., 2013). Psychological factors may present a risk for a medical disease, or they may magnify or adversely affect a medical condition. Studies in recent years have contributed to the growing body of evidence demonstrating links between mental disorders and cardiovascular disease. Major depressive disorder is now seen as a risk factor in the occurrence of coronary heart disease (Charlson, Stapelberg, Baxter, et al., 2011). Depression has been identified as a risk factor for cancer (Gross, Gallo, & Eaton, 2010).

Chronic stressors affect components of the immune system in detrimental ways. Research in the field of psychoneuroimmunology (the study of how emotions and brain function affect

| TABLE 23-1 | **SOMATIC SYMPTOM DISORDERS** | | |
|---|---|---|---|
| **DISORDER** | **AGE OF ONSET** | **GENDER PREDILECTION** | **CO-MORBIDITIES** |
| Somatic symptom disorder | Adolescence to 30s | Women: 80%; men: 20% | Major depression<br>Anxiety disorder<br>Personality disorder |
| Conversion disorder | Any age | Twice as frequent in women | Major depression<br>Anxiety disorder<br>Schizophrenia |
| Illness anxiety disorder | 20–30 years | Equal prevalence in women and men | Depressive disorder<br>Anxiety disorder<br>Other somatic symptom disorders |

**Source:** Adapted from Sadock, B.J., & Sadock, V.A. (2008). *Kaplan & Sadock's concise textbook of clinical psychiatry* (3rd ed.). Philadelphia: Lippincott Williams & Wilkins.

### Falling Out

Dante is a 22-year-old Jamaican immigrant who lives in Toronto. He drives a cab during the day and attends school in the evening. He wants to become an accountant, and his goal is to attain the first college degree in his family. Life moves by quickly in a blur of passengers and fares, textbooks, teachers, and tests. He has made few friends and is isolated from his family, who are still in the Caribbean. He is lonely, but describes himself as being too busy to be lonely.

At the end of another long day, Dante hastily turns in the keys to his cab to the manager, exits the garage onto the rush-hour-filled sidewalk, and begins a near-jog as he hurries to get to his first class. A wave of dizziness hits him and casts him into a slow-motion world, blackness surrounds him, and he falls to the ground. Dante hears the sounds of the street, people walking, and horns blaring. A baby cries somewhere close by. A man's voice says, "What's wrong with you? Get up and out of the way." Dante tries to respond, but he cannot lift a finger, let alone stand up.

What Dante experienced is known as *falling out* (or *blacking out*), a culture-bound syndrome that occurs in people from Caribbean countries. It is characterized by a sudden collapse followed by an inability to see or move. The individual is aware of what is happening around him, and his eyes remain open. Falling out may be a variant of conversion or dissociative disorder.

**Source:** Adapted from Hales, R.E., Yudofsky, S.C., & Gabbard, G.O. (2008). *Textbook of psychiatry* (5th ed.). Washington, DC: American Psychiatric Publishing.

the immune system) has provided insights into the relationship between psychological and physiological health in human immunodeficiency virus (HIV) and other diseases (Temoshok, Waldstein, Wald, et al., 2008). This research explains the negative impact of perceived stress on HIV disease progression, primarily as a function of immunosuppression mediated by elevated cortisol. In an analysis of more than 300 research articles, Segerstrom and Miller (2004) suggest that psychological stressors may be associated with suppression of both cellular and humoral responses. Being able to reduce the stress within this patient population is important because we can potentially positively affect not only the quality of life but also the illness trajectory of persons living with HIV. A variety of other medical disorders have been studied with regard to the effects of stress on the course of the illness. In fact, anyone experiencing a serious medical condition needs a variety of supports and may benefit from learning new coping skills (Temoshok, Waldstein, Wald, et al., 2008).

The relationship between stress and changes in physical and mental health was first introduced by Hans Selye (1956). Selye's description of the *general adaptation syndrome* (see Chapter 12) and Cannon's 1914 identification of the *fight-or-flight response* (see Chapter 12) provided insight into the biological and molecular reactions to stressors in the sympathetic nervous

system, the pituitary–adrenocortical axis, and the immune system. Extensive studies have left little doubt that psychosocial stress affects the course and severity of illness (Table 23-2).

## ETIOLOGY

Somatizations are a complex biopsychosocial phenomenon, with many factors influencing the onset and course of the illnesses. A link between somatization and traumatic experiences is frequently reported (Aragona, Catino, Pucci, et al., 2010). Additionally, patients with somatic disorders are more sensitive to negativity, less resilient in response to stress, and more prone to catastrophic thinking and negative interpretation of life events (Miller, 2009). In early development of somatic disorders, stress has been implicated as a triggering factor, most often stemming from parents and the pressure to perform a behaviour. Somatization is often the "tip of the iceberg" that calls attention to a psychiatric disorder necessitating mental health treatment. Unfortunately, many untreated children risk continuous somatization as adults (Silber, 2011).

### Biological Factors

Remember that research into anxiety disorders has demonstrated structural changes in the brain that may result from prolonged stress or trauma, as well as imbalances in neurotransmitters. In the case of anxiety disorders, these abnormalities create altered feeling and thinking processes, whereas the processes of perception and interpretation of bodily sensations remain fairly intact. It is not known why the brains of some patients change to develop an anxiety disorder, and others change to develop a somatic symptom disorder. However, the neurochemistry of the brain in people who have somatic symptom disorders is abnormal. Any abnormality in the structure of the brain or the function of the neurotransmitters can lead to a misinterpretation of ordinary events. For example, the brain may misunderstand (or amplify the significance of) a stimulus, such as identifying a minor gas pain as a serious abdominal injury (somatization). The brain may also overreact in its analysis of the stimulus, deciding that the same minor gas pain is a sign of colon cancer (illness anxiety) and then hope that death comes quickly.

Han, Pae, Lee, and colleagues (2008) studied patients with a somatic symptom disorder, and from baseline to end of treatment, somatic symptoms were significantly decreased after treatment with a selective serotonin reuptake inhibitor (SSRI). Although further research is warranted, treatment with antidepressants has been found to have beneficial effects in individuals with somatic symptoms.

### Genetic Factors

Somatic symptom disorders tend to run in families, occurring in 10% to 20% of first-degree female relatives of women with a somatic symptom disorder (Sadock & Sadock, 2008). Twin studies show an increased risk of conversion disorder in monozygotic twin pairs. First-degree biological relatives of people with a somatic symptom disorder are more likely to have chronic pain, depressive disorder, and alcohol dependence.

| TABLE 23-2 | COMMON MEDICAL CONDITIONS NEGATIVELY AFFECTED BY STRESS | | | |
|---|---|---|---|---|
| **MEDICAL CONDITION** | **INCIDENCE** | **GENETIC AND BIOLOGICAL CORRELATES** | **COMMON PRECIPITATING FACTORS** | **POTENTIAL HOLISTIC THERAPIES USED IN ADDITION TO MEDICAL MANAGEMENT** |
| Cardiovascular disease (e.g., coronary heart disease) | Rates higher in Caucasian males until age 60 years | Risk factors: family history of cardiac disease, hypertension, increased serum lipid levels, obesity, sedentary lifestyle, cigarette smoking<br>Psychosocial risk factors: stress, depression, loneliness<br>High anxiety risk in patient with prior cardiac events | Sudden stress preceded by a period of losses, frustration, and disappointments (often resulting in myocardial infarction) | Relaxation training, stress management, group social support, and psychosocial intervention<br>Support groups for type-A personalities |
| Peptic ulcer (caused by *Helicobacter pylori* infection) | Occurs in 12% of men, 6% of women (more prevalent in industrialized societies) | Infection with *H. pylori* is associated with 95% to 99% of peptic ulcers<br>Both peptic and duodenal ulcers cluster in families, but separately from each other | Periods of social tension and increased life stress<br>Losses<br>Postmenopause | Biofeedback to alter gastric acidity<br>Cognitive-behavioural approaches to reduce stress (stress management) |
| Cancer | Men: most common in lung, prostate, colon, and rectum<br>Women: most common in breast, uterus, colon, and rectum<br>Death rate higher in men than in women | Genetic evidence suggesting dysfunction of cellular proliferation<br>Familial patterns of breast cancer, colorectal cancer, stomach cancer, melanoma | Prolonged and intensive stress<br>Stressful life events (e.g., separation from or loss of significant other 2 years before diagnosis)<br>Feelings of hopelessness, helplessness, and despair (depression) | Relaxation (e.g., meditation, autogenic training, self-hypnosis)<br>Visualization<br>Psychological counselling<br>Support groups<br>Massage therapy<br>Stress management |
| Tension headache | Occurs in 80% of population when under stress<br>Begins at end of workday or early evening | | Associated with anxiety and depression | Psychotherapy for chronic tension headaches<br>Learning to cope or avoiding tension-creating situations or people<br>Relaxation and stress management techniques<br>Cognitive restructuring techniques |
| Essential hypertension | Rates higher in males until age 60 years | Risk factors: family history of cardiac disease and hypertension | Life changes and traumatic life events<br>Stressful job (e.g., air-traffic controller) | Behavioural feedback, stress reduction techniques, meditation, yoga, hypnosis<br>**Note:** Pharmacological treatment considered primary for treatment of hypertension. |

## Psychological Factors
### Psychodynamic Theories

Since the late nineteenth century, psychoanalytic theory has dominated medical thinking about conversion disorder (Stone, Vuilleumier, & Friedman, 2010). Psychoanalytic theorists believe that psychosomatic complaints of pain, illness, or loss of physical function are related to repression of a conflict or unwelcome experiences (usually of an aggressive or sexual nature) and that the transformation of anxiety into a physical symptom is symbolically related to the conflict (Nicholson Stone, & Kanaan, 2011). For example, in conversion disorder, conversion symptoms permit the individual to communicate a need for special treatment or consideration from others.

Illness anxiety disorder is considered by many clinicians to have psychodynamic origins. These clinicians suggest that anger, aggression, or hostility that had its source in past losses or disappointments are expressed as a need for help and concern from others. Other clinicians suggest that illness anxiety is a defence against guilt or low self-esteem (van Dijke, 2012). In the view of many patients, the somatic symptoms serve as deserved punishment.

### Behavioural Theory

Behaviourists suggest that people with somatic symptoms learn methods of communicating helplessness. These "helpless" behaviours are used to get their needs met. The symptoms become more intense when they are reinforced by attention from others. For example, since Canadian primary care providers and nurses are taught to be attentive and responsive to a patient's reports of pain, the patient's behaviours are inadvertently reinforced. In some cases, because of the stigma and prejudice that accompany the reporting of psychological symptoms, patients may feel that they receive more attentive care by reporting only their physical symptoms. Behaviourists also identify potential secondary gains from somatic-related disorders. Secondary gains are those benefits derived from the symptoms alone; for example, in the sick role, the patient is not able to perform the usual family, work, and social functions and receives extra attention from loved ones. Other potential benefits relating to somatic symptoms include avoiding activities the individual considers distasteful, obtaining financial benefit, and gaining some advantage in interpersonal relationships due to the symptom.

### Cognitive Theory

Cognitive theorists believe that the patient with somatic symptoms focuses on body sensations, misinterprets their meaning, and then becomes excessively alarmed by them.

### Environmental Factors

We know that adverse childhood events result in lifelong problems, including somatic disorders (van Dijke, 2012). The Adverse Childhood Experiences (ACE) Study (Fuller-Thomson, Sulman, Brennenstuhl, et al., 2011) surveyed more than 16 000 adults and discovered that childhood trauma exposure accounted for negative outcomes across a variety of diagnoses

in later life, including multiple somatic symptoms of diabetes, heart disease, cancer, gastrointestinal conditions, and immune functioning. Childhood maltreatment has been associated with elevated levels of C-reactive protein, a biomarker of inflammation that may play a role in autoimmune diseases in adults 20 years later (Dube, Fairweather, Pearson, et al., 2009). The Research Highlight provides more information on the connection between childhood trauma and subsequent somatization.

### RESEARCH HIGHLIGHT
#### Childhood Trauma and Somatic Preoccupation

**Source**: Sansone, R., Wiederman, M., Tahir, N.A., et al. (2009). A re-examination of childhood trauma and somatic preoccupation. *International Journal of Psychiatry in Clinical Practice, 13*(3), 227–231. doi:10.1080/13651500802621551.

**Problem**
Studies of childhood abuse have typically concentrated on the area of psychological outcomes; however, a number of studies suggest that abuse in childhood is related to somatic preoccupation in adulthood. In past studies, each type of trauma was not examined for its individual contribution to adult somatic problems.

**Purpose of Study**
The aim of this study is to explore five types of childhood trauma—(1) physical, (2) sexual, (3) emotional, (4) witness to violence, and (5) physical neglect—to determine each type of trauma's unique contribution, if any, to somatic preoccupation in adulthood.

**Methods**
Participants were male and female outpatients (N = 36 males and 77 females), between the ages of 18 and 87 years, who were being seen for nonemergent medical care in an outpatient internal medicine setting located in an American midwestern medium-sized city.

Participants were asked, "Prior to age 12, did you ever experience any of five types of trauma?" with yes/no options.

**Key Findings**
- Physical and emotional abuse showed significant associated relationships with somatic preoccupation in adulthood.
- Sexual abuse, the witnessing of violence, and physical neglect were not associated with subsequent somatization.

**Implications for Nursing Practice**
Patients in general medical settings with high levels of somatic symptoms may have been victims of childhood abuse. An awareness of this association will facilitate more mental health assessments within the general physical exam and history. These individuals have a history of extreme discomfort and emotional distress. Compassion and empathy will go a long way in reducing their emotional and physical pain.

### Cultural Factors

The type and frequency of somatic symptoms vary across cultures (Brown & Lewis-Fernandez, 2011). The sensation of burning hands and feet, worms in the head, or ants under the skin is more common in Africa and southern Asia than in North America. Fainting is a symptom commonly associated with culture-specific religious and healing rituals. Somatic symptom disorder, which is rarely seen in men in North America, is often reported in Greek and Puerto Rican men, suggesting that cultural customs permit these men to somatize as an acceptable approach to dealing with life stress. Somatization related to post-traumatic stress and depression was the most prevalent psychiatric symptom in North Korean defectors to South Korea (Kim, Lee, Kim, et al., 2011). West Indians (Caribbean) attribute somatic symptoms to chronic overwork and the irregularity of daily living, citing symptoms such as dizziness, fatigue, joint pain, and muscle tension. Patients from Korea may explain some distress to *Hwa-Byung* (see Chapter 7), a syndrome of both somatic and depressive symptoms commonly attributed to suppressed anger or rage (Edwards, Stern, Clarke, et al., 2010).

In some cultures, certain physical symptoms are believed to result from the casting of spells. Spellbound individuals often seek the help of traditional healers in addition to modern medical staff. The medical health care provider may diagnose a non–life-threatening somatic symptom disorder, whereas the traditional healer may offer an entirely different explanation and prognosis. The individual might not show improvement until the traditional healer removes the spell.

In contemporary Western culture, the past few decades have seen unprecedented growth and comfort; however, levels of health have not increased. Core values such as materialism, consumerism, and individualism may be damaging to people's sense of well-being and health, inciting a high incidence of somatization.

Abraham Maslow's hierarchy of needs theorizes that humans are inclined to shift attention to higher-level needs (social, intellectual, spiritual) once lower-level needs of food, shelter, and clothing are attained. However, the Western consumer culture has become extremely adept at persuading people to remain fixated upon materialism, resisting movement to higher-level needs such as love, belonging, and respect for others (Schumaker, 2007). This current culture of individualism with decreased interest in family and group needs negatively impacts supportive development of communities, socialization, and overall mental and physical health, including somatic responses of individuals.

Patients across cultures with somatic symptoms often offer clues about their underlying concerns and want more emotional support from their health care provider in comparison to what is given other patients, and they are most satisfied with their care when their health care provider shares their understanding of the presenting problems and treatment options (Edwards, Stern, Clarke, et al., 2010). New Canadians frequently experience multiple traumatic events, both intentional and unintentional, preimmigration as well as postimmigration. A study of asylum seekers reported 79% had experienced a traumatic event such as witnessing killings, being assaulted, or suffering torture and captivity. It is important for primary care providers evaluating immigrants to be aware of the possible link between somatization symptoms reported by the patient and

undisclosed traumatic experiences (Aragona, Catino, Pucci, et al., 2010).

## APPLICATION OF THE NURSING PROCESS

### ASSESSMENT

Assessment of patients with somatic symptom disorders is a complex process that requires careful and complete documentation. This section outlines several areas that are important in the assessment of a patient with a suspected somatic symptom disorder.

> ### 📋 ASSESSMENT GUIDELINES
>
> #### Somatic Symptom Disorders
> 1. Assess for nature, location, onset, characteristics, and duration of the symptom(s).
> 2. Assess the patient's ability to meet basic needs.
> 3. Assess risks to safety and security needs of the patient as a result of the symptom(s).
> 4. Determine whether the symptoms are under the patient's voluntary control.
> 5. Identify any secondary gains the patient is experiencing from symptom(s).
> 6. Explore the patient's cognitive style and ability to communicate feelings and needs.
> 7. Assess type and amount of medication the patient is using.

Assessment should begin with the collection of data about the nature, location, onset, character, and duration of the symptom or symptoms. A thorough medical, emotional, and psychosocial history is also essential. Assessment of nutrition, fluid balance, and elimination needs should be a high priority as patients with somatic symptom disorders often complain of gastrointestinal distress, diarrhea, constipation, and anorexia.

### Physical Symptoms

A useful assessment tool to understand the degree of somatization is the Patient Health Questionnaire–15 (PHQ), a somatic symptom severity scale for the purpose of diagnosis (see Figure 23-1). The questionnaire inquires about 15 somatic symptoms (stomach pain, back pain, headache, chest pain, dizziness, fainting, palpitations, shortness of breath, bowel complaints, nausea, fatigue, sleep problems, pain in joints or limbs, menstrual pain, and problems during sexual intercourse) that account for more than 90% of physical complaints reported in the primary care setting by asking patients to rate the severity of symptoms during the previous four weeks on a three-point scale (Korber, Frieser, Steinbrecher, et al., 2011).

In addition, information should be sought about the patient's ability to meet his or her own basic needs. Rest, comfort, activity, and hygiene needs may be altered as a result of patient problems such as fatigue, weakness, insomnia, muscle tension, pain, and avoidance of diversional activities (hobbies). Safety

| During the past four (4) days how much have you been bothered by . . . | | | | |
|---|---|---|---|---|
| | | Not bothered at all | Bothered a little | Bothered a lot |
| 1. | Stomach pain | 0 | 1 | 2 |
| 2. | Back pain | 0 | 1 | 2 |
| 3. | Pain in your arms, legs, or joints | 0 | 1 | 2 |
| 4. | Menstrual cramps or other problems with your periods (women) | 0 | 1 | 2 |
| 5. | Headaches | 0 | 1 | 2 |
| 6. | Chest pain | 0 | 1 | 2 |
| 7. | Dizziness | 0 | 1 | 2 |
| 8. | Fainting spells | 0 | 1 | 2 |
| 9. | Feeling your heart pound or race | 0 | 1 | 2 |
| 10. | Shortness of breath | 0 | 1 | 2 |
| 11. | Pain or problems during sexual intercourse | 0 | 1 | 2 |
| 12. | Constipation, loose bowels, or diarrhea | 0 | 1 | 2 |
| 13. | Nausea, gas, or indigestion | 0 | 1 | 2 |
| 14. | Feeling tired or having no energy | 0 | 1 | 2 |
| 15. | Trouble sleeping | 0 | 1 | 2 |

Scores of 5 or less indicate mild somatization, 10 or less are moderate somatization, and 15 or more are considered severe indications of somatization.

**FIGURE 23-1** Patient Health Questionnaire Somatic Symptom—Short Form (PHQ-SSS) **Source:** Adapted from Kroenke, K., Spitzer, R.L., Williams, J.B.W., et al. (2010). The patient health questionnaire somatic, anxiety, and depressive symptom scales: A systematic review. *General Hospital Psychiatry, 32*(4), 345–359. doi:10.1016/j.genhosppsych.2010.03.006. Copyright 2010, with permission from Elsevier.

and security needs may be threatened by patient experiences of blindness, deafness, loss of balance, and anaesthesia of various parts of the body.

During assessment, it is important to determine whether symptoms are under the patient's voluntary control. Somatic symptoms *are not* under the individual's voluntary control. Although the relationship between symptoms and interpersonal conflicts may be obvious to others, the patient is not aware of it.

Often, patients with conversion disorder report having a sudden loss of function of a body part: "I woke up this morning and couldn't move my arm." Patients with somatic symptom disorder or illness anxiety disorder usually discuss their symptoms in dramatic terms. They may use colourful metaphors and exaggerations: "The pain was searing, like a hot sword drawn across my forehead"; "My symptoms are so rare that I've stumped hundreds of doctors."

### Psychosocial Factors

Psychosocial factors are relevant to somatic symptoms, and the way a patient thinks and feels can have a profound effect on

recovery. For example, strong emotions such as fear, anger, sadness, confusion, and guilt can impact a patient's physical, emotional, and spiritual recovery. Patients may feel overwhelmed and alone, and friends and family members may feel helpless and at a loss emotionally.

When working with a person with a somatic symptom disorder, the nurse must complete a psychosocial assessment in tandem with a thorough physical workup and mental status examination (see Table 23-3).

### Coping Skills

Assessing how a patient has dealt with adversity in the past provides information about the availability of coping skills. Health care workers can also support the patient in gaining additional coping skills that may help him or her better manage.

### Spirituality and Religion

Nurses and other health care workers are becoming increasingly aware of the role spirituality or religion plays in many patients' lives and its importance as a source of peace. Support from a

| TABLE 23-3 | PSYCHOSOCIAL ASSESSMENT OF PATIENTS WITH MEDICAL CONDITIONS |
|---|---|
| **AREAS TO ASSESS** | **SPECIFIC QUESTIONS TO ASK** |
| | **SOCIAL SUPPORTS AND CULTURAL ISSUES** |
| Family | What were the effects of the patient's illness, treatments, and recovery on the family in the past? |
| Friends | Who can the patient share painful feelings with? |
| | Does the patient have friends to joke and laugh with? |
| | Are there people the patient believes would stand by him or her? |
| Religious or spiritual beliefs | Does the patient find comfort and support in spiritual practices? |
| | Is the patient a member of a spiritual or religious group in the community (e.g., church, temple, other place of worship)? |
| | Does the patient find inner peace and strength in religious or spiritual practices? |
| | *The following statements may be used in performing a spiritual assessment of a patient:* |
| | • I [often/sometimes/seldom] believe that life has value, meaning, and direction. |
| | • I [often/sometimes/seldom] feel a connection with the universe. |
| | • I [often/sometimes/seldom] believe in a power greater than myself. |
| | • I [often/sometimes/seldom] believe that my actions make a difference. |
| | • I [often/sometimes/seldom] believe that my actions express my true self. |
| Cultural beliefs | Does the patient use specific culture-oriented treatments or remedies for his or her condition? |
| | Do the patient's cultural beliefs allow for adequate treatment by Western medical standards? |
| Work | Are there colleagues at work the patient can count on for support? |
| | **COEXISTING PHYSICAL CONDITIONS AFFECTING PSYCHOSOCIAL WELL-BEING** |
| Physical pain | Is the patient in pain? |
| | How does the patient cope with the pain? |
| | Is the pain disabling? |
| | Are there pain-reducing techniques that might help? |
| Major illness | Does the patient have a co-occurring major illness that will negatively affect his or her current condition? |
| | Is the patient undergoing treatments that are affecting daily life more than expected? |
| | Are there interventions that would help the patient better cope with the sequelae of the illness and treatments? |
| | Has the patient been hospitalized in the past? |
| | How many times? |
| | For what? |
| | How did the patient cope? |
| Addictions and mental health | Does the patient have a co-occurring mental health problem (e.g., depression, anxiety, compulsions)? |
| | Has the patient suffered a mental illness in the past? |
| | Does the patient participate in any compulsive behaviour (e.g., smoking, overworking, excessive spending, gambling, cybersex)? |
| | Does the patient abuse substances (e.g., alcohol, drugs [illicit, over-the-counter, prescription])? |

priest, pastor, rabbi, imam, or other religious leader may be indicated, especially in a case of spiritual distress. Religious beliefs and practices are forces that can promote resilience. Practising healthy coping depends upon the capacity to create meaning from life experiences.

### Secondary Gains

The nurse should try to identify secondary gains the patient may be receiving from the symptoms. If a patient derives personal benefit from the symptoms, giving up the symptoms is more difficult unless the patient can achieve the same benefits through healthier avenues, such as learning to communicate more adaptively and to connect with others—skills the clinician can help the patient learn. One approach to identifying the presence of secondary gains is to ask the patient questions such as the following:

• What are you unable to do now that you used to be able to do?
• How has this problem affected your life?

### Cognitive Style

In general, patients with somatic symptom disorders may misinterpret physical stimuli and distort the reality of their symptoms. For example, sensations a "normal" individual would interpret as a slight headache might suggest a brain tumour to a patient with illness anxiety disorder.

### Ability to Communicate Feelings and Emotional Needs

Patients with somatic symptom disorders have difficulty communicating their emotional needs. Although they are able to describe their physical symptoms, they frequently do not verbalize feelings, especially those related to anger, guilt, and dependence. The somatic symptom may be the patient's chief means of communicating emotional needs. Psychogenic blindness or hearing loss may represent the symbolic statement "I can't face this knowledge." For example, after a woman overheard friends discussing her husband's sexual infidelity, she developed total deafness.

### Dependence on Medication

Individuals experiencing many somatic complaints often become dependent on medication to relieve pain, relieve anxiety, or induce sleep. Primary care providers prescribe anxiolytic agents for patients who seem highly anxious and concerned about their symptoms. Patients often return to the primary care provider for prescription renewal or seek treatment from numerous primary care providers as the effectiveness of these types of medications is short-lived. It is important that the nurse assess the type and amount of medications being used, including nonprescription medication or substances.

### Self-Assessment

Nurses and other health care providers often find working with patients with somatic symptom disorders to be difficult and unsatisfying. In the absence of a physiological basis for the patient's symptoms, they may resent this patient's taking up valuable time that might better be spent on a "sick" patient. Negative feelings occur whether the patient is being cared for in a medical setting—whose staff tend to feel more comfortable working with patients with physical illnesses that can be measured or identified with a blood test or some type of scan—or by psychiatric staff, who tend to prefer working with disorders of emotion or thought.

It is helpful to remember that the symptom the patient is experiencing feels real to him or her, even though the objective data may not support a physiological basis for it. It is important for the clinician not to convey, by word or body language, frustration over the difficult and time-consuming task of trying to find a physical base for a somatic disorder. Clinicians should also avoid the temptation to perform unnecessary, repetitive, or extensive testing in an attempt to demonstrate to the patient or family that the presenting complaint is of somatic origin (Silber, 2011). Such actions are easily interpreted by patients as the clinician trying to "prove" to them that they are "faking it" when indeed the person does really experience the physical symptom.

Staff members may also experience anger when they feel as though a patient has used somatic symptoms to manipulate the environment and the people within it. Patients with somatic symptom disorders exhibit remarkable resistance to change. They have a steadfast conviction that something is physically wrong. Some may suggest that the "right doctor or nurse" would be able to figure out what is really wrong with them. They cling to unrealistic beliefs about the origin of the somatic symptoms, despite objective evidence to the contrary. As a result, clinicians feel helpless and frustrated because the patient will not agree to the recommended treatment. As you plan the care for people with somatic symptom disorder, a useful strategy is to set goals with staged outcomes (i.e., small, attainable steps) to offset feelings of helplessness or ineffectuality for both the clinician and the patient.

It is helpful for health care providers, no matter the setting, to discuss emotional reactions to patients in conferences with other members of the health care team. Sharing these feelings facilitates critical reflections and helps the clinician develop an awareness of counter-transference issues that will negatively impact patient care.

## DIAGNOSIS

Patients with somatic symptom disorders present with various problems. *Ineffective coping* is frequently diagnosed. Causal statements might include the following:
- Chronic symptomatology of psychological origin
- Suppression of feelings
- Decreased use of social support
- Inability to meet role expectations
- Dependence on pain relievers or anxiolytics

Table 23-4 describes signs and symptoms and potential nursing diagnoses for somatic symptom disorders.

## OUTCOMES IDENTIFICATION

Because shared decision-making promotes goal attainment, patients should participate in identifying desired outcomes. Outcome criteria must be realistic and attainable. Structuring outcomes in small steps helps the patient and the nurse see concrete evidence of progress. The following are examples of possible outcomes for a patient with a somatic symptom disorder (Ackley & Ladwig, 2011):
- Patient will exhibit sensitivity to self-needs and those of others.
- Patient will resume performance of work, family, and social role behaviours.
- Patient will identify ineffective coping patterns.
- Patient will make realistic appraisal of strengths and weaknesses.
- Patient will assertively verbalize feelings such as anger, shame, or guilt.

## PLANNING

Because patients with somatic symptom disorders are rarely admitted to psychiatric care settings for treatment, long-term interventions usually take place on an outpatient basis. Short-term treatment may be initiated if the patient is admitted to a medical-surgical unit. Stays on medical units are usually short, and discharge occurs as soon as diagnostic tests are completed and negative results are received.

| TABLE 23-4 | POTENTIAL NURSING DIAGNOSES FOR SOMATIC SYMPTOM DISORDERS | |
|---|---|---|
| **SIGNS AND SYMPTOMS** | **NURSING DIAGNOSES** | |
| Inability to meet occupational, family, or social responsibilities because of symptoms | Ineffective coping | |
| Inability to participate in usual community activities or friendships because of psychogenic symptoms | Ineffective role performance Impaired social interaction | |
| Dependence on pain relievers | Powerlessness | |
| Distortion of body functions and symptoms | Disturbed body image | |
| Presence of secondary gains by adoption of sick role | Pain, acute or chronic | |
| Inability to meet family role function and need for family to assume role function of the somatic individual | Interrupted family processes Ineffective sexuality pattern | |
| Assumption of some of the roles of the somatic parent by the children | Impaired parenting | |
| Shifting of the sexual partner's role to that of caregiver or parent and of the patient's role to that of recipient of care | Risk for caregiver role strain | |
| Feeling of inability to control symptoms or understand why he or she cannot find help | Chronic low self-esteem | |
| Development of negative self-evaluation related to losing body function, feeling useless, or not feeling valued by significant others | Spiritual distress | |
| Inability to take care of basic self-care needs related to conversion symptoms (paralysis, seizures, pain, fatigue) Inability to sleep due to psychogenic pain | Self-care deficit Disturbed sleep pattern | |

Somatization is common in primary care, but providers are generally not confident about managing it and often prescribe unnecessary interventions (Walters, Tylee, Fisher, et al., 2007). For approximately 25% to 50% of symptoms seen in primary health care, there is no evidence of physical disease (Van

Ravenzwaaij, Hartman, Ravesteijn, et al., 2010). A top priority stated in the report *Changing Directions, Changing Lives: The Mental Health Strategy for Canada* (Mental Health Commission of Canada, 2012) is to identify and integrate mental health needs into primary care settings. Given that multiple health care providers are often involved in the care of patients with somatic symptom disorder, good communication among treating clinicians is essential to maintain a consistent approach both for the patient and for the clinicians (Feinstein, 2011). Because of the frequency of co-morbidities between somatic disorders and major depression and anxiety in primary care, an integrated model of care among mental health and medical clinicians is essential (Steinbrecher, Koerber, Frieser, et al., 2011). In an ideal situation, a multidisciplinary team of clinicians would include an advanced-practice nurse who could provide consultation to health care providers outside of psychiatry.

One of the many advantages of integrating mental health services into primary health care settings is less stigmatization of treatment for mental illness and of people with mental disorders. Because primary health care services are not associated with any specific health conditions, this level of care seems far more "acceptable," and therefore accessible, for most users and families (World Health Organization, 2007). This accessibility may be one of the reasons for the high incidence of primary clinic visits for physical symptoms that do not have an underlying medical cause. Many primary care centres have psychiatric mental health nurses as part of the regular treatment team as they can bring a strong perspective in managing both physical and mental health needs in integrated care settings.

## IMPLEMENTATION

Establishing a therapeutic relationship is the first step in delivering effective nursing care. A therapeutic relationship provides a foundation for overcoming the patient's resistance to the concept that no physical cause for the symptom exists and for curbing the patient's tendency to go from caregiver to caregiver.

Six key recommendations have been made for developing effective relationships with and treatment for patients with somatic symptom disorders (Kenny & Egan, 2011):
1. Provide continuity of care.
2. Avoid unnecessary tests and procedures.
3. Provide frequent, brief, and regular office visits.
4. Always conduct a physical exam.
5. Avoid making disparaging comments such as "Your symptoms are all in your head."
6. Set reasonable therapeutic goals such as maintaining function despite ongoing pain.

To be successful, therapeutic interventions must address patient needs. The primary goal for people with somatic symptom disorders is to help them identify ways to get needs met without resorting to somatization. The secondary gains derived from illness behaviours become less important to the patient when underlying needs can be met directly. *Reattribution treatment*, a specific treatment approach for somatization (see Box 23-1), helps toward this goal.

| BOX 23-1 | REATTRIBUTION TREATMENT TO LINK PHYSICAL COMPLAINTS AND PSYCHOLOGICAL DISTRESS |
|---|---|

*Reattribution treatment* is a structured intervention designed to provide a simple explanation of somatic symptoms to patients. Health care providers with reattribution skills help patients feel understood and help them make the link between physical complaints and psychological distress.

Reattribution has four stages:

**Stage 1: Feeling Understood**
The health care provider uses empathetic listening skills in taking the history of physical, emotional, spiritual, and social factors of the presenting symptoms, including patient beliefs about and perceptions of the cause of illness, times when it is worse, and what helps improve symptoms. This stage includes a brief, focused physical exam.

**Stage 2: Broadening the Agenda**
The health care provider gives feedback of assessment findings, discusses the implications of the findings, and acknowledges the patient's distress.

**Stage 3: Making the Link**
The health care provider uses empowering explanations for symptoms—for example, "You may have a heightened sensitivity to particular stressors that is affected by genetics, your personal experiences, and the environment." This comment is patient-centred and does not blame the patient for the symptoms (Fuller-Thomson, Sulman, Brennenstuhl, et al., 2011).

**Stage 4: Negotiating Further Treatment**
The health care provider and the patient collaboratively create a treatment plan that includes regular follow-up visits and short-term and long-term goals.

**Source:** Adapted from Walters, P., Tylee, A., Fisher, J., et al. (2007). Teaching junior doctors to manage patients who somatise: Is it possible in an afternoon? *Medical Education, 41*, 995–1001. doi:10.1111/j.1365-2923.2007.02833.x. Copyright © 2007, John Wiley and Sons.

## Psychosocial Interventions

People who have distressing symptoms are vulnerable to a variety of psychosocial stresses. How they cope with these stresses may make the difference between living with an acceptable quality of life and experiencing despair, withdrawal, helplessness, hopelessness, and suicidal ideation. Nurses are in a position to assess and understand patients' psychosocial stressors, identify needed coping skills, and teach stress-management techniques. Nurses can play an important role not only in managing patients' immediate care but also in helping patients improve their ability to cope and increase their quality of life during the course of somatic disorders.

Effective coping skills that can be taught are many and varied (e.g., assertiveness training, cognitive reframing, problem-solving skills, and social supports). A nurse is in a key position to assess, educate, or provide referrals to a patient to enable

healthier ways of looking at and dealing with illness. Consider referring the patient for instruction in relaxation techniques such as reiki, meditation, guided imagery, breathing exercises, and others, or teach the patient some techniques yourself. Behavioural techniques, such as progressive muscle relaxation and biofeedback (which nurses can get special training to perform), are also useful. Relaxation techniques, stress-management skills, and supportive education should be part of patient care, regardless of the medical diagnosis.

The following interventions have all been shown to positively affect a patient's recovery:
- Educating the patient about specific treatments
- Referring the patient to community support groups (or systems)
- Teaching patients more effective coping skills that take into consideration patients' values, preferences, and lifestyle
- Focusing on a patient's strengths and reinforcing coping skills that work (e.g., prayerfulness, participation in hobbies, relaxation techniques)

The Nursing Interventions Classification (NIC) offers several categories pertinent to caring for patients with somatic symptom disorders: Promotion of self-care activities, Assertiveness training, Family involvement promotion, Limit setting, Self-awareness enhancement, and Self-esteem enhancement (Bulechek, Butcher, Dochterman, et al., 2012). The presence of somatization may impair the patient's ability to perform self-care activities, requiring nursing intervention. In general, interventions use a matter-of-fact approach to support the highest level of self-care the patient is capable of. For patients manifesting paralysis, blindness, or severe fatigue, an effective nursing approach is to support them while expecting them to feed, bathe, or groom themselves (e.g., the patient who demonstrates paralysis of an arm can be expected to eat using the other arm; the patient experiencing blindness can be told at what numbers on an imaginary clock the food is located on the plate). These strategies are effective in reducing secondary gain. The use of assertiveness techniques gives patients a direct means of getting needs met and thereby decreases the need for somatic symptoms. Teaching an exercise regimen, such as doing range-of-motion exercises for 15 to 20 minutes daily and regular walks, if possible, can help the patient feel in control, can increase endorphin levels, and may help decrease anxiety.

Table 23-5 provides basic-level interventions for somatic symptom disorders.

## Pharmacological Interventions

Researchers are currently investigating the effectiveness of medications for the treatment of somatic symptom disorders. Medication trials with antidepressants (including serotonin norepinephrine reuptake inhibitors (SNRIs), such as venlafaxine (Effexor XR) and duloxetine (Cymbalta), and a noradrenergic and specific serotonergic antidepressant, such as mirtazapine (Remeron), have been effective in reducing the somatic symptoms, but further controlled trials are needed to determine the most effective antidepressants (Garcia-Martin, Miranda, & Soutullo, 2012). Tricyclic antidepressants (TCAs) and SSRIs have also been helpful for some patients with somatic

| TABLE 23-5 | BASIC-LEVEL INTERVENTIONS FOR SOMATIC SYMPTOM DISORDERS |
|---|---|
| **INTERVENTION** | **RATIONALE** |
| Offer explanations and support during diagnostic testing. | Reduces anxiety while ruling out organic illness |
| After physical complaints have been investigated, avoid further reinforcement (e.g., do not take vital signs each time patient complains of palpitations). | Directs focus away from physical symptoms |
| Spend time with patient at times other than when patient summons nurse to voice physical complaint. | Rewards non–illness-related behaviours and encourages repetition of desired behaviour |
| Observe and record frequency and intensity of somatic symptoms. (Patient or family can give information.) | Establishes a baseline and later enables evaluation of effectiveness of interventions |
| Do not imply that symptoms are not real. | Acknowledges that psychogenic symptoms are real to the patient |
| Shift focus from somatic complaints to feelings or to neutral topics. | Conveys interest in patient as a person rather than in patient's symptoms; reduces need to gain attention via symptoms |
| Assess secondary gains "physical illness" provides for patient (e.g., attention, increased dependency, and distraction from another problem). | Allows these needs to be met in healthier ways and thus minimizes secondary gains |
| Use matter-of-fact approach to patient exhibiting resistance or covert anger. | Avoids power struggles; demonstrates acceptance of anger and permits discussion of angry feelings |
| Have patient direct all requests to primary nurse. | Reduces manipulation |
| Help patient look at effect of illness behaviour on others. | Encourages insight; can help improve family relationships |
| Show concern for patient while avoiding fostering dependency needs. | Shows respect for patient's feelings while minimizing secondary gains from "illness" |
| Reinforce patient's strengths and problem-solving abilities. | Contributes to positive self-esteem; helps patient realize that needs can be met without resorting to somatic symptoms |
| Teach assertive communication. | Provides patient with a positive means of getting needs met; reduces feelings of helplessness and need for manipulation |
| Teach patient stress reduction techniques, such as meditation, relaxation, and mild physical exercise. | Provides alternative coping strategies; reduces need for medication |

symptom disorders by reducing depressive symptoms and hence somatic responses but also indirectly by altering nerve circuits that affect not only mood but fatigue, pain perception, gastrointestinal distress, and other somatic symptoms (Kroenke, 2007). Patients may also benefit from short-term use of anti-anxiety medication, which must be monitored carefully because of the risk for dependence.

## Health Teaching and Health Promotion

Some patients who somatize as a way of coping with anxiety may benefit from education about body functions. The type and depth of teaching is determined by the information the patient already understands. Others may know extensively about their physical illness and demonstrate all of the potential symptoms. In these situations, the teaching would focus on accurately assessing and interpreting the body's responses to digestion, stress, fatigue, and excitement.

## Case Management

"Doctor shopping" is common among patients with somatic symptom disorders. They go from physician to physician, clinic to clinic, or hospital to hospital, hoping to establish a physical basis for their distress. Repeated computed tomographic (CT) scans, magnetic resonance imaging (MRI), and other diagnostic tests are often documented in the medical record. Case management can help limit health care costs associated with such visits. The case manager can recommend to the primary care provider that the patient be scheduled for brief appointments every four to six weeks at set times, rather than on demand, and that laboratory tests be avoided unless they are absolutely necessary. The patient who establishes a relationship with the case manager often feels less anxiety because the patient has someone to contact and knows that someone is "looking after them."

## Advanced-Practice Interventions

Advanced-practice nurses may use various types of psychotherapy or provide consultation to primary care providers who treat patients with somatic symptom disorders. Because nursing has as a major focus viewing the patient in a holistic way, the advanced-practice nurse can lead the health care team in assessing each patient's unique biological, environmental, psychological, spiritual, and sociocultural needs to develop the most

## TABLE 23-6 ADVANCED-PRACTICE INTERVENTIONS FOR SOMATIC SYMPTOM DISORDERS

| DISORDER | COURSE | INTERVENTIONS |
|---|---|---|
| Somatic symptom disorder | Chronic and relapsing | Consistent primary care provider with regular patient visits, limited tests<br>Group therapy<br>Cognitive-behavioural therapy |
| Illness anxiety disorder | Chronic and relapsing, but 50% of patients improve | Cognitive-behavioural therapy<br>Insight-oriented therapy<br>Group therapy<br>Psychopharmacological management for co-morbid conditions<br>Stress management |
| Conversion disorder | Usually acute onset; resolves quickly | Suggest that the conversion symptom will gradually improve<br>Behavioural therapy<br>Insight-oriented therapy<br>Hypnosis<br>Antianxiety drugs |
| Psychological factors affecting medical condition | Acute and chronic; variable resolution | Treat psychiatric symptoms<br>Tailor treatment to address both the psychological symptom and the medical condition |
| Factitious disorder | Highly treatment-resistant | Confrontation is counterproductive<br>Emphasis on management over cure<br>Legal interventions may be necessary in the case of Munchausen's by proxy |

**Source:** Adapted from Braun, I.M., Greenberg, D.B., Smith, F.A., et al. (2010). Functional somatic symptoms, deception syndromes, and somatoform disorders. In T.A. Stern, G.L. Fricchione, N.H. Cassem, et al. (Eds.), *Massachusetts General Hospital handbook of general hospital psychiatry* (6th ed.) (pp. 173–187). St. Louis, MO: Mosby.

comprehensive, individualized plan of care to alleviate the distress of somatic symptoms.

Cognitive-behavioural therapy (CBT) is the most consistently supported treatment for the full spectrum of somatic disorders. CBT helps patients find ways to reframe their thoughts and gain control of their situation and break what can become a self-fulfilling cycle of pain, despair, and health-seeking behaviours (Kroenke, 2007). Refer to Chapter 3 for a more complete explanation of CBT. Table 23-6 provides a summary of advanced-practice interventions.

Managing both psychiatric and physical symptoms can be a challenge for general medical nurses. Psychiatric liaison nurses, a subspecialty of psychiatric mental health nursing initiated in the early 1960s, can bridge that gap. Usually, the psychiatric liaison nurse has a master's degree and a background in psychiatric and medical-surgical nursing. He or she functions as a consultant assisting other nurses in managing psychiatric symptoms and as a clinician working directly to help the patient deal more effectively with physical and emotional problems. The psychiatric liaison nurse first meets with the nurse who initiated the consultation and then reviews the patient's medical records, talks with the physicians, and interviews the patient. After the patient interview, the liaison nurse discusses the assessment and suggestions with the referring nurse. If a psychiatric consultation is warranted, the psychiatric liaison nurse initiates the consultation by contacting the patient's physician.

A case conference is sometimes needed to enhance communication and consistency in the care of a particular patient.

## EVALUATION

Evaluation of patients with somatic symptom disorders is a simple process when measurable behavioural outcomes have been written clearly and realistically. For these patients, however, you might often find that goals and outcomes are only partially met. Patients are likely to report the continuing presence of somatic symptoms, but they often say they are less concerned about the symptoms. Families frequently report relatively high satisfaction with outcomes, even without total eradication of the patient's symptoms.

## FACTITIOUS DISORDERS

Factitious disorders—disorders in which patients intentionally and consciously feign illnesses—result in disability and immeasurable costs to the health care system. Whereas most people with somatic disorders do not consciously control symptoms, people with factitious disorders consciously pretend to be ill to get emotional needs met and attain the status of "patient" (Sadock & Sadock, 2008). The term *factitious* is derived from the Latin word meaning "artificial or contrived." Patients with this disorder artificially, deliberately, and dramatically fabricate symptoms or self-inflict injury, with the goal of assuming a sick role. Examples of contrived illnesses include bleeding, fever, hypoglycemia, seizures, and even cancer and HIV (Smith, 2008).

## CLINICAL PICTURE

Factitious disorders are either self-directed or other-directed. There are two subtypes of self-directed factitious disorders. Individuals with the first subtype usually do not "doctor shop" (i.e., go from one primary care provider to another). They visit the same person time and again and are known by the health care personnel. The patient may get admitted to the hospital through the emergency department, where he or she dramatically describes the illness using proper medical terminology that can be quite convincing. The patient is often reluctant for professionals to speak with family members, friends, or previous health care providers. Once admitted, the patient is frequently demanding and requests specific treatments and interventions. Negative test results are often followed by new or additional symptoms. If the health care team sets limits and does not follow through with requests, the patient may become angry and accuse the staff of incompetence and maltreatment.

The second subtype of self-directed factitious disorder is referred to as **Munchausen's syndrome**, named for Baron Karl Friedrich Hieronymus von Münchausen (1720–1797), an eighteenth-century German cavalry officer with a reputation for fabricating exaggerated tales. Munchausen's syndrome is notable for the way patients go from one primary care provider or hospital to another, seeking attention. Serious complications and sepsis may result from self-injections of toxins such as *E. coli*. Patients may have "criss-crossed" or "railroad-track" abdomens due to scars from exploratory surgeries to investigate unexplained symptoms. In the extreme, amputations may even result from this disorder.

The most insidious form of factitious disorders is factitious disorder imposed on another (other-directed factitious disorder), commonly called *Munchausen's syndrome by proxy*, in which a caregiver deliberately feigns illness in a vulnerable dependent. People with this disorder are not motivated by awards such as insurance money or other compensation; they are motivated by attention, excitement, and the perpetuation of relationships with health care providers of that dependent. The disorder results in unnecessary medical visits and potentially harmful medical procedures. Examples of actions taken by people with this disorder include inducing premature delivery by rupturing the amniotic sac with a fingernail, putting a pillow over a child's face, and introducing microorganisms into a child's wound. Falsification of illnesses can result in extreme pain, surgical procedures, and even death of dependents.

### Malingering

While not a specific mental disorder, **malingering** is related to the factitious disorders. Malingering is a consciously motivated act to deceive for material gain (Sadock & Sadock, 2008). People may fabricate an illness or exaggerate symptoms so as to become eligible for disability compensation, commit fraud against insurance companies, obtain prescription medications, evade military service, or receive a reduced prison sentence. Reported pains (e.g., back pain, headache, or toothache) are vague and hard for clinicians to prove or disprove.

## EPIDEMIOLOGY

Epidemiological studies estimate an incidence rate of factitious disorders at 0.8% to 1.3%. Explanations for the low incidence rate include the belief that a large number of cases are missed due to frequent denial of factitious-disorder behaviours, the challenge of differentiating between real and feigned illness, and the fact that many patients flee the health care setting (Hagglund, 2009). Contrary to studies' results, factitious disorder is now thought to account for up to 6% of contacts with health care providers.

The diagnosis of factitious disorder should be considered in complicated patients, especially those with a history of emotional or physical distress, excessive dependence, or resistance to discharge (Williams, 2012).

Malingering is thought to be more common in men than in women (Smith, 2008). Among the criminal population, the rates may be as high as 10% to 20% (Sadock & Sadock, 2008). It is nearly impossible to determine the prevalence of malingering, owing to the concealment of its origins.

## CO-MORBIDITY

People with factitious disorders tend to focus on physiological problems, although some patients may also try to convince clinicians that they have a psychiatric disorder. Patients may describe symptoms of depression, dissociation, conversion, and psychoses and seek treatment for these problems (Sadock & Sadock, 2008). According to some reports, substance abuse, borderline personality disorders, and sexual disorders are frequently present along with a normal to high intelligence quotient (IQ) and an intimate knowledge of the health care system (Ardesrani, Zairoddin, Shahpouri, et al., 2009). Malingering is associated with antisocial, narcissistic, and borderline personality disorders.

## ETIOLOGY

### Biological Factors

Brain dysfunction, specifically impaired information processing, has been identified as a possible source of the symptoms of factitious disorders (Sadock & Sadock, 2008). No other biological abnormalities have been proposed at this time.

### Psychological Factors

It is difficult to determine or understand the psychological basis of these disorders because of the patient's intention to skew the facts. There is some evidence that people with these disorders suffered abuse and neglect as children and may have been hospitalized more frequently than is typical (Sadock & Sadock, 2008). These hospitalizations may have been perceived as a refuge from a chaotic home life. It has also been suggested that patients with factitious disorders may have a masochistic side and feel a need to be punished through painful procedures.

## APPLICATION OF THE NURSING PROCESS

### ASSESSMENT

Many of the principles of care for somatic-related disorders apply to factitious disorders. Often, determining whether a patient's signs and symptoms are conscious or unconscious (i.e., whether they constitute a somatic symptom disorder or a factitious disorder) is a challenge for clinicians, particularly those in the position to diagnose psychiatric disorders. Your role as a nurse, whether you work in psychiatry, mental health, or any other setting, is to carefully assess the patient and document your care. A general principle in treating people with a factitious disorder is to avoid confrontation, which may result in the patient's defensiveness, elusiveness, or exit from the treatment facility prior to the completion of treatment (Smith, 2008).

#### Self-Assessment

Nurses who work with patients with factitious disorders are often angry and resentful. Because people with factitious disorders cause their symptoms, they are wasting health care dollars, taking away resources from people who really need them, and wasting the nurse's time. These counter-transference reactions should be acknowledged and can be addressed through discussions with other members of the treatment team and careful treatment planning. Nurses often superficially conclude that, if the patient with a factitious disorder would stop making him- or herself ill, the patient's problems would be resolved. It is important to consider, however, that factitious disorders may cause real problems that can be overlooked.

### DIAGNOSIS

In addition to the physical symptoms (e.g., pain, lacerations, ingestion of a foreign object), emotions such as anxiety, depression, and despair are frequent concerns for health care providers. Health care workers are also required to address their own feelings related to possible manipulation by patients with this disorder. Table 23-7 lists common potential nursing diagnoses related to the psychological components of factitious disorders.

### OUTCOMES IDENTIFICATION

To evaluate the effectiveness of treatment, outcome criteria are established. Relevant categories of the *Nursing Outcomes Classification (NOC)* (Moorhead, Johnson, Maas, et al., 2012) include *Personal resiliency*, *Anxiety self-control*, and *Self-esteem*. Refer to Table 23-8 for examples of short-term *NOC* indicators for the patient with a factitious disorder.

### PLANNING

For patients with either type of factitious disorder, and particularly other-directed factitious disorder, the nurse must consider

| TABLE 23-7 | POTENTIAL NURSING DIAGNOSES FOR FACTITIOUS DISORDERS |
|---|---|
| **SIGNS AND SYMPTOMS** | **NURSING DIAGNOSES** |
| Crisis, high levels of anxiety | *Ineffective coping* |
| | *Anxiety* |
| | *Self-mutilation* |
| Anger and aggression; child, elder, or spouse abuse | *Risk for other-directed violence* |
| | *Ineffective coping* |
| | *Impaired parenting* |
| | *Disabled family coping* |
| Depression | *Hopelessness* |
| | *Risk for suicide* |
| | *Self-mutilation* |
| | *Chronic low self-esteem* |
| | *Spiritual distress* |
| Difficulty in relationships, manipulation | *Ineffective coping* |
| | *Impaired social interaction* |
| | *Defensive coping* |
| | *Interrupted family processes* |
| Failure to follow prescribed medical procedure or medication regimen | *Ineffective therapeutic regimen management* |
| | *Nonadherence* |

| TABLE 23-8 | NOC OUTCOMES RELATED TO FACTITIOUS DISORDER |
|---|---|
| **NURSING OUTCOME AND DEFINITION** | **SHORT-TERM INDICATORS** |
| *Personal resiliency:* positive adaptation and function of an individual following significant adversity or crisis | Expresses emotion |
| | Seeks emotional support |
| | Uses strategies to promote safety |
| | Takes responsibility for own actions |
| | Identifies available community resources |
| *Anxiety self-control:* personal action to eliminate or reduce feelings of apprehension, tension, or uneasiness from an unidentifiable source | Monitors intensity of anxiety |
| | Plans coping strategies for stressful situations |
| | Uses effective coping strategies |
| *Self-esteem:* personal judgement of self-worth | Verbalization of self-acceptance |
| | Description of self |
| | Acceptance of compliments from others |
| | Feelings about self-worth |

**Source:** Data from Moorhead, S., Johnson, M., Maas, M.L., et al. (Eds.). (2012). *Nursing outcome classification (NOC)* (5th ed.). St. Louis, MO: Mosby.

safety. Patients who may purposefully inflict damage on themselves or others must be carefully monitored, and suspicious activities should be reported to and discussed by the health care team. It is essential that the nurse share any information that may prevent a person or a vulnerable and unsuspecting dependent from undergoing unnecessary surgery or treatments.

## IMPLEMENTATION

After determining that the physical symptoms have been intentionally and consciously generated, the health care team will shift the focus to determining the secondary gains possible from the feigned illness. Nurses will need to use their therapeutic communication skills in order to develop a trusting relationship to further explore the ineffective coping of individuals with factitious disorders.

## EVALUATION

Interventions are determined to be effective when patients remain safe, conflicts have been explored, new coping strategies have permitted the patient to function at a higher level, and stress is handled adaptively without the desire or need for the pretense of a physiological disorder.

## DISSOCIATIVE DISORDERS

Dissociative disorders are a group of disorders precipitated by significant adverse experiences or traumas resulting in the unconscious altering of mind–body connections. Dissociation is an unconscious defence mechanism that protects the individual against overwhelming anxiety and stress through an emotional separation; however, this separation results in disturbances in memory, consciousness, self-identity, and perception.

Patients with dissociative disorders are able to assess a situation realistically, rather than for what they want it to be or fear that it might be. They do not have hallucinations or delusions (meaning they have "intact reality testing"), but they may have flashbacks or see images that are triggered by current events that are related to the past trauma. Mild, fleeting dissociative experiences are relatively common to all of us; for example, we may be listening to someone and suddenly realize that we have not heard part or all of what was said. These common experiences are distinctly different from the processes of pathological dissociation.

Pathological dissociation is involuntary and results in failure of control over one's mental processes and the integration of conscious awareness (Spiegel, Loewenstein, Lewis-Fernandez, et al., 2011). With pathological dissociation, pieces of a memory become fragmented. For example, normally, when people remember an experience, they can recall the people who were there, maybe a significant smell (like cooking turkey), maybe singing, and maybe an uncle who wore a bright red suit. However, when memories become fragmented, as in pathological dissociation, a person may recall a sound or smell but not be able to link these sensations to the actual event, instead feeling as though there is something familiar about the smell or sound

but not knowing why. If the pieces of memory are associated with a traumatic experience, the fragments can leave the person fearful, confused, or both. If the memory was very traumatic, the fragments may cause the person to re-enact, as well as re-experience, trauma without consciously knowing why.

Symptoms of dissociation may be either *positive* or *negative*. Positive symptoms refer to unwanted additions to mental activity, such as flashbacks; negative symptoms refer to deficits, such as memory problems or the inability to sense or control different parts of the body. It is thought that dissociation decreases the immediate subjective distress of the trauma (a self-protective mechanism) and also continues to protect the individual from full awareness of the disturbing event. Continued dissociative symptoms, however, can interfere with activities of daily living and relationships.

In the case of abused or neglected children, dissociation can be interpreted as somewhat protective, allowing the child to continue to be attached to abusive or neglectful caretakers. This instinctive mechanism highlights the importance of attachments and relationships in allowing the child to grow socially, intellectually, and cognitively. If abuse or neglect has occurred, memories of it become compartmentalized and often do not intrude into awareness until later in life during a stressful situation or in trying to develop another significant relationship.

## CLINICAL PICTURE

Dissociative disorders include (1) depersonalization/derealization disorder, (2) dissociative amnesia, and (3) dissociative identity disorder.

### Depersonalization/Derealization Disorder

Depersonalization/derealization disorder may cause a person to feel mechanical, dreamy, or detached from the body. Some people suffer episodes of these problems that come and go, while others have episodes that begin with stressors and eventually become constant. People with this disorder may experience episodes of depersonalization or derealization or both. When experiencing depersonalization, individuals feel as though they are observers of their own body or mental processes—there is an internal feeling of disconnect. Similarly, with derealization, there is a recurring feeling that one's surroundings are unreal or distant—an external or outside feeling of disconnect. These feelings are not consciously controlled by the patients with dissociative disorders and are reported to be very distressing to those who experience them.

---

**VIGNETTE**

Marguerite describes becoming very troubled by perceived changes in her appearance when she looks in a mirror. She thinks that her image looks wavy and indistinct. Soon after, she describes feeling as though she is floating in a fog, with her feet not actually touching the ground. Questioning reveals that Marguerite's son has recently confided to her that he tested positive for HIV and that she is extremely worried about him.

## Dissociative Amnesia

Dissociative amnesia is marked by the inability to recall important autobiographical information, often of a traumatic or stressful nature, that is too pervasive to be explained by ordinary forgetfulness. While autobiographical memory is available (i.e., stored within the brain), the person is not accessible (i.e., the memory cannot be retrieved). When memories are stored, information about the situation (*retrieval cues*) is also stored. This additional information can be about the environment (smell, place, colour) or about a feeling (happy, sad, mad) or about an activity at the time (walking, crying, sitting, studying). Seeing or thinking about these retrieval cues helps us recall the memory. For example, have you ever got up from watching television and gone into the kitchen to do something but then forgotten what you were going to do once you got to the kitchen? But then you go back and sit down in front of the television and you remember? You have just accessed a memory using a retrieval cue.

In contrast, a patient with generalized amnesia is unable to recall information about his or her entire lifetime. The generalized amnesia may be *localized* (the patient is unable to remember all events in a certain period) or *selective* (the patient is able to recall some but not all events in a certain period). For the person with generalized amnesia, the information is neither available nor accessible, contrary to dissociative amnesia.

A subtype of dissociative amnesia, also usually precipitated by a traumatic event, is dissociative fugue. This disorder is characterized by sudden, unexpected travel away from the customary locale and an inability to recall one's identity and information about some or all of the past. The word *fugue* comes from the Latin word for *flight*. In rare cases, an individual with dissociative fugue assumes a whole new identity. During a fugue state (individuals are in a different location, unable to recall personal information about themselves or their past), individuals show no signs of illness and tend to lead rather simple lives, rarely calling attention to themselves. Only the memories tied to their identities are lost. If the person experiencing the fugue state knows how to drive, use the computer, make meals, and use a public transit system, he or she retains that knowledge. After a few weeks to a few months, the person may become confused about his or her identity or remember the former identity and then become amnesic for the time spent in the fugue state. The fictional character Jason Bourne portrayed in *The Bourne Identity* (Crowley, Gladstein, & Liman, 2002) was found by a fisherman after being badly wounded. Jason Bourne could remember nothing about his life until one day he "woke up." Although fictional, the *Bourne Identity* protagonist is named after Ansel Bourne, one of the first-ever documented cases of dissociative fugue. Ansel Bourne was a Rhode Island minister who, in January 1887, suddenly "disappeared" and travelled to Pennsylvania, where he worked selling stationery. After approximately three months, he "woke up," did not know where he was, and still thought that it was January (Kenny, 1986).

## Dissociative Identity Disorder

The essential feature of dissociative identity disorder (DID) is the presence of two or more distinct personality states that alternately and recurrently take control of behaviour. It is believed that severe sexual, physical, or psychological trauma in childhood predisposes an individual to the development of DID. Each alternate personality (alter), or subpersonality, has its own pattern of perceiving, relating to, and thinking about the self and the environment. Each alter is a complex unit with its own memories, behaviour patterns, and social relationships that dictate how the person acts when that personality is dominant. If the original or primary personality is religious and moralistic, the subpersonality or subpersonalities are often pleasure-seeking and nonconforming. The alters may also behave as individuals of a different sex, race, or religion.

Dissociative identity disorder appears to be associated with two dissociative identity states (alternate personalities): (1) a state in which the individual blocks access and responses to traumatic memories so as to be able to function daily and (2) a state fixated on traumatic memories. The primary personality, or *host*, is usually not aware of the subpersonalities and is perplexed by lost time and unexplained events. Experiences such as finding unfamiliar clothing in the closet, being called a different name by a stranger, and not having childhood memories are characteristic of DID. Subpersonalities are often aware of the existence of each other to some degree. Transition from one personality to another occurs during times of stress and may range from a dramatic to a barely noticeable event. Some patients experience the transition when awakening. Shifts may last from minutes to months, although shorter periods are more common.

The alternate personalities also impact physiological functioning. For example, regional cerebral blood-flow patterns and autonomic and subjective reactions are displayed differently for each alternate personality when the individual is exposed to trauma-related stimuli (Reinders, Nijenhuis, Quak, et al., 2006). The dominant hand and the voice may be different, and intelligence and electroencephalographic findings may also change.

## EPIDEMIOLOGY

Although mental health care providers in Canada believe that dissociative disorders are rare, depersonalization disorder prevalence rates range from about 1% to 3%, which is comparable to disorders such as schizophrenia, bipolar disorder, and obsessive-compulsive disorder (Spiegel, Loewenstein, Lewis-Fernandez, et al., 2011). Dissociative amnesia is also fairly common, with a prevalence of about 2% to 7%. However, Piper and Merskey, Canadian psychiatrists (2004), have indicated that "DID is best understood as a culture-bound and often iatrogenic condition" (p. 592).

## CO-MORBIDITY

Psychiatric co-morbidities are extremely common for people with dissociative disorders. Patients with dissociative disorders usually seek treatment for another problem such as anxiety or depression (International Society for the Study of Trauma and Dissociation, 2012; Spiegel, Loewenstein, Lewis-Fernandez, et al., 2011).

## ETIOLOGY

Physical, sexual, or emotional abuse and other traumatic life events are associated with children's or adults' experiencing dissociative symptoms (Schlozman & Nonacs, 2008). Regardless of the age at which the dissociative symptoms start, their purpose is to reduce disturbing feelings and protect the person from full awareness of the trauma.

### Biological Factors

Research suggests that the limbic system is involved in the development of dissociative disorders. Animal studies show that early, prolonged emotional detachment from the caretaker negatively affects the development of the limbic system, which is where traumatic memories are processed; therefore, trauma negatively interferes with the normal development of the limbic system. Individuals with dissociative disorders have increased activation of the orbital frontal cortex, which inhibits activation of the amygdala and insular cortex as well as the hippocampal areas, where traumatic memories are stored (Speigel, Loewenstein, Lewis-Fernandez, et al., 2011). Refer to Chapter 3 for more detailed information related to the functions of these areas of the brain.

### Genetics

Although genetic variability is thought to play a role in stress reactivity, dissociation is thought to be largely due to extreme stress or environmental factors.

### Psychological Factors

Learning theory suggests that dissociative disorders can be explained as learned methods for avoiding stress and anxiety. Dissociation is one of the most primitive ego defence mechanisms. The pattern of avoidance occurs when an individual deals with an unpleasant event by consciously deciding not to think about it. The more anxiety-provoking the event is, the greater is the need to avoid thinking about it. As the individual increasingly depends on this coping strategy, dissociation becomes easier, and it becomes more likely that this defence mechanism will be the individual's predominant means of reacting to stress.

### Environmental Factors

The environmental factors related to a person developing a dissociative disorder are exposures to traumatic events, including any experience that is overwhelming to the person, such as a motor vehicle accident, combat experience, emotional or verbal abuse, incest, neglectful or abusive caregivers, and imprisonment.

### Cultural Factors

Certain disorders appear to develop only in specific cultures. These disorders are known as culture-bound disorders or syndromes. These syndromes include *piblokto*, seen in First Nations people of the Arctic (Inuit); frenzy witchcraft, which the Navajo are vulnerable to; and amok, experienced by First Nations people living in the Western Pacific. These disorders manifest in the form of individuals' experiencing a high level of activity, a trancelike state, then running or fleeing, followed by exhaustion, sleep, and amnesia regarding the episode. When these symptoms are observed in individuals native to the corresponding geographical areas, they must be differentiated from symptoms of dissociative disorders versus a culture-bound syndrome.

## APPLICATION OF THE NURSING PROCESS

### ASSESSMENT

For a diagnosis of a dissociative disorder to be made, other medical and neurological illnesses, substance use, and other coexisting (co-morbid) psychiatric disorders must be ruled out as the cause of the patient's symptoms. Specific information about identity, memory, consciousness, life events, mood, suicide risk, and the impact of the disorder on the patient and the family are important dimensions to assess. The assessment should include objective data from physical examination, electroencephalography, imaging studies, and specific questions to identify dissociative symptoms. Assessment tools are important because a psychiatric interview will often miss the presence of dissociation because the individual does not know what he or she does not know—that is, by definition, dissociative periods involve lapses of memory of which the person may not even be aware.

Several scales have been developed to assess dissociation, including the Dissociative Experience Scale (DES) (Bernstein & Putnam, 1986), the Structured Clinical Interview for Dissociative Disorders (SCID-D) (Schlozman & Nonacs, 2008), the Somatoform Dissociation Questionnaire (SDQ) (available from http://www.enijenhuis.nl/sdq.html), and the Dissociative Disorders Interview Schedule (DDIS) (available from http://www.empty-memories.nl/dis_89/ross_structuredinterview.pdf).

### General Assessment

For general guidelines for assessment of a patient with a dissociative disorder, see the Assessment Guidelines box.

### ASSESSMENT GUIDELINES

**Dissociative Disorders**

1. Assess identity and memory.
   a. Assess for signs of dissociation.
   b. Assess for a history of a similar episode in the past with benign outcomes.
2. Establish whether the person suffered abuse, trauma, or loss as a child.
3. Evaluate mood and level of anxiety.
4. Identify support systems through a psychosocial assessment.
5. Identify relevant psychosocial distress issues by performing a basic psychosocial assessment.
6. Assess for a history of self-harm.

## Identity and Memory

Assessing patients' ability to identify themselves requires more than asking them to state their names. The nurse should consider the following when assessing memory:

- Can the patient remember recent and past events?
- Is the patient's memory clear and complete or partial and fuzzy?
- Is the patient aware of gaps in memory (e.g., lack of memory for events such as a graduation or a wedding)?
- Do the patient's memories place the self with a family, in school, in an occupation?

Patients with amnesia and fugue may be disoriented with regard to time and place, as well as person. Relevant assessment questions include these:

- Do you ever lose time or have blackouts?
- Do you find yourself in places with no idea how you got there?

## History

The nurse must gather information about events in the person's life. Has the patient sustained a recent injury, such as a concussion? Does the patient have a history of epilepsy, especially temporal lobe epilepsy? Does the patient have a history of early trauma, such as physical, mental, or sexual abuse? Additional pertinent questions include these:

- Have you ever found yourself wearing clothes you cannot remember buying?
- Have you ever had strange people greet and talk to you as though they were old friends?
- Does your ability to engage in things such as athletics, artistic activities, or mechanical tasks seem to change?
- Do you have differing sets of memories about childhood?

## Mood and Anxiety

Many patients with dissociative disorders seek treatment, not for their dissociations but for concerns they have related to symptoms of depression or anxiety. A complete mental status examination should be conducted to determine the degree of co-morbid symptoms related to changes in mood. See Chapters 14 and 15 for more detailed information related to the assessment of mood.

## Impact on Patient and Family

All of the dissociative disorders impact both the patient and the patient's family. For example, people with depersonalization disorder are often fearful that others may perceive their appearance as distorted and may avoid being seen in public. If they exhibit consistently high levels of anxiety, the family is likely to find it difficult to keep relationships stable. By comparison, people who experience fugue states often function adequately in their new identities by choosing simple, undemanding occupations and having few intimate social interactions. Patients with amnesia, in contrast to those with fugue, may be more dysfunctional. Their perplexity often renders them unable to work, and their memory loss impairs normal relationships. Families often direct considerable attention toward the patient

but may exhibit concern over having to assume roles that were once assigned to the patient. Finally, patients with dissociative identity disorder often have both family and work problems. Families find it difficult to accept the seemingly erratic behaviours of the patient. Employers dislike the lost time that may occur when alternate identities are in control.

## Suicide Risk

Whenever a patient's life has been substantially disrupted, the patient may have thoughts of suicide. The nurse gathering data should be alert for expressions of hopelessness, helplessness, or worthlessness and for verbalization or other behaviour that indicates the intent to engage in self-destructive or self-mutilating behaviours.

## Self-Assessment

It is natural for nurses to experience feelings of scepticism while caring for patients who are diagnosed with dissociative disorders. Believing in the authenticity of the symptoms the patient is displaying can be difficult, and feeling confused and bewildered by the presence of dissociative symptoms is not unusual. Some nurses even experience feelings of fascination and get caught up in the intrigue of caring for a patient with dissociative symptoms.

Most people with dissociative disorders have experienced a significant trauma or have been in relationships in which trust was betrayed. As a result, developing a therapeutic relationship with these patients can be a slower process than with patients who have other mental illnesses. Nurses may, therefore, feel inadequate and frustrated by their efforts.

Because a patient's dissociative symptoms may occur unexpectedly, staff must remain hypervigilant and prepare for the unexpected, including the possibility of a suicide attempt. Such demands can eventually lead to great fatigue. Caring for a patient with dissociative disorder can generate anxiety in nursing staff in any of the following situations:

- A patient who has regained memory develops panic-level anxiety related to guilt feelings
- A patient becomes assaultive because of extreme confusion or panic-level anxiety
- A patient attempts self-harm by acting out against the primary personality or other personalities

If the patient manifesting symptoms of a dissociative disorder has been involved in the commission of a crime, the medical record is likely to be a court exhibit. You may experience concern over that fact or be angry if you believe the patient is faking illness to avoid being found guilty of the crime.

Supervision should always be available for nursing staff and clinicians caring for a patient with a dissociative disorder. By discussing feelings and the plan of care with the treatment team or peers, the nurse can better provide objective and appropriate care for the patient.

## DIAGNOSIS

Potential nursing diagnoses for patients with dissociative disorders are suggested in Table 23-9.

| TABLE 23-9 | POTENTIAL NURSING DIAGNOSES FOR DISSOCIATIVE DISORDERS |
|---|---|
| **SIGNS AND SYMPTOMS** | **NURSING DIAGNOSES** |
| Amnesia or fugue related to a traumatic event<br>Symptoms of depersonalization; feelings of unreality or body-image distortions | *Disturbed personal identity*<br>*Disturbed body image* |
| Alterations in consciousness, memory, or identity<br>Abuse of substances related to dissociation<br>Disorganization or dysfunction in usual patterns of behaviour (absence from work, withdrawal from relationships, changes in role function) | *Ineffective coping*<br>*Ineffective role performance* |
| Disturbances in memory and identity<br>Interrupted family processes related to amnesia or erratic and changing behaviour | *Interrupted family processes*<br>*Impaired parenting* |
| Feeling of being out of control of memory, behaviours, and awareness<br>Inability to explain actions or behaviours when in altered state | *Anxiety*<br>*Spiritual distress*<br>*Risk for other-directed violence*<br>*Risk for self-directed violence* |

## OUTCOMES IDENTIFICATION

*NOC* (Moorhead, Johnson, Maas, et al., 2012) outcomes potentially appropriate for patients with dissociative disorders include *Identity*, *Role performance*, *Coping*, *Anxiety self-control*, *Self-mutilation restraint*, and *Aggression self-control*. Specific examples of indicators that the outcomes are being achieved are as follows:
- Patient will verbalize clear sense of personal identity.
- Patient will report decrease in stress.
- Patient will report comfort with role expectations.
- Patient will use coping strategies for stressful situations.
- Patient will refrain from injuring self.

## PLANNING

Planning for the delivery of specific nursing care is influenced by both the setting (community or inpatients) and the presenting problem. However, a phase-oriented treatment model is recommended for any setting and includes the

following (International Society for the Study of Trauma and Dissociation, 2012):

Phase 1: Establishing safety, stabilization, and symptom reduction

Phase 2: Confronting, working through, and integrating traumatic memories

Phase 3: Integrating identity and rehabilitating

The nurse will most often encounter the patient in times of crisis (i.e., when the patient is suicidal or expressing homicidal behaviour), and in times of crisis, the care plan will focus on Phase 1 strategies to ensure safety and crisis intervention. Basic nursing interventions should be implemented. Phases 2 and 3 are advanced interventions, so clinicians using these interventions require special training.

## IMPLEMENTATION

Nursing interventions are aimed at offering emotional support during the recall of painful experiences, providing a sense of safety, and encouraging an optimal level of functioning. *NIC* topics that offer relevant interventions include *Anxiety reduction*, *Coping enhancement*, *Self-awareness enhancement*, *Self-esteem enhancement*, and *Emotional support*. Refer to Table 23-10 for examples of basic-level interventions.

### Milieu Management

When the patient is in a crisis that requires hospitalization, providing a safe environment is fundamental. Other desirable characteristics of the environment are quietness, simplicity, structure, and supportiveness. Confusion and noise increase anxiety and the potential for depersonalization, delayed return of memory, or shifts among subpersonalities. Inpatient group therapy is not as helpful as task-oriented therapy, such as occupational and art therapy, which give an opportunity for self-expression. Attendance at community or unit milieu meetings relieves feelings of isolation.

### Health Teaching and Health Promotion

Stress management and coping skills are important areas of health education for people with dissociative disorders. Normalizing experiences by explaining that symptoms are adaptive responses to past overwhelming events is important. Often, the victim of childhood trauma feels as if he or she is a bad person and grows up with the false negative belief that the abuse was deserved punishment.

Another important intervention strategy is to teach grounding techniques that help the person focus on the present and help to counter dissociative symptoms. Examples of grounding techniques include the following: stomping one's feet on the ground, taking a shower, holding an ice cube, exercising, breathing deeply, counting beads, and touching fabric or upholstery on a chair. Patients can also be taught to keep a daily journal to increase their awareness of feelings and to identify triggers of their dissociative symptoms. If a patient has never written a journal, the nurse should suggest beginning with five to ten minutes of daily writing.

## TABLE 23-10   NURSING INTERVENTIONS FOR DISSOCIATIVE DISORDERS

| INTERVENTION | RATIONALE |
|---|---|
| Ensure patient safety by providing safe, protected environment and frequent observation. | Patient's sense of bewilderment may lead to inattention to safety needs |
| Provide undemanding, simple routine. | Reduces anxiety |
| Confirm identity of patient and orientation to time and place. | Supports reality and promotes ego integrity |
| Encourage patient to do things for self and make decisions about routine tasks. | Enhances self-esteem by reducing sense of powerlessness and reduces secondary gain associated with dependence |
| Assist with other decision making until memory returns. | Lowers stress and prevents patient from having to live with the consequences of unwise decisions |
| Support patient during exploration of feelings surrounding the stressful event. | Helps lower the defence of dissociation used by patient to block awareness of the stressful event |
| Do not flood patient with data regarding past events. | Memory loss serves the purpose of preventing severe to panic levels of anxiety from overtaking and disorganizing the individual |
| Allow patient to progress at own pace as memory is recovered. | Prevents undue anxiety and resistance |
| Provide support during disclosure of painful experiences. Do not force the patient to disclose. | Can be healing, while minimizing feelings of isolation. Forced disclosure can retraumatize the patient |
| Help patients see consequences of using dissociation to cope with stress. | Increases insight and helps patient understand own role in choosing behaviours |
| Accept patient's expression of negative feelings. | Conveys permission to have negative or unacceptable feelings |
| Teach stress-reduction methods. | Provides alternatives for anxiety relief |
| If patient does not remember significant others, work with involved parties to re-establish relationships. | Helps patient experience satisfaction and relieves sense of isolation |

## Pharmacological Interventions

There are no specific medications used to treat patients with dissociative disorders, but medications are often prescribed for the presenting symptoms (International Society for the Study of Trauma and Dissociation, 2012). In the acute care setting, intravenous benzodiazepines may be used to decrease intense anxiety; subsequently, the nurse may witness dramatic memory retrieval in patients with dissociative amnesia or fugue. Other medications sometimes prescribed are antidepressants, anxiolytics, and antipsychotics. As is the case whenever medications are prescribed, substance-use disorders and potential suicidal risk must be assessed carefully prior to selecting a safe and appropriate medication.

## Advanced-Practice Interventions

Advanced-practice nurses and other skilled, licensed mental health care providers use cognitive-behavioural therapy, psychodynamic psychotherapy, exposure therapy, neurofeedback, ego state therapies, somatic therapies, and medication to treat patients with dissociative disorders. Advanced training is needed to treat these patients effectively, and ongoing supervision of the therapist is suggested. Somatic therapy, another advanced-practice intervention, is described in more detail below.

## Somatic Therapy

Dissociation causes people to experience a distressing fragmentation of consciousness and a sense of separation from themselves. Disturbances of perception, sensation, autonomic regulation, and movement are common among those who have suffered significant trauma because trauma is often stored physically in the body.

Verbal and body psychotherapies are seen as complementary interventions. Dance movement therapists work with traumatized dissociative patients in emotional recovery (Koch & Harvey, 2012). A specific type of somatic psychotherapy, sensorimotor psychotherapy, combines talking therapy with body-centred interventions and movement to address the dissociative symptoms inherent in trauma (Ogden, Minton, & Pain, 2006). This type of therapy is integrated into phase-oriented trauma treatment to facilitate symptom reduction and stability, to integrate the traumatic memory, and to restore the person's ability to stay in the present moment. This therapy is based on the premise that the body, mind, emotions, and spirit are interrelated, and a change at one level results in changes at the others. Being aware, focusing on the present, and recognizing touch as a means of communicating are some of the principles of this therapy. During psychotherapy sessions, the patient is asked to describe physical sensations he or she is experiencing. The goal is to safely disarm the pathological defence mechanism of dissociation and replace it with other resources, especially body awareness and mindfulness.

# EVALUATION

Overall, treatment effectiveness for dissociative disorders is achieved by a reduction of the dissociation (International Society for the Study of Trauma and Dissociation, 2012). Treatment is considered successful when

- Patient safety has been maintained
- Anxiety has been reduced
- Conflicts have been explored
- New coping strategies have permitted the patient to function at a better level
- Difficulties in relationships and at work have been reduced
- Stress is handled adaptively, without the use of dissociation

## CASE STUDY AND NURSING CARE PLAN 23-1

### *Somatic Symptom Disorder*

*Cara, age 49, a recently divorced mother of twin teenage daughters, works as a copy editor for a local newspaper and has been trying to sell her house in order to downsize after her daughters graduate from high school next year. She has a two-year history of numerous physical complaints—insomnia, fatigue, muscle aches, irritable bowel syndrome, and occasional paroxysmal arterial tachycardia (PAT); she feels "nervous most of the time"; and she leaves the house only to go to work or to do grocery shopping. She attends work regularly but has no real social life as she is often "too tired to go out."*

*She has been referred to a variety of specialists, but there continues to be no evidence of organic origins of her ailments. Today, she presented in the local emergency department with tachycardia and shortness of breath. All diagnostic tests were normal.*

*Cara agreed to attend an outpatient mental health intensive outpatient program (IOP) three mornings each week. After attending IOP for two days, she has not made much progress and states concern about a possible job loss if she does not return to work as soon as possible. She says that she feels happy at times when at home but is very frustrated that her fatigue and physical symptoms are continuing. She says that nothing seems to help her, that she is not sure what she is doing here, and that her future looks bleak. Most staff members have reported frustration that Cara is helpful with other patients but not actively engaged in working on any of her own issues and that she continually states that her mood is fine but her body is a "major problem."*

### ASSESSMENT

**Self-Assessment**

Ms. Silverthorn, a registered nurse, has three years of experience in this intensive outpatient program. She recognizes that she has mixed feelings toward Cara. On the one hand, the patient is interesting, talkative, and charming as she discusses her happy childhood. On the other, she is refusing to identify any psychological concerns and consistently prods staff to see if she can "graduate" from this program and go back to work. Staff members feel Cara negates any of their suggestions. Ms. Silverthorn realizes she has to carefully monitor her emotional reactions to Cara and adopt a persistent matter-of-fact approach to encourage the patient to be more assertive, self-aware, and independent. Ms. Silverthorn plans to actively support Cara in creating her discharge plan.

| **Objective Data** | **Subjective Data** |
|---|---|
| • Results of all diagnostic tests are negative. | • "I don't know what I'm doing here." |
| • Onset of symptoms coincides with her divorce and impending loss of daughters as their high school graduations are approaching. | • She says her mood is fine, but her body is a "major problem." |
| • There is no prior history of somatic or psychiatric disorders. | |

### DIAGNOSIS

1. *Complicated grieving* related to loss of significant other (spouse) and anticipatory losses of children and home
**Supporting Data**
- Patient has difficulty communicating needs or emotions.
- Patient reports recent and impending losses with lack of emotion or concern.

2. *Social isolation* related to fatigue and pain
**Supporting Data**
- Patient has minimal support system.
- Patient reports frequent fatigue and loss of social interests.

*Continued*

## CASE STUDY AND NURSING CARE PLAN 23-1—cont'd

### Somatic Symptom Disorder

## OUTCOMES IDENTIFICATION

Long-term goal: Patient will identify and express emotions without physical symptoms.

## PLANNING

The initial plan is to encourage Cara to explore feelings related to recent and impending losses and develop a support system.

## IMPLEMENTATION

The personalized plan for Cara is as follows:

| Short-Term Goals | Intervention | Rationale | Evaluation |
|---|---|---|---|
| 1. Patient will identify levels of anxiety in at least three situations and encounters with other patients and staff. | 1. Develop a relationship with the patient that includes a mutually agreed-upon contract that details expected changes in behaviours. | 1. A contract provides a concrete means to keep track of patient's actions and enhances self-direction and independent actions. | 1. After spending three weeks in the intensive outpatient mental health program, Cara developed a trusting relationship with one staff member and two patients. |
| 2. Patient will seek support from staff and patients when feelings of anxiety become difficult to handle or physical symptoms increase. | 2. Educate the patient about sharing feelings of loss with staff, friends, and family members. | 2. Communication and expression of feelings with family and friends helps to alleviate stress and often provides a more supportive environment. | 2a. Ms. Silverthorn made several attempts to engage Cara in discussion of feelings, losses, and conflicts to no avail until she arranged for a family meeting with Cara, her daughters, and her former husband. Cara was able to express her anxiety and occasional anger about the loss of her role as wife and the impending loss of her daughters when they attend college away from home.<br><br>2b. Cara also became more active in expressing her grief, particularly in the assertiveness and anger-management classes, and actively sought out Ms. Silverthorn on three occasions to discuss her feelings. |
| 3. Patient will make a list with contacts and phone numbers of community resources of interest to her and make plans to attend a community event within a week. | 3. Identify available support systems. | 3. Patients are more successful handling stressful life events if they have adequate support. | 3. Cara decided to take piano lessons and also enrolled in some of her town's adult-education classes. |
| 4. Patient will remain free of injury throughout the hospitalization. | 4. Assess for suicidal ideation. | 4. Suicidal ideation may occur in response to depression or hopelessness over medical conditions. | 4. Cara made no attempts to self-injure while in the hospital. |

## EVALUATION

Many of Cara's symptoms have decreased; in particular, there have been no further episodes of tachycardia. However, Cara states she is still hindered by some fatigue and muscle pain but much less so than previously. She admits she has not fully adhered to her exercise and healthy-eating plan, and occasionally she still feels furious with herself for not coping as well as she would like in social situations. Cara feels that the assertiveness training was particularly helpful to her as she has realized how her passivity and bottled-up anger could have contributed to her physical symptoms and distress. Cara will continue to see her nurse therapist weekly to work on assertiveness skills, identification of and expression of feelings, and living a healthier lifestyle.

## KEY POINTS TO REMEMBER

- Somatic symptom disorders are characterized by the presence of multiple real physical symptoms for which there is no evidence of medical illness.
- Dissociative disorders involve a disruption in consciousness with a significant impairment in memory, identity, or perceptions of self.
- Somatic symptom and dissociative disorders are believed to be responses to psychological stress, although the patient shows no insight into the potential stressors.
- Patients with somatic symptom and dissociative disorders often have co-morbid psychiatric illness—primarily depression, anxiety, or substance abuse.

- The course of these disorders may be brief, with acute onset and spontaneous remission, or chronic, with a gradual onset and prolonged impairment.
- Because these patients may not seek psychiatric treatment, the nurse does not usually see them in the acute psychiatric setting, except during a period of crisis such as suicidal risk.
- The nursing assessment is especially important to clarify the history and course of past symptoms, as well as to obtain a complete picture of the current physical and mental status.
- Although these patients do respond to crisis intervention, they usually require referral for longer-term treatment to attain sustained improvement in level of functioning.

## CRITICAL THINKING

1. A patient with suspected somatic symptom disorder has been admitted to the medical-surgical unit after an episode of chest pain with possible electrocardiographic changes. She frequently complains of palpitations, asks the nurse to check her vital signs, and begs staff to stay with her. Some nurses take her pulse and blood pressure when she asks. Others evade her requests. Most staff members try to avoid spending time with her.
   a. How would you feel as a nurse in this situation? Consider why staff might wish to avoid her.
   b. Design interventions to cope with the patient's behaviours. Give rationales for your interventions.

2. A patient is admitted to a medical-surgical unit. She has been admitted to the unit many times. The reasons for the admissions vary. Some have been for gastrointestinal problems; others for breathing difficulty; others for unexplained tachycardia and for unexplained fainting and seizures. She has undergone many tests, and all have come back normal. She tells you about her children. She discloses to you that her own childhood was extremely difficult. Both her parents were physically abusive and she was sexually abused by an older male cousin.
   a. What factors are most important in planning care for this patient?
   b. What type of abuse is most likely linked to her somatic preoccupation?

## CHAPTER REVIEW

1. A patient states she has been ill for several months with stomach pain, headache, and dizziness. A review of records shows that she has been tested repeatedly for various conditions, yet no clinical diagnosis has been found. She states her pain is "10 out of 10" on a scale of 1 to 10. She has been treated in the past for anxiety and depression. Which condition should the nurse anticipate?
   1. Illness anxiety disorder
   2. Somatic symptom disorder
   3. Conversion disorder
   4. Factitious disorder

2. The nurse is caring for a patient who has experienced the onset of a headache and has no history of headaches. When talking with the nurse, the patient states, "I am sure this is a brain tumour." Which condition should the nurse anticipate?
   1. Illness anxiety disorder
   2. Somatic symptom disorder
   3. Conversion disorder
   4. Factitious disorder

3. A patient presents to the emergency department with a sudden onset of lower paralysis. Although the patient's wife is hysterical, the patient himself is calm and unemotional. All organic causes for the paralysis have been ruled out. Which condition should the nurse anticipate?
   1. Illness anxiety disorder
   2. Somatization
   3. Conversion disorder
   4. Factitious disorder

4. A patient has been diagnosed with Munchausen's syndrome. Which behaviour should the nurse anticipate?
   1. Tendency to frequent the same caregiver and use the emergency department at night
   2. Exaggeration of symptoms with the intent of becoming eligible for disability compensation
   3. Inability to recall important information related to a recent rape attempt
   4. Attempts to make oneself ill and going from one hospital to another to call attention to oneself

5. The nurse is planning care for a patient with a somatic symptom disorder. Which intervention(s) would be appropriate? Select all that apply.
    1. Have patient direct requests to varying nurses so they will become familiar with the patient's needs.
    2. Objectively explain that the patient's symptoms are not real.
    3. Teach assertive communication.
    4. Shift focus from somatic concerns to feelings.
    5. Spend time with patient only when summoned.

## Evolve WEBSITE

**Post-Test** interactive review

*Visit the Evolve Web site for Chapter Review Answers and Rationales, Critical Thinking Answer Guidelines, and additional resources related to the content in this chapter: http://evolve.elsevier.com/Canada/Varcarolis/psychiatric/*

## REFERENCES

Ackley, B.J., & Ladwig, G.B. (2011). *Nursing diagnosis handbook: An evidence-based guide to planning care* (9th ed.). St. Louis, MO: Mosby/Elsevier.

Aragona, M., Catino, E., Pucci, D., et al. (2010). The relationship between somatization and posttraumatic symptoms among immigrants receiving primary care services. *Journal of Traumatic Stress, 23*(5), 615–622.

Ardesrani, S.M.S., Zairoddin, A.R., Shahpouri, H.R., et al. (2009). Comorbidity of factitious disorders and intellectual disability: A case report. *Iranian Journal of Psychiatry and Behavioral Sciences, 3*(2), 44–46.

Bernstein, E.M., & Putman, F.W. (1986). Development, reliability, and validity of a dissociation scale. *Journal of Nervous and Mental Disorders, 174*(12), 727–735. doi:10.1097/00005053-198612000-00004.

Brown, R.J., & Lewis-Fernandez, R. (2011). Culture and conversion disorder: Implications for DSM-5. *Psychiatry: Interpersonal & Biological Processes, 74*(3), 187–206. doi:10.1521/psyc.2011.74.3.187.

Bulechek, G.M., Butcher, H.K., Dochterman, J.M., et al. (2012). *Nursing interventions classification (NIC)* (6th ed.). St. Louis, MO: Mosby.

Charlson, F.J., Stapelberg, N.J.C., Baxter, A.J., et al. (2011). Should global burden of disease estimates include depression as a risk factor for coronary heart disease? *BMC Medicine, 9*(47). doi:10.1186/1741-7015-9-47.

Crowley, P., Gladstein, R.N., Liman, D., et al. (Producers), & Liman, D. (Director). (2002). *The Bourne Identity* [Motion picture]. United States: Universal Pictures.

Dickson, B., Hay-Smith, E.J.C., & Dean, S.G. (2009). Demonised diagnosis: The influence of stigma on interdisciplinary rehabilitation of somatoform disorder. *New Zealand Journal of Physiotherapy, 37*(3), 115–121.

Dols, A., Rhebergen, D., Eikelenboom, P., et al. (2012). Hypochondriacal delusion in an elderly woman recovers quickly with electroconvulsive therapy. *Clinical and Practice, 2*(11), 21–22. doi:10.4081/cp.2012.e11.

Dube, S., Fairweather, D., Pearson, W.S., et al. (2009). Cumulative childhood stress and autoimmune diseases in adults. *Psychosomatic Medicine, 71*(2), 243–250.

Edwards, T., Stern, A., Clarke, D.D., et al. (2010). The treatment of the patient with medically unexplained symptoms in primary care: A review of the literature. *Mental health in family medicine, 7,* 209–221.

Feinstein, A. (2011). Conversion disorder: Advances in our understanding. *Canadian Medical Association Journal, 183*(8), 915–920. doi:10.1503/cmaj.110490.

Fink, P. (2010). The outcome of health anxiety in primary care: A two-year follow up study on health care costs and self-rated health. *PloS ONE, 5*(3). Retrieved from http://www.plosone.org/article/info%3Adoi%2F10.1371%2Fjournal.pone.0009873.

Fuller-Thomson, E., Sulman, J., Brennenstuhl, S., et al. (2011). Functional somatic syndromes and childhood physical abuse in women: Data from a representative community-based sample. *Journal of Aggression, Maltreatment and Trauma, 20,* 445–469.

Garcia-Martin, I., Miranda-Vicario, E.M., & Soutullo, C.A. (2012). Duloxetine in the treatment of adolescents with somatoform disorders: A report of two cases. *Actas espanolas de psiquiatra, 20*(3), 165–168.

Greenberg, D.B., Braun, I.M., & Cassem, N.H. (2008). Functional somatic symptoms and somatoform disorders. In T.A. Stern, J.F. Rosenbaum, M. Fava, et al. (Eds.), *Massachusetts General Hospital comprehensive clinical psychiatry* (pp. 319–330). St. Louis, MO: Mosby.

Gross, A., Gallo, J.J., & Eaton, W.W. (2010). Depression and cancer risk: 24 years of follow up of the Baltimore epidemiologic catchment area sample. *NIH Cancer Causes Control, 21*(2), 191–199.

Hagglund, L. (2009). Challenges in the treatment of factitious disorder: A case study. *Archives of Psychiatric Nursing, 23*(1), 58–64.

Hale, D., & Reck, A. (2010). Somatoform disorder: Understanding hypochondriasis and somatization. *Journal of Health Sciences and Practice, 1*(9), 1–7.

Han, C., Pae, C.U., Lee, B.H., et al. (2008). Venlafaxine versus mirtazapine in the treatment of undifferentiated somatoform disorder: A 12-week prospective, open-label, randomized, parallel-group trial. *Clinical Drug Investigation, 28*(4), 251–261.

Huang, H., & McCarron, R.M. (2011). Medically unexplained symptoms: Evidence-based interventions. *Current Psychiatry, 10*(7), 17.

International Society for the Study of Trauma and Dissociation. (2012). Guidelines for treating dissociative identity disorder in adults (3rd rev.). *Journal of Trauma and Dissociation, 12*(2), 115–187. doi:10.1080/15299732.2011.537247.

Kenny, M. (1986). *Passion of Ansel Bourne* (Smithsonian Series in Ethnographic Inquiry, Vol 5). New York: Smithsonian.

Kenny, M., & Egan, J. (2011). Somatization disorder: What clinicians need to know. *Psychologist, 37*(4), 93–96.

Kim, H.H., Lee, Y.J., Kim, H.K., et al. (2011). Prevalence and correlates of psychiatric symptoms in North Korean Defectors. *Psychiatry Investigation, 8*(3), 179–185.

Koch, S.C., & Harvey, S. (2012). Dance/movement therapy with traumatized dissociative patients. In S.C. Koch, T. Fuchs, M. Summa et al. (Eds.), *Body memory, metaphor and movement* (pp. 369–386). Philadelphia: John Benjamins Publishing.

Konnopka, A., Löbner, M., Luppa, M., et al. (2012). Psychiatric comorbidity as predictor of costs in backpain patients undergoing disc surgery: A longitudinal observational study. *BioMed Central Musculoskeletal Disorders, 13,* 165. doi:10.1186/1471-2474-13-165.

Korber, S., Frieser, D., Steinbrecher, N., et al. (2011). Classification characteristics of Patient Health Questionnaire-15 Screening for somatoform disorders in a primary care setting. *Journal of Psychosomatic Research, 71,* 142–147.

Kroenke, K. (2007). Efficacy of treatment of somatoform disorders: A review of randomized controlled trials. *Psychosomatic Medicine, 69*(9), 881–888.

Landa, A., Peterson, B., & Fallon, B. (2012). Somatoform pain: A developmental theory and translational research review. *Psychosomatic Medicine, 74*(7), 717–727. doi:10.1097/PSY.0b013e3182688e8b.

Lemal, M., & den Bulck, J.V. (2009). Television news exposure is related to fear of breast cancer. *Preventative Medicine, 48,* 189–192.

MacDonald, P. (2011). Dealing with health anxiety. *Practice Nurse, 41*(16), 38.

Mental Health Commission of Canada. (2012). *Changing directions, changing lives: The mental health strategy for Canada.* Retrieved from strategy.mentalhealthcommission.ca/pdf/strategy-images-en.pdf.

Miller, M. (2009). *Treating somatoform disorders.* Harvard Mental Health Letter. Retrieved from http://www.health.harvard.edu/newsletters/harvard_mental_health_letter/2009/November.

Moorhead, S., Johnson, M., Maas, M., et al. (2012). *Nursing outcomes classification (NOC)* (5th ed.). St. Louis, MO: Mosby.

Nicholson, T., Stone, J., & Kanaan, R.A.A. (2011). Conversion disorder: A problematic diagnosis. *Journal of Neurology, Neurosurgery and Psychiatry, 82,* 1267–1273.

Noyes, R., Longley, S.L., Langbehn, D.R., et al. (2010). Hypochondriacal symptoms associated with a less therapeutic physician patient relationship. *Psychiatry, 73*(1), 57–69.

Ogden, P., Minton, K., & Pain, C. (2006). *Trauma and the body: A sensorimotor approach to psychotherapy.* New York: Norton.

Piper, A., & Merskey, H. (2004). The persistence of folly: A critical examination of dissociative identity disorder. Part I: The excesses of an improbable concept. *Canadian Journal of Psychiatry, 49*(8), 592–600. Retrieved from http://publications.cpa-apc.org/browse/documents/3.

Reinders, A.A.T.S., Nijenhuis, E.R.S., Quak, J., et al. (2006). Psychobiological characteristics of dissociative identity disorder: A symptom provocation study. *Biological Psychiatry, 60,* 730–740. doi:10.1016/j.biopsych.2005.12.019.

Sadock, B.J., & Sadock, V.A. (2008). *Kaplan & Sadock's concise textbook of clinical psychiatry* (3rd ed.). Philadelphia: Lippincott Williams & Wilkins.

Schlozman, S.C., & Nonacs, R.M. (2008). Dissociative disorders. In T.A. Stern, J.F. Rosenbaum, M. Fava, et al. (Eds.), *Massachusetts General Hospital comprehensive clinical psychiatry* (pp. 481–486). St. Louis, MO: Mosby.

Schumaker, J.F. (2007). *In search of happiness: Understanding an endangered state of mind.* Westport, CT: Praeger.

Segerstrom, S.C., & Miller, G.E. (2004). Psychological stress and the human immune system: A meta-analytical study of 30 years of inquiry. *Psychological Bulletin, 130*(4), 601–630. doi:10.1037/0033-2909.130.4.601.

Selye, H. (1956). What is stress. *Metabolism: Clinical and Experimental, 5*(5), 525–530. Retrieved from http://www.metabolismjournal.com/.

Shidhaye, R., Mendenhall, E., Sumathipala, K., et al. (2013). Association of somatoform disorders with anxiety and depression in women in low and middle income countries: A systematic review. *International Review of Psychiatry, 259*(1), 65–76. doi:10.3109/09540261.2012.748651.

Silber, T.J. (2011). Somatization disorders: Diagnosis, treatment and prognosis. *Pediatrics in Review, 32*(2), 56–64. doi:10.1542/pir.32-2-56.

Smith, F.A. (2008). Factitious disorders and malingering. In T.A. Stern, J.F. Rosenbaum, M. Fava, et al. (Eds.), *Massachusetts General Hospital comprehensive clinical psychiatry* (pp. 331–336). St. Louis, MO: Mosby.

So, J. (2008). Somatization as a cultural idiom of distress: Rethinking mind and body in a multicultural society. *Counseling Psychology Quarterly, 21*(2), 167–174. doi:10.1080/09515070802066854.

Soltis-Jarrett, V.M. (2010). His-story or her-story: Deconstruction of the concepts of somatization towards a new approach in advanced nursing practice care. *Perspectives in Psychiatric Care, 47*(4), 183–193. doi:10.1111/j.1744-6163.2010.00288.x.

Spiegel, D., Loewenstein, R., Lewis-Fernandez, R., et al. (2011). Dissociative disorders in DSM-5. *Depression and Anxiety, 28,* 824–852. doi:10.1002/da.20874.

Steinbrecher, N., Koerber, S., Frieser, D., et al. (2011). The prevalence of medically unexplained symptoms in primary care. *Psychosomatics, 52,* 263–271. doi:10.1016/j.psym.2011.01.007.

Stone, J., Vuilleumier, P., & Friedman, J.H. (2010). Conversion disorder: Separating the "how" from "why." *Neurology, 74,* 190–191.

Temoshok, L., Waldstein, S.R., Wald, R.L., et al. (2008). Type C coping, alexithymia, and heart rate reactivity are associated independently and differentially with specific immune mechanisms linked to HIV progression. *Brain, Behaviour, and Immunity, 22*(5), 781–792. doi:10.1016/j.bbi.2008.02.003.

van Dijke, A. (2012). Dysfunctional affect regulation in borderline personality disorder and in somatoform disorder. *European Journal of Psychotraumatology, 3,* 19566. doi:10.3402/ejpt.v3i0.19566.

Van Ravenzwaaij, J., Hartman, T.C., Ravesteijn, H., et al. (2010). Explanatory models of medically unexplained symptoms: A qualitative analysis of the literature. *Mental Health in Family Medicine, 7,* 223–231.

Walters, P., Tylee, A., Fisher, J., et al. (2007). Teaching junior doctors to manage patients who somatise: Is it possible in an afternoon? *Medical Education, 41,* 995–1001.

Webb, T. (2010). Medically unexplained symptoms. *Therapy Today, 21*(3). Retrieved from http://www.therapytoday.net/article/15/49/categories/.

Williams, L. (2012). Factitious disorder in a psychogeriatric patient. *General Hospital Psychiatry, 34*(4), 5–6.

World Health Organization. (2007). *Integrating mental health services into primary health care.* Mental Health Policy, Planning and Service Development Sheet. Geneva, Switzerland: Author.

# Trauma Interventions

# CHAPTER

# 24

# Crisis and Disaster

*Sonya L. Jakubec*

## KEY TERMS AND CONCEPTS

adventitious crisis, 494
coping, 492
coping methods, 492
crisis, 492
crisis intervention, 492
critical incident stress debriefing (CISD), 500
disasters, 494
maturational crisis, 493

mental health emergency, 494
mental health first aid (MHFA), 497
phases of crisis, 494
primary care, 499
secondary care, 500
situational crisis, 494
tertiary care, 500
trauma, 494

## OBJECTIVES

1. Differentiate among the three types of crisis.
2. Delineate six aspects of crisis relevant for nurses involved in crisis intervention.
3. Understand areas of assessment and approaches to assessment during crisis.
4. Discuss four common problems in the nurse–patient relationship encountered by beginning nurses when starting crisis intervention. Discuss resolutions to these problems.

5. Compare and contrast the differences among primary, secondary, and tertiary intervention, including appropriate intervention strategies.
6. Identify modalities of crisis intervention.
7. List at least five resources in the community that could be used as referrals for a patient in crisis.

## ⊖volve WEBSITE

*Visit the Evolve website for Flashcards, Case Studies, and additional testing resources related to the content in this chapter:* http://evolve.elsevier.com/Canada/Varcarolis/psychiatric/　Pre-Test　interactive review

In a matter of a few hours, a wildfire destroys entire neighbourhoods in Slave Lake, Alberta, taking the homes of many. Floods in Quebec and Manitoba leave hundreds homeless and without their livelihoods. A young man is killed by a bullet intended for a neighbourhood drug dealer in a drive-by shooting; the deceased young man's family recently emigrated from Sudan, where several other family members had been killed or injured during years of war. A 35-year automotive manufacturing employee is laid off and, after months of desperately trying to pay his family's bills, finds his family and himself homeless. A

young nursing student discovers she is pregnant, and the father of the baby abandons her. A retired executive relocates to her cottage, quickly discovering she lacks hobbies, purpose, and a social network.

What do these situations have in common? Each scenario could be the precipitant of a crisis—leaving individuals, families, or whole communities struggling to cope with the impact of the event.

Everyone experiences crises, which are not in themselves a mental illness but rather are representative of a struggle for

**491**

equilibrium and adaptation. Crisis and disaster experiences do, however, create vulnerable populations and conditions that require mental health services (Kanel, 2012). A crisis is an acute state of psychological imbalance resulting in poor coping with evidence of distress and functional impairment. The primary cause of a crisis is an intensely felt threat or a stressful event (Registered Nurses' Association of Ontario, 2002). Two necessary conditions for a crisis identified by Roberts (2005) are (1) the individual's perception of the event as the cause of considerable upset, disruption, or both and (2) the individual's inability to resolve the disruption by previously used coping mechanisms (p. 778).

Crisis both threatens personality organization and presents an opportunity for personal growth and development. Successful crisis resolution results from the development of adaptive coping methods, reflects ego development, and suggests the employment of physiological, psychological, and social resources. Crisis, or rather *coping* with crisis, is an essential component of individual growth and development. Coping can be defined as "finding ways to accomplish goals despite obstacles and challenges" (Goldner, Palma, Jenkins, et al., 2011, p. 197). Coping methods are the thinking, behavioural, and emotional processes individuals use to support functioning in the face of stressors (Registered Nurses' Association of Ontario, 2006).

Crises are acute and time-limited, usually lasting four to six weeks. They are associated with events that precipitate overwhelming emotions of increased tension, helplessness, and disorganization. As shown in Figure 24-1, resolution from the state of crisis depends on the following three factors:

1. The realistic perception of the event
   - People vary in the way they absorb, process, and use information from the environment (Aguilera, 1998).
2. Adequate situational supports
   - Situational supports include nurses, other health care providers, and community members who use *crisis intervention* to assist those in crisis. Crisis intervention is a process focused on resolution of the immediate problem through personal, social, and environmental resources. The goals of early intervention are (Registered Nurses' Association of Ontario, 2002, p. 15):
     - Stabilization of the situation
     - Rapid resolution of the crisis experience
     - Prevention of further deterioration or trauma
     - Achievement of (at least) pre-crisis level of functioning
     - Promotion of effective problem solving and realistic understanding of the experience
     - Facilitation of a sense of self-reliance and belief in one's ability to return to independence and apply new coping skills to future challenges

In general, interventions are responsive to the situation, timing, environment, and resources available. Modalities may include mental health first aid, including early identification and comfort measures; telephone support; home visits or mobile response interventions; reflection and goal setting to promote coping; or even emergency psychiatric

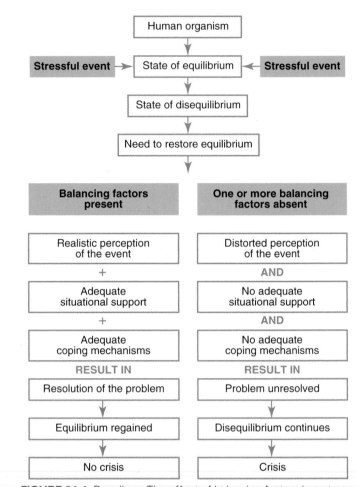

**FIGURE 24-1** Paradigm: The effect of balancing factors in a stressful event. **Source:** Aguilera, D.C. (1998). *Crisis intervention: Theory and methodology* (8th ed.). St. Louis, MO: Mosby.

services and hospitalization (British Columbia Ministry of Health, 2002; Goldner, Palma, Jenkins, et al., 2011).

3. Adequate coping mechanisms
   - Coping skills are acquired through a variety of sources, such as cultural responses, modelling behaviours of others, and life opportunities that broaden experience and promote new adaptive coping responses (Aguilera, 1998). Many factors compromise a person's ability to cope with a crisis event—for example, the number of other stressful life events the person is currently coping with, the presence of other unresolved losses, the presence of coexisting psychiatric or medical problems, the presence of excessive fatigue or pain, and the quality and quantity of a person's usual coping skills.

## THE DEVELOPMENT OF CRISIS THEORY

An early crisis theorist, Erich Lindemann, studied the grief reactions of relatives of victims who died in the 1942 fire at Boston's Coconut Grove nightclub. His research formed the foundation of crisis theory and intervention. Lindemann (1944) concluded that while acute grief is a normal reaction to a distressing situation, preventive interventions could eliminate or decrease the serious psychological consequences of the anxiety associated with crisis. He believed that the same interventions helpful in bereavement would prove helpful in crises.

In the 1960s, Gerald Caplan advanced crisis theory and intervention strategies. Since then, clinicians and theorists have further extended our understanding of crisis and interventions. The significant impact of crisis on individual and population health has been well articulated. Mental health first aid training, early intervention, and support crisis intervention are all priorities for strategic action in Canada's evolving national mental health strategy (Mental Health Commission of Canada, 2011). Donna Aguilera and Janice Mesnick provided a classic framework for nurses for crisis assessment and intervention, and Aguilera continues to set a standard in the practice of crisis assessment and intervention, including examination of the individual's reactions, education, coping, and problem solving. Albert R. Roberts's seven-stage model of crisis intervention (see Figure 24-2) provides another useful model for addressing the suffering experienced in acute situational crises, as well as in acute stress disorder.

More recently, in an effort to establish consensus on mass disaster intervention principles, Hobfoll, Watson, Bell, and colleagues (2007) identified five essential, empirically supported elements of mass trauma interventions that promote (1) a sense of safety, (2) calming, (3) a sense of self-efficacy and collective efficacy, (4) connectedness, and (5) hope.

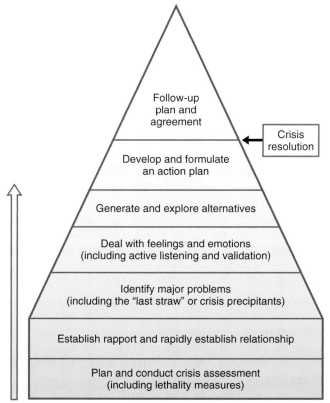

**FIGURE 24-2** Roberts's seven-stage model of crisis intervention.

The effects of a mass disaster like the 2003 disease pandemic severe acute respiratory syndrome (SARS), the sexual assault of a young man in a rural area, or the fatal motor vehicle accident of a young Australian tourist en route to a ski hill all represent the need for crisis assessment and intervention at the community level. Regardless of the type of crisis and whether traumatized individuals are victims, families, rescue workers, or witnesses, those with access to crisis assessment and intervention are more likely to feel safe, supported, and able to make sense of their response to the disaster, as compared to those without such access (Health Canada, 2010; Hobfoll, Watson, Bell, et al., 2007).

Components of crisis assessment and intervention are derived from established crisis theory and evidence base. An understanding of three areas of crisis theory enables application of the nursing process: (1) types of crisis, (2) phases of crisis, and (3) aspects of crisis that have relevance for nurses.

## Types of Crisis

There are three basic types of crisis situation: (1) developmental or maturational crises; (2) situational crises; and (3) disasters, or adventitious crises. Disadvantaged and stigmatized people, such as those with pre-existing mental health problems, substance abuse, or limited external resources, are especially vulnerable to crisis (Saunders, 2007).

### Maturational Crisis

A process of maturation occurs across the life cycle. Erik Erikson conceptualized the process by identifying eight stages of ego growth and development (see Table 3-2). Each stage represents a time during which physical, cognitive, instinctual, and sexual changes prompt an internal conflict or crisis, which results in either psychosocial growth or regression. Therefore, each developmental stage represents a maturational crisis (that is, a critical period of increased vulnerability and heightened potential—a turning point).

When a person arrives at a new stage, formerly used coping styles are no longer effective, and new coping mechanisms have yet to be developed. Thus, for a time, the person is without effective defences. This deficit often leads to increased tension and anxiety, which may manifest as variations in the person's normal behaviour. Examples of events that can precipitate a maturational crisis include leaving home during late adolescence, marriage, the birth of a child, retirement, and the death of a parent. Successful resolution of these maturational tasks leads to the development of basic human qualities.

Erikson (1959) believed that the way these crises are resolved at one stage affects the ability to pass through subsequent stages, because each crisis provides the starting point for movement toward the next stage. If a person lacks support systems and adequate role models, successful resolution may be difficult or may not occur. Unresolved problems in the past and inadequate coping mechanisms then adversely affect what is learned in each developmental stage. Experiencing severe difficulty during a maturational crisis may disrupt progression through the maturational stages and warrant professional intervention. For example, Steve developed addictive behaviours in early adolescence and may, therefore, lack adult coping and problem-solving skills when dealing with a situational (financial) crisis as a result of gambling debts at age 25.

## Situational Crisis

A situational crisis arises from events that are extraordinary, external rather than internal, and unanticipated (Roberts, 2005). Examples of precipitating events to a situational crisis are job loss or change, the death of a loved one, an unplanned pregnancy, financial troubles, relationship breakup, and severe physical or mental illness. Whether or not these events precipitate a crisis depends on factors such as the degree of support available from caring friends, family members, and others; general emotional and physical status; and the ability to understand and cope with the meaning of the stressful event. As in all crises, the stressful event involves loss or change that threatens a person's self-concept, self-esteem, and sense of security.

## Adventitious Crisis

An adventitious crisis crises result from events not part of everyday life, such as a natural disaster (e.g., flood, fire, earthquake) or a national disaster (e.g., acts of terrorism, war, riots, airplane crashes). Disasters are those events that threaten (physically or psychologically) the well-being of citizens. Adventitious crises may also result from a violent crime (e.g., rape, assault or murder in the workplace or school, bombing in public areas, spousal or child abuse). Experiencing or witnessing such events that threaten an individual's very survival (physical or psychological) is referred to as trauma. An important development in the field of adventitious crisis theory has been the recognition of just how differently people respond to and are impacted by disaster. It is known that traumatizing events may overwhelm an individual's usual coping skills and be of such intensity that lasting psychological harm occurs, including the potential for post-traumatic stress disorder (PTSD) (Goldner, Palma, Jenkins, et al., 2011). For more information on PTSD and interventions, see Chapter 13. PTSD is among several post-trauma disorders that also include acute stress disorder, dissociative disorder, and depression.

While certain people may be more vulnerable to crisis than others, the need for intervention for all people who experience crisis cannot be overemphasized. Situational and adventitious crises can challenge the basic assumptions that underlie individuals' world views. Roberts (2005) proposed that "a person's vulnerability to a stressful event depends on the newness, intensity, and duration of the stressful event" (p. 687). Vulnerability also depends on the number of crises experienced simultaneously. Consider a 51-year-old woman who may be going through a midlife transition (maturational) when her husband dies suddenly of cancer (situational).

## Phases of Crisis

Caplan (1964) first identified four distinct phases of crisis:

### Phase 1

A person confronted by a conflict or problem that threatens the self-concept responds with increased feelings of anxiety. The increase in anxiety stimulates the use of problem-solving techniques and defence mechanisms in an effort to solve the problem and lower anxiety.

### Phase 2

If usual defensive responses fail and the threat persists, anxiety continues to rise and produces feelings of extreme discomfort. Individual functioning becomes disorganized. Trial-and-error solutions in an effort to restore a normal balance begin.

### Phase 3

If the trial-and-error attempts fail, anxiety can escalate to the severe or panic level, and the person may mobilize automatic relief behaviours, such as withdrawal and flight. Some form of resolution (e.g., compromising needs or redefining the situation to reach an acceptable solution) may be made in this stage.

### Phase 4

If the problem remains unresolved and new coping skills are ineffective, then an individual may transition into a mental health emergency—a state of overwhelming anxiety that can lead to serious personality disorganization, depression, confusion, and behavioural disturbances. In a mental health emergency, there are urgent issues of safety, potentially because of risk for self-care limitations (e.g., lack of nutrition, exposure to physical risks), self-harm behaviour (e.g., substance abuse, risk of suicide), or violence against others (Goldner, Palma, Jenkins, et al., 2011).

## APPLICATION OF THE NURSING PROCESS

Because people typically experience increased stress and anxiety in medical, surgical, and psychiatric hospital settings, as well as in community settings, nurses are often positioned to implement mental health first aid (see page 497) and crisis intervention. Crisis theory defines aspects of crisis that are basic to crisis intervention and relevant to the nursing process (see Box 24-1).

## ASSESSMENT

### General Assessment

As shown in Figure 24-1, a person's equilibrium may be adversely affected by one or more of the following: (1) an unrealistic perception of the precipitating event, (2) inadequate situational supports, and (3) inadequate coping mechanisms (Aguilera, 1998). It is crucial for nurses to assess these factors during a crisis. Data gained from the assessment guides the nurse and the patient in planning realistic and meaningful goals and interventions.

The steps of the nursing assessment follow:

1. Promote a sense of safety by assessing the patient's potential for suicide or homicide.

    If the patient is suicidal, homicidal, or unable to take care of personal needs, hospitalization should be considered (Aguilera, 1998). Sample questions to ask include:
    - Do you feel you can keep yourself safe?
    - Have you thought of killing yourself or someone else? If yes, have you thought of how you would do this?

## BOX 24-1   FOUNDATION FOR CRISIS INTERVENTION

- A crisis is self-limiting and usually resolves within four to six weeks.
- At the resolution of a crisis, the patient will emerge at one of three different functional levels:
  - A higher level of functioning
  - The same level of functioning
  - A lower level of functioning
- The goal of crisis intervention is to return the patient to at least the precrisis level of functioning.
- The level of crisis resolution depends on the patient's actions and others' interventions.
- During a crisis, people are often more receptive than usual to outside intervention. With intervention, the patient can learn new approaches to the problem.
- The patient in a crisis situation is assumed to be mentally healthy and to have previously functioned well but is currently in a state of disequilibrium.
- Crisis intervention deals only with the patient's present problem and resolution of the immediate crisis (i.e., the here and now).
- The nurse must take an active, even directive, role in intervention, which is in contrast to conventional therapeutic intervention that stresses a more nondirective role.
- Early intervention increases the potential for a good prognosis.
- The patient is encouraged to set realistic, focused goals and interventions with the nurse.

### VIGNETTE

A 25-year-old woman named Caitlin is brought to the emergency department by police after being beaten by her husband. Caitlin is seen by the emergency physician and then interviewed by the emergency department's psychiatric mental health nurse. The nurse calmly introduces herself and tells Caitlin she would like to spend some time with her. The nurse says, "It looks as if things are pretty overwhelming. Is that how you're feeling?" The nurse makes the observation that things must be very bad if Caitlin stays with an abusive husband. Caitlin sits slumped in a chair, her hands in her lap, head hanging down, and tears in her eyes.

After establishing that the patient poses no danger to self or others, the nurse assesses three main areas: (1) the patient's perception of the precipitating event, (2) the patient's situational supports, and (3) the patient's personal coping skills.

2. Assess the patient's perception of the precipitating event.

The nurse's task is now to assess the individual or family and the problem. The more clearly the problem can be defined, the more likely effective solutions will be identified. Sample questions that may facilitate assessment include:

- Has anything particularly upsetting happened to you within the past few days or weeks?
- What was happening in your life before you started to feel this way?

- What leads you to seek help now?
- Describe how you are feeling right now.
- How does this situation affect your life?
- How do you see this event affecting your future?
- What would need to be done to resolve this situation?

### VIGNETTE

**Nurse:** "Caitlin, tell me what has happened."
**Caitlin:** "I can't go home. … No one cares. No one believes me. I can't go through it again."
**Nurse:** "Tell me what you can't go through again."
(Caitlin cries, shaking with sobs. The nurse sits quietly for a while and then speaks.)
**Nurse:** "Tell me what is so troublesome. Let's look at it together."
After a while, Caitlin tells the nurse that her husband, Dan, has been beating her regularly, particularly after drinking. The beatings have progressively become more violent, and Caitlin states, "I'm afraid I'll end up dead."

3. Assess the patient's situational supports.

Next, the nurse determines resources available to the patient. The following are sample questions:

- Who do you live with?
- Who do you talk to when you feel overwhelmed?
- Who can you trust?
- Who is available to help you?
- Do you belong to a spiritual community?
- Where do you go to school or to other community-based activities?
- During difficult times in the past, who did you want most to help you?
- Who is the most helpful?

### VIGNETTE

**Nurse:** "Caitlin, who can you go to? Do you have any other family?"
**Caitlin:** "No. My family is in another province. Dan and I are pretty much alone."
**Nurse:** "Do you have anyone you can talk to?"
**Caitlin:** "I really don't have any friends. Dan's jealousy makes it difficult for me to have friends. He doesn't like anyone that I would want as a friend."
**Nurse:** "What about co-workers?"
**Caitlin:** "My co-workers are nice, but I can't tell them things like this. They wouldn't believe me anyway."
The nurse learns that Caitlin feels successful at her job and work is a refuge from her troubles. Getting good job reviews also has another reward: it is the only time Dan says anything nice about her.

4. Assess the patient's personal coping skills.

Finally, the nurse evaluates the patient's anxiety level and identifies his or her established coping patterns. Common coping mechanisms may be overeating, drinking, smoking, withdrawing, seeking out someone to talk to, yelling, fighting, or engaging in other physical activity (Behrman & Reid, 2002). Sample questions to ask include:

- What do you usually do to feel better?
- Did you try it this time? If so, what was different?
- What do you think might happen now?
- What helped you through difficult times in the past?
- What role does your culture play in handling situations like this? (See the Considering Culture box.)

## CONSIDERING CULTURE
### How Acknowledging Culture Supports Crisis Resolution

Consider your client who has lost his job with the closure of the local paper mill and presents in crisis at a rural health centre, or your First Nations client at the clinic on a reserve who has experienced the stillbirth of her third child, or the new-immigrant woman you are assessing in the psychiatric emergency department of a large urban hospital who has attempted suicide following a relationship breakdown. While rapid resolution of the crisis is the goal, there are many reasons a nurse should consider culture during such a crisis intervention. Culture can influence one's interpretation of and the meaning attributed to a disaster or crisis event. Culture can also influence an individual's personal coping or a community's reaction to an event. Despite the significance of culture on the assessment and intervention process, the immediacy of crisis intervention nursing often results in cultural factors and issues of cultural identity being overlooked in favour of efficient assessment and interventions. Ignoring the important role of culture, however, may get in the way of effective and efficient crisis resolution.

Acknowledging the client's personal history and context, as well as the distinct history, context, and cultures of the client and nurse (i.e., occupation, income, age, gender, nationality, physical abilities, language, ethnic heritage, sexual orientation, education, and so on), allows for more rapid development of the trust and rapport necessary to communicate both verbally and nonverbally for assessment and intervention. Addressing context and culture in this way assists the nurse to convey acceptance and trust to assist with the immediate problems.

After the symptoms of crisis are stabilized and controlled, knowledge of the client's culture can assist in identifying important resources available for follow-up care, such as family, religious community, or cultural heritage agencies, which can provide continuing support after the symptoms are controlled. In short, culture is crucial to the three balancing factors to a crisis: perception of the event, coping, and support. A nurse's capacity to acknowledge the client's context, history, and culture will enhance crisis intervention and support resolution and good client outcomes. See also Chapter 7 and Chapter 11.

**Source:** Dykeman, B.F. (2005). Cultural implications of crisis intervention. *Journal of Instructional Psychology, 32*(1), 45–48.

### VIGNETTE
**Nurse:** "What do you think would help your situation?"
**Caitlin:** "I don't want to be in an abusive marriage. I just don't know where to turn."
The nurse tells Caitlin that she wants to work with her to find a solution and that she is concerned for Caitlin's safety and well-being.

## Self-Assessment

Nurses' self-awareness when dealing with a patient in crisis is crucial. It is important for them to recognize their own anxiety level and negative feelings to prevent patients from closing off their expression of painful feelings.

There may be times when nurses feel they cannot deal effectively with a patient's situation. When this happens, the nurse should ask a colleague to work with the individual rather than limiting the required assessment and intervention in order to avoid troublesome feelings. Asking for support and supervision will help the nurse separate his or her own needs from the patient's and identify ways to address uncomfortable or painful personal issues to care more effectively for patients in crisis.

Beginning nurses in crisis intervention often face problems long identified in practice that must be dealt with before they can become comfortable and competent in the role of a crisis counsellor. Four of the more common problems are (Wallace & Morley, 1970, pp. 1484–1487):

1. The nurse's needs are placed before those of the patient.
2. The nurse sets unrealistic goals for patients.
3. The nurse has difficulty dealing with the issue of suicide.
4. The nurse has difficulty terminating the nurse–patient relationship.

Essential aspects of the therapeutic relationship include strong verbal and nonverbal communication skills, responsiveness to patient needs, attention to diversity and power relations, and genuine empathy for the lived experience of the patient. As examined in Chapter 10, these aspects of therapeutic relationships are even more pronounced in crisis situations, in which rapid decisions and more extreme emotions are expected. It is crucial that the nurse engages in ongoing self-reflection and self-awareness and that expert supervision be available as an integral part of crisis intervention nursing.

Even experienced nurses can become overwhelmed when witnessing severe suffering, catastrophic loss of human life (e.g., acts of war, plane crashes, workplace shootings), or mass destruction of people's homes and belongings (e.g., floods, fires, earthquakes). Mental health care providers may experience psychological distress from working with traumatized populations, a phenomenon called *secondary traumatic stress* or *vicarious traumatization* (Dunkley & Whelan, 2006). Supervision and critical incident stress debriefing (see page 500) are strategies that support nurses' ability to cope with overwhelming violent and disastrous situations (Registered Nurses' Association of Ontario, 2002).

## DIAGNOSIS

The North American Nursing Diagnosis Association International (NANDA-I) provides nursing diagnoses that can be considered for patients experiencing anxiety and anxiety disorders. When a person is in crisis, the nursing diagnosis of *Ineffective coping* is often useful (Herdman, 2012). This diagnosis is not to suggest that people in crisis are inadequate or do not have coping abilities, but because anxiety may escalate to moderate or severe levels in times of crisis, the ability to solve problems

## 📋 ASSESSMENT GUIDELINES
### Crisis

1. Identify whether the patient's response to the crisis warrants psychiatric treatment or hospitalization to minimize decompensation (e.g., suicidal or violent behaviour, psychotic thinking).
2. Identify whether the patient is able to identify the precipitating event.
3. Assess the patient's understanding of his or her present situational supports.
4. Identify the patient's usual coping styles, determining coping mechanisms suited to the present situation.
5. Determine any cultural beliefs or spiritual practices that should be responded to in assessing and intervening in this patient's crisis.
6. Assess whether this situation is one in which the patient needs primary (education, environmental manipulation, or new coping skills), secondary (crisis intervention), or tertiary (rehabilitation) interventions.

may be impaired. *Ineffective coping* may be experienced as an inability to meet basic needs, inability to meet role expectations, alteration in social participation, use of inappropriate defence mechanisms, or impairment of usual patterns of communication. The "related to" component of the diagnosis will vary according to the individual patient. Table 24-1 identifies potential nursing diagnoses for people in crisis and provides signs and symptoms that might be present to support the diagnosis.

In the preceding vignettes, the assessment of Caitlin's perception of the precipitating event, situational supports, and personal coping skills provides the nurse enough data to formulate two diagnoses and set goals and plan interventions with Caitlin.

---

**VIGNETTE**

Caitlin's nurse formulates the following nursing diagnoses:
- *Anxiety (moderate or severe)* related to mental and physical abuse, as evidenced by ineffectual problem solving and feelings of impending doom
- *Compromised family coping* related to the constant threat of violence

---

## OUTCOMES IDENTIFICATION

Relevant outcomes of the *Nursing Outcomes Classification (NOC)* (Moorhead, Johnson, Maas, et al., 2008) for a person experiencing a crisis include *Coping, Decision making, Role performance,* and *Stress level.* The planning of realistic outcomes is done with the patient and family so as to determine outcomes congruent with the patient's cultural and personal values. Without the patient's involvement, the outcome criteria (i.e., goals at the end of four to eight weeks) may be irrelevant or unacceptable solutions to that patient's crisis. Table 24-2 lists selected *NOC* outcomes with intermediate and short-term indicators for a patient in crisis.

Mental health first aid (MHFA) is the help provided to a person developing a mental health problem or experiencing a

---

| TABLE 24-1 POTENTIAL NURSING DIAGNOSES FOR CRISIS INTERVENTION | |
|---|---|
| **SIGNS AND SYMPTOMS** | **NURSING DIAGNOSIS** |
| Inability to meet basic needs, decreased use of social support, inadequate problem solving, inability to attend to information, isolation | *Ineffective coping* <br> *Risk for compromised resilience* |
| Denial, exaggerated startle response, flashbacks, horror, hypervigilance, intrusive thoughts and dreams, panic attacks, feeling numb, substance abuse, confusion, incoherence | *Post-trauma syndrome* <br> *Rape-trauma syndrome* <br> *Anxiety (moderate, severe, panic)* <br> *Acute confusion* <br> *Sleep deprivation* |
| Minimizes symptoms, delays seeking care, displays inappropriate affect, makes dismissive comments when speaking of distressing events | *Ineffective denial* |
| Overwhelmed, depressed, states has nothing in life worthwhile, self-hatred, feelings of being ineffectual, sees limited alternatives, feels strange, perceives a lack of control | *Risk for suicide* <br> *Chronic low self-esteem* <br> *Disturbed personal identity* <br> *Hopelessness* <br> *Powerlessness* |
| Has difficulty with interpersonal relationships, isolated, has few or no social supports | *Social isolation* <br> *Impaired social interaction* |
| Changes in family relationships and functioning, difficulty performing family caregiver role | *Interrupted family processes* <br> *Caregiver role strain* |

## TABLE 24-2   *NOC* OUTCOMES FOR PATIENT IN CRISIS

| NURSING OUTCOME AND DEFINITION | INTERMEDIATE INDICATORS | SHORT-TERM INDICATORS |
|---|---|---|
| *Coping:* Personal actions to manage stressors that tax an individual's resources | Modifies lifestyle as needed<br>Uses effective coping strategies<br>Reports decrease in physical symptoms of stress<br>Reports decrease in negative feelings | Identifies effective coping patterns<br>Identifies ineffective coping patterns<br>Reports decrease in stress<br>Uses personal support system<br>Verbalizes need for assistance |
| *Decision making:* Ability to make judgements and choose between two or more alternatives | Chooses among alternatives | Identifies relevant information<br>Identifies alternatives<br>Weighs alternatives |
| *Role performance:* Congruence of an individual's role behaviour with role expectations | Able to meet role expectations | Performs family role behaviours<br>Describes role changes with illness or disability<br>Describes role changes with older-adult dependents, new family member, or family member who is leaving home<br>Performs family, parental, intimate, community, work, or friendship role behaviours |
| *Stress level:* Severity of manifested physical or mental tension resulting from factors that alter an existing equilibrium | Able to modulate stress level | Reduction in elevated blood pressure<br>Reduction in increased radial pulse rate<br>Reduction in symptoms of upset stomach<br>Reduced level of restlessness<br>Improved sleep<br>Reduction in interruption of thought process<br>Reduced forgetfulness<br>Infrequent cognitive mistakes<br>Improved ability to concentrate on tasks<br>Decrease in emotional outbursts |

**Source:** Based on Moorhead, S., Johnson, M., Maas, M., et al. (2008). *Nursing outcomes classification (NOC)* (4th ed.). St. Louis, MO: Mosby.

mental health crisis. We know that physical first aid is administered to an injured person before medical treatment can be obtained; likewise, MHFA is given until appropriate treatment is found or until the crisis is resolved, and it is often life saving. Many laypeople in communities are receiving this training that, like physical first aid, is found to support early intervention and disease prevention by preserving life when there is a danger or threat to life, to promote recovery and good mental health, and to provide comfort to those experiencing mental health problems.

The MHFA approach and the training of people in MHFA represent a growing area of health promotion in Canada (Mental Health Commission of Canada, 2011). Overall, this approach aims to provide skills and knowledge to help people manage developing mental health problems in themselves, family members, friends, or co-workers. It does not attempt to train amateur therapists but, rather, teaches people to (1) recognize the signs and symptoms of mental health problems, (2) provide initial help, and (3) guide a person toward appropriate professional help. Lessons learned about MHFA from Australia and Scotland (see Research Highlight box), in particular, are being drawn upon for current initiatives by the Mental Health Commission of Canada (Mental Health Commission of Canada, 2011).

> **VIGNETTE**
>
> The nurse consults a social worker about Caitlin, and the three meet together. All agree that Caitlin should not return to her home. Caitlin and the nurse then establish goals and plan interventions. The goals are as follows:
> - Caitlin will return to her precrisis state within two weeks.
> - With the support of the staff, Caitlin will find a safe environment.
> - With the support of the staff, Caitlin will have at least two outside supports available within 24 hours.
> - Caitlin will receive continued evaluation and support until the immediate crisis is over (six to eight weeks).

## PLANNING

Nurses are called upon to plan and intervene in a variety of crisis intervention modalities, such as disaster nursing, mobile crisis units, group work, mental health first aid training, health education and crisis prevention, victim outreach programs, and crisis lines or telephone outreach. The nurse may be involved in planning interventions for individuals (e.g., cases of physical abuse), groups (e.g., students after a classmate's suicide or shooting), or communities (e.g., disaster nursing after fires, shootings, or airplane crashes). Data from the answers to the

**RESEARCH HIGHLIGHT**

### Mental Health First Aid: Lessons From Drought-Affected Rural Australia

**Source:** Sartore, G.M., Kelly, B., Stain, H.J., et al. (2008). Improving mental health capacity in rural communities: Mental health first aid delivery in drought-affected rural New South Wales. *Australian Journal of Rural Health, 16,* 313–318. doi:10.1111/j.1440-1584.2008.01005.x.

#### Problem
Crisis mental health care in rural communities with few services and resources can be challenging, particularly when a large population may be impacted.

#### Purpose of Study
Mental health first aid (MHFA) training was part of a strategy to improve capacity among farming communities for early intervention for mental health problems. This strategy was viewed as particularly important in those regions affected by drought and wildfire and often lacking in professional mental health systems.

#### Methods
A pre- and post-survey of 99 participants from 12 New South Wales towns was administered before and after delivery of MHFA training, emphasizing the role of front-line workers from agriculture-related services.

#### Key Findings
Participants' abilities to identify high-prevalence disorders and promote evidence-informed interventions for both high- and low-prevalence disorders, and their confidence in providing appropriate help and referrals, all increased following MHFA training.

#### Implications for Nursing Practice
The conclusion from the study was that MHFA training is an effective part of a strategy to improve early intervention in rural communities by using local networks to provide mental health support. Nurses play an important teaching, training, and health-promoting role to support MHFA training, particularly in rural or resource-poor communities.

following questions guide the nurse in determining immediate actions (Aguilera, 1998):
- How much has this crisis affected the patient's life? Can the patient still go to work? Attend school? Care for family members?
- How is the state of disequilibrium affecting significant people in the patient's life (e.g., wife, husband, children, other family members, boss, boyfriend, girlfriend)?

## IMPLEMENTATION

Crisis intervention is a function of the basic-level nurse and has two initial goals:
1. Patient safety. External controls may be applied for protection of the patient in crisis if the patient is suicidal or homicidal.

2. Anxiety reduction. Anxiety-reduction techniques are used so inner resources can be mobilized.

During the initial interview, the patient in crisis first needs to gain a feeling of safety. Solutions to the crisis may be offered so the patient is aware of various options. Feelings of support and hope will temporarily diminish anxiety. The nurse needs to play an active role by indicating that help is available, conveyed by the competent use of crisis intervention skills and genuine interest and support. The availability of help is not conveyed by the use of false reassurances and platitudes, such as "Everything will be all right." Crisis intervention requires a creative and flexible approach through the use of traditional and nontraditional therapeutic methods. The nurse may act as educator, advisor, and role model, always keeping in mind that it is the patient who solves the problem, not the nurse. The following are important assumptions when working with a patient in crisis:
- The patient is in charge of his or her own life.
- The patient is able to make decisions.
- The crisis counselling relationship is one between partners.

The nurse helps the patient refocus to gain new perspectives on the situation. The nurse supports the patient during the process of finding constructive ways to solve or cope with the problem. It is important for nurses to be mindful of how difficult it is for the patient to change behaviours. Table 24-3 offers guidelines for nursing interventions and corresponding rationales.

> **VIGNETTE**
> After talking with the nurse and the social worker, Caitlin seems open to going to a safe house for battered women. She also agrees to talk to a counsellor at a mental health centre. The nurse sets up an appointment at which she, Caitlin, and the counsellor will meet. The nurse will continue to see Caitlin twice a week.

### Counselling
#### Primary Care
Psychotherapeutic crisis interventions are directed toward three levels of care: (1) primary, (2) secondary, and (3) tertiary. Primary care promotes mental health and reduces mental illness to decrease the incidence of crisis. On this level, the nurse can:
1. Work with a patient to recognize potential problems by evaluating the patient's experience of stressful life events
2. Teach the patient specific coping skills, such as decision making, problem solving, assertiveness skills, meditation, and relaxation skills
3. Assist the patient in evaluating the timing or reduction of life changes to decrease the negative effects of stress as much as possible

The third intervention may involve working with a patient or client such as a government or a health services department to plan environmental changes, make important interpersonal decisions, and rethink changes in occupational roles. Health Canada plays an important role in mass-disaster planning and

| TABLE 24-3 | GUIDELINES FOR CRISIS INTERVENTION |
|---|---|
| **INTERVENTION** | **RATIONALE** |
| Assess for suicidal or homicidal thoughts or plans. | Safety is always the first consideration. |
| Take initial steps to make patient feel safe and less anxious. | A person who feels safe and less anxious is able to more effectively problem-solve solutions with the nurse. |
| Listen carefully (e.g., make eye contact, give frequent feedback to verify and convey understanding, summarize what patient says). | A person who believes someone is really listening is more likely to believe that someone cares about his or her situation and help may be available. This belief offers hope. |
| Crisis intervention calls for directive and creative approaches. Initially, the nurse may make phone calls to arrange babysitters, schedule a visiting nurse, find shelter, or contact a social worker. | A person who is confused, frightened, or overwhelmed may be temporarily unable to perform usual tasks. |
| Identify needed social supports (with patient's input) and mobilize the priority. | A person's need for shelter, help with care for children or older-adult dependents, medical workup, emergency medical attention, hospitalization, food, safe housing, and self-help groups is determined. |
| Identify needed coping skills (e.g., problem solving, relaxation, assertiveness, job training, newborn care, self-esteem building). | Increasing coping skills and learning new ones can help with current crisis and help minimize future crises. |
| Involve patient in identifying realistic, acceptable interventions. | The person's involvement in planning increases his or her sense of control, self-esteem, and compliance with the plan. |
| Plan regular follow-up (e.g., phone calls, clinic visits, home visits) to assess patient's progress. | Plan is evaluated to see what works and what does not. |

prevention—for instance, with H1N1 pandemic flu planning and G8 meetings on disaster planning in Kananaskis and Toronto—and has recorded many lessons learned for future disaster planning (Health Canada, 2010).

## Secondary Care

Secondary care includes intervention during an acute crisis to prevent prolonged anxiety from diminishing personal effectiveness and personality organization. The nurse's primary focus is to ensure the safety of the patient. After safety issues are dealt with, the nurse works with the patient to assess the patient's problem, support systems, and coping styles. Desired goals are explored and interventions planned. This level of care lessens the time a patient is mentally disabled during a crisis. Secondary care occurs in hospital units, emergency departments, clinics, and mental health centres, usually during daytime hours.

## Tertiary Care

Tertiary care provides support for those who have experienced a severe crisis and are now recovering from a disabling mental state. Social and community facilities that offer tertiary intervention include rehabilitation centres, sheltered workshops, day hospitals, and outpatient clinics. Primary goals are to facilitate optimal levels of functioning and prevent further emotional disruptions. People with severe and persistent mental problems are often extremely susceptible to crisis, and community facilities provide the structured environment that can help prevent problem situations. Box 24-2 lists *Nursing Interventions*

*Classification (NIC)* (Bulechek, Butcher, & Dochterman, 2008) interventions for responding to a crisis.

***Critical incident stress debriefing.*** A critical incident stress debriefing (CISD) is a group-level crisis intervention carried out very soon following a traumatic event. Individuals involved in or witnessing the event (e.g., those in a school, workplace, or emergency responder group) are brought together in a safe and confidential environment to talk about what happened, discuss feelings and behavioural responses, and obtain health education about the crisis process for early intervention purposes. Generally, the discussion is guided by a professional or trained peer. CISD has its proponents and critics. There is evidence both promoting CISD as an important strategy to prevent PTSD (Everly & Mitchell, 1999) and criticizing the approach as either having no benefit (van Emmerik, Kamphius, Hulsbosch, et al., 2002) or even increasing rates of PTSD in certain individuals (Bledsoe, 2002). Everly, Flannery, and Eyler (2002) responded to such critics that CISD is not intended to be implemented in isolation; it should be implemented as part

---

**VIGNETTE**

The nurse performs secondary crisis intervention and meets with Caitlin twice weekly for four weeks. At first, Caitlin is motivated to work with the social worker and the nurse to find another permanent place to live. The nurse suggests Caitlin see a counsellor in the outpatient clinic after the crisis is over so that she can talk about some of her pain. Caitlin becomes ambivalent and is already thinking she will return to her husband.

## BOX 24-2 CRISIS INTERVENTION

*Definition of crisis intervention:* Use of short-term counselling and other interventions to help the patient cope with a crisis and resume precrisis state of functioning modalities. Interventions may include:

- Crisis lines—telephone support provided by trained volunteers (for first aid and support) or professionals (for assessment, triage, and referral)
- Mobile crisis outreach—outreach crisis response services often provided by collaborative teams including police or other first responders
- Urgent or walk-in crisis care—services through which people can present their crisis needs to professionals for assessment, intervention, and referral
- Psychiatric emergency care—services such as emergency mental health care in hospital triage; assessment; crisis counselling; emergency medical treatment, often for brief-stay admissions

Activities:

- Provide an atmosphere of support.
- Avoid giving false reassurances.
- Provide a safe haven.
- Determine whether the patient presents a safety risk to self or others.
- Initiate necessary precautions to safeguard the patient or others at risk for physical harm.
- Encourage expression of feelings in a nondestructive manner.
- Assist in identification of the precipitants and dynamics of the crisis.

- Encourage patient to focus on one implication at a time.
- Assist in identification of personal strengths and abilities that can be used in resolving the crisis.
- Assist in identification of past and present coping skills and their effectiveness.
- Assist in development of new coping and problem-solving skills, as needed.
- Assist in identification of available support systems.
- Link the patient and family with community resources, as needed.
- Provide guidance about how to develop and maintain support system(s).
- Introduce the patient to people (or groups) who have successfully undergone the same experience.
- Assist in identification of alternative courses of action to resolve the crisis.
- Assist in evaluation of the possible consequences of the various courses of action.
- Assist the patient to decide on a particular course of action.
- Assist in formulating a time frame for implementation of the chosen course of action.
- Evaluate with the patient whether the crisis has been resolved by the chosen course of action.
- Plan with the patient how adaptive coping skills can be used to deal with crises in the future.

**Sources:** Adapted from British Columbia Ministry of Health. (2002). *Best practices in mental health: Crisis response and emergency services.* Retrieved from http://www.health.gov.bc.ca/library/publications/year/2000/MHABestPractices/bp_crisis_response.pdf.; and Bulechek, G.M., Butcher, H.K., & Dochterman, J.M. (2008). *Nursing interventions classification (NIC)* (5th ed.). St. Louis, MO: Mosby.

of a broad approach to crisis intervention that includes formal assessment and referrals for individual and family counselling and a range of other supports (Goldner, Palma, Jenkins, et al., 2011).

## EVALUATION

Guided by nursing best practice guidelines, the nurse might consider asking the following in the evaluation of interventions (Registered Nurses' Association of Ontario, 2002, p. 28):

- Did the patient carry out the crisis plan, and what was the outcome?
- Does the patient have a plan to work toward meeting, through alternative actions, his or her goals?
- Does the patient require additional or alternative links to community resources and supports?

*NOC* includes a built-in measurement for each outcome and for the indicators that support the outcome. Each indicator is measured on a five-point Likert scale, which helps the nurse evaluate the effectiveness of the crisis intervention. This evaluation is usually performed four to eight weeks after the initial interview, although it can be done earlier (e.g., by the end of the visit, the anxiety level has decreased from 1 = severe to 3 =

moderate). If the intervention has been successful, the patient's level of anxiety and ability to function should be at precrisis levels. A patient may wish to follow up on additional areas of concern and get referrals to other agencies for more long-term work. Crisis intervention frequently serves to prepare a patient for further treatment.

### VIGNETTE

Caitlin returns to her husband five weeks after the battering episode. She has convinced herself that he has changed his behaviour, even though he has not sought any help to control his anger.

Caitlin continues to see the nurse, as planned; however, Caitlin is aloof and distant. After six weeks, Caitlin and the nurse decide that the crisis is over. The nurse evaluates Caitlin as being in a moderate amount of emotional pain, but Caitlin feels she is doing well. The nurse's assessment indicates that Caitlin has other serious issues (e.g., low self-esteem, childhood abuse), and the nurse strongly suggests that she could benefit from further counselling. The decision, however, belongs to Caitlin, who says she is satisfied with the way things are and again states that if she has any future problems, she will return to the women's shelter counsellor.

## RESEARCH HIGHLIGHT

### Crisis-Service Needs for Urban and Rural Areas—One Size Does Not Fit All

**Source:** Forchuk, C., Jensen, E. Martin, M.L., et al. (2010). Psychiatric crisis services in three communities. *Canadian Journal of Community Mental Health, 29*(Suppl. 5), 73–86. Retrieved from http://cjcmh.metapress.com/openurl.asp?genre=article&issn=0713-3936&volume=29&supp=5&spage=73.

#### Problem
An evaluation of psychiatric crisis services is needed to determine the unique characteristics of rural versus urban settings and the distinct facilitators and barriers each setting poses to crisis workers and services.

#### Purpose of Study
The study set out to evaluate three models of crisis service (i.e., police as part of a specialized crisis mental health team, mental health workers as part of a police team, and an informal structure of support between police and mental health crisis services) for both urban and rural communities.

#### Methods
A qualitative study, gathering information through observations and focus groups of service providers, of the three models of crisis service for both urban and rural communities was conducted in Ontario.

#### Key Findings
The analysis of data from focus groups and observations showed that, while all communities valued their crisis services, all identified limitations in responsiveness and access, as well as systems-related issues. In both rural and urban areas, rapid access to psychiatric beds when hospitalization was indicated was seen as important. In rural areas, transportation was of particular concern, and safe transportation of clients in crisis became a police role.

Rural mental health workers took on broad generalist practitioner roles and often had to be able to address complex and challenging situations independently. In urban areas, transportation was more readily available, and mental health team members had more specialized roles, including crisis intervention expertise.

#### Implications for Nursing Practice
The study emphasizes that "one size does not fit all" and recommends that crisis programs serving rural communities adapt a model that integrates a well-seasoned mental health care worker—someone with generalist skills—with police service teams that have the ability to travel in rural areas. In urban areas, the team's research findings indicate that it's preferable for police to be affiliated with a team of specialized mental health workers.

## CASE STUDY AND NURSING CARE PLAN 24-1

### Crisis

Gurpreet Sidhu, the psychiatric clinical nurse specialist, is called to the neurological unit. She is told that Alexzy, a 43-year-old man with Guillain-Barré syndrome, is demonstrating challenging behaviours, and the staff has requested a consult. The disease has caused severe muscle weakness to the point that Alexzy is essentially paralyzed; however, he is able to breathe on his own.

The nurse manager says that Alexzy is hostile and sexually abusive, and his abusive language, demeaning attitude, and angry outbursts are having an adverse effect on the unit as a whole. The staff nurses state that they feel ineffective and angry and have tried to be patient and understanding; however, Alexzy's difficult behaviours have persisted. The situation has affected the morale of the staff and, the nurses believe, the quality of their care.

Alexzy, a new Canadian from Eastern Europe, was employed as a taxicab driver. Six months before his hospital admission, he had given up drinking after years of episodic alcohol abuse. His fiancée visits him every day. He needs a great deal of assistance with every aspect of his activities of daily living: he has to be turned and repositioned every two hours and is fed through a gastrostomy tube.

### ASSESSMENT

Gurpreet gathers data from Alexzy, the nursing staff, and Alexzy's fiancée.

#### Perception of the Precipitating Event
During the initial interview, Alexzy speaks to Gurpreet angrily, using profanity and making lewd sexual suggestions. He also expresses anger about needing a nurse to "scratch my head and help me blow my nose." He cannot figure out how his illness suddenly developed. He says the doctors told him that it was too early to know for sure if he would recover completely but that the prognosis was good.

#### Support System
Gurpreet speaks with Alexzy's fiancée. Alexzy's relationships with his fiancée, within his Eastern European cultural group, and with his taxi company co-workers are strong. Neither Alexzy nor his fiancée has much knowledge of supportive agencies.

#### Personal Coping Skills
Alexzy comes from a strongly male-dominated subculture, in which the man is expected to be a strong leader. His independence and power to affect the direction of his life is central to his perception of being acceptable as a man.

*Continued*

## CASE STUDY AND NURSING CARE PLAN 24-1—cont'd

*Crisis*

Alexzy feels powerless, out of control, and enraged. He is handling his anxiety by displacing these feelings onto the environment—namely, the staff and his fiancée. This redirection of anger temporarily lowers his anxiety and distracts him from painful feelings. When he intimidates others, he feels temporarily in control and experiences an illusion of power. He uses displacement to relieve his painful levels of anxiety.

Alexzy's unconscious use of displacement is maladaptive and does not resolve the issues causing his distress. His anxiety continues to escalate. Furthermore, his behaviour leads others to avoid him, further increasing his sense of isolation and helplessness.

**Self-Assessment**

Gurpreet meets with the staff twice. The staff members discuss feelings of helplessness and lack of control stemming from their feelings of rejection by Alexzy. They talk of their anger about Alexzy's demeaning behaviour and frustration about the situation. Gurpreet points out to the staff that Alexzy's feelings of helplessness, lack of control, and anger at his situation are the same feelings the staff are experiencing. His displacement of his feelings of helplessness and frustration by intimidating the staff gives Alexzy a brief feeling of control. It also distracts him from his own feelings of helplessness.

The nurses become more understanding of the motivation for the behaviour Alexzy employs to cope with moderate to severe levels of anxiety. The staff begins to focus more on the patient, less on personal reactions, and decides on two approaches to try as a group. First, they will not take Alexzy's behaviour personally. Second, Alexzy's displaced feelings will be refocused back to him.

On the basis of her assessment, Gurpreet identifies three main problem areas of importance and formulates the nursing diagnoses.

## DIAGNOSIS

1. *Ineffective coping* related to inadequate coping methods, as evidenced by inappropriate use of defence mechanisms (displacement)

**Supporting Data**
- Anger directed toward staff and fiancée
- Profanity and crude sexual remarks aimed at staff
- Isolation related to staff withdrawal
- Continued escalation of anxiety

2. *Powerlessness* related to lack of control over his health care environment, as evidenced by frustration over inability to perform previously uncomplicated tasks

**Supporting Data**
- Anger over nurses' having to "scratch my head and help me blow my nose"
- Minimal awareness of available supports in larger community

3. *Ineffective coping* related to exhaustion of staff's supportive capacity toward patient, as evidenced by staff withdrawal and limited personal communication with patient

**Supporting Data**
- Staff feels ineffective.
- Morale of staff is poor.
- Nurses believe that the quality of their care has been adversely affected.

## OUTCOMES IDENTIFICATION

Gurpreet speaks to Alexzy and tells him she would like to spend 15 minutes with him every morning to talk about his concerns. She suggests that he might be able to handle his feelings in alternative ways and notes that they can also explore community resources. Alexzy gruffly agrees, saying, "You can visit me if it will make you feel better." They make arrangements to meet each morning at 0730 hrs.

The following outcomes are set:

| Nursing Diagnosis | Short-Term Goal |
|---|---|
| 1. *Ineffective coping* related to inadequate coping methods, as evidenced by inappropriate use of defence mechanisms (displacement) | 1. Alexzy will be able to name and discuss at least two feelings about his illness and lack of mobility by the end of the week. |
| 2. *Powerlessness* related to lack of control over health care environment, as evidenced by frustration over inability to perform previously uncomplicated tasks | 2. Alexzy will be able to name two community organizations that can offer him information and support by the end of 2 weeks. |
| 3. *Ineffective coping* related to exhaustion of staff's supportive capacity toward patient, as evidenced by staff withdrawal and limited personal communication with patient | 3. Staff and nurse consultant will discuss reactions and alternative nursing responses to Alexzy's behaviour twice within the next 7 days. |

*Continued*

**CASE STUDY AND NURSING CARE PLAN 24-1—cont'd**

*Crisis*

## PLANNING

Gurpreet creates a nursing care plan and shares it with the staff.

**Nursing diagnosis:** *Ineffective coping* related to inadequate coping methods, as evidenced by inappropriate use of defence mechanisms (displacement)

**Outcome:** By discharge, Alexzy will state that he feels more comfortable discussing difficult feelings.

| Short-Term Goal | Intervention | Rationale | Evaluation |
|---|---|---|---|
| 1. By the end of the week, Alexzy will be able to name and discuss at least 2 feelings about his illness and lack of mobility. | 1a. Nurse will meet with patient daily for 15 minutes at 0730 hrs. | 1a. Night is usually the most frightening for patient; in early morning, feelings are closer to surface. | **GOAL MET** Within 7 days, Alexzy speaks to nurse more openly about feelings. |
| | 1b. When patient lashes out, nurse will remain calm. | 1b. Patient perceives that nurse is in control of her feelings. This belief can reassure patient and increase patient's sense of security. | |
| | 1c. Nurse will consistently redirect and refocus anger from environment back to patient (e.g., "It must be difficult to be in this situation"). | 1c. Refocusing feelings offers patient opportunity to cope effectively with his anxiety and decreases need to act out. | |
| | 1d. Nurse will come on time each day and stay for allotted time. | 1d. Consistency sets stage for trust and reinforces that patient's anger will not drive nurse away. | |

**Nursing diagnosis:** *Powerlessness* related to lack of control over health care environment, as evidenced by frustration over inability to perform previously uncomplicated tasks

**Outcome:** By discharge, Alexzy will contact at least one community support source.

| Short-Term Goal | Intervention | Rationale | Evaluation |
|---|---|---|---|
| 1. By the end of the 2 weeks, Alexzy will name and discuss at least 2 community organizations that can offer information and support. | 1a. Nurse will spend time with patient and fiancée. Role and use of specific agencies will be discussed. | 1a. Both patient and fiancée will have opportunity to ask questions of nurse. | **GOAL MET** By the end of 10 days, Alexzy and his fiancée can name 2 community resources they are interested in. At the end of 6 weeks, Alexzy has contacted the Guillain-Barré Society. |
| | 1b. Nurse will introduce 1 agency at a time. | 1b. Gradual introduction allows time for information to sink in and minimizes feeling of being pressured or overwhelmed. | |
| | 1c. Nurse will not push patient to contact any of the agencies. | 1c. Patient is able to make own decisions once he has appropriate information. | |

## IMPLEMENTATION

Nurse Gurpreet goes into Alexzy's room at 0730 hrs the following morning and sits by his bedside. At first, Alexzy's comments are hostile.

| Dialogue | Therapeutic Tool or Comment |
|---|---|
| **Nurse:** "Alexzy, I'm here as we discussed. I'll be spending 15 minutes with you every morning. We could use this time to talk about some of your concerns." | Nurse offers herself as a resource, gives information, and clarifies her role and patient expectations. Night is Alexzy's most difficult time. In the early morning, he will be the most vulnerable and open for therapeutic intervention and support. |
| **Alexzy:** "Listen, sweetheart, my only concern is how to get a little sexual relief, get it?" | |
| **Nurse:** "Being hospitalized and partially paralyzed can be overwhelming for anyone. Perhaps you wish you could find some relief from your situation." | Nurse focuses on the process "need for relief," not the sexual content, and encourages discussion of feelings. Sexual issues often challenge new nurses, and discussing their feelings and appropriate interventions with an experienced professional is important for their growth and the quality of the care they give. |
| **Alexzy:** "What do you know, Ms. Know-it-all? I can't even scratch my nose without getting one of those fools to do it for me ... and half the time those bitches aren't even around." | |

*Continued*

## CASE STUDY AND NURSING CARE PLAN 24-1—cont'd

### Crisis

| Dialogue | Therapeutic Tool or Comment |
|---|---|
| **Nurse:** "It must be difficult to have to ask people to do everything for you."<br><br>**Alexzy:** "Yeah. … The other night a fly kept landing on my face. I had to shout for 5 minutes before one of those bitches came in, just to take the fly out of the room."<br><br>**Nurse:** "Having to rely on others for everything can be a terrifying experience for anyone. It sounds extremely frustrating for you."<br><br>**Alexzy:** "Yeah. … It's a bitch … like a living hell." | Nurse restates what the patient says in terms of his feelings and continues to refocus away from the environment back to the patient.<br><br>Nurse acknowledges that frustration and anger would be a natural response for anyone in this situation. This response encourages the patient to talk about these feelings instead of acting them out. |

Gurpreet continues to spend time with Alexzy. He gradually talks more about his feelings and shows less hostility toward the staff. As he begins to feel more in control, he becomes less defensive about others' caring for him. After two weeks, Gurpreet decreases her visits to twice a week. Alexzy is beginning to experience gross motor movements but is not walking yet. He still displaces much of his frustration and lack of control onto the environment, but he is better able to acknowledge the reality of his situation. He can also identify and briefly talk about his feelings.

| Dialogue | Therapeutic Tool or Comment |
|---|---|
| **Nurse:** "What's happening? Your face looks tense this morning, Alexzy."<br><br>**Alexzy:** "I had to wait 10 minutes for a bedpan last night."<br><br>**Nurse:** "And you're angry about that."<br><br>**Alexzy:** "Well, there were only 2 nurses on duty for 30 people, and the nursing assistant was on his break. … You can't expect them to be everywhere, but still …"<br><br>**Nurse:** "It may be hard to accept that people can't be there all the time for you."<br><br>**Alexzy:** "Well … that's the way it is in this place." | Nurse observes the patient's clenched fists, rigid posture, and tense facial expression.<br><br>Nurse verbalizes the implied.<br><br>Nurse validates the difficulty of accepting situations one does not like when one is powerless to make changes. |

### EVALUATION

After six weeks, Alexzy is able to get around with assistance, and his ability to perform his activities of daily living is increasing. Although Alexzy still feels angry and overwhelmed at times, he is able to identify more of his feelings and acts them out less often, and he is able to talk to his fiancée about his feelings and lashes out at her less. He is looking forward to going home, and his boss is holding his old job.

Alexzy makes arrangements for a meeting with the Guillain-Barré Society, and he is thinking about Alcoholics Anonymous but believes he can handle this problem himself.

Staff members feel more comfortable and competent in their relationships with Alexzy. The goals have been met. Alexzy and Gurpreet agree that the crisis is over and terminate their visits. Alexzy is given the number of the crisis line and encouraged to call if he has questions or feels the need to talk.

## ▌KEY POINTS TO REMEMBER

- A crisis is not a pathological state but a struggle for emotional balance.
- Crises offer opportunities for emotional growth but can also lead to personality disorganization.
- There are three types of crisis: maturational, situational, and adventitious.
- Crises are usually resolved within four to six weeks.
- Assessment involves reviewing the balancing factors of the patient's perception of the problem, usual coping mechanisms, and situational supports.
- Social support and intervention can promote successful resolution.

- Resolution of a crisis takes three forms: a patient emerges at a higher level, at the precrisis level, or at a lower level of functioning.
- Crisis therapists take an active and directive approach with the patient in crisis.
- The patient is an active participant in setting goals and planning possible solutions.
- Crisis intervention is usually aimed at the mentally healthy patient who generally is functioning well but is temporarily overwhelmed and unable to function.
- The steps in crisis intervention are consistent with the steps of the nursing process.

- Specific qualities in the nurse that can facilitate effective intervention are a caring attitude, flexibility in planning care, an ability to listen, and an active, directive approach.
- The basic goals of crisis intervention are to reduce the individual's anxiety level and to support the effort to return the patient to his or her precrisis level of functioning.
- Crisis intervention therapy is short term—from one to six weeks—and focuses on the present problem only.
- Modalities of crisis intervention depend on the situation and services available at the time and locale (e.g., mental health first aid, which may be provided by professionals or community members; crisis lines; mobile response teams; urgent clinics; in-hospital emergency psychiatric care, including medical and other interventions).
- The goals of mental health first aid are much like those of physical first aid: to assist in early intervention, health promotion, protection from harm, and application of comfort until other measures are obtained.
- A critical incident stress debriefing is a group approach that helps groups of people who have been exposed to a crisis situation.

## CRITICAL THINKING

1. List the three important areas of crisis assessment once safety concerns have been identified. Give examples of two questions in each area that need to be answered before planning can take place.

2. Carley, a 21-year-old nursing student, tells her clinical instructor that her father (age 50 years) has just lost his job. Her father has been drinking heavily for years, and Carley is having difficulty coping. Because of her father's alcoholism and the increased stress in her family, Carley wants to leave school. Her mother has multiple sclerosis and thinks Carley should quit school to take care of her.
    a. How many different types of crisis are going on in this family? Discuss each crisis from the viewpoint of each individual family member.
    b. If you were providing crisis counselling for this family, what areas would you assess? What kinds of questions would you ask to evaluate each member's individual needs and the needs of the family as a unit (perception of events, social supports, coping styles)?
    c. Formulate some tentative goals you might set in conjunction with the family.
    d. Identify specific referral agencies in your area that would be helpful if members of this family were willing to expand their use of outside resources and stabilize the situation.
    e. How would you set up follow-up visits for this family? Would you see the family members together, alone, or in combination during the crisis period (four to six weeks)? How would you decide whether follow-up counselling was indicated?

3. Why is it important for nurses to promote mental health first aid (MHFA) training in rural or resource-poor communities?

4. What are some of the unique characteristics of rural versus urban settings and the distinct facilitators and barriers each setting poses for crisis workers and services?

## CHAPTER REVIEW

1. Jack had a psychotic episode when he was 15 years old. He did not respond well to treatments available at the time and continued to have a significant number of residual symptoms. At the age of 42, he began taking olanzapine (Zyprexa), which significantly reduced his remaining symptoms, allowing him to leave his group home and live independently for the first time. However, once his mental health became more stable and he was living in his own apartment, he was unsure of what to do with his time, how to go about getting a job, and how to meet his sexual and companionship needs appropriately. What type of crisis situation is represented by this case?
    1. Maturational crisis
    2. Situational crisis
    3. Adventitious crisis
    4. Phase 4 crisis

2. Rashid witnessed a car suddenly careen. out of control and onto the sidewalk where he and his best friend were walking. Rashid's friend pushed him out of the way at the last second but was struck and killed instantly. Rashid was treated for minor injuries and released but was referred for mental health evaluation because he was very distraught over the death of his friend. Which response should be used first during your assessment of Rashid?
    1. "Tell me about what happened that day."
    2. "What would you like to accomplish during your treatment?"
    3. "Do you think you are coping well with this very tragic event?"
    4. "Tell me what has been going through your mind since the accident."

3. Rashid confides that he feels so guilty that his friend died while pushing him to safety that he has found himself having overwhelming impulses to kill himself by crashing his car, which he almost did yesterday. Which intervention would be most therapeutic?
   1. Admit Rashid to an inpatient mental health unit to assure his safety until his condition can improve.
   2. Work with Rashid's family to ensure that he does not have access to a car, and set up emergency counselling sessions.
   3. Persuade Rashid to agree to remain safe pending counselling, as admitting him would only further traumatize him.
   4. Consult with a psychiatrist or prescribing physician so that Rashid can be started immediately on antianxiety and antidepressant medications.

4. Justine Lee, a mother of two teenagers and a nurse with 15 years of experience in the crisis centre, fails to show up for work several days in a row not long after providing crisis intervention to area high school students following a shooting at their school. Co-workers complain that she is not taking her share of crisis calls. As Justine's manager, you attempt to address the issue, but she responds irritably and denies that anything is wrong. Justine most likely:
   1. Is becoming burned out on crisis work
   2. Is experiencing vicarious traumatization
   3. Has developed a hidden substance abuse problem
   4. Has lost her objectivity, owing to having children of her own

5. Suzanne experiences a crisis after witnessing the brutal assault of her friend during a robbery in their office tower parkade. Which outcome is the most appropriate for Suzanne?
   1. Suzanne reports greater satisfaction with her life within two months.
   2. Suzanne attends all treatment sessions specified in her treatment plan.
   3. Within three weeks, Suzanne reports that she no longer feels distressed.
   4. Suzanne returns to her precrisis level of functioning within two weeks.

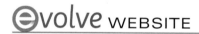 WEBSITE

Post-Test interactive review

*Visit the Evolve Web site for Chapter Review Answers and Rationales, Critical Thinking Answer Guidelines, and additional resources related to the content in this chapter: http://evolve.elsevier.com/Canada/Varcarolis/psychiatric/*

## REFERENCES

Aguilera, D.C. (1998). *Crisis intervention: Theory and methodology* (8th ed.). St. Louis, MO: Mosby.

Behrman, G., & Reid, W.J. (2002). Post-trauma intervention: Basic tasks. *Brief Treatment and Crisis Intervention, 2,* 39–48. doi:10.1093/brief-treatment/2.1.39.

Bledsoe, B. (2002). Critical incident stress management (CISM): Benefit or risk for emergency services? *Prehospital Emergency Care, 7,* 272–279.

British Columbia Ministry of Health. (2002). *Best practices in mental health: Crisis response and emergency services.* Retrieved from http://www.health.gov.bc.ca/library/publications/year/2000/MHABestPractices/bp_crisis_response.pdf.

Bulechek, G.M., Butcher, H.K., & Dochterman, J.M. (2008). *Nursing interventions classification (NIC)* (5th ed.). St. Louis: Mosby, MO.

Caplan, G. (1964). *Symptoms of preventive psychiatry.* New York: Basic Books.

Dunkley, J., & Whelan, T. (2006). Vicarious traumatisation: Current status and future directions. *British Journal of Guidance and Counselling, 34,* 107–116. doi:10.1080/03069880500483166.

Erikson, E.H. (1959). *Identity and the life cycle.* New York: International Universities Press.

Everly, G.S., Flannery, R.B., & Eyler, V.A. (2002). Critical incident stress management (CISM): A statistical review of the literature. *Psychiatric Quarterly, 73,* 171–182. doi:10.1023/A:1016068003615.

Everly, G.S., & Mitchell, J.T. (1999). *Critical incident stress management (CISM): A new era and standard of care in crisis intervention* (2nd ed.). Ellicott City, MD: Chevron Publishing.

Goldner, E.M., Palma, J., Jenkins, E., et al. (2011). *A concise introduction to mental health in Canada.* Toronto: Canadian Scholar's Press.

Health Canada. (2010). *Psychosocial emergency preparedness and response.* Retrieved from http://www.hc-sc.gc.ca/ewh-semt/occup-travail/empl/psychosoc-eng.php.

Herdman, T.H. (Ed.). (2012). *NANDA International nursing diagnoses: Definitions & classification, 2012–2014.* Oxford, UK: Wiley-Blackwell.

Hobfoll, S., Watson, P., Bell, C., et al. (2007). Five essential elements of immediate and mid-term mass trauma intervention: Empirical evidence. *Psychiatry, 70*(4), 283–315.

Kanel, K. (2012). *A guide to crisis intervention* (4th ed.). Belmont, CA: Brooks/Cole.

Lindemann, E. (1944). Symptomatology and management of acute grief. *American Journal of Psychiatry, 101*(9), 141–148.

Mental Health Commission of Canada. (2011). *Together we can: Annual report 2010–2011.* Ottawa: Author. Retrieved from http://www.mentalhealthcommission.ca/English/node/468.

Moorhead, S., Johnson, M., Maas, M., et al. (2008). *Nursing outcomes classification (NOC)* (4th ed.). St. Louis, MO: Mosby.

Registered Nurses' Association of Ontario. (2002). *Crisis intervention.* Toronto: Author.

Registered Nurses' Association of Ontario. (2006). *Crisis intervention.* Toronto: Author.

Roberts, A.R. (2005). *Crisis intervention handbook: Assessment, treatment, and research* (3rd ed.). New York: Oxford.

Saunders, J.M. (2007). Vulnerable populations in an American Red Cross shelter after Hurricane Katrina. *Perspectives in Psychiatric Care, 43*, 30–37. doi:10.1111/j.1744-6163.2007.00103.x.

van Emmerik, A., Kamphius, J., & Hulsbosch, A., et al. (2002). Single session debriefing after psychological trauma: A meta-analysis. *The Lancet, 360*, 766–771.

Wallace, M.A., & Morley, W.E. (1970). Teaching crisis intervention. *American Journal of Nursing, 70*(7), 1484–1487.

# Suicide

*Sharon L. Moore, Sherri Melrose*

## KEY TERMS AND CONCEPTS

copycat suicide, 515

death by suicide, 509

lethality, 517

postvention, 520

primary intervention, 519

SAD PERSONS scale, 518

secondary intervention, 519

suicidal behaviour, 509

suicidal ideation, 511

suicide, 509

survivors of suicide, 509

tertiary intervention, 520

## OBJECTIVES

1. Describe the profile of suicide in Canada, noting psychosocial and cultural factors that affect risk.
2. Identify three common precipitating events.
3. Describe risk factors and warning signs for suicide, including coexisting psychiatric disorders.
4. Name the most frequent coexisting psychiatric disorders.
5. Use the SAD PERSONS scale to assess suicide risk.
6. Describe three expected reactions a nurse may have when beginning work with suicidal patients.
7. Give examples of primary, secondary, and tertiary (postvention) interventions.
8. Describe basic-level interventions that take place in the hospital or community.
9. Identify key elements of suicide precautions and environmental safety factors in the hospital.

## ⊖volve WEBSITE

*Visit the Evolve website for Flashcards, Case Studies, and additional testing resources related to the content in this chapter: http://evolve.elsevier.com/Canada/Varcarolis/psychiatric/* Pre-Test  interactive review

Sadly, it is the rare individual who has yet to encounter, directly or indirectly, the significant public health problem that is suicide. Approximately every 40 seconds, a human life ends as a result of suicide (World Health Organization, 2010). Nursing students and practising nurses at all levels encounter individuals suffering from the pain and hopelessness that all too frequently culminate in the act of some type of suicidal behaviour. These individuals can be identified in inpatient settings, outpatient treatment settings, and in the community. Studies have shown that almost 90% of people who die by suicide had a health service in the year before their death (Morrison & Laing, 2011).

Nurses at the primary, secondary, and tertiary levels of intervention can play a crucial role in the care of these patients, their families, and the survivors of suicide (family and friends of a person who has died by suicide). Suicide is a permanent solution to an often temporary problem and is largely preventable, yet all too often, efforts are directed only toward individuals who are at immediate risk. It is critical for the health care community to become advocates for suicide prevention and to begin to mobilize the community in reducing and preventing factors that may contribute to suicide (American Association of Suicidology, n.d.; Canadian Association for Suicide Prevention, n.d.; International Association for Suicide Prevention, n.d.).

This chapter uses definitions that represent more current thinking in reference to suicide and suicidal behaviours. The words suicide or death by suicide are used to describe the act of taking one's own life. The term suicidal behaviour is used to describe potentially self-injurious actions with a nonfatal outcome for which there is evidence that a person intended to kill him- or herself (Standing Senate Committee on Social Affairs, Science and Technology, 2004). Examples of suicidal behaviours include self-harm, suicidal ideation, desire to hasten death, risky behaviour, and suicide threats. Suicidal behaviour may or may not result in injury. Sommer-Rotenburg (1998) noted that several terms used in association with suicide added to the stigma and alienation that survivors of suicide experienced. Reinforced by the Canadian Coalition for Seniors' Mental Health (2006), terms such as *committed suicide, failed suicide,* and *successful suicide* are avoided. Words like *commit* and *attempt* evoke connotations of criminality, and as such are inappropriate and potentially stigmatizing to suicidal individuals and those touched by suicide. Likewise,

> the term "completed suicide" connotes a sense of incompleteness for those who engaged in nonfatal self-harm behaviour and sends a potentially destructive message to those engaging in such behaviour. The term "successful suicide" is similarly problematic, as it implies that those who survive self-harm behaviour have somehow failed. ... Additionally, the notion of success and failure ignores the ever-present ambivalence among individuals contemplating and engaging in suicidal behaviour. (Canadian Coalition for Seniors' Mental Health, 2006, p. 8)

Changing the language that we use to describe suicide and suicidal behaviours is a first step in addressing the ways in which nurses can sensitively and empathically begin working with individuals who are suicidal.

This chapter presents the facts about suicide and discusses approaches for assessment and care of suicidal patients and their loved ones.

## EPIDEMIOLOGY

According to Statistics Canada (2013), in 2009, 3890 people committed suicide. The suicide mortality rate for both sexes and all ages was 11.5 per 100 000. Males were three times more likely to commit suicide than females. However, the rate of male suicide has been generally decreasing since 1999. The highest rates of suicide were in those aged 40 to 59. However, suicide was the leading cause of death for people aged 15 to 34. After the age of 35, the rate of suicide actually decreased, while other causes of death became more common (Statistics Canada, 2012). By province, rates for both sexes and all ages ranged from 8.5 per 100 000 in Ontario to 12.5 per 100 000 in Quebec. Among the territories, rates ranged from 5.1 per 100 000 in the Yukon to 27.8 per 100 000 in Nunavut (Statistics Canada, 2012).

"Research from general population surveys show that the rates of suicide related behaviours not resulting in a fatal outcome may be up to 100 times higher than rates of suicide" (Canadian Association for Suicide Prevention, 2009, p. 19). In 2009–2010, approximately 17 482 overnight hospitalizations—the equivalent of 135 333 hospital days—occurred as a result of self-harm among Canadians age 15 and older. This figure represents 65 hospitalizations for every 100 000 Canadians age 15 and older (Canadian Institute for Health Information, 2011).

 **RESEARCH HIGHLIGHT**

*Understanding Self-Harm and Suicidal Behaviour*

**Source:** Santa Mina, E.E. (2010). Self-harm intentions: Can they be distinguished based upon a history of childhood physical and sexual abuse? *Canadian Journal of Nursing Research, 42*(4), 122–143. Retrieved from http://cjnr.mcgill.ca/.

**Problem**

Better assessments and more precise interventions are needed for people who engage in self-harming and suicidal behaviours.

**Purpose of Study**

The purpose of this study was to determine if adults presenting to an inner-city Canadian hospital with self-harm or suicidal behaviour had experienced physical and sexual abuse during their childhood. The researchers believed that better understanding of the link between childhood physical and sexual abuse and self-harm or suicidal intentions could lead to more precise assessments and interventions.

**Methods**

A nonexperimental, comparative design was used to compare the experiences of clients who were admitted to mental health inpatient and emergency units who had self-harming behaviour with and without a history of childhood physical and sexual abuse. A convenience sample of 83 participants, who gave informed consent and completed self-reporting instruments (mainly questionnaires) within three days of the episode of self-harming behaviour.

**Key Findings**

Findings revealed that a history of childhood physical and sexual abuse was not a distinguishing factor in self-harm intention. Both men and women reported multiple reasons for the episode of self-harm. These included trying to achieve a feeling of peace through suicide (60%), but many others reported that their reason did not include wanting to die (38%).

**Implications for Nursing Practice**

Regardless of gender, self-harm method, or known abuse history, patients need to be assessed for their intentions behind the self-harming behaviours. It is only through a fully informed assessment that interventions can be tailored to specific patient needs.

Men are more likely to die by suicide, tending to use more lethal methods such as hanging and firearms, while women are more likely to survive a suicide attempt, frequently using less immediate lethal methods such as drugs, poisons, and gases (Canadian Association for Suicide Prevention, 2009). Older men are at especially high risk for suicide, having a rate more than double the national average (Canadian Coalition for Seniors' Mental Health, 2006). Almost 2.5 million Canadians are impacted by suicide each year, based on a conservative estimate that for every death by suicide six people are affected in some way. Families, friends, schools, workplaces, and health care and mental health care providers are profoundly affected by suicide (Canadian Association for Suicide Prevention, 2009).

It is important to consider that the number of suicides may actually be double or triple the reported statistics due to under-reporting in general (Rocket, 2010). Purposefully aiming a car at a bridge abutment and crashing may look like an accident. But, in fact, many reported accidents, homicides, and deaths ruled as "undetermined" are actually suicides.

Although death by suicide in the Canadian Forces is lower than in the general population, veterans who leave active service in the military are at high risk for suicidal behaviour (Zamorski, 2010). Studies have indicated that Canadian veterans can experience a greater incidence of depression, alcohol abuse (Shields, White, & Egan, 2009), and post-traumatic stress disorder (Richardson, Thompson, Boswall, et al., 2010) than those who were not in the military. Male war veterans are twice as likely to die from suicide as nonveteran males (Kaplan, Huguet, McFarland, et al., 2007), and female war veterans aged 18 to 34 are three times as likely to die from suicide as nonveteran females (McFarland, Kaplan, & Huguet, 2010). The *Life After Service Studies*, a joint research venture of Veterans Affairs Canada (VAC), the Department of National Defence/Canadian Forces (DND/CF), and Statistics Canada, continues to examine Canadian veterans' mental health issues as they transition to civilian life (Pedlar, 2010).

## Racial and Ethnic Statistics

Aboriginal peoples (First Nations, Inuit, and Métis) in Canada are especially vulnerable to death by suicide. The rate of suicide among some First Nations communities is two times greater than that of the rest of Canada. "From the ages of 10 to 29, Aboriginal youth on reserves are 5 to 6 times more likely to die of suicide than their peers in the general population. Over a third of all deaths among Aboriginal youth are attributable to suicide" (Aboriginal Healing Foundation, 2007).

The rate in northern Canada is even higher: "Between 1999 and 2007, approximately 40% of the 553 reportable deaths investigated by the coroner's office in Nunavut have involved suicidal deaths of young men" (Canadian Association for Suicide Prevention, 2009, p. 25). In Canada, the highest rate of death by suicide occurs among the Inuit. The National Aboriginal Health Organization (2006) reported that the rates rose from 79 per 100 000 cases between 1989 and 1993 to 119 per 100 000 cases between 1999 and 2003, "appallingly higher" than the general population in Canada. "Inuit of Nunatsiavut, formerly known as Labrador (239 per 100 000 suicides) and Nunavik (181 per 100 000) have the highest annual rates per population" (p. 4). While the rates of death by suicide for Inuit women are lower than for men, they are still significantly higher than that of the Canadian general population.

In response, in 2005, Health Canada, the Assembly of First Nations (AFN), and the Inuit Tapiriit Kanatami (ITK) established the First Nations and Inuit Mental Wellness Advisory Committee (MWAC) to develop community-based solutions to mental health issues such as the disproportionate rate of suicide among First Nations youth. One MWAC initiative, the Alianait Inuit-Specific Mental Wellness Task Group (IMWTGA), is mandated to explore mental wellness issues in the context of the distinct circumstances and culture of Inuit. "The word

*alianait* is an expression of joy in the Inuktitut language and the choice of this term illustrates the strength-based approaches taken by Inuit" (Kral, Wiebe, Nisbet, et al., 2009, p. 301). Another MWAC initiative, the National Aboriginal Youth Suicide Prevention Strategy (NAYSPS) is a multimillion-dollar federal strategy providing funds to support community-based research and capacity building for suicide-prevention plans. NAYSPS posits that suicide-prevention initiatives should be evidence-informed; support for community-based approaches should be provided by publicly funded agencies; support must be culturally appropriate; all levels of prevention must be offered; youth should be involved in the process; varying levels of community readiness have to be considered; suicide prevention is the responsibility of all people, communities, agencies, organizations, and governments; and the promotion of life and well-being is as important as suicide prevention. In 2010, the Centre for Suicide Prevention in Calgary published an online Aboriginal Youth Suicide Prevention course called "River of Life" (http://riveroflifeprogram.ca/) in contribution to international approaches to addressing youth suicide.

## Risk Factors

Suicide is not a psychiatric disorder per se; rather, self-harm is the manifestation of inner pain, hopelessness, and helplessness suffered by people experiencing suicidal ideation, also known as suicidal thoughts. These thoughts can range from a fleeting idea about one's own death (or about not being here) that does not include the act of killing oneself to a detailed plan, including the final act of killing oneself. In Canada, in 2009–2010, approximately seven in ten hospitalizations for self-harm included a mental health illness diagnosis. The percentages of hospitalizations for self-harm attributable to specific psychiatric disorders are listed in Table 25-1.

It is estimated that 90% of people who die by suicide are experiencing depression, another mental health illness, or a substance use disorder, all of which are potentially treatable

| TABLE 25-1 | PERCENTAGE OF HOSPITALIZATIONS FOR SELF-HARM ATTRIBUTABLE TO PSYCHIATRIC DISORDERS |
|---|---|
| DISORDERS | PERCENTAGE |
| Affective illnesses (major depression and bipolar disorder) | 23% |
| Substance-related disorders | 12% |
| Anxiety disorders | 11% |
| Disorders of personality and behaviour | 6% |
| Schizophrenia | 3% |
| Multiple mental health–related diagnoses (coexisting disorders) | 14% |

**Source:** Data from Canadian Institute for Health Information.

(Institute of Marriage and Family Canada, 2009). About 15% of patients who have major depression or bipolar disorder (during the depressed phase) will die by suicide (Brendel, Lagomasino, Perlis, et al., 2008). Loss of relationships, financial difficulty, and impulsivity are contributing factors in this population.

Suicide risk is 50 times higher among patients with schizophrenia than among the general population, especially during the first few years of the illness, and suicide is the number-one leading cause of early death of those with the illness. About 40% of all patients—and 60% of males—with schizophrenia attempt suicide at least once. Up to 10% of these patients die by suicide, usually related to depressive symptoms rather than to command hallucinations or delusions. The more risk factors that are present, the higher the risk for suicide (see Figure 25-1).

Patients with alcohol or substance use disorders also have a higher suicide risk. Co-morbidity of substance abuse and depression or antisocial personality disorder is also associated with increased risk. Up to 15% of those with alcohol or substance abuse die by suicide (Sadock & Sadock, 2008).

Keep in mind that suicide is not necessarily synonymous with a mental health disorder. The act of purposeful self-destruction represented by taking one's own life is usually accompanied by intensely conflicted feelings of pain, hopelessness, guilt, and self-loathing, coupled with the belief that there are no solutions and that things will not improve. Self-harming actions have been associated with the feeling that there is no one to turn to for support (Muehlenkamp, Brausch, Quigley et al., 2013). People who survive serious suicide attempts often report that it is these feelings that fuelled the sense of isolation

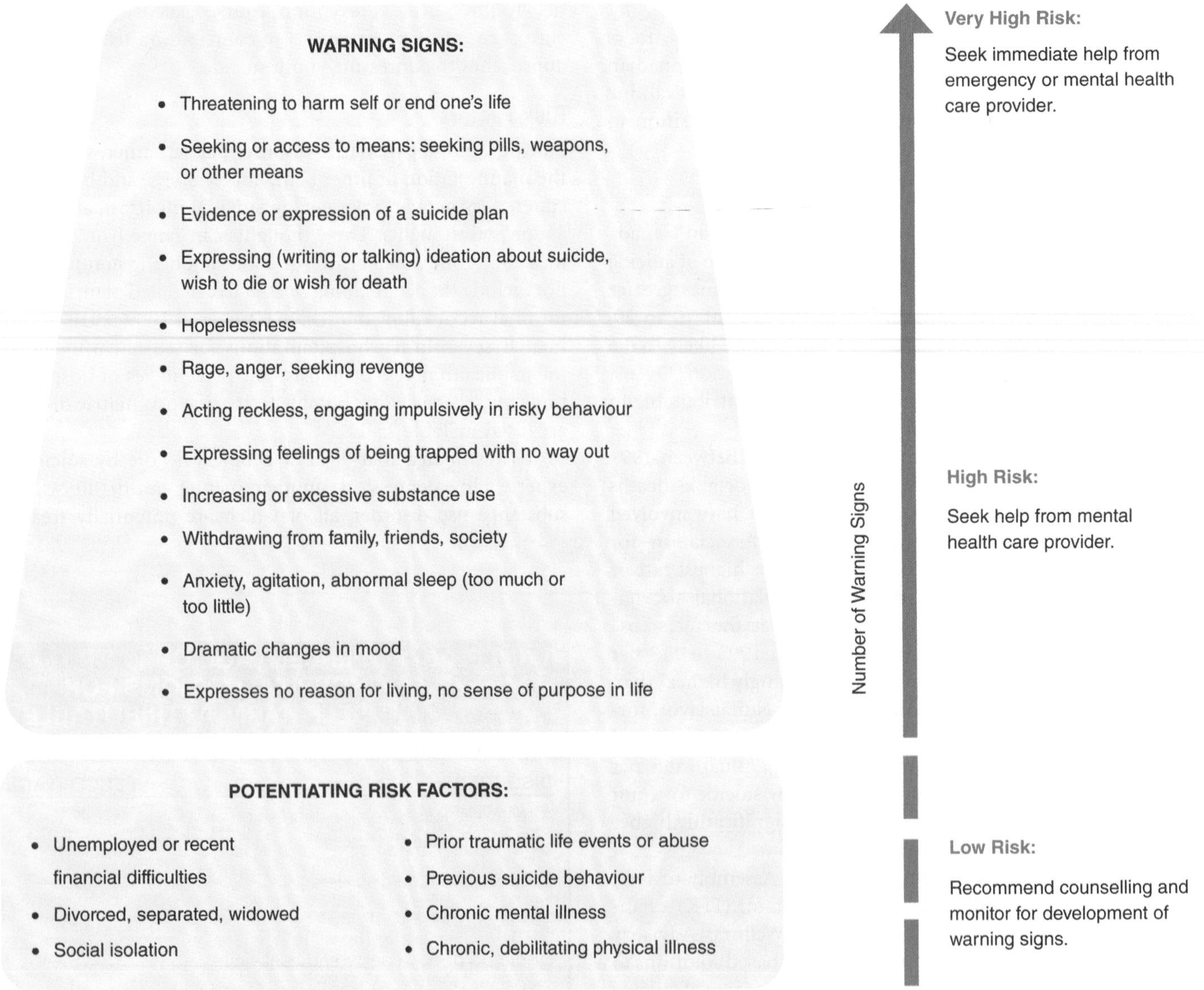

**WARNING SIGNS:**

- Threatening to harm self or end one's life
- Seeking or access to means: seeking pills, weapons, or other means
- Evidence or expression of a suicide plan
- Expressing (writing or talking) ideation about suicide, wish to die or wish for death
- Hopelessness
- Rage, anger, seeking revenge
- Acting reckless, engaging impulsively in risky behaviour
- Expressing feelings of being trapped with no way out
- Increasing or excessive substance use
- Withdrawing from family, friends, society
- Anxiety, agitation, abnormal sleep (too much or too little)
- Dramatic changes in mood
- Expresses no reason for living, no sense of purpose in life

**Very High Risk:**
Seek immediate help from emergency or mental health care provider.

**High Risk:**
Seek help from mental health care provider.

Number of Warning Signs

**POTENTIATING RISK FACTORS:**

- Unemployed or recent financial difficulties
- Divorced, separated, widowed
- Social isolation
- Prior traumatic life events or abuse
- Previous suicide behaviour
- Chronic mental illness
- Chronic, debilitating physical illness

**Low Risk:**
Recommend counselling and monitor for development of warning signs.

**FIGURE 25-1** Illustration of the accumulation of potentiating risk factors and warning signs on risk for suicide. **Source:** Perlman, C.M., Neufeld, E., Martin, L., et al. (2011). *Suicide risk assessment inventory: A resource guide for Canadian health care organizations.* Toronto: Ontario Hospital Association and Canadian Patient Safety Institute. Retrieved from http://www.oha.com/KnowledgeCentre/ Documents/Final%20-%20Suicide%20Risk%20Assessment%20Guidebook.pdf.

and despair. They describe an all-consuming psychic pain that shuts out thoughts of the loved ones and heartache they will leave behind. To understand this phenomenon, imagine the pain of your hand on a hot stove burner. At that moment, you are unlikely to think of anything but putting an immediate end to the pain. Emotional pain can render the individual void of thought and without even enough motivation to leave a suicide note. Antoon Leenars, a Canadian psychologist and researcher who has studied suicide notes extensively, has stated that only between 12% and 37% of people who died by suicide left suicide notes (Canadian Association for Suicide Prevention, 2009).

Besides psychiatric disorders, other risk factors associated with the psychic pain that can trigger suicidal behaviour include victimization by bullying, pathological gambling, incarceration, and nonheterosexuality. Researchers have established connections between being bullied and suicidal thoughts among children (Kim & Levanthal, 2008) and a positive correlation between adolescent bullying victims and suicide, with girls more strongly affected than boys (Klomek, Sourander, & Gould, 2010). Suicide rates among Canadian girls aged 10 to 19 have risen in the past two decades (Skinner & McFaull, 2012). The term *bullycide* was coined by Marr and Field (2000) to refer to suicidal behaviour in response to bullying.

Researchers have also established connections between pathological gambling and suicidal ideation, bipolar disorder, personality disorders, anxiety disorder, major depression, and substance use disorders (Alberta Health Services, 2009; Newman & Thompson, 2007). The Canada Safety Council (2006) estimated that over 200 Canadians experiencing problems related to gambling end up taking their own lives every year. Séguin, Boyer, Lesage, and colleagues (2010) found that pathological gamblers who completed suicide rarely sought mental health services the month prior to their suicide and were less likely than nonpathological gamblers to seek treatment in the previous year.

Further, researchers have established that many inmates living in prisons are at high risk for suicide and self-harming incidents, particularly during the initial phase of imprisonment and when on remand (Correctional Service of Canada, 2009). In a review of the implementation of Canada's *Mental Health Strategy* in federal prisons, Service (2010) identified that 11% of offenders were diagnosed with a mental illness, 21.3% were prescribed psychiatric medication, and 14.5% of male offenders had a past psychiatric hospitalization. Female offenders are twice as likely as male offenders to have a mental illness diagnosis. Service's review concluded that "the mental health needs of offenders exceed the capacity, services and supports of the federal correctional authority to meet the growing demand" (p. 3).

Researchers have established that suicidal behaviour is significantly higher in nonheterosexual populations (Chakraborty, McManus, Brugha, et al., 2011; King, Semlyen, Tai, et al., 2008). Among youth, lesbian, gay, bisexual, transgender, and those questioning their sexuality are at higher risk for suicide than their heterosexual peers (Suicide Prevention Resource Center, 2008). Nonheterosexual youth who are homeless, have run away, are living in foster care, or are involved in the juvenile justice system have fewer supports and are therefore at even

greater risk (Suicide Prevention Resource Center, 2008). Although most mortality data do not include sexual orientation, nonheterosexual youth are believed to experience suicidal ideation and engage in suicidal behaviour to a greater extent than heterosexual adolescents and young adults. The stigma and discrimination associated with their sexual orientation elevate risk and lower protective factors among this group.

Refer to Box 25-1 for a description of significant psychosocial risk and protective factors for suicide and Box 25-2 for warning signs.

---

**BOX 25-1 SUICIDE RISK FACTORS AND PROTECTIVE FACTORS**

**Risk Factors**
- Suicidal ideation with intent
- Lethal suicide plan
- History of previous suicide attempt
- Co-occurring psychiatric illness
- Co-occurring medical illness
- History of childhood abuse
- Family history of suicide
- Lack of social support
- Unemployment
- Recent stressful life event (e.g., death, other loss)
- Hopelessness
- Helplessness
- Panic attacks
- Feeling of shame or humiliation
- Impulsivity
- Aggressiveness
- Loss of cognitive function (e.g., loss of impulse control)
- Access to firearms and other highly lethal means
- Substance abuse (without formal disorder)
- Impending incarceration
- Low frustration tolerance
- Sexual orientation issues
- Social isolation

**Protective Factors**
- Sense of responsibility to family (e.g., spouse, children)
- Pregnancy
- Religious beliefs
- Satisfaction with life
- Positive social support
- Access to health care
- Effective coping skills
- Effective problem-solving skills
- Intact reality testing
- Connection with others
- Sense of purpose and meaning in life

**Sources:** Canadian Association for Suicide Prevention. (2009). *The CASP national suicide prevention strategy* (2nd ed.). Winnipeg: Author. Retrieved from http://www.suicideprevention.ca/wp-content/uploads/2009/10/2010strategy-final-september.pdf; Lakeman, R., & FitzGerald, M. (2008). How people live with or get over being suicidal: A review of qualitative studies. *Journal of Advanced Nursing, 64,* 114–126. doi:10.1111/j.1365-2648.2008.04773.x; and Moore, S.L., Metcalf, B., & Schow, E. (2006). The quest for meaning in aging. *Geriatric Nursing, 27,* 293–299. doi:10.1016/j.gerinurse.2006.08.012.

## BOX 25-2  WARNING SIGNS

The American Association of Suicidology (AAS) uses the mnemonic IS PATH WARM to assist people in recognizing and identifying the warning signs of suicide.

**SUICIDE WARNING SIGNS**

I   Ideation
S   Substance use
P   Purposelessness
A   Anxiety or agitation
T   Trapped
H   Hopelessness or helplessness
W   Withdrawal
A   Anger
R   Recklessness
M   Mood changes

The presence of any warning sign may signify that someone is thinking about suicide. The presence of more than one warning sign indicates a higher risk for suicide. The presence of one or more warning signs should signal the need to begin a dialogue into a person's circumstances and a follow-up with a more in-depth suicide risk assessment.

**Source:** American Association of Suicidology. (n.d.). *Know the warning signs.* Retrieved from http://www.suicidology.org/stats-and-tools/suicide-warning-signs.

## ETIOLOGY

### Biological Factors

Researchers continue to study biological factors in order to better understand and screen for suicidal behaviour, although none of the biological markers identified to date are sensitive or precise enough for use in the clinical setting. Failures in neurotransmitter and neuroendocrine systems, such as the serotonergic, noradrenergic, dopaminergic, and hypothalamic–pituitary–adrenocortical (HPA) systems, have been investigated (Ganz, Braquehais, & Sher, 2010) but have not yet yielded any evidence strong enough to significantly change clinical practice. For example, evidence suggests a potentially causal association between suicidal behaviour and the serotonin neurotransmission system (Carballo, Akamnonu, & Oquendo, 2008). Further, low cerebrospinal fluid 5-hydroxyindoleacetic acid (5-HIAA, the main serotonin metabolite) is considered a promising biological predictor of suicidal behaviour (Ganz, Braquehais, & Sher, 2010).

In the context of acute stress response to life events, dysregulation of HPA axis function, particularly nonsuppression of the HPA axis by dexamethasone, may also be involved in suicidal behaviour (Currier & Mann, 2009). Another consideration is

 **RESEARCH HIGHLIGHT**

### Post-Suicide Stress: Nurses Need Support

**Source:** Takahashi, C., Chida, F., Nakamura, H., et al. (2011). The impact of inpatient suicide on psychiatric nurses and their need for support. *BMC Psychiatry, 11,* 2–8. doi:10.1186/1471-244X-11-38.

**Problem**

Although nurses working in psychiatric hospitals and wards are prone to encounter death by suicide, support for their post-suicide stress may not be available.

**Purpose of Study**

The research was conducted to examine post-suicide stress in nurses and the availability of suicide-related mental health care services and education.

**Methods**

Experiences with inpatient suicide were investigated using an anonymous, self-reported questionnaire, which was, along with the Impact of Event Scale—Revised (IES-R) administered to 531 psychiatric nurses.

**Key Findings**

The rate of nurses who had encountered patient suicide was 55.0%. The mean IES-R score was 11.4. The proportion of respondents at a high risk (≥25 on the 88-point IES-R score) for post-traumatic stress disorder (PTSD) was 13.7%. However, only 15.8% of respondents indicated that they had access to post-suicide mental health care programs. The survey also revealed a low rate of nurses who reported attending in-hospital seminars on suicide prevention or mental health care for nurses (26.4% and 12.8%, respectively). These results indicated that nurses

exposed to inpatient suicide suffer significant mental distress. However, the low availability of systematic post-suicide mental health care programs for such nurses and the lack of suicide-related education initiatives and mental health care for nurses are problematic. The situation is likely related to the fact that there are no formal systems in place for identifying and evaluating the psychological effects of patient suicide in nurses and to the pressures stemming from the public perception of nurses as suppliers rather than recipients of health care.

**Implications for Nursing Practice**

Involvement with people who engage in suicidal behaviour is a significantly distressing event, for nurses as well as for all those involved in the individual's life. Opportunities to debrief and discuss the impact of suicide are critical. While individual counselling, grief support groups, and educational opportunities are often available to family members, post-suicide mental health care geared specifically to the needs of nurses and other health care providers may not be accessible. Health care workers may feel their responsibility is to provide rather than receive help for their own distress. Knowing that our colleagues as well as our patients' family members are at high risk for post-traumatic stress following experiences with death by suicide, we must provide opportunities for all suicide survivors to talk about what happened. Our peers may be in need of more support than we imagine. Asking questions sensitively can frequently open the door for people to talk about the often overwhelming feelings of fear, grief, anger, puzzlement, and even condemnation of suicidal feelings or behaviours that they may be experiencing after involvement with suicidal behaviour.

the involvement of protein kinase A (PKA), a crucial enzyme in the adenylyl cyclase signal transduction pathway, which regulates gene transcription, cell survival, and plasticity. When stress affects PKA's synaptic and structural plasticity, an association with suicide has been identified (Dwivedi & Pandey, 2011).

## Psychosocial Factors

Sigmund Freud originally theorized that suicide resulted from unacceptable aggression toward another person that is turned inward. Karl Menninger added to Freud's thought by describing three parts of suicidal hostility: the wish to kill, the wish to be killed, and the wish to die (Sadock & Sadock, 2008). Aaron Beck identified a central emotional factor underlying suicide intent: hopelessness. Certain cognitive styles that contribute to higher risk are rigid all-or-nothing thinking, inability to see different options, and perfectionism (Lester, 2012). Maladaptive perfectionist thinking, in which anything less than perfect is unacceptable, can leave individuals vulnerable to depression and suicide (Melrose, 2011).

Recent theories of suicide have focused on the lethal combination of suicidal fantasies accompanied by loss (e.g., of love, self-esteem, job, freedom due to imminent incarceration), rage or guilt, or identification with a suicide victim (copycat suicide). A copycat suicide follows a highly publicized suicide of a public figure, an idol, or a peer in the community. Adolescents are at especially high risk for copycat suicide, owing to their immature prefrontal cortex, the portion of the brain that controls the executive functions involving judgement, frustration tolerance, and impulse control.

Athletes, at both elite and amateur levels, can feel constant pressure to perform. Loss of status in their sport, steroid use, or an injury such as postconcussion syndrome can leave them susceptible to suicidal fantasies. Persistent pain has been found to increase depression in retired professional athletes (Schwenk, Gorenflo, Dopp, et al., 2007). When professional athletes die by suicide, the resulting media attention can be used to shine a spotlight on suicide prevention (Centre for Suicide Prevention, 2011).

## Cultural Factors

Cultural factors, including religious beliefs, family values, and attitude toward death, can influence suicide rates. And yet, as Leong and Leach (2008) observed, "Pain is pain. ... The suicidal mind is the suicidal mind ... whether in any cultural group" (p. 3). In Canada, white males have the highest number of deaths by suicide. As previously mentioned, groups with the highest rate of suicide are Inuit and Aboriginal people. However, individuals within a particular culture may have different personal beliefs from those attributed to the group. "Within-group variables, such as acculturation, racial identity, extrinsic religiosity, gay identity development and gender identity ... impact empirical literature on cultural influences on suicide," and findings are often critiqued for their subjectivity (Leach, 2006, p. 3).

Of particular importance in caring for patients who are experiencing the pain of suicidal behaviour is an understanding of the relational concept of cultural safety. According to the Registered Nurses' Association of Ontario (2009) *Best Practice* *Guidelines*, cultural safety is about more than respecting differences; it is about demonstrating "acceptance and respect for the 'culture' of the client and for the associated differences, in addition to advocating for change in response to policies and practices that may be experienced as 'unsafe' by the client" (p. 26). Both nurses and patients bring to the therapeutic relationship their own culturally centric values and beliefs about suicide. By virtue of nurses' perceived position of power, their own values, however inadvertently, can impact patients' feeling of safety, a situation nurses must be aware of. "The nurse needs to recognize that both the client (as individual, family and/or community) and the provider are 'bearers of culture'—a 1 : 1

## CONSIDERING CULTURE

### Factors: Cultural Safety

Grounded in the principle of safety as a nursing expectation and standard, cultural safety seeks to overcome situations wherein people from one cultural group feel demeaned, disempowered, or "unsafe" as a consequence of the actions of a more dominant group from another culture. From a critical-theory perspective, culture is a complex, dynamic, political, historical, and relational process that shifts over time and one that has significantly been influenced by our social, professional, and gendered location (Registered Nurses' Association of Ontario, 2008). Cultural safety is not about ethnocultural differences, customs, and practices. Rather, cultural safety calls us to view our way of providing nursing care through a lens of critical consciousness and to question the inherent power differentials in the health care systems we learn and work in.

Originating in New Zealand, the concept of cultural safety emerged as indigenous Maori nurse leaders began to link the poor health outcomes of Maori people, in part, to the cultural inappropriateness and insensitivity of health care providers, who were descendents of European settlers, the dominant culture (Syme, Josewiski, & Kendall, 2010). In essence, "cultural safety analyzes power imbalances, institutional discrimination, colonization, and colonial relationships" (National Aboriginal Health Organization, 2009, p. 3). The approach continues to gain international recognition, primarily in relation to indigenous peoples' experiences with mainstream health care, and is particularly relevant in caring for patients with suicidal behaviour in Canada's multicultural context. Health care providers must remember that, although knowledge of practices that may be associated with different cultural groups can be valuable in assessing some suicidal behaviour, this same knowledge can also be construed as stereotyping, labelling, and marginalizing patients.

**Sources:** National Aboriginal Health Organization. (2009). *Cultural competency and safety in First Nations, Inuit and Métis health care* [Fact Sheet]. Ottawa: Author; Registered Nurses' Association of Ontario. (2009, January). *Assessment and care of adults at risk for suicidal ideation and behaviour.* Toronto: Author; and Syme, V., Josewiski, V., & Kendall, E. (2010). *Cultural safety: An overview* [Report to the First Nations, Inuit and Métis Advisory Committee and Mental Health Commission of Canada]. Retrieved from http://www.mooddisorderscanada.ca/documents/Publications/CULTURAL%20SAFETY%20AN%20OVERVIEW%20%28draft%20mar%202010%29.pdf

relationship is always bicultural. It requires an examination of how each individual is located within historical, social, economic and political processes" (Registered Nurses' Association of Ontario, 2009, p. 26).

## Societal Factors

No discussion about current societal attitudes and trends would be complete without an examination of the way in which suicide is viewed in a general context. In Canada, both euthanasia and assisted suicide are against the law. Regarding euthanasia, the "General: Consent to Death" section of the Criminal Code (1985) states: "No person is entitled to consent to have death inflicted on him, and such consent does not affect the criminal responsibility of any person by whom death may be inflicted on the person by whom consent is given" (c. C-46, s. 14). Regarding assisted suicide, the "Suicide: Counselling or Aiding Suicide" section states: "Everyone who (a) counsels a person to commit suicide, or (b) aids or abets a person to commit suicide, whether suicide ensues or not, is guilty of an indictable offence and liable to imprisonment for a term not exceeding fourteen years" (Criminal Code, 1985, s. 241). However, not all cases result in charges, prosecution, or imprisonment (D'Orazio, 2010).

Efforts to decriminalize euthanasia and assisted suicide have been under way for many years. In 1993, the Supreme Court of Canada ruled on Sue Rodriguez's landmark case. Ms. Rodriguez's claim addressed how section 241(b) of the Canadian Criminal Code infringed on sections 7 ("Life, Liberty and Security"), 15(1) ("Equality of Rights"), and 12 ("Cruel and Unusual Punishment") of the Canadian Charter of Rights and Freedoms (*Rodriguez v. British Columbia*, 1992). Although she lost her case, Rodriguez did take her life with help from a physician, who was not criminally charged.

Internationally, legislative debates continue about euthanasia and assisted suicide. In some countries, the law is not the same in all jurisdictions. In the United States, Oregon's *Death With Dignity Act* of 1997 legally allows adult Oregon residents diagnosed with a terminal illness that will lead to death within six months to obtain a physician-assisted suicide. The patient must be thoroughly screened by a physician and deemed to be both terminally ill and psychiatrically sound. However, concern has been raised that as many as 25% of the patients in Oregon who have been assisted to die actually had clinical depression (Ganzini, Goy, & Dobscha, 2008). The Netherlands allows for this practice in nonterminal cases of "lasting and unbearable" suffering (Appel, 2007). Belgium authorizes physician-assisted suicide for nonterminal cases when suffering is deemed to be "constant and cannot be alleviated." And no country has laws as liberal as Switzerland, in which assisted suicide has been legal since 1918 and allows nonresidents to terminate their lives without a physician involved in the process (Appel, 2007).

The ethical and moral dilemmas in this evolving trend are clear. Questions continue to be posed about whether chronic and serious mental illness is no different in the depth and breadth of suffering from chronic and serious physical illness (Appel, 2007). Ethicists question whether the "slippery slope" of legally sanctioned suicide will result in abuse of vulnerable groups such as the clinically depressed (Battin, van der Heide,

Ganzini, et al., 2007; Finlay & George, 2011). Until more effective treatment or a cure is found, some individuals who obtain little or no benefit from existing psychiatric treatments may choose to end suffering. At the core of the argument supporting assisted suicide are the twin goals of minimizing human suffering and maximizing individual autonomy.

## APPLICATION OF THE NURSING PROCESS

The process of suicide risk assessment is comprehensive and requires identifying specific risk factors, taking a psychosocial and medical history, and interacting with the patient during the interview. The nurse usually completes this assessment in conjunction with other clinicians since comparison of data from two interviewers is often a significant element of the evaluation.

Not all patients who show suicidal ideation or who engage in suicidal behaviour truly want to die. Suicidal behaviour can include a variety of behaviours, including self-harm either with or without clear intent to cause bodily harm or death. Any previous suicidal behaviour is a risk factor for suicide—about half of all people who kill themselves have a history of some form of suicidal behaviour. Especially prevalent in the adolescent and young adult populations, self-harm (usually in the form of cutting) is most often done with the intent to either alleviate psychic pain or to pierce the psychic numbness these individuals describe (Cleaver, 2007; Heisel, Moore, Bowman, et al., 2010). They do not engage in this behaviour as a means of seeking attention and will often go to great lengths to conceal the evidence. Self-harm often carries a lethal risk for death or permanent injury. It is important for nurses to try to understand what is behind the behaviour as it is often a sign that the individual is trying to communicate his or her pain and despair.

Nonacute suicidal or self-destructive thoughts and feelings can be treated in the outpatient setting. Alternative services available to suicidal patients include crisis intervention, community mental health services, assertive community treatment (ACT), addiction treatment, social services, and legal assistance. These types of interventions are evidence-informed and cost effective, as well as individualized and realistic—all essential aspects of the person-centred recovery model (American Nurses Association, American Psychiatric-Mental Health Nurses Association, & International Society of Psychiatric-Mental Health Nurses, 2007). The Mental Health Commission of Canada (2009) advocates for a mental health system that focuses on recovery and hope, choice, responsibility, dignity, and respect.

## ASSESSMENT

*The Suicide Risk Assessment Guide: A Resource for Health Care Organizations* (Perlman, Neufeld, Martin, et al., 2011) is a general guide to help health care organizations with understanding and standardizing the practice of high-quality suicide risk assessment. The guide emphasized the importance of thorough documentation in assessing suicide. Box 25-3 provides a sample of recommended documentation, summarizing eight important points to include in nursing assessments.

## BOX 25-3 SAMPLE OF RECOMMENDED DOCUMENTATION

1. The overall level of suicide risk

The level of risk should be clearly documented, along with information to support this assertion, which can include the following:
   - The types of assessment tools used to inform risk assessment
   - Details from clinical interviews and from communication with others (e.g., the person's family and friends, other professionals), including:
     - The circumstances and timing of the event
     - Method chosen for suicide
     - Degree of intent
     - Availability of resources to carry out plan
     - Description of actions taken by the health care provider or family members
     - Consequences of previous suicidal ideation or self-harming behaviours (e.g., Were there any permanent injuries?)

2. Prior history of suicide attempt(s) and self-harming behaviour
   - The prior care or intervention plan that was in place
   - The length of time since previous suicide attempt(s) or self-harming behaviour(s)
   - The rationale for not being admitted to a more intensive environment or discharged to a less restrictive environment, and what safety plans were put into place
   - Details about family concerns and how these were addressed

3. Details about all potentiating risk factors, warning signs, and protective factors

4. The degree of suicide intent

The degree of intent may include, for example, what the person thought or hoped would happen.

5. The person's feeling and reaction following suicidal behaviour

Record, for example, whether the person feels a sense of relief or regret at being alive.

6. Evidence of an escalation in potential lethality of self-harm or suicidal behaviours

Document whether the person has begun to consider, plan, or use increasingly lethal means (e.g., from cutting to hanging, seeking a gun).

7. Similarity of person's current circumstances to those surrounding previous suicide attempt(s) or self-harming behaviour(s)

8. History of self-harm or suicidal behaviour(s) among family or friends or significant loss of family or friends

This history should include anniversary dates of these events as risk may be elevated at such times.

**Source:** Centre for Addiction and Mental Health. (2011). *Suicide prevention and assessment handbook.* Toronto: Author. Retrieved from http://www.camh.ca/en/hospital/health_information/a_z_mental_health_and_addiction_information/suicide/Documents/sp_handbook_final_feb_2011.pdf.

Organizations should also develop standard protocols for the location of documentation regarding suicide risk within the patient's record so that documentation is consistently located and, therefore, easily identified by others within the organization or by those involved in the care of the person.

### Verbal and Nonverbal Clues

Almost all people considering suicide send out clues, especially to people they think of as supportive. Nurses and other health care workers often fit into this category. There may be overt or covert verbal clues and nonverbal signals. Examples include:
- Overt statements
  - "I can't take it anymore."
  - "Life isn't worth living anymore."
  - "I wish I were dead."
  - "Everyone would be better off if I died."
- Covert statements
  - "It's okay now. Soon everything will be fine."
  - "Things will never work out."
  - "I won't be a problem much longer."
  - "Nothing feels good to me anymore and probably never will."
  - "How can I give my body to medical science?"

Most often, it is a relief for people contemplating suicide to finally talk to someone about their despair and loneliness. Asking about suicidal thoughts does not "give a person ideas" and is, in fact, a professional responsibility similar to asking about chest pain in cardiac conditions. Talking openly leads to a decrease in isolation and can increase problem-solving alternatives for living. People who contemplate suicide, act on their suicidal thoughts, and even those who regret the "failure" of their actions are often extremely receptive to talking about their suicide crisis. Specific questions to ask about suicidal ideation include the following (Meerwijk, van Meijel, van den Bout, et al., 2010):
- Have you ever felt that life was not worth living?
- Have you been thinking about death recently?
- Have you been feeling so bad that you have thought about taking your own life?
- Did you ever think about suicide?
- Have you ever tried to end your life?
- Do you have a plan for what you would do to end your own life?
- If so, what is your plan?

### Lethality of Suicide Plan

The evaluation of a suicide plan is extremely important in determining the degree of suicidal risk. Five main elements must be considered when evaluating lethality (the degree of suicidal risk) (Toth, Schwartz, & Kurka, 2007):
1. Presence of risk factors for suicide
2. Degree of suicidal ideation
3. Intent to carry out suicide plan
4. Means and availability of resources to carry out selected method of suicide
5. Degree of hope for improvement of psychological state

People who have definite plans for the time, place, and means are at high risk.

People experiencing psychotic episodes are at high risk—regardless of the specificity of details—because their impulse control and judgement are grossly impaired. A person suffering psychosis is particularly vulnerable when depressed or having command hallucinations. Regardless of whether the nurse considers a patient high or low risk, *all* threats of suicide should be taken seriously, and a suicide risk assessment should be completed.

## Assessment Tools

Many tools have been developed to aid a health care worker in assessing suicidal potential. Patterson, Dohn, Bird, and colleague (1983) devised an assessment aid with the acronym *SAD PERSONS* to evaluate ten major risk factors for suicide (Table 25-2). The SAD PERSONS scale is a simple and practical guide for triaging potentially suicidal patients, particularly in an emergency department environment. Ten categories are described in the assessment tool, and the person being evaluated is assigned one point for each applicable characteristic. The total point score for the individual correlates with an action scale that assists health care workers to determine whether hospital admission is advisable. If a patient scores in the 3- to 4-point range, it is then necessary for a psychiatric or mental health care provider to conduct a full mental status examination and interview.

The SAD PERSONS tool has its shortcomings. It does not address whether or not the patient is taking either illicit or prescribed drugs that may have a significant impact on him or her, and it is also dated (from 1983). There is a need for a uniform and evidence-informed screening tool that can be used in clinical environments (Price, 2007).

Prescription medications such as antidepressants should be evaluated for their contribution to suicide risk. Health Canada advisories warn against the use of selective serotonin reuptake inhibitor (SSRI) antidepressants in pregnant women and children and young adults up to age 24 due to their potential to increase the risk for suicide. Health Canada monitors the safety of these and other psychiatric medications and posts ongoing alerts on its website. Some patients taking psychiatric medications develop extreme restlessness and agitation (akathisia) that can make life intolerable and thereby increase the risk for suicide. The impulsivity associated with mania, and the regret that may be felt because of acts committed during a manic state, may also increase suicidal risk factors. Health care practitioners need to be aware that there are several medications that can induce a manic state (e.g., antidepressants, steroids) and ensure that responses to medications are carefully monitored and screening for suicide potential is completed (Harvard Medical School, 2007).

## Self-Assessment

All health care professionals who work with suicidal people need to collaborate with other clinicians. Fear, grief, anger, puzzlement, and condemnation of suicidal feelings or intent are common feelings. If these intense emotional responses are not acknowledged, counter-transference may limit effective intervention. Understanding the suicidal patient, as well as acknowledging, understanding, and accepting the emotions that arise from working with and caring for these patients, is essential.

| TABLE 25-2 | SAD PERSONS SCALE | |
|---|---|---|
| S | Sex | 1 if male |
| A | Age | 1 if 25 to 44 years or 65+ years |
| D | Depression | 1 if present |
| P | Previous attempt | 1 if present |
| E | Ethanol use | 1 if present |
| R | Rational thinking loss | 1 if psychotic for any reason |
| S | Social supports lacking | 1 if lacking, especially recent loss |
| O | Organized plan | 1 if plan with lethal method |
| N | No spouse | 1 if divorced, widowed, separated, or single male |
| S | Sickness | 1 if severe or chronic |

### GUIDELINES FOR ACTIONS

| POINTS | CLINICAL ACTION |
|---|---|
| 0–2 | Send home with follow-up |
| 3–4 | Closely follow up; consider hospitalization |
| 5–6 | Strongly consider hospitalization |
| 7–10 | Hospitalize or commit |

**Source:** From Patterson, W.M., Dohn, H.H., Bird, J., et al. (1983). Evaluation of suicidal patients: The SAD PERSONS scale. *Psychosomatics, 24*(4), 343–345, 348–349.

## ASSESSMENT GUIDELINES

### *Suicide*

1. Assess risk factors, including history of suicide (in family, friends), degree of hopelessness and helplessness, and lethality of plan.
2. If there is a history of a suicide attempt, assess intent, lethality, and injury.
3. Determine whether the patient's age, medical condition, psychiatric diagnosis, or current medications put the patient at higher risk.
4. Further assessment is necessary if the patient suddenly goes from sad or depressed to happy and peaceful. Often, a decision to kill oneself gives a feeling of relief and calm.
5. If the patient is to be managed on an outpatient basis, also assess social supports and helpfulness of significant others.

## IMPLEMENTATION

Nursing interventions for suicide take place at three different levels: primary, secondary, and tertiary. Because improving *overall* community mental health can reduce the incidence of suicide more effectively than extensive efforts directed at identifying imminently suicidal individuals, more attention focused on primary interventions that involve communitywide participation can improve outcomes at the community level (Ortiz, 2006).

### Primary Intervention

Primary intervention includes activities that provide support, information, and education to prevent suicide (Box 25-4). The foundation of any intervention for suicide or suicidal behaviours is establishing a therapeutic relationship. Understanding and appreciating clients' unique situations and treating

individuals with respect and openness are essential. Nurses who remain informed, empathic, and nonjudgemental are well positioned to initiate interventions at both the individual and community levels. Primary intervention can be practised in a wide variety of community settings, such as schools, homes, churches, hospitals, and work settings. Elementary school children are screened using evidence-informed tools that focus on both risk factors and warning signs (Joe & Bryant, 2007). Several high schools are adopting suicide prevention curricula that involve elements of education, peer support and referral, and discussions about risk factors and warning signs (Ciffone, 2007).

### Secondary Intervention

Secondary intervention is treatment of the actual suicidal crisis. It is practised in clinics, hospitals, and jails and on telephone hotlines. Involving the entire community, especially in primary and secondary interventions, is essential to reducing

---

### BOX 25-4  GOALS OF THE NATIONAL STRATEGY FOR SUICIDE PREVENTION

In 2009, the Canadian Association for Suicide Prevention (2009), released the second edition of the *Blueprint for a National Suicide Prevention Strategy* (the first edition having been released in 2004). It was developed out of the belief that many suicidal behaviours are potentially preventable and that it is the collective responsibility of Canadians to work together toward prevention, intervention, and postvention.

Six principles guided the development of the national strategy (Canadian Association for Suicide Prevention, 2009, p. 9):
1. Suicide prevention is everyone's responsibility.
2. Canadians respect our multicultural and diverse society and accept responsibility to support the dignity of human life.
3. Suicide is an interaction of biological, psychological, social and spiritual factors and can be influenced by societal attitudes and conditions.
4. Strategies must be humane, kindly, effective, caring and should be:
   a. Evidence or experience based
   b. Active and informed
   c. Respectful of community and culture-based knowledge
   d. Inclusive of research, surveillance, evaluation, accountability, and reporting
   e. Reflective of evolving knowledge and practices
5. Many suicides are preventable by knowledgeable, caring, compassionate, and committed communities.
6. We must have the courage to confront the stigma of suicide and the patience to address mental health literacy on both a national and local level.

#### Awareness and Understanding Goals
1. Promote awareness in every part of Canada that suicide and suicide-related behaviour is our problem and is preventable.
2. Develop broad-based support for suicide prevention, intervention, and postvention.
3. Develop and implement a strategy to reduce stigma, to be associated with all suicide prevention, intervention, and bereavement activities.
4. Increase media knowledge regarding suicide.

#### Prevention, Intervention and Postvention Goals
1. Develop, implement, and sustain community-based suicide prevention, intervention, and postvention programs, respecting diversity and culture at local, regional, and provincial or territorial levels.
2. Reduce the availability and lethality of suicide methods.
3. Increase training for recognition of risk factors, warning signs and at-risk behaviours and for provision of effective intervention and postvention, targeting key gatekeepers, volunteers, and professionals.
4. Develop and promote effective clinical and professional practice (effective strategies, standards of care) to support patients, families, and communities.
5. Improve access and integration with strong linkages between the continuum-of-care components/services/families.
6. Prioritize intervention and service delivery for high-risk groups while respecting local, regional, and provincial or territorial uniqueness.
7. Increase crisis intervention and support.
8. Increase services and support to those bereaved by suicide or who have attempted suicide.
9. Increase the number of primary prevention activities.

#### Knowledge Development and Transfer
1. Improve and expand surveillance systems.
2. Promote and support the development of effective evaluation tools.
3. Promote and develop suicide-related research.
4. Increase opportunities for reporting.

#### Funding and Support
1. Increase funding and support for all activities connected with the CASP Blueprint for a Canadian National Suicide Prevention Strategy (2nd edition).
2. Ensure access to appropriate and adequate health, wellness and recovery services for all Canadians in keeping with the *Canada Health Act.*

**Source:** Canadian Association for Suicide Prevention. (2009). *The CASP national suicide prevention strategy* (2nd ed., pp. 10–16). Winnipeg: Author. Retrieved from http://www.suicideprevention.ca/wp-content/uploads/2009/10/2010strategy-final-september.pdf.

suicides. Oftentimes, secondary interventions are the determinants of life or death, and nurses with good crisis intervention skills are in a position to use, role model, and teach these skills to others.

## Tertiary Intervention

Tertiary intervention (or postvention) refers to interventions with the family and friends of a person who has died by suicide. Postvention aims to both reduce the traumatic after-effects and explore effective means of addressing survivor problems using primary and secondary interventions. Nurses understand grief or loss well and are in a position to refer, consult, and collaborate in the best interests of those left behind, a vital service since the suicide rate increases for those left behind (Vessier-Batcher & Douglas, 2006). Survivors of suicide are in immediate need of supportive avenues for coping with such complicated grief. A recent Canadian study out of the University of Calgary offers support for an intervention protocol for suicide bereavement that consists of peer supporters and professionals working collaboratively to offer cost-effective, patient-centred services (Barlow, Waegemakers Schiff, Chugh, et al., 2010).

## Milieu Management
### Suicide Precautions

In accordance with unit policies and procedures, the patient is observed continuously by nursing staff. Refer to Table 25-3 for a general description of suicide precautions. This intense attention from the nurse provides for safety and allows for constant reassessment of risk. Monitoring flow sheets for suicide precautions are more clinically useful if they include a description of affect as well as behaviour. For example, instead of noting "Patient watching television," the nurse can describe the patient's affect at each observation interval (e.g., hostile, fearful, calm). Flow sheets should also indicate clear accountability for staff starting and ending their periods of observation. In addition to

observing the patient, the nurse is responsible for monitoring the environment for safety hazards. Review Box 25-5 for guidelines on how to minimize physical risks in the milieu.

Studies show that acute care of suicidal patients is usually effective. Suicide risk is highest in the first few days of admission

**BOX 25-5   ENVIRONMENTAL GUIDELINES FOR MINIMIZING SUICIDAL BEHAVIOUR ON THE PSYCHIATRIC UNIT**

- Conduct frequent environmental tours of all areas of the unit, including patient bathrooms and other private spaces.
- Provide plastic eating utensils.
- Do not assign patient to a private room, and ensure the door remains open at all times.
- Jump-proof and hang-proof the bathrooms by installing break-away shower rods and recessed shower nozzles.
- Keep electrical cords to a minimal length.
- Install unbreakable glass in windows. Install tamper-proof screens or partitions too small to pass through. Keep all windows locked.
- Lock all utility rooms, kitchens, adjacent stairwells, and offices. All nonclinical staff (e.g., housekeepers, maintenance workers) should receive instructions to keep doors locked.
- Take all potentially harmful gifts (e.g., flowers in glass vases) from visitors before allowing them to see patients.
- Go through personal belongings with patient present, and remove all potentially harmful objects (e.g., belts, shoelaces, metal nail files, tweezers, matches, razors, perfume, shampoo).
- Ensure that visitors do not bring in or leave potentially harmful objects in patient's room (e.g., matches, nail files).
- Search patient for harmful objects (e.g., drugs, weapons, sharp objects, cords) on return from pass.

**TABLE 25-3   SUICIDE PRECAUTIONS WITH CONSTANT ONE-TO-ONE OBSERVATION**

| STAFF ASSESSMENT | POSSIBLE PATIENT SYMPTOMS | NURSING RESPONSIBILITIES |
|---|---|---|
| Patient with suicidal ideation or delusions of self-mutilation who, according to assessment by unit staff, presents clinical symptoms that suggest a clear intent to follow through with the plan or delusion | • Patient is currently verbalizing a clear intent to harm self.<br>• Patient shows no insight into existing problems.<br>• Patient has poor impulse control.<br>• Patient has already attempted suicide in the recent past by a particularly lethal method (e.g., hanging, gun, carbon monoxide poisoning). | 1. Conduct one-to-one nursing observation and interaction 24 hours a day (never let patient out of staff's sight).<br>2. Maintain arm's length observation at all times.<br>3. Chart patient's whereabouts and record mood, verbatim statements, and behaviour every 15 to 30 minutes per protocol.<br>4. Ensure that meal trays contain no glass or metal silverware.<br>5. When patient is sleeping, patient's hands should always be in view, not under the bedcovers.<br>6. Carefully observe patient swallow each dose of medication.<br>7. Respectfully maintain observation even when patient is in the bathroom.<br>8. The nurse and physician should explain to the patient what they will be doing and why; both document this explanation in the chart. |

and during times of staff rotation, particularly rotation of psychiatric residents. Assessment of suicidal risk must be an ongoing process; assessment should be performed particularly before a change in level of observation or upon sudden improvement or worsening of symptoms.

## Counselling

Counselling skills, including interviewing, crisis care, and problem-solving techniques, are used in both the inpatient and outpatient settings. The key element is establishing a working alliance to encourage the patient to engage in more realistic problem solving. Helpful staff characteristics include warmth, sensitivity, interest, and consistency. Once patients leave the hospital, the nurse may see them in the clinic, in a partial hospital program, or in home care.

Talking openly and honestly about suicide and the feelings a patient is having is an important part of the process of ongoing assessment and intervention. Encouraging patients to consult with their physician, community mental health worker, or emergency department if they are experiencing suicidal ideation can be a first step in helping to link them with appropriate resources. While the use of "no-suicide contracts" has been a past practice in mental health work, they are now discouraged as there is limited evidence to support the value of such contracts.

## Health Teaching and Health Promotion

The nurse teaches the patient about psychiatric diagnoses, medications and complementary therapies, and age-related crises. Teaching regarding community resources, coping skills, stress management, and communication skills is also important. When possible, the family or significant others are included to strengthen the patient's support system. A focus on personal strengths and positive thoughts and emotions (e.g., hope) is essential (Harvard Medical School, 2008). Talk therapy, in addition to medications, should be incorporated.

## Case Management

Case management is an important aspect of nursing care for the suicidal patient. The patient's perception of being alone without supports often blinds the person to the real support figures who are present. Reconnecting the patient with family and friends is a major focus, whether in the hospital or the community. Aftercare referral may be given and may include information on the following resources: substance treatment centres, crisis hotlines, support groups for patients or families, and recreational activities to enhance socialization and self-esteem. Encouraging the patient to get reacquainted with a previous spiritual support system can also be beneficial.

## Pharmacological Interventions

A significant nursing intervention to assist the suicidal patient in regaining self-control is the careful administration of medication. All medications given to high-risk patients are monitored carefully, although lethal overdose is nearly impossible with SSRIs, unlike the risky tricyclic antidepressants and monoamine oxidase inhibitors. Mouth checks may be used to be sure patients are not saving (hoarding) medications in the hospital; in the community, provision of a limited day supply or family supervision is required.

Antidepressants should be ordered for patients who have depressive or anxiety disorders, with an emphasis on administering an adequate dosage and providing appropriate clinical evaluation when using SSRIs. Close monitoring must occur during the two- to three-week post-initiation period, when energy increases can lead to acting on suicidal ideation, and during times of dosage adjustment. Astute nursing care involves careful patient (and family, if appropriate) teaching about the identified benefits and risks of antidepressant therapy.

There is clear evidence that long-term lithium treatment for bipolar disorder and major depression significantly reduces suicide and suicide attempts. Some studies have shown a reduced suicide rate among patients with schizophrenia receiving clozapine. Thus far, no clinical studies have examined the effect of antianxiety treatment on suicide risk.

An alternative somatic treatment for acute suicidal risk is electroconvulsive therapy (ECT). Evidence suggests that ECT decreases acute suicidal ideation. Refer to Chapter 14 for further discussion of ECT.

## Postvention for Survivors of Suicide

A discussion of suicidal patients is incomplete without noting the issues surrounding a death by suicide. Surviving family and friends can experience overwhelming guilt and shame, compounded by the difficulty of discussing the frequently taboo subject of suicide (Peters, Murphy, & Jackson, 2013). The usual social supports of neighbours and church are sometimes lacking for these mourners.

Evidence collected in a systematic review that investigated differences in suicide survivors' mental health and grief reactions compared to those of other bereaved groups found no significant differences. However, when "specific aspects of the suicide survivors' grief are considered, the evidence clearly shows significant differences compared with all of the survivor groups regarding the following variables: rejections, shame, stigma, concealing the cause of death, and blaming" (Sveen & Walby, 2008, p. 25). See Box 25-6 for suggestions survivors have made to health care providers who want to be sure to meet the survivors' needs.

Staff members who have cared for a suicide victim are similarly traumatized by suicide. Staff may also experience symptoms of PTSD, with guilt, shock, anger, shame, and decreased self-esteem. Group support is essential as the treatment team conducts a thorough psychological postmortem assessment. The event is carefully reviewed to identify the potential overlooked clues, faulty judgements, or changes that are needed in employer protocols.

Most facilities have a clear policy about communication with families after suicide. Although some lawyers advise having no contact except through them, others recommend designating a spokesperson who can address the feelings of the family without discussing the details of the patient's care. Referrals should be given to family members to try to assist them in dealing with their grief and to address any emotional problems that develop, especially in adolescents. The Calgary Health Region (2006) has published a practical guidebook for people who have lost someone to suicide. British Columbia (Centre for Applied Research in Mental Health and Addiction, 2007) and Ontario (Centre for Addiction and Mental Health, 2011) have adapted that booklet, tailoring the practical information to their own provincial resources. These booklets are all available online.

As for documentation, all staff members need to ensure that the record is complete and that any late entries are identified. Courts require that the patient be periodically evaluated for suicidal risk, that the treatment plan provide for high-level security, and that staff members follow the individual treatment plan. Despite adherence to institution protocols, treatment plans, and the appropriate standards of practice, suicides do occasionally still happen, especially with patients in the community. Human behaviour is simply not predictable.

## EVALUATION

Evaluation of a suicidal patient is ongoing. The nurse must be constantly alert to changes in the suicidal person's mood, thinking, and behaviour. The nurse also looks for indications that the patient is communicating thoughts and feelings more readily and that the patient's social network is widening. For example, it is a positive sign if the person is able to talk about his or her feelings and engage in problem solving with the nurse. Is the patient increasing his or her social activities and expanding his or her interests? The nurse must remember that suicidal behaviour is the result of interpersonal turmoil. If an episode of major depression is the main admitting diagnosis and a serious suicidal gesture resulted from this depression, both problems are initially assessed and treated. When the patient is no longer an acute suicide risk, treating the depression becomes the main focus of care. Essentially, the nurse evaluates each short-term goal and establishes new ones as the patient progresses toward the long-term goal of resolving suicidal ideation.

Once stabilized, the patient may qualify for transfer to an intensive outpatient (IOP) treatment program, which involves continuing treatment after discharge, or a partial hospitalization program (PHP), which allows patients to go home in the evening to practise new coping skills. Community-based support groups are also available and are both effective and free of charge. Nurses need to be knowledgeable about, and proactive in, referring patients to these support groups.

## ■ KEY POINTS TO REMEMBER

- Suicide is a significant public health problem in Canada.
- Suicide is everyone's business.
- Specific biological, psychosocial, and cultural factors are known to increase the risk for suicide.
- Most suicidal patients can be helped by treatment of a coexisting psychiatric disorder.
- Certain medical conditions and psychiatric diagnoses are associated with increased risk for suicide.
- Suicidal ideation must be taken seriously, even if the person has a history of multiple attempts.
- The nurse can have a real impact on suicide prevention through primary, secondary, and tertiary interventions.
- Nursing care of the suicidal patient is challenging but rewarding: patients' desperate feelings evoke intense reactions in staff, but most people with suicidal ideation respond to treatment and do not complete suicide.
- If a patient dies by suicide, family, friends, and health care workers are traumatized and need support, possibly including referrals for mental health intervention.

# CRITICAL THINKING

1. Locate and review the suicide protocol at your hospital unit or community centre. Are there any steps you anticipate having difficulty carrying out? Discuss these difficulties with your peers or clinical group.

2. Knowing that nurses can suffer postsuicide stress and that they need support when those in their care are involved in suicidal behaviour, do you believe help is available for nurses? What sort of support do you feel would be most helpful to you in this situation? How would you respond to another staff member who expresses guilt over completed death by suicide of a patient on your unit?

3. Identify three common and expected emotional reactions that a nurse might have when initially working with people who are suicidal.
   a. How do you think you might react?
   b. What actions could you take to deal with the event and obtain support?

4. In addition to psychiatric mental health nursing practice areas, are there other practice areas in which nursing assessments for self-harm would strengthen client care? How does knowing the reason for a patient self-harming make a difference in planning care?

# CHAPTER REVIEW

1. Which assessment statement(s) would be appropriate for a patient who may be suicidal?
   Select all that apply.
   1. Do you ever think about suicide?
   2. Are you thinking of hurting yourself?
   3. Do you sometimes wish you were dead?
   4. Has it ever seemed like life is not worth living?
   5. If you were to kill yourself, how would you do it?
   6. Does it seem as though others might be better off if you were dead?

2. Jon, 15 years old, asks the community health nurse what the greatest health risk for his age group is. How should the nurse respond?
   1. Suicide
   2. Substance abuse
   3. Eating disorders
   4. Unintentional injuries

3. Ms. Rallyea, 58 years old, is admitted with severe clinical depression and started on antidepressant medications. Her mood has remained low and she has not initiated conversation. On her fifteenth day of hospitalization, she informs the nurse she is feeling great and energetic. What should the nurse do?
   1. Notify the social worker of the improvement to schedule a discharge planning conference.
   2. Invite Ms. Rallyea to talk and ask her if she is thinking of hurting herself.
   3. Report to the team that the antidepressant medication is effective.
   4. Chart the mood change and share the observation at the team meeting the next day.

4. A nurse has great difficulty distancing herself from the care of a client when she leaves work. What should the nurse do?
   1. Recognize that she is too compassionate.
   2. Request that the client be assigned to another nurse.
   3. Share her concern with the patient.
   4. Confide in a colleague she trusts.

## evolve WEBSITE

**Post-Test** interactive review

*Visit the Evolve Web site for Chapter Review Answers and Rationales, Critical Thinking Answer Guidelines, and additional resources related to the content in this chapter: http://evolve.elsevier.com/Canada/Varcarolis/psychiatric/*

# REFERENCES

Aboriginal Healing Foundation. (2007). *Suicide among Aboriginal people in Canada*. Ottawa: Author.
Alberta Health Services. (2009). *Problem gambling, mental health and suicide: A literature review*. Edmonton: Author. Retrieved from http://www.albertahealthservices.ca/Researchers/if-res-problem-gambling-mental-health-suicide.pdf.
American Association of Suicidology. (n.d.). *Translating suicide research into practice*. Retrieved from http://www.suicidology.org/web/guest/current-research.
American Nurses Association, American Psychiatric-Mental Health Nurses Association, & International Society of Psychiatric-Mental Health Nurses.

(2007). *Psychiatric mental health nursing: Scope and standards of practice*. Silver Spring, MD: American Nurses Association.
Appel, J.M. (2007). A suicide right for the mentally ill? A Swiss case opens a new debate. *Hastings Center Report, 37*, 21–23. doi:10.1353/hcr.2007.0035.
Barlow, C.A., Waegemakers Schiff, J., Chugh, U., et al. (2010). An evaluation of a suicide bereavement peer support program. *Death Studies, 34*, 915–930. doi:10.1080/07481181003761435.
Battin, M., van der Heide, A., Ganzini, L., et al. (2007). Legal physician-assisted dying in Oregon and the Netherlands: Evidence concerning the impact on patients in "vulnerable" groups. *Journal of Medical Ethics, 33*, 591–597. doi:10.1136/jme.2007.022335.

Brendel, R.W., Lagomasino, I.T., Perlis, R.H., et al. (2008). The suicidal patient. In T.A. Stern, J.R. Rosenbaum, M. Fava, et al. (Eds.), *Massachusetts General Hospital comprehensive clinical psychiatry* (pp. 733–745). St. Louis, MO: Mosby.

Calgary Health Region. (2006). *Hope and healing: A practical guide for survivors of suicide*. Calgary: Alberta Health Services. Retrieved from http://www.albertahealthservices.ca/InjuryPrevention/hi-ip-pipt-chc-hope-and-healing-nr-booklet.pdf.

Canada Safety Council. (2006). *Canadian roulette*. Ottawa: Author.

Canadian Association for Suicide Prevention. (n.d.). *Research and publications*. Retrieved from http://www.suicideprevention.ca/.

Canadian Association for Suicide Prevention. (2009). *The CASP national suicide prevention strategy* (2nd ed.). Winnipeg: Author. Retrieved from http://www.suicideprevention.ca/wp-content/uploads/2009/10/2010strategy-final-september.pdf.

Canadian Charter of Rights and Freedoms, Part I of the *Constitution Act, 1982*, being Schedule B to the *Canada Act 1982* (UK), 1982, c. 11. Retrieved from http://laws.justice.gc.ca/eng/charter/.

Canadian Coalition for Seniors' Mental Health. (2006). *National guidelines for seniors' mental health: The assessment of suicide risk and prevention of suicide*. Toronto: Author. Retrieved from http://www.ccsmh.ca/en/guidelinesdownload.cfm.

Canadian Institute for Health Information. (2011). *Health indicators 2011*. Ottawa: Author.

Carballo, J.J., Akamnonu, C.P., & Oquendo, M.A. (2008). Neurobiology of suicidal behavior. An integration of biological and clinical findings. *Archives of Suicide Research, 12*, 93–110. doi:10.1080/13811110701857004.

Centre for Addiction and Mental Health. (2011). *Hope and healing after suicide. A practical guide for people who have lost someone to suicide in Ontario*. Retrieved from http://knowledgex.camh.net/amhspecialists/resources_families/Documents/hope_and_healing.pdf.

Centre for Applied Research in Mental Health and Addiction. (2007). *Hope and healing: A practical guide for survivors of suicide*. Retrieved from http://www.comh.ca/publications/resources/pub_hh/HopeandHealing.pdf.

Centre for Suicide Prevention. (2011). The media and high-profile suicides. *Info Exchange, 2*, 1–4. Retrieved from http://suicideinfo.ca/LinkClick.aspx?fileticket=_IL3FiefxUA%3d&tabid=552.

Chakraborty, A., McManus, S., Brugha, T., et al. (2011). Mental health of the non-heterosexual population of England. *British Journal of Psychiatry, 198*(2), 143–148. doi:10.1192/bjp.bp.110.082271.

Ciffone, J.C. (2007). Suicide prevention: An analysis and replication of a curriculum-based high school program. *Social Work, 52*(1), 41–49.

Cleaver, K. (2007). Characteristics and trends of self-harming behaviour in young people. *British Journal of Nursing, 16*(3), 148–152.

Correctional Service of Canada. (2009). *Forum on corrections research*. Ottawa: Author.

Criminal Code, R.S.C. 1985, c. C-46. (2011). Retrieved from http://laws-lois.justice.gc.ca/eng/acts/C-46/page-103.html#s-241.

Currier, D., & Mann, J. (2009). Stress, genes and the biology of suicidal behaviour. *Psychiatric Clinics of North America, 31*, 247–269. doi:10.1016/j.psc.2008.01.005.

D'Orazio, O. (2010, December 29). *De-criminalize euthanasia and assisted suicide, says law prof. Canadian Lawyer Magazine*. Retrieved from http://www.canadianlawyermag.com/de-criminalize-euthanasia-and-assisted-suicide-say-law-prof.html.

Dwivedi, Y., & Pandey, G. (2011). Elucidating biological risk factors in suicide: Role of protein kinase A. *Progress in Neuro-Psychopharmacology & Biological Psychiatry, 35*, 831–841. doi:10.1016/j.pnpbp.2010.08.025.

Finlay, I., & George, R. (2011). Legal physician-assisted suicide in Oregon and the Netherlands: Evidence concerning the impact on patients in vulnerable groups—another perspective on Oregon's data. *Journal of Medical Ethics, 37*, 171–174. doi:10.1136/jme.2010.037044.

Ganz, D., Braquehais, M.D., & Sher, L. (2010). Secondary prevention of suicide. *PLoS Medicine, 7*, 1–4. doi:10.1371/journal.pmed.1000271.

Ganzini, L., Goy, E., & Dobscha, S.K. (2008). Prevalence of depression and anxiety in patients requesting physicians' aid in dying: A cross-sectional survey. *British Medical Journal, 337*, 1–5. doi:10.1136/bmj.a1682.

Harvard Medical School. (2007). Antidepressants and suicide. *Harvard Mental Health Letter, 24*(1), 1–4.

Harvard Medical School. (2008). Positive psychology in practice. *Harvard Mental Health Letter, 24*(11), 1–3.

Heisel. M.J., Moore, S.L., Bowman, J., et al. (2010, September 27). *Evaluating knowledge transfer, recall, attitudes and clinical care provision of mental health clinicians working with older adults at-risk for suicide*. Workshop presented at the conference of the Canadian Coalition for Seniors' Mental Health, *Connecting Research and Education to Care in Senior's Mental Health*. Halifax, NS.

Institute of Marriage and Family Canada. (2009). *Canadian suicide statistics*. Retrieved from http://archive.imfcanada.org/default.aspx?go=article&aid=1191&tid=8.

International Association for Suicide Prevention. (n.d.). *Resources: Suicide prevention and research*. Retrieved from http://www.iasp.info/resources/Suicide_Research_and_Prevention/.

Joe, S., & Bryant, H. (2007). Evidence-based suicide prevention screening in schools. *Children & Schools, 29*(4), 219–227.

Kaplan, M., Huguet. N., McFarland, B.H., et al. (2007). Suicide among male veterans: A prospective population-based study. *Journal of Epidemiology and Community Health, 61*, 619–624. doi:10.1136/jech.2006.054346.

Kim, Y., & Levanthal, B. (2008). Bullying and suicide: A review. *International Journal of Adolescent Medicine and Health, 20*, 133–154. doi:10.1515/IJAMH.2008.20.2.133.

King, M., Semlyen, J., Tai, S.S., et al. (2008). A systematic review of mental disorder, suicide, and deliberate self-harm in lesbian, gay and bisexual people. *BMC Psychiatry, 8*, 70. doi:10.1186/1471-244X-8-70.

Klomek, A., Sourander, A., & Gould, M. (2010). The association of suicide and bullying in childhood to young adulthood: A review of cross-sectional and longitudinal research findings. *Canadian Journal of Psychiatry, 55*(5), 282–288.

Kral, M., Wiebe, P., Nisbet, K., et al. (2009). Canadian Inuit community engagement in suicide prevention. *International Journal of Circumpolar Health, 68*(3), 292–308.

Leach, M. (2006). *Cultural diversity and suicide: Ethnic, religious, gender and sexual orientation perspectives*. Binghamton, NY: Haworth Press.

Leong, F., & Leach, M. (2008). *Suicide among racial and ethnic minority groups: Theory, research and practice*. New York: Routledge.

Lester, D. (2012). The role of irrational thinking in suicidal behaviour. *Comprehensive Psychology, 1*(8), 1–9. doi:10.2466/12.02.07.16.CP.1.8.

Marr, N., & Field, T. (2000). *Bullycide: Death at playtime*. Didcot, UK: Success Unlimited.

McFarland, B.H., Kaplan, M.S., & Huguet, N. (2010). Self-inflicted deaths among women with U.S. military service: A hidden epidemic? *Psychiatric Services, 61*(12), 1177.

Meerwijk, E., van Meijel, B., van den Bout, J., et al. (2010). Development and evaluation of a guideline for nursing care of suicidal patients with schizophrenia. *Perspectives in Psychiatric Care, 46*(1), 65–73. doi:10.1111/j.1744-6163.2009.00239.x.

Melrose, S. (2011). Perfectionism and depression: Vulnerabilities nurses need to understand. *Nursing Research and Practice, 2011*, 1–7. doi:10.1155/2011/858497.

Mental Health Commission of Canada. (2009). *Toward recovery and well-being: A framework for a mental health strategy for Canada*. Ottawa: Author. Retrieved from http://www.mentalhealthcommission.ca/English/Pages/Reports.aspx.

Morrison, K.B., & Laing, L. (2011). Adults' use of health services in the year before death by suicide in Alberta (Statistics Canada, Cat. no. 82-003-XPE). *Health Reports, 22*(3), 1–8.

Muehlenkamp, J., Brausch, A., Quigley, K., et al. (2013). Interpersonal features and functions of nonsuicidal self-injury. *Suicide and Life-Threat Behavior, 43*(1), 67–80. doi:10.1111/j.1943-278X.2012.00128.x.

National Aboriginal Health Organization. (2006). *Suicide prevention: Inuit traditional practices that encouraged resilience and coping*. Ottawa: Author. Retrieved from http://www.naho.ca/documents/it/2006_Suicide_Prevention-Elders.pdf.

Newman, S., & Thompson, A. (2007). The association between pathological gambling and attempted suicide: Findings from a national survey in Canada. *Canadian Journal of Psychiatry, 52*(9), 605–612.

Ortiz, M. (2006). Staying alive! A suicide prevention overview. *Journal of Psychosocial Nursing and Mental Health Services, 44*(12), 43–49.

Patterson, W.M., Dohn, H.H., Bird, J., et al. (1983). Evaluation of suicidal patients: The SAD PERSONS scale. *Psychosomatics, 24*(4), 343–345, 348–349.

Pedlar, D. (2010, November). *Life after service: Veterans research and the life course.* Presented at the meeting of Canadian Military & Veteran Health Research Forum, Kingston, ON. Retrieved from http://www.queensu.ca/conferences/mvhr/images/pdf/presentations/Pedlar_David_16_MVHR2010.pdf.

Perlman, C.M., Neufeld, E., Martin, L., et al. (2011). *Suicide risk assessment inventory: A resource guide for Canadian health care organizations.* Toronto: Ontario Hospital Association and Canadian Patient Safety Institute. Available at http://www.oha.com/KnowledgeCentre/Documents/Final%20-%20Suicide%20Risk%20Assessment%20Guidebook.pdf.

Peters, K., Murphy, G., & Jackson, D. (2013). Events prior to completed suicide: Perspectives of family members. *Issues in Mental Health Nursing, 34*(5), 309–316. doi:10.3109/01612840.2012.751639.

Price, N. (2007). Improving emergency care for patients who self harm. *Emergency Nurse, 15*(8), 30–36.

Registered Nurses' Association of Ontario. (2009, January). *Assessment and care of adults at risk for suicidal ideation and behaviour: Best practice guidelines.* Toronto: Author.

Richardson, J., Thompson, J.M., Boswall, M., et al. (2010). Horror comes home: Veterans with posttraumatic stress disorder. *Canadian Family Physician, 56*(5), 430–433.

Rocket, I. (2010). Counting suicides and making suicide count as a public health problem. *Journal of Crisis Intervention and Suicide Prevention, 31,* 227–230. doi:10.1027/0227-5910/a000071.

Rodriguez v. British Columbia (Attorney General), 1993 CanLII 75 (SCC), [1993] 3 SCR 519. Retrieved from http://canlii.ca/t/1frz0.

Sadock, B.J., & Sadock, V.A. (2008). *Kaplan and Sadock's concise textbook of clinical psychiatry* (3rd ed.). Philadelphia: Lippincott Williams & Wilkins.

Schwenk, T., Gorenflo, D., Dopp, R., et al. (2007). Depression and pain in retired professional football players. *Medicine & Science in Sports & Exercise, 39,* 599–605. doi:10.1249/mss.0b013e31802fa679.

Séguin, M., Boyer, R., Lesage, A., et al. (2010). Suicide and gambling: Psychopathology and treatment seeking. *Psychology of Addictive Behaviours, 24,* 541–547. doi:10.1037/a0019041.

Service, J. (2010). *Under warrant: A review of the implementation of the Correctional Service of Canada's "Mental Health Strategy."* Kanata, ON: John Service Consulting. Retrieved from http://www.oci-bec.gc.ca/cnt/rpt/oth-aut/oth-aut20100923-eng.aspx.

Shields N., White, M., & Egan, M. (2009). Battlefield blues: Ambivalence about treatment among military veterans with depression. *Canadian Family Physician, 55*(8), 799–802.

Skinner, R., & McFaull, S. (2012). Suicide among children and adolescents in Canada: Trends and sex differences, 1980–2008. *Canadian Medical Association Journal, 184*(9), 1029–1034. doi:10.1503/cmaj.111867.

Sommer-Rotenburg, D. (1998). Suicide and language. *Canadian Medical Association Journal, 159*(3), 239–240. Retrieved from http://www.ncbi.nlm.nih.gov/pmc/articles/PMC1229556/?tool=pmcentrez.

Standing Senate Committee on Social Affairs, Science and Technology (2004, November). Concepts and definitions. In *Mental health, mental illness and addiction: Overview of policies and programs in Canada. Report 1.* Retrieved from http://www.parl.gc.ca/Content/SEN/Committee/381/soci/rep/report1/repintnov04vol1part2-e.htm.

Statistics Canada. (2012). *Mortality, summary: List of causes (Cat. no. 84F0209X).* Retrieved from http://www.statcan.gc.ca/pub/84f0209x/84f0209x2009000-eng.pdf.

Statistics Canada. (2013). *Health at a glance. Suicide rates: An overview* (Cat. no. 82-624-X). Retrieved from http://www.statcan.gc.ca/pub/82-624-x/2012001/article/11696-eng.htm.

Suicide Prevention Resource Center. (2008). *Suicide risk and prevention for lesbian, gay, bisexual, and transgender youth.* Newton, MA: Education Development Center, Inc.

Sveen, C., & Walby, F. (2008). Suicide survivors' mental health and grief reactions: A systematic review. *Suicide & Life-Threatening Behaviour, 38*(1), 13–29. doi:10.1521/suli.2008.38.1.13.

Toth, M., Schwartz, R., & Kurka, S. (2007). Strategies for understanding and assessing suicide risk in psychotherapy. *Annals of the American Psychotherapy Association, 10*(4), 18–25. Retrieved from http://www.annalsofpsychotherapy.com/index.php.

Vessier-Batcher, M., & Douglas, D. (2006). Coping with complicated grief in survivors of homicide and suicide decedents. *Journal of Forensic Nursing, 2,* 25–32. doi:10.1111/j.1939-3938.2006.tb00050.x.

World Health Organization. (2010). *Suicide prevention (SUPRE).* Retrieved from http://www.who.int/mental_health/prevention/suicide/suicideprevent/en/index.html.

Zamorski, M.A., (2010). *Report of the Canadian Forces expert panel on suicide prevention* (Report no. 2010-2001). Ottawa: Canadian Forces Health Services Group.

# Anger, Aggression, and Violence

*Melodie B. Hull*

## KEY TERMS AND CONCEPTS

aggression, 527
bullying, 530
de-escalation techniques, 532
locus of control (LOC), 528

rage, 527
trauma-informed care, 529
violence, 527

## OBJECTIVES

1. Compare and contrast three theories that explore the determinants for anger, aggression, and violence.
2. Distinguish between the emotions of anger and rage and the behavioural manifestations of aggression and violence.
3. Identify precipitators to anger, aggression, or violence.

4. Compare and contrast interventions for a patient with healthy coping skills with those for a patient with marginal coping behaviours.
5. Identify four principles of de-escalation with a moderately angry patient.
6. Describe two criteria for the use of seclusion or restraint.

## ⊖volve WEBSITE

*Visit the Evolve website for Flashcards, Case Studies, and additional testing resources related to the content in this chapter:* http://evolve.elsevier.com/Canada/Varcarolis/psychiatric/   Pre-Test   interactive review

Anger, aggression, and violence are the subject of daily news headlines. Anger is a normal, natural emotion occurring on a continuum, stemming from a wide variety of feelings that are sometimes misinterpreted as anger (e.g., jealousy, confusion). Evidence of the scope and prevalence of the problem can been seen in an expanding list of terminology used to describe specific types of aggression. For example, *road rage* is a dangerous aggressive response to anger that is accompanied by cursing, offensive gestures, and cutting off of others while driving. Road rage is rampant in high-stress industrialized societies. *Air rage* is manifested as objectionable behaviour, aggressive utterances, threats, and violence within the confines of an aircraft. *Workplace violence* includes lashing out at work. Hospitals are potential sites for this particular type of violence.

## CLINICAL PICTURE

Once the anger response is triggered, it can escalate into positive or negative aggression, even violence. Not everyone responds to anger with aggression and violence. A healthy and appropriate release of anger might lead to a clearing of the air between people or provide a signal to the person expressing it that an anger-provoking stressor is present. Understanding the emotion, its etiology, and its psychological and behavioural manifestations are keys to accurate assessment, intervention, and treatment. Box 26-1 provides examples of feelings that may precipitate anger.

Anger is an emotional response. It can be released appropriately or inappropriately, suppressed over periods of time, or

## BOX 26-1 FEELINGS THAT MAY PRECIPITATE ANGER

- Discounted, ignored, or rejected
- Embarrassed, humiliated
- Frightened
- Guilty
- Hurt
- Inadequate
- Insecure
- Unheard
- Overwhelmed, out of control of the situation
- Threatened
- Tired
- Vulnerable

controlled in its release. It does not always lead to violence. It can be used as a motivator or an aid in survival (Kassinove & Tafrate, 2006). For some people, anger is a coping response to embarrassment, jealousy, or fear of rejection or replacement. Personal appraisals of self-worth and self-efficacy also factor into the anger response.

*Rage* is an uncontrollable, violent state of anger and is quite uncommon. Once the person has begun expressing rage, he or she cannot think clearly or logically, and psychosocial or cognitive-behavioural interventions are not possible. Rage must dissipate on its own. Protective strategies are necessary both for the person in a state of rage and for those around him or her.

*Aggression* is an emotion that results in a verbal or physical attack. *Aggression* is often used synonymously with *violence*, although not quite accurately. Aggression is not always inappropriate. Instrumental aggression is sometimes necessary for self-protection or to achieve a goal. Reactive or hostile aggression is violence. Causality for reactive or hostile aggression can

### VIGNETTE

Solange is a 41-year-old woman with a diagnosis of bipolar disorder. She has a history of eight hospital admissions to acute care psychiatry over the past 20 years. She is experiencing a manic episode and has been admitted as an involuntary patient to the psychiatric unit of a general hospital. Being admitted against her wishes frustrates and angers her. She attempts to intimidate the staff with verbal aggression and threats. She refuses to take her mood-stabilizing medications. She exhibits hyperactivity, racing thoughts, poor judgement, distractibility, pressured speech, and sleep deprivation. She has very low frustration tolerance and reacts spontaneously and impulsively to stressors. Solange feels trapped. She is able to voice her feelings of being overwhelmed and out of control, but she is quite incapable of dealing with these feelings. Nursing interventions require setting clear and consistent limits on her behaviours to promote a low-stimulus environment. Seclusion is ordered when Solange is unable to exhibit self-control of her behaviour.

be multifactorial. States of high arousal, hyperexcitability, psychosis, or confusion are all possible precipitators to acts of violence.

*Violence* includes the intent to harm. It can be directed at self, others, or objects. The Criminal Code of Canada, Section 265(1) (2011), includes violence under its definition of *assault*: physical or verbal. Violence includes psychological and emotional abuse, damage to property, suicide, and self-harm. Violence is almost always an objectionable act. Exceptions include the work of armed forces and police officers.

Workplace violence is not uncommon in health care. Nurses are at highest risk due to the amount of contact they have with patients. In 2005, an estimated 29% of nurses experienced physical assault, and 44% emotional abuse from patients (Canadian Institute of Health Information, 2005). Not all workplace aggression or violence stems from patients, visitors, or family members; 44% of all Canadian nurses have experienced hostility from their co-workers, whereas in the general workforce, fewer than 30% have had the same experience (Canadian Institute of Health Information, 2005). In the last two decades, employers, unions, and policy-makers have moved to a zero-tolerance position on all types of workplace violence (Canadian Federation of Nurses Unions, 2008).

## EPIDEMIOLOGY

As a nurse, you will deal with violent behaviour. The National Trauma Registry of Canada (Canadian Institute of Health Information, 2008) identified physical assault as the third leading cause of injury-specific admission to hospital from 2005 to 2006, and subsequent reports show a continuation of this trend (Canadian Institute of Health Information, 2008). The Centers for Disease Control and Prevention (2008) suggests that the widespread incidence of aggression and violence indicates that these are common components of social interactions in many environments, including hospitals. Box 26-2 identifies milieu characteristics that are conducive to violence. Violence in health care settings is most frequent in the psychiatric unit and emergency department and on geriatric units (Chandler, 2008).

## CO-MORBIDITY

Kassinove and Tafrate (2006) stated that anger can coexist with depression, anxiety, psychosis, personality disorders, brain

## BOX 26-2 MILIEU CHARACTERISTICS CONDUCIVE TO VIOLENCE

- Overcrowding
- Staff inexperience
- Provocative or controlling staff
- Poor limit setting
- Arbitrary revocation of privileges
- Language or other communication barriers
- Cultural barriers

injury, or organicity. More recently, researchers have explored the co-morbidity of aggression and violence in people with post-traumatic stress disorder and substance abuse disorders (Sirotich, 2008).

Anger and hostility affect physical well-being and are risk factors for hypertension and cardiovascular disease (Kassinove & Tafrate, 2006). While there may be a time and a place to temporarily suppress anger, suppression of anger has been shown to increase diastolic blood pressure and heart rate (Jorgensen & Kolodziej, 2007). Suppressed anger has also been shown to increase a person's perception of pain (Burns, Holly, Quartana, et al., 2008).

There is some evidence of an association between violence and mental disorders, but the greater association is between violence and co-morbid alcohol or drug abuse. Patients with acute mental illnesses who have co-occurring diagnoses or are in withdrawal are more at risk for violent acting out (Arboleda-Florez, Holley, Crisanti, et al., 1996).

## ETIOLOGY

### Biological Factors

A biological predisposition to respond to life events with irritability, low frustration tolerance, and anger may be a function of genetics or of early neurological development.

Neurological conditions such as certain brain tumours, dementias, and temporal lobe epilepsy are associated with anger and aggression. Traumatic brain injury can result in changes to personality, including increased violence, severe behavioural disorders, and low levels of frustration tolerance.

The limbic system is responsible for the mediation of primitive emotions and behaviours necessary for survival. Within it, the amygdala mediates anger experiences, causing the person to judge events as either aversive or rewarding (Rabinak & Maren, 2010). In animal studies, stimulation of the amygdala produces rage responses, whereas lesions in the same structure produce docility (Neisewander, 2004).

Selye's (1976) *general adaptation syndrome* can be applied to the natural anger response. When a response occurs to an anger-provoking stressor, the alarm stage is initiated. Neurotransmitters are released, and the ability to think with reason and good judgement diminishes and is replaced by the self-protective mechanisms of fight or flight. *Fight* is the aggressive response to a threat; its goal is to remove or extinguish the dangerous or noxious stimuli. *Flight* is the flee response. Once a fight-or-flight response is initiated, the neurochemical processes in the body need time to dissipate. It is not prudent to engage a client who is already in an agitated or hostile state in any manner that may continue the escalation of emotion or lead to further misinterpretation of the situation.

Serotonin, dopamine, norepinephrine, gamma-aminobutyric acid (GABA), glutamate, and acetylcholine all have an impact on anger and aggression (Siever, 2008). Studies have shown a relationship between impulsive aggression and low levels of serotonin (Gross & Sanders, 2008). Dopamine has also been linked to aggressive outbursts (de Almeida, Ferrari, Parmigiani, et al., 2005). Depressed patients with impulsivity and anger issues may have decreased dopamine receptors (Dougherty, Bonab, Ottowitz, et al., 2006).

The brain's temporal lobes share some memory function with the limbic system. Memory of previous insult or assault is important in the cognitive appraisal of a threat and can play a determining role in the expression of anger. The temporal lobes are also the source of complex partial seizures, which may give rise to aggressive behaviour (Ito, Okazaki, Takahashi, et al., 2007).

Prefrontal cortex damage is also implicated in aggressive behaviour (Siever, 2008). Individuals with antisocial personality disorder have been shown to have less grey matter in their prefrontal cortices (Narayan, Narr, Kumari, et al., 2007). The prefrontal cortex is the last part of the brain to mature; this maturation occurs in late adolescence or early adulthood. This later development is significant in that anger, aggression, impulse control, judgement, and reasoning are all functions of the prefrontal cortex (Harmon-Jones & Sigelman, 2001). In EEG analyses, a positive correlation has been found between left frontal lobe activity and anger (Coccaro, McCloskey, Fitzgerald, et al., 2007; Harmon-Jones, 2007).

Steroid hormones can influence the ability to cope with or express anger, particularly in pubescent, adolescent, and young adult males who experience surges in testosterone. Mehta and Beer (2010) assert that testosterone creates a propensity toward aggression by reducing impulse control and the self-regulation mechanism in the brain. Preliminary results of other research reveal that higher levels of testosterone in pubescent boys and men are positively associated with impulsivity and aggression (Borod, 2000).

### Psychological Factors

Development of the perception of emotions plays a crucial role in the psychology of anger. Behaviourists hold that emotions are learned responses to environmental stimuli (Skinner, 1953). When a stimulus is perceived as a threat, this thought leads to the emotional and physiological arousal necessary to take action (Selye, 1976). A perceived assault on areas of personal domain (e.g., values, moral code, self-esteem) can lead to anger (Beck, 1976).

In 1966, Rotter identified **locus of control (LOC)** as an inherent factor in our experience and expression of mood (Ellis, Abrams, & Dengelegi-Abrams, 2008). Today, we might refer to LOC as *personal power*. Menninger (2007) asserts that the struggle for control over our lives is fundamental in every person. If that control is threatened, we experience trauma, and it is from that trauma that anger, aggression, and violence may originate. A person who believes he or she has a strong, positive locus of control believes that any rewards and successes that occur are the result of self-efficacy. Nursing interventions often reflect LOC as we strive to empower patients in their own care. However, a person who perceives an external locus of control believes that negative outcomes and circumstances are inevitable—that it is not his own fault when bad things occur. This person sees him- or herself as a victim of life. The results are ineffective coping and anger.

Cognitive therapist Ellis (1973) asserts that our own irrational thinking, as well as our appraisals about how the world

## RESEARCH HIGHLIGHT

### Self-Reported Aggression and the Perception of Anger in Facial Expression Photos

**Source:** Hall, C. (2006). Self-reported aggression and the perception of anger in facial expression photos. *Journal of Psychology, 140*, 255–267. doi:10.3200/JRLP.140.3.255-267.

#### Problem

A person can perceive anger in others that can then trigger aggressive behaviour.

#### Purpose of Study

This study set out to determine whether photographs of faces trigger aggression.

#### Methods

Using photographs of faces, a correlation between perception of anger in others and one's own aggression was discovered.

#### Key Findings

Hall found that individuals who identified themselves as high on levels of overall aggression also misidentified and misinterpreted expressions of anger in others.

#### Implications for Nursing Practice

When a facial expression made by another is perceived to be directed personally at the individual interpreting it, the fight-or-flight response is triggered. These additional thoughts lead to escalating behaviour that can erupt into violence unless the situation is defused through successful interventions.

should be and how others should behave in relation to us, personally leaves us frustrated, dissatisfied, and angry. A person who believes he or she should be loved and accepted by absolutely everyone at all times is demonstrating irrational or faulty thinking. Anger, hostile aggression, and violence are not uncommon behaviours used by these individuals to deal with any perceived sense of rejection, devaluing, or disrespect.

Cognitive-behaviourists Beck, Emery, and Greenberg (2005) believe dysfunctional anger is rooted in our predispositions, beliefs, memories, learning, and interpretations of self and others in relation to self. Our personal self-appraisal of efficacy and confidence determines how we deal with all situations, including perceived threats. A patient who is kept waiting in a clinic for long periods of time without explanation may interpret this situation as neglect and a lack of respect. Anger may escalate when the initial appraisal is followed by thoughts such as "They have no right to treat me this way. I am a person, too." For some individuals, escalation can be rapid. In contrast, patients who are less predisposed to anger might interpret the wait as a sign that the clinic is busy. These patients might be frustrated by the situation, but in the absence of anger, they might access and utilize strategies such as asking how much longer the wait is likely to be, finding distractions in the environment, or rescheduling the appointment. For patients who have been suppressing anger, this situation might be the trigger that suddenly releases pent-up anger, even though the situation has little or nothing to do with the original causes of the anger.

Long-term suppression of anger may decrease the ability to deal effectively with new anger-provoking stimuli, and there is some suggestion that chronic anger suppression can potentiate a sudden outburst of built-up anger (Ellis, 1990). This built-up anger is often misdirected when released.

### Sociological Factors

Social learning theory asserts that children learn aggression by imitating others and that people repeat behaviour that is rewarded (Bandura, 1973). Children exposed to television and video-game violence learn that violence is an option for resolving conflict and that those violent acts have no real negative consequences. This theory asserts that children who experience violence in the home have an increased propensity for aggression, hostility, and suspension from school (Solomon, Bradshaw, Wright, et al., 2008).

Although all people experience the emotion of anger, it is not expressed in the same way across cultures. Biologically and psychologically based anger responses are inextricably entwined with folkways (group habits that are common to a society or culture) that mediate the actual expression of anger. In a multicultural context, this difference in expression of anger provides a challenge to both nurses and patients. Language difficulties and culturally based acceptance of how anger is and can be expressed can easily confound a person's abilities to experience and deal successfully with an anger-producing situation. In Western cultures, the functionality of anger is acknowledged and accepted. The expression of anger is a way to protect rights, personal freedoms, and self-esteem. Anger is seen as a means to find clarity. In some other cultures, the overt expression of anger is often seen as contrary to seeking harmony within relationships; it is in opposition to the sense of order and authority of society (Safdar, Friedlmeier, Mastumoto, et al., 2009).

The Considering Culture box below provides an example about the culture of bullying in schools.

## APPLICATION OF THE NURSING PROCESS

### ASSESSMENT

#### General Assessment

Most reactions to stimuli come from previous experiences; therefore, identifying patient triggers to anger and aggression through a comprehensive history is essential. Initial and ongoing assessment of the patient can reveal problems before they escalate to anger and aggression. When patients are experiencing anger, it may manifest as increased demands, irritability, frowning, redness of the face, pacing, twisting of the hands, or clenching and unclenching of the fists. Speech may be increased in rate and volume or may be slowed, pointed, and quiet. Any change in behaviour from what is typical for that patient must be addressed. The Assessment Guidelines box on page 531 highlights various predictors and precipitators.

An older concept of providing care has recently been reintroduced. Trauma-informed care refers to care focused on the

### The Culture of Bullying in Schools

Bullying is a repetitive behaviour that sustains an imbalance of power. It includes any negative activity intended to bother or harm someone, including verbal actions that are demeaning and intimidating by teasing, gossiping, insulting, or threatening. It can be done in person, by phone, by letter, or online. The physical actions of bullying include all forms of assault.

In a 2003 Canadian study, approximately 8% of students between the ages of 12 and 19 reported being bullied, while a similar number of students identified themselves as the bullies and admitted to bullying on a weekly basis. Victims are more likely than those not experiencing bullying to feel unsafe at school, have lower GPAs, and feel sad most days. They may develop anxiety disorders, depression, or suicidal thoughts. Suicide can be and has been the result of incessant bullying.

Psychologically, bullies seem to lack empathy, have poor interpersonal skills, and have no respect for authority. Bullies are more likely to develop enduring aggressive behaviour styles and persistent negative attitudes. Scholastically, they are less focused than other students (Public Safety Canada, 2010). In a health care setting, whether adults or youths, bullies have the potential for aggressive verbal and physical acting out against staff.

**Source:** Public Safety Canada. (2010). Bullying prevention: Nature and extent of bullying in Canada. In *Building the evidence—bullying prevention*. April 2008BP-1. National Crime Prevention Centre Publications. Retrieved from http://publications.gc.ca/collections/collection_2010/sp-ps/PS4-42-20-2008-eng.pdf.

patient's past experiences of violence or trauma and the role it currently plays in their lives. When a history of trauma is present, it is important for the nursing team to be aware and to avoid any situations that may retraumatize the patient. Consider the following examples:

- A woman who was raped may be retraumatized by being catheterized for a medical procedure.
- A Canadian veteran who was wounded and held prisoner may be retraumatized if confined to a hospital bed in traction.
- A psychiatric patient who has been a victim of assault may be retraumatized by the angry, aggressive outbursts of a co-patient on the unit (Chandler, 2008).

These traumatic histories can impede a patient's ability to self-soothe, resulting in negative coping responses and creating a vulnerability to coercive interventions by staff.

### Self-Assessment

Nurses may have their own histories with anger, aggression, and violence, and these experiences can influence their ability to intervene safely and effectively in a similar incident. Nurses should reflect on self-assessment of personal responses to anger and aggression, including choice of words, tone of voice, and nonverbal communication. It is essential to be aware of personal dynamics that may trigger nontherapeutic emotions and reactions with specific patients. Finally, the nurse must assess situational factors (e.g., fatigue, insufficient staff) that may decrease normal competence in the management of complex patient problems. Self-assessment promotes calm responses to patient anger and potential aggression. These responses are further supported by the creation of an environment that encourages staff to express feelings, use humour, and develop a professional support system.

## DIAGNOSIS

Some patients have coping skills that are adequate for day-to-day events, but they may be overwhelmed by the stresses of illness or hospitalization. Others may have a maladaptive coping pattern that is marginally effective for them, but consists of coping strategies that are unhealthy and may potentiate anger and aggression. When the nursing assessment identifies the potential for anger or aggression, *Ineffective coping* (overwhelmed or maladaptive), *Stress overload*, *Risk for self-directed violence*, and *Risk for other-directed violence* are relevant nursing diagnoses (Herdman, 2012).

## OUTCOMES IDENTIFICATION

Having clearly defined outcome criteria is important for identifying the behaviours that staff can encourage. These outcomes should be identified in initial planning, prior to intervening.

The *Nursing Outcomes Classification (NOC)* outlines specific outcome criteria for use with angry and aggressive patients (Moorhead, Johnson, Maas, et al., 2008). Table 26-1 lists outcome indicators for aggression self-control.

## PLANNING

Planning interventions requires a sound assessment of history, present coping skills, and the patient's willingness and capacity to learn alternative and nonviolent ways of handling angry feelings. Additionally, the nurse needs to consider if:

- The situation calls for:
  - Psychoeducational approaches to teach the patient new skills for handling anger
  - Immediate intervention to prevent overt violence (e.g., de-escalation techniques, restraint or seclusion, medications)
- The environment provides:
  - Privacy for the patient
  - Enough space for patients
  - A healthy balance between structured and quiet time
  - Adequate personnel to safely and effectively deal with potentially violent situations
- Staff skills call for:
  - Education in verbal de-escalation techniques
  - Education about positive and consistent approaches to patients
  - Education for appropriate use of restraints

## ASSESSMENT GUIDELINES
*Anger, Aggression, or Violence*

### ASSESSMENT FOR ADAPTIVE VERSUS MALADAPTIVE EXPRESSION OF ANGER

Demographic assessment:
- History of difficulty with anger management
- History of ineffective coping
- Difficulty expressing or dealing with emotions
- Diagnosis of borderline, histrionic, or antisocial personality disorder
- Diagnosis of dementia or brain injury
- Puberty and adolescence (mood swings, hormonal surges, peer pressures)

### PRE-ASSAULTIVE ASSESSMENT OF MENTAL STATE
Feelings of ...
- Frustration, fear, anxiety, embarrassment, shame, or rejection
- Irritability, hypersensitivity to perceived criticism, or attempts by others to control

Voicing ...
- Lack of control over life or situation
- Defiance
- Need for support of anger from others

Behaviours indicative of ...
- Hyperactivity, impulsivity, withdrawal
- Confusion, delusions
- Intoxication or other impairment
- Rumination, sullenness, or pacing

### ASSAULTIVE STAGE—RISK ASSESSMENT
Voicing ...
- Verbal abuse (profanity, argumentativeness, threats)
- Loud voice; change of pitch; or very soft voice, forcing others to strain to hear
- Negative or hostile response in the context of limit setting by the nurse

Thinking (cognition or decision-making) ...
- Diminishing ability to recognize the anger
- Diminishing ability or desire to diffuse own anger
- Inability to differentiate between assertiveness and aggressive expressions of anger
- Plan, wish, or intent to harm and capacity or means to do so
- Possession of a weapon or object that may be used as a weapon (fork, knife, rock)

Behaviours ...
- Hyperactivity most important predictor of imminent violence (pacing, restlessness)
- Increasing anxiety and tension (clenched jaw or fist, rigid posture, fixed or tense facial expression, mumbling to self, shortness of breath, sweating, and rapid pulse)
- Intense or avoidant eye contact
- Assault (hitting, punching, striking, throwing, intimidating, threatening)

### ASSESSMENT FOR AGGRESSION OR VIOLENCE

Demographic assessment:
- History of violence is the best predictor of future violence
- Male gender
- Age of 14 to 24 years
- Low socioeconomic status
- Substance abuse
- Inadequate support system
- Prison time
- History of limited coping skills increases risk for using violence

## IMPLEMENTATION

Ideally, intervention begins prior to any sign of escalation of anger. This intervention includes developing a trusting relationship with the patient by having numerous brief, nonthreatening, nondirective interactions to get to know the patient. In certain settings (e.g., crisis units, emergency departments), episodes of patient anger and aggression can be predicted; therefore, education and practice of verbal and nonverbal interventions with patients and staff are essential. Cultural competency is an essential part of staff education.

### Psychosocial Interventions

As the nurse determines a patient's emotional state, intervention begins. During this process, the nurse listens to the patient's story and acknowledges his or her needs. Summarizing what

| TABLE 26-1 | *NOC* OUTCOME INDICATORS FOR AGGRESSION SELF-CONTROL | |
| --- | --- | --- |
| **NURSING OUTCOME AND DEFINITION** | **INTERMEDIATE INDICATORS** | **SHORT-TERM INDICATORS** |
| Aggression self-control: Self-restraint of assaultive, combative, or destructive behaviours toward others | Maintains self-control without supervision<br>Upholds contract to restrain aggressive behaviours | Identifies when angry or frustrated<br>Vents negative feelings appropriately<br>Expresses needs in a nondestructive manner<br>Refrains from striking others<br>Refrains from destroying property<br>Uses specific techniques to control anger or frustration<br>Identifies situations that precipitate hostility |

**Source:** Data from Moorhead, S., Johnson, M., Maas, M.L., et al. (2008). *Nursing outcome classification (NOC)* (4th ed.). St. Louis, MO: Mosby.

the patient has said demonstrates the nurse's empathy, compassion, and acceptance of the patient. Acceptance of the patient does not indicate an acceptance of aggressive or violent behaviour. It is important to clearly and simply state expectations for the patient's behaviour. In some situations, the anger may not be resolved before the risk for violence arises.

Approaching an angry patient can be unnerving or frightening. The goal is to facilitate the expression of anger in an adaptive, nonviolent manner.

When approaching the patient, convey a calm, relaxed, open, nonthreatening, and caring demeanour. The ability to maintain a calm exterior while feeling inner distress comes with experience.

Pay attention to the environment. If the patient is in a state of low arousal, choose a quiet place to talk, but one that is visible to other staff. This approach is most beneficial in helping a patient regain control. If the patient is in a state of moderate arousal, pacing up and down a corridor together while the patient vents can be effective. The use of advanced communication skills to de-escalate the situation can help dissipate pent-up energy fuelled by the release of neurotransmitters and hormones. This technique is helpful when the patient is unable to use the flight response and may feel trapped. Box 26-3 lists some principles underlying de-escalation techniques.

Personal space changes when the body and mind are in a heightened state of arousal. Patients in the pre-assaultive stage need much more space. Do not crowd the patient in or attempt to touch him or her. Allow the patient enough personal space so that you are not perceived as intrusive but not so much space that the patient cannot speak in a normal voice. Always stay about 30 cm (1 foot) farther than the patient can reach with his or her arms or legs.

An angry patient may invade your space with verbal abuse and profanity. This means of communicating may be the only way the patient can express his or her feelings. As uncomfortable as this kind of communication may make you feel, you cannot take the patient's words personally or respond in kind. During an escalating situation is not the time to forbid the patient to communicate in this way or to end the conversation because of the patient's verbal abusiveness. The patient who is about to lose emotional control should not be abandoned. For the protection of the patient and others, the nurse needs to

| BOX 26-3 | DE-ESCALATION TECHNIQUES: PRACTICE PRINCIPLES |
| --- | --- |

- Respond as early as possible
- Assess for personal safety
- Maintain calmness for self and patient
- Use a calm, clear tone of voice
- Assess the patient and the situation for stressors and stress indicators
- Maintain the patient's self-esteem and dignity
- Establish what the patient considers to be needed
- Invest time; be goal oriented
- Remain honest
- Maintain a large personal space
- Avoid verbal struggles
- Make the options clear
- Utilize a nonaggressive posture
- Use genuineness and empathy
- Be assertive, not aggressive

**Source:** Mason, T., & Chandley, M. (1999). *Management of violence and aggression.* Philadelphia: Churchill Livingstone.

remain engaged while a preplanned crisis intervention begins to unfold.

As escalation increases, the patient's ability to process stimuli decreases. Keep your voice audible, but at a lower volume than the patient's. Eventually, the patient will match it and begin to listen more closely. Ensure that you are speaking at an appropriate level and not whispering. Choose your words carefully, speak in short sentences, be clear and concise, and listen to the patient's response. Use open-ended statements and questions to elicit the patient's thoughts. Avoid punitive, threatening, accusatory, or challenging statements.

Honestly verbalize the patient's options and encourage the individual to assume responsibility for choices made. During the pre-assaultive stage, you may want to give two options, such as "Do you want to go to your room or to the quiet room for a while?" This approach decreases the sense of powerlessness that often precipitates violence. This type of question is quite appropriate in the pre-assaultive stage, but not during the assaultive stage. At the pre-assaultive stage, the patient's lack of clarity in thinking and poor decision making become key elements in the intervention. Now, open-ended questions create too much confusion. You might say, "Some quiet time in your room might help now" or "The quiet room is free." Again, be sure your voice is calm and confident, with a tone that demonstrates that these statements to the patient are options, not directions.

At the assaultive stage, when aggression is deemed likely, seclusion, restraint, or pharmacological means of de-escalation may be necessary to ensure the safety of patients and staff. These measures should be used only when other interventions have failed. Canadian care facilities are mandated by policies that dictate the use of the least restrictive means to care for patients whenever possible. Nurses are also guided by position statements set out by their regulatory bodies.

### Staff Safety

Staff should know who is working with a potentially violent patient, keep an eye on the interaction, and be prepared to intervene if the situation escalates. At that time, other patients should be moved away from the incident, and the environment around the specific patient should be free from any object that could be used as a weapon. On psychiatric units, policies and procedures for working as a team in a critical incident of violence (or potential for violence) are in place. All staff should become familiar with the protocols. Discussing and rehearsing the protocols ensures confidence, safety, security, and trust. Facility policies and Workers' Compensation Boards dictate that dangling earrings, necklaces, and similar jewellery should never be worn on duty.

### Considerations for Engaging the Angry or Aggressive Patient

Prior to engaging an angry or aggressive patient, ensure that sufficient staff members are available for support. Avoid confrontation with the patient. If security personnel are called to stand by, keep them in the background until they are needed to assist.

Do not stand directly in front of the patient or in front of a doorway; this position could be interpreted as confrontational. Instead, stand slightly off to the side. Encourage the patient to have a seat. An angry person may sit. An aggressive person will not.

If a patient's behaviour begins to escalate, provide feedback. "You seem to be very upset." Such an observation allows exploration of the patient's feelings and may lead to de-escalation of the situation. If the patient validates what you have said, invite him or her to sit down and talk about it. It is best to use a closed-ended statement here. "Let's sit down and talk about it."

Call a Code White if you believe the aggression and violence are going to require additional help (Workers' Compensation Board of British Columbia, Occupational Health and Safety Agency for Healthcare, & Health Association of BC, 2002). In many hospitals, nurses with experience dealing with anger, aggression, and violence and who have completed special training may be designated as *Code White responders*. In British Columbia, this role may fall to the psychiatric nurse clinician in the emergency department. When a Code White is called, the Code White nurse attends an incident occurring in the facility. Upon arrival on the scene, the staff initiating the call defers to the expertise of the Code White nurse.

Generally, the first staff member on the scene is the only person who should talk to the patient. That person takes the lead while other staff maintain an unobtrusive presence. They may be directed to call for additional help, prepare a seclusion room, gather restraints, or prepare to give medications.

PLEASE NOTE: Code White policies and procedures are not in place in all jurisdictions nationally. Also, the procedures may differ. It is important to check with the employer or institution regarding that institution's policies and procedures.

### Pharmacological Interventions

When a patient is showing increased signs of anxiety or agitation, it is appropriate to offer antianxiety or antipsychotic medication to alleviate symptoms. When used in conjunction with psychosocial interventions and de-escalation techniques, these medications may prevent a violent incident. The following Drug Treatment box identifies medications of choice, routes, and indications. Note: Some medications are given concurrently for optimal therapeutic effect.

It is the nurse's role to assess for appropriateness of prn (as needed) medications. Many patients feel traumatized by the use of intramuscular injections; therefore, oral medications should always be the first choice (Gilburt, Rose, & Slade, 2008). Nurses must educate the patient about the medication, the reason it is being given, and potential adverse effects, even if the patient is out of control.

The long-term treatment of anger, aggression, and violence is based on treating the underlying psychiatric disorder. Selective serotonin reuptake inhibitors (SSRIs), lithium, anticonvulsants, benzodiazepines, atypical antipsychotics, and beta blockers are all used successfully for specific patient populations. Anger and aggression related to attention deficit disorder or attention deficit hyperactivity disorder may be reduced through the use of psycho-stimulants. The Drug Treatment box on page 535 provides an overview of the drugs used to treat chronic aggression.

### Health Teaching and Health Promotion

A nurse can model appropriate responses and ways to cope with anger, teach a variety of methods to appropriately express anger, and educate patients regarding coping mechanisms, identification of personal triggers, de-escalation techniques, and self-soothing skills to manage emotions. These skills include removing themselves from a situation or taking a personal time out. Working with patients to explore their own psychological and somatic responses to anger or anger-provoking stimuli enhances self-awareness related to personal triggers and facilitates learning about how to intervene and to exert self-management skills during these stressful events. Box 26-4 provides an example of confrontational assertion when dealing with angry and aggressive people.

### Case Management

A multidisciplinary approach is important for a patient with behavioural issues. Consistency and planning are key to the patient's success. Intervention strategies should be discussed during treatment team meetings and then with the patient,

## DRUGS TREATMENTS USED FOR EMERGENCY MANAGEMENT OF VIOLENT BEHAVIOUR

| GENERIC (TRADE) | ROUTES | INDICATIONS |
|---|---|---|
| **ANTIANXIETY AGENTS (BENZODIAZEPINES)** | | |
| Lorazepam (Ativan) | PO, SL, IM, IV | Drug of choice in this class<br>Use with caution with hepatic dysfunction |
| Alprazolam (Xanax) | PO | Paradoxical (opposite response) with personality disorders and older adults |
| Diazepam (Valium) | PO, IM, IV | Rapid onset of calming and sedating<br>Long half-life; use with caution in older adults |
| **CONVENTIONAL ANTIPSYCHOTICS** | | |
| Haloperidol | PO, IM, IV | Favourable adverse-effect profile<br>Due to risk for neuroleptic malignant syndrome, keep hydrated, check vital signs, and test for muscle rigidity |
| Loxapine (Loxapac) | PO, IM, SC | Decreases abnormal excitement in the brain; decreases agitation and aggression<br>Incompatible with other medications in a syringe<br>Avoid or minimize use with the frail elderly |
| Chlorpromazine | PO, PR, IM | Very sedating<br>Injections can cause pain; watch for hypotension |
| **ATYPICAL ANTIPSYCHOTICS** | | |
| Risperidone (Risperdal) | PO, IM | Calms while treating underlying condition<br>Watch for hypotension<br>Increased risk for stroke in older adults |
| Olanzapine (Zyprexa, Zyprexa Zydis) | PO, IM, SL | Useful in patients who are unresponsive to haloperidol<br>Calms while treating underlying condition<br>Avoid when using lorazepam<br>Increased risk for stroke in older adults |
| Zuclopenthixol acetate (Clopixol-Acuphase) | IM | Rapid acting to decrease psychotic symptoms and excitability<br>Watch for drowsiness<br>Avoid if prior alcohol consumption or substance abuse is suspected |
| **COMBINATIONS** | | |
| Haloperidol, lorazepam (Ativan), and benztropine | IM | Commonly used in the acute setting<br>Men who are young and athletic are at increased risk for dystonia<br>Consider akathisia (sensations of inner restlessness that manifest as an inability to sit or remain seated) if agitation increases |
| Loxapine (Loxapac) and lorazepam (Ativan), and benztropine | IM, PO | Consider this combination if patient has difficulty taking haloperidol<br>Loxapine must be given PO while lorazepam and benztropine may be given PO or IM |

**Sources:** Data adapted from Canadian Pharmacists Association. (2011). *Compendium of pharmaceuticals and specialties: The Canadian drug reference for health professionals.* Ottawa: Author; Gross, A.F., & Sanders, K.M. (2008). Aggression and violence. In T.S. Stern, J.F. Rosenbaum, M. Fava, et al. (Eds.), *Massachusetts General Hospital comprehensive clinical psychiatry* (pp. 895–905). St. Louis, MO: Mosby; and Martinez, M., Marangell, L.B., & Martinez, J.M. (2008). Psychopharmacology. In R.E. Hales, S.C. Yudofsky, & G.O. Gabbard (Eds.), *Textbook of psychiatry.* Arlington, VA: American Psychiatric Publishing.

before implementation. A discharge plan outlining follow-up, anger management classes, and counselling is essential.

### Milieu Management

Behaviours rarely occur in a vacuum. A thorough, proactive examination of the environment is important when considering the potential for anger and aggression on a unit. It is hard to determine how the stimulation of any unit might affect someone whose anxiety is extremely high or who is delusional or confused.

Patients' ability to cope with their acute illness is confounded by unfamiliar environments full of unfamiliar and often unpredictable co-patients. Feelings of frustration, fear, anxiety, and confusion can escalate to aggression and acting out. Frequent rounds on the unit are important as part of the ongoing assessment of the milieu.

If an escalating patient has enough self-control, sometimes taking a time out in his or her room is sufficient to enable the person to regain composure. Some inpatient psychiatric units, group homes, residential care facilities, and correctional centres offer a therapeutic quiet room. The room is partially lit and has relaxing music and comfortable furniture that promote feelings of security and safety. Patients who identify their own need for time out in a therapeutic quiet room are able to use it of their

## DRUGS TREATMENTS USED FOR LONG-TERM MANAGEMENT OF CHRONIC AGGRESSION

| CLASS | POPULATION | CONSIDERATIONS |
|---|---|---|
| Selective serotonin reuptake inhibitors (SSRIs) | Antisocial personality disorder, schizophrenia, dementia, brain injury | Reduces irritability, impulsivity, and aggression<br>Stabilizes mood<br>Use cautiously with bipolar disorder |
| Lithium | Antisocial personality disorder, prison inmates, intellectual disability, brain injury | TSH levels measured prior to treatment<br>Due to anti-aggressive properties, blood levels can be lower than those necessary to treat mania |
| Anticonvulsants | Prison inmates, antisocial personality disorder, borderline personality disorder, substance use, attention deficit disorder, brain injury, schizophrenia, and intermittent explosive disorder (IED; rages) | Significantly reduces impulsive aggression<br>Similar doses with bipolar disorder<br>Multiple drug interactions<br>Periodic blood levels<br>Monitor CBC and LFTs |
| Gabapentin | Anxiety disorder, personality disorders | No interactions with other anticonvulsants |
| Benzodiazepines | Anxiety disorder | Potential for abuse, dependence, and withdrawal<br>May cause paradoxical aggression |
| Atypical antipsychotics | Schizophrenia, psychosis, mania, borderline personality disorder, intellectual disability | Clozapine superior to other atypical antipsychotics<br>Fewer adverse effects and greater adherence than with conventional antipsychotics<br>Risperidone reduces irritability in autistic disorder |
| Beta blockers | Schizophrenia, brain injury, dementia, intellectual disability | Propranolol (Inderal) contraindicated with asthma, COPD, and type 1 diabetes<br>Sedation adverse effects may explain anti-aggressive effects |
| Psychostimulants | ADD/ADHD in children and adults | Potential for addiction and abuse |

ADD/ADHD, Attention deficit disorder/attention deficit hyperactivity disorder; CBC, complete blood count; COPD, chronic obstructive pulmonary disease; LFTs, liver function tests; TSH, thyroid-stimulating hormone.

**Source:** Data from Canadian Pharmacists Association. (2011). *Compendium of pharmaceuticals and specialties: The Canadian drug reference for health professionals.* Ottawa: Author; First, M.B., & Tasman, A. (2004). *DSM-IV-TR Mental disorders: Diagnosis, etiology and treatment.* Hoboken, NJ: Wiley; Gross, A.F., & Sanders, K.M. (2008). Aggression and violence. In T.S. Stern, J.F. Rosenbaum, M. Fava, et al. (Eds.), *Massachusetts General Hospital comprehensive clinical psychiatry* (pp. 895–905). St. Louis, MO: Mosby; Scott, C.L., Quanbeck, C.D., & Resnick, P.J. (2008). Assessment of dangerousness. In R.E. Hales, S.C. Yudofsky, & G.O. Gabbard (Eds.), *Textbook of psychiatry* (pp. 1655–1672). Arlington, VA: American Psychiatric Publishing; and Stahl, S.M. (2008). *Stahl's essential psychopharmacology* (3rd ed.). New York: Cambridge University Press.

### BOX 26-4 CONFRONTATIONAL ASSERTION

*Assertiveness* is standing up for your personal rights and expressing thoughts, feelings, and beliefs in honest and appropriate ways that do not violate another person's rights. It involves respect, not deference. The goals of assertiveness are communication and mutually giving and receiving respect.

Confrontational assertion can be used when someone says one thing and does another.

Components to think about before you proceed with confrontational assertion include the following:
- Identify the feeling(s) you have. (e.g., Do you feel strongly enough about it to initiate an encounter?)
- Identify what you want the outcome of the encounter to be.
- Rehearse what you want to say. Stick to the behaviour and do not attack the person.
- Initiate the encounter.
- Give feedback.

**Source:** Adapted from Gooding, L. (n.d.). *Assertiveness: A key to success.* Retrieved from http://lonestar.edu/blogs/lgooding/files/2009/10/assertiveness-a-key-to-success.pdf.

own volition. In many institutions, quiet rooms are locked and used as seclusion rooms. The decision to lock the door is based on the patient's risk assessment and the discretion of the multidisciplinary team.

### Use of Restraints or Seclusion

Seclusion or restraint is used only if the patient presents a clear danger to self or others. Restraints of any type should be used only when alternatives fail to protect the patient and others from harm (see Research Highlight box).

Brickell, Nicholls, Procyshyn, and colleagues (2009) define three types of patient restraints:
1. Environmental restraint: Seclusion is an example of an environmental restraint. The patient's locomotion is restricted by confinement to a defined area or locked room. The situation is temporary, the patient is alone, and there is no furniture or other amenities in the room.
2. Physical or mechanical restraints: These are techniques or devices used to physically restrict or subdue whole or partial body movements (e.g., posey belts, four-point restraints, geriatric chairs).

## RESEARCH HIGHLIGHT
### *Reducing the Use of Restraints*

**Source:** Sclafani, M.J., Humphrey, F.J., Repko, S., et al. (2008). Reducing patient restraints: A pilot approach using clinical case review. *Perspectives in Psychiatric Care, 44*, 32–39. doi:10.1111/j.1744-6163.2008.00145.x.

### Problem
The excessive reliance on mechanical restraints to minimize disruptive patient behaviours is being met with increasing initiatives to reduce their use. In North America, initiatives at various levels of government, as well as federal regulations and accreditation standards, have resulted in strong advocacy for restraint elimination. There is also increasing awareness on the part of service providers and their unions regarding the damaging effects restraints have on patients, clinicians, and caretakers.

### Purpose of Study
The purpose of this study was to implement alternatives to the use of mechanical restraints and evaluate the effectiveness of these approaches in contrast to approaches that had relied on the significant use of restraints.

### Methods
A group of interdisciplinary consultants used a variety of approaches in working with both the unit staff and two selected patients at an acute psychiatric hospital. Both patients had a history of violent behaviours that resulted in the frequent use of mechanical restraints. This pilot study focused on enhancing clinical care provided to patients who are dually diagnosed with mental illness and developmental disabilities. Staff education and training, in conjunction with patient-centred approaches, significantly decreased the use of restraints.

### Key Findings
- During the 16-month period of this pilot study, there was a steady decline in the use of restraints, from 36 episodes per month to 0.
- The use of patient coaching (helping people discover and improve their coping skills) and group and individual problem-solving approaches significantly decreases the need to use mechanical restraints.
- Staff education and training that focus on person-centred approaches, positive reinforcements, and strength-based treatment assist in creating more humane living conditions and a therapeutic milieu for patients.

### Implications for Nursing Practice
Nurses served as an integral part of both the consultation team and the unit staff in this pilot study. The study revealed the success of the interdisciplinary team working together to understand the needs of a particular population and to intervene more effectively. Evidence-informed strategies can significantly improve the care of vulnerable patients, as well as strengthen the cohesion and effectiveness of the staff.

---

## BOX 26-5 ADDITIONAL GUIDELINES FOR USE OF MECHANICAL RESTRAINT OR SECLUSION

**Indications for Use**
- To protect the patient from self-harm
- To prevent the patient from assaulting others

**Legal Requirements**
- Multidisciplinary involvement
- Appropriate health care provider's signature according to provincial and territorial law
- Patient advocate or relative notification
- Restraint or seclusion discontinuation as soon as possible

**Documentation Describes**
- Patient's behaviour leading to restraint or seclusion
- Nursing interventions used and the patient's responses (including least restrictive measures used prior to restraint or seclusion)
- Evaluation of the interventions used and patient's response

**Plan of Care for Restraint Use or Seclusion Implementation**
- Ongoing evaluations by nursing staff and appropriate health care providers
- Method of reintegration into the unit milieu
- Evidence of least restrictive measures used prior to restraint or seclusion
- Critical Incident or Unusual Occurrence Report form completed

**Clinical Assessments**
- Patient's mental state at time of restraint or seclusion (i.e., pre-assaultive, assaultive, post-assaultive)
- Physical exam for medical problems possibly causing behaviour changes
- Need for restraints or seclusion

**Observation and Ongoing Assessment**
- Staff in constant or close attendance
- Written record completed every 15 minutes
- Range of movement frequently assessed if limbs are restrained
- Vital signs monitored
- Circulation assessed: blood flow observed in hands or feet
- Observation to ensure that restraint is not rubbing or causing friction on skin
- Provision for nutrition, hydration, and elimination

**Release Procedure**
- Patient able to follow commands and stay in control
- Termination of restraints or seclusion
- Debriefing with patient

---

3. Chemical restraints: Chemical restraint is achieved through the use of medications, with the sole intent of managing behaviour.

Additional guidelines for the use of mechanical restraints are given in Box 26-5.

Prior to seclusion, a patient must be assessed for contraindications, including pregnancy, chronic obstructive pulmonary disorder (COPD), head or spinal injury, seizure disorder, abuse, history of surgery or fracture, morbid obesity, and sleep apnea. A patient can be secluded or restrained with an order from a psychiatrist or physician in accordance with a provincial or territorial mental health act.

Staff work as a team when secluding a patient. The team leader briefly describes the rationale for seclusion and directs the team. One nurse prepares the seclusion room while others promote safety and privacy by clearing the area of onlookers. A nurse prepares prn or stat medication. Options are provided to the patient, including taking a time out, accepting medication orally, or walking with the nursing team into the seclusion room. When these options fail, the staff intervenes to physically restrain the patient and escort him or her into seclusion. The patient may be required to change into pyjamas, and medication may be administered despite patient objections. One by one, team members back out of the room, locking the door behind them. Close or constant observation protocols are initiated per hospital policy. The patient remains in seclusion until assessed as being less at risk for harm to self or others.

Following seclusion of a patient, the treatment team should debrief the incident, and when seclusion is discontinued, the nurse and patient should also debrief. It is important to identify precipitating factors, explore coping resources, and develop a plan of action for a time when another incident is likely to occur. Questions to be answered during the team debriefing might include:

- Could we have done anything that would have prevented the violence? If yes, how will we ensure this approach is taken another time?
- Did we respond as a team? Were team members acting according to the policies and procedures of the unit? If not, what could we do another time?
- How do staff members feel about this patient now and about the incident that occurred?

Feelings of fear and anger must be discussed and worked through; otherwise, staff may deal with the patient in a punitive and nontherapeutic manner. Employee morale, productivity, use of sick leave time, transfer requests, and absenteeism are all affected by patient violence, especially if a staff member has been injured. Staff members must feel supported by their peers as well as by the organizational policies and procedures established to maintain a safe environment.

- Is there a need for additional staff education regarding how to respond to violent patients?
- How did the actual restraining process go? What could be done differently?
- If injury occurred, has it been reported and cared for?

Incidents that require the use of seclusion or restraints provoke anxiety for the staff and may trigger their stress responses. Skills in nonviolent crisis intervention techniques are critical. Nurses should not be put into positions such as these without this additional training. Many health authorities, care facilities, and health institutions across Canada provide this training at the time of hiring and intermittently during employment.

Reintegration to the unit occurs when the patient is assessed as being able to handle increasing amounts of stimulation. Reintegration should be gradual. If the process proves to be too much for the patient and increased agitation results, the individual is returned to the seclusion room or another quiet area or restraints are reapplied. Prior to release from restraint or seclusion, patients must be able to follow directions and control behaviours. With restraints, a structured reintegration is the best approach. Begin by removing one of the four-point restraints, then another, and so on. Close observation of the patient is essential as the restraints are removed and for several hours following. If the patient is unable to manage his or her behaviour, further seclusion or restraint may be necessary.

It is important to acknowledge that psychiatric patients are not the only patients who exhibit anger and have the potential for aggression and violence.

## Caring for Patients in General Hospital Settings
### Patients With High Anxiety Related to Hospitalization
Caring for hospitalized patients who exhibit signs of anxiety begins with listening to the patient's story and helping the patient identify immediate goals. Mild anxiety can be moderated by the provision of comfort items before they are requested (beverage, deck of cards, access to TV). This kind of response can build rapport and reassure the patient. Anxiety can also be minimized by reducing ambiguity. This strategy includes clear and concrete communication. An interaction providing clarity about what the nurse can and cannot do is most usefully ended by offering something within the nurse's power to provide (i.e., leaving the patient with a "yes").

Interventions for anxiety might also include the use of distractions such as magazines, action comics, and video games. Generally, distractions that are colourful and do not require sustained attention work best, although the choice of distraction varies according to the patient's interests and abilities. When a patient is anxious, frustrated, angry, or fearful, pacing with the patient up and down the corridor can be a helpful strategy. Continue to converse with the patient as you do so.

Patients with a high level of baseline anxiety and limited coping skills are helped when their interactions with the treatment team are predictable. This predictability may include speaking with the physician at a specific time each day and providing consistency in nursing assignments. Individuals from outside the unit, such as a chaplain or a volunteer, may help by giving the patient more attention.

### Patients With Healthy Coping Skills Who Are Overwhelmed
A patient loses autonomy and control when hospitalized, which can cause a great deal of related distress. When this stress is combined with the uncertainty of illness, a patient may respond in ways that are not usual for him or her. A careful nursing assessment, with history and information from family members, helps evaluate whether a patient's anger is a usual or an unusual way for that patient to manage stress.

Interventions for patients whose usual coping strategies are healthy involve finding ways to re-establish or substitute similar means of dealing with the hospitalization. This problem solving occurs in collaboration with the patient, in interactions that demonstrate that the nurse acknowledges the patient's distress, validates it as understandable under the circumstances, and indicates a willingness to search for solutions. Validation includes making an apology to the patient when appropriate, such as when a promised intervention (e.g., changing a dressing by a certain time) has not been delivered or sympathizing with the patient about the "horrible food" and assisting him or her to make tastier choices on the menu.

Patients who have become angry may be unable to moderate this emotion enough to problem-solve with their nurses; others may be unable to communicate the source of their anger. Often, the nurse—knowing the patient and the context of the anger—can make an accurate guess at what feeling is behind the anger and help name it for the patient. Doing so can lead to a sense of being understood and dissipation of the anger, resulting in a calmer discussion of the event.

---

**VIGNETTE**

Jagwinder, a 21-year-old patient who had been in an automobile accident, was admitted to the medical unit with a pelvic fracture and is bedridden. Since admission, he has yelled at each nurse who walks by his room, using expletives to demand that the nurse enter and attend to his needs.

*Intervention:* The nurse assigned to the patient for the evening stops in his doorway after he yells at her and assertively states, "Jagwinder, it is inappropriate to yell and swear at the staff. If you would like our attention, please address us courteously." She continues on her way and Jagwinder is left to process the message. He is unable to offer a retort or to engage the nurse in argument. He is initially angry and profane in response. However, the nurse will not return to him. Should he repeat this behaviour on her next encounter with him, she will repeat her original message, consistently setting limits on his behaviour. She will not engage in conversation with him until he is prepared to act and speak appropriately. At each negative encounter, the patient is left to think about his behaviour.

*Response:* Jagwinder eventually comes to realize how to get the attention he needs in a more appropriate manner. He gains insight and modifies his behaviour. His anger and frustration triggered by not getting his needs met immediately begin to dissipate. When the nurse meets with him, she engages him in the primary topic of his concern, followed by a debriefing of his inappropriate behaviour. Together they explore how to communicate his needs more effectively, more appropriately, and more assertively. They discuss his anger and frustration with hospitalization and explore his pattern of coping. At each step of the encounter, the nurse applies principles of behavioural therapy to her intervention strategies.

---

## Patients With Marginal Coping Skills

Patients whose coping skills were marginal before hospitalization need a different set of interventions from those who have basically healthy ways of coping. They are poorly equipped to use alternatives when initial attempts to cope are unsuccessful or are found to be inappropriate. Such patients frequently manifest anxiety that moves quickly to anger and on to aggression. For some, anger and intimidation are primary coping strategies used to obtain short-term goals of control or mastery. For others, the anger occurs when their limited or primitive attempts at coping are unsuccessful, and alternatives are unknown. For these patients, anger and violence are particular risks in inpatient settings.

The potential for violence is especially true for hospitalized patients with chemical dependence, who may be anxious about being cut off from the substance to which they are addicted. They may have well-founded concerns that any physical pain will be inadequately addressed. Many chemically dependent patients may see the source of their discomfort and anxiety as being outside themselves (i.e., impaired locus of control); relief must therefore also come from an outside source (e.g., the nurse, medication). These patients exhibit frustration intolerance and can be quite verbally aggressive. An understanding of the patient's lived experience with addiction helps the nurse and other staff determine a course of action for dealing with hostile aggression and the potential for violent acting out (see Chapter 19). Most hospitals have a withdrawal protocol that ensures that patients do not go through withdrawal without medication. Medication administration needs to be provided promptly and consistently to communicate to patients that nurses can be trusted. Attention to patients' need for the medication can be very anxiety relieving for those patients with a chemical-dependency problem. Precautionary measures may be in place on the hospital unit to limit certain visitors, to protect the sobriety or withdrawal and maintenance protocols for chemically dependent patients.

Interventions for patients who externalize blame requires firm and consistent limit setting on inappropriate behaviours. Anger may be communicated by verbal abuse targeting the staff. If attempts to teach alternative methods of coping and communicating are unsuccessful, three interventions can be used:

1. Leave the room as soon as the verbal abuse begins. Inform the patient that you, the nurse, will return in a specific amount of time (e.g., 20 minutes) when the situation is calmer. A matter-of-fact, neutral demeanour is important because fear, indignation, and arguing are gratifying to many verbally abusive patients. Alternatively, if the nurse is in the midst of a procedure and cannot leave immediately, she or he can break off conversation and eye contact, completing the procedure quickly and matter-of-factly before leaving the room. The nurse avoids chastising, threatening, or responding punitively to the patient.

2. Withdraw your attention from the abuse. Withdrawal of attention to verbal or emotional abuse is successful only if a second intervention is also used. This step requires attending positively to, and thus reinforcing, nonabusive communication by the patient. Interventions can include discussing non–illness-related topics, responding to requests, and providing emotional support, particularly when the patient is calm and approachable. This technique is quite effective when used in conjunction with the third one.

3. Schedule routine interactions. Patients who are verbally abusive may respond best to the predictability of routine, such as scheduled contacts with the nurse (every 30 or 60 minutes). Use of such contacts provides nursing attention that is not contingent on the patient's behaviour; therefore,

it does not reinforce the abuse. Of course, the patient's illness or injury may sometimes require nursing visits for assessment or intervention outside the scheduled contact times. These visits can be carried out in a calm, brief, matter-of-fact manner. For patients with marginal coping skills, once anxiety is moderated, nursing interventions include teaching alternative behaviours and coping strategies.

Implementing appropriate interventions can be difficult when the nurse is feeling threatened. Remaining matter-of-fact with patients who habitually use anger and intimidation can be difficult as they are often skillful at making personal and pointed statements. It is important to remember that patients do not know their nurses personally and thus have no basis on which they can make judgements. Nurses can discuss their feelings and beliefs with other staff members or with the critical incident debriefing team.

## Caring for Patients in Inpatient Psychiatric Settings
### Patients Who Are Acutely Psychotic
Assault on inpatient psychiatric units is of worldwide concern. On a psychiatric unit, the potential for hostile aggression and violence is most often demonstrated by those who are acutely psychotic, in a manic phase, substance dependent, or being held under the authority of a mental health act.

## Caring for Patients With Cognitive Deficits in Long-Term Residential Care Settings
### Patients With Cognitive Deficits
Patients (or residents) with cognitive deficits are particularly at risk for acting aggressively. Such deficits may result from delirium, dementia, or brain injury (see Chapter 18). Traditional approaches to disorientation and to the agitation it can cause rely heavily on reality orientation and medication. Reality orientation consists of providing the correct information to the patient about place, date, and current life circumstances. For many patients, this orientation is comforting because it reminds them of pertinent information and helps them feel in touch with their world. For others, reality orientation does not work. Because of their cognitive disorder, they can no longer "enter into our reality"; they become frightened and more agitated and may become aggressive. Sometimes the patient with a cognitive disorder experiences such severe agitation and aggression that it is referred to as a *catastrophic reaction*. The patient may scream, strike out, or cry because of overwhelming fear. Adopting a calm and unhurried manner is the best approach.

Patients who misperceive their setting or life situation may be calmed by validation therapy. Some disoriented older patients believe that they are young and feel the need to return to important tasks that were a significant part of those earlier years. For example, a woman may insist that she must go home to take care of her babies. Telling the patient that her babies have grown up and there is no home to return to is nontherapeutic and results in increased agitation. It is often more helpful to reflect back to the patient the feelings behind her demand and to show understanding and concern for her worry. During the conversation, the nurse can comment on what appears to be underlying

**VIGNETTE**
Ken is a 32-year-old patient with a diagnosis of schizophrenia who has lived in a group home for ten years. He is well maintained on his medications and attends daily programs and recreation at a local psychosocial clubhouse. He has a delusion that the Canadian Security Intelligence Service (CSIS) is listening in on him because he has some intimate knowledge of nuclear weapons design. When well, he continues to suffer from delusions and auditory hallucinations, but they are less intense and less intrusive, and they do not interfere with his daily living or ability to cope. Currently, Ken is experiencing an exacerbation of his symptoms. He is increasingly paranoid, and this paranoia has led to admission to an acute psychiatric inpatient unit. Ken is yelling at the nurses and accusing them of being part of the conspiracy against him. He believes they will force him to take medications that will erase his knowledge about the secret weapon. He insists that he must remain alert, vigilant, and self-protective.

*Intervention:* Ken is escalating, and the potential for violence is determined. The staff prepare to intervene. James, a nurse, engages Ken in the hallway. The nurse acknowledges Ken's concerns for his safety. (The use of skillful communication facilitates development of rapport, respect, and trust.) To help Ken settle, James offers him a prn medication or one-to-one time to talk with the staff. He gives the patient time to process the options. James continues to set limits and attempts to de-escalate the situation with Ken. Sensing that the patient is unable to use reason at the moment, the nurse signals the care team and they prepare for an intervention of seclusion. James advises Ken and also gives him one more opportunity to take medication to help him settle.

*Response:* Despite Ken's altered thought content, he is able to understand the potential for being secluded. When the nurse offers him medication to settle, Ken makes some choices. He chooses not to be put in seclusion, commenting that he believes the room is "bugged." He adds that he prefers to take a tablet form of medication rather than liquid or capsule. The nurse is able to provide a tablet. James has been able to meet the need for safety and security for everyone on the unit through the pre-emptive strategies of listening, setting limits, offering options, and providing space and time for the patient to process the information. These actions also allowed Ken to maintain a sense of control.

**VIGNETTE**
Mrs. Green, an 81-year-old woman with a diagnosis of Alzheimer's disease, always becomes agitated during her morning care; her caregivers have come to dread this time. Careful observation of antecedents to the episodes of agitation reveals a pattern. Mrs. Green is initially calm when care begins; however, one staff person gives morning care to the patient and her roommate at the same time, moving between the two. Observation of the process reveals that the patient becomes distracted by cues being given to her roommate and often startles when the caregiver returns to her. As this process continues over several minutes, Mrs. Green becomes increasingly distressed and then agitated.

When a change is made to ensure patient care is provided on an individual basis, Mrs. Green becomes receptive to the nursing care provided.

the patient's distress, thereby validating it. For example, when working with Mrs. Green in the vignette, the nurse may note that Mrs. Green misses her children and that she gets lonely at times:

> **Nurse:** "Mrs. Green, you miss your children, and this can be a lonely place."

The nurse shows interest in aspects of the patient's life, thereby establishing herself as a safe, understanding person. Mrs. Green finds more focus and is less overwhelmed by the stimulus occurring in her environment. The patient often becomes calmer and more open to redirection. As patients reminisce in this fashion, they often bring themselves into the present.

> **Mrs. Green:** "Of course, they're all grown and doing well on their own now."

Refer to Chapter 18 for a more detailed discussion of interventions for people with cognitive impairments. Refer to Chapter 30 for a more detailed discussion of the use of validation and reminiscent therapeutic modalities for older adults.

## EVALUATION

Evaluation of the nursing care plan (NCP) is essential for patients with a potential for anger, aggression, and violence. Evaluation provides information about the extent to which the interventions have achieved the outcomes. The initial NCP may have included assessment of the environmental stimuli that precede a patient's agitation. Once stimuli are identified, interventions specific to those stimuli are developed. Results of the interventions are evaluated and documented and the NCP is revised.

## KEY POINTS TO REMEMBER

- Angry emotions and aggressive, violent actions are difficult targets for nursing intervention, and self-awareness of personal responses to angry or threatening patients is essential.
- Nurses benefit from an understanding of how to intervene with an angry, aggressive, or violent patient.
- Understanding precipitating factors that can lead to an escalation of aggression facilitates care planning for individuals in a variety of situations.
- The expression of anger can lead to negative physiological changes.
- Psychosocial, cognitive, sociocultural, and biological theories provide explanations for anger and aggression.
- A patient's past aggressive behaviour is the most important indicator of future aggressive episodes.

- A variety of interventions are used to help patients de-escalate and maintain control, depending on their coping abilities, cognitive and mental status, and potential for violence.
- Administration of antipsychotics, mood stabilizers, and anti-anxiety medications may be indicated.
- Seclusion or restraints may be necessary to ensure safety for the patient and others on the unit.
- Clear protocols for the safe use of seclusion or restraints and for the humane management of care during this time are essential.
- The nurse is expected to have a clear understanding of policies, protocols, and legalities related to anger, aggression, and violence, as well as how to intervene.

## CRITICAL THINKING

1. Jennifer admits a 24-year-old man with a diagnosis of mania to an inpatient unit. She notes that the patient is irritable, has trouble sitting during the interview, and has a history of assault.
   a. Identify appropriate responses the nurse can make to the patient.
   b. What interventions should be built into the care plan?
   c. Identify at least three long-term outcomes to consider when planning care.

2. What are the two indicators for the use of seclusion and restraint rather than verbal interventions? Provide rationale.

3. Enter into a debate on the use of restraint and seclusion with your clinical group or in class. Choose a side and defend it, even if you do not necessarily agree with it. Use these topics:

   a. There are always better alternatives to seclusion and restraint.
   b. Seclusion and restraint are underutilized—people who have tried to limit their use have gone too far.
   c. Using chemical restraint with medication is preferable to seclusion and restraint.

4. Jordan is a 26-year-old male who is prone to alcohol and drug abuse. He likes to fight and initiate fights. He prides himself in his strength and aggressive personality. When another person looks directly at Jordan for more than just a few seconds, based on research, how is he likely to interpret the person's staring?

## CHAPTER REVIEW

1. Which statement about violence and nursing is accurate?
   1. Unless working in psychiatric or mental health settings, nurses are unlikely to experience patient violence.
   2. About three in ten nurses will face an injury due to patient violence during their careers.
   3. Emergency, psychiatric, and step-down units have the highest rates of violence towards staff.
   4. Violence primarily affects inexperienced or unskilled staff who cannot calm their patients.

2. A nurse working with a patient who describes himself as "always angry" should assess the patient for which problem(s)? Select all that apply.
   1. Pain
   2. Dementia
   3. Tachycardia
   4. Hypertension
   5. Traumatic brain injury

3. Which statement(s) by a patient indicate an increased likelihood of violent behaviour? Select all that apply.
   1. "People push me, but they can only push me so far."
   2. "I have a right to feel angry, and right now I am angry."
   3. "You are really stupid. I'd get better nursing care from a monkey."
   4. "A man has to do what a man has to do when somebody crosses him."
   5. "This is frustrating; I wish people would leave me alone. That's what would help me."

4. A nurse, Sarah, responds to loud, angry voices coming from the day room, where she finds that Mr. Christopher is pacing and shouting that he "isn't going to take this (expletive) anymore." Which reaction by Sarah is likely to be helpful in de-escalating the situation with Mr. Christopher?
   1. Acts calm, quiet, and in control.
   2. States, "You are acting inappropriately and must calm yourself now."
   3. Matches the patient's volume level so that he is able to hear over his own shouting.
   4. Stands close to the patient so she can intervene physically, if needed, to protect others.

5. Andrea, a patient, is anxiously waiting her turn to speak with a nurse. The nurse is very busy, however, and asks Andrea if she can wait a few minutes so she can finish her task. The nurse is distracted and forgets her promise temporarily, and 45 minutes pass before the nurse remembers and approaches Andrea. On seeing the nurse, Andrea accuses the nurse of lying and refuses to speak with her. Which response by the nurse is most likely to be therapeutic at this time?
   1. "You seem angry that I didn't speak with you when I promised I would."
   2. "Look, I'm sorry for being late, but screaming at me is not the best way to handle it."
   3. "You are too angry to talk right now. I'll come back in 20 minutes and we can try again."
   4. "Why are you angry? I told you that I was busy and would get to you soon as I could."

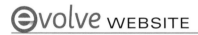 WEBSITE

**Visit the Evolve Web site for Chapter Review Answers and Rationales, Critical Thinking Answer Guidelines, and additional resources related to the content in this chapter:** *http://evolve.elsevier.com/Canada/Varcarolis/psychiatric/*

Post-Test interactive review

## REFERENCES

Arboleda-Florez, J., Holley, H., Crisanti, A., et al. (1996). *Mental illness and violence: Proof or stereotype?* (Cat. No. H39-346/1996E). Ottawa: Minister of Supply and Services Canada.

Bandura, A. (1973). *Aggression: A social learning analysis.* New York: Prentice Hall.

Beck, A. (1976). *Cognitive therapy and the emotional disorders.* New York: International Universities Press.

Beck, A., Emery, G., & Greenberg, R. (2005). *Anxiety disorders and phobias* (15th Anniversary Edition). New York: Basic Books.

Borod, J.C. (2000). *The neuropsychology of emotion.* New York: Oxford University Press.

Brickell, T., Nicholls, T., Procyshyn, R., et al. (2009). *Patient safety in mental health.* Edmonton: BC Mental Health and Addictions Services.

Burns, J.W., Holly, A., Quartana, P., et al. (2008). Trait anger management style moderates effects of actual ("state") anger regulation on symptom-specific reactivity and recovery among chronic low back pain patients. *Psychosomatic Medicine, Journal of Biobehavioural Medicine, 70*(8), 898–905.

Canadian Federation of Nurses Unions. (2008). *A position statement on psychological violence in the workplace (also known as "bullying").*

Retrieved from http://www.nursesunions.ca/sites/default/files/Bullying_Position_Statement.pdf.

Canadian Institute for Health Information. (2005). *A summary of highlights from the 2005 national survey of the work and health of nurses* (Cat. No. 83-003-XPE). Retrieved from http://www.cihi.ca/CIHI-ext-portal/pdf/internet/NURSING_NSWHN_SUMMARY2005_EN.

Canadian Institute for Health Information. (2008). *Analysis in brief: National trauma registry: 2007 injury hospitalizations highlights report.* Retrieved from http://www.cihi.ca/CIHI-ext-portal/pdf/internet/PDF_NTR_BL_HIGHLIGHTS_FEB08_EN.

Centers for Disease Control and Prevention. (2008). *Adverse health conditions and health risk behaviors associated with intimate partner violence, morbidity and mortality weekly report.* Retrieved from http://www.cdc.gov/mmwr/PDF/wk/mm5705.pdf.

Chandler, G. (2008). From traditional inpatient to trauma-informed treatment: Transferring control from staff to patient. *Journal of the American Psychiatric Nurses Association, 14*(5), 363–371. doi:10.1177/1078390308326625.

Coccaro, E.F., McCloskey, M.S., Fitzgerald, D.A., et al. (2007). Amygdala and orbitofrontal reactivity to social threat in individuals with impulsive aggression. *Biological Psychiatry, 62*(2), 168–178.

Criminal Code, R.S.C. 1985, c. C-46 (2011), s. 265. Retrieved from http://laws-lois.justice.gc.ca/eng/acts/C-46/.

de Almeida, R.M.M., Ferrari, P.F., Parmigiani, S., et al. (2005). Escalated aggressive behavior: Dopamine, serotonin and GABA. *European Journal of Pharmacology, 526*(1–3), 51–64. doi:10.1016/j.ejphar.2005.10.004.

Dougherty, D.D., Bonab, A.A., Ottowitz, W.E., et al. (2006). Decreased striatal D1 binding as measured using PET and [$^{11}$C]SCH 23,390 in patients with major depression with anger attacks. *Depression and Anxiety, 23*(1–3), 175–177. doi:10.1002/da.20168.

Ellis, A. (1973). *Humanistic psychotherapy: The rational-emotive approach.* New York: McGraw-Hill.

Ellis, A. (1990). *Anger: How to live with and without it.* New York: Citadel Press.

Ellis, A., Abrams, M., & Dengelegi-Abrams, L. (2008). *Personality theories: Critical perspectives.* New York: Sage.

Gilburt, H., Rose, D., & Slade, M. (2008). The importance of relationships in mental health care: A qualitative study of service users' experiences of psychiatric hospital admission in the UK. *BMC Health Services Research, 8,* 1–12. doi:10.1186/1472-6963-8-92.

Gross, A.F., & Sanders, K.M. (2008). Aggression and violence. In T.S. Stern, J.F. Rosenbaum, M. Fava, et al (Eds.), *Massachusetts General Hospital comprehensive clinical psychiatry* (pp. 895–905). St. Louis, MO: Mosby.

Harmon-Jones, E. (2007). Trait anger predicts relative left frontal cortical activation to anger-inducing stimuli. *International Journal of Psychophysiology, 66*(2), 154–160. doi:10.1016/j.ijpsycho.2007.03.020.

Harmon-Jones, E., & Sigelman, J. (2001). State anger prefrontal brain activity: Evidence that insult-related relative left-prefrontal activation is associated with experienced anger and aggression. *Journal of Personality and Social Psychology, 80*(5), 797–803. doi:10.1037/0022-3514.80.5.797.

Herdman, T.H. (Ed.). (2012). *NANDA International nursing diagnoses: Definitions & classification, 2012–2014.* Oxford, UK: Wiley-Blackwell.

Ito, M., Okazaki, M., Takahashi, S., et al. (2007). Subacute postictal aggression in patients with epilepsy. *Epilepsy Behaviour, 10*(4), 611–614.

Jorgensen, R.S., & Kolodziej, M.E. (2007). Suppressed anger, evaluative threat, and cardiovascular reactivity: A tripartite profile approach. *International Journal of Psychophysiology, 66*(2), 102–108. doi:10.1016/j.ijpsycho.2007.03.015.

Kassinove, H., & Tafrate, R.F. (2006). Anger-related disorders: Basic issues, models, and diagnostic considerations. In E.L. Feindler (Ed.), *Anger-related disorders: A practitioner's guide to comparative treatments* (pp. 1–27). New York: Springer.

Mehta, P.H., & Beer, J. (2010). Neural mechanisms of the testosterone-aggression relation: The role of orbitofrontal cortex. *Journal of Cognitive Neuroscience, 22*(10), 2357–2368.

Menninger, W.W. (2007). Uncontained rage: A psychoanalytic perspective on violence. *Bulletin of the Menninger Clinic, 71*(2), 115–131. doi:10.1521/bumc.2007.71.2.115.

Moorhead, S., Johnson, M., Maas, M.L., et al. (2008). *Nursing outcome classification (NOC)* (4th ed.). St. Louis, MO: Mosby.

Narayan, V.M., Narr, K.L., Kumari, V., et al. (2007). Regional cortical thinning in subjects with violent antisocial personality disorder or schizophrenia. *American Journal of Psychiatry, 164*(9), 1418–1427. doi:10.1176/appi.ajp.2007.06101631.

Neisewander, J. (2004). Amygdala. In W.E. Craighead, & C.B. Nemeroff (Eds.), *The concise Corsini encyclopedia of psychology and behavioral science* (3rd ed., Vol. 1, pp. 49–51). Hoboken, NJ: John Wiley and Sons.

Rabinak, C.A., & Maren, S. (2010). Amygdala. In I.B. Weiner & W.E. Craighead (Eds.), *The concise Corsini encyclopedia of psychology and behavioral science* (4th ed., Vol. 1, pp. 49–51). Mississauga, ON, Canada: John Wiley and Sons.

Safdar, S., Friedlmeier, W., Mastumoto, D., et al. (2009). Variations of emotional display rules within and across cultures: A comparison between Canada, USA, and Japan. *Canadian Journal of Behavioural Science, 41*(1), 1–10. doi:10.1037/a0014387.

Selye, H. (1976). *The stress of life.* New York: McGraw-Hill.

Siever, L.J. (2008). Neurobiology of aggression and violence. *American Journal of Psychiatry, 165,* 429–442. doi:10.1176/appi.ajp.2008.07111774.

Sirotich, F. (2008). Correlates of crime and violence among persons with mental disorder: An evidence-based review. *Brief Treatment and Crisis Intervention, 8*(2), 171–194. doi:10.1093/brief-treatment/mhn006.

Skinner, B. (1953). *Science and human behaviour.* New York: Macmillan.

Solomon, B.S., Bradshaw, C.P., Wright, J., et al. (2008). Youth and parental attitudes toward fighting. *Journal of Interpersonal Violence, 23*(4), 544–560. doi:10.1177/0886260507312947.

Workers' Compensation Board of British Columbia, Occupational Health and Safety Agency for Healthcare (OSAH), & Health Association of BC. (2002). *Guidelines: Code White response (a component of prevention and management of aggressive behaviour in health care).* Richmond, BC: Author.

# Interpersonal Violence: Child, Older Adult, and Intimate Partner Abuse

*Judi Sateren, Verna Benner Carson*
*Adapted by Susan L. Ray*

## KEY TERMS AND CONCEPTS

crisis situation, 551
ecological model, 547
economic abuse, 544
emotional abuse, 544
family violence, 543
neglect, 544
perpetrators, 548
physical abuse, 544

primary prevention, 560
safety plan, 558
secondary prevention, 561
sexual abuse, 544
survivor, 549
tertiary prevention, 561
typology of interpersonal violence, 543
vulnerable person, 549

## OBJECTIVES

1. Define interpersonal violence.
2. Identify three indicators of (a) physical abuse, (b) sexual abuse, (c) psychological or emotional abuse, and (d) deprivation or neglect.
3. Discuss the ecological model of violence in terms of etiology of abuse (e.g., stresses on the perpetrator, vulnerable person, and environment that could escalate anxiety to the point at which abuse becomes the relief behaviour).
4. Compare and contrast three characteristics of a perpetrator with three characteristics of a vulnerable person.

5. Describe four areas to assess when interviewing a person who has experienced abuse.
6. Formulate four nursing diagnoses for the survivor of abuse, and list supporting data from the assessment.
7. Write out a safety plan with the essential elements for a victim of intimate partner abuse.
8. Compare and contrast primary, secondary, and tertiary levels of intervention, giving two examples of intervention for each level.
9. Discuss three psychotherapeutic modalities useful in working with abusive families.

## ⊖volve WEBSITE

*Visit the Evolve website for Flashcards, Case Studies, and additional testing resources related to the content in this chapter:* http://evolve.elsevier.com/Canada/Varcarolis/psychiatric/ Pre-Test interactive review

According to the World Health Organization (WHO) (Krug, Dahlberg, Mercy, et al., 2002), interpersonal violence refers to violence between individuals and is subdivided into family and intimate partner violence and community violence. The former category includes child abuse, intimate partner violence, and older adult abuse, while the latter is broken down into acquaintance and stranger violence and includes youth violence, assault by strangers, violence related to property crimes, and violence in workplaces and other institutions. Figure 27-1 illustrates this typology of interpersonal violence, which is further broken down into four modes in which violence may be inflicted: physical abuse, sexual abuse, psychological or emotional abuse, and deprivation or neglect. Recently, economic abuse has been identified as a fifth mode in which violence can be inflicted. Interpersonal family violence includes child abuse, intimate partner abuse, and older adult abuse and can involve all five modes.

To be effective in working with victims, the nurse needs an understanding of the conditions for violence, the types of abuse,

**543**

**FIGURE 27-1** Typology of interpersonal violence. **Source**: Krug, E.G., Dahlberg, L.L.,
Mercy, J.A., et al. (Eds.). (2002). *World report
on violence and health.* Geneva, Switzerland:
World Health Organization. Retrieved from
http://www.who.int/violence_injury_
prevention/violence/world_report/en/.

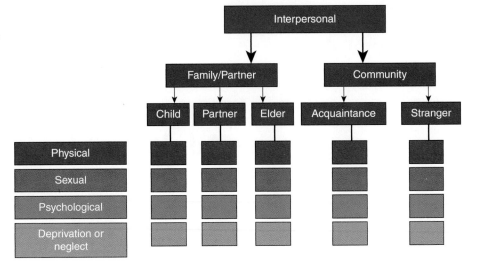

and the modes in which violence may be inflicted. Fundamental
to this entire discussion is self-understanding (see the Self-
Assessment section later in the chapter).

## CLINICAL PICTURE

### Types of Abuse

Five specific modes of abuse have been identified: (1) physical
abuse, (2) sexual abuse, (3) psychological or emotional abuse,
(4) deprivation or neglect, and (5) economic abuse. Physical
abuse is the infliction of physical pain or bodily harm (e.g.,
slapping, punching, hitting, choking, pushing, restraining,
biting, throwing, burning). Sexual abuse is any form of sexual
contact or exposure without consent or in circumstances in
which the victim is incapable of giving consent. Sexual abuse of
adults is usually referred to as *sexual assault* or *rape* and is discussed in Chapter 28. Emotional abuse is the infliction of
mental anguish and can take the form of any of the following:

- Terrorizing an individual through verbal threats
- Demeaning an individual's worth or putting the person
  down
- Directing blatant or subtle hostility and hatred toward an
  individual—or omitting positive behaviours such as warmth
  and affection
- Persistently ignoring an individual and her or his needs
- Humiliating or consistently belittling and criticizing an
  individual
- Isolating, or withholding support and companionship
- Threatening an individual with abandonment or institutionalization (e.g., nursing home, psychiatric hospital)
  Neglect, the failure to provide basic needs for a dependent,
can take several forms:
- Physical neglect is failure to provide for basic needs, such as
  shelter and food, or to protect from harm.
- Emotional neglect is failure to attend to basic emotional
  needs and nurturing.
- Educational neglect is failure to provide a child with experiences, including formal education necessary for intellectual
  growth and development.

- Medical neglect is failure to provide basic medical, dental, or
  psychiatric care.
  Economic abuse is the withholding of financial support or
the illegal or improper exploitation of funds or other resources
for one's personal gain.
  The five modes of abuse are described in more detail below.

### Physical Abuse

Covert indicators of violence could include minor accidents—
especially falls and a series of minor complaints, such as low
energy, fatigue, sleep problems, pain, swollen joints, sore
muscles, faintness, dizziness, memory loss, difficulty concentrating, ringing in ears, indigestion, and appetite loss (Ford-
Gilboe, Varcoe, & Merrit-Gray, 2010). Overt signs of battering
include bruises, scars, burns, and other wounds in various
stages of healing, particularly around the head, face, chest, arms,
abdomen, back, buttocks, and genitalia. Injuries that should
arouse the nurse's suspicion are listed in Box 27-1.

If the explanation does not match the injury or if the patient
minimizes the seriousness of the injury, abuse may be suspected. Ask directly, but in a nonthreatening manner, if the
injury has been caused by someone close to them. Observe the
nonverbal response, such as hesitation or lack of eye contact, as
well as the verbal response. Then ask specific questions such as
"When was the last time it happened? How often does it happen?
In what ways are you hurt?" Inconsistent explanations serve as
a warning that further investigation is necessary. Vague explanations should alert the nurse to possible abuse ("She fell from a
chair"; "The hot water was turned on by mistake"). The key to
identification is a high index of suspicion.

Nonspecific bruising in older children is a common sign of
abuse. Any bruises on an infant younger than 6 months of age
should be considered suspicious. *Shaken baby syndrome*, one of
the most serious types of child abuse, is the result of the brain
moving in the opposite direction as the baby's head (King,
MacKay, & Sirnick, 2003). A baby who has been shaken may
present with respiratory problems, bulging fontanels, and
central nervous system damage, resulting in seizures, vomiting,
and coma.

**COMMON PRESENTING PROBLEMS OF VICTIMS OF ABUSE**

**Emergency Department**
- Bleeding injuries, especially to head and face
- Internal injuries, concussions, perforated eardrum, abdominal injuries, severe bruising, eye injuries, strangulation marks on neck
- Back injuries
- Broken or fractured jaw, arms, pelvis, ribs, clavicle, legs
- Burns from cigarettes, appliances, scalding liquids, acids
- Psychological trauma, anxiety, attacks of hyperventilation, heart palpitations, severe crying spells, suicidal tendencies
- Miscarriage

**Ambulatory Care Settings**
- Perforated eardrum, twisted or stiff neck and shoulder muscles, headache
- Depression, stress-related conditions (e.g., insomnia, violent nightmares, anxiety, extreme fatigue, eczema, loss of hair)
- Talk of having "problems" with spouse; describing person as very jealous, impulsive, or an alcohol or drug abuser
- Repeated visits with new complaints
- Bruises of various ages and specific shapes (fingers, belt)

**Any Setting**
- Signs of stress due to family violence: emotional, behavioural, school, or sleep problems and increase in aggressive behaviour
- Injuries in a pregnant woman
- Recurrent visits for injuries attributed to being "accident prone"

## Sexual Abuse

There are a variety of emotional and behavioural consequences of sexual abuse, including depression, anxiety, suicide, aggression, chronic low self-esteem, and PTSD (Draughon & Urbancic, 2010). Childhood sexual abuse is a significant factor in the development of depression in many women (Draughon & Urbancic, 2010). Girls are at higher risk for sexual abuse, although boys may be less likely to report it, and, therefore, it is less recognized and less treated (Ramsey & Abrams, 2010).

## Emotional Abuse

Emotional abuse may exist on its own or as a result of co-occurring physical or sexual abuse. Emotional abuse has devastating effects on children. Although it is less obvious and more difficult to assess than physical violence, studies have shown that those who were emotionally abused as children show higher rates of anxiety, depression, interpersonal sensitivity, and dissociation (Draughon & Urbancic, 2010).

## Neglect

Neglected children and older adults often appear undernourished, dirty, and poorly clothed. Neglect is also manifested by inadequate medical care, such as lack of immunizations or untreated medical conditions. Adults who were neglected in

childhood are more likely to report current symptoms of anxiety, depression, somatization, paranoia, and hostility than those who were physically abused but did not suffer neglect (Draughon & Urbancic, 2010).

## Economic Abuse

Economic abuse results when the abuser has complete control over the victim's money and other economic resources or activities, thereby reducing the victim to complete dependence for money to meet personal needs. Economic abuse can include limiting access to funds and credit; controlling access to health care, employment, and education; and deciding without regard to the victim how the money is to be spent or saved (Fawole, 2008).

## Cycle of Violence

Dr. Donald Dutton studied the relationship of borderline personality organization (BPO) to the characteristics of both chronic and intermittent family abusers. Dutton (2007) identified three BPO characteristics: (1) an unstable sense of self with dependency and fear of abandonment, (2) unstable interpersonal relationships with manipulation, and (3) intense and impulsive behaviours, as relating to the cycle of violence perpetrators use to control their partners.

The *cycle of violence*, first proposed by Walker (1979), includes three recurring phases of violence. These phases are characterized by periods of intense violence that tend to increase in severity and frequency, alternating with periods of safety, hope, and trust. Phase I of the borderline, or *cyclic*, personality consists of an internal buildup of tensions as a result of the abuser not knowing how to verbalize inner feelings of dysphoria. The abuser converts dysphoria into abuse through the assertion that it is the partner's fault for not being able to soothe the abuser's bad feelings (Dutton, 1998, 2007). The *tension-building stage* is characterized by relatively minor incidents, such as pushing, shoving, and verbal abuse. During this time, the victim often ignores or accepts the abuse for fear that more severe abuse will follow. Abusers then rationalize that their abusive behaviour is acceptable. As the tension escalates, both participants may try to reduce it. The abuser may try to reduce the tension with the use of alcohol or drugs, and the victim may try to reduce the tension by minimizing the importance of the incidents ("I should have had the house neater … dinner ready"). The abuser may become increasingly demanding. The splitting characteristics of BPO become evident, as the abuser sees the partner as "all bad"—unloving, unfaithful, and malevolent (Dutton, 1998, 2007). During the *acute battering stage*, the unexpressed rage builds until the abuser with BPO releases the built-up tension by brutal beatings. Severe injuries can and do result, driving the victim further away and increasing the abuser's feelings of abandonment. Consequently, the abuser promises anything to get the victim back. The opposite side of splitting here becomes evident, as the abuser describes the victim as "all good" (Dutton, 1998, p. 96). This phase coincides with the *honeymoon stage*, which may be characterized by kindness and loving behaviours. The abuser, at least initially, feels remorseful and apologetic and may bring presents, make promises, and tell the victim how

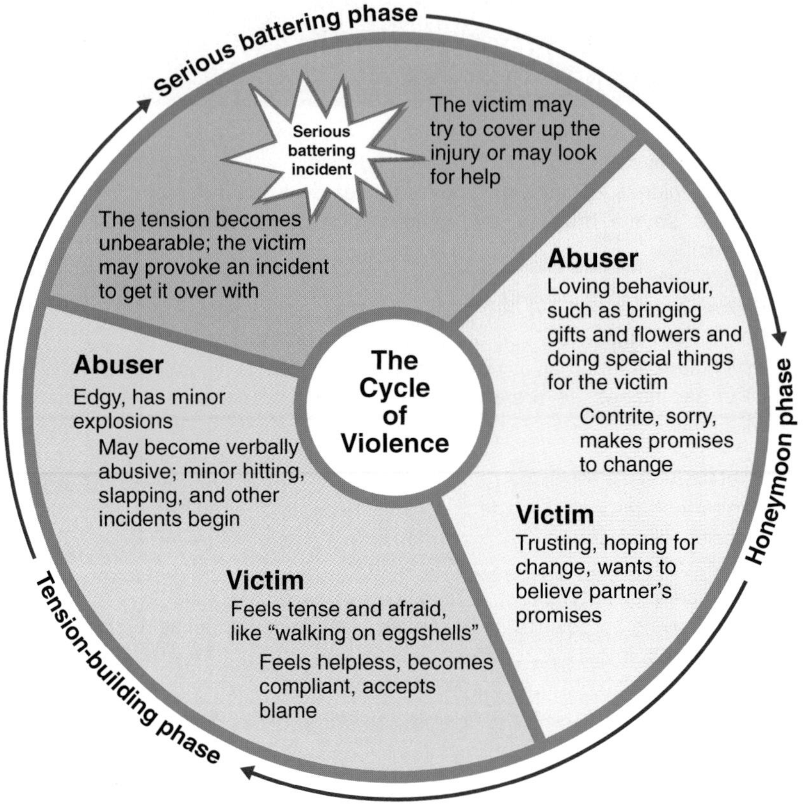

**FIGURE 27-2** The cycle of violence. **Source:** Redrawn from YWCA of Annapolis and Anne Arundel County, 1517 Ritchie Highway, Arnold, MD 21012.

much she or he is loved and needed. The victim usually believes the promises, feels needed and loved, and drops any legal proceedings or plans to leave that may have been initiated during the acute battering stage.

Unfortunately, without intervention, the cycle will repeat itself. Over time, the periods of calmness and safety become briefer, and the periods of anger and violence increase. With each repeat of the pattern, the victim's self-esteem becomes more and more eroded. The victim either believes the violence was deserved or accepts the blame for it. This self-blame can lead to feelings of depression, hopelessness, immobilization, and self-deprecation. Figure 27-2 illustrates the cycle of violence.

## EPIDEMIOLOGY

Abuse within families is among the most important Canadian public health issue and is therefore a significant nursing concern. The abusive behaviours exist within a context in which their purpose is to gain power and control and to induce fear. Abusive behaviour may involve one or more of the types of violence already described and may be inflicted upon a child, an intimate partner, an older adult or other populations. While the true prevalence of child, older adult, and intimate partner abuse is unknown (because of under-reporting and variability in reporting methods, instruments, sites, and reporters), it is clear that abuse is a significant problem.

### Child Abuse

In 2008, the Canadian Incidence Study (CIS) of Reported Child Abuse and Neglect (Public Health Agency of Canada, 2010)

estimated 85 440 substantiated child-abuse investigations that year (14.19 investigations per 1000 children). Thirty-four percent identified exposure to intimate partner violence as the primary type of abuse and another 34% identified neglect as the overriding concern, followed by physical abuse (20%), emotional abuse (9%), and sexual abuse (3%). There was some variation by age and sex in the incidence of investigated abuse with rates being highest for infants. The rate of family-related sexual offences was more than four times higher for girls than for boys, and the rate of physical assault was similar for girls and boys (Statistics Canada, 2009). According to the CIS (Public Health Agency of Canada, 2010), 94% of substantiated investigations involved children whose primary caregiver was a biological parent, and 2% lived with a primary caregiver who was a parent's partner or an adoptive parent.

Aboriginal children were identified as a key group to examine because of concerns about their over-representation in the foster care system (Trocmé, MacLaurin, Fallon, et al., 2006). The rate of substantiated child abuse investigations was four times higher in Aboriginal child investigations than non-Aboriginal child investigations.

### Intimate Partner Abuse

Spousal abuse is also referred to as *intimate partner violence (IPV)* and *domestic violence (DV)*. According to Statistics Canada (2009), of the 19 million Canadians who had a current or former spouse, 6% reported being physically or sexually victimized by their partner or spouse in the preceding five years. Spousal violence was more likely to occur between ex-spouses or -partners than current spouses or partners. According to the

Canadian Centre for Justice (2009), females accounted for 83% of spousal abuse that is reported to the police, compared to 17% for men. Females were also more likely than males to report multiple victimizations in cases of spousal abuse, at 57% and 40% respectively. Canadians living in common-law relationships were approximately three times more likely than their married counterparts to report having experienced at least one incident of spousal violence in the previous 12 months. Those who self-identified as gay or lesbian were more than twice as likely as heterosexuals to report having experienced spousal violence, while those who self-identified as bisexual were four times more likely than heterosexuals to self-report spousal violence. Household income and education levels were found to have had little impact on experiencing spousal violence. Those who self-identified as an Aboriginal person were almost twice as likely as those who did not to report being the victim of spousal violence (10% versus 6%) (Canadian Centre for Justice Statistics, 2009).

## Older Adult Abuse

The rate of violent victimization for older adults was less than half that for adults aged 55 to 64 and more than eight times lower than the rate for adults aged 25 to 34 (Statistics Canada, 2009). Lower rates of family violence among older adults compared to their younger counterparts may be linked to differences in their living situations. Older adults aged 75 years and older are more likely to live alone or in an institutional setting than older adults under age 75 are (Turcotte & Schellenberg, 2007). Although the overall rate of violent victimization was higher for older adult men than for older adult women, family-related violent victimization was higher among older adult women. Older adult men were more likely to be victimized by an acquaintance or a stranger than a family member.

## CO-MORBIDITY

Common long-term psychological and social effects of abuse include depression, suicidal ideation, chronic post-traumatic stress symptoms, dissociation, interpersonal disturbances, substance abuse, and revictimization (Bonomi, Anderson, Rivara, et al., 2007; Dube, Anda, Whitfield, et al., 2005; Fergusson, Boden, & Horwood, 2008). Family violence is common in the childhood histories of juvenile offenders, runaways, violent criminals, prostitutes, and those who in turn are violent toward others. Exposure to abuse has been associated with decrements in children's optimal development in the areas of social behaviour, academic performance, physical health, and mental health (Graham-Bermann, Gruber, Girz, et al., 2009; Skopp, McDonald, Jouriles, et al., 2007).

The increased occurrence of prolonged childhood sexual abuse in girls may contribute to the increased prevalence of stress disorders reported in women (Carter-Snell & Hegadoren, 2003). When health care providers do not routinely assess for history of childhood sexual abuse, symptoms arising in times of crisis may be labelled as adult psychopathological disorders and not understood as possible post-traumatic stress responses

---

### BOX 27-2 LONG-TERM EFFECTS OF FAMILY VIOLENCE

- People involved in family violence are found to have a higher incidence of:
  - Depression
  - Suicidal feelings
  - Self-contempt
  - Inability to trust
  - Inability to develop intimate relationships in later life
- Victims of severe violence are also at higher risk for experiencing recurring symptoms of post-traumatic stress disorder (PTSD):
  - Flashbacks
  - Dissociation—out-of-body experiences
  - Poor self-esteem
  - Compulsive or impulsive behaviours (e.g., substance abuse, excessive spending, gambling, and promiscuity)
  - Multiple somatic complaints
- Children who witness violence in their homes are at greater risk for developing behavioural and emotional problems throughout their lives.
- After the age of 5 or 6, children who witness violence at home show an indication of identifying with the aggressor and losing respect for the victim.
- Some mental and behavioural conditions are associated with childhood abuse or witnessing of abuse:
  - Depressive disorders
  - Post-traumatic stress disorder
  - Somatic complaints
  - Low self-esteem
  - Phobias (agoraphobia, social and specific phobias)
  - Antisocial behaviours
  - Potential for future child or spousal abuse
- Adolescent victims or witnesses of abuse are more likely to have behavioural symptoms such as:
  - Failing grades
  - Difficulty forming relationships
  - Increased incidence of theft, police arrest, and violent behaviours
  - Seductive or promiscuous behaviours
  - Running away from home

---

(Carter-Snell & Hegadoren, 2003). Box 27-2 identifies some of the long-term effects of family violence.

## ETIOLOGY

### The Ecological Model

The WHO adopted an "ecological model" in its *World Report on Violence and Health* to help understand the multilevel, multifaceted nature of violence (Krug, Dahlberg, Mercy, et al., 2002). As an analytical tool, the ecological model (see Figure 27-3) recognizes and identifies personal history and characteristics of the victim or perpetrator, other family members, the immediate social context (often referred to as *community factors*), and the characteristics of the larger society. In contrast to simplistic explanations, the ecological model emphasizes that it is a *combination* of factors, acting at different levels, that

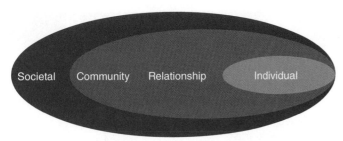

**FIGURE 27-3** The ecological model of violence. **Source:** Krug, E.G., Dahlberg, L.L., Mercy, J.A., et al. (Eds.). (2002). *World report on violence and health.* Geneva, Switzerland: World Health Organization. Retrieved from http://www.who.int/violence_injury_prevention/violence/world_report/en/.

influence the risk and resiliency for violence and the potential for recurrence of abuse. The various factors relevant to the different levels of the ecological model will also be affected by the context of the settings that children interact with—in their home and family environment, at school, in institutions and workplaces, as well as in their community and broader society.

### Environmental Factors

Violence and abuse occur across all segments of Canadian society. While some risk factors may be unique to a particular type of violence, the various types of violence more commonly share a number of risk factors. Prevailing cultural norms, poverty, social isolation, and such factors as alcohol abuse, substance abuse, and access to firearms are risk factors for more than one type of violence (Krug, Dahlberg, Mercy, et al., 2002).

The occurrence of abuse requires the following participants and conditions:
- A perpetrator
- Someone who, by age or situation, is vulnerable (e.g., child, woman, older adult, mentally ill or physically challenged person)
- A crisis situation

### Perpetrator

Perpetrators, those who initiate violence, often consider their own needs to be more important than anyone else's and look to others to meet their needs. The term *perpetrator* applies to any member of a household who is violent toward another member (e.g., children, siblings, same-sex partners, extended family members). Risk factors for those who may become abusive to their children are summarized in Box 27-3.

Control and power are acted out by perpetrators of abuse in all stages of the cycle of violence. The abuse of power and control is the foundational etiology of relationship violence (see Figure 27-4), with additional ecological risk and resiliency factors determining the typology. Because of extreme pathological jealousy, many perpetrators of relationship violence refuse to allow their partners to work outside the home; others demand that their partners work in the same place as they do so they can monitor activities and friendships. Many accompany their partners to and from all activities and forbid them

### BOX 27-3   CHARACTERISTICS OF ABUSIVE PARENTS

- A history of abuse, neglect, or emotional deprivation as a child
- Family authoritarianism: a commitment to raising children as they were raised by their own parents
- Low self-esteem, feelings of worthlessness, depression
- Poor coping skills
- Social isolation (may be suspicious of others): few or no friends, little or no involvement in social or community activities
- Involvement in a crisis situation: unemployment, divorce, financial difficulties
- Rigid, unrealistic expectations of child's behaviour
- History of severe mental illness
- Violent temper outbursts
- Looking to child for satisfaction of need for love, support, and reassurance (often unmet because of parenting deficits in family of origin)
- Projection of blame onto the child for parents' "troubles" (e.g., step-parent may project hostility toward new mate onto a child)
- Lack of effective parenting skills
- Inability to seek help from others
- Perception of the child as bad or evil
- History of drug or alcohol abuse
- Feeling of little or no control over life
- Low tolerance for frustration
- Poor impulse control

to have personal friends or participate in recreational activities outside the home. Even after imposing such restrictions, perpetrators often accuse their partners of infidelity. Many perpetrators maintain their control and possessiveness by controlling the family finances so tightly that there is barely enough money for daily living. Typically, perpetrators believe in male supremacy—being in charge and being dominant. Messages of male dominance are reinforced via observations of the partner dyad, parent–child interactions, peer group experiences, and the influence of the media (Internet, television, movies, comics, computer games).

Culturally driven violence against women is a growing problem in Canada's immigrant communities (Papp, 2010). However, it is important to recognize that a wide variety of cultural norms in Canadian society dictate the dynamics of relationships between intimate partners and child-rearing practices. Learning about the cultural backgrounds of patients can assist health care providers in identifying risk factors and culturally appropriate interventions.

Parental substance abuse is associated with a more than twofold increase in the risk of exposure to both childhood physical and sexual abuse (Walsh, MacMillan, & Jamieson, 2003). Abbey, Zawacki, Buck, and colleagues (2004) found three factors related to alcohol abuse and violence: (1) alcohol-induced cognitive impairment, (2) users' expectation that alcohol increases aggression, and (3) sociocultural beliefs that people are unaccountable for their behaviour while intoxicated.

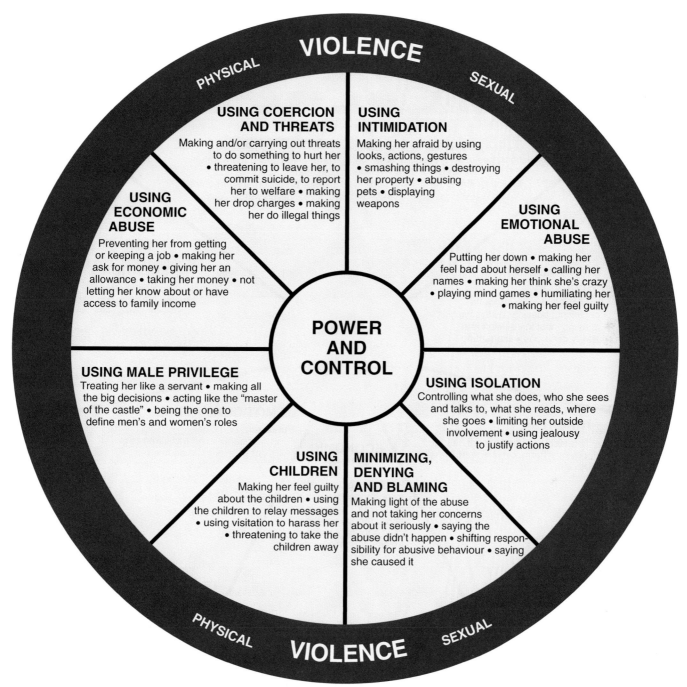

**FIGURE 27-4** The Duluth "Power and Control" wheel. **Source:** Redrawn from Domestic Abuse Intervention Programs, 202 East Superior Street, Duluth, MN 55802. Retrieved from http://www.theduluthmodel.org/training/wheels.html.

The belief that intoxicated behaviour will be judged less harshly may lead perpetrators to justify their behaviour by blaming their actions on alcohol or other substances.

### Vulnerable Person

The **vulnerable person** is an adult or child who, as a result of illness, physical condition, or experiences, is at greater risk than the general population for being harmed. The term **survivor** recognizes the recovery and healing process that follows victimization and does not have the connotation of passivity that *victim* has.

***Women.*** Pregnancy may trigger or increase violence. The Public Health Agency of Canada (2004) reported the prevalence of abuse during pregnancy to be 5.7% to 6.6% based on two major studies done in Saskatoon and Toronto. A past history of abuse is one of the strongest predictors of abuse during pregnancy. Other risk factors include social instability (e.g., young, unmarried, failed to complete high school, unemployed, having an unplanned pregnancy), an unhealthy lifestyle (e.g., unhealthy diet, alcohol use, illicit drug use, emotional problems), and physical and psychological health problems (including prescription drug use).

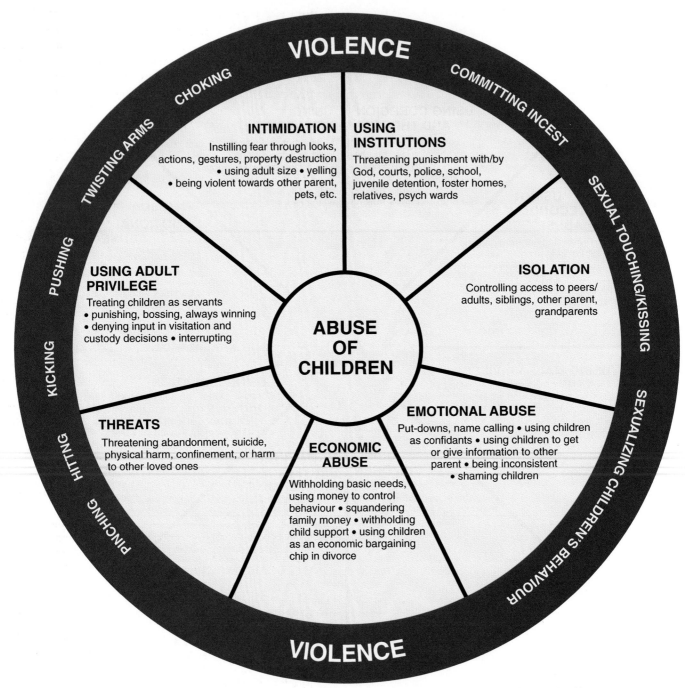

**FIGURE 27-5**  The Duluth "Abuse of Children" wheel. **Source:** Redrawn from Domestic Abuse Intervention Programs, 202 East Superior Street, Duluth, MN 55802. Retrieved from http://www.theduluthmodel.org/training/wheels.html.

*Children.* The Canadian Incidence Study (Public Health Agency of Canada, 2010) found that, in 46% of substantiated child-abuse investigations, at least one child functioning issue was indicated. Academic difficulties were the most frequently reported functioning concern (23%), with 11% involving intellectual or developmental disabilities. The second most common was depression, anxiety, or withdrawal (19%). Fifteen percent of cases involved child aggression, while 14% involved attachment issues. Eleven percent of investigations involved children experiencing attention deficit disorder (ADD) or attention

deficit hyperactivity disorder (ADHD). The increased risk for abuse could be due to the added stress of caring for a child with functioning difficulties as well as the differences between the parents' expectations of their child and the reality of who the child is. As with relationship violence more broadly, the abuse of power and control and particular risks for child abuse are described in the Duluth model (see Figure 27-5).

*Older adults.* Older adult abuse is recognized as a serious problem in Canada. In 2007, 1938 incidents of family violence against older adults were reported to police, representing more than one third of all violent incidents committed against older adults (Statistics Canada, 2009). Risk factors for older adult abuse include cognitive disability (e.g., Alzheimer's disease) or other mental illness, poor physical health, impairment in the activities of daily living (ADLs), dependency on the caregiver, isolation, stressful events, and a history of intergenerational conflict between the older adult and the caregiver (Fulmer, Sengstock, Blankenship, et al., 2010).

### Crisis Situation

Anyone may be at risk for abuse in a *crisis situation*—a situation that puts stress on a family that includes a violent member. In the CIS (Public Health Agency of Canada, 2010) report, 78% of substantiated child-abuse cases reported at least one primary caregiver risk factor. The most frequently noted concerns for primary caregivers were being a victim of domestic violence (46%), having few social supports because of frequent moves (39%), and having mental health issues (27%). Refer to Chapter 24 for more on crisis and crisis intervention.

## APPLICATION OF THE NURSING PROCESS

## ASSESSMENT

Assessment includes standard clinical assessment procedures that will vary depending on the population, setting, and stage of acuity or crisis related to abuse or violence. Basic guidelines include using a compassionate manner with attention to the details of the signs and symptoms of violence, as well as coping, supports, and current states of crises, including suicidal or homicidal ideation (see Assessment Guidelines box).

### General Assessment

It has been increasingly recommended that routine universal screening for violence be implemented within all manner of health care settings (Jack, Jamieson, Wathen, et al., 2008;

 **ASSESSMENT GUIDELINES**

### *Family Violence*

During assessment and counselling, maintain an interested and empathetic manner. Assess:
- Presenting signs and symptoms of victims of abuse
- Potential indicators of vulnerable parents who might benefit from education and instruction in effective coping techniques
- Physical, sexual, or emotional abuse, neglect, and economic maltreatment of older adults
- Family coping patterns
- Patient's support system
- Drug or alcohol use
- Suicidal or homicidal ideas
- Post-traumatic stress

If the patient is a child or older adult, identify the protective services in your province that must be notified.

Registered Nurses' Association of Ontario, 2005). The nurse is often the first point of contact for people experiencing abuse and thus is in an ideal position to contribute to prevention, detection, and effective intervention. Organizations need to develop policies that support nursing practice while considering the unique setting where the screening is to take place, patient needs, and outcomes (Perinatal Partnership Program of Eastern and Southeastern Ontario, 2004).

Effective programs to assess and intervene with violence target specific populations based on the risk and resiliency factors described as part of the clinical picture. Pregnant women are just one population considered at risk for violence and abuse (see Research Highlight box).

 **RESEARCH HIGHLIGHT**

### *Population at Risk—Maternal Exposure to Domestic Violence*

**Source:** Shah, P.S., & Shah, J. (2010). Maternal exposure to domestic violence and pregnancy and birth outcomes: A systematic review and meta-analysis. *Journal of Women's Health, 19*(11), 2017–2031. doi:10.1089/jwh.2010.2051.

**Problem**
The Knowledge Synthesis Group on Determinants of Preterm/Low-Birth-Weight Births has identified that women's exposure to domestic violence has implications for the woman, for the fetus, and for society.

**Purpose of Study**
The study aimed to identify risk factors for prenatal domestic violence in order to intervene before the fetus is at risk.

**Methods**
A systematic review and meta-analysis of 30 studies was conducted. The analysis focused on identifying the birth outcomes of women who experienced domestic violence.

**Key Findings**
This group concluded that the experience of domestic violence is under-reported and that effective programs are required to identify domestic violence and intervene during pregnancy.

**Implications for Nursing Practice**
Nurses need to screen for domestic violence, particularly during pregnancy.

### Interview Process and Setting

Important and relevant information about the family situation can be incorporated into a routine health history process. Because many victims of violence do not disclose abuse the first time they are asked, nor do they recognize violence as a health issue, screening for abuse among women and their families should occur not only on the initial health history but also each time the health history is updated (Registered Nurses' Association of Ontario, 2005). For screening strategies, refer to Woman Abuse: Screening, Identification and Initial Response at http://rnao.ca/bpg/guidelines/woman-abuse-screening-identification-and-initial-response.

1. **Within the last year**, have you been hit, slapped, kicked, pushed, shoved, or otherwise physically hurt by someone?  YES    NO

   If YES, who? (Circle all that apply)

   Intimate partner    Care provider    Health professional    Family member    Other

   Please describe: _____    _____

2. **Within the last year**, has anyone forced you to have sexual activities?    YES    NO

   If YES, who? (Circle all that apply)

   Intimate partner    Care provider    Health professional    Family member    Other

   Please describe: _____    _____

3. **Within the last year**, has anyone prevented you from using a wheelchair, cane, respirator, or other assistive devices?    YES    NO

   If YES, who? (Circle all that apply)

   Intimate partner    Care provider    Health professional    Family member    Other

   Please describe: _____    _____

4. **Within the last year**, has anyone you depend on refused to help you with an important personal need, such as taking your medicine, getting to the bathroom, getting out of bed, bathing, getting dressed, or getting food or drink?    YES    NO

   If YES, who? (Circle all that apply)

   Intimate partner    Care provider    Health professional    Family member    Other

   Please describe: _____    _____

**FIGURE 27-6**    Abuse assessment screen. **Source:** McFarlane, J., Hughes, R.B., Nosek, M.A., et al. (2001). Abuse assessment screen—disability (AAS-D): Measuring frequency, type, and perpetrator of abuse toward women with physical disabilities. *Journal of Women's Health & Gender-Based Medicine, 10*, 861–866. doi:10.1089/152460901753285750. The publisher for this copyrighted material is Mary Ann Liebert, Inc. publishers.

Screening tools use specific terminology that describe the *actions* of abusers rather than using general terminology like "abuse." Therefore, screening questions need to be clear and examples of abusive behaviour may be needed to help the patient understand what constitutes abusive behaviour. There are validated tools that can be used in screening (e.g., the Abuse Assessment Screen [AAS], the Abuse Assessment Screen—Disability [AAS-D], and the Woman Abuse Screening Tool [WAST]), or nurses can develop their own style, keeping in mind these principles (Registered Nurses' Association of Ontaraio, 2005). The Abuse Assessment Screen developed by the Nursing Research Consortium on Violence and Abuse (McFarlane, Hughes, Nosek, et al., 2001) has been used extensively to assist in the routine identification of intimate partner abuse (Figure 27-6).

Guiding principles for screening for abuse will assist the nurse in implementing effective interventions. The adapted mnemonic tool **ABCD-ER**, explained in Box 27-4, outlines the principles.

In the case of suspected child abuse or neglect, it is better to ask about methods of disciplining children rather than to use the words *abuse* or *violence*. Questions that are open-ended and require a descriptive response can be less threatening and elicit more relevant information than questions that are direct or can be answered with *yes* or *no* (see Chapter 11):

- What arrangements do you make when you have to leave your child alone?
- How do you discipline your child?
- When your infant cries for a long time, how do you get him or her to stop?
- What about your child's behaviour bothers you the most?

Areas to include in any abuse assessment (child, older adult, IPV) include the following: (1) violence indicators, (2) levels of anxiety and coping responses, (3) family coping patterns, (4) support systems, (5) suicide potential, (6) homicide potential, and (7) drug and alcohol use. The vignette on page 554 illustrates the key points in assessing a woman in crisis at the initial interview, as well as suggested follow-up.

### Maintaining Accurate Records

Documentation is an integral aspect of safe, effective nursing practice and must be comprehensive and legible and accurately reflect screening practice (College of Registered Nurses of Nova Scotia, 2012; Northwest Territories Health and Social Services,

## BOX 27-4  THE MNEMONIC TOOL ABCD-ER

**A—Attitude** and **Approachability** of the health care provider:
- Treat the patient with respect, dignity, and compassion.
- Be sensitive to differences in age, culture, language, ethnicity, and sexual orientation.
- State clearly that abuse is not the fault of the victim but the responsibility of the abuser.
- Reinforce that no one has the right to use physical, sexual, or emotional abuse to control another person's actions.
- Reinforce that physical and sexual abuse are against the law in Canada.
- Convey a nonthreatening, nonjudgemental stance in words, facial expressions, and body language.
- Express concern for the patient's safety.
- Acknowledge the strength the patient has shown in surviving abuse and disclosing it to you.
- Offer support.
- Avoid excessive criticism of the abuser.

**B—Belief** in the person's account of his or her own experience of abuse:
- Show by your words and your actions that you believe the patient's disclosure.
- Remember that the fear of not being believed silences many victims of abuse. Abusers may also convince victims that no one will believe them if they disclose the abuse.
- Help the patient to understand that most of us try to block out memories that are too painful to deal with. A patient disclosing retrospective abuse may not even be sure of exactly what happened or where.
- Reassure and encourage the patient to have confidence in her or his own perceptions of the abuse.

**C—Confidentiality** is essential for disclosure:
- Interview in private, without the patient's partner or family members present.
- Use a professional interpreter if one is required, not a friend or family member.
- Tell the patient directly about the policies and procedures used in your practice or institution to protect patient confidentiality.
- Assure the patient that you will not release the information unless he or she gives written permission.
- Outline the exceptions to this pledge of confidentiality: (1) where child abuse or neglect is in question; (2) where the health care provider has reason to fear for the safety of a third party; and (3) where a file is subpoenaed by a court order.
- Let the patient know that you are documenting the information disclosed so that it will help you provide appropriate medical services and referrals and so that it will be available to help the patient later if she or he should provide you with permission to share it.

**D—Documentation:**
- Document consistently and legibly.

- Distinguish between your observations and the patient's reports.
- Record information on the first, the worst, and the most recent abusive incident.
- If more than one person has abused the patient, distinguish between the abusers and the specific injuries or health effects of each incident.
- Indicate the frequency of abusive incidents, as well as any increase or decrease in frequency and seriousness.
- Avoid subjective statements and speculations that might undermine the patient's credibility.
- Use the patient's own words, in quotation marks, as frequently as possible.
- Use diagrams and photographs where possible to document physical injuries.

**E—Education:**
- Educate about abuse and its health effects.
- Help the patient to understand that she or he is not alone.
- Attempt to engage the patient in long-term continuity of care by offering appropriate referrals and follow-up.
- Know about available community resources and help the patient choose the services he or she needs when ready to seek assistance.
- Display posters, brochures, and other available information about abuse in your office or institution.
- Provide the female patient with information about the abused women's helpline and the male patient with information about the crisis hotline.

**R—Respect and Recognition:**
- Respect the integrity and autonomy of the patient's life choices.
- Recognize that the patient must deal with the abuse at her or his own pace directed by her or his own decisions.
- Recognize that an abused person is an expert about his or her own abuse and abuser.
- Affirm the patient's strengths and survival skills.
- Do not try to tell the patient what to do but help him or her understand the options available; the patient must choose the options that will meet his or her own goals and priorities.
- Offer referrals to other specialized services and follow-up with you.
- Do not label the patient resistant or nonadherent if she or he decides not to accept your advice; make it clear you respect the patient's right to choose and will continue your support as her or his caregiver.
- Make sure any medications you offer to help the patient deal with stress or sleep problems do not impair the patient's ability to act appropriately on his or her own behalf.
- Help the patient to recognize that she or he cannot control the actions of others; the patient can choose only her or his own actions.

**Source:** Adapted from Middlesex-London Health Unit. (2000). *Task force on the health effects of woman abuse—Final report*. London, ON: Author.

2009), as it may be used by the justice system as evidence during legal proceedings (Rozovsky & Inions, 2003). According to the Registered Nurses' Association of Ontario (2005), the health care record needs to include the following:

- A safety check
- Direct quotations of what the victim describes
- Direct observations made by the nurse
- Referrals discussed and made and information given

The record should be nonbiased, containing direct observations by the nurse. Nonbiased terms such as "chooses," "declines," or "patient states" are more appropriate than judgemental terms like "alleges" or "victim" (Middlesex-London Health Unit, 2000). For example, it would be better to record "Patient states, 'My partner beat me'" (nonjudgemental) than "Victim alleges he was assaulted by partner" (judgemental).

Referral services and secondary intervention would include more detailed documentation such as the following (Middlesex-London Health Unit, 2000):

- Relevant health history
- History of abuse, including the first, worst, and most recent incident
- Where and when the abuse took place
- Name of and relationship to abuser
- Detailed description of injuries (e.g., a body map to indicate size, colour, shape, areas, and types of injuries, with explanations [see Figure 27-6] and photos if taken)
- Physical evidence of sexual abuse, when possible
- All health care provided and information or referrals to resources provided

When no disclosure of abuse is made, the nurse should document "no disclosure to abuse screening."

Legal, ethical, and professional requirements guide the management of patient records (College of Nurses of Ontario, 2008; Personal Health Information Protection Act, 2004; Rozovsky & Inions, 2003). Policies and procedures concerning access to the patient's health information need to be developed as part of the screening protocol in all health care settings (Registered Nurses' Association of Ontario, 2005). The patient needs to be informed prior to screening that the interaction will be documented, that the record will be kept confidential, and that it can serve as evidence should legal action be initiated. Even if further intervention or legal action does not occur at this time, the record is begun, and the next provider will be aware of the problem and be in a better position to offer support. The vignette illustrates some of the issues related to assessment that are important for reporting and documentation for a patient experiencing family violence.

## Self-Assessment

Self-reflection assists nurses in all areas of practice to identify the values and biases that underscore their approach and interventions in response to those experiencing abuse (Registered Nurses' Association of Ontario, 2005). Strong negative feelings can cloud one's judgement and interfere with objective assessment and intervention, no matter how well we try to cover or deny personal bias. Common responses of health care providers to violence are listed in Table 27-1.

---

**VIGNETTE**

Petra Darnell is brought to the emergency department by ambulance in obvious distress with swollen eyes, lips, nose, and lacerations to her face. She tells the nurse that her husband had been in bed asleep for hours before she joined him. On getting into bed, she attempted to redistribute the blankets. Suddenly he started punching her in the face and began to throw her against the wall. She called out to her 11-year-old son to call the police. The police arrived, called an ambulance, and took Mr. Darnell to jail. The nurse takes Mrs. Darnell to an individual examination room (to emphasize confidentiality) for a full assessment. Mrs. Darnell describes the relationship as "stormy" and "bad for a long time."

"He is always putting me down and yelling at me," she states. He started hitting her five years earlier when she became pregnant with her second and last child. The beatings have increased in intensity over the past year, and this emergency department visit is the fifth this year. Tonight is the first time she has ever called the police.

Mrs. Darnell has visibly lost control. Periods of crying alternate with periods of silence. She appears apathetic and depressed. The nurse remains calm and objective. After Mrs. Darnell has finished talking, the nurse explores alternatives designed to help her reduce the danger once she is discharged. "I'm concerned that you will be hurt again if you go home. What options do you have?" Acknowledging the escalating intensity of the violence, Mrs. Darnell is able to make arrangements with a shelter to take in her and her two children until after she has secured a restraining order. The nurse charts the abuse referrals. The keeping of careful and complete records helps ensure that Mrs. Darnell will receive proper follow-up care and will assist Mrs. Darnell when and if she pursues legal action.

---

Since nursing is largely made up of women and women are more commonly the targets of abuse, it has been suggested that many nurses have experienced or are experiencing violence at the hands of their intimate partners (Registered Nurses' Association of Ontario, 2005). Nurses need to become aware of their reactions by gaining insight into their own somatic signals of distress (Robinson, Clements, & Land, 2003). Supervision and multidisciplinary team conferences can be especially helpful in clarifying reactions, neutralizing intense emotions, and reducing feelings of isolation and discomfort.

## Level of Anxiety and Coping Responses

Nonverbal responses to the assessment interview can be indicative of the victim's anxiety level (see Chapter 13). Agitation and anxiety bordering on panic are often present in victims of violence. Abused individuals live under conditions of chronic stress, which can lead to health effects such as heart disease or heart attack, arthritis, fibromyalgia, asthma, stroke (Ford-Gilboe, Varcoe, & Merrit-Gray, 2010), and cervical cancer (Coker, Hopenhayn, DeSimone, et al., 2009). Coping mechanisms to endure living in violent and terrifying situations may take the form of flawed beliefs or myths (Table 27-2).

| TABLE 27-1 | COMMON RESPONSES OF HEALTH CARE PROVIDERS TO VIOLENCE |
|---|---|
| **RESPONSE** | **SOURCE** |
| Anger | Anger may be felt toward the person responsible for the abuse, toward those who allowed it to happen, and toward society for condoning its occurrence through attitudes, traditions, and laws. |
| Embarrassment | The victim may be a symbol of something close to home: the nurse may have experienced abuse. |
| Confusion | One's view of the family as a haven of safety and privacy is challenged. |
| Fear | A small percentage of perpetrators are dangerous to others. |
| Helplessness | The nurse may want to do more, eliminate the problem, or cure the victim, perpetrator, or both. |
| Discouragement | Discouragement may result if no long-term solution is achieved. |
| "Blame the victim" mentality | Health care workers can get caught up in "blaming the victim" for behaviours they see as provoking the abuse. There is never an excuse for abuse, and no one has the right to hurt another person. "Blaming the victim" can occur when health care providers feel overwhelmed. Supervision is essential for therapeutic intervention. |

| TABLE 27-2 | MYTH VERSUS FACT: FAMILY ABUSE |
|---|---|
| **MYTH** | **FACT** |
| Ninety-five percent of intimate partner abuse victims are women. | Recent surveys report 40% of men had partners who hit them first, and 66% of men had partners who were also violent (Statistics Canada, 2009). |
| The victim's behaviour often causes violence. | The victim's behaviour is *not* the cause of the violence. Violence is the abuser's pattern of behaviour, and the victim cannot learn how to control it. |
| Intimate partner abuse is a minor problem. | There is a *real* danger that victims may be killed by abusive partners. |
| Victims of intimate partner abuse could leave if they really wanted to. | Numerous factors influence a decision to stay or leave, including fear of injury or death, financial dependence, and welfare of children. |
| Family abuse is most prevalent in poorly educated people from poor, working-class backgrounds. | Abuse occurs in families of all socioeconomic, religious, cultural, and educational backgrounds. |
| Family matters are private, and families should be allowed to take care of their own problems. | Intervention in family abuse is justified; abuse always escalates in frequency and intensity, can end in death, and is passed on to future generations. |
| Victims of abuse tacitly accept the abuse by trying to conceal it, by not reporting it, or by failing to seek help. | When attempting to disclose their situation, many victims are met with disbelief, which discourages them from persevering. |
| Myths victims commonly believe the following: "I can't live without him (her)." "If I hadn't done _____, it wouldn't have happened." "He (She) will change." "I stay for the sake of the children." | These myths are coping mechanisms used to allay panic in a situation of random and brutal violence. They give the illusion of control and rationality. |
| Alcohol and stress are the major causes of physical and verbal abuse. | There are no excuses—abuse is not acceptable behaviour. Abuse is a learned behaviour, not an uncontrollable reaction. People are abusive because they have acquired the belief that violence and aggression are acceptable and effective responses to real or imagined threats. |

## Family Coping Patterns

Consistent with a view of the intergenerational nature of the conditions and contexts of trauma, all forms of violence occurring in families of origin are predictive of future relationship violence (Franklin & Kercher, 2012). Altering the pattern of violence against women can affect child abuse because the main predictor of violence toward children is violence toward their mothers. However, it is important for the nurse to be nonjudgemental and to assess family strengths as well as styles of coping and stressors. Attitudes about child-rearing and discipline, including how parents were disciplined as children, may provide insight into violence and abuse in the home.

Living with and caring for children and older adults can cause frustration, anger, and stress (Draughon & Urbancic, 2010; Fulmer, Sengstock, Blankenship, et al., 2010). If there

## BOX 27-5 FACTORS TO ASSESS DURING A HOME VISIT

**For a Child**

- Responsiveness to infant's signals
- Caregiver's facial expressions in response to infant
- Playfulness of caregiver with infant
- Nature of physical contact during feeding and other caretaking activities
- Temperament of infant
- Caregiver's history of harsh discipline or abuse as a child
- Parental attitudes:
  - Feelings of inadequacy as a parent
  - Unrealistic expectations of child
  - Fear of "doing something wrong"
  - Attribution of negative qualities to newborn
  - Misdirected anger
  - Continued evidence of isolation, apathy, anger, frustration
  - Adult conflict
- Environmental conditions:
  - Sleeping arrangements
  - Child management
  - Home management
  - Use of supports (formal and informal)
- Need for immediate services for situational (e.g., economics, child care), emotional, or educational information:
  - Information about hotlines, babysitters, homemakers, parent groups
  - Information about child development
  - Information about child care and home management services

**For an Older Adult**

- Absence of or lack of access to basic necessities (e.g., food, water, medications)
- Unsafe housing
- Lack of or inadequate utilities, ventilation, space
- Poor physical hygiene
- Lack of necessary assistive devices (e.g., hearing aids, eyeglasses, wheelchair)
- Medication mismanagement (outdated prescriptions, unmarked bottles)

is no relief, the caregiver may become overwhelmed, lose control, and abuse the child or the older adult. Box 27-5 is a useful guide for assessing the risk for child or older adult abuse in the home.

### Support Systems

In the case of older adult abuse, risk factors include dependency on the caregiver for basic needs, isolation, limited or lack of access to support systems, and a history of intergenerational conflict between the older adult and the caregiver (Fulmer, Sengstock, Blankenship, et al., 2010). Assessment of the support system is crucial to identification of risk and resiliency factors. Children's support-system options are especially limited, as are those of people who are physically and mentally challenged. Assessment for support systems should focus on intrapersonal,

interpersonal, and community resources (e.g., the school system for school-aged victims).

### Suicide Potential

A suicide attempt may be the presenting symptom in the emergency department. With sensitive questioning conducted in a caring manner, the nurse can elicit the history of violence. A person experiencing violence may feel desperate to leave yet be trapped in a detrimental relationship, and suicide may seem like the only option. The threat of suicide may also be used by an emotionally abusive person in an attempt to manipulate the victim into caving in to demands ("Don't leave me or I'll kill myself"; "I took all my pills. ... I said I would the next time you were late").

Often, the means of attempted suicide is overdose with a combination of alcohol and other central nervous system depressants, or sleeping medications that have been prescribed in previous visits to physicians' offices, clinics, or emergency departments. Refer to Chapter 25 for more on suicide.

### Homicide Potential

At a minimum, the nurse should inquire about the patient's current safety risks and possible safety strategies. Because victims of abuse often underestimate the risk, using a tool such as the Danger Assessment (Campbell, Webster, & Glass, 2009) can be useful in helping victims to think about risk (for more information, see http://www.dangerassessment.org).

Individuals victimized by violence should be asked if they have ever felt like killing the perpetrator and, if so, whether they have the current desire and means to do so. If the answer is yes, intervention is required.

### Drug and Alcohol Use

There is a high rate of co-occurrence of victimization and substance abuse among women (Logan, Walker, Cole, et al., 2002). A person experiencing violence may self-medicate with alcohol or other drugs as a way of escaping an intolerable situation. The drugs are usually central nervous system depressants (e.g., benzodiazepines) prescribed by physicians in response to the patient's presentation with vague complaints, which are often stress-related (e.g., insomnia, gastrointestinal upsets, anxiety). The degree of intoxication can be determined by history, physical examination, and blood alcohol level. Refer to Chapter 19 for information on how to assess for a chronic alcohol or drug problem.

## DIAGNOSIS

Nursing diagnoses are focused on the underlying causes and symptoms of family violence.

Table 27-3 lists potential nursing diagnoses for abuse.

The identification of desired outcomes and the design of nursing interventions that facilitate achieving those outcomes should be developed as much as possible in collaboration with the survivor and a primary support person. These outcomes should be continually reassessed and revised as new information about the survivor's needs emerges. A

| TABLE 27-3 | POTENTIAL NURSING DIAGNOSES FOR FAMILY VIOLENCE |
|---|---|
| **SIGNS AND SYMPTOMS** | **POTENTIAL NURSING DIAGNOSES** |
| Bruises, cuts, broken bones, lacerations, scars, burns, wounds in various phases of healing, particularly when explanations do not match injury or explanations are vague | *Risk for injury* <br> *Acute pain* <br> *Chronic pain* <br> *Risk for infection* <br> *Impaired skin integrity* <br> *Risk for post-traumatic stress* |
| Isolation, fear, feelings of shame, low self-esteem, feelings of worthlessness, depression, feelings of helplessness | *Powerlessness* <br> *Ineffective coping* <br> *Fear* <br> *Risk for self-directed violence* <br> *Chronic low self-esteem* <br> *Situational low self-esteem* <br> *Hopelessness* <br> *Spiritual distress* |
| Vaginal–anal bruises, sores, discharge, peritoneal pain, positive venereal-disease test results | *Rape-trauma syndrome* <br> *Risk for infection* |

| TABLE 27-4 | *NOC* OUTCOMES FOR FAMILY ABUSE |
|---|---|
| **NURSING OUTCOME AND DEFINITION** | **SHORT-TERM AND INTERMEDIATE INDICATORS** |
| *Abuse cessation:* Evidence that the victim is no longer hurt or exploited | Evidence that physical abuse has ceased <br> Evidence that emotional abuse has ceased <br> Evidence that sexual abuse has ceased |
| *Abuse recovery: Physical:* Extent of healing of physical injuries due to abuse | Timely treatment of injuries <br> Healing of physical injuries <br> Resolution of physical health problems |
| *Abuse recovery: Financial:* Extent of control of monetary and legal matters following financial exploitation | Control of social security and pension income <br> Protection of financial resources <br> Control of withdrawal of money from account(s) |
| *Abusive behaviour self-restraint:* Self-restraint of abusive and neglectful behaviours toward others | Obtains needed treatment <br> Controls impulses <br> Discusses the abusive behaviour |

**Source:** Data from Moorhead, S., Johnson, M., Maas, M., et al. (2008). *Nursing outcomes classification (NOC)* (4th ed.). St. Louis: Mosby.

comprehensive plan can also guide the actions of the multidisciplinary team.

## OUTCOMES IDENTIFICATION

The *Nursing Outcomes Classification (NOC)* (Moorhead, Johnson, Maas, et al., 2008) identifies the following indicators for the outcome of *Abuse cessation*, defined as "evidence that the victim is no longer hurt or exploited":

- Physical abuse has ceased.
- Emotional abuse has ceased.
- Sexual abuse has ceased.
- Financial exploitation has ceased.

*NOC* offers other abuse-specific outcomes, including *Abuse protection, Abuse recovery, Abuse recovery: Emotional, Abuse recovery: Financial, Abuse recovery: Physical,* and *Abuse recovery: Sexual.* In addition, outcomes focused on improved coping, self-esteem, social support, and pain control, to name a few, are appropriate for these patients.

Table 27-4 provides some specific outcome criteria, along with short-term and intermediate indicators for victims of child, intimate partner, and older adult abuse, as well as for the abuser.

## PLANNING

Nurses and other health care workers encounter abuse frequently, not only in health care settings but also in their communities and families. Most hospitals and community centres provide protocols for dealing with child, intimate partner, or older adult abuse, but these protocols may or may not meet all the needs of a given patient.

Unless the case is one of child abuse in which the child has been removed from the home, most interventions performed after necessary emergency care will take place within the community. Plans should centre on the patient's safety first. The nurse must ascertain whether the survivor is in danger for his or her life, either from suicide or homicide, and, if there are children involved, whether they are in danger (Ford-Gilboe, Varcoe, & Merrit-Gray, 2010). Whenever it is possible or in the best interests of the patient, plans should be discussed with the patient. Planning should also take into consideration the needs of the abuser(s) (e.g., parents, caretakers, spouse, or partner) if he or she is willing to learn alternatives to abuse and violence.

## IMPLEMENTATION

### Reporting Abuse

There is no mandatory obligation to report woman abuse to the police. It is the woman's right to choose if she wishes to have police involvement, and she must consent to this involvement prior to the nurse's initiating contact with authorities (Registered Nurses' Association of Ontario, 2005). According to provincial or territorial legislation, any suspected or actual cases of child abuse must be reported to the official social service agency. For example, under Alberta's *Child, Youth and Family*

*Enhancement Act* (2012), any person who has "reasonable and probable grounds" to believe that a child is being harmed or is in danger of being abandoned, neglected, physically injured, emotionally injured, or sexually abused must report the situation to authorities.

Child witnesses to abuse may be reportable to the provincial or territorial social service agency, as proximity to such events can represent a condition of harm for the child (Registered Nurses' Association of Ontario, 2005). Nurses are advised to consult their local social service agency to discuss individual situations, and all health care organizations need to have a protocol in place with their local social service agency.

The Canadian Criminal Code provides the legislation necessary to deal with physical, sexual, and financial abuse of older adults (Lai, 2008). Additionally, provincial and territorial legislation addresses abuse and reporting. For example, some jurisdictions in Canada now enforce mandatory reporting of abuse of older adults, but specific reporting requirements and penalties for failing to report abuse vary (Department of Justice Canada, 2007; Human Resources and Skills Development Canada, 2011). Nova Scotia and Newfoundland have general mandatory reporting requirements in their adult protection legislation, placing a general social responsibility on all citizens to report suspected abuse or neglect (Lai, 2008; Nova Scotia Department of Seniors, 2012). Alberta, Manitoba, and Ontario now have special legislation for the protection of persons in care, and laws in Prince Edward Island, New Brunswick, Saskatchewan, and British Columbia provide for voluntary reporting for specific forms of abuse and neglect of older adults (Human Resources and Skills Development Canada, 2011).

Competency may be a consideration in a situation of older adult abuse. Competent older adults have the right to self-determination. Unless the individual is found to be incompetent, help can be offered but cannot be forced upon the person. In Canada, there is no general test of competency. The definition of *competency* varies across legislations, institutions, agencies, and provinces and territories (McDonald & Collins, 2000). However, it can be generally defined as a person's ability to understand the situation he or she is in and the decisions that have to be made about that situation (McDonald & Collins, 2000). The legal determination of incompetency is a last resort since it dramatically changes the rights of an individual. For this reason, it is important that the least restrictive approaches be taken before attempting to have an older adult declared incompetent.

Nurses must be cognizant of the cultural diversity of the populations with whom they work (see Chapter 7). *Cultural diversity* in this instance is used broadly and may be derived from one's race, ethnicity, class, religious or spiritual beliefs, age, ability, or sexual orientation (Registered Nurses' Association of Ontario, 2005). *Culture* refers to "the processes that happen between individuals and groups within organizations and society, and that confer meaning and significance" (Varcoe & Rodney, 2009, p. 123). The nurse must be aware of the cultural issues of those experiencing abuse, as such issues may affect the survivor's response to violence and to intervention. The nurse is responsible for developing a communication plan to make the survivor an informed partner in the provision of care. Nurses need to check their provincial practice standards for the provision of culturally sensitive care.

## Counselling

Counselling includes crisis intervention measures. It is important to emphasize that people have a right to live without fear of violence, physical harm, or assault. Powerful statements such as "Abuse is never right "and "No one deserves to be abused" will display unconditional acceptance and positive regard (Ford-Gilboe, Varcoe, & Merrit-Gray, 2010).

All individuals experiencing abuse should be counselled about developing a safety plan, a plan for a rapid escape when abuse recurs. Nurses should be aware that safety is never guaranteed, nor can the most detailed safety plan ensure that the violence will end (Registered Nurses' Association of Ontario, 2005). The victim experiencing violence is ultimately the only one who can reliably predict the risks and the likelihood for further violence, and, therefore, the best plan is the victim's own plan, one that is viewed by the victim as achievable and one that the victim has a personal commitment to follow (Middlesex-London Health Unit, 2000). The nurse should suggest packing the items listed in Box 27-6 ahead of time. The packed bag should be kept in a place where the perpetrator will not find it.

If the abused person chooses to leave, shelters or safe houses (for both sexes) are available in many communities in Canada. They are open 24 hours a day and can be reached through crisis hotline information numbers, hospital emergency departments, YWCAs, or the local office of the National Council of Women in Canada. Besides offering protection for individuals and families in crisis, many of these shelters and safe houses offer important education, counselling, and transitional housing services. Patients should be given the number of the nearest available shelter, even if they decide for the present to stay with their partners. Referral phone numbers may be kept for years before the decision to call is made. Having the number and a contact person all that time contributes to thinking about options.

## Case Management

Nurses working in outpatient and community mental health settings have the opportunity to coordinate community, medical, criminal justice, and social services to provide comprehensive assistance to families in crisis. Strategies must encompass needs for household necessities, child care, stability in providing basic needs, economic stability, physical and emotional safety, counselling, legal protection, career development or job training, education, ongoing support groups, and health care. Safe and affordable housing is often crucial to the person's ability to break free (Pavao, Alvarez, Baumrind, et al., 2007). A nurse functioning in a case manager role can assist the patient in choosing the best options and coordinating the interventions of several agencies. Box 27-7 lists selected *NIC* interventions for *Abuse protection support* for children, intimate partners, and older adults (Bulechek, Butcher, & Dochterman, 2008).

## BOX 27-6   PERSONALIZED SAFETY GUIDE

**Suggestions for Increasing Safety While in the Relationship**

- I will have important phone numbers available to my children and myself.
- I can tell _____ and _____ about the violence and ask them to call the police if they hear suspicious noises coming from my home.
- If I leave my home, I can go to (list four places) _____, _____, _____, or _____.
- I can leave extra money, car keys, clothes, and copies of documents with _____.
- If I leave, I will bring items _____ (e.g., ID, birth certificates, social insurance card, school and medical records, health insurance card, money, bank books, credit cards).
- To ensure safety and independence, I can keep my cellphone battery charged or have another phone available, open my own savings account, rehearse my escape route with a support person, and review my safety plan on _____ (date).

**Suggestions for Increasing Safety When the Relationship Is Over**

- I can change the locks and install steel or metal doors, a security system, smoke detectors, and an outside lighting system.
- I will inform _____ and _____ that my partner no longer lives with me and ask them to call the police if he or she is observed near my home or my children.
- I will tell people who take care of my children the names of those who have permission to pick them up. The people who have permission are _____, _____, and _____.
- I can tell _____ at work about my situation and ask _____ to screen my calls.
- I can avoid stores, banks, and _____ that I used when living with my battering partner.
- I can obtain a restraining order from _____. I can keep it on or near me at all times, as well as have a copy with _____.
- If I feel down and ready to return to a potentially abusive situation, I can call _____ for support or attend workshops and groups to gain support and strengthen my relationships with other people.

**Important Phone Numbers**

- Police _____
- Crisis Hotline _____
- Family _____
- Friends _____
- Shelter _____

## Milieu Management

Interventions are geared toward stabilizing the home situation and maintaining an abuse-free environment. Some mental health programs have caseworkers or clinicians who visit the home instead of requiring the family to go to the agency. Providing and maintaining a therapeutic environment in the home ideally involves three levels of help for abusive families:

1. Provides the family with economic support, job opportunities, and social services
2. Arranges social support in the form of a public health nurse, day care teacher, schoolteacher, social worker, respite worker, or any other potential contact person who has a good relationship with the family
3. Encourages and provides family therapy

### Promotion of Self-Care Activities

Nurses can help victims of abuse find hope and view themselves as "survivors," which emphasizes agency and choices, identifies strengths, and attributes more responsibility to them over aspects of their lives that are under their control (Dunn & Powell-Williams, 2007). Reimagining their own capacities to choose and act may empower survivors to find options and ultimately take steps to leave the abusive relationship. Ford-Gilboe, Wuest, and Merrit-Gray (2005) found that women were able to promote the health of their families after leaving an abusive partner. Therefore, offering hope, identifying strengths, and displaying confidence that the person can take care of him- or herself are important aspects of nursing care. Referrals regarding crisis counselling, emergency housing, or financial assistance, as well as legal and vocational counselling, should be made available to each patient. Referrals to parenting resources that explore alternative approaches to physical discipline of children in their care may also be appropriate.

### Health Teaching and Health Promotion

Health teaching and promotion include meeting with the individual, caregiver, and family to discuss the cycle of violence, associated risk factors, and situations that might trigger violence. Other nursing interventions can include teaching about healthy relationships and healthy sexuality, which may be especially important to children who have no role models.

Nurses who work on maternity units and in public health departments are often in a position to identify risk factors for abuse and initiate appropriate interventions, including education about effective parenting, caregiving, and coping techniques, as well as information for nurturing healthy relationships. Information about these interventions should be shared with the patient's health care team for appropriate monitoring and follow-up in the community. Assessment of risk and resiliency factors is essential to the implementation of health-promoting activities. For example, parents who are at particular risk for abusing a child include the following:

- New parents whose behaviour toward the infant is rejecting, hostile, or indifferent
- Teenage parents who require special help in handling the baby, have difficulty discussing their expectations of caring for the child, or lack support systems
- Parents with cognitive deficits, for whom careful, explicit, and repeated instructions on caring for the child and recognizing the infant's needs are indicated
- Parents who grew up watching their mothers being abused (a significant risk factor for perpetuation of family violence)

| BOX 27-7 | INTERVENTIONS FOR ABUSE PROTECTION SUPPORT FOR CHILDREN, INTIMATE PARTNERS, AND OLDER ADULTS |
|---|---|

**Abuse Protection Support: Children**

*Definition of* abuse protection support: children: Identification of high-risk, dependent child relationships and actions to prevent possible or further infliction of physical, sexual, or emotional harm or neglect of basic necessities of life.

Activities*:

- Identify mothers who have a history of late (four months or later) or no prenatal care.
- Identify parents who have had another child removed from the home or have placed previous children with relatives for extended periods.
- Identify parents with a history of domestic violence or a mother who has a history of numerous "accidental" injuries.
- Determine whether a child demonstrates signs of physical abuse, including numerous injuries in various stages of healing; unexplained bruises and welts; unexplained pattern, immersion, and friction burns; facial, spiral, shaft, or multiple fractures; unexplained facial lacerations and abrasions, and so on.
- Encourage admission of child for further observation and investigation as appropriate.
- Monitor parent–child interactions and record observations.
- Report suspected abuse or neglect to proper authorities in compliance with mandatory reporting laws.

**Abuse Protection Support: Intimate Partners**

*Definition of* abuse protection support: intimate partners: Identification of high-risk, dependent domestic relationships and action to prevent possible or further infliction of physical, sexual, or emotional harm or exploitation of a domestic partner.

Activities*:

- Screen for risk factors associated with domestic abuse (e.g., history of domestic violence, abuse, rejection, excessive criticism, or feelings of being worthless and unloved; difficulty

trusting others or feeling disliked by others; feeling that asking for help is an indication of personal incompetence; high physical care needs; intense family care responsibilities; substance abuse; depression; major psychiatric illness; social isolation; poor relationships between domestic partners; multiple marriages; pregnancy; poverty; unemployment; financial dependence; homelessness; infidelity; divorce; or death of a loved one).

- Document evidence of physical or sexual abuse using standardized assessment tools and photographs.
- Listen attentively to individual who begins to talk about own problems.
- Encourage admission to a hospital for further observation and investigation, as appropriate.
- Provide positive affirmation of worth.

**Abuse Protection Support: Older Adults**

*Definition of* abuse protection support: older adults: Identification of high-risk, dependent older adult relationships and actions to prevent possible or further infliction of physical, sexual, or emotional harm; neglect of basic necessities of life; or exploitation.

Activities*:

- Identify older patients who perceive themselves to be dependent on caretakers due to impaired health status, functional impairment, limited economic resources, depression, substance abuse, or lack of knowledge of available resources and alternatives for care.
- Identify family caretakers who have a childhood history of abuse or neglect.
- Monitor patient–caretaker interactions and record observations.
- Report suspected abuse or neglect to proper authorities in compliance with mandatory reporting laws.

*Partial list.
Adapted from Bulechek, G.M., Butcher, H.K., & Dochterman, J.M. (2008). *Nursing interventions classification (NIC)* (pp. 97–104). St. Louis, MO: Mosby.

Nurses can often recognize when children are at risk and make referrals to community resources, including emergency child care facilities, emergency telephone numbers, numbers of 24-hour crisis centres or hotlines, and respite programs for parents to have some relief from child care. Community and public health nurses can make home visits to identify risk factors for abuse in the crucial first few months of life, during which the style of parent–child interactions is established. See Box 27-5 for important factors for the community health nurse to assess during a home care visit. Such observations made by nurses in clinic and public health settings are fundamental in case finding and evaluation.

## Prevention of Abuse
### Primary Prevention

Primary prevention consists of measures taken to prevent the occurrence of abuse. Identifying individuals and families at high risk, providing health teaching, and coordinating supportive services to prevent crises are examples of primary

prevention. Specific strategies include (1) reducing stress, (2) reducing the influence of risk factors, (3) increasing social support, (4) increasing coping skills, and (5) increasing self-esteem. In particular, reducing the risk of the different forms of child abuse can contribute to reducing the repeated conditions and patterns of violence and abuse from generation to generation (Butchart, Harvey, & Fürniss, 2006). The most promising strategies for preventing child abuse include home visitation and parent education programs (Mikton & Butchart, 2009).

Community and public health nurses are in a unique position to assess family functioning in the home over time, which allows for assessment of changes. They are also in an excellent position to connect those at risk (such as people with addictions) to appropriate resources in the community that can meet their needs. All nurses can advocate for social policy change to improve the coordination of health, justice, and social services, thereby enhancing the health care response to abuse (Registered Nurses' Association of Ontario, 2005).

## Secondary Prevention

Secondary prevention involves early intervention in abusive situations to minimize their disabling or long-term effects. Nurses can establish universal screening programs in all health care settings for individuals at risk, assist in treating any injuries resulting from abuse, and coordinate community referrals to provide continuity of care (Registered Nurses' Association of Ontario, 2005). Stress, depression, low self-esteem, and social isolation can be addressed by providing supportive psychotherapy, psychoeducation, support groups, pharmacotherapy, and contact information for community resources. Caregiver burden can be reduced by arranging assistance in caregiving, nursing, or housekeeping or, if necessary, by placing the person in a different home or health care facility (Freysteinson, 2011). For some, support through criminal proceedings may be important to prevent revictimization. Refer to the Trauma Toolkit from the British Columbia Centre of Excellence for Women's Health for further information on trauma-informed care: http://www.coalescing-vc.org/virtualLearning/documents/trauma-informed-online-tool.pdf. The recently established Sheldon Kennedy Child Advocacy Centre, based in Calgary, Alberta, is another organization concerned with all levels of child abuse prevention, including community education and training to prevent revictimization and interrupt the potential cycle of violence from generation to generation. The vignette illustrates a successful secondary prevention effort.

## Tertiary Prevention

Tertiary prevention, which often occurs in mental health care settings, involves nurses' facilitating the healing and rehabilitative process by counselling individuals and families, providing support for groups of survivors, and assisting survivors of violence to achieve their optimal level of safety, health, and well-being. Services targeted at parents who have been reported for child abuse and neglect and had such reports substantiated are an example of tertiary prevention (Harder, 2005).

## Advanced-Practice Interventions

### Individual Psychotherapy

The goals of individual therapy for a survivor are empowerment, the ability to recognize and choose productive life options, and the development of a solid sense of self. Survivors of abuse may choose individual therapy to address symptoms of depression, anxiety, somatization, or PTSD. Many of the psychological symptoms shown by women who have been abused can be understood as complex survival strategies and responses to violence. This constellation of symptoms, such as fear and a perceived inability to escape, has been referred to as battered woman syndrome (American Heritage Medical Dictionary, 2007).

Nurses must address the guilt, shame, and stigmatization experienced by survivors of abuse (Draucker, Martsolf, Ross, et al., 2009). It is helpful for nurses to understand that the patient's feelings and behaviours may reflect those of the grieving process since the survivor has experienced numerous losses as a result of the abusive relationship.

---

**VIGNETTE**

George, aged 4 years, is brought into the physician's office by 25-year-old Asha, the child's nanny, with second-degree burns on his right hand. Asha is the nanny for George and his younger brother, Tyrone, aged 2, and older brother Logan, aged 6. Asha appears apprehensive and says she is very concerned. Asha tells the nurse that the children have told her in the past that their mother has threatened them with burning if they do not behave. George told her that his mother once held his hands on a cold stove element and told him that if he was bad, she would turn it on and burn him. Asha is shocked that George's mother would do such a thing, but at the same time, she says she feels guilty for "telling on Ms. J."

Asha also states that the older brother, Logan, told her what happened to George but was afraid that if his mother found out, she would burn him also. Asha says she is aware that the mother hits the children, but she did not believe that anyone would burn her own child. The nurse reports the incident to the physician, and the mother is called and asked to come to the office. Meanwhile, the nurse asks Asha to stay with George while she examines him. George appears frightened and in pain.

**Nurse:** "Tell me about your hand, George." *(George looks down and starts to cry.)* "It's OK if you don't want to talk about it, George."

**George:** *(Does not look at the nurse and speaks softly.)* "My mommy burned my hand on the stove."

**Nurse:** "Tell me what happened before that."

**George:** "Mommy was mad because I didn't put my toys away."

**Nurse:** "What does your mommy usually do when she gets mad?"

**George:** "She yells mostly. Sometimes she hits us. Mommy is going to be so mad at Logan for telling."

**Nurse:** "Tell me about the hitting."

**George:** "Mommy hits us a lot since Daddy left." *(George starts to cry to himself.)*

On examination, the nurse notices on George's right palm a ringed pattern of burns resembling the burner on an electric stove. There are blisters on his fingers. George appears well nourished and properly dressed. He is at his approximate developmental age except for some language delay. Because of the physical evidence and history, there is strong suspicion of child abuse. The provincial social service agency is notified, and the family situation is evaluated for possible placement of George in foster care. The initial evaluation concludes that there is no indication of serious potential harm to the child and that George should return home. The mother, who is initially defensive, starts to cry and states, "I can't cope with being alone, and I don't know where to turn."

Nursing interventions centre on caring for George's immediate health needs, finding supports for the mother to help her cope with crises, providing a counselling referral for the mother to learn alternative ways of expressing anger and frustration, informing the mother of parents' groups, providing referrals to play groups or day care for the children to help increase their feelings of self-esteem and security, and providing a break and instruction in parenting for the mother.

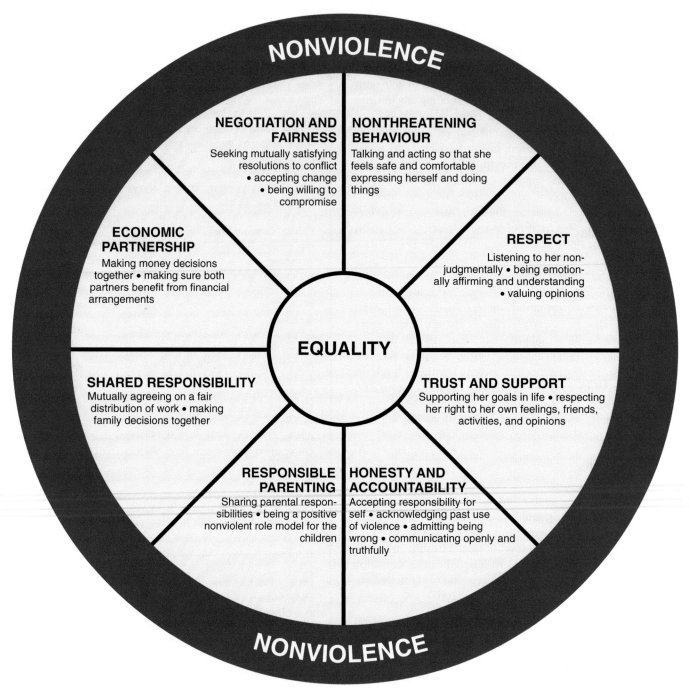

**FIGURE 27-7** The Duluth "Equality" wheel. **Source:** Redrawn from Domestic Abuse Intervention Programs, 202 East Superior Street, Duluth, MN 55802. Retrieved from http://www.theduluthmodel.org/training/wheels.html.

Programs for perpetrators of abuse are still associated with the justice system and are mandated interventions rather than voluntary and desirable community services for batterers. Although court-mandated treatment tends to be the most effective for perpetrators, it is critical that the domestic violence movement make assistance for perpetrators of abuse more readily available so as to shift societal norms to encourage and promote voluntary help-seeking behaviours (Campbell, Neil, Jaffe, et al., 2010). The perpetrator needs to seek help for issues concerning power and control. Refer to the Duluth model "Power and Control" wheel (Figure 27-4) and "Equality" wheel

(Figure 27-7), which are standard frameworks for violence education.

Nurses engaged in therapy with perpetrators of abuse have a duty to warn potential victims if they conclude that the perpetrator is a danger. Refer to Chapter 8 for a more detailed discussion of the duty to warn and duty to protect.

### Family Psychotherapy

Because abuse is a symptom of a family in crisis, each member of the family system needs attention. Also, because change in one member of the family system affects the whole system, all

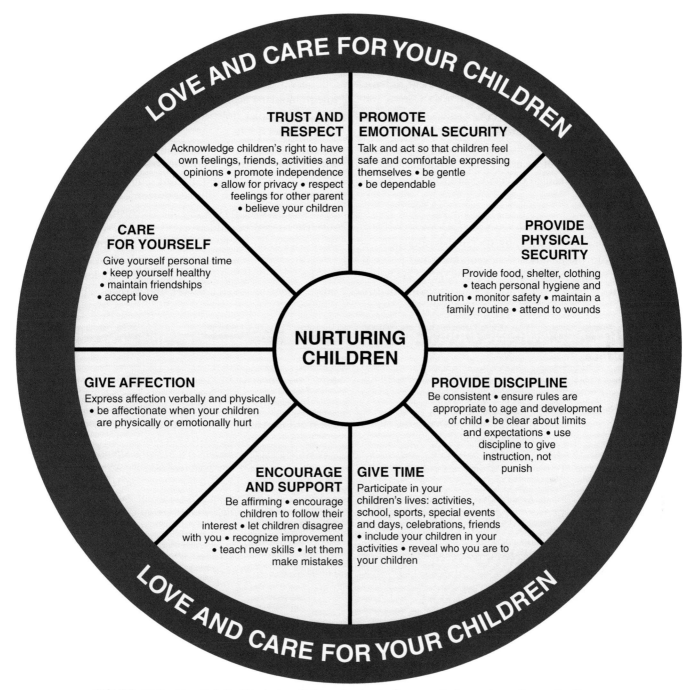

**FIGURE 27-8** The Duluth "Nurturing Children" wheel. **Source:** Redrawn from Domestic Abuse Intervention Programs, 202 East Superior Street, Duluth, MN 55802. Retrieved from http://www.theduluthmodel.org/training/wheels.html.

members need support and understanding. Dialectical behaviour therapy (DBT) has been proven to be effective in treating individuals and families with histories of abuse by teaching emotion regulation, interpersonal skills, mindfulness, and distress tolerance skills (Feigenbaum, 2007). Family or marital therapy should take place *only* if the perpetrator has had individual therapy and has demonstrated change as a result and if both parties agree to participate.

Expected outcomes are that the perpetrator will recognize destructive patterns of behaviour and learn alternative responses. Intermediate goals are that members of the family will openly communicate and learn to listen to each other. Refer to the

Duluth Model "Nurturing Children" wheel (Figure 27-8), which is a standard framework for the care of children in families with histories of abuse. Refer to Chapter 36 for a more detailed discussion of family therapy.

### Group Psychotherapy

Group therapy offers a powerful way to counter self-denigrating beliefs and to confront issues of secrecy and stigmatization while decreasing isolation, improving self-esteem, and increasing the potential for realistic problem solving (Draughon & Urbancic, 2010). Also, the therapeutic factor of universality, or the discovery that others have had similar experiences, may be beneficial, especially for child survivors. DBT has been used in groups with abusers to teach emotion regulation, interpersonal, mindfulness, and distress tolerance skills (Van Wel, Kockmann, Blum, et al., 2006).

Emotion regulation skills are taught to manage intense labile moods; interpersonal skills, to develop assertiveness and problem-solving skills; mindfulness, for meditation; and distress tolerance skills, to learn how to tolerate and accept distress as a part of normal life (Feigenbaum, 2007). Group therapy can help create a community of healing and restoration. Refer to Chapter 35 for a more detailed discussion of group therapy.

## EVALUATION

The failure of interventions with abusive families often are due to problems within the health, social, economic, and political systems. Nurses must act at all levels by lobbying for (1) better education about violence and abuse, (2) resources in health care settings to support more effective responses to violence and abuse, (3) better collaboration across all sectors, and (4) the development of policies on understanding the dynamics of violence in such areas as social assistance and child welfare (Ford-Gilboe, Varcoe, & Merrit-Gray, 2010). Nurses can play a powerful role in lobbying against factors that promote violence (such as media that depict violence, gender or racial inequity, and devaluing of older adults).

The evaluation of brief interventions can be based on whether the survivor acknowledges the violence, is willing to accept intervention, and removes him- or herself from the abusive situation. The ultimate outcome of long-term interventions and follow-up is to end the violence and to empower the survivor to lead a productive and safe life without the haunting memories of abuse. Because abuse is a symptom of a family in crisis, diagnosis, interventions, and evaluation should be carried out by a multidisciplinary team that includes a physician, a nurse, a social worker, a lawyer, and perhaps a psychiatrist.

---

## CASE STUDY AND NURSING CARE PLAN 27-1

### Family Violence

Mrs. Tran, a recently widowed 84-year-old woman, moved to her son's apartment three months ago. She had been living in her third-floor walk-up in the city. Because of her declining health, crime in the neighbourhood, and the need to climb three flights of stairs, with her son Chien's encouragement, she went to live with him. He and his wife, Kim, who have been married for almost 20 years, have five children 6 to 18 years of age, all living in a rather cramped three-bedroom apartment.

Mrs. Tran is being cared for by a nurse from the Victoria Order of Nurses (VON), who monitors her blood pressure and adjusts her medication. Over a series of visits, the nurse, Ms. Grohl, notices that Mrs. Tran is looking unkempt, pale, and withdrawn. While taking her blood pressure, Ms. Grohl observes bruises on Mrs. Tran's arms and neck. When questioned about the bruises,

Mrs. Tran appears anxious and nervous. She says that she slipped in the bathroom. Mrs. Tran becomes increasingly apprehensive and stiffens in her chair when her daughter-in-law Kim comes into the room to ask when the next visit is. The nurse notices that Kim avoids eye contact with Mrs. Tran.

When the injuries are brought to Kim's attention, she responds by becoming angry and agitated, blaming Mrs. Tran for causing so many problems. She will not explain the reason for the change in Mrs. Tran's behaviour or the origin of the bruises to the nurse. She merely comments, "I have had to give up my job since my mother-in-law came here. It's been difficult and crowded ever since she moved in. The kids are complaining. We are having trouble making ends meet since I gave up my job. And my husband is no help at all."

### ASSESSMENT

#### Self-Assessment
Ms. Grohl has worked in a number of situations with violent families, but this is the first time she has encountered older adult abuse. She discusses her reactions with the other team members. She is especially angry at Kim, although she is able to understand the daughter-in-law's frustration. The team concurs with Ms. Grohl that there seems to be potential for positive change in this family. If abuse does not abate, more drastic measures will need to be taken and legal services contacted.

| Objective Data | Subjective Data |
| --- | --- |
| Physical symptoms of violence (bruises, unkempt appearance, withdrawn attitude) | Mrs. Tran states she slipped in the bathroom, but physical findings do not support this explanation. |
| Stressful, crowded living conditions | Kim states, "It's been difficult and crowded ever since she moved in." |
| No eye contact between Mrs. Tran and her daughter-in-law | |
| Economic hardships leading to stress | Mrs. Tran exhibits withdrawn and apprehensive behaviour in the presence of Kim. |
| No support for the daughter-in-law from the rest of the family for care of Mrs. Tran | |

### DIAGNOSIS

On the basis of the data, the nurse formulates the following nursing diagnoses:
1. *Risk for injury* related to increase in family stress, as evidenced by signs of violence

*Continued*

## CASE STUDY AND NURSING CARE PLAN 27-1—cont'd

### *Family Violence*

**Supporting Data**
- Statement by Mrs. Tran that she slipped in the bathroom, but physical findings do not support this explanation
- Physical symptoms of violence (bruises, unkempt appearance, withdrawn attitude)
- Stressful, crowded living conditions

2. *Ineffective coping* related to helplessness, as evidenced by inability to meet role expectations
**Supporting Data**
- Unkempt, anxious, depressed
- Withdrawn and apprehensive behaviour

3. *Risk for other-directed violence* related to increased stressors within a short period, as evidenced by probable older adult abuse and feelings of helplessness verbalized by the primary caregiver
**Supporting Data**
- Kim states, "It's been difficult and crowded ever since she moved in."
- No eye contact between Kim and Mrs. Tran
- Signs and symptoms of physical abuse on Mrs. Tran
- Kim says, "My husband is no help at all."

4. *Caregiver role strain* related to extreme feelings of being overwhelmed and feeling helpless
**Supporting Data**
- Family not helping with care of mother-in-law; burden of care on Kim
- Economic hardships, leading to stress when Kim gave up her job to care for Mrs. Tran

## OUTCOMES IDENTIFICATION

Abuse cessation: Evidence that the victim is no longer hurt or exploited
  *Short-term indicators:*
- Evidence that physical abuse has ceased
- Evidence that emotional abuse has ceased

## PLANNING

Ms. Grohl discusses several possible outcomes with members of her team, giving attention to the priority of outcomes and to whether they are realistic in this situation. She also plans to report the older adult abuse to law enforcement and to work with Mrs. Tran, Kim, and the rest of the family to improve this situation for everyone.

## IMPLEMENTATION

Mrs. Tran's plan of care is personalized as follows:
  **Nursing diagnosis:** Risk for injury related to increase in family stress, as evidenced by signs of violence
  **Outcome:** Abuse cessation

| Short-Term Goal | Interventions | Rationale | Evaluation |
|---|---|---|---|
| 1. On each visit made by the nurse, the patient will state that abuse has decreased, using a scale from 1 to 5 (1 being the least abuse). | 1a. Follow provincial laws and guidelines for reporting older adult abuse. | 1a. Provides maximum protection under the law Provides data for future use | **GOAL MET** Patient states that after family talked to the nurse and planned strategies, physical abuse no longer occurs. |
|  | 1b. Assess severity of signs and symptoms of abuse. | 1b. Accurate charting (body map, pictures with permission, verbatim statements) helps follow progress and provides legal data. |  |

*Continued*

**CASE STUDY AND NURSING CARE PLAN 27-1—cont'd**

*Family Violence*

| Short-Term Goal | Interventions | Rationale | Evaluation |
|---|---|---|---|
| | 1c. Do a careful home assessment to identify other areas of abuse and neglect. Identify community resources that could help the older adult and caregivers. | 1c. Check for inadequacy of food, presence of vermin, blocked stairways, medication safety issues, and so on—all indicate abuse and neglect. | |
| | 1d. Identify community resources that could help the older adult and caregivers to manage care at home. | 1d. Determining the kinds of problems in the home and identifying available resources help with planning appropriate intervention. | |
| | 1e. Discuss with patient factors leading to abuse and concern for safety. | 1e. Allows for identification of family stressors and potential areas for intervention. Validates that situation is serious and increases patient's knowledge base | |
| 2. Within 2 weeks, patient will be able to identify at least two supportive services to deal with emergency situations. | 2. Discuss with patient supportive services such as crisis hotlines and 911 to call in case of emergency situations. | 2. Maximizes patient's safety through use of support systems | **GOAL MET** Patient has been talking to two old friends she had stopped talking to because of shame and depression. She has called the crisis hotline once to get information on transportation to the older adult centre in town. |
| 3. Within 3 weeks, family members will be able to identify difficult issues that increase their stress levels. | 3. Discuss with family members their feelings, and identify at least four areas that are most difficult for the various family members. | 3. Listening to each family member and identifying unmet needs helps both family and nurse identify areas that require changing and appropriate interventions. | **GOAL MET** Family members identify areas of increased stress, such as overwork, lack of free time, lack of privacy, and financial difficulties. |
| 4. Within 3 weeks, family will seek out community resources to help with anger management, need for homemaker support, and other needs. | 4. Identify potential community supports, skills training, respite places, homemakers, financial aids, and so on that might help meet family's unmet needs. | 4. When stressed, individuals solve problems poorly and do not know about or cannot manage to organize outside help. Finances may be controlled by the perpetrator or become unmanageable in the crisis stages of abuse. | **GOAL MET** The daughter-in-law is glad to get out of the house for anger-management classes, and the son states he will try to take on more responsibility, but he often feels guilty and angry, too. Reluctantly, he and his wife agree to try a support group with other caregivers in similar situations. |

## EVALUATION

Eight weeks after Ms. Grohl's initial visit, Mrs. Tran appears well groomed, friendly, and more spontaneous in her conversation. She comments, "Things are better with my daughter-in-law." No bruises or other signs of physical violence are noticeable. She is considerably more outgoing and has even taken the initiative to contact an old friend. Mrs. Tran has talked openly to her son and daughter-in-law about stress in the family. Mrs. Tran says that she went for a walk when her daughter-in-law Kim appeared tense and returned to find that the tension had lessened. Neither Mrs. Tran nor her family has initiated plans for alternative housing.

## KEY POINTS TO REMEMBER

- Abuse can occur in any family and can be predicted with some accuracy by examining the risk and resiliency factors related to the characteristics of perpetrators, vulnerable people, and crisis situations in which violence is likely.
- Abuse can be physical, sexual, psychological or emotional, or economic or caused by deprivation or neglect.
- The cycle of violence includes three recurring phases of violence (tension building, acute battering, and honeymoon stages), which often increase in severity and frequency.
- Assessment includes identifying indicators of abuse, levels of anxiety, coping mechanisms, support systems, and suicide and homicide potential, as well as alcohol and drug abuse.

- Reporting abuse to the police is a matter of provincial legislation. Nurses should be aware that in the case of abuse of adults, violence is something that competent adults must choose to self-report. Nurses are responsible for reporting abuse of children, dependent adults, and older adults to authorities, though the particular standards of reporting vary among provinces and territories. Awareness of these standards is the responsibility of the nurse.
- Interventions for victims or perpetrators of violence depend on the level of crisis and are focused on planning strategies to remove the individual and family members from violent situations and preventing abuse from recurring. Support and crisis intervention are key nursing interventions.

## CRITICAL THINKING

1. A colleague who has witnessed a child being abused states, "I don't think it's any of our business what people do in the privacy of their own homes."
   a. What would you be legally required to do?
   b. What are your ethical responsibilities?

2. Congratulations! You successfully convinced your colleagues to assess routinely for abuse. Now they want to know how to do it. How would you go about teaching them to assess for child abuse? Intimate partner abuse? Older adult abuse?

3. Your health care organization's routine health screening form for adolescents, adults, and older adults has just been changed to include questions about family abuse. How would you respond to patients who indicate on this form that abuse occurs in their home?

4. Write out a safety plan that could be adopted by individuals who are being abused.
   a. Identify at least four referrals in your community for an abused person.
   b. Identify two referrals in your community for a violent person, partner, or parent.

5. What would the nurse screen for when a young, visibly upset pregnant woman attends a prenatal outpatient clinic with multiple bruises on her upper arms?

## CHAPTER REVIEW

1. A man becomes frustrated when his children cry repeatedly and shoves his wife into the refrigerator. His wife explains to the neighbour, who witnessed this, that "I should have made the children go to bed earlier so they wouldn't be so cranky." This event is an example of:
   1. Masochism
   2. Emotional abuse
   3. Tension reduction
   4. Secondary prevention

2. Which statement(s) about perpetrators and victims of abuse is accurate? Select all that apply.
   1. Approximately 40% of victims of intimate partner and family abuse are male.
   2. Abusive behaviour is usually the result of intoxication or stress.
   3. Perpetrators tend to respond best to treatment if it is court ordered.
   4. Victims do not report abuse, because they tacitly are accepting of it.

5. Victims of abuse stay in the relationship because they really do not want to leave.
6. Disruptive behaviour may make older adults with dementia vulnerable to abuse.

3. A staff nurse, Chandra, is assisting a 30-year-old victim of domestic violence in the emergency department. The patient suffered numerous bruises and abrasions, is reluctant to be examined, seems very ashamed, and is very fearful that the Children's Aid Society will take custody of her young daughter, who has not been assaulted and is safe, if the police become involved. Which intervention is indicated?
   1. Report the assault to the police since reporting of domestic violence is mandatory.
   2. Probe the patient for information to use as evidence in prosecuting the perpetrator.
   3. Press the patient to disrobe so that she can be examined for signs of hidden injuries.
   4. Guide and assist the patient to develop a safety plan for rapid escape should abuse recur.

4. Ms. Patel, a student nurse, is assigned to a patient recovering from injuries received during an episode of domestic violence, the third such assault for which she has received treatment. Ms. Patel left home at age 17 to escape an abusive father. Which statements about this situation are accurate? Select all that apply.
   1. Ms. Patel may be prone to blame the patient for her injuries and abuse.
   2. Ms. Patel's personal experiences give her special insight into the needs of this patient.
   3. Ms. Patel's experiences are likely to make her more empathic toward victims.
   4. Caring for victims of abuse will help Ms. Patel cope with her own abuse experiences.
   5. Ms. Patel may experience overwhelming anguish as a result of caring for abuse victims.
   6. Ms. Patel would likely benefit from clinical supervision related to caring for abuse victims.

5. Perpetrators of domestic violence tend to (select all that apply):
   1. Belong to lower socioeconomic groups and be poorly educated
   2. Have relatively poor social skills and have grown up with poor role models
   3. Believe they, if male, should be dominant and in charge in relationships
   4. Force their mates to work and expect them to support the family
   5. Be controlling and willing to use force to maintain their power in relationships
   6. Prevent their mates from having relationships and activities outside the family

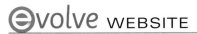 WEBSITE

Post-Test   interactive review

*Visit the Evolve Web site for Chapter Review Answers and Rationales, Critical Thinking Answer Guidelines, and additional resources related to the content in this chapter:* http://evolve.elsevier.com/Canada/Varcarolis/psychiatric/

## REFERENCES

Abbey, A., Zawacki, T., Buck, P.O., et al. (2004). Sexual assault and alcohol consumption: What do we know about their relationship and what types of research are still needed? *Aggression & Violent Behaviour, 9,* 271–303. doi:10.1016/S1359-1789(03)00011-9.

*American heritage medical dictionary.* (2007). Boston: Houghton Mifflin Company.

Bonomi, A.E., Anderson, M.L., Rivara, F.P., et al. (2007). Health outcomes in women with physical and sexual intimate partner violence exposure. *Journal of Women's Health, 16,* 987–997. doi:10.1089/jwh.2006.0239.

Bulechek, G.M., Butcher, H.K., & Dochterman, J.M. (2008). *Nursing interventions classification (NIC)* (5th ed.). St. Louis, MO: Mosby.

Butchart, A., Harvey, A.H., & Fürniss, T. (2006). *Preventing child maltreatment: A guide to taking action and generating evidence.* Geneva, Switzerland: World Health Organization. Retrieved from http://www.who.int/violence_injury_prevention/violence/activities/child_maltreatment/en/index.html.

Campbell, J.C., Webster, D.W., & Glass, N.E. (2009). The danger assessment: Validation of a lethality risk assessment instrument for intimate partner femicide. *Journal of Interpersonal Violence, 24,* 653–674. doi:10.1177/0886260508317180.

Campbell, M., Neil, J.A., Jaffe, P.G., et al. (2010). Engaging abusive men in seeking community intervention: A critical research & practice priority. *Journal of Family Violence, 25,* 413–422. doi:10.1007/s10896-010-9302-z.

Canadian Centre for Justice Statistics. (2009). *Family violence in Canada: A statistical profile.* Ottawa: Statistics Canada.

Carter-Snell, C., & Hegadoren, K. (2003). Stress disorder and gender: Implications for theory and research. *Canadian Journal of Nursing Research, 35*(2), 34–55.

Coker, A.L., Hopenhayn, C., DeSimone, C.P., et al. (2009). Violence against women raises the risk of cervical cancer. *Journal of Women's Health, 18,* 1179–1185. doi:10.1089/jwh.2008.1048.

College of Nurses of Ontario. (2008). *Practice standard: Documentation.* Toronto: Author.

College of Registered Nurses of Nova Scotia. (2012). *Documentation guidelines for registered nurses.* Halifax: Author. Retrieved from http://www.crnns.ca/documents/DocumentationGuidelines.pdf.

Department of Justice Canada. (2007). Abuse of older adults: A fact sheet from the Department of Justice Canada. *Family Violence Initiative.* Retrieved from http://www.justice.gc.ca/eng/pi/fv-vf/index.html.

Draucker, C., Martsolf, D., Ross, R., et al. (2009). The essence of healing from sexual violence: A qualitative metasynthesis. *Research in Nursing and Health, 32,* 366–378. doi:10.1002/nur.20333.

Draughon, J., & Urbancic, J.C. (2010). Childhood sexual abuse. In J. Humphrey & J.C. Campbell (Eds.), *Family violence and nursing practice* (2nd ed., pp. 319–346). New York: Springer.

Dube, S.R., Anda, R.F., Whitfield, C.L., et al. (2005). Long-term consequences of childhood sexual abuse by gender of victim. *American Journal of Preventive Medicine, 28,* 430–438. doi:10.1016/j.amepre.2005.01.015.

Dunn, J.L., & Powell-Williams, M. (2007). "Everybody makes choices." *Violence Against Women, 13,* 977–1001. doi:10.1177/1077801207305932.

Dutton, D.G. (1998). *The abusive personality.* New York: Guilford Press.

Dutton, D.G. (2007). *The abusive personality: Violence and control in intimate relationships* (2nd ed.). New York: Guilford Press.

Fawole, O.I. (2008). Economic violence to women and girls: Is it receiving the necessary attention? *Trauma Violence Abuse, 9,* 167–177. doi:10.1177/1524838008319255.

Feigenbaum, J. (2007). Dialectical behaviour therapy: An increasing evidence base. *Journal of Mental Health, 16,* 51–68. doi:10.1080/09638230601182094.

Fergusson, D.M., Boden, J.M., & Horwood, L.J. (2008). Exposure to childhood sexual and physical abuse and adjustment in early adulthood. *Child Abuse and Neglect, 32,* 607–619. doi:10.1016/j.chiabu.2006.12.018.

Ford-Gilboe, M., Varcoe, C., & Merrit-Gray, M. (2010). Intimate partner violence and nursing practice. In J. Humphrey & J.C. Campbell (Eds.), *Family violence and nursing practice* (2nd ed., pp. 115–153). New York: Springer.

Ford-Gilboe, M., Wuest, J., & Merritt-Gray, M. (2005). Strengthening capacity to limit intrusion: Theorizing family health promotion in the aftermath of women abuse. *Qualitative Health Research, 15,* 477–501. doi:10.1177/1049732305274590.

Franklin, C.A., & Kercher, G.A. (2012). The intergenerational transmission of intimate partner violence: Differentiating correlates in a random community sample. *Journal of Family Violence, 27*(3), 187–199. doi:10.1007/s10896-012-9419-3.

Freysteinson, W. (2011). Opening Pandora's box: A comprehensive approach to home violence prevention. *Home Health Care Management & Practice, 23,* 6–12. doi:10.1177/1084822309360381.

Fulmer, T., Sengstock, M.C., Blankenship, J., et al. (2010). Elder mistreatment. In J. Humphrey & J.C. Campbell (Eds.), *Family violence and nursing practice* (2nd ed., pp. 347–365). New York: Springer.

Graham-Bermann, S.A., Gruber, G., Girz, L., et al. (2009). Factors discriminating among profiles of resilient coping and psychopathology in children exposed to domestic violence. *Child Abuse & Neglect, 33,* 648–660. doi:10.1016/j.chiabu.2009.01.002.

Harder, J. (2005). Prevention of child abuse and neglect: An evaluation of a home visitation parent aide program using recidivism data. *Research on Social Work Practice, 15,* 246–256. doi:10.1177/1049731505275062.

Human Resources and Skills Development Canada. (2011). *Elder abuse modules.* Ottawa: Author. Retrieved from http://www.hrsdc.gc.ca/eng/seniors/funding/pancanadian/elder_abuse.shtml.

Jack, S., Jamieson, E., Wathen, N.C., et al. (2008). The feasibility of screening for intimate partner violence during postpartum home visits. *Canadian Journal of Nursing Research, 40*(2), 150–170.

King, W.J., MacKay, M., & Sirnick, A. (2003). Shaken baby syndrome in Canada: Clinical characteristics and outcomes of hospital cases. *Canadian Medical Association Journal, 168*(2), 155–159.

Krug, E.G., Dahlberg, L.L., Mercy, J.A., et al. (Eds.), (2002). *World report on violence and health.* Geneva, Switzerland: World Health Organization. Retrieved from http://www.who.int/violence_injury_prevention/violence/world_report/en/.

Lai, S. (2008). Elder abuse and policing issues: A review of the literature. *United Senior Citizens of Ontario. Community mobilization empowering seniors against victimization.* Retrieved from http://www.uscont.ca/wp-content/uploads/2012/12/elder_abuse_and_policing_issues.pdf.

Logan, T.K, Walker, R., Cole, J., et al. (2002). Victimization and substance abuse among women: Contributing factors, interventions, and implications. *Review of General Psychology, 6,* 325–397. doi:10.1037/1089-2680.6.4.325.

McDonald, L., & Collins, A. (2000). *Abuse and neglect of older adults: A discussion paper* (Cat. No. H72-21/162-1998E). Retrieved from http://dsp-psd.pwgsc.gc.ca/Collection/H88-3-30-2001/pdfs/violence/abuse_e.pdf.

McFarlane, J., Hughes, R.B., Nosek, M.A., et al. (2001). Abuse Assessment Screen—Disability (AAS-D): Measuring frequency, type, and perpetrator of abuse toward women with physical disabilities. *Journal of Women's Health & Gender-Based Medicine, 10,* 861–866. doi:10.1089/152460901753285750.

Middlesex-London Health Unit. (2000). *Task force on the health effects of woman abuse—Final report.* London, ON: Author.

Mikton, C., & Butchart, A. (2009). Child maltreatment prevention: A systematic review of reviews. *Bulletin of the World Health Organization, 87,* 353–361. doi:10.2471/BLT.08.057075.

Moorhead, S., Johnson, M., Maas, M., et al. (2008). *Nursing outcomes classification (NOC)* (4th ed.). St. Louis, MO: Mosby.

Northwest Territories Health and Social Services. (2009). *Northwest Territories community health nursing administrative policies & guidelines.* Yellowknife: Author. Retrieved from http://www.hss.gov.nt.ca/sites/default/files/nwt_community_health_nursing_administrative_policies_and_guidelines.pdf.

Nova Scotia Department of Seniors. (2012). *Understanding senior abuse: A toolkit for community champions.* Halifax: Communications Nova Scotia.

Papp, A. (2010). *Culturally driven violence against women: A growing problem in Canada's immigrant communities.* Retrieved from http://www.fcpp.org/files/1/Culturally-Driven%20Violence%20Against%20Women.pdf.

Pavao, J., Alvarez, J., Baumrind, N., et al. (2007). Intimate partner violence and housing stability. *American Journal of Preventative Medicine, 32*(2), 143–146. doi:10.1016/j.amepre.2006.10.008.

Perinatal Partnership Program of Eastern and Southeastern Ontario. (2004). *Women abuse in the perinatal period: Guidelines for care providers.* Ottawa: Author.

Personal Health Information Protection Act (Ontario), S.O. 2004, c. 3, Schedule A.

Public Health Agency of Canada. (2004). *Physical abuse during pregnancy.* Retrieved from http://www.phac-aspc.gc.ca/rhs-ssg/factshts/pdf/abusepreg_e.pdf.

Public Health Agency of Canada. (2010). *Canadian incidence study of reported child abuse and neglect—2008: Major findings.* Ottawa: Author. Retrieved from http://www.phac-aspc.gc.ca/publicat/cisfr-ecirf/pdf/cis_e.pdf.

Ramsey, S.H., & Abrams, D.E. (2010). A primer on child abuse and neglect law. *Juvenile and Family Court Journal, 61,* 1–31. doi:10.1111/j.1755-6988.2009.01036.x.

Registered Nurses' Association of Ontario. (2005). *Woman abuse: Screening, identification and initial response.* Toronto: Author.

Robinson, J.R., Clements, K., & Land, C. (2003). Workplace stress among psychiatric nurses: Prevalence, distribution, correlates, & predictors. *Journal of Psychosocial Nursing & Mental Health Services, 41*(4), 32–41.

Rozovsky, L.E., & Inions, N.J. (2003). *Canadian health information: A practical legal and risk management guide* (3rd ed.). Markham, ON: Butterworths.

Skopp, N.A., McDonald, R., Jouriles, E.N., et al. (2007). Partner aggression and children's externalizing problems: Maternal and partner warmth as protective factors. *Journal of Family Psychology, 21,* 459–467. doi:10.1037/0893-3200.21.3.459.

Statistics Canada. (2009). *Family violence in Canada: A statistical profile* (Cat. No. 85-224-X). Ottawa: Author. Retrieved from http://www.statcan.gc.ca/pub/85-224-x/85-224-x2009000-eng.htm?

Trocmé, N., MacLaurin, B., Fallon, B., et al. (2006). *Mesnmimk Wasatek: Understanding the overrepresentation of First Nations children in Canada's child welfare system: An analysis of the Canadian incidence study of reported child abuse and neglect (CIS-2003).* Toronto, ON: Centre of Excellence in Child Welfare.

Turcotte, M., & Schellenberg, G. (2007). Portrait of seniors in Canada (Cat. no. 89-519-XIE). Ottawa: Statistics Canada.

Van Wel, B., Kockmann, I., Blum, N., et al. (2006). STEPPS group treatment for borderline personality disorder in the Netherlands. *Annals of Clinical Psychiatry, 18,* 63–67. doi:10.1080/10401230500464760.

Varcoe, C., & Rodney, P. (2009). Constrained agency: The social structure of nurses' work. In B.S. Bolaria & H. Dickinson (Eds.), *Health, illness and health care in Canada* (4th ed., pp. 122–151). Scarborough, ON: Nelson Thomson Learning.

Walker, L.E. (1979). *The battered woman* (2nd ed.). New York: Springer.

Walsh, C., MacMillan, H.L., & Jamieson, E. (2003). The relationship between parental substance abuse and child maltreatment: Findings from the Ontario Health Supplement. *Child Abuse & Neglect, 27,* 1409–1425. doi:10.1016/j.chiabu.2003.07.002.

# CHAPTER

# 28

# Sexual Assault

*Margaret Jordan Halter, Verna Benner Carson*
*Adapted by Angela Hyden and Sonya L. Jakubec*

## KEY TERMS AND CONCEPTS

aggravated sexual assault, 570
blame, 578
controlled style of coping, 575
expressed style of coping, 575
intrusive thoughts, 574

rape-trauma syndrome, 573
secondary victimization, 571
sexual assault, 570
sexual assault nurse examiners (SANEs), 575

## OBJECTIVES

1. Define sexual assault and aggravated sexual assault.
2. Describe the profile of the survivor and the perpetrator of sexual assault.
3. Distinguish between the acute and long-term phases of the rape-trauma syndrome, and identify some common reactions during each phase.
4. Discuss a trauma-informed approach and describe three related practices.

5. Reflect on one's own thoughts and feelings and consider the myths about sexual assault and its impact on survivors.
6. Identify five areas to assess and six overall guidelines for nursing interventions related to sexual assault.
7. Discuss the long-term psychological effects of sexual assault.
8. Identify three outcome criteria that would signify successful interventions for a person who has suffered a sexual assault.

## ⊖volve WEBSITE

*Visit the Evolve website for Flashcards, Case Studies, and additional testing resources related to the content in this chapter: http://evolve.elsevier.com/Canada/Varcarolis/psychiatric/*  [ Pre-Test ][ interactive review ]

In 2012 and 2013, several Indian, American, and Canadian accounts of young women being sexually assaulted by multiple perpetrators raised international concern. In some of these cases, further violation occurred through the display of electronic images of these assaults, and the resulting peer humiliation led to the hopelessness, desperation, and suicide of the victims. While horrific and extreme, these outcomes have reinforced the seriousness and life-threatening consequences of sexual violence. These accounts demonstrate some of the most contemptible violations that can be perpetrated by one human being on another. In this chapter, we will further explore the epidemiology, the consequences of, and the treatment approaches for sexual assault. Sexual assault, a legal term that refers to any sexual activity for which consent is not obtained or freely given, is also referred to as *sexual violence*. Sexual harassment and stalking, also criminal behaviours that are

sexual in nature, are, however, not classified as assault. Sexual assault violates the sexual integrity of the victim and can result in a range of injury from no injury to serious injury. Using a weapon, threatening, or even endangering the life of the victim during a sexual attack are all defined as sexual assault; however, sexual assault or violence is more often much less extreme yet nonetheless equally traumatic (Brennan & Taylor-Butts, 2008).

Sex offenders may commit acts of sexual violence against children, which are considered sexual abuse (see Chapter 27). These offences are termed *sexual interference, invitation to sexual touching, incest,* and *sexual exploitation* in the criminal justice system. Aggravated sexual assault is another legal term that is used when, during a sexual assault, the life of the survivor is endangered or the assault results in injury (Brennan & Taylor-Butts, 2008).

Regardless of the descriptor or legal framework of a sexual assault, it is an act of violence. The Canadian Nurses Association's (2008) position statement on violence outlines the serious implications violence has on the physical and mental health of individuals, families, and society. In particular, research has demonstrated the significant mental health impacts of sexual assault. Sexual assault is not about sex but, rather, is an exertion of power and control over another individual. Children, older adults, women, and men can all be victims of sexual assault.

Nurses are often among the first to encounter patients who have been sexually assaulted and are instrumental not only in providing them with holistic care but also in helping to preserve evidence that could lead to prosecution of the perpetrator(s). It is essential that nurses be adequately informed about their roles and responsibilities with regard to these patients.

Sexual assault is a multidimensional problem and calls for a public health approach that emphasizes the primary prevention of sexual violence (i.e., stopping it from occurring in the first place). Until recently, this approach has been relatively neglected in the field, with the majority of resources directed toward secondary or tertiary prevention (World Health Organization & London School of Hygiene and Tropical Medicine, 2010).

This chapter will address issues surrounding sexual assault and the mental health impacts of this traumatic abuse of power and control. Throughout this chapter, survivors of sexual assault will be referred to using the female pronoun in recognition of the fact that women are significantly more frequently the victims of sexual assault. However, the principles discussed apply to anyone who has been sexually assaulted, male or female.

## EPIDEMIOLOGY

Sexual assault is a topic people are reluctant to discuss because it is attached to much anguish, blame, shame, and desperation. The silence, however, has far-reaching impacts—it is estimated that 90% of sexual assaults in Canada go unreported. Nonetheless, over 22 000 sexual assaults were reported nationwide in 2010, according to Statistics Canada (2013).

Everyone is at risk for sexual assault—it crosses all socioeconomic groups; ages, from infant to older adult; genders; sexual orientations; abilities; and cultural groups (Association of Alberta Sexual Assault Services, 2010). Recent research studies, though, have identified particular risk and resiliency factors to mental health post-assault. In particular, it has been noted that rates of post-traumatic stress disorder (PTSD) are two to three times higher for survivors of sexual assault than for any other trauma, including other crimes, motor vehicle accidents, and even disasters (Foa & Street, 2001; Kessler, Davis, & Kendler, 1997). Women who have been sexually assaulted have rates of health care utilization as much as four to five times higher than nonassaulted women and higher rates of chronic disease, particularly if they have mental health effects such as PTSD, depression, or substance abuse (Max, Rice, Finkelstein, et al., 2004).

Another important pattern of disease resulting from sexual assault is the concern for secondary victimization. Secondary victimization results when survivors experience further stress or trauma when seeking help, through practices such as victim blaming, insensitive communication techniques, delays in care, disbelief, shame, stigmatization, or minimization of the experience by others (Campbell, 2008; Campbell, Wasco, Ahrens, et al., 2001; Campbell, 2005). Because of the high rate of the above-mentioned patterns, understanding sexual assault and its effects, prevention, and treatment is an important mental health and public health concern.

The Criminal Code of Canada was amended in 1983 to replace the crimes of rape and indecent assault with three new sexual assault offences, focusing on the violent rather than sexual aspects of sexual assault. These changes are in keeping with the view that sexual assault is an abuse of power and control. Legislative changes also reinforced that a spouse could be charged with sexual assault and that both males and females could be considered victims of sexual assault (Brennan & Taylor-Butts, 2008).

Data collected from the General Social Survey (GSS) and Uniform Crime Reporting Survey (UCR) (Brennan & Taylor-Butts, 2008) outline the characteristics and prevalence of sexual assault in Canada. Fewer than one in ten incidents of sexual assault is reported to the police. Rates of sexual assault are higher among females. The 2004 GSS revealed that the incidence of sexual assault of females was almost five times that of males. The rate of sexual assault for Canadians aged 15 to 24 was almost 18 times greater than the rate for Canadians aged 55 years and older. The majority (82%) of the sexual assaults reported involved an offender who was a friend or acquaintance of the victim, with stranger assaults accounting for 18% of incidents. Just over half (51%) of sexual assault incidents occurred in a commercial establishment; 31% in a residence or surrounding location; 12% in a street or other public place; and 6% in another location.

Data from the GSS indicated that most sexual assault survivors obtained support from friends (72%), family (41%), co-workers (33%), or doctors or nurses (13%), rather than report the sexual assault to the police (Brennan & Taylor-Butts, 2008), illustrating the importance of mental health first aid (see Chapter 24), as well as professional training and support. The majority of sexual assaults are considered less severe forms (as opposed to aggravated sexual assault), though this descriptor does not lessen the anguish experienced following any sexual assault.

The rate of reported sexual assault among Aboriginal people is 70 incidents per 1000 people, compared to 23 per 1000 among non-Aboriginal people (Perreault, 2011). Aboriginal women are known to have significantly higher rates of sexual assault and are more likely to be hospitalized for their injuries (Statistics Canada, 2013). Violence and sexual assault in Aboriginal communities are very complex issues and require multidimensional approaches, such as trauma-informed practices (Harris & Fallot, 2001). Culture (see Chapter 7) is an important consideration of services provided, and without attention, patients may experience secondary victimization.

### Profile of Sexual Perpetrators

Females are statistically more likely to be sexually assaulted, and males are most likely to be the perpetrator or perpetrators.

Police-reported data state that 97% of persons accused of sexual offences were male. As mentioned, a large majority of reported sexual assaults were committed by a friend or acquaintance of the victim. While we may think of the stranger lurking in the shadows in parking lots as the typical perpetrator, rape by a stranger is not typical: survivors typically know the person who sexually assaulted them. Police-reported data have indicated that 68% of aggravated sexual assaults occur at or near a residence (Brennan & Taylor-Butts, 2008), including at the victim's or perpetrator's home, at a house party, or in an outdoor party setting.

## CLINICAL PICTURE

### Relationships Between Victims and Perpetrators

The terms *intimate partner violence* and *spousal abuse* (see Chapter 27), *date rape, acquaintance rape,* and *drug-facilitated sexual assault* describe the relationship between the victim and perpetrator. In Canada, spousal sexual assault became against the law in 1983. Whether it is spousal abuse or date rape, in such cases, the perpetrator is known to, and presumably trusted by, the person who is sexually assaulted (Butler & Welch, 2009).

The psychological and emotional outcomes of sexual assault seem to vary depending on the level of intimacy and the relationship between the victim and the perpetrator. Sexual distress (including post-assault sexual problems such as dysfunction and pain) is more common among women who have been sexually assaulted by intimate partners; PTSD symptoms are common among those assaulted by someone they know; and fear and anxiety are more common in those assaulted by strangers. Depression has been found to be common among survivors, whether the perpetrators were known to them or not (Carter-Snell & Jakubec, 2013).

Drug-facilitated sexual assault has been increasingly recognized over the past 15 to 20 years. Many drugs, including alcohol (the most commonly used date rape drug), can be used alone or in combination to facilitate sexual assault (see Table 28-1). Often, these drugs are given to an unknowing victim. Once the

| TABLE 28-1 | DRUGS ASSOCIATED WITH DATE RAPE | | |
|---|---|---|---|
| **DRUG, ALTERNATIVE NAMES, AND STATUS IN CANADA** | **FORM, MECHANISM OF ACTION, AND ONSET** | **EFFECT ON VICTIM** | **OVERDOSE SYMPTOMS AND TREATMENT** |
| GHB (gamma-hydroxybutyrate) Also known as *G, easy lay, liquid ecstasy, salty water, soap, cherry meth,* and *scoop* Often made in illegal labs, resulting in the purity and strength of the final product being unpredictable | Liquid, white powder, or pill with a salty taste Schedule III central nervous system depressant A metabolite of gamma-aminobutyric acid (GABA) Onset within 5–20 minutes; duration, from 1–12 hours, is dose related | Produces relaxation, euphoria, and disinhibition Causes incoordination, confusion, deep sedation, and amnesia Tolerance and dependence exhibited by agitation, tachycardia, insomnia, anxiety, tremors, and sweating | *Symptoms:* Respiratory depression, seizures, nausea, vomiting, bradycardia, hypothermia, agitation, delirium, unconsciousness, and coma *Treatment:* Intubation for severe respiratory distress; atropine for bradycardia, and benzodiazepines for seizure activity; vomiting should be induced when possible |
| Rohypnol (flunitrazepam)* Also known as *forget-me pill, roofies* Mexico and other Latin American countries are the main illegal source of supply for North America | Pill that dissolves in liquids Schedule IV potent benzodiazepine; 10 times stronger than diazepam Impact is within 10–30 minutes and lasts 2–12 hours | More potent when combined with alcohol; causes sedation, psychomotor slowing, muscle relaxation, and amnesia Dependence and tolerance may develop | Overdose unlikely *Treatment:* Airway protection and gastrointestinal decontamination |
| Ketamine Also known as *big K, kit-kat, Special K, wonk, horsey P* A rapid-acting anaesthetic drug used mainly by veterinarians and sometimes in human surgery | Liquid or a white powder An anaesthetic frequently used in veterinary practice; also a hallucinogenic substance related to phenylcyclohexyl piperidine (PCP) Onset within 30 seconds intravenously and 20 minutes orally; duration only 30–60 minutes; amnesia effects may last longer | Causes dissociative reaction, with a dreamlike state leading to deep amnesia and analgesia and complete compliance of the victim May become confused, paranoid, delirious, combative, with drooling and hallucinations | *Treatment:* Airway maintenance and use of anticholinergics such as atropine and benzodiazepines |

*Two other benzodiazepines—clonazepam (Clonapam) and alprazolam (Xanax)—are also used.
**Sources:** Data adapted from Lehne, R.A. (2010). *Pharmacology for nursing care* (7th ed.). Philadelphia: Saunders; Health Canada. (2013). *Drugs of abuse and addiction.* Retrieved from http://healthycanadians.gc.ca/health-sante/addiction/index-eng.php; and U.S. Department of Health and Human Services. (2008). *Date rape drugs.* Retrieved from http://www.womenshealth.gov/publications/our-publications/fact-sheet/date-rape-drugs.pdf.

drugs are ingested, victims lose their ability to ward off attackers, develop amnesia, and become unreliable witnesses. Because the symptoms mimic those of alcohol intoxication, survivors are not always screened for these drugs, resulting in underreporting of drug-facilitated sexual assault (Butler & Welch, 2009). As nurses, we must remember that whether a person willingly or unwillingly consumes alcohol or drugs and is subsequently sexually assaulted, it is not the victim's fault. The Criminal Code of Canada (1985) states that consent cannot be given by a person who is unconscious or intoxicated.

## Psychological Effects of Sexual Assault

Most people who are sexually assaulted suffer severe and long-lasting emotional trauma. Long-term psychological effects of sexual assault may include depression, suicide, anxiety, and fear; difficulties with daily functioning; low self-esteem; sexual dysfunction; and somatic complaints. Survivors of incest may experience a negative self-image, depression, eating disorders, personality disorders, self-destructive behaviour, and substance abuse. A history of sexual abuse in psychiatric patients is associated with a characteristic pattern of symptoms that may include depression, anxiety disorders, chemical dependency, suicide attempts, self-mutilation, compulsive sexual behaviour, and psychosislike symptoms (Carter-Snell & Jakubec, 2013; Read, Hammersley, & Rudegeair, 2007). Reviews of the literature have summarized that timely intervention; trauma-informed approaches, such as having some control over the legal process; and the availability of positive support systems (both social and professional) provide resiliency to the psychological impacts of sexual assault (Carter-Snell & Jakubec, 2013).

## Rape-Trauma Syndrome

Rape-trauma syndrome is a variant of PTSD and consists of an acute phase and a long-term reorganization process that occurs after an actual or attempted sexual assault. Each phase has separate symptoms, discussed below. See Chapter 13 for a more detailed discussion of PTSD.

## Acute Phase

The acute phase of rape-trauma syndrome occurs immediately after the assault and may last two to three weeks. At this stage, patients usually are seen by emergency-department personnel and, if available, the sexual assault nurse examiner (SANE), who are most involved in dealing with initial reactions. During this phase, there is a great deal of disorganization in the person's life, and somatic symptoms are common. This disorganization can be described in terms of impact, somatic, and emotional reactions (Box 28-1).

The survivor's most common initial reactions are shock, numbness, and disbelief. Outwardly, the person may appear self-contained and calm and may make remarks such as "It doesn't seem real" or "I don't believe this really happened to me." Sometimes, cognitive functions may be impaired, and the traumatized person may appear extremely confused and have difficulty concentrating and making decisions. Alternatively, the person may become hysterical or restless or may cry or even smile. These reactions to crisis are typical and may shift in

---

### BOX 28-1 ACUTE PHASE OF RAPE-TRAUMA SYNDROME

**Impact Reaction**

*Expressed Style*

Overt behaviours:
- Crying, sobbing
- Smiling, laughing, joking
- Agitation, anger, hysteria
- Volatility, lability, restlessness
- Confusion, incoherence, disorientation
- Tenseness

*Controlled Style*

Ambiguous appearances and reactions:
- Confusion, incoherence, disorientation
- Lack of affective response
- Calm, subdued appearance
- Shock, numbness, confusion, freezing, disbelief
- Distractibility, difficulty making decisions

**Somatic Reaction**

Evidenced within first several weeks after a rape:
- Physical trauma
  - Bruises (breasts, throat, or back)
  - Soreness
- Skeletal muscle tension
  - Headaches
  - Sleep disturbances
  - Grimaces, twitches
- Gastrointestinal symptoms
  - Abdominal pains
  - Nausea
  - Loss of appetite
  - Diarrhea
- Genitourinary Symptoms
  - Vaginal itching or discharge
  - Pain or discomfort

**Emotional Reaction**
- Fear of physical violence and death
- Denial
- Anxiety
- Shock
- Humiliation
- Fatigue
- Embarrassment
- Desire for revenge
- Self-blame
- Decreased self-esteem
- Shame
- Guilt
- Anger

**Source:** Adapted from Burgess, A.W. (1995). Rape trauma syndrome: A nursing diagnosis. *Occupational Health Nursing, 33*(8), 405; and Burgess, A.W., & Holstrom, L.L. (1974). The rape victim in the ER. *American Journal of Nursing, 73*(10), 1740.

presentation and reflect cognitive, affective, and behavioural disruptions resulting from the trauma.

People who have experienced an emotionally overwhelming event may find it too painful to discuss. Examples of this response are found in statements such as "I don't want to talk about it" or "I just want to forget what happened." Behaviours that minimize the magnitude of the event include reluctance to seek medical attention and failure to follow up with legal counsel.

### Long-Term Reorganization Phase

The long-term reorganization phase of rape-trauma syndrome occurs two or more weeks after the sexual assault. Nurses who care for survivors during the acute phase can help them anticipate and prepare for the reactions they are likely to experience during this later phase, which include the following:

- Intrusive thoughts of the sexual assault that break into the survivor's conscious mind both during the day and during sleep. These thoughts commonly include visions of violence toward the assailant, flashbacks (re-experiencing of the traumatic event), or dreams with violent content contributing to insomnia and incite emotions such as anger.
- Increased activity, such as moving, taking trips, changing telephone numbers, and making frequent visits to old friends. This activity stems from the fear that the assailant will return.
- Increased emotional lability, including intense anxiety, mood swings, crying spells, and depression.

Fears and phobias develop as a defensive reaction to the sexual assault. Typical phobias include the following:

- Fear of the indoors if the assault occurred indoors
- Fear of the outdoors if the assault occurred outdoors
- Fear of being alone (common for most women after an assault)
- Fear of crowds (women may believe any person in the crowd might be a rapist)
- Fear of sexual encounters and activities

Many women experience acute disruption of their sex lives with their partners. Sexual assault is especially disruptive for those with no previous sexual experience.

As mentioned, the consequences of sexual assault may be severe, debilitating, and long term. Intervention and support for the survivor can help prevent some of the complications of anxiety, depression, suicide, difficulties with daily functioning and interpersonal relationships, sexual dysfunction, and somatic complaints.

## APPLICATION OF THE NURSING PROCESS

### A TRAUMA-INFORMED APPROACH

Harris and Fallot (2001) stated that a trauma such as a sexual assault changes the world view of survivors so dramatically so as to shift the way they construct their sense of themselves and others. This trauma and the lasting effects then further inform other life choices and may guide the development of coping strategies that may help or hinder the growth and well-being of

| BOX 28-2 | PRACTICES USED IN A TRAUMA-INFORMED APPROACH |

- Supporting patients in understanding the connections between their experience of trauma and their maladaptive or adaptive strategies for coping
- Ensuring patients have choices about and control over their treatment options
- Using collaborative ways of determining needs and plans and handling distress with sincere attempts to share power, decrease hierarchy, and build trust
- Adapting screening and intake procedures so that patients are not required to disclose trauma before they are ready nor have to repeatedly tell their stories
- Recognizing the range of emotional responses and symptoms that patients may experience and identifying these as symptoms or adaptations to extreme life experiences rather than problem behaviours or extremes of personality
- Facilitating the development and use of coping skills, culturally safe healing strategies, and mechanisms for personal empowerment (which may or may not involve seeking police or legal action or survivor's support)

**Source:** Adapted from Canadian Centre on Substance Abuse. (2012). The essentials of trauma informed care. Retrieved from http://www.cnsaap.ca/SiteCollectionDocuments/PT-Trauma-informed-Care-2012-01-en.pdf.

the patient. In this way, the impact of trauma may be felt throughout an individual's life in areas of functioning both related to and far removed from the trauma.

Using a trauma-informed approach in the care of patients who have experienced sexual assault appropriately responds to the deep and profound impact of trauma (see Chapter 26). This approach emphasizes the physical, psychological, and emotional safety of both patients and caregivers, and creates opportunities for patients to rebuild a sense of control and empowerment. A trauma-informed approach can include a range of specific practices (Box 28-2).

## ASSESSMENT

Many sexual assault survivors do not report their sexual assault to the police and approximately only 13% report it to doctors or nurses (Brennan & Taylor-Butts, 2008).

The Emergency Nurses Association position statement on care of sexual assault victims (2010a) suggests the following interventions:

- Using a nonjudgemental and empathic approach
- Rapidly assessing the needs and support required to prevent further trauma
- Treating and documenting injuries
- Providing a private environment (e.g., limiting personnel to those health care providers examining the patient, a translator if needed, and a specially trained advocate if indicated and consented to by the patient)
- Assisting with or conducting the physical examination

- Collecting evidence, with appropriate documentation and technique
- Assessing for sexually transmitted infections (STIs) (including obtaining pertinent laboratory tests such as human immunodeficiency virus [HIV] testing, hepatitis profiles, and others) and treating STIs
- Conducting pregnancy risk evaluation and prevention
- Providing crisis intervention and arranging follow-up counselling

## General Assessment

With consent, the SANE should talk with the survivor, the family or friends who accompany the survivor, and the police to gather as much data as possible for assessing the crisis. The nurse then assesses the survivor's (1) level of anxiety, (2) coping mechanisms, (3) available support systems, (4) signs and symptoms of emotional trauma, and (5) signs and symptoms of physical trauma. Information obtained from the assessment is then analyzed, and nursing diagnoses are formulated.

### Level of Anxiety

A patient experiencing severe to panic levels of anxiety will not be able to problem-solve or process information. Providing support, reassurance, and appropriate therapeutic techniques can lower the patient's anxiety and facilitate mutual goal setting and the assimilation of information. Refer to Chapters 13 and 24 for more detailed discussions of the levels of anxiety and therapeutic interventions for crises.

### Coping Mechanisms

The same coping skills that have helped the survivor through other difficult problems in her lifetime will be used in adjusting to life after the sexual assault. In addition, new ways of getting through the difficult times may be developed for both the short- and long-term adjustment. Active and outwardly observable behavioural responses include crying, withdrawing, smoking, abusing alcohol and drugs, talking about the event, becoming extremely agitated, confused, disoriented, incoherent, and even laughing or joking. These behaviours are examples of an expressed style of coping (see Box 28-1).

Cognitive coping mechanisms are the thoughts people have that help them deal with high anxiety levels. A positive cognitive response might be "At least I am alive and will get to see my children again." Not-so-positive responses may become generalized as a way to sum up the situation—"It's my fault this happened; my mother warned me about working in such a trashy place"—and may develop into an ego-damaging refrain. If such thoughts are verbalized, the nurse will know what the survivor is thinking. If not, the nurse can ask questions such as "What are you thinking and feeling?" or "What can I do to help you in this difficult situation?" or "What has helped in the past?"

### Available Support Systems

The availability, size, and usefulness of a survivor's social support system must be assessed. Often, partners or family members do not understand the survivor's feelings about the sexual assault, and they may not be the best supports available. Pay careful attention to verbal and nonverbal cues of the survivor that may communicate the strength of her social network.

---

**VIGNETTE**

Sam, age 18, is brought to the emergency department by a concerned neighbour. She was found wandering aimlessly outside her house, sobbing and muttering, "He had no right to do that to me." Because of Sam's distraught appearance and her statement, the triage nurse suspects sexual assault and asks Sam if she would like to see the sexual assault nurse examiner (SANE). Sam agrees and is brought to a private area and introduced to the SANE, Ms. Davies. After respectful, non-judgemental questioning, Sam divulges that her boyfriend forced her to have sex with him. Following the assessment and treatment, plans for discharge are discussed. Sam has nowhere to go because her family is away, and she does not want anyone called. Her neighbour, MaiLin, told the nurse earlier that Sam can stay with her family.

**Nurse:** "Earlier, your neighbour, MaiLin, told me that you are welcome to spend the weekend with her family."
**Sam:** (loudly, sharply, with eyes wide) "Oh no, I couldn't do that."
**Nurse:** "You don't like that idea?"
**Sam:** (wringing a tissue in her hands, head hanging, voice soft) "I can't go in her house anymore."
**Nurse:** "Something about being in that house disturbs you?"
**Sam:** "MaiLin's husband, Don" (deep sigh, pause) "used to ... uh ... take advantage of me when I would babysit their children."
**Nurse:** "Take advantage?"
**Sam:** "Yes ... " (sobbing) "He used to try to get me to have sex with him. He said he'd blame it on me if I told anyone."
**Nurse:** "What a frightening experience that must have been for you."
**Sam:** "Yes."
**Nurse:** "I can see why you would not want to spend the night there. Let's explore other options."

A suitable place to stay is finally arranged. Sam is given counselling referrals that will help her deal with the process of reorganization after this current rape experience. Her counsellor will explore her feelings about past sexual abuse she has suffered at the hands of her neighbour when she is ready.

---

## Signs and Symptoms of Emotional Trauma

Nurses work with sexual assault survivors most frequently in the emergency department soon after the sexual assault has occurred. Sexual assault is a psychological emergency and should receive immediate attention. Many emergency departments in urban areas provide the services of sexual assault nurse examiners (SANEs) specially trained to meet the needs of sexual assault survivors. They are trained to assess the extent of psychological and emotional trauma that may not be readily apparent, especially if the person uses the controlled style of coping, a contained response, during the acute phase of the rape trauma (see Box 28-1).

Whether a SANE or another nursing or medical professional is conducting the assessment and evidence collection, a nursing history should be obtained and carefully recorded. When taking a history, the nurse determines only the details of the assault that will be helpful in addressing the immediate physical and psychological needs of the survivor. The nurse allows the survivor to talk at a comfortable pace; poses questions in non-judgemental, descriptive terms; and refrains from asking "why" questions. The survivor frequently finds relating the events of the sexual assault traumatic and embarrassing.

If suicidal thoughts are expressed, the nurse assesses what precautions are needed by asking direct questions, such as "Are you thinking of harming yourself?" and "Have you ever tried to kill yourself before or since this attack occurred?" If the answer is yes, the nurse conducts a thorough suicide assessment, as described in Chapter 25.

### Signs and Symptoms of Physical Trauma

It is essential that nurses provide psychological support while collecting and preserving legal evidence such as hair, skin, and semen samples that may be crucial for conviction of the perpetrator. The most characteristic physical signs of sexual assault are injuries to the face, head, neck, and extremities. Any physical injuries should be carefully documented, both in narrative and pictorial form using preprinted body maps, hand-drawn copies, or photographs.

The nurse takes a brief gynecological history, including the date of the last menstrual period and the likelihood of current pregnancy, and assesses for a history of sexually transmitted infection. If the survivor has never undergone a pelvic examination, the steps of the examination will need to be explained. The nurse plays a crucial role in giving support and minimizing the trauma of the examination because the survivor may experience it as another violation of her body. Recognizing this, the nurse can explain the examination procedure in a way that will be reassuring and supportive. Allowing the survivor to participate in all decisions affecting care is essential to a trauma-informed approach and helps her regain a sense of control over her life.

The survivor has the right to refuse either a legal or a medical examination. Consent forms must be signed before photographs are taken, a pelvic examination occurs, and any other procedures that might be needed to collect evidence and provide treatment are carried out. The correct preservation of body fluids and swabs is essential because DNA samples may identify the perpetrator. A shower and fresh clothing should be made available to the survivor as soon as possible after the examination and collection of specimens.

Providing prophylactic treatment for syphilis, chlamydiosis, and gonorrhea—according to guidelines of the Centers for Disease Control and Prevention (2007)—is common practice. HIV exposure is often a concern of sexual assault survivors. This concern should always be addressed, and the sexual assault survivor given the information needed to evaluate the likelihood of risk. With this information, the person can make informed choices about HIV testing tand safer-sex practices until testing can be done.

Depending on circumstances, the risk for pregnancy should be considered along with treatment options. The morning-after pill can be offered for up to 72 hours after the assault (Kagan-Krieger & Rehfeld, 2000).

All data are carefully documented, including verbatim statements by the survivor, detailed observations of emotional and physical status, and all results of the physical examination. All laboratory tests performed are noted and findings recorded as soon as they are available. One of the greatest concerns is that crucial evidence may be lost or overlooked. The Emergency Nurses Association position statement on forensic evidence collection (2010b) underscores the role of the nurse in collecting and securing medical and legal evidence.

### Self-Assessment

Nurses' attitudes influence the physical and psychological care received by sexual assault survivors. Knowing the myths and facts surrounding sexual assault can increase your awareness of your personal beliefs and feelings regarding sexual assault. If you examine personal feelings and reactions before encountering a sexual assault survivor, you will be better prepared to give empathic and effective care. Examining your feelings about abortion is also important, because a patient might choose to abort a pregnancy that results from assault. Table 28-2 compares sexual assault myths and facts.

### 📋 ASSESSMENT GUIDELINES

#### Sexual Assault

1. Assess psychological trauma, and document the patient's verbatim statements.
2. Assess level of anxiety. If in a severe to panic level of anxiety, the patient will not be able to problem-solve or process information.
3. Assess physical trauma and document per institutional, provincial or territorial, and Royal Canadian Mounted Police (RCMP) protocols. Use a preprinted body map, and ask permission and obtain written consent to take photographs.
4. Assess the survivor's available support system. Often, partners or family members do not understand the trauma of sexual assault, and they may not be the best supports to draw on at this time.
5. Identify community supports (e.g., crisis centres, support groups, therapists) that work in the area of sexual assault.
6. Encourage the patient to talk about the experience, but do not press the patient to tell.

## DIAGNOSIS

The nursing diagnosis *Rape-trauma syndrome* applies to the physical and psychological effects of a sexual assault. It includes an acute phase of disorganization of the survivor's lifestyle and a long-term phase of reorganization (see page 574).

## TABLE 28-2  MYTH VERSUS FACT: RAPE

| MYTH | FACT |
|---|---|
| Rape is caused by lust or uncontrollable sexual urges and the need for sexual gratification. | Rape is an act of physical violence and domination that is not motivated by sexual gratification. |
| Women fantasize about being raped. | No woman fantasizes about being raped. Fantasies about aggressive sex may be controlled and turned off if they become threatening. Sexual assault is a traumatic, painful, and terrifying experience. |
| Only "bad" women get raped. | Women of all ages, cultural backgrounds, social classes, and of all sexual orientations are equally likely to become victims of sexual assault. |
| When a woman dresses provocatively, she's inviting sexual attention and "asking for it". | Suggesting that women provoke sexual assault by the way they dress transfers blame from the perpetrator to the victim. If a woman is sexually assaulted, it is NOT her fault. No one ever "asks" or deserves to be sexually assaulted regardless of how they dress or behave. |
| Rape only occurs outside and at night. | Many rapes occur during the day and in the victims' homes. 80% of sexual assaults occur in the home and 49% occur in broad daylight. Rape can and does occur anytime and anyplace. |
| Men can't be sexually assaulted. | Men are sexually assaulted. Any man can be sexually assaulted regardless of size, strength, appearance or sexual orientation. |
| Only homosexual men are sexually assaulted. | Heterosexual, gay and bisexual men are equally likely to be sexually assaulted. Being sexually assaulted has nothing to do with your current or future sexual orientation. |
| Only homosexuals sexually assault other men. | Most men who sexually assault other men are heterosexual. This fact helps to highlight another reality that sexual assault is about violence, anger and control over another person, not lust or sexual attraction. |
| Erection or ejaculation during sexual assault means "you really wanted it" or "enjoyed it" or consented to it. | Erection and ejaculation are physiological responses that may result from mere physical contact or even extreme stress. These responses do not imply that the victim wanted or enjoyed the assault and do not indicate anything about the victim's sexual orientation. Some rapists are aware how erection and ejaculation can confuse the sexual assault victim, manipulating their victims to the point of erection or ejaculation to increase their feelings of control and to discourage reporting of the crime. |
| It is impossible to sexually assault a man. | Young boys or adult males can be victims of rape/sexual assault. |
| Men do NOT experience the same degree of emotional pain associated with sexual assault like women do. If a man experiences emotional pain, he should be able to deal with it. | All survivors may experience flashbacks, rage, depression or anxiety when the traumatic experience is not acknowledged and treated. Survivors of trauma may turn to alcohol or drugs to cope with overwhelming feelings. |

**Sources:** Created with data from http://www.d.umn.edu/cla/faculty/jhamlin/3925/myths.html; http://rwu.edu/campus-life/health-counseling/counseling-center/sexual-assault/rape-myths-and-fac; http://well.wvu.edu/articles/rape_myths_and_facts; http://www.secasa.com.au/pages/myths-about-male-rape/; http://www.vwsac.com/help-male-survivor.html; http://www.torontopolice.on.ca/sexcrimes/sas/statistics.php

## OUTCOMES IDENTIFICATION

The long-term outcome includes the absence of any residual symptoms after the trauma. The *Nursing Outcomes Classification (NOC)* identifies additional outcomes appropriate for the rape survivor: *Abuse protection, Abuse recovery: Emotional, Abuse recovery: Sexual, Coping, Personal resiliency, Sexual functioning,* and *Stress level* (Moorhead, Johnson, Maas, et al., 2008). Some of the suggested indicators for these outcomes include the following:

- Patient will demonstrate positive interpersonal relationships.
- Patient will demonstrate adequate social interactions.
- Patient will demonstrate healing of physical injuries.
- Patient will demonstrate evidence of appropriate opposite- or same-sex relationships.
- Patient will verbalize accurate information about sexual functioning.
- Patient will express comfort with body.
- Patient will express sexual interest.
- Patient will report increased psychological comfort.
- Patient will report a decrease in physical symptoms of stress.

## PLANNING

Unless the survivor has sustained serious physical injury, treatment is offered, and the patient is released. However, because the ramifications of sexual assault are experienced for an extended time after the acute phase, the plan of care includes information for follow-up care. The survivor needs information about available community supports and how to access them. Nurses may also encounter sexual assault survivors in other settings when they are no longer in acute distress but still dealing with the aftermath of assault. Such settings include inpatient facilities, the community, and the home. A comprehensive plan of care addresses the continuing needs of the sexual assault survivor in any setting.

## IMPLEMENTATION

The occurrence of sexual assault can be the most devastating experience in a person's life and constitutes an acute adventitious (unexpected) crisis. Typical crisis reactions reflect cognitive, affective, and behavioural disruptions. For survivors to return to their previous level of functioning, it is necessary for them to fully mourn their losses, experience anger, and work through their fears. Box 28-3 provides *Nursing Interventions Classification (NIC)* interventions for rape-trauma syndrome (Bulechek, Butcher, & Dochterman, 2008).

| BOX 28-3 | INTERVENTIONS FOR RAPE-TRAUMA SYNDROME |
| --- | --- |

*Definition of* interventions for rape-trauma syndrome: Provision of emotional and physical support immediately following a reported sexual assault.

Activities:
- Provide support person to stay with patient.
- Explain legal proceedings available to patient.
- Explain sexual assault protocol, and obtain consent to proceed through protocol.
- Document whether patient has showered, douched, or bathed since incident.
- Document mental state, physical state (clothing, dirt, and debris), history of incident, evidence of violence, and prior gynecological history.
- Determine presence of cuts, bruises, bleeding, lacerations, or other signs of physical injury.
- Implement forensic evidence collection kit (e.g., label and save soiled clothing, vaginal secretions, and vaginal hair combings).
- Secure samples for legal evidence.
- Implement crisis intervention counselling.
- Offer medication to prevent pregnancy, as appropriate.
- Offer prophylactic antibiotic medication against sexually transmitted infection (STI).
- Discuss HIV post-exposure prophylaxis.
- Give clear, written instructions about medication use, crisis support services, and legal support.
- Offer follow-up services for STI results and counselling services.
- Document according to agency policy.

**Source:** Adapted from Bulechek, G.M., Butcher, H.K., & Dochterman, J.M. (Eds.). (2008). *Nursing interventions classification (NIC)* (5th ed.). St. Louis, MO: Mosby.

### Counselling

The most effective approach for counselling in the emergency department or crisis centre is to provide nonjudgemental care and optimal emotional support. Confidentiality is crucial. The most helpful things the nurse can do are to listen and to let the survivor talk. A survivor who feels understood is no longer alone and feels more in control of the situation. It is especially important to help the survivor and significant others to separate issues of vulnerability from blame—attachment of personal responsibility for the assault onto the victim. Although the person may have made choices that made her more vulnerable, she is not to blame for the sexual assault. She may, however, decide to avoid some of those choices in the future (e.g., walking alone late at night or using alcohol excessively). Focusing on one's behaviour (which is controllable) allows the survivor to believe that similar experiences can be avoided in the future.

In many rural and urban communities across Canada, community-based organizations, health care providers, and grassroots organizations have brought forward concerns that the needs of survivors of sexual assault were not being met in emergency departments. Care provided was often delayed by long wait times, and nurses and physicians were not adequately trained to meet the unique needs of the survivor. Many communities have responded to these concerns. For instance, in 1984, Canada's first hospital-based sexual assault centre was opened at Women's College Hospital in Toronto. The mandate of such sexual assault and domestic violence treatment centres is to address the medical, emotional, social, forensic, and legal needs of women, men, and children who have been recently sexually assaulted or who are survivors of domestic abuse in a prompt, professional, and compassionate manner (Ontario Network Sexual Assault/Domestic Violence Treatment Centres, n.d.). Since the first one was opened, similar sexual assault care centres have been introduced in many different formats throughout Canada, including individual centres serving vast rural communities. Other examples of regional sexual assault organizations include the Northern Society for Domestic Peace in Smithers, British Columbia, and the Avalon Sexual Assault Centre in Halifax, Nova Scotia.

If the survivor consents, involve supportive family or friends and discuss with them the nature and trauma of sexual assault, as well as the possible delayed reactions that may occur. One survivor expressed the aftermath of her assault as follows: "It takes a few days to hit you. It was bad. It was really rough for my husband. I needed to be reassured. I needed to be told that there was nothing I could have done to prevent it. Understanding helps."

Social support effectively moderates somatic symptoms and subjective health ratings. The survivor who is able to confide comfortably in one or two friends or family members, especially immediately after the assault, is likely to experience fewer somatic manifestations of stress. In many cases, family and friends need support and reassurance as much as the survivor does. This is especially true for those from traditional cultures, particularly those cultures that believe that sexual assault brings shame to the entire family. The longstanding cultural myth that women are the property of men still prevents some people from empathizing with the woman's severe psychic injury and from being supportive. In these cases, the woman is devalued instead.

## Promotion of Self-Care Activities

When preparing the survivor for discharge, the nurse provides a printout of all referral information and follow-up instructions, detailing potential physical concerns and emotional reactions, legal matters, referrals to community agencies and counselling, and ways that family and friends can help. Providing this information in print is important because the amount of verbal information the patient can retain will likely be limited due to high levels of anxiety. Written material can be referred to repeatedly over time.

## Follow-Up Care

The emotional state and psychological needs of the survivor should be reassessed by telephone or personal contact within 24 to 48 hours of discharge from the hospital. Repeat referrals should be made for resources or support services. Effective crisis intervention and continuity of care require outreach activities and services beyond the emergency medical setting.

Survivors may avoid seeking treatment from psychiatric mental health care providers because medical treatment is more socially sanctioned, and they are likely to be experiencing physical symptoms of stress. Thus, the outpatient nurse can make a more focused assessment of stress-related symptoms, depression, or both and ascertain the need for mental health referral. Reporting symptoms and seeking medical treatment are adaptive coping behaviours and can be reinforced as such.

Follow-up visits should occur at least two, four, and six weeks after the initial evaluation; however, this frequency requires the consent of the survivor. At each visit, the survivor should be assessed for psychological progress, the presence of an STI, and pregnancy. Follow-up treatments for potential HIV exposure may also be administered if required. Case Study and Nursing Care Plan 28-1 on pages 580–582 describes the care of a patient who has been sexually assaulted.

## Advanced-Practice Interventions

### Sexual Assault Nurse Examiners

Internationally, forensic nursing is becoming a specialty, and the largest subspecialty of forensic nursing is caring for the sexual assault survivor. This role is filled by the sexual assault nurse examiner. Training to become a SANE requires knowledge and skill in the areas of testing and treatment for sexually transmitted infections; collection of forensic evidence; assessment of injuries; documentation; typical survivor responses and crisis intervention; collaboration with community agencies, such as police and women's shelters; and physical assessment and examination to determine the effects of the sexual assault (Kagan-Krieger & Rehfeld, 2000).

*Survivors.* Most of those who have been sexually assaulted are eventually able to resume their previous lifestyle and level of functioning after supportive services and crisis counselling. However, many continue to experience emotional trauma, including flashbacks, nightmares, fear, phobias, and other symptoms associated with the trauma and with the related stress disorder PTSD (see Chapter 13). Some people who survive sexual assault may be susceptible to a psychotic episode or an emotional disturbance so severe that hospitalization is required. Others whose emotional lives may be overburdened with multiple internal and external pressures may require individual psychotherapy.

Depression and suicidal ideation too frequently follow sexual assault. Depression is more common in those who do not disclose the assault to significant others because they have concerns about being stigmatized, have children living at home, or have a pending civil lawsuit. Any exposure to stimuli related to the traumatic event may activate a reliving of the traumatic state.

People who have been sexually assaulted are likely to benefit from group therapy or support groups. These modalities may be particularly beneficial for survivors from cultures that are group oriented rather than individualistic and for women who derive much of their self-definition from cultural norms. Group therapy can make the difference between a person's coming out of the crisis at a lower level of functioning and that person's gradually adapting to the experience with an increase in coping skills.

*Perpetrators.* As stated previously, sexual assault is an act of violence and an abuse of power and control. This abuse is not necessarily indicative of a particular mental health problem; however, psychotherapy is essential for perpetrators of sexual assault to gain consciousness and change behaviours. Unfortunately, most perpetrators do not acknowledge the need for behavioural change, and no single method or program of treatment has been found to be completely effective. The nurse's awareness of his or her own feelings and reactions will be crucial to avoid interference with the therapeutic process.

# EVALUATION

Sexual assault survivors are considered to be recovered if they are relatively free of any signs or symptoms of PTSD; that is, if they are
- Sleeping well with very few instances of episodic nightmares or broken sleep
- Eating as they were before the assault (patients may respond to the crisis of rape by undereating or overeating)
- Calm and relaxed or only mildly suspicious, fearful, or restless
- Getting support from family and friends (some strain might still be present in relationships, but it should be minimal)
- Generally positive about themselves (on occasion, doubts about self-worth may occur)
- Free from somatic reactions (if mild symptoms persist and minor discomfort is reported, the survivor should be able to talk about it and feel in control of the symptoms)
- Showing a return to pre–sexual assault sexual functioning and interest

In general, the closer the survivor's lifestyle is to the pattern that was present before the sexual assault, the more complete the recovery has been.

## RESEARCH HIGHLIGHT

### Differences Between Single and Multiple Perpetrator Sexual Assaults

**Source:** Morgan, L., Brittain, B., & Welch, J. (2012). Multiple perpetrator sexual assault: How does it differ from assault by a single perpetrator? *Journal of Interpersonal Violence, 27*(12), 2415–2436.

#### Problem

Multiple perpetrator sexual assaults (MPSAs), commonly referred to as "gang rapes," have been reported in several high-profile cases in India, the United States, and Canada in recent years. Little is known about the characteristics of MPSAs compared to those of single perpetrator sexual assaults (SPSAs).

#### Purpose of Study

Understanding MPSAs as distinct from SPSAs can isolate characteristic features of the perpetrators, the victims, and the nature of these assaults.

#### Methods

This study compared characteristics of 135 cases of MPSAs and 139 cases of SPSAs from a London, UK, sexual assault centre over a four-year period.

#### Key Findings

Victims of MPSAs were found to be younger, be more likely to report previous self-harm, be non-White, and have sustained injuries in the assault than victims of SPSA. The perpetrators of MPSAs were younger, less likely to be White, and more likely to be strangers to the victim than in cases of SPSA. The nature of the assaults was also distinct, with more completed and multiple rapes in MPSA. These perpetrators were more likely than perpetrators of SPSAs to meet the victim in an outside location before carrying out the assault in a place of residence that was not the victim's.

#### Implications for Nursing Practice

The implications of these discoveries contribute to knowledge for future directions for crime prevention, specifically targeted education programs for youth, and assistance provided to survivors of MPSA. Because survivors of MPSA tend to present with more injuries, it follows that STI prevention would be considered an important component of follow-up treatment strategies.

## CASE STUDY AND NURSING CARE PLAN 28-1

### Sexual Assault

*Jenna Smith is a 23-year-old Australian working at a Canadian ski hill hotel on a temporary working visa. One evening when not on shift at the hotel, she goes out with some friends and workmates for a night of bowling and drinks at a club afterwards. Later in the evening, Jenna is tired and ready to go back home. A man, Ryan, who joined the group at the club, offers to take her home. She has seen Ryan at other parties before but does not know much about him, though he is fun to be around and is an acquaintance of one of her workmates. Not in the habit of going home alone with men she does not know, she hesitates. Their mutual friend, whom she trusts, encourages her to accept the ride, stating that he "seems like a nice man."*

*Ryan drives Jenna home. He then asks if he can come into her house to use the bathroom before driving the long distance back to his house. She reluctantly agrees and sits on the living room couch. After using the bathroom, Ryan sits next to Jenna and begins to kiss her and fondle her breasts. As she protests, Ryan becomes more forceful in his advances. Jenna is confused and frightened. She manages to get away from him briefly, but he begins grabbing, squeezing, and biting her. He tells her gruffly, "If you don't do what I say, I'll break your neck." She screams, but he proceeds to sexually assault her. Ryan becomes nervous that the noise will alert the neighbours and races out of the house.*

*A neighbour does in fact arrive just after Ryan flees. The neighbour calls the police and then brings Jenna to the local hospital emergency department for a physical examination, crisis intervention, and support. In the emergency department, Jenna is visibly shaken. She keeps saying, over and over, "I shouldn't have let him take me home. I should have fought harder; I shouldn't have let him do this."*

*The nurse takes Jenna to a quiet cubicle. She does not want Jenna to stay alone and asks the neighbour to stay with her. The*

*nurse then notifies the doctor and the SANE. When the nurse comes back, she tells Jenna that she would like to talk to her before the doctor comes. Jenna looks at her neighbour and then down. The nurse asks the neighbour to wait outside for a while and says she will call her later.*

**Jenna:** *"It was horrible. I feel so dirty."*

**Nurse:** *"You have had a traumatic experience. Do you want to talk about it?"*

**Jenna:** *"I feel so ashamed. I never should have let that man take me home."*

**Nurse:** *"You think that if you hadn't gone home with a stranger this wouldn't have happened?"*

**Jenna:** *"Yes ... I shouldn't have let him do it to me anyway. I shouldn't have let him rape me."*

**Nurse:** *"You mentioned that he said he would break your neck if you didn't do as he said."*

**Jenna:** *"Yes, he said that ... he was going to kill me. It was awful."*

**Nurse:** *"It seems you did the right thing in order to stay alive."*

*As the nurse continues to talk with her, Jenna's anxiety level seems to lessen. The nurse talks to Jenna about the kinds of experiences survivors may have after a sexual assault and explains that the reactions she might have two or three weeks from now are normal in these circumstances. The nurse continues to collect the necessary information. She says that the doctor will want to examine Jenna and explains the procedure to her. She then asks Jenna to sign a consent form. While preparing Jenna for examination, the nurse notices bite marks and bruises on both breasts. She also notes Jenna's lower lip, which is cut and bleeding. The nurse keeps detailed notes on her observations and draws a body map of the injuries. After the examination, Jenna is given clean clothes and a place to shower.*

*Continued*

## CASE STUDY AND NURSING CARE PLAN 28-1—cont'd

### *Sexual Assault*

## ASSESSMENT

### Self-Assessment

The nurse has worked with sexual assault survivors before and has helped develop the hospital protocol. It took a while for her to be able to remain both neutral and responsive, because her own anger at perpetrators had initially interfered. She also remembers a time when a woman came in stating that she was assaulted but was so calm, smiling, and polite that the nurse initially did not believe her story. She had not at that point examined her own feelings or dealt with the popular societal myths regarding sexual assault. It was only later, when she had talked to more experienced health care personnel, that she learned that crisis reactions can seem bizarre, confusing, and contradictory.

The nurse learned that staying with the survivor, encouraging her to express her reactions and feelings, and listening are effective methods of reducing feelings of anxiety. Once the nurse learned through supervision and peer discussion to let go of her personal anger at the attacker and her ambivalence toward the survivor, her care and effectiveness improved greatly. All of this growth took time and support from more experienced nurses and other members of the health care team.

| Objective Data | Subjective Data |
|---|---|
| • Crying and sobbing | • "He was going to kill me." |
| • Bruises and bite marks on each breast | • "It was horrible. I feel so dirty." |
| • Lip cut and bleeding | • "I shouldn't have let him rape me." |
| • Sexual assault reported to the police | |

## DIAGNOSIS

The nurse formulates the following diagnosis:

*Rape-trauma syndrome*

### Supporting Data

• "I shouldn't have let him rape me."
• "He was going to kill me."
• Crying and sobbing
• Bruises and bite marks on both breasts
• Rape reported to the police
• "It was horrible. I feel so dirty."

## OUTCOMES IDENTIFICATION

**Overall outcome:** Abuse recovery: Emotional
**Short-term indicator:** Jenna will demonstrate appropriate affect for the situation.
**Intermediate indicator:** Jenna will demonstrate confidence. Short-term and intermediate outcome indicators are measured on a five-point Likert scale from 1 (none) to 5 (extensive).

## PLANNING

The nurse plans to provide emotional and physical support to Jenna while she receives care in the emergency setting and to make sure that Jenna is aware of the importance of follow-up care.

## IMPLEMENTATION

Jenna's plan of care is personalized as follows.

| Short-Term Goal | Intervention | Rationale |
|---|---|---|
| 1. Jenna will demonstrate appropriate affect by discharge from the emergency department. | 1a. Remain neutral and nonjudgemental, and assure survivor of confidentiality. | 1a. Lessens feelings of shame and guilt and encourages sharing of painful feelings. |
| | 1b. Do not leave survivor alone. | 1b. Deters feelings of isolation and escalation of anxiety. |
| | 1c. Allow patient negative expressions and behavioural self-blame while using reflective techniques. | 1c. Fosters feelings of control. |
| | 1d. Assure survivor she did the right thing to save her life. | 1d. Decreases burden of guilt and shame. |
| | 1e. When anxiety level is down to moderate, encourage problem solving, choice, and power in decision making. | 1e. Increases survivor's feeling of control in her own life. (When in severe anxiety, a person cannot problem-solve.) |

*Continued*

CASE STUDY AND NURSING CARE PLAN 28-1—cont'd

*Sexual Assault*

| Short-Term Goal | Intervention | Rationale |
|---|---|---|
| | 1f. Tell survivor of common reactions experienced by people in long-term reorganization phase (e.g., phobias, flashbacks, insomnia, increased motor activity). | 1f. Helps survivor anticipate reactions and understand them as part of recovery process. |
| | 1g. Explain emergency-department procedure to survivor. | 1g. Lowers anticipatory anxiety. |
| | 1h. Explain physical examination. | 1h. Allows for questions and concerns; survivor may be too traumatized and may refuse. |
| | 1i. Stay with survivor during physical examination. A SANE can perform examination. | 1i. Physical examination may be experienced as a second assault. Nurse provides comfort and support. |

### EVALUATION

Jenna is able to express her feelings in the emergency department, as well as understand the feelings she may experience as she moves through the reorganization phase. The indicator is achieved at a level of 3 (moderate).

## KEY POINTS TO REMEMBER

- Sexual assault is a common and often under-reported crime of violence in Canada.
- Females are far more likely to be survivors of sexual assault and tend to know their perpetrators. Sexual assault of males tends to be under-reported, owing to the humiliation and stigma attached to such victimization.
- Psychoactive substances play a major role in sexual assault, and alcohol is the most commonly used date rape drug. Other disinhibiting and amnesic substances also play a role in forcible sex acts.
- A sexual assault survivor experiences a wide range of feelings, which may or may not be exhibited to others.
- Feelings of fear, degradation, anger and rage, helplessness, and nervousness; sleep disturbances; disturbed relationships; flashbacks; depression; and somatic complaints are all common following sexual assault.
- The circumstances of the initial medical evaluation may be frightening and stressful. Police interrogation, repeated questioning by health care providers, and the physical examination itself all have the potential to add to the trauma of the sexual assault.
- The SANE can serve to minimize repetition of questions and support the survivor as she goes through the entire ordeal.
- Survivors require long-term health care that can include counselling to minimize long-term effects of the sexual assault and assist in early return to a normal living pattern.
- Telephone and online resources are available to assist sexual assault survivors.

## CRITICAL THINKING

1. Isaac, 18 years of age, is brutally beaten and sexually assaulted by a group of young men at a university party where Isaac was intoxicated and unconscious. After he regained consciousness, he tried to walk home but fell and was found semiconscious by a passerby and taken to the emergency department. Isaac has three large bruises around the occipital area of his head and several on his chest and buttocks. He has sustained a cracked rib, which he splints when walking. In assessment, he has a visible two-centimetre anal tear and is wincing in pain that he states is an 8 out of 10. Ms. Lynkowski, a SANE, works with Isaac using the hospital's sexual assault protocol. Isaac appears stunned and confused and has difficulty focusing on what the nurse says. He states repeatedly, "This is crazy, this can't be happening. … I can't believe this has happened to me. … Oh, my God, I can't believe this."
   a. What areas of Isaac's assessment should be given highest priority by Ms. Lynkowski and her staff while he is in the emergency department?
   b. Chart the signs and symptoms of Isaac's physical and emotional trauma and verbatim statements in as much detail as you can.
   c. What are some of the pivotal issues that need to be addressed in terms of assessing Isaac's signs and symptoms of physical trauma? Although the risk of pregnancy is not present, what other real physical risks need to be assessed?
   d. What are some of the signs and symptoms of rape-trauma syndrome? Of the controlled style of coping?
   e. Identify the short-term outcome criteria for Isaac that ideally would be met before he leaves the emergency department.
   f. What information does Isaac need to have regarding potential signs and symptoms that may occur in the near future? Why is this important for him to understand at present?
   g. Identify specific indicators that will be met if Isaac recovers with minimal trauma from the event. How would you evaluate these criteria?

# CHAPTER REVIEW

1. The nurse is caring for a patient in the emergency department who was sexually assaulted just hours earlier. Which behaviours should the nurse expect if the patient was exhibiting controlled-style reactions?
   1. Shock, numbness
   2. Volatility, anger
   3. Crying, sobbing
   4. Smiling, laughing

2. The nurse is caring for a patient who has just been sexually assaulted. Which is the appropriate initial nursing response?
   1. "I will get you the number for the crisis intervention specialist."
   2. "May I get your consent to test you for pregnancy and HIV?"
   3. "You are safe here."
   4. "I need to look at your bruises and cuts."

3. A patient who has been sexually assaulted has chosen to accept pregnancy prophylaxis medication but states she does not believe in abortion. What information can you, as a nurse, give that will help with her decision?
   1. "Emergency contraception is not an abortion pill and will not work if you are already pregnant. That is the reason we perform a pregnancy test."
   2. "Just take a few days to consider your options."
   3. "Here is the number to your local sexual health clinic. They can explain it to you."
   4. "I won't give you the pregnancy prophylaxis medication then."

4. The nurse is working at a telephone hotline centre when a sexual assault survivor calls. If the sexual assault survivor states she is fearful of going to the hospital, what is the appropriate nursing response?
   1. "You don't need to go to the hospital if you don't want to."
   2. "I'm here to listen to you, and we can talk about your feelings."
   3. "Did you do something to make the other person attack you?"
   4. "Why are you afraid to seek medical attention?"

5. The nurse is caring for a patient who is in the long-term reorganization phase of rape-trauma syndrome. Which symptom(s) should the nurse anticipate? Select all that apply.
   1. Development of fear of locations that resemble the rape location
   2. Emergence of acceptance of the rape
   3. Dreams with violent content
   4. A shift from anxiety to calm
   5. Onset of phobia of being alone

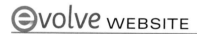 WEBSITE

Post-Test  interactive review

*Visit the Evolve Web site for Chapter Review Answers and Rationales, Critical Thinking Answer Guidelines, and additional resources related to the content in this chapter:* http://evolve.elsevier.com/Canada/Varcarolis/psychiatric/

# REFERENCES

Association of Alberta Sexual Assault Services. (2010). *Our message to Albertans: Sexual assault affects every one of us.* Retrieved from http://aasas.ca/index.php/main/page//our-message-to-albertans-2010-09-21-13-09-08.

Brennan, S., & Taylor-Butts, A. (2008). *Statistics Canada Canadian Centre for Justice Statistics profile series: Sexual assault in Canada 2004 and 2007* (Cat. No. 85F0033M). Ottawa: Statistics Canada. Retrieved from http://www.statcan.gc.ca/pub/85f0033m/85f0033m2008019-eng.pdf.

Bulechek, G.M., Butcher, H.K., & Dochterman, J.M. (2008). *Nursing interventions classification (NIC)* (5th ed.). St. Louis, MO: Mosby.

Butler, B., & Welch, J. (2009). Drug-facilitated sexual assault. *Canadian Medical Association Journal, 180,* 493–494. doi:10.1503/cmaj.090006.

Campbell, R. (2005). What really happened? A validation study of rape survivors' help-seeking experiences with the legal and medical systems. *Violence & Victims, 20*(1), 55–69.

Campbell, R. (2008). The psychological impact of rape victims' experiences with the legal, medical and mental health systems. *American Psychologist, 63*(8), 702–717.

Campbell, R., Wasco, S.M., Ahrens, C.E., et al. (2001). Preventing the "second rape": Rape survivors' experiences with community service providers. *Journal of Interpersonal Violence, 16*(12), 1239–1259.

Canadian Nurses Association. (2008). *Joint position statement: Workplace violence.* Retrieved from http://www2.cna-aiic.ca/CNA/documents/pdf/publications/JPS95_Workplace_Violence_e.pdf.

Carter-Snell, C., & Jakubec, S.L. (2013). Exploring influences on women's mental health after interpersonal violence. *International Journal of Child, Youth and Family Studies, 1,* 72–99. Retrieved from http://journals.uvic.ca/index.php/ijcyfs/article/view/11844/3413.

Centers for Disease Control and Prevention. (2007). *Understanding sexual violence fact sheet.* Retrieved from http://www.cdc.gov/ncipc/pub-res/images/SV%20Factsheet.pdf.

Criminal Code of Canada, R.S.C. 1985, c. C-46.

Emergency Nurses Association. (2010a). *Emergency Nurses Association position statements: Care of sexual assault and rape victims in the emergency department.* Retrieved from http://www.ena.org/SiteCollectionDocuments/Position%20Statements/SexualAssaultRapeVictims.pdf.

Emergency Nurses Association. (2010b). *Emergency Nurses Association position statements: Forensic evidence collection.* Retrieved from http://www.ena.org/SiteCollectionDocuments/Position%20Statements/Forensic%20Evidence.pdf.

Foa, E.B., & Street, G.P. (2001). Women and traumatic events. *Journal of Clinical Psychiatry, 62,* 29–34.

Harris, M., & Fallot, R.D., (2001). Using trauma theory to design service systems. *New Directions for Mental Health Services, 89,* 1–103.

Kagan-Krieger, S., & Rehfeld, G. (2000). The sexual assault nurse examiner. *Canadian Nurse, 96*(6), 20–24.

Kessler, R.C., Davis, C.G., & Kendler, K.S. (1997). Childhood adversity and adult psychiatric disorder in the U.S. national comorbidity survey. *Psychological Medicine, 27*(5), 1101–1119.

Max, W., Rice, D.P., Finkelstein, E., et al. (2004). The economic toll of intimate partner violence against women in the United States. *Violence & Survivors, 19*(3), 259–272.

Moorhead, S., Johnson, M., Maas, M.L., et al. (Eds.). (2008). *Nursing outcome classification (NOC)* (4th ed.). St. Louis, MO: Mosby.

Ontario Network of Sexual Assault/Domestic Violence Treatment Centres. (n.d.). *Our centres: Mandate.* Retrieved from http://www.satcontario.com/en/home.php.

Perreault, S. (2011). Violent victimization of Aboriginal people in the Canadian provinces, 2009 (Cat. No. 85-002-X). *Juristat.* Ottawa: Statistics Canada. Retrieved from http://www.statcan.gc.ca/pub/85-002-x/2011001/article/11415-eng.pdf.

Read, J., Hammersley, P., & Rudegeair, T. (2007). Why, when and how to ask about childhood abuse. *Advances in Psychiatric Treatment, 13,* 101–110. doi:10.1192/apt.bp.106.002840.

Statistics Canada. (2013). Measuring violence against women: Statistical trends (Cat. No. 85-002-X). *Juristat.* Retrieved from http://www.statcan.gc.ca/pub/85-002-x/2013001/article/11766-eng.pdf.

World Health Organization & London School of Hygiene and Tropical Medicine. (2010). *Preventing intimate partner and sexual violence against women: Taking action and generating evidence.* Geneva, Switzerland: World Health Organization. Retrieved from http://www.who.int/violence_injury_prevention/publications/violence/9789241564007_eng.pdf.

# UNIT 6

# Interventions for Distinct Populations

# 29

# Disorders of Children and Adolescents

*Elizabeth Hite Erwin, Cherrill W. Colson*
*Adapted by Robert J. Meadus*

## KEY TERMS AND CONCEPTS

assent, 589
attention deficit–hyperactivity disorder (ADHD), 599
bibliotherapy, 596
conduct disorder, 603
consent, 589
dissent, 589
mutual storytelling, 596
neurodevelopmental disorders, 597

oppositional defiant disorder, 602
pica, 608
play therapy, 595
principle of least restrictive intervention, 594
rumination disorder, 609
temperament, 589
therapeutic games, 596

## OBJECTIVES

1. Explore factors contributing to child and adolescent mental disorders, and develop intervention strategies for this population.
2. Explain characteristics associated with resiliency.
3. Identify characteristics of positive mental health and development in children and adolescents.
4. Discuss holistic assessment of a child or adolescent.

5. Explore areas in the assessment of suicide for children and adolescents.
6. Compare and contrast at least six treatment modalities for children and adolescents.
7. Describe clinical features and behaviours of at least three child and adolescent mental disorders.
8. Formulate three nursing diagnoses, stating patient outcomes and interventions for each.

## ⊖volve WEBSITE

*Visit the Evolve website for Flashcards, Case Studies, and additional testing resources related to the content in this chapter:* http://evolve.elsevier.com/Canada/Varcarolis/psychiatric/    Pre-Test  interactive review

Many children and adolescents may struggle with a disabling mental illness, but most go unnoticed and unidentified (Mental Health Commission of Canada, 2012). Until *Changing Directions, Changing Lives: The Mental Health Strategy for Canada* was released by the Mental Health Commission of Canada (MHCC) in 2012, the mental health needs of young people in Canada had not received much attention.

Mental health disorders in children and adolescents are associated with disturbances in psychological, physiological, academic, and social functioning. The economic, social, and personal costs to society associated with childhood- and adolescent-onset mental disorders are tremendous because the

illness occurs during important developmental periods, has frequent recurrences, and persists into adulthood (Belfer, 2008). Stigma and misconceptions can cause patients and families to attempt to conceal the conditions or even limit help seeking and professional care (Gulliver, Griffiths, & Christensen, 2010). The commission also reports that stigma, a silent public health epidemic, can be addressed through "contact-based education" (Mental Health Commission of Canada, 2012)—that is, meeting and talking with people and families who experience mental health problems.

Childhood and adolescence are distinct developmental periods during which significant changes in physical, cognitive, and social functioning occur. As such, childhood is defined in terms of early (1–4 years) and middle childhood (5–10 years), while adolescence is described in terms of the sub-phases of early (11–14 years), middle (15–17 years), and late (18–21 years) (Hagan, Shaw, & Duncan, 2008). Important mental disorders that can occur in children and adolescents include mood disorders, anxiety disorders, schizophrenia, and substance abuse. Anxiety and depression as they relate to this age group are discussed in this chapter. These disorders, as well as the others discussed in this chapter, are more difficult to diagnose in younger children because of limited language skills and cognitive and emotional development. Additionally, children undergo more rapid psychological, neurological, and physiological changes over a briefer period than adults do. The rapidity and complexity of this development must be taken into consideration during assessment for mental health disorders. Clinicians and parents often wait to see whether symptoms are the result of a developmental lag or trauma response that will eventually correct itself; therefore, intervention may be delayed—for instance, until the child reaches school age. Usually, a number of factors influence a child's or adolescent's mental health, so a variety of interventions are needed to improve psychological, social, physical, educational, and spiritual well-being.

Meeting the mental health needs of youth and their families is a challenge for the nurse because need is steadily increasing while funding and access to care are decreasing and existing services remain fragmented or lacking in many communities. Considering all the developmental changes and associated vulnerabilities and resiliencies that occur during childhood and adolescence, it is clear that this is an optimal time to target prevention and intervention.

This chapter describes the nurse's role in assessment and interventions for selected mental health disorders, as well as broad treatment modalities that are implemented through the nursing process with this population and their families.

## EPIDEMIOLOGY

One in five children and adolescents in Canada suffers from a major mental illness that causes significant impairments at home, at school, with peers, and in the community. Some of these mental health disorders have a likelihood of recurrence and chronicity in young adulthood; in fact, 80% of adults with mental illness experienced problems in childhood or early adolescence. Epidemiology data suggest that about 14% to 25% of Canadian children and youth meet the diagnostic criteria for at least one mental disorder (Boyle & Georgiades, 2009). It is estimated that two thirds of young people with mental health problems are not receiving needed services. Suicide ranks as the second leading cause of death for youth aged 10 to 19 years, and suffocation was the predominant means of committing suicide among young Canadians. Suicide rates in Canada are increasing among female youth but decreasing among male children and adolescents (Skinner & McFaull, 2012).

Suicide is a significant problem for some Aboriginal youth whose communities lack the necessary protective benefits and appropriate sources of support, including professional and nonprofessional help. It is reported that Aboriginal youth have a suicide rate that is five to six times greater than that of non-Aboriginal youth (Canadian Association for Suicide Prevention, 2009).

### RESEARCH HIGHLIGHT

#### Depression Impact on Adolescents

**Source:** McCann, T.V., Lubman, D.I., & Clark, E. (2012). The experience of young people with depression: A qualitative study. *Journal of Psychiatric and Mental Health Nursing, 19*(4), 334–340.

**Problem**

Adolescence itself can be a stressful time for youth. The presence of a mental health disorder during this developmental stage presents a major challenge for young people who are preparing for transition into adulthood. Understanding how depression impacts the lives of young people will provide knowledge that aids development and implementation of nursing interventions specific to this population.

**Purpose of Study**

The purpose of this research study was to examine the lived experience of young people diagnosed with depression.

**Methods**

A phenomenological interpretative approach was used in semi-structured, audio-recorded interviews with 26 youth aged 16 to 22 who described their experience of what it was like to have depression.

**Key Findings**

Four themes identified in the data reflecting the experience of living with depression were (1) struggling to make sense of their situation, (2) spiralling down, (3) withdrawing, and (4) contemplating self-harm or suicide. While *struggling to make sense of their situation*, the participants questioned why they were different and not the same as others in their peer group. The youth *spiralling down* expressed how the illness became more prominent and engulfed their lives. They described the onset of illness symptoms and not knowing what to do to reverse the situation. For theme three, *withdrawing*, the adolescents reported distancing themselves from others because of fear and stigma of being labelled mentally ill. This distancing allowed them time to reflect but contributed to their feelings of loneliness and isolation. The final theme, *contemplating self-harm or suicide*, involved how they reacted to their situation. Some youth reported engagement in risk-taking behaviours such as drug and alcohol use, suicidal behaviour, contemplation of suicide, and sexually promiscuous behaviours.

**Implications for Nursing Practice**

Nurses who have knowledge and understanding of how adolescents experience and cope with depression are better able to assess these patients' coping abilities and promote enhancement of healthy coping skills. They can also promote within this youth population initiatives to counteract stigma and to seek mental health care.

The Canadian government's recognition of childhood and adolescent mental health problems and efforts toward identifying effective treatments were reported in the senate report *Out of the Shadows at Last* (Standing Senate Committee on Social Affairs, Science and Technology, 2006). Based on a key recommendation of this senate committee, the Mental Health Commission of Canada (MHCC) was formed and, in close consultation with people living with mental health problems and illnesses, families, stakeholder organizations, governments, and experts, identified child and youth mental health services as a critical component to improving mental health outcomes of Canadians. However, barriers to assessment, treatment, prevention, and early intervention remain, including the following:

- Lack of clarity about conditions for screening children
- Lack of coordination among multiple systems
- Lack of resources and long wait times for services
- Shortage of mental health care professionals
- Lack of a child and youth mental health framework

More research is needed to understand the reasons for the underutilization and early termination of mental health care services, and funding is needed to improve access to and coordination among existing resources to provide programs for these young people (Canadian Institutes of Health Research, 2010).

## CO-MORBIDITY

Children and adolescents with mental health disorders often meet the criteria for more than one diagnostic category. Attention deficit–hyperactivity disorder (ADHD), a prominent co-morbid condition, occurs in 90% of individuals with juvenile-onset bipolar disorder, 90% of children with oppositional defiant disorder, and 50% of those with conduct disorder. Childhood depression has a high incidence of co-morbidity: 20% to 80% of children with depression have conduct or oppositional disorders, 30% to 75% have anxiety disorders, and 5% to 60% display symptoms of ADHD (Reinhardt & Reinhardt, 2013). Multiple services are often needed by those with coexisting diagnoses, such as special education evaluation and services, after-school services, family counselling, and behaviour management.

## RISK FACTORS

Mental illness can become serious or severe and persistent if early detection and effective intervention are not implemented. A child with a parent with depression is at risk for developing an anxiety disorder, mood disorder, conduct disorder, or substance use disorder. The parent's inability to model effective coping strategies can lead to learned helplessness, the creation of anxiety or apathy, and an inability to master the environment. A child with a conduct disorder may develop an antisocial personality. In fact, two thirds of youth in the juvenile justice system have one or more diagnosable mental disorders (Teplin, Welty, Abram, et al., 2012).

Children who have been abused or neglected are at great risk for developing emotional, intellectual, and social problems as a result of their traumatic experiences (Public Health Agency of Canada, 2008). Exposure to intimate partner violence and neglect are two of the most prevalent forms of child abuse in Canada. According to the Public Health Agency of Canada (2008), 235 842 child-maltreatment–related investigations were conducted in Canada in 2008. Of those, 20% were related to physical abuse; 9%, emotional maltreatment; and 3%, sexual abuse. Other studies suggest more children suffer abuse and neglect than is reported to child protection services, with girls more frequently victims of sexual abuse. While boys are also sexually abused, the numbers are underreported due to shame and stigma. The nurse must understand that sexual abuse ranges from fondling to forcing a child to observe or participate in lewd acts to sexual intercourse. All instances of sexual abuse are devastating to a child who lacks the mental capacity or emotional maturation to consent to this type of a relationship.

Witnessing violence also is traumatizing and a well-documented risk factor for many problems, including depression, anxiety, nightmares, intrusive thoughts, hypervigilance, aggressive and delinquent behaviour, drug use, academic failure, and low self-esteem (Meltzer, Doos, Vostanis, et al., 2009). Children who have been abused also are at risk for identifying with the aggressor, and they may act out, bully others, become abusers in adulthood, or otherwise develop dysfunctional patterns in close interpersonal relationships.

Among adolescents, gang involvement is a growing problem. Estimates from the Royal Canadian Mounted Police (2006) suggest there are over 300 gangs and 7,000 gang members across Canada. Primarily, youths aged 11 to 13, a time of particular vulnerability, are solicited to become gang members because decision-making capacities are limited, and they may look up to older peers for status and belonging. Certain risk factors seem to predispose a person to gang membership, including past trauma, learning disability, poor school performance, poverty, and family disorganization (Esbensen, Peterson, Taylor, et al., 2009). Gang members often inflict violence on others, including vandalism, theft, and aggression. Many end up in the juvenile court system, where they exhibit mental health problems that may remain untreated.

All Canadian provinces and territories have child protection legislation, and all instances of suspected abuse of a minor child are required to be reported to the local child protection services. Further, the Government of Canada in 2001 passed legislation that came into effect in 2008 to help protect youth from nonexploitative sexual activity by raising the age of consent for sexual activity from 14 to 16 years (Parliament of Canada, 2001). This legislation brought the age of consent in line with that of other countries such as the United States and Australia. Depending upon the province or territory, a *child* is defined as a young person up to age 16 to 19, and the age of majority is 18 or 19 years. Box 29-1 discusses the decision-making terms *consent, assent,* and *dissent* as they relate to children.

It is important for nurses working in youth detention, school, and community settings to assess for post-traumatic stress disorder (PTSD) and safety of environment for young people who have been traumatized or who have experienced abuse or a

<table>
<tr><td>BOX 29-1</td><td>INCLUDING THE CHILD IN HEALTH CARE DECISION MAKING</td></tr>
</table>

Nurses working with children and youth need to recognize the young person's right to self-determination and participation in decision making related to health care and research. **Consent** is an expression of autonomy. It represents a person's capacity to understand information and voluntarily to act on this information. For example, a person may give consent (agree) to participate in a research study, or he or she may withhold consent (refuse) to participate in a particular health care treatment. Provincial and territorial legislation stipulates the age of majority—the age at which a person may give his or her own consent. Although not legally binding, including the child in the decision-making process shows respect for the child and gives the child a sense of ownership about what is happening. Despite children's lacking the capacity to consent, they still may be able to express their wishes in a meaningful way (*assent* or *dissent*). **Assent** refers to the child's agreement to participate; **dissent** indicates a child's refusal to participate in the suggested health care or research study (Lambert & Glacken, 2011). Including the child in health care decision making supports the child's growth and development. However, a disagreement between the child and the legally recognized decision maker (i.e., a parent or guardian) creates complex, ethical dilemmas for members of the health care team. In these situations, requesting an ethics consult, often provided by a clinical ethicist, is appropriate.

**Source:** Lambert, V., & Glacken, M. (2011). Engaging with children in research: Theoretical and practical implications of negotiating informed consent/assent. *Nursing Ethics, 18*(6), 781–801.

history of violence. Interventions should focus on teaching coping skills to deal with trauma, supporting efforts to achieve socially appropriate goals, and facilitating integration into healthy social support systems.

## ETIOLOGY

Mental illness in children and adolescents, as in adults, is caused by multiple factors, and distinguishing among the genetic, psychosocial, and environmental factors makes diagnosis challenging. Increasing numbers of children are born with or develop disordered brain function related to malnutrition, human immunodeficiency virus (HIV) infection, fetal alcohol syndrome, drug addiction, and brain injury. In addition, they are exposed to environmental stressors in the family, school, peer group, or community that have an impact on their social, emotional, cognitive, psychological, and spiritual development (Fryers & Brugha, 2013).

The degree of a child's vulnerability to mental illness changes over time. The resiliency of the child and the presence of positive environmental factors (e.g., parental role models, a healthy school environment) enable a child to learn and adapt. Positive influences can decrease vulnerability to mental disorders or improve functioning to the fullest possible level if a disorder exists.

### Biological Factors
#### Genetic

Hereditary factors are implicated in a number of mental disorders, including autism, bipolar disorders, schizophrenia, attention-deficit problems, and intellectual developmental disorder. Because not all genetically vulnerable children develop mental disorders, it is assumed that resilience and a supportive environment are key factors in avoiding the development of mental disorders. According to Lahiri, Sokol, Erickson, et al., (2013), some disorders (e.g., autism spectrum disorder [ASD], fragile X syndrome) have a direct genetic link.

### Brain Development and Biochemicals

Dramatic changes occur in the brain during childhood and adolescence, including a declining number of synapses (they peak at age 5), myelination of brain fibres, changes in the relative volume and activity level in different brain regions, and interactions of hormones. Myelination increases the speed of information processing, improves the conduction speed of nerve impulses, and enables faster reactions to occur. Myelination of fibres in the cortex of the brain occurs most rapidly during childhood but continues until well after puberty (Giedd, Lalonde, Celano, et al., 2009). The teen years are also marked by changes in the frontal and prefrontal cortex regions, leading to improvements in executive functions, organization and planning skills, and inhibiting responses (Sullivan, Pfefferbaum, Rohlfing, et al., 2011). These changes, including cerebellum maturation and hormonal changes, reflect the emotional and behavioural fluctuations characteristic of adolescence. Early adolescence is typically characterized by low emotional regulation and intolerance for frustration; emotional and behavioural control usually increase over the course of adolescence.

Alterations in neurotransmitters have also been implicated as playing a role in causing child and adolescent disorders. Decreased norepinephrine and serotonin levels are related to depression and suicide, and elevated levels are related to mania and pathological fear. Abnormalities in dopamine receptors and dopamine transporters are implicated in ADHD, certain addictions, and schizophrenia (Sadock & Sadock, 2008).

### Temperament

Temperament, according to Hanington, Ramchandani, and Stein (2010), is the style of behaviour habitually used to adapt to the demands and expectations of the environment. Varying temperaments are present in infants, are modified by maturation, and develop in the context of the social environment (Gemelli, 2008). All people have temperaments, and the fit between the child and parent's temperament is critical to the child's development. The parent's role in shaping that relationship is of primary importance, and, when needed, the nurse can teach parents ways to modify their behaviours to improve interactions with their children. If there is incongruence between parent and child temperament and the parent is unable to respond positively to the child, there is a risk of insecure attachment, developmental problems, and future mental disorders.

By the time children enter grade school, any inclination to use and abuse drugs in later life will show in their temperament and behaviour traits (e.g., traits such as shyness, aggressiveness, and rebelliousness). External risk factors for such abuse include substance use among peers, parental drug use, and involvement in legal problems such as truancy or vandalism. Researchers have also identified childhood protective factors that shield some children from drug use, including self-control, parental monitoring, academic achievement, anti–drug use policies, and strong neighbourhood attachment (National Institute on Drug Abuse, 2008).

### Resilience

Most children with risk factors for the development of mental illness develop normally. The term *resilience* has been used to denote the relationship between a child's constitutional endowment and success negotiating stressful environmental factors. Studies have shown that a resilient child has the following characteristics (Cicchetti, 2010):

- Adaptability to changes in the environment
- Ability to form nurturing relationships with other adults when the parent is not available
- Ability to distance self from emotional chaos
- Good social intelligence
- Good problem-solving skills

Other studies have also identified the cushioning effects of family stability in the face of poverty and adversity. The nurse's role is to identify and foster these qualities to prevent at-risk children from developing emotional and mental problems.

### Environmental Factors

To a greater degree than adults, children are dependent on others. During childhood, the main context is the family. Parents model behaviour and provide the child with a view of the world. If parents are abusive, rejecting, or overly controlling, the child may suffer detrimental effects at the developmental point(s) at which the trauma occurs. There is strong evidence that a number of familial risk factors correlate with childhood psychiatric disorders, including severe marital discord, low socioeconomic status, large families and overcrowding, parental criminality, parental mental disorders, and foster-care placement.

External factors in the environment can either support or put stress on children and adolescents and shape their development. Young people are vulnerable in an environment in which systems (e.g., schools, court systems) and people (e.g., parents, counsellors) have power and control (Gonzalez, Boyle, Kyu, et al., 2012).

### Cultural Factors

Children and youth in ethnic minority groups may be at risk for a variety of mental health problems. Economics, service availability, cultural beliefs, values, and attitudes of health care providers toward young people may impact help seeking (Stewart, Simmons, & Habibpour, 2012). In addition, because of the lack of same-culture role models, children in some minority groups experience increased risk. Differences between the cultural expectations of family and peers, presence of stresses, and lack of support within the dominant culture may have profound effects on these children and increase the risk of mental, emotional, and academic problems. Nurses working with children and adolescents from diverse backgrounds require an increased awareness of their own biases, as well as the patient's needs. The social and cultural context of the patient and family, including factors as such as age, ethnicity, gender, sexual orientation, world view, religiosity, and socioeconomic status should be taken into consideration when assessing and planning care.

## CHILD AND ADOLESCENT PSYCHIATRIC MENTAL HEALTH NURSING

Child and adolescent psychiatric mental health nurses use evidence-informed knowledge to provide care that is responsive to the patient and family's specific problems, strengths, personality, sociocultural context, and preferences.

Although the number of young people with acute mental illness in our society is increasing, inpatient and residential treatment time among this population has steadily decreased. Treatment for children often consists of brief hospitalization followed by interventions conducted in a wide spectrum of community support settings, including day treatment programs, partial hospitalization programs, clinics, schools, and psychiatric home care. To be considered eligible for inpatient hospitalization, the child or adolescent typically must be an imminent danger to self or others. In short-term inpatient facilities, the nurse has less time to form a therapeutic relationship with the child and family, making it more difficult to facilitate lasting behavioural changes. Residential and group home facilities for long-term placement are more difficult to secure because availability is often scarce, the cost is high, and consistent evidence of their effectiveness in reducing symptoms and improving long-term functioning is lacking (Shepperd, Doll, Gowers, et al., 2009).

As psychiatric care moved from inpatient facilities to the community, child and adolescent psychiatric mental health nurses became an integral part of these programs. Advanced-practice registered nurses, including clinical nurse specialists, nurse counsellors, and nurse practitioners, have established outpatient practices, school-based primary prevention, and other innovative treatment programs for young people. Research on interventions for young people at risk for developing mental illness is also being carried out in nontraditional settings such as homeless shelters, group homes, and mentoring programs, as well as online.

### Assessing Development and Functioning

A child or adolescent with mental illness is one whose progressive personality development and functioning is hindered or arrested due to biological, psychosocial, or spiritual factors, resulting in functional impairments. In comparison, a child or adolescent who does not have a mental illness matures with only minor regressions, coping with the stressors and developmental tasks of life. Learning and adapting to the environment and bonding with others in a mutually satisfying way are signs

## 🌐 CONSIDERING CULTURE

### *Hostility Toward Lesbian, Gay, Bisexual, and Transgendered Adolescents*

On October 18, 2011, in Ottawa, A.Y. Jackson High School student Jamie Hubley, 15 years of age, committed suicide. Jamie, who was openly gay, reported on his blog months before he died that he suffered continuous and constant bullying because of his sexuality. According to his father, an Ottawa city councillor, Jamie had been bullied throughout elementary school and into high school. At the time of his suicide, he was experiencing depression and receiving care from health care providers. Reaction to Jamie's death was brought forward in the House of Commons by MPs, highlighting the need for bullying and other forms of intolerance toward others to end. This event illuminates the difficulties schools and communities may have in coping with the needs of youth with emotional and behavioural difficulties and can open dialogue for nurses about how to increase community readiness to work with lesbian, gay, bisexual, and transgendered (LGBT) youth.

Statistics on hate crimes in Canada indicate that about 1 in 10 has been related to sexual orientation, and 75% of those crimes were marked by violence (Statistics Canada, 2010). Teenagers and children as young as 10 may experience feelings of identification with or sexual attraction to the same gender. Young people often disclose these feelings to friends, and they may be met with social rejection, anger, ridicule, bullying, and violence. Studies have shown that LGBT youth are at risk for a variety of negative outcomes, including dramatically increased suicidality, mental health problems, high-risk behaviours, poorer school outcomes, and homelessness. Externally, LGBT youth are subject to higher rates of violence and victimization than heterosexual youth are.

A nursing diagnosis that may apply is *Readiness for enhanced community coping* related to adapting and problem solving to meet the demands or needs of the community (in this case, the school) for the management of current stressors. Better community adapting and problem solving would lead to improved communication among community members and larger organizations. In addition to providing counselling for LGBT youth, nurses could play a key role in the following:

- Educating schools and parents about the needs of LGBT youth in an effort to change attitudes
- Helping the community apply for and obtain funds for additional programs for LGBT youths
- Encouraging communication and collaboration among community members on these issues
- Serving as advocates for LGBT youth

In its landmark document *Changing Directions, Changing Lives: The Mental Health Strategy for Canada*, the Mental Health Commission of Canada (2012) identified this population as a priority. Stemming from one of the six key strategic directions was a recommendation for increased services and more knowledge and understanding among the public and among health care providers about the impact of discrimination and stigma for LGBT individuals.

**Sources:** Mental Health Commission of Canada. (2012). *Changing directions, changing lives: The mental health strategy for Canada.* Calgary: Author; Statistics Canada. (2010). *Gay pride ... by the numbers.* Retrieved from http://www42.statcan.gc.ca/smr08/2011/smr08_158_2011-eng.htm; and Woods, M. (2011, October 18). Bullied son of Ottawa city councillor commits suicide. *Toronto Star.* Retrieved from http://www.thestar.com/news/canada/2011/10/18/bullied_son_of_ottawa_city_councillor_commits_suicide.html.

---

### BOX 29-2 CHARACTERISTICS OF A MENTALLY HEALTHY CHILD OR ADOLESCENT

- Trusts others and sees his or her world as being safe and supportive
- Correctly interprets reality—makes accurate perceptions of the environment and his or her ability to influence it through actions (e.g., self-determination)
- Behaves in a way that is developmentally appropriate and does not violate social norms
- Has a positive, realistic self-concept and developing identity
- Adapts to and copes with anxiety and stress using age-appropriate behaviour
- Can learn and master developmental tasks and new situations
- Expresses self in spontaneous and creative ways
- Develops and maintains satisfying relationships

of mental health (Box 29-2). The degree of mental health or illness can be viewed on a continuum, with one's level on the continuum changing over time. Many mental illnesses are chronic but can be managed effectively with evidence-informed treatments.

## Data Collection

Methods of collecting data include interviewing, screening, testing (neurological, psychological, intelligence), observing, and interacting with the child or adolescent. Histories are taken from multiple sources, including parents, other caregivers, the child or adolescent, and other adults, such as teachers, when possible. Structured questionnaires and behaviour checklists can be completed by parents and teachers. A genogram can document family composition, history, and relationships (see Chapter 36). Numerous assessment tools are available, and with education, nurses can use them to effectively monitor symptoms and behavioural changes.

The observation–interaction part of a mental health assessment begins with a semi-structured interview in which the nurse meets with the child or adolescent alone and asks about the home environment, parents, and siblings and the school environment, teachers, and peers. In this format, the young person is free to describe current problems and give information about his or her developmental history. Play activities, such as games, drawings, and puppets, are used for younger children who cannot respond to a direct approach. The initial interview is key to observing interactions among the child, caregiver, and siblings (if available) and building trust and rapport. The nurse needs to be cognizant of being nonthreatening in approach and

## BOX 29-3   TYPES OF ASSESSMENT DATA

**History of Present Illness**
- Chief complaint
- Development and duration of problems
- Help sought and results
- Effect of problem on child's life at home and school
- Effect of problem on family and siblings' lives

**Developmental History**
- Pregnancy, birth, neonatal data
- Developmental milestones
- Description of eating, sleeping, and elimination habits and routines
- Attachment behaviours
- Types of play
- Social skills and friendships
- Sexual activity
- Spiritual beliefs

**Developmental Assessment**
- Psychomotor skills
- Language skills
- Cognitive skills
- Interpersonal and social skills
- Academic achievement
- Behaviour (response to stress, to changes in environment)
- Problem-solving and coping skills (impulse control, delay of gratification)
- Energy level and motivation
- Self-concept
- Drug and alcohol use

**Neurological Assessment**
- Cerebral functions
- Cerebellar functions

- Sensory functions
- Reflexes
  *Note:* Functions can be observed during developmental assessment and while playing games involving a specific ability (e.g., "Simon says touch your nose").

**Medical History**
- Review of body systems
- Traumas, hospitalizations, operations, and child's response
- Illnesses or injuries affecting central nervous system
- Medications (past and current)
- Allergies

**Family History**
- Illnesses in related family members (e.g., seizures, mental disorders, drug and alcohol abuse, diabetes, cancer)
- Background of family members (occupation, education, social activities, religion)
- Family relationship (separation, divorce, deaths, contact with extended family, communication, support system)

**Mental Status Assessment**
- General appearance
- Activity level
- Coordination and motor function
- Affect
- Speech
- Manner of relating
- Intellectual functions
- Thought processes and content
- Risk assessment
- Characteristics of play

using language appropriate to the young person's cognitive capabilities and verbal skills.

### Assessment Data

The type of data collected to assess mental health depends on the setting, the severity of the presenting problem, and the availability of resources. Agency policies determine which data are collected, but a nurse should be prepared to make an independent judgement about what to assess and how to assess it. In all cases, a physical examination is part of a complete assessment for serious mental health problems. Box 29-3 identifies essential assessment data.

*Developmental Assessment.* The developmental assessment provides information about the child or adolescent's maturational level. These data are then reviewed in relation to the child's chronological age to identify developmental strengths or deficits. The Denver II Developmental Screening Test is a popular assessment tool. For adolescents, tools may be tailored to specific areas of assessment, such as neuropsychological, physical, hormonal, and biochemical. One tool to assess risk is the Youth Risk Behaviour Survey for children and adolescents.

Abnormal findings in the developmental and mental status assessments may be related to stress and adjustment problems or to more serious disorders. Children may outgrow a difficulty, but nurses need to evaluate behaviours indicative of stress or minor regressions, as well as those indicative of more serious psychopathology, and identify the need for further evaluation, intervention, or referral. Stress-related behaviours or minor regressions may be handled by working with parents or caregivers. However, as young people develop maladaptive coping behaviours and use these behaviours over time, they are at risk for developing mental health disorders. Serious psychopathology requires evaluation by an advanced-practice nurse in collaboration with clinicians specializing in child and adolescent health.

*Mental Status Examination.* Assessment of mental status of children and youth is similar to that of adults. It provides information about the mental state at the time of the examination and identifies problems with thinking, feeling, and behaving. Broad categories to assess include safety, general appearance, socialization, activity level, speech, coordination and motor function, affect, manner of relating, intellectual function, thought processes and content, and characteristics of play. It is also important to obtain information not only from the child or adolescent but from others (e.g., parents, teachers, health care providers) who have been involved with the young person.

**Risk Assessment.** Suicide is the second leading cause of death in adolescence (Statistics Canada, 2012); therefore, assessment of suicidality is an essential nursing skill. Some children and youths make idle threats about killing themselves, but to determine the cause of the distress and the risk for violence, the nurse must use active listening when interacting with any young person expressing the wish to hurt self or others. The number-one predictor of suicidal risk is a past suicide attempt. Areas to explore when assessing suicidal risk include the following:

- Past and current suicidal thoughts, threats, or attempts
- Existence of a plan, lethality of the plan, and accessibility of any necessities for carrying out the plan
- Feelings of hopelessness; changes in level of energy
- Circumstances, state of mind, and motivation
- Viewpoints about suicide and death (e.g., Has a family member or friend attempted suicide?)
- Depression and other moods or feelings (e.g., anger, guilt, rejection)
- History of impulsivity, poor judgement, or decreased decision making
- Drug or alcohol use
- Prescribed medications and any recent adherence issues

Additional questions may be asked of teens, including those about risk-taking and acting-out behaviours, artwork with a violent theme, interests in music or books with morbid themes, and recent changes in behaviour or social life (e.g., eating, sleeping, isolating, loss of a relationship).

Assessing lethality of a young child's suicide plan is complicated by the distorted concept of death, immature ego functions, and an immature understanding of lethality. For instance, a child who is highly suicidal may believe a few aspirin will cause death. The incorrect judgement about the lethality does not diminish the seriousness of the intent. Another child simply seeking attention may threaten to jump off a bridge believing this action would not be fatal. Some teens may make a pact to kill themselves or become upset after a friend has committed suicide or died accidentally (Swanson & Colman, 2013). Early intervention is essential, and parents need to understand that suicidal thoughts or self-harming behaviour (e.g., burning, cutting, reckless driving, binge drinking) must be taken seriously and evaluated by mental health care providers as an emergency. Suicide prevention among children and youths is also reflected in several of the strategic directions in the *Mental Health Strategy for Canada* (Mental Health Commission of Canada, 2012).

**Cultural Factors.** Mental health care providers recognize the importance of culture in evaluating psychiatric disorders, especially when working with families. The *DSM-5* identifies culture-bound syndromes of mental illness that are not diagnostic categories in Western medicine (see Chapter 7). Sensitivity to cultural influences in mental illness is a necessity to show respect for cultural preferences in providing individualized care and to avoid behaviour stereotyping and incorrect assessment.

The use of "nonstandard" English dialects can make speech difficult to assess and can contribute to stereotyping. To facilitate accuracy in assessment, a young person should be interviewed in his or her native language to fully understand any problems (Ackley & Ladwig, 2008).

## General Interventions

The interventions described in this section below can be used by nurses in a variety of clinical and nonclinical settings. Many of the modalities can encompass activities of daily living, learning activities, multiple forms of play and recreational activities, and interactions with adults and peers.

### Family Therapy

The family is seen as critical to improving the function of a young person with a psychiatric illness; therefore, family counselling is often a key component of treatment used by nurses. There are many models of family therapy (see Chapter 36), but the focus of all is on promoting, improving, and maintaining family functioning. Following assessment, the nurse works with family members to identify specific goals and provides education on ways to achieve the goals for the family or subunits within the family (e.g., parental, sibling). Homework assignments are often used for family members to practise newly learned skills outside the therapeutic environment.

In addition to therapy involving a single family, multiple-family therapy provides useful interaction for participants to learn how other families solve problems and build on strengths, develop insight and improve judgement about their own family, learn and practise new information, and develop lasting and satisfying relationships with other families (Wright & Leahey, 2012).

### Group Therapy

Nurses use group therapy as an integral component of their practice to promote therapeutic change among children and adolescents. Group therapy (see Chapter 35) for younger children takes the form of play to introduce ideas and work through issues. For preschool and grade-school children, it combines play, learning skills, and talk about the activity. The child learns social skills by taking turns and sharing with peers. For adolescents, group therapy involves learning skills and talking, focusing largely on peer relationships and working through specific problems. Adolescent group therapy might use a popular media event or personality as the basis for a group discussion. Groups have been used effectively to deal with specific issues in a young person's life (e.g., bereavement, depression, physical abuse, substance use, dating, chronic illnesses like juvenile diabetes) (Jacobson & Mufson, 2012).

### Behavioural Therapy

Behavioural therapy involves rewarding desired behaviour to reduce maladaptive behaviours. In a healthy relationship, a child's developmentally appropriate behaviours are validated by a significant adult (*operant conditioning*). Behaviour management in psychiatry is classified according to the level of restrictiveness and intrusiveness. To ensure that the civil and legal rights of individuals are not violated, and effective treatment is provided, techniques are selected according to the principle of least restrictive intervention. This principle requires that more restrictive interventions be used only after less restrictive interventions to manage the behaviour have been attempted. Intrusive techniques (such as physical restraints) are implemented to manage behaviour and maintain safety only when very severe or dangerous behaviours (i.e., those that may result in injury to the patient or others) are exhibited.

Most child and adolescent treatment settings use a behaviour modification program to motivate and reward age-appropriate behaviours. One popular method is the point or level system, in which points are awarded for desired behaviours, and increasing levels of privileges can be earned. The value for specific behaviours and privileges for each level are spelled out, and points earned each day are recorded. Older youth can be made responsible for keeping their own point sheet and for requesting points for their behaviours. Children who work on individual behavioural goals (e.g., seeking help in problem solving) can earn additional points. Points are used to obtain a specific reward, which can be part of the system or be negotiated on an individual or group basis (Mohr, Martin, Olson, et al., 2009).

### Cognitive-Behavioural Therapy

As discussed in Chapter 3, cognitive-behavioural therapy (CBT) is an evidence-informed treatment approach based on the premise that negative and self-defeating thoughts lead to psychiatric pathology and that learning to replace these thoughts with more accurate appraisals results in improved functioning. Researchers and clinicians have discovered that CBT is also useful in treating children and youth with depression, anxiety, obsessive-compulsive disorder, and self-harming tendencies (Benjamin, Puleo, Settipani, et al., 2011).

### Milieu Management

Milieu management is the mechanism for structuring inpatient, residential, and day treatment programs. The nurse collaborates with other health care providers in structuring and maintaining the therapeutic environment to achieve the following:
- Provide physical and psychological security
- Promote growth and mastery of developmental tasks
- Ameliorate mental health disorders and promote well-being

The physical milieu for inpatient or residential care is designed to provide a safe, comfortable place to live, play, and learn, with areas for both private time and group activity. There may be a gym, outdoor playground, swimming pool, recreational facilities, and even pets. A daily schedule sets the structure for what activities will occur (e.g., school, therapy sessions, outings, family or home visits). The nurse and multidisciplinary team share and articulate a philosophy regarding how to provide physical and psychological security, promote personal growth, and work with problematic behaviours. This philosophy is reflected in the policies of the facility and is typically written in a handbook given to patients and families upon admission. The child or adolescent's behaviour, emotions, and cognitive processes are the focus of the therapeutic interventions in the

| BOX 29-4 | THERAPEUTIC FACTORS IN THE MILIEU |
|---|---|

- Safe, therapeutic environment with roles, boundaries, and limits
- Reduction of stressors
- Structure for coping with stress
- Ability to express feelings without fear of rejection or retaliation
- Availability of emotional support and comfort
- Assistance with reality testing and support for weak or missing ego functions
- Interventions for impulsive, aggressive, or inappropriate behaviours
- Opportunities for learning and testing new adaptive behaviours and mastering developmental tasks
- Consistent, constructive feedback from trained and supportive adult staff
- Reinforcement of positive behaviours and development of self-esteem
- Corrective emotional experiences
- Availability of role models for making healthy identifications and positive attachments
- Opportunities to develop peer relationships and practise handling peer pressure
- Opportunities to be spontaneous and creative
- Opportunities to explore issues related to self-esteem and identity formation

milieu. The therapeutic factors operating in the milieu's structure, activities, and interactions with staff are listed in Box 29-4.

***Seclusion and Restraint.*** Hospitalized patients are often a high risk to themselves, and effective use of prevention strategies for dangerous behaviour begins at intake. Nurses have an important role in the promotion of a culture of patient safety through assessment and intervention. Promoting a therapeutic environment for all patients involves the following (De Hert, Dirix, Demunter, et al., 2011):
- Actively engaging the patient and family in treatment planning to avoid the use of seclusion or restraint
- Maintaining adequate staffing patterns with motivated staff experienced in working with patients who have been violent, abused, or both
- Accurately assessing the acuity of the individuals and group makeup of the unit
- Using positive and less restrictive alternatives (e.g., de-escalation strategies, time-space interviews)

Controversy continues over the use of locked seclusion and physical restraint in managing dangerous behaviour, and evidence suggests both are psychologically harmful and can be physically harmful. Deaths have resulted, primarily by asphyxiation due to physical holds during restraints (De Hert, Dirix, Demunter, et al., 2011). However, at times, a child's behaviour is so destructive or dangerous that physical restraint or seclusion is needed. All nurses who might be involved in therapeutic holding or physical restraint of children and adolescents must receive education and training to decrease the risk for injury to themselves and the child. This intervention requires prompt, firm, nonretaliatory protective restraint that is gentle and safe. Children are released as soon as they are no longer dangerous, usually a few minutes, and most facilities strive to avoid all intensive interventions that restrict movement, such as holds and restraints.

The decision to restrain or seclude a child is made by the nurse who is working with the patient. A physician, nurse practitioner, or other advanced-level practitioner must authorize this action, either at the same time or after the fact. All patients in seclusion or restraints must be monitored constantly. Vital signs, including pulse and blood pressure, and range of motion in extremities must be monitored every 15 minutes. Hydration, elimination, comfort, and other psychological and physical needs should also be monitored. The patient's family should be informed of any incident of seclusion or restraint, and they should be encouraged to discuss the event with their child and reinforce the treatment plan to reduce the likelihood of future incidents (Masters, 2009).

Debriefings with staff post-incident help to strengthen the nurse–patient relationship, which may have been disrupted, and also enable staff to learn from the event to prevent it from happening in the future. Debriefings are important to determine if injury has occurred and identify whether the situation could have been avoided by using less restrictive alternatives. Research emphasizes the need for further reduction and eventual elimination of the use of restraints and seclusion as best practice in the clinical specialty of child and adolescent mental health (Azeem, Aujla, Rammerth, et al., 2011).

**Quiet Room.** A unit may have an unlocked *quiet room* for a child who needs an area with decreased stimulation for regaining and maintaining self-control. Variations on the quiet room include the *feelings room*, which is carpeted and supplied with soft objects that can be punched and thrown, and the *freedom room*, which contains items for relaxation and meditation, like music and yoga mats. The child is encouraged to express freely and work through feelings of anger or sadness in privacy and with staff support. When a child has difficulty being in touch with or expressing feelings, staff members provide practice sessions and act as role models.

**Time Out.** Asking or directing a child or adolescent to take a *time out* from an activity is another method for intervening to halt disruptive behaviours or encourage self-control. It has been reported to be a less restrictive alternative to seclusion (Bowers, Ross, Owiti, et al., 2012). Taking a time out may require going to a designated room or sitting on the periphery of an activity until self-control is regained and the episode is reviewed with a staff member. The child's individual behavioural goals are considered in setting limits on behaviour and using time-out periods. If they are overused or used as an automatic response to a behavioural infraction, time outs lose their effectiveness.

## Mind–Body Therapies

Mind–body therapies have been used in Western society for years as a treatment modality for a variety of physical and psychological disorders. These approaches focus on interactions between the mind and the body, using the mind to affect physical reactions and promote emotional health. Hypnotherapy, guided imagery, meditation, music therapy, and yoga have been shown to be effective for children and youth with mental health problems such as phobias, self-harming behaviour, anxiety, and eating disorders (Spinazzola, Rhodes, Emerson, et al., 2013). In a pilot study, Goldbeck and Ellerkamp (2012) reported that multimodal music therapy (MMT)—a combination of music therapy and cognitive-behavioural therapy—was superior to treatment as usual for children with anxiety disorders.

### ⚙ INTEGRATIVE THERAPY

#### *Yoga for Adolescents*

Low self-esteem contributes to feelings of depression, suicide, teen pregnancy, and other health-related problems of adolescence. To live a healthy and safe life, teens need to feel good about themselves and be confident. This study demonstrated that a 16-week yoga course, occurring as part of a physical education program for grade eight students, enhanced their self-esteem. The psychological benefits of yoga in general include an increase in somatic and kinesthetic awareness, positive mood, well-being, and self-acceptance and decreases in negative feelings. It also has physical benefits in improving strength and flexibility.

Before teaching yoga, the nurse must assess for any physical limitation to yoga, obtain parental consent, and encourage children to progress safely, listening to their bodies and not forcing movements that might be painful.

**Source:** Bridges, K., & Madlem, M. (2007). Yoga, physical education, and self-esteem: Off the court and onto the mat for mental health. *Californian Journal of Health Promotion. 5*(2), 13–17.

## Play Therapy

Play is often described as the work of childhood through which the child learns to master impulses and adapt to the environment. A choice of play materials can be offered to the child to aid self-expression, assess developmental and emotional status, determine diagnosis, and institute therapeutic interventions. Clinicians can also use imaginary or pretend play with young children to gain an understanding of their world (Yanof, 2013). Melanie Klein (1955) and Anna Freud (1965) were the first to use play as a therapeutic tool in their psychoanalysis of children in the 1920s and 1930s. Axline (1969) identified the guiding principles of play therapy, which are still used by mental health care providers:

- Accept the child as he or she is and follow the child's lead.
- Establish a warm, friendly relationship that helps the child express feelings.
- Recognize the child's feelings and reflect them back so the child can gain insight into the behaviour.
- Accept the child's ability to solve personal problems.
- Set limits only to provide reality and security.

The many forms of play therapy can be used individually or in groups. The term *play therapy* usually refers to a one-to-one session the therapist has with a child in a playroom. Most playrooms are equipped with a range of developmentally appropriate toys, including art supplies, clay or play dough, dolls and dollhouses, hand puppets, toys, building blocks, and trucks and cars. The dolls, puppets, and dollhouse provide the child with opportunities to act out conflicts and situations involving the family, work through feelings, and develop more adaptive ways of coping. The following vignette shows how play therapy can help a child cope with a significant loss.

> **VIGNETTE**
>
> Hannah, a 6-year-old, begins having nightmares and refusing to go to school after her grandmother, who was also her babysitter, dies. Her parents do not let her attend the funeral, thinking it will upset her. Hannah becomes fearful and preoccupied with the death. In play sessions, she repeatedly uses dolls to act out her grandmother's hospitalization, death, and funeral. She then pretends to bury her grandmother in a small, coffinlike box. Her parents have told Hannah that "Grandma has gone to heaven." Hannah demonstrates the concept by removing "Grandma" from the box and placing her high up on a bookshelf in the playroom, looking down on the rest of the doll family.

***Mutual Storytelling.*** Mutual storytelling is a psychodramatic technique developed by Gardner (1971) to help young children express themselves verbally. The child is asked to make up a story with a beginning, middle, and ending. At the end of the story, the child is asked to state the lesson or moral of the story. The nurse determines the psychodynamic meaning of the story and selects one or two of its important themes. Using the same characters and a similar setting, the nurse retells the story, providing a healthier resolution. The lesson of the story is also reformulated to help the child become consciously aware of the better resolution. If the child has trouble starting a story, the nurse can assist by beginning the story with "Once upon a time in a faraway land there lived a …" and then asking the child to continue. After the child has identified the main characters, the nurse may need to keep prompting with comments such as "and then …" until the story is completed. The story can be recorded as audio or video, which allows for a review to reinforce the learning. A similar technique called multisensory storytelling is used with children and youth. This approach involves a combination of verbal and sensory technology (games, storytelling, video, computer animation) with emphasis on sensory experience and social engagement (Penne, ten Brug, Munde, et al., 2012).

***Therapeutic Games.*** The use of therapeutic games is ideal for children who have difficulty talking about their feelings and problems. Playing a game with a child facilitates the development of a therapeutic alliance and provides an opportunity for conversation. The game might be as simple as checkers, but specific therapeutic games are more effective in eliciting children's fears and fantasies. Gardner (1979) developed a series of therapeutic games for children, one of which, Board of Objects, can be used with children 4 to 8 years of age. The game pieces are small items (people, animals, various objects) that are placed on a checkerboard. The players roll coloured dice. If a red side lands face up, the player selects an object. To get a reward chip, the player must say something about the object; if the player tells a story about the object, he or she gets two reward chips.

The child's statement or story can be used in a therapeutic interchange (e.g., to communicate empathy or make a statement suggesting a more adaptive way to cope with a difficult situation). In the end, the player with the most chips (usually the child) wins.

A board game appropriate for latency-age children (6 to 12 years) is Gardner's (1986) Talking, Feeling, and Doing Game. The player throws dice to advance his or her playing piece along a pathway of different-coloured squares. Depending on the colour landed upon, the player draws a talking, feeling, or doing card, which gives instructions or asks a question. A reward chip is given when the player responds appropriately. For example, a feeling card might read, "All the girls in the class were invited to a birthday party except one. How did she feel?" If this game is played with more than one child, the nurse can elicit additional responses and engage the whole group in the therapeutic interchange. The nurse may stack the deck to make sure that cards relating to the child's problems will be selected.

***Bibliotherapy.*** Bibliotherapy involves using literature for children or adolescents to help the child express feelings in a supportive environment, gain insight into feelings and behaviour, and learn new ways to cope with difficult situations. When children listen to or read a story, they unconsciously identify with the characters and experience a catharsis of feelings. The books selected by the nurse should reflect the situations or feelings the child is experiencing. It is important to assess not only the needs of the child but also the child's readiness for the particular topic and the child's level of understanding. A children's librarian has access to a large collection of stories and knows which books are written specifically to help children deal with particular subjects; however, the nurse should read the book first to be sure the content is age appropriate and fits with the treatment plan and be prepared to discuss it with the patient. Whenever possible, the nurse consults with the family to make sure the books do not violate the family's belief systems. A choice of several books is offered, and a book is never forced on the child.

***Therapeutic Drawing.*** Many children and adolescents love to draw and paint and will spontaneously express themselves in artwork. Their drawings capture the thoughts, feelings, and tensions they may not be able to express verbally, are unaware of, or are denying. For some, however, this modality may be too threatening or not engaging. Children and adolescents can be encouraged to draw themes, such as people, families, themselves, or more abstract themes, such as feelings. To use this modality, the nurse needs to be familiar with the drawing capabilities expected of children at particular developmental levels, and additional training is recommended. In the next vignette, the art therapist and the nurse use a family art session to identify family dynamics and begin interventions.

## Psychopharmacology

Medication is usually not used as the first line of defence in treatment of children and youth with mental health disorders. Evidence of the safety and efficacy of medication use in this population is lacking (Egberts, Mehler-Wex, & Gerlach, 2011). Medicating children typically works best when combined

Yotam, an intelligent 15-year-old with obsessive-compulsive behaviours and severe insecurity, lives with his parents and younger sister. In an art session, all family members are given paper on an easel and asked to draw themselves and the other members of the family. Yotam draws his parents and sister as being the same size and standing together shoulder to shoulder. He draws himself as a tiny figure in a box that appears to be suspended in space. When questioned, he reports feeling as though he were trapped in a falling elevator and disconnected from the family.

The family is surprised that he feels isolated (he is a normal size in their drawings). After completing a series of drawings and discussing them, the family is asked to draw a joint picture that requires them to work together. The picture they draw shows a smiling family standing by a house near a tree and a fence. The picture suggests that the family does view Yotam as separate and different, for although he is standing beside the family, he is placed behind the fence. This observation is discussed, and as an intervention, the family is given the task of finding ways to make Yotam feel included.

with another treatment such as cognitive-behavioural therapy (Sadock & Sadock, 2008). Medications that target specific symptoms can make a real difference in a family's ability to cope and in quality of life, and they can enhance the child or adolescent's potential for growth. The Drug Treatment box on page 598 lists some child and adolescent disorders and identifies some of the medications used in the treatment of these disorders.

## NEURODEVELOPMENTAL DISORDERS

Neurodevelopmental disorders (NDDs) are a complex group of diseases that cause abnormal functions of the brain or central nervous system. Children and youth with these types of disorders show impairment in language, speech, learning, memory, and motor skills (Li, Zhao, & Gao, 2013). These attributes inhibit the child's ability to participate in age-appropriate activities and introduce the need for specific programs for the child and family. A population-based study reported that 5% of Canadian children had a disability, and, of these, 74% were classified as neurodevelopmental disorders (Mâsse, Miller, Shen, et al., 2013). The disorders discussed in this section of the chapter include some of the most common child and adolescent neurodevelopmental disorders.

## INTELLECTUAL DISABILITIES

Intellectual developmental disorder (intellectual disability), previously called *mental retardation*, is characterized by developmental deficits in intellectual and adaptive functioning. The young child's level of disability severity occurs on a continuum that ranges from mild to moderate, severe, and profound. Impairment in children includes deficits in problem solving, reasoning, judgement, communication, self-care activities, and social participation (Burack, Hodapp, Iarocci, et al., 2012).

## COMMUNICATION DISORDERS

Communication disorders occur during the early developmental period of the child and are manifested by difficultly in language-skills acquisition, which impacts academic achievement, social achievement, and self-activities. The main indicators of this condition are speech and language disorders, which affect a child's ability to communicate. The child has speech-related deficits in both expressive and receptive ability, which may be evident by the inability to make vocal sounds or a disturbance in fluency. As a result, the child may stutter. The child has little or no vocabulary growth, limiting the ability to initiate or maintain engagement with others (Carlsson, Norrelgen, Kjellmer, et al., 2013). Nurses who work in a variety of settings have knowledge of appropriate developmental milestones and can serve as an important resource for children and families in early identification and referral.

## AUTISM SPECTRUM DISORDER

Autism spectrum disorder (ASD) is a complex neurobiological and developmental disability that is evident during a child's first three years of life. However, few children are diagnosed before reaching school age. It is reported that one in every 88 children born today has ASD (Autism Society Canada, 2013). This disorder affects the normal development of the brain in social interaction and communication skills. People with ASD typically have difficulties in verbal and nonverbal communication, social interactions, and leisure or play activities. These communication difficulties can include delays in babbling, echolalia (the pathological repeating of another's words), and nonmeaningful sentences. Severity is determined by the level of communication impairments and repetitive, stereotyped behaviours (Barbaro, Ridgway, & Dissanayake, 2011). While problems with left hemispheric functions (e.g., language, logic, reasoning) are evident, music and visual–spatial activities may, in rare cases, be enhanced, as in *savant syndrome* (Ursano, Kartheiser, & Barnhill, et al., 2008).

The concordance rate for identical twins is 70% to 90% (Smoller, Sheidley, & Tsuang, 2008), indicating a genetic component to ASD. Autism is four times more common in boys than girls (Sadock & Sadock, 2008). It has no racial, ethnic, or social boundaries and is not influenced by family income, educational levels, or lifestyles.

Although there is currently no universally recommended screening program for detecting ASD, Autism Society Canada (2013) has advocated for screening to be made available in Canada. Early diagnosis, identification, and intervention for children with ASD are critical to promoting better developmental outcomes for affected children and their families (Barbaro, Ridgway, & Dissanayake, 2011). Unfortunately, many families who have a child with ASD may not know it. Often, symptoms are first noticed when the infant fails to be interested in others or to be socially responsive through eye contact and facial expressions. Some children show improvement during development, but puberty can be a turning point toward either improvement or deterioration.

## DRUG TREATMENT OF CHILD AND ADOLESCENT DISORDERS AND SYMPTOMS

| DISORDER OR SYMPTOM | TYPE OF DRUG | EXAMPLES AND COMMENTS |
|---|---|---|
| Neurodevelopmental disorders | Antipsychotics | Risperidone (Risperdal) reduces hyperactivity, fidgetiness, and labile affect.<br>Olanzapine (Zyprexa) reduces hyperactivity, social withdrawal, use of language, and depression. |
| Autism spectrum disorder | Antipsychotics<br>Propranolol hydrochloride<br>Selective serotonin reuptake inhibitors (SSRIs) | Haloperidol (Haldol) can reduce irritability and labile affect.<br>Propranolol hydrochloride (Inderal) reduces rage outbursts, aggression, and severe anxiety.<br>Clomipramine (Anafranil) may help treat anger and compulsive behaviour. |
| Attention deficit–hyperactivity disorder (ADHD) | Stimulants<br><br>Antidepressants<br><br><br><br>α-adrenergic agonists | Methylphenidate hydrochloride (Ritalin, Biphentin)<br>Amphetamine (Adderall XR)<br>Both improve symptoms of ADHD.<br>Nortriptyline hydrochloride (Aventyl)<br>Bupropion hydrochloride (Wellbutrin)<br>Fluoxetine hydrochloride (Prozac)<br>All produce improvements in issues of hyperactivity, attention, and global functioning.<br>Clonidine hydrochloride (Catapres) can be used for aggressiveness, impulsivity, and hyperactivity in patients with ADHD. |
| Conduct disorders | Antipsychotics<br>Stimulants<br>Antidepressants<br>Mood stabilizers<br><br>α-adrenergic agonists | Risperidone decreases aggression.<br>Methylphenidate decreases antisocial behaviours.<br>Bupropion improves symptoms of conduct disorder.<br>Carbamazepine (Tegretol) and lithium both have demonstrated efficacy in decreasing aggression.<br>Clonidine hydrochloride may help with impulsive and disordered behaviours. |
| Panic and school phobia | SSRIs<br><br>Tricyclic antidepressants (TCAs) | Citalopram (Celexa), fluoxetine, and paroxetine (Paxil) decrease symptoms of anxiety.<br>Imipramine (Impril) is commonly used. |
| Obsessive-compulsive disorder (OCD) | SSRIs<br><br>TCAs<br>Atypical anxiolytics | Fluoxetine hydrochloride and paroxetine (Paxil) decrease symptoms of anxiety.<br>Clomipramine decreases symptoms of anxiety.<br>Buspirone hydrochloride (Bustab) is used as adjunct treatment for refractory OCD. |
| Separation anxiety disorder | TCAs<br>SSRIs | Imipramine decreases symptoms of anxiety.<br>Fluoxetine hydrochloride decreases symptoms of anxiety. |
| Social phobia | TCAs<br>Anxiolytics | Imipramine decreases symptoms of anxiety.<br>Buspirone hydrochloride decreases symptoms of anxiety. |
| Post-traumatic stress disorder (PTSD) | Atypical antipsychotics | Risperidone is used to control the flashbacks and aggression in PTSD. |
| Insomnia | Antihistamines | Diphenhydramine (Benadryl) causes the adverse effect of mild sedation. |
| Major depression and dysthymia | SSRIs<br>TCAs<br><br>Atypical antidepressants | Fluoxetine is effective in decreasing depressive symptoms.<br>No significant differences have been found between responses to TCAs and placebo.<br>Venlafaxine (Effexor XR): One small study reported no difference between venlafaxine and placebo. |
| Psychotic symptoms | Antipsychotics | Quetiapine (Seroquel) and Risperidone are effective in reducing positive psychotic symptoms. |

**Source:** Adapted from Preston, J.D., O'Neal, J.H., & Talaga, M.C. (2010). *Handbook of clinical psychopharmacology for therapists* (6th ed.). Oakland, CA: New Harbinger Publications.

Without intensive intervention, individuals with severe ASD may not be able to live and work independently, and only about one third achieve partial independence with restricted interests and activities. Managing the care of a child with ASD can be very stressful for parents and families. It is important for nurses to support and educate families in the provision of health care services that are critical in assessment, detection, and intervention for these young children. Nurses from a variety of practice settings may be involved in providing care and must use a family-centred approach.

The core presenting symptoms of ASD (Barbaro, Ridgway, & Dissanayake, 2011) include the following:

- Impairment in communication and imaginative activity
  - Language delay or absence of language
  - Stereotypical or repetitive use of language
  - Lack of spontaneous make-believe or imaginative play
  - Failure to imitate others' activities or words
- Impairment in social interactions
  - Lack of responsiveness to or interest in social activities
  - Limited eye-to-eye contact and facial responses
  - Indifference or aversion to affection and physical contact
  - Inability to share enjoyment, interest, or achievement with others
  - Failure to develop friendships or cooperative or imaginative play with peers
- Markedly restricted, stereotypical patterns of behaviour, interest, and activities
  - Rigid adherence to routines and rituals with catastrophic reactions to changes in the environment (e.g., eat only certain-textured foods)
  - Stereotypical and repetitive motor mannerisms (hand or finger flapping, spinning, head banging, hand biting)
  - Preoccupation with repetitive activities (flicking light switches, pouring water, twirling string)

## ATTENTION DEFICIT–HYPERACTIVITY DISORDER

Children with attention deficit–hyperactivity disorder (ADHD) show an inappropriate degree of inattention, impulsiveness, and hyperactivity, all of which interfere with functioning or development. Some children can have attention deficit disorder without hyperactivity (ADD). Preschoolers with ADHD exhibit excessive gross motor activity that becomes less pronounced as the child matures. The disorder is most often detected when the child has difficulty adjusting to elementary school. Attention problems and hyperactivity contribute to low frustration tolerance, temper outbursts, labile moods, poor school performance, peer rejection, and low self-esteem (Sadock & Sadock, 2008).

For a diagnosis of ADHD or ADD, symptoms must be present in at least two settings (e.g., at home and school). Children with ADHD often meet the diagnostic criteria for more than one mental disorder. They may also be diagnosed as having oppositional defiant disorder (see page 602) or conduct disorder (see page 603). Presenting symptoms of ADHD include the following:

- Inattention
  - Has difficulty paying attention during tasks (especially those requiring sustained attention) or play, even if they are enjoyable activities
  - Has difficulty listening, even with prompts and redirection
  - Is easily distracted, loses things, and is forgetful in daily activities
  - Does not pay attention to social cues
- Hyperactivity
  - Fidgets, climbs, is unable to sit still or play quietly
  - Acts as if "driven by a motor" and is constantly "on the go"
  - Talks excessively
- Impulsivity
  - Blurts out answers before the question has been completed
  - Has difficulty waiting for own turn or being patient
  - Interrupts, intrudes in others' conversations and games

## SPECIFIC LEARNING DISORDER (SLD)

This disorder in children is identified during the school-age years and varies in severity from mild to moderate to severe. One prominent feature is impairment in academic skills such as reading (dyslexia), mathematics (dyscalculia), and written expression (dysgraphia) acquisition. The prevalence of this disorder is 5% to 15% among school-age children and is more common in males than females (Peterson & Pennington, 2012). This disorder is lifelong, so early assessment, intervention, and support are important for the child and the family. Nurses are instrumental in teaching parents and children how to manage and live with the disorder. Also, ongoing assessment will involve other professionals with expertise in the areas of specific learning disorder and psychological and cognitive assessment.

The educational and occupational outcomes for individuals with specific learning disorders include high drop-out rates, low graduation rates, failure to attend post-secondary facilities, and higher rates of unemployment (Stein, Blum, & Barbaresi, 2011). Children and youth with SLD may require accommodation in school and their work environment. The Learning Disabilities Association of Canada, an important advocacy group for this population, provides education and support to families, teachers, and health care providers. These children and their families receive assistance through provincial and territorial school-based services and also through a disability tax credit offered by the federal government.

## MOTOR DISORDERS

Motor coordination is important for children as they negotiate their world. These disorders present in the early developmental period, interfering with gross motor and fine motor skills. Developmental coordination disorder is diagnosed before 5 years of age when acquisition of motor skills or coordination is below what is expected for young children achieving motor milestones such as sitting, crawling, or walking (Zwicker, Missiuna, Harrris, et al., 2012). These disorders are chronic and cause impairment in activities of daily living.

Two prevalent motor disorders are *stereotypic movement disorder* and *Tourette's disorder*. Stereotypic movement disorder is demonstrated by repetitive and stereotypic motor behaviour (e.g., body rocking, head nodding, hand shaking, waving). These movements are usually seen in young children during the first three years of age, and behaviours may occur many times during the day and last seconds, minutes, or longer. The stereotypic self-injury behaviours (e.g., head banging, self-biting, eye poking) may persist for years. The repetitive motor behaviour interferes with social, academic, or other daily activities (Jankovic & Kurlan, 2011). In assessment, the nurse needs to be aware that simple stereotypic movements are common in infancy and childhood (e.g., rocking) but usually resolve with age.

Interventions focus on changing behaviour, promoting safety, and preventing injury. Protective clothing (e.g., helmet, gloves) may be recommended for children who are prone to self-harm behaviour, as well as behaviour modification techniques including distraction and replacement. Psychotropic medications may be prescribed to reduce self-harm occurrences (Ougrin, Tranah, Leigh, et al., 2012).

Tourette's disorder (TD) usually presents itself before 18 years of age. The disorder is characterized by the presence of multiple motor tics (sudden, repetitive motor movements) and one or more vocal tics that repeat many times throughout the day. Tics disorders typically begin between 4 and 6 years of age, and diagnosis is based upon the presence of motor or vocal tics or both for more than one year. Tics are classified as either simple (e.g., eye blinking, grunting) or complex (e.g., sexual or obscene gestures [copropraxia]). A child or adolescent with tics may experience impairment in social and academic relationships as a result of feeling ashamed and self-conscious and of being ridiculed or bullied by peers (Meucci, Leonardi, Zibordi, et al., 2009). Other symptoms associated with Tourette's disorder are obsessions, compulsions, hyperactivity, distractibility, and impulsivity.

Prevalence estimates in school-age children range from 3 to 8 per 1000, with males more commonly affected than females (Bloch & Leckman, 2009). The disorder is usually permanent, but periods of remission may occur, and symptoms often diminish during adolescence and sometimes disappear by young adulthood. Common co-morbidities of TD include ADHD, obsessive-compulsive disorder, and depressive, bipolar, or substance use disorders (Jankovic & Kurlan, 2011).

The first-line treatment for Tourette's disorder is behaviour therapy rather than drug treatment. Pharmacological treatment is recommended only if tics are distressing and interfering with daily activities (Pringsheim, Doja, Gorman, et al., 2012). A comprehensive behavioural intervention for tics (CBIT) refers to habit-reversal training, which helps the patient to self-monitor current tics and then use a competing muscular response that is incompatible with the tic (Piacentini, Woods, Scahill, et al., 2010). The Canadian guidelines for treatment of tic disorders supports the use of behavioural therapy, particularly habit-reversal therapy (HRT) and exposure and response prevention (ERP), for both adults and children. However, the use of deep brain stimulation or transcranial magnetic stimulation as treatment options is not recommended. Due to a lack of evidence to support their effectiveness, these treatments are considered experimental and are recommended only for adults in severe cases (Steeves, McKinlay, Gorman, et al., 2012).

## APPLICATION OF THE NURSING PROCESS

### ASSESSMENT

Assessment is the first stage of the nursing process. Assessing for developmental milestones, child–parent relationship, and mental status is critical when initiating care for patients with NDDs.

### ASSESSMENT GUIDELINES
#### Neurodevelopmental Disorders

- Assess for developmental delays, uneven development, or loss of acquired abilities. Use baby books and diaries, photographs, films, or videotapes.
- Assess the quality of the parent–child relationship for evidence of bonding, anxiety, tension, and quality of caregiver–child temperaments.
- Be aware that children with behavioural and developmental problems are at risk for abuse, and be knowledgeable about community programs providing support services for parents and children, including parent education, counselling for parents and children, and after-school programs.

### ASSESSMENT GUIDELINES
#### Attention Deficit–Hyperactivity Disorder (ADHD)

- Observe for level of physical activity, attention span, talkativeness, frustration tolerance, impulse control, and the ability to follow directions.
- Assess social skills, friendship history, problem-solving skills, and school performance. Academic failure and poor peer relationships lead to low self-esteem, depression, and further acting out.
- Assess for associated co-morbidities, such as depression.

### DIAGNOSIS

The child with a neurodevelopmental disorder has severe impairments in social interactions and communication skills, often accompanied by stereotypical behaviour, interests, and activities. The stress on the family can be severe, owing to the chronic nature of the disease. The severity of the impairment is evident in the degree of responsiveness to or interest in others, the presence of associated behavioural problems (e.g., head banging), and the ability to bond with peers. Table 29-1 lists potential nursing diagnoses.

### OUTCOMES IDENTIFICATION

*Nursing Outcomes Classification (NOC)* (Moorhead, Johnson, Maas, et al., 2008) identifies a number of outcomes appropriate for the child with NDD. Table 29-2 presents examples of *NOC* outcomes and supporting indicators that target developmental competencies and coping skills.

| TABLE 29-1 | POTENTIAL NURSING DIAGNOSES FOR DISORDERS OF CHILDHOOD AND ADOLESCENCE | |
|---|---|

| SIGNS AND SYMPTOMS | NURSING DIAGNOSIS |
|---|---|
| Lack of responsiveness or interest in others, lack of empathy, or unwillingness to share | *Impaired social interaction*<br>*Risk for impaired parent or child attachment* |
| Severe behaviour problems, creating stress on family members | *Risk for caregiver role strain*<br>*Interrupted family processes*<br>*Chronic sorrow*<br>*Spiritual distress* |
| Lack of cooperation or imaginative play with peers | *Activity intolerance* |
| Disruptive, hostile behaviour, leading to difficulty in making or keeping friends | *Situational low self-esteem* |
| Language delay or absence, stereotyped or repetitive use of language | *Impaired verbal communication* |
| Inability to feed, bathe, dress, or toilet self at age-appropriate level | *Delayed growth and development* |
| Head banging, face slapping, hand biting | *Risk for trauma* |
| Catastrophic reactions (e.g., severe temper tantrums, rage reactions) | *Risk for other-directed violence* |
| Impulsiveness, anger, and aggression | *Risk for self-mutilation* |
| Thoughts or verbalizations regarding self-harm | *Risk for self-directed violence* |
| Frequent disregard for bodily needs | *Self-care deficit (bathing, dressing, feeding, and toileting)*<br>*Risk for situational low self-esteem* |
| Conflict with authority, refusal to comply with requests | *Powerlessness*<br>*Readiness for enhanced power* |
| Failure to follow age-appropriate social norms | *Ineffective coping* |
| Blaming of others for problems or for causing his or her actions | *Defensive coping*<br>*Impaired individual resilience* |
| Fear of being separated from parent (e.g., going to school or to a party) | *Anxiety*<br>*Relocation stress syndrome* |
| Depression | *Stress overload*<br>*Spiritual distress* |
| Refusal to attend school | *Ineffective coping*<br>*Readiness for enhanced parenting* |
| Inability to concentrate, withdrawal, difficulty in functioning, feeling down, change in vegetative symptoms | *Risk for suicide* |
| Re-experiences of past trauma (dreams, illusions, flashbacks) | *Post-trauma syndrome*<br>*Rape-trauma syndrome* |
| Fear of objects, people, or situations | *Anxiety* |

## IMPLEMENTATION

Currently, two therapies reported to be effective interventions for ASD are applied behavioural analysis (ABA) and intensive behavioural intervention (IBI). These therapies are expensive, not available in all provinces and territories, and not routinely publicly funded. However, the federal government offers a variety of income support for individuals with autism and their parents through the *Income Tax Act* and Canada Plan Disability Benefits (Standing Senate Committee on Social Affairs, Science and Technology, 2007). These supports are usually insufficient to meet the demands of individuals with autism and their families.

Treatment plans include behaviour management plans with a reward system and education of parents for providing structure, rewards, consistency in rules, and expectations at home in order to shape and modify behaviour and foster the development of socially appropriate skills. It is important that the nurse recognize and capitalize on the individual's and family's strengths and incorporate them into the plan of care. Pharmacological agents such as risperidone (Risperdal), clomipramine (Anafranil), and desipramine are used with some

| TABLE 29-2 | *NOC* OUTCOMES FOR NEURODEVELOPMENTAL DISORDERS | |
|---|---|---|
| **NURSING OUTCOME AND DEFINITION** | **INTERMEDIATE INDICATORS** | **SHORT-TERM INDICATORS** |
| *Child development: 3 Years:* Milestones of physical, cognitive, and psychosocial progression by 3 years of age | Speech understood by strangers | Gives own first name |
| *Child development: 4 Years:* Milestones of physical, cognitive, and psychosocial progression by 4 years of age | Engages in creative play | Draws person with 3 parts |
| *Child development: 5 Years:* Milestones of physical, cognitive, and psychosocial progression by 5 years of age | Follows simple rules of interactive games with peers | Recognizes most letters of the alphabet |
| *Communication: Expressive:* Expression of meaningful verbal or nonverbal messages | Directs messages appropriately | Uses spoken language; vocal |
| *Play participation:* Use of activities by a child from 1 year through 11 years of age to promote enjoyment, entertainment, and development | Expresses emotions during play activities | Expresses satisfaction with play activities |

**Source:** Moorhead, S., Johnson, M., Maas, M., et al. (2008). *Nursing outcomes classification (NOC)* (4th ed.). St. Louis: Mosby.

success in conjunction with ongoing psychiatric medication management.

Interventions for ADHD include administration of pharmacological agents for the inattention and hyperactive-impulsive behaviours, behaviour modification, family counselling, and play therapy for young children. As the child ages, special education programs to address the academic difficulties and cognitive-behavioural therapy may also be appropriate. Children and teens in specialized programs (e.g., day treatment programs) may receive additional services, such as recreational or art therapy.

Paradoxically, the mainstay of treatment for ADHD is the use of psychostimulant drugs. Responses to these drugs can be dramatic and can quickly increase attention and task-directed behaviour while reducing impulsivity, restlessness, and distractibility (Lehne, 2010). Methylphenidate (Ritalin) is the most widely used psychostimulant because of its safety and simplicity of use. However, there is a risk for abuse and misuse. Unfortunately, the medication has gained a reputation as a street drug. A common adverse effect of stimulant ADHD medications is insomnia (Lehne, 2010). To combat this effect, treating with the minimal effective dose is essential, as is administering the medication no later than 1600 hrs. Other adverse effects include headache, abdominal pain, and lethargy. Growth retardation secondary to appetite suppression has been associated with the use of stimulants, although studies have provided contradictory findings.

A nonstimulant selective norepinephrine reuptake inhibitor (SNRI), atomoxetine (Strattera), is approved for childhood and adult ADHD. Although not as effective in improving symptoms as the stimulants, this drug eliminates the risk for abuse. Therapeutic responses develop slowly, and full improvement may take up to three weeks (Lehne, 2010). The most common adverse effects are gastrointestinal disturbances, reduced appetite, weight loss, dizziness, fatigue, and insomnia. It may also cause a small increase in blood pressure and heart rate. Rarely, serious allergic reactions occur.

The dosing schedule of stimulant and nonstimulant medications is important. Drug preparations vary in their onset of action and duration of action, so dosing may be only once a day (in the morning) or up to three times a day. Because once-a-day dosing is easier and avoids the uncertainty and potential stigma of taking medications at school, long-acting medications tend to be more attractive. See the following Drug Treatment box for a summary of the Canadian-approved medications used to treat ADHD.

# DISRUPTIVE, IMPULSE-CONTROL, AND CONDUCT DISORDERS

## OPPOSITIONAL DEFIANT DISORDER

Oppositional defiant disorder is a recurrent pattern of negativistic, disobedient, hostile, defiant behaviour toward authority figures without going so far as to seriously violate the basic rights of others (Winther, Carlsson, & Vance, 2013). Children with this disorder exhibit persistent stubbornness and argumentativeness, limit testing, unwillingness to give in or negotiate, touchiness and quick annoyance, and refusal to accept blame for misdeeds. The behaviours lead to significant impairment in home or social relationships and school or occupational functioning. Children and adolescents with oppositional defiant disorder justify their behaviour as a response to unreasonable demands or situations.

This disorder is usually evident before 8 years of age and, until puberty, is more common in males; after that point, the prevalence is equal for males and females. This disorder may vary in severity from mild to moderate to severe, and the severity is determined by the symptoms and setting (e.g., at home, at school, with peers, or at work). Symptoms may be confined

## DRUG TREATMENT OF PATIENTS WITH ADHD

| CLASSIFICATION | TRADE NAME | INDICATIONS | DURATION | SCHEDULE |
|---|---|---|---|---|
| Methylphenidate hydrochloride | Ritalin | Ages 6–12 | 3–5 hours | 2 or 3 times a day |
| *Extended or sustained release* | Ritalin SR | Ages 6–12 | 6–8 hours | 1 or 2 times a day |
| | Biphentin | Ages 6 and older | 10–12 hours | Once a day |
| | Concerta | Ages 6–65 | Up to 14 hours | Once a day |
| Dextroamphetamine sulfate *Short acting* | Dexedrine | Ages 3–16 | 4–6 hours | 2 or 3 times a day |
| *Intermediate acting* | Dexedrine Spansules SRC | Ages 6–16 | 6–10 hours | 1 or 2 times a day |
| Lisdexamfetamine dimesylate | Vyvanse | Ages 6–12 | 10–12 hours | Once a day |
| Amphetamine mixture *Extended release* | Adderall XR | Ages 6 and older | 10–12 hours | 1 or 2 times a day |
| Atomoxetine hydrochloride *Extended release* | Strattera | Ages 6–65 | 24 hours | Once a day |

**Source:** Data from Huffman, J.C., & Stern, T.A. (2008). Side effects of psychotropic medications. In T.S. Stern, J.F. Rosenbaum, M. Fava, et al. (Eds.), *Massachusetts General Hospital comprehensive clinical psychiatry* (pp. 705–720). St. Louis: Mosby; and Lehne, R.A. (2010). *Pharmacology for nursing care* (7th ed.). Philadelphia: Saunders.

to only one setting (mild), be present in at least two settings (moderate), or appear in three or more settings (severe). Children and youth with this diagnosis have an increased risk for problems (e.g., antisocial behaviour, impulse-control issues, substance use, anxiety, depression) as they transition into adulthood (Burke, 2012).

## CONDUCT DISORDER

Conduct disorder is characterized by a persistent pattern of antisocial behaviour in which children and adolescents have no concern for the rights of others and a disregard for appropriate societal norms or rules. Children with this disorder also display callous–unemotional traits (e.g., lack of empathy or guilt, shallow affect) (Kolko & Pardini, 2010) and bullying, threatening, or intimidating behaviour. It is one of the most frequently diagnosed disorders of childhood and adolescence, and the behaviours associated with conduct disorder are commonly observed within settings frequented by this population (e.g., school, home, community). Complications associated with conduct disorder are academic failure, school suspensions and dropouts, juvenile delinquency, drug and alcohol abuse and dependency, and juvenile court involvement. Psychiatric disorders that frequently coexist with conduct disorder are anxiety, depression, ADHD, learning disabilities, and substance dependency.

There are four types of conduct disorder: (1) aggression toward people and animals, (2) property destruction, (3) theft, and (4) serious violations of rules. There are two subtypes of conduct disorder—child onset and adolescent onset—both of which can occur in mild, moderate, or severe forms. Predisposing factors are ADHD, oppositional child behaviours, parental rejection, inconsistent parenting with harsh discipline, early institutional living, chaotic home life, large family size, absent mother or father, mother or father who abuses alcohol,

antisocial and drug-dependent family members, and association with delinquent peers.

*Childhood-onset conduct disorder* occurs prior to age 10 years and is found mainly in males who are physically aggressive, have poor peer relationships, show little concern for others, and lack feelings of guilt or remorse. These children frequently misperceive others' intentions as hostile and believe their aggressive responses are justified. Violent children also often display antisocial reasoning, such as "He deserved it," when rationalizing aggressive behaviours (Frick, 2012). Children with childhood-onset conduct disorder attempt to project a strong image, but they actually have low self-esteem. They also display limited frustration tolerance, irritability, and temper outbursts. Individuals with childhood-onset conduct disorder are more likely to have problems that persist through adolescence and, without intensive treatment, develop antisocial personality disorder in the adult years.

In *adolescent-onset conduct disorder*, youths tend to act out misconduct with their peer group (e.g., early onset of sexual behaviour, substance abuse, risk-taking behaviours). Males are apt to fight, steal, vandalize, and have discipline problems in school, whereas girls tend to lie, be truant, run away, abuse substances, and engage in prostitution. The male-to-female ratio is not as high as for the childhood-onset type, indicating more girls become aggressive during this period of development (Thornton, Frick, Crapanzano, et al., 2013).

### Bullying

Bullying, as a concept, is broadly defined in terms of behaviour and its impact on those who are bullied. Globally, the occurrence of child and adolescent bullying in society has become a universal concern and is recognized as a major public health problem. Children and youth with disruptive, impulse-control, or conduct disorder may display aggressive behaviour toward others. Bullying is identified as an abuse of power that involves three components: harm, repetition, and unequal power. It is manifested in several ways, often called *physical* (e.g., hitting, kicking), *verbal* (e.g., threats, derogatory remarks or names), *relational* (e.g., social exclusion, spreading of rumours), and *cyberbullying* (i.e., bullying carried out through electronic means) (Klomek, Sourander, & Gould, 2010).

In Canada, the rates of bullying are reported to be higher than in many other countries (Lamb, Pepler, & Craig, 2009). Children who are victims of bullying experience low self-esteem, see themselves as socially incompetent, have more physical health problems, may go through depression, and may experience suicidal ideation. Research has also reported that the bullies themselves are more prone to substance misuse and to becoming involved in antisocial behaviours as teens and adults (Gini & Pozzoli, 2009).

Nurses should be aware that children who are being bullied may not report problems unless asked directly (Vernberg, Nelson, Fonagy, et al., 2011). It is imperative that nurses and parents or other caregivers be knowledgeable of specific signs that may indicate bullying. Some reported behaviours are sleep disturbances, unexplained cuts or bruises, tearfulness, requesting to change schools, fear of walking to and from school, and self-harm behaviours (Weston, 2009). Nurses play an important role in detecting early symptoms and signs through assessment and screening and need to work with the patient, family, and members of the school system to offset difficulties for these children and adolescents. A great resource for bullied children and their families is a government Web site that aims to stop bullying called *Bullying Canada* at http://www.bullyingcanada.ca/content/239900.

## APPLICATION OF THE NURSING PROCESS

### ASSESSMENT

When clinicians are assessing for the presence of a behavioural disorder, it is important to gather information from the perspective of the child and from that of the parent or guardian. Determining how the child and parent interact with each other as well as how the child interacts with peers, extended family, and authority figures yields valuable assessment data.

### DIAGNOSIS

Children and adolescents with oppositional defiant disorder or conduct disorder display disruptive behaviours that are impulsive, angry or aggressive, and often dangerous. They are often in conflict with others, do not follow rules, do not follow age-appropriate social norms, and have inappropriate ways of meeting their needs. Refer to Table 29-1 for potential nursing diagnoses.

### OUTCOMES IDENTIFICATION

*NOC* identifies a number of outcomes appropriate for the child experiencing hyperactivity, severe inattention, or difficulty controlling his or her impulses. These symptoms are most commonly seen in children with the neurodevelopmental disorder ADHD and in children who have any of the disruptive, impulse-control, and conduct disorders (e.g., oppositional defiant disorder, conduct disorder, intermittent explosive disorder). Table 29-3 lists a sampling of *NOC* outcomes and supporting indicators that target hyperactivity, impulse self-control, the development of self-identity and self-esteem, positive coping skills, and family functioning.

## IMPLEMENTATION

Interventions for severe oppositional defiant and conduct disorders focus on correcting the faulty personality (ego and superego) development, which include firmly entrenched patterns, such as blaming others and denial of responsibility for actions. Children and adolescents with these disorders also must generate more mature and adaptive coping mechanisms and prosocial goals, a process that is gradual and cannot be accomplished during short-term treatment. In the case of conduct disorder, inpatient hospitalization for crisis intervention, evaluation, and treatment planning, as well as transfer to therapeutic foster care, a group home, or long-term residential treatment, is often needed. Oppositional youths are generally treated on an outpatient basis, using individual, group, and family therapy, with much of the focus on parenting issues.

Unfortunately, studies indicate that many children who are simply placed in group homes and in some residential programs do not maintain improvements following discharge. However, intensive programs such as multisystemic therapy and therapeutic foster care and the use of interprofessional, community-based treatment teams for children with serious emotional and behavioural disturbances have been found to improve outcome and reduce offences over the long term (Besier, Fegert, & Goldbeck, 2009). These types of programs are more promising in improving positive adjustment, decreasing negative behaviours, and improving family stability.

To control the aggressive behaviours, a wide variety of pharmacological agents have been tried, including antipsychotics, lithium, anticonvulsants, and antidepressants, with limited effect (Calles Jr., 2011). Cognitive-behavioural therapy is used to change the pattern of misconduct by fostering the development of internal controls and working with the family to improve coping and support. Development of problem solving, conflict resolution, empathy, and social skills is an important component of the treatment program.

Families are actively engaged in therapy and given support in using parenting skills to provide nurturance and set consistent limits. They are taught techniques for behaviour modification, monitoring medication for effects, collaborating with teachers to foster academic success, and setting up a home environment that is consistent, structured, and nurturing and promotes achievement of normal developmental milestones. If families are abusive, drug dependent, or highly disorganized, the child may require out-of-home placement. The following nursing interventions are helpful when working with parents and caregivers:

- Explore the impact of the child's behaviours on family life and the impact of the other members' behaviour on the child.
- Assist the immediate and extended family to access available and supportive individuals and systems.

## 📋 ASSESSMENT GUIDELINES

### Disruptive, Impulse-Control, and Conduct Disorders

- Assess the quality of the relationship between the child or adolescent and parents or caregivers for evidence of bonding, anxiety, tension, and quality of fit between temperaments, all of which can contribute to the development of disruptive behaviours.
- Assess parents' or caregivers' understanding of growth and development, effective parenting skills, and handling of problematic behaviours; a lack of knowledge and poor parenting contribute to the development of these problems.
- Assess cognitive, psychosocial, and moral development for lags or deficits because immaturity in developmental competencies results in disruptive behaviours.
- Assess for involvement in the justice system, which may suggest a lack of impulse control or a disregard for the rights of others.
- Assess parenting practices for rules, roles, and responsibilities in the family, relationships with siblings and extended family, history of conflict, and presence of support system (e.g., extended family members, clergy, after-school program).
- Assess the school history for problems and strengths in school, grades, occupational goals, disciplinary problems, and placements.

### Oppositional Defiant Disorder

- Identify issues that result in power struggles and triggers for outbursts; note when they begin and how they are handled.

- Assess the child's or adolescent's view of his or her behaviour and its impact on others at home, at school, and with peers. Explore feelings of empathy and remorse.
- Explore how the child or adolescent can exercise control and take responsibility, problem-solve for situations that occur, and plan to handle things differently in the future. Assess barriers to change, motivation to change, and potential rewards to engage patient.

### Conduct Disorder

- Assess the seriousness, types, and initiation of disruptive behaviour and how it has been managed.
- Assess anxiety, aggression and anger levels, motivation, and the ability to control impulses.
- Assess moral development, problem solving, belief system, and spirituality for the ability to understand the impact of hurtful behaviour on others, to empathize with others, and to feel remorse.
- Assess the ability to form a therapeutic relationship and engage in honest and committed therapeutic work leading to observable behavioural change (e.g., signing a behavioural contract, drug testing, living according to "house rules").
- Assess for substance use (past and present).

| TABLE 29-3 | *NOC* OUTCOMES FOR ATTENTION DEFICIT–HYPERACTIVITY DISORDER AND DISRUPTIVE, IMPULSE-CONTROL, AND CONDUCT DISORDERS | |
| --- | --- | --- |
| **NURSING OUTCOME AND DEFINITION** | **INTERMEDIATE INDICATORS** | **SHORT-TERM INDICATORS** |
| *Hyperactivity level:* Severity of patterns of inattention of impulsivity in a child from 1 year through 17 years of age | Inappropriate aggressive behaviour decreases | Active listening |
| *Impulse self-control:* Self-restraint of compulsive or impulsive behaviours | Self-control maintenance without supervision | Identification of harmful impulsive behaviours |
| *Self-esteem:* Personal judgement of self-worth | Expression of feelings about self-worth | Acceptance of self-limitations |
| *Coping:* Personal actions to manage stressors that tax an individual's resources | Reports of psychological comfort increase | Identification of effective coping patterns |
| *Family normalization:* Capacity of the family system to maintain routines and develop strategies for optimal functioning when a member has a chronic illness or disability | Maintenance of usual parenting expectations for affected child; help sought from a health care provider as appropriate | Acknowledgement of impairment and its potential to alter family routines |

**Source:** Data from Ackley, B., & Ladwig, G. (2008). *Nursing diagnosis handbook: An evidence-based guide to planning care.* St. Louis: Mosby; and Moorhead, S., Johnson, M., Maas, M., et al. (2008). *Nursing outcomes classification (NOC)* (4th ed.). St. Louis: Mosby.

- Discuss how to make home a safe environment, especially in regard to weapons and drugs; attempt to talk separately to family members whenever possible.
- Discuss realistic behavioural goals and how to set them; problem-solve potential problems.

- Teach behaviour modification techniques. Practise the techniques through role play, with the parents in different problem situations that might arise with their child.
- Give support and encouragement as parents learn to apply new techniques.

## BOX 29-5 TECHNIQUES FOR MANAGING DISRUPTIVE BEHAVIOURS

**Behavioural contract:** A verbal or written agreement between the patient and nurse or other parties (e.g., family, treatment team, teacher) about behaviours, expectations, and needs. The contract is periodically evaluated and reviewed and typically coupled with rewards and other contingencies, positive and negative.

**Counselling:** Verbal interactions, role playing, and modelling to teach, coach, or maintain adaptive behaviour and provide positive reinforcement. It is most effective for motivated youth and those with well-developed communication and self-reflective skills.

**Modelling:** A method of learning behaviours or skills by observation and imitation that can be used in a wide variety of situations. It is enhanced when the modeller is perceived to be similar (e.g., age, interests) and attending to the task is required.

**Role playing:** A counselling technique in which the nurse, the patient, or a group of youngsters act out a specified script or role to enhance the understanding of that role, learn and practise new behaviours or skills, and practise specific situations. It requires well-developed expressive and receptive language skills.

**Planned ignoring:** When behaviours are determined by staff not to be dangerous but are attention seeking, they may be ignored. Additional interventions may be used in conjunction (e.g., positive reinforcement for on-task actions).

**Use of signals or gestures:** Use a word, a gesture, or eye contact to remind the child to use self-control. To help promote behavioural change, this technique may be used in conjunction with a behavioural contract and a reward system. An example is placing your finger to your lips and making eye contact with a child who is talking during a quiet drawing activity.

**Physical distance and touch control:** You could move closer to the child for a calming effect, perhaps putting an arm around the child (with permission). Evaluate the effect of this, because some children may find such an action more agitating and may need more space and less physical closeness. This technique also may involve putting the nurse or a staff member between certain children who have a history of conflict.

**Redirection:** A technique used following an undesirable or inappropriate behaviour to engage or re-engage an individual in an appropriate activity. It may involve the use of verbal directives (e.g., setting firm limits), gestures, or physical prompts.

**Additional affection:** Giving a child planned emotional support for a specific problem or engaging in an enjoyable activity. It can be used to redirect a child away from an undesirable activity as well. This might be involvement in an activity, such as a game of basketball or working on a puzzle. This shows acceptance of the child while ignoring the behaviour and can increase rapport in the nurse–patient relationship.

**Use of humour:** Use well-timed, appropriate kidding about some external, nonpersonal (to the child) event as a diversion to help the child save face and relieve feelings of guilt or fear.

**Clarification as intervention:** Breaking down a problem situation that a child experiences can help the child understand the situation, other people's roles, and his or her own motivation for the behaviour. This technique can be done verbally or using worksheets, depending on the age and functional level of the child.

**Restructuring:** Changing an activity in a way that will decrease the stimulation or frustration (e.g., shorten a story or change to a physical activity). Restructuring requires flexibility and planning in advance to have an alternative in mind in case the activity is not going well.

**Limit setting:** Giving direction, stating an expectation, or telling a child what to do or where to go. Limit setting should be done firmly, calmly, without judgement or anger, preferably in advance of any problem behaviour occurring and consistently when in a treatment setting among multiple staff members. An example would be "I would like for you to stop turning the light on and off."

**Simple restitution:** Refers to a procedure in which an individual is required or expected to correct the adverse environmental or relational effects of his or her misbehaviour by restoring the environment to its prior state, making a plan to correct his or her actions with the nurse, and implementing the plan (e.g., apologizing to the persons harmed, fixing the chairs that are upturned). Simple restitution is not punitive in nature, and there are typically additional activities involved (e.g., counselling).

**Physical restraint:** Therapeutic holding to control and protect the child from his or her own impulses to act out and hurt self or others.

---

- Provide education about medications.
- Refer parents or caregivers to a local self-help group.
- Advocate for special-education services if needed.

Techniques for managing disruptive behaviours are listed in Box 29-5.

## ANXIETY DISORDERS

According to Beesdo-Baum and Knappe (2012), the developmental period of childhood through adolescence poses many challenges for children. As a result, an anxiety disorder, such as separation anxiety disorder, specific phobia, social anxiety disorder, or adjustment disorder, may develop. Separation anxiety disorder and generalized anxiety disorder are discussed in more detail below.

The prevalence of anxiety disorders is higher than virtually all other mental disorders of childhood and adolescence (Keeley & Storch, 2009). The one-year prevalence in children ages 9 to 17 is 13%. Not all anxiety is abnormal in childhood or adolescence, and a number of fears are a part of normal development. Young people may worry about grades, peer problems, or family issues. Anxiety becomes problematic when the child or adolescent fails to move beyond the fears associated with a particular problem or when the anxiety interferes with functioning over an extended period of time.

There is evidence of genetic contributions to anxiety disorders (Hollander & Simeon, 2008). However, genetic predisposition does not mean a disorder will develop. From a prevention standpoint, early intervention and support can be effective. Cognitive theorists propose that anxiety is the result of dysfunctional efforts to make sense of life events.

The physiological, behavioural, and cognitive characteristics of anxiety in youth are clinically similar to those in adults. Selective serotonin reuptake inhibitors (SSRIs) have demonstrated efficacy for the treatment of childhood social anxiety disorder (Masi, Pfanner, Mucci, et al., 2012). Studies have shown that cognitive-behavioural therapy (CBT) in combination with medication offers more benefit than either therapy alone (Lee, Dupuis, Jones, et al., 2013).

## SEPARATION ANXIETY DISORDER

Separation anxiety disorder is recognized as one of the most common anxiety disorders in childhood. Children and adolescents with separation anxiety disorder become excessively anxious when separated from or anticipating separation from their home or parental figures. The fear or anxiety in children is usually persistent and excessive and results in impairment in social, academic, or occupational functioning (Allen, Lavallee, Herren, et al., 2010). Separation anxiety disorder may develop after a significant stress, such as the death of a relative or pet, an illness, a move or change in schools, or a physical or sexual assault. The prevalence in children is estimated to be 4%, with a higher incidence among females. It is common in first-degree biological relatives of an affected individual, and the incidence may be higher in children whose mothers have a panic disorder. Although remission rates are high, the disorder can persist and lead to panic disorder with agoraphobia. A depressed mood often accompanies the anxiety.

Characteristics of separation anxiety disorder identified in this population are the following (Allen, Lavallee, Herren, et al., 2010):

- Excessive distress when separated or anticipating separation from home or parental figures
- Excessive worries one will be lost, that parents will be harmed, or that the home will be violated or damaged
- Fear of being home alone or in situations without significant adults
- Refusal to sleep unless near a parental figure or refusal to sleep away from home
- Refusal to attend school or other activities without parents
- Physical or somatic symptoms of anxiety

## GENERALIZED ANXIETY DISORDER (GAD)

The child or youth with generalized anxiety disorder has excessive worry or anxiety over routine activities such as school, family, or sports. The individual finds it difficult to control the worry and experiences physiological symptoms such as headache, muscle tension, sleep disturbance, fatigue, difficulty concentrating, heart palpitations, and restlessness. This disorder occurs in about 10% of children and adolescents with an average age of onset about 8.5 years. Children with GAD tend to need and seek reassurance about all performance activities or other things they are worried about. In considering a diagnosis, a complete assessment is recommended to rule out other explanations for symptoms that may not be related to anxiety (Keeton, Kolos, & Walkup, 2009).

## APPLICATION OF THE NURSING PROCESS

### ASSESSMENT

Children generally report their experiences of anxiety honestly but may be a bit hesitant to elaborate on their worries. The clinician needs to use a sensitive and caring approach with an anxious child.

> ### 📋 ASSESSMENT GUIDELINES
> #### Anxiety Disorders
>
> - Assess the quality of the parent–child relationship for evidence of anxiety, conflicts, and quality of fit between their temperaments.
> - Assess relationships among other family members.
> - Observe parent–child interactions to determine patterns.
> - Assess for recent stressors and their severity, duration, and proximity to the child.
> - Assess parent or caregiver understanding of developmental norms, parenting skills, and handling of problematic behaviours.
> - Assess the child's developmental level, and determine whether regression has occurred.
> - Assess for symptoms of anxiety and coping style.
>
> #### Separation Anxiety Disorder
> Assess the child's previous and current ability to separate from parents or caregivers. (The separation or individuation process may not be completed, or the child may have regressed.)

### DIAGNOSIS

The chief characteristic of anxiety disorders is disabling anxiety. Refer to Table 29-1 for potential nursing diagnoses.

### OUTCOMES IDENTIFICATION

*NOC* identifies a number of outcomes appropriate for children with an anxiety disorder. The two most relevant outcomes focus on decreasing the anxiety level of the child or adolescent and increasing the child's ability to control anxiety (Table 29-4).

### IMPLEMENTATION

The nursing interventions for an anxious child or adolescent include the following:

- Help prevent the child or adolescent from experiencing panic levels of anxiety by acting as a parental surrogate, providing a safe environment, and providing for biological and psychosocial needs.
- Accept regression, but give emotional support and praise to enable progression, healing, and reintegration into activities of daily living.
- Increase self-esteem and feelings of competence in the ability to perform, achieve, and influence the present and future.

| TABLE 29-4   *NOC* OUTCOMES FOR ANXIETY DISORDERS | | |
|---|---|---|
| **NURSING OUTCOME AND DEFINITION** | **INTERMEDIATE INDICATOR** | **SHORT-TERM INDICATOR** |
| *Anxiety level:* Severity of manifested apprehension, tension, or uneasiness arising from an unidentifiable source | School achievement and performance in activities of daily living | Problem behaviours (e.g., avoidance) with peers, family members, or other community members |
| *Anxiety self-control:* Personal actions to eliminate or reduce feelings of apprehension, tension, or uneasiness from an unidentifiable source | Controls anxiety response and demonstrates return of basic problem-solving skills | Monitors intensity of anxiety |

**Source:** Data from Ackley, B., & Ladwig, G. (2008). *Nursing diagnosis handbook: An evidence-based guide to planning care.* St. Louis: Mosby; and Moorhead, S., Johnson, M., Maas, M., et al. (2008). *Nursing outcomes classification (NOC)* (4th ed.). St. Louis: Mosby.

- Help the child or adolescent accept and work through traumatic events without the use of cognitive distortions or unrealistic fears.
- Teach and practise positive self-talk and reframing to reduce cognitive distortions.
- Teach coping skills (e.g., deep breathing, counting to 10, exercise, guided imagery, listening to music, distraction) to manage feelings.

Children and adolescents with anxiety disorders are most often treated on an outpatient basis, using cognitive-behavioural techniques in individual, group, or family therapy. Medications such as antidepressants, antianxiety agents, and beta blockers are also used. Cognitive therapy focuses on the underlying fears and concerns, and behaviour modification is used to shape behaviour and reinforce self-control behaviours. Children who refuse to start school are introduced gradually into the school environment, with a supportive adult present for part of the day. When adolescents develop school phobia, the goal is to return them to the classroom at the earliest possible date and give parents support in setting limits on truancy.

Refer to the Drug Treatment box on page 598 for a summary of medications used in the treatment of childhood and adolescent clinical and developmental disorders.

## OTHER DISORDERS OF CHILDREN AND ADOLESCENTS

### DEPRESSIVE DISORDERS AND BIPOLAR AND RELATED DISORDERS

The most frequently diagnosed mood disorders (disorders whose primary symptoms relate to changes in mood) in children and adolescents are major depressive disorder, persistent depressive disorder, and bipolar I or II disorder. Symptoms of depressive or bipolar disorders in young people may be similar to the symptoms in adults (see Chapters 14 and 15), with feelings of sadness, pessimism, hopelessness, and anhedonia (inability to experience happiness); social withdrawal; and suicidal ideation. Children may have somatic complaints, be critical of themselves and others, and feel unloved. Adolescents may have psychomotor agitation or retardation and hypersomnia (Maughan, Collishaw, & Stringaris, 2013). Both children and

adolescents often manifest irritability leading to aggressiveness. They are less likely than adults to have psychotic symptoms.

Factors associated with child and adolescent depression are physical and sexual abuse or neglect; homelessness; parental problems, including marital discord, death, divorce or separation, or separation from parents; learning disabilities; chronic illness; and conflicts with others such as peers. The complications of depression are school failure and dropout, substance abuse, sexual acting out, pregnancy, running away, illegal behaviour, and suicide.

## POST-TRAUMATIC STRESS DISORDER

Children exposed to traumatic events such as receiving acute injuries from accidents or witnessing significant harm to others may develop a trauma- or stressor-related disorder (Carrion & Kletter, 2012). After an assessment for personal exposure to an extreme traumatic stressor, further information is needed about any evidence of internalized or externalized symptoms. These symptoms may include anxiety, dissociative symptoms, emotional re-experience of the trauma, and avoidance. It is also important to explore the child's understanding of the meaning of the event and feelings of safety and security. Children whose symptoms last longer than one month will be diagnosed with post-traumatic stress disorder, a disorder that can occur at any age. Young children may engage in repetitive play in which themes of the traumatic event are expressed. The child may experience frightening dreams without recognizable content. Younger children with PTSD tend to exhibit behaviours indicative of internalized anxiety. In older children and adolescents, the anxiety is more often externalized. There may be co-morbid disorders such as depression and anxiety and behaviours such as self-mutilation, depending on the severity and longevity of the trauma that precipitated the PTSD (Hornor, 2013).

## FEEDING AND EATING DISORDERS

Feeding and eating disorders include pica, rumination disorder, and avoidant/restrictive food intake disorder (Bryant-Waugh, Markham, Kreipe, et al., 2010). Anorexia nervosa and bulimia nervosa, which also can occur in childhood and adolescence, are described in detail in Chapter 17. Pica is the persistent eating of nonnutritive substances without an aversion to eating food. Infants and toddlers may eat paint, plaster, string, or cloth. This behaviour is frequently associated with an intellectual disorder. Rumination disorder is the repeated regurgitation and rechewing of food without apparent nausea, retching, or gastrointestinal problems. In avoidant/restrictive food intake disorder, the child fails to eat adequate amounts of food, despite availability, and there is no medical condition or intellectual disability. However, because the child fails to gain weight or undergoes a significant weight loss, he or she can develop nutritional problems that lead to developmental delays.

Interventions for these disorders include working with the family to provide a safe and well-monitored environment that prohibits placing unsafe items in the child's mouth and ensures removal of unsafe items; working with associated care providers (e.g., pediatricians and nutritionists); and providing praise and support for parents and caregivers as they manage the child's behaviour.

## ■ KEY POINTS TO REMEMBER

- One in five children and adolescents in Canada suffers from a major mental illness that causes significant impairments at home, at school, with peers, and in the community.
- Factors known to affect the development of mental and emotional problems in children and adolescents include genetic influences, biochemical (prenatal and postnatal) factors, temperament, psychosocial developmental factors, social and environmental factors, and cultural influences.
- The characteristics of a resilient child include an adaptable temperament, the ability to form nurturing relationships with surrogate parental figures, the ability to distance the self from emotional chaos in parents and family, and good social intelligence and problem-solving skills.
- Children experience a number of psychiatric disorders. The most commonly diagnosed child psychiatric disorders are anxiety disorders, depressive disorders, bipolar and related disorders, and impulse-control disorders.
- Treatment of childhood and adolescent disorders requires a multimodal approach in almost all instances, and family involvement is seen as critical to improvement in outcomes.
- Nurses can be important advocates for children with severe emotional and behavioural disorders.
- Cognitive-behavioural therapies, social skills groups, family therapy, parent training in behavioural techniques, and individual therapy focused on self-esteem issues have been found useful.
- Skills training may focus on a variety of areas, depending on the child's or adolescent's presenting symptoms, and require an individualized assessment to determine each child's need.

## ■ CRITICAL THINKING

1. Owen, a 4-year-old boy, has been diagnosed with a neurodevelopmental disorder—autism.
   a. Describe the specific behavioural data you would find on assessment in terms of (1) communication, (2) social interactions, (3) behaviours and activities.
   b. Name at least three realistic outcomes for a child with NDD.
   c. Which interventions are the most important for a child with NDD? Identify at least six.
   d. What kinds of support should the family receive?

2. Natasha is a 7-year-old girl in grade two who has been diagnosed with ADHD.
   a. What clinical behaviours might she be exhibiting at home and in the classroom? Give behavioural examples for her (1) inattention, (2) hyperactivity, and (3) impulsivity.
   b. Identify at least six intervention strategies one might use for Natasha, including medication management.
   c. Describe the concept of time out.

3. Saed is an 8-year-old boy who has been diagnosed with conduct disorder.
   a. Explain to one of your classmates his probable behaviours in terms of (1) aggression toward others, (2) destruction of property, (3) deceitfulness, and (4) violation of rules.
   b. What are three outcomes for this child? What is the overall prognosis for children with this disorder?
   c. What are four ways you could support Saed's parents? Where could you refer this family within your own community?

4. Jasmine is a 16-year-old who is attending an appointment with her nurse–therapist at the local community health clinic. Jasmine has been diagnosed with depression.
   a. Based on current research, what themes would you expect to hear as Jasmine describes her experiences of depression?
   b. As you complete a mental status exam, what area of assessment is essential?

## CHAPTER REVIEW

1. The nurse is assessing a teenage patient for suicidal risk. Which patient response requires immediate further nursing assessment?
   1. "The idea of death really scares me."
   2. "I smoked only one time in my life."
   3. "My mom keeps a bunch of pills in her nightstand."
   4. "I've never tried to kill myself before."

2. The nurse meets with the parents of a child diagnosed with conduct disorder. What advice from the nurse is most appropriate?
   1. "Use time out as a way to control any unacceptable behaviour."
   2. "Ignore his head banging. He is just trying to get attention."
   3. "Allow the child to come up with a list of play activities."
   4. "Encourage the child to talk when he is around others."

3. The nurse is caring for a 9-year-old patient who will be entering a freedom room. Which activity should the nurse anticipate the child would engage in?
   1. Listening to a CD
   2. Throwing pillows
   3. Sitting in the periphery of the room
   4. Punching soft objects

4. A 7-year-old male who has not met earlier normal expectations in cognitive and language development and who has difficulty establishing friendships with other schoolchildren develops a fascination with the water fountain in his neighbourhood. Which condition should the nurse anticipate?
   1. Intellectual developmental disorder
   2. Major depressive disorder
   3. Tourette's disorder
   4. Autism spectrum disorder

5. The school nurse is assessing Than, who has been coming to the office the past week with cuts and bruises for treatment. What must the nurse include in his assessment?
   1. Assess for suicidal ideation
   2. Offer professional advice about his reasons for the visits
   3. Question Than directly about bullying
   4. Anticipate the need for an antianxiety agent

## evolve WEBSITE

**Post-Test** interactive review

*Visit the Evolve Web site for Chapter Review Answers and Rationales, Critical Thinking Answer Guidelines, and additional resources related to the content in this chapter:* http://evolve.elsevier.com/Canada/Varcarolis/psychiatric/

## REFERENCES

Ackley, B.J., & Ladwig, G.B. (2008). *Nursing diagnosis handbook: An evidence-based guide to planning care.* St. Louis: Mosby.

Allen, J.L., Lavallee, K.L., Herren, C., et al. (2010). DSM-IV criteria for childhood separation anxiety disorder: Informant, age, and sex differences. *Journal of Anxiety Disorders, 24*(8), 946–952. doi:10.1016/j.janxdis.2010.06.022.

Autism Society Canada. (2013). *What is autism spectrum disorder?* Retrieved from http://www.autismsocietycanada.ca/DocsAndMedia/ASC_Internal/info_ascwhatisautisminfosheet_27_june_07_e.pdf.

Axline, V. (1969). *Play therapy.* New York: Ballantine Books.

Azeem, M.W., Aujla, A., Rammerth, M., et al. (2011). Effectiveness of six core strategies based on trauma informed care in reducing seclusion and restraints at a child and adolescent psychiatric hospital. *Journal of Child & Adolescent Psychiatric Nursing, 24*(1), 11–15. doi:10.1111/j.1744-6171.2010.00262.x.

Barbaro, J., Ridgway, L., & Dissanayake, C. (2011). Developmental surveillance of infants and toddlers by maternal and child health nurses in an Australian community-based setting: Promoting the early identification of autism spectrum disorders. *Journal of Pediatric Nursing, 26*(4), 334–347. doi:10.1016/j.pedn.2010.04.007.

Beesdo-Baum, K., & Knappe, S. (2012). Developmental epidemiology of anxiety disorders. *Child and Adolescent Psychiatric Clinics of North America, 21*(3), 457–478. doi:10.1016/j.chc.2012.05.001.

Belfer, M.L. (2008). Child and adolescent mental disorders. The magnitude of the problem across the globe. *Journal of Child Psychology and Psychiatry and Allied Disciplines, 49*(3), 226–236.

Benjamin, C.L., Puleo, C.M., Settipani, C.A., et al. (2011). History of cognitive-behavioral therapy in youth. *Child and Adolescent Psychiatric Clinics of North America, 20*(2), 179–189. doi:10.1016/j.chc.2011.01.011.

Besier, T., Fegert, J.M., & Goldbeck, L. (2009). Evaluation of psychiatric liaison-services for adolescents in residential group homes. *European Psychiatry, 24*, 483–489. doi:10.1016/j.eurpsy.2009.02.006.

Bloch, M.H., & Leckman, J.F. (2009). Clinical course of Tourette syndrome. *Journal of Psychosomatic Research, 67*(6), 497–501. doi:10.1016/j.jpsychores.2009.09.002.

Bowers, L., Ross, J., Owiti, J., et al. (2012). Event sequencing of forced intramuscular medication in England. *Journal of Psychiatric and Mental Health Nursing, 19*(9), 799–806. doi:10.1111/j.1365-2850.2011.01856.x.

Boyle, M.H., & Georgiades, K. (2009). Perspectives on child psychiatric disorder in Canada. In J. Cairney & D. Streiner (Eds.), *Mental disorders in Canada: An epidemiological perspective.* Toronto: University of Toronto Press.

Bryant-Waugh, R., Markham, L., Kreipe, R.E., et al. (2010). Feeding and eating disorders in childhood. *International Journal of Eating Disorders, 43*(2), 98–111. doi:10.1002/eat.20795.

Burack, J.A., Hodapp, R.M., Iarocci, G., et al. (2012). *The Oxford handbook of intellectual disability and development.* New York: Oxford University Press.

Burke, J.D. (2012). An affective dimension within oppositional defiant disorder symptoms among boys: Personality and psychopathology outcomes into early adulthood. *Journal of Child Psychology and Psychiatry, 53*(11), 1176–1183. doi:10.1111/j.1469-7610.2012.02598.x.

Calles, J.L., Jr. (2011). Psychopharmacologic control of aggression and violence in children and adolescents. *Pediatric Clinics of North America*, *58*, 73–84. doi:10.1016/j.pcl.2010.11.002.

Canadian Association for Suicide Prevention. (2009). *The CASP blueprint for a Canadian national suicide prevention strategy* (2nd ed.).Winnipeg. Retrieved from http://suicideprevention.ca/wp-content/uploads/2009/12/SuicidePreventionBlueprint0909.pdf.

Canadian Institutes of Health Research. (2010). *Access & wait times in child and youth mental health: A background paper.* Retrieved from http://www.excellenceforchildandyouth.ca/sites/default/files/policy_access_and_wait_times.pdf.

Carlsson, L.H., Norrelgen, F., Kjellmer, L., et al. (2013). Coexisting disorders and problems in preschool children with autism spectrum disorders. *Scientific World Journal*, *2013*, 1–6. doi:10.1155/2013/213979.

Carrion, V.G., & Kletter, H. (2012). Posttraumatic stress disorder: Shifting toward a developmental framework. *Child and Adolescent Psychiatric Clinics of North America*, *21*(3), 573–591. doi:10.1016/j.chc.2012.05.004.

Cicchetti, D. (2010). Resilience under conditions of extreme stress: A multilevel perspective. *World Psychiatry*, *9*(3), 145–154.

De Hert, M., Dirix, N., Demunter, H., et al. (2011). Prevalence and correlates of seclusion and restraint use in children and adolescents: A systematic review. *European Child and Adolescent Psychiatry*, *20*(5), 221–230. doi:10.1007/s00787-011-0160-x.

Egberts, K.M., Mehler-Wex, C., & Gerlach, M. (2011). Therapeutic drug monitoring in child and adolescent psychiatry. *Pharmacopsychiatry*, *44*(6), 249–253. doi:10.1055/s-0031-1286291.

Esbensen, F.A., Peterson, D., Taylor, T.J., et al. (2009). Similarities and differences in risk factors for violent offending and gang membership. *Australian and New Zealand Journal of Criminology*, *42*(3), 310–335.

Freud, A. (1965). *Normality and pathology in childhood: Assessments of development.* New York: International Universities Press.

Frick, P.J. (2012). Developmental pathways to conduct disorder: Implications for future directions in research, assessment, and treatment. *Journal of Clinical Child & Adolescent Psychology*, *41*(3), 378–389. doi:10.1080/15374416.2012.664815.

Fryers, T., & Brugha, T. (2013). Childhood determinants of adult psychiatric disorder. *Clinical Practice & Epidemiology in Mental Health*, *9*, 1–50. doi:10.2174/1745017901309010001.

Gardner, R.A. (1971). *Therapeutic communication with children: The mutual story-telling technique.* New York: Jason Aronson.

Gardner, R.A. (1979). Helping children cooperate in therapy. In J.D. Noshpitz & S.I. Harrison (Eds.), *Basic handbook of child psychiatry: Therapeutic interventions* (pp. 414–432). New York: Basic Books.

Gardner, R.A. (1986). The talking, feeling and doing game. In C.E. Schaefer & S.E. Reid (Eds.), *Game play: Therapeutic use of childhood games* (pp. 41–72). New York: Wiley.

Gemelli, R.J. (2008). Normal child and adolescent development. In R.E. Hales, S.C. Yudofsky, & G.O. Gabbard (Eds.), *Textbook of psychiatry* (5th ed., pp. 245–300). Washington, DC: American Psychiatric Publishing.

Giedd, J.N., Lalonde, F.M., Celano, M.J., et al. (2009). Anatomical brain magnetic resonance imaging of typically developing children and adolescents. *Journal of the American Academy of Child and Adolescent Psychiatry*, *48*(5), 465–470. doi:10.1097/chi.0b013e31819f2715.

Gini, G., & Pozzoli, T. (2009). Association between bullying and psychosomatic problems: A meta-analysis. *Pediatrics*, *123*, 1059–1065. doi:10.1542/peds.2008-1215.

Goldbeck, L., & Ellerkamp, T. (2012). A randomized controlled trial of multimodal music therapy for children with anxiety disorders. *Journal of Music Therapy*, *49*(4), 395–413.

Gonzalez, A., Boyle, M.H., Kyu, H.H., et al. (2012). Childhood and family influences on depression, chronic physical conditions, and their comorbidity: Findings from the Ontario child health study. *Journal of Psychiatric Research*, *46*(11), 1475–1482. doi:10.1016/j.jpsychires.2012.08.004.

Gulliver, A., Griffiths, K.M., & Christensen, H. (2010). Perceived barriers and facilitators to mental health help-seeking in young people: A systematic review. *BMC Psychiatry*, *10*(113), 2–9. doi:10.1186/1471-244X-10-113.

Hagan, J.F., Shaw, J.S., & Duncan, P.M. (Eds.). (2008). *Bright futures: Guidelines for health supervision of infants, children, and adolescents* (3rd ed.). Elk Grove Village, IL: American Academy of Pediatrics. Retrieved from http://brightfutures.aap.org/pdfs/Guidelines_PDF/1-BF-Introduction.pdf.

Hanington, L., Ramchandani, P., & Stein, A. (2010). Parental depression and child temperament: Assessing child to parent effects in a longitudinal population study. *Infant Behavior & Development*, *33*, 88–95. doi:10.1016/j.infbeh.2009.11.004.

Hollander, E., & Simeon, D. (2008). Anxiety disorders. In R.E. Hales, S.C. Yudofsky, & G.O. Gabbard (Eds.), *Textbook of psychiatry* (5th ed., pp. 505–607). Arlington, VA: American Psychiatric Publishing.

Hornor, G. (2013). Posttraumatic stress disorder. *Journal of Pediatric Health Care*, *27*(3), e29–e38. doi:10.1016/j.pedhc.2012.07.020.

Jacobson, C.M., & Mufson, L. (2012). Interpersonal psychotherapy for depressed adolescents adapted for self-injury (IPT-ASI): Rationale, overview, and case summary. *American Journal of Psychotherapy*, *66*(4), 349–374.

Jankovic, J., & Kurlan, R. (2011). Tourette syndrome: Evolving concepts. *Movement Disorders*, *26*(6), 1149–1156. doi:10.1002/mds.23618.

Keeley, M.L., & Storch, E.A. (2009). Anxiety disorders in youth. *Journal of Pediatric Nursing*, *24*(1), 26–40. doi:10.1016/j.pedn.2007.08.021.

Keeton, C.P., Kolos, A.C., & Walkup, J.T. (2009). Pediatric generalized anxiety disorder: Epidemiology, diagnosis, and management. *Pediatric Drugs*, *11*(3), 171–183. doi:10.2165/00148581-200911030-00003.

Klein, M. (1955). The psychoanalytic play technique. *American Journal of Orthopsychiatry*, *25*, 223–237.

Klomek, A.B., Sourander, A., & Gould, M. (2010). The association of suicide and bullying in childhood to young adulthood: A review of cross-sectional and longitudinal research findings. *Canadian Journal of Psychiatry*, *55*(5), 282–288.

Kolko, D.J., & Pardini, D.A. (2010). ODD dimensions, ADHD, and callous–unemotional traits as predictors of treatment response in children with disruptive behavior disorders. *Journal of Abnormal Psychology*, *119*(4), 713–725. doi:10.1037/a0020910.

Lahiri, D.K., Sokol, D.K., Erickson, C., et al. (2013). Autism as early neurodevelopmental disorder: Evidence for a sappa-mediated anabolic pathway. *Frontiers in Cellular Neuroscience 21*, 1–17. doi:10.3389/fncel.2013.00094.

Lamb, J., Pepler, D.J., & Craig, W. (2009). Approach to bullying and victimization. *Canadian Family Physician*, *55*, 356–360.

Lee, T.C., Dupuis, A., Jones, E., et al. (2013). Effects of age and subtype on emotional recognition in children with anxiety disorders: Implications for cognitive-behavioural therapy. *Canadian Journal of Psychiatry*, *58*(5), 283–290.

Lehne, R.A. (2010). *Pharmacology for nursing care* (7th ed.). Philadelphia: Saunders.

Li, J., Zhao, G., & Gao, X. (2013). Development of neurodevelopmental disorders: A regulatory mechanism involving bromodomain-containing proteins. *Journal of Neurodevelopmental Disorders*, *5*(5), 1–11.

Masi, G., Pfanner, C., Mucci, M., et al. (2012). Pediatric social anxiety disorder: Predictors of response to pharmacological treatment. *Journal of Child and Adolescent Psychopharmacology*, *22*(6), 410–414. doi:10.1089/cap.2012.0007.

Mâsse, L.C., Miller, A.R., Shen, J., et al. (2013). Patterns of participation across a range of activities among Canadian children with neurodevelopmental disorders and disabilities. *Developmental Medicine & Child Neurology*, *55*(8), 729–736. doi:10.1111/dmcn.12167.

Masters, K. (2009). Risk management: Part 1: Seclusion and restraint. *Audio Digest Psychiatry*, *38*(6). Retrieved from http://www.cme-ce-summaries.com/psychiatry/ps3806.html.

Maughan, B., Collishaw, S., & Stringaris, A. (2013). Depression in childhood and adolescence. *Journal of the Canadian Academy of Child and Adolescent Psychiatry*, *22*(1), 35–40.

Meltzer, H., Doos, L., Vostanis, P., et al. (2009). The mental health of children who witness domestic violence. *Child and Family Social Work*, *14*(4), 491–501. doi:10.1111/j.1365-2206.2009.00633.x.

Mental Health Commission of Canada. (2012). *Changing directions, changing lives: The mental health strategy for Canada.* Calgary: Author.

Meucci, P., Leonardi, M., Zibordi, F., et al. (2009). Measuring participation in children with Gilles de la Tourette syndrome: A pilot study with ICF-CY. *Disability and Rehabilitation, 31*(S1), s116–s120. doi:10.3109/09638280903317773.

Mohr, W.K., Martin, A., Olson, J.N., et al. (2009). Beyond point and level systems: Moving toward child-centered programming. *American Journal of Orthopsychiatry, 79*(1), 8–18. doi:10.1037/a0015375.

Moorhead, S., Johnson, M., Maas, M., et al. (2008). *Nursing outcomes classification (NOC)* (4th ed.). St. Louis: Mosby.

National Institute on Drug Abuse. (2008). *Preventing drug abuse among children and adolescents.* Retrieved from http://www.nida.nih.gov/Prevention/risk.html.

Ougrin, D., Tranah, T., Leigh, E., et al. (2012). *Journal of Child Psychology and Psychiatry, 53*(4), 337–350. doi:10.1111/j.1469-7610.2012.02525.x.

Parliament of Canada. (2001). *Canada's legal age of consent to sexual activity.* Ottawa: Author. Retrieved from http://www.parl.gc.ca/content/LOP/researchpublications/prb993-e.htm.

Penne, A., ten Brug, A., Munde, V., et al. (2012). Staff interactive style during multisensory storytelling with persons with profound intellectual and multiple disabilities. *Journal of Intellectual Disability Research, 56*(2), 167–178. doi:10.1111/j.1365-2788.2011.01448.x.

Peterson, R.L., & Pennington, B.F. (2012). Developmental dyslexia. *Lancet, 379*(9830), 1997–2007. doi:10.1016/S0140-6736(12)60198-6.

Piacentini, J., Woods, D.W., Scahill, L., et al. (2010). Behavior therapy for children with Tourette disorder: A randomized controlled trial. *Journal of the American Medical Association, 303*(19), 1929–1937. doi:10.1001/jama.2010.607.

Pringsheim, T., Doja, A., Gorman, D., et al. (2012). Canadian guidelines for the evidence-based treatment of tic disorders: Pharmacotherapy. *Canadian Journal of Psychiatry, 57*(3), 133–143.

Public Health Agency of Canada. (2008). *Canadian incidence study of reported child abuse and neglect 2008.* Retrieved from http://www.phac-aspc.gc.ca/cm-vee/csca-ecve/2008/.

Reinhardt, M.C., & Reinhardt, C.A.U. (2013). Attention deficit–hyperactivity disorder, comorbidities, and risk situations. *Jornal de Pediatria, 89*(2), 124–130. doi:10.1016/j.jped.2013.03.015.

Royal Canadian Mounted Police. (2006). *RCMP environmental scan: Feature focus: Youth gangs and guns.* Retrieved from http://www.rcmp-grc.gc.ca/pubs/yg-ja/gangs-bandes-eng.pdf.

Sadock, B.J., & Sadock, A. (2008). *Kaplan & Sadock's concise textbook of clinical psychiatry* (3rd ed.). Philadelphia: Lippincott Williams & Wilkins.

Shepperd, S., Doll, H., Gowers, S., et al. (2009). Alternatives to inpatient mental health care for children and young people [Review]. *Cochrane Library, 15*(2), 1–25.

Skinner, R., & McFaull, S. (2012). Suicide among children and adolescents in Canada: Trends and sex differences, 1980–2008. *Canadian Medical Association Journal, 184*(9), 1029–1034. doi:10.1503/cmaj.111867.

Smoller, J.W., Sheidley, B.R., & Tsuang, M.T. (2008). *Psychiatric genetics: Applications in clinical practice.* Arlington, VA: American Psychiatric Publishing.

Spinazzola, J., Rhodes, A.M., Emerson, D., et al. (2013). Application of yoga in residential treatment of traumatized youth. *Journal of the American Psychiatric Nurses Association, 17*(6), 431–444. doi:10.1177/1078390311418359.

Standing Senate Committee on Social Affairs, Science and Technology. (2006). *Out of the shadows at last: Transforming mental health, mental illness and addiction services in Canada.* Retrieved from http://www.parl.gc.ca/39/1/parlbus/commbus/senate/com-e/soci-e/rep-e/rep02may06-e.htm.

Standing Senate Committee on Social Affairs, Science and Technology. (2007). *Pay now or pay later: Autism families in crisis.* Retrieved from http://www.parl.gc.ca/Content/SEN/Committee/391/soci/rep/repfinmar07-e.htm.

Statistics Canada. (2012). *Study: Suicide rates, an overview, 1950 to 2009.* Retrieved from http://www.statcan.gc.ca/daily-quotidien/120725/dq120725a-eng.htm.

Steeves, T., McKinlay, B.D., Gorman, D., et al. (2012). Canadian guidelines for the evidence-based treatment of tic disorders: Behavioural therapy, deep brain stimulation, and transcranial magnetic stimulation. *Canadian Journal of Psychiatry, 57*(3), 144–151.

Stein, D.S., Blum, N.J., & Barbaresi, W.J. (2011). Developmental and behavioral disorders through the life span. *Pediatrics, 128*(2), 364–373. doi:10.1542/peds.2011-0266.

Stewart, S.M., Simmons, A., & Habibpour, E. (2012). Treatment of culturally diverse children and adolescents with depression. *Journal of Child and Adolescent Psychopharmacology 22*(1), 72–79. doi:10.1089/cap.2011.0051.

Sullivan, E.V., Pfefferbaum, A., Rohlfing, T., et al. (2011). Developmental change in regional brain structure over 7 months in early adolescence: Comparison of approaches for longitudinal atlas-based parcellation. *NeuroImage, 57*(1), 214–224. doi:10.1016/j.neuroimage.2011.04.003.

Swanson, S.A., & Colman, I. (2013). Association between exposure to suicide and suicidality outcomes in youth. *Canadian Medical Association Journal, 185*(10), 870–877. doi:10.1503/cmaj.121377.

Teplin, L.A., Welty, L.J., Abram, K.M., et al. (2012). Prevalence and persistence of psychiatric disorders in youth after detention: A prospective longitudinal study. *Archives of General Psychiatry, 69*(1), 1031–1043. doi:10.1001/archgenpsychiatry.2011.2062.

Thornton, L.C., Frick, P.J., Crapanzano, A.M., et al. (2013). The incremental utility of callous–unemotional traits and conduct problems in predicting aggression and bullying in a community sample of boys and girls. *Psychological Assessment, 25*(2), 366–378. doi:10.1037/a0031153.

Ursano, A.M., Kartheiser, P.H., & Barnhill, L.J. (2008). Disorders usually first diagnosed in infancy, childhood, or adolescence. In R.E. Hales, S.C. Yudofsky, & G.O. Gabbard (Eds.), *Textbook of psychiatry* (5th ed., pp. 861–920). Washington, DC: American Psychiatric Publishing.

Vernberg, E.M., Nelson, T.D., Fonagy, P., et al. (2011). Victimization, aggression, and visits to the school nurse for somatic complaints, illnesses, and physical injuries. *Pediatrics, 127*(5), 842–848. doi:10.1542/peds.2009-3415.

Weston, F. (2009). Working with children who have been bullied. *British Journal of School Nursing, 5*(4), 172–176.

Winther, J., Carlsson, A., & Vance, A. (2013). A pilot study of a school-based prevention and early intervention program to reduce oppositional defiant disorder/conduct disorder. *Early Intervention in Psychiatry*, 1–9. doi:10.1111/eip.12050.

Wright, L.M., & Leahey, M. (2012). *Nurses and families: A guide to family assessment and intervention* (6th ed.). Philadelphia: F.A. Davis.

Yanof, J.A. (2013). Play technique in psychodynamic psychotherapy. *Child and Adolescent Psychiatric Clinics of North America, 22*(2), 261–282. doi:10.1016/j.chc.2012.12.002.

Zwicker, J.G., Missiuna, C., Harris, S.R., et al. (2012). Developmental coordination disorder: A review and update. *European Journal of Paediatric Neurology, 16*(6), 574–578. doi:10.1016/j.ejpn.2012.05.005.

# Psychosocial Needs of the Older Adult

*Leslie A. Briscoe, Evelyn Yap*
*Adapted by Cheryl L. Pollard*

## KEY TERMS AND CONCEPTS

adult support program, 628
ageism, 622
caregiver burden, 622

## OBJECTIVES

1. Discuss facts and myths about aging.
2. Describe mental health disorders that may occur in older adults.
3. Analyze how ageism may affect attitudes and willingness to care for older adults.
4. Explain the importance of a comprehensive geriatric assessment.
5. Describe the role of the nurse in different settings of care.
6. Discuss the importance of pain assessment, and identify three tools used to assess pain in older adults.

## ⊖volve WEBSITE

*Visit the Evolve website for Flashcards, Case Studies, and additional testing resources related to the content in this chapter:* *http://evolve.elsevier.com/Canada/Varcarolis/psychiatric/*    Pre-Test  interactive review

---

The aging of the population is a global phenomenon occurring at a record-breaking rate, especially in developing countries around the world. The Canadian economy, as well as health and social services, is affected by this marked increase in the proportion of older adults in the population. In 2010, the percentage of adults older than 65 was 15%; by the year 2036, 23% of the population in Canada will consist of individuals older than 65 years of age (Statistics Canada, 2010a). Among older adults, the fastest-growing subgroups are minorities, the poor, and those aged 85 years and older.

An outline of some major developmental theories of aging is provided in Box 30-1. Although these theories provide the framework for formulating appropriate nursing interventions for caring for older adults, there is no specific theory that encompasses all the developmental stages.

In addition to dealing with the developmental milestones associated with aging, as people live longer, they are more likely to deal with chronic illness and disability. At least 80% of individuals older than age 65 have one chronic condition; many older people have more than one. The likelihood of developing one or more chronic illnesses increases notably with age: individuals 75 years of age and older are the most prone to chronic illnesses and functional disabilities. After age 85, there is a one-in-three chance of developing dementia, immobility, incontinence, or another age-related disability (Statistics Canada, 2010a).

Statistics indicate that women generally outlive men. This disparity has significant ramifications for society at large and for the health care system in particular. Not only do women constitute the largest proportion of older adults; they also use health care services more frequently than men and seek services earlier, even for minor conditions. Most provincial governments recognize an impending crisis as health care costs soar, resources dwindle, and the baby boomers age (Statistics Canada, 2010a).

Chronological age is considered an arbitrary indicator of function because there are significant variables that contribute to the capabilities of older adults. Surveys focusing on how

## BOX 30-1 MAJOR THEORIES OF AGING

**Biological**

Aging is influenced by molecular, cellular, or physiological systems and processes.

- *Gene theory:* Harmful genes become active in later life.
- *Error theory:* Error in protein synthesis results in impaired cellular function.
- *Free radical theory:* Reactive molecules damage DNA.
- *Wear-and-tear theory:* Internal and external stressors harm cells.
- *Programmed aging theory:* Biological or genetic clock plays out on genes.
- *Neuroendocrine theory:* There is neurohormonal regulation of life until death.
- *Immunological theory:* Immune system diversifies with age.

**Psychological**

- *Kohlberg's theory:* Crises and turning points in adult life are moral dilemmas.
- *Piaget's theory:* Cognitive operations in youth influence aging.
- *Erikson's theory:* Integrity is built on morality and ethics.
- *Bandura's theory:* Self-efficacy is essential for longevity.
- *Sullivan's theory:* Interpersonal responses influence behaviour.
- *Freud's theory:* Control of instinctual responses decreases with age.
- *Psychobiological theory:* Neurotransmitters modulate behaviours, emotions, and thoughts.
- *Dialectical theory:* Crises and transitions release positive and negative forces that lead to developmental progress.
- *Behavioural theory:* Learning determines the organization of behaviour.

**Psychosocial**

- *Maslow's theory:* Self-actualization and the evolution of developmental needs occur as the individual ages.
- *Disengagement theory:* Mutual withdrawal occurs between the aging person and others.
- *Activity theory:* Actions, roles, and social pursuits are important for satisfactory aging.
- *Continuity theory:* Life satisfaction and activity are expressions of enduring personality traits.

**Source:** Adapted from Hess, P. (2004). Theories of aging. In P. Ebersole, P. Hess, & A.S. Luggen (Eds.), *Toward healthy aging: Human needs and nursing response* (6th ed.). St. Louis: Mosby.

members, and independence) and co-morbid illness (Cremens, 2008). Polypharmacy also contributes to health problems, especially since there is a gradual reduction in renal, hepatic, and gastric function—all of which are needed to metabolize and degrade medications.

Aging is a complex psychological and physical process. Box 30-2 provides some facts and myths about aging that influence how society perceives the older adult.

## BOX 30-2 FACTS AND MYTHS ABOUT AGING

**Facts**

- The senses of vision, hearing, touch, taste, and smell decline with age.
- Muscular strength decreases with age. Muscle fibres atrophy and decrease in number.
- Regular sexual expressions are important to maintain sexual capacity and effective sexual performance.
- At least 50% of restorative sleep is lost as a result of the aging process.
- Older adults are major consumers of prescription drugs because of the high incidence of chronic diseases in this population.
- Older adults have a high incidence of depression.
- Many individuals experience difficulty when they retire.
- Older adults are prone to become victims of crime.
- Older widows appear to adjust better than younger ones.

**Myths**

- Most adults past the age of 65 have dementia.
- Sexual interest declines with age.
- Older adults are unable to learn new tasks.
- As individuals age, they become more rigid in their thinking and set in their ways.
- The aged are well off and no longer impoverished.
- Most older adults are infirm and require help with daily activities.
- Most older adults are socially isolated and lonely.

## MENTAL HEALTH ISSUES RELATED TO AGING

The Mental Health Strategy of Canada (Mental Health Commission, 2012) has made several recommendations that relate to mental health issues in Canada's aging population. These strategies include identifying and treating mental illnesses early, decreasing age discrimination, and helping older adults continue to engage in meaningful activities.

### Late-Life Mental Illness

Older adults who develop late-life mental illness are less likely than young adults to be accurately diagnosed and receive mental health treatment. Psychiatric issues such as depression, memory loss, and prolonged grieving are not a normal part of aging and should be diagnosed and treated. Treating psychiatric disorders prolongs the individual's ability to remain independent and increases his or her ability to take the lead in personal decision making.

older adults see themselves reveal that nearly half of people 65 years and older consider themselves to be middle-aged or young, and only 15% of people aged 75 years and older consider themselves "very old" (Ebersole, Hess, & Luggen, 2004). A common classification for people 65 and older is as follows:

- Young old—65 to 75 years
- Middle old—75 to 85 years
- Old old—85 to 100 years
- Elite old (centenarians)—100+ years of age

Aging is accompanied by increased rates of medical and psychiatric illnesses. This increase is brought about in part by increasingly stressful life events (e.g., the loss of a spouse, family

### Chinese Immigrants' Growing Old in Canada

Canada has a rapidly aging population, and this population is becoming more ethnically diverse. People who come to Canada in later life have unique challenges that have typically been overlooked. Statistics Canada (2008) reported that 24% of the Canadian population identified themselves as Chinese, accounting for the second largest visible-minority population in the country. It is critical that nurses recognize the diversity among the Chinese in Canada. These individuals come from diverse origins and speak many different dialects. Nurses need to avoid making broad-based cultural assumptions.

Chow (2010) investigated the health care needs, general well-being, and life satisfaction of older-adult Chinese immigrants and explored the views of Chinese Canadians on various health-related issues. A sample of 147 Chinese older adults was drawn from residential complexes located in Calgary, Alberta, that were occupied exclusively by older adults of Chinese origin. Interviews using a structured questionnaire were conducted by trained bilingual interviewers. The interviews took an average of 30 minutes to complete.

The results suggest that higher levels of physical well-being are significantly associated with increased physical mobility, country of origin (Hong Kong emigrants), increased education, and a self-perception of financial security. Better reports of psychosocial health are significantly associated with being female, being married, having a higher level of education, and having resided in Canada longer.

Several areas have been suggested for further research, including comparing the health status of foreign-born Chinese older adults to those who were born in Canada and comparing the health status of Chinese older adults who co-reside with adult children.

**Sources:** Chow, H.P. (2010). Growing old in Canada: Physical and psychological well-being among elderly Chinese immigrants. *Ethnicity & Health 15*(1), 61–72; Statistics Canada. (2008, April 2). 2006 census: Ethnic origin, visible minorities, place of work and mode of transportation. *The Daily*, 1–9.

## Depression

Depression is not a normal part of aging and is often under-identified because of co-morbid medical conditions. Depression is often confused with dementia, and delirium is often misdiagnosed as dementia. A careful, systematic assessment is necessary to properly distinguish among the three.

This assessment must determine the following:
- Onset of mental-status change and course of illness
- Level of consciousness
- Attention span

All three illnesses are treatable if properly identified. Delirium and dementia are discussed in significantly more detail in Chapter 18; therefore, they are not discussed further in this chapter. Chapter 18 also provides more information on distinguishing among depression, dementia, and delirium.

Selective serotonin reuptake inhibitors (SSRIs) are the first-line treatment for depression; this category is often helpful if anxiety, worry, or rumination is problematic. If pain or diabetic neuropathy is a co-morbid condition, serotonin norepinephrine reuptake inhibitors (SNRIs) are often prescribed. Tricyclic antidepressants (TCAs) are used for those with chronic pain. Treatment-resistant depression can be treated with psychostimulants such as methylphenidate (Concerta); such monoamine oxidase inhibitors (MAOIs) are older treatments but remain effective.

***Depression and suicide risk.*** In 2007, within the demographic group of older adults, the highest rate of suicide was among those Canadians between the ages of 80 and 84 years: 11.6 per 100 000 (Statistics Canada, 2010b). The rate of suicide for males within this age group was 23.5 per 100 000 (Statistics Canada, 2010d), compared to 3.8 per 100 000 for females (Statistics Canada, 2010c). The factors that impact the risk of suicide within this demographic are mental illness and addictions, personality factors, medical illness, negative life events, difficult transitions, lack of social support, and functional impairment (Canadian Coalition for Seniors' Mental Health, 2006). Approximately 70% of people who commit suicide suffer with depression. The risk for suicide is even higher if the depression is accompanied by psychosis (Cremens, 2008). Early identification of and treatment for depression, therefore, are key measures for suicide prevention. Other factors that can lead to suicide are feelings of hopelessness, uselessness, and despair. For older adults, suicide may be seen as a final gesture of control at a stage when independence is at risk or activities are limited. Severe medical illness, functional disability, alcohol abuse, history of suicide attempts, co-morbid anxiety, and psychotic depression are added risk factors for suicide (Dharmarajan & Norman, 2003). Unlike younger persons, whose suicidal gestures may be a cry for help, older adults more frequently have a real desire to die.

Even though the suicide rate among older adults is high, suicide in this group is probably under-reported. Suicide is often not listed on the death certificate, even if it is suspected. The numbers also do not reflect those who passively or indirectly commit suicide by abusing alcohol, starving themselves, overdosing or mixing medications, stopping life-sustaining drugs, or simply losing the will to live. Unfortunately, primary care providers continue to under-recognize and undertreat; many are slow to refer older adults to mental health care providers despite evidence that treatment of depression is cost-effective and decreases the amount of health care expenditures utilized (Canadian Coalition for Seniors' Mental Health, 2006). Review Chapter 25 for an in-depth discussion of suicide.

## Anxiety Disorders

Cassidy and Rector (2008) identified anxiety disorders in late life as the "Silent Geriatric Giant." Older adults often have multiple physical complaints, medication problems, pain, and sleep disturbances, as well as psychiatric illness. Anxiety is twice as prevalent as dementia and four to eight times as common as major depressive disorders. Again, accurate diagnosis of the anxiety disorder is difficult. The most common sources of anxiety are phobias and generalized anxiety disorder (Cremens, 2008). Co-morbid conditions, including depression, bipolar disorder, dementia, and alcoholism, may contribute to anxiety.

Anxiety disorders may have been present earlier in life but had not significantly impaired functioning. Once the stress of aging, retirement, loss, or physical frailty occurs, the previous coping strategies may no longer be effective. Older adults with anxiety often have physical complaints or describe fears of illness. Treatment for anxiety disorders typically includes an SSRI. Antianxiety agents are also used, but they should be used cautiously since they may result in confusion, oversedation, and paradoxical agitation. Anxiety disorders are discussed in greater detail in Chapter 13.

### Substance Abuse

People of any age can abuse any type of substance. Regardless of age, substance abuse has social, psychological, and physical consequences. Almost 80% of Canadians consume alcohol at least once a year (Health Canada, 2011). Although heavy drinking tends to decline with age, it continues to be a serious problem that can create particular problems for older adults. The risk factors for heavy drinking in older adults are being male and single, having less than a high-school education, having a low income, and smoking (Karlamangla, Zhou, Reuben, et al., 2006). Identifying alcohol and substance abuse is often difficult because personality and behavioural changes frequently go unrecognized in older adults.

The stressful or reactive factors that precipitate late-onset substance abuse are often related to environmental conditions and may include retirement, widowhood, and loneliness. These stressors in the older adult, who may have retired, may not drive, and may be isolated from family and friends, are often greater than the problems faced by the middle-aged adult, who has to manage a job or career and care for a family and household. Work and family responsibilities may help keep a potential alcoholic from drinking too much. Once these demands are gone and the structure of daily life is disrupted, there is little impetus to remain sober. Another factor that may lead to late-onset substance abuse is chronic pain. Chronic pain is discussed in more detail later in this chapter.

Caution is required when medicating the older adult who abuses alcohol. Central nervous system toxicity from psychoactive drugs increases with aging. Ingestion of antidepressants or tranquilizers can be particularly harmful because their effect is further potentiated by alcohol. The toxicity of other drugs (e.g., acetaminophen) is enhanced by alcohol and by the age-related decrease in clearance (Luggen, 2004).

Whenever there is a suspicion or indication that an older adult is abusing alcohol, the health care provider should conduct a screening test. The CAGE-AID screening tool (Wagenaar, Mickus, & Wilson, 2001) (Box 30-3) and the MAST-G (Box 30-4) are instruments commonly used to assess high-risk drinking in older adults.

Signs of alcohol abuse in younger individuals (e.g., alcohol-induced pancreatitis or liver disease, blackouts, major trauma) occur infrequently in older adults. Instead, the older adult who abuses alcohol displays vague geriatric syndromes of contusions, malnutrition, self-neglect, depression, and falls (Wagenaar, Mickus, & Wilson, 2001). Diarrhea, urinary incontinence, decreased functional status, failure to thrive, and

---

### BOX 30-3

**CAGE-AID Screening Tool**

**C**—Have you ever felt you ought to **C**ut down on your drinking (drug use)?

**A**—Have people **A**nnoyed you by criticizing your drinking (drug use)?

**G**—Have you ever felt bad or **G**uilty about your drinking (drug use)?

**E**—Have you ever had a drink (used drugs) first thing in the morning (**E**ye-opener) to steady your nerves or get rid of a hangover?

**AID**—**A**dapt to **I**nclude **D**rugs.

One positive answer indicates a possible problem; two positive answers indicate a probable problem.

apparent dementia may also be present. Although confusion and disorientation in an older patient are often associated with dementia or Alzheimer's disease, they could be caused by other factors, including alcohol abuse. Assessment of these conditions is necessary to differentiate the normal physiological changes of aging from those due to excessive drinking.

Treatment plans should emphasize social therapies. Older adults who abuse alcohol tend to be more passive than younger adults who abuse alcohol and may benefit from interpersonal involvement with professional health care personnel. Older people respond well to emotional and social support, and family therapy should be encouraged. Group therapy with other middle-aged and older adults with alcoholism, as well as self-help groups like Alcoholics Anonymous, can also be effective.

The Canadian Network of Substance Abuse and Allied Professionals (Fandrey, 2007) supports the following six recommendations, developed by the Center for Substance Abuse Treatment (CSAT)—Treatment Improvement Protocol for Older Adults (TIP) Consensus Panel, when working with seniors:

1. Age-specific group treatment that is supportive and nonconfrontational and aims to build or rebuild the patient's self-esteem
2. A focus on coping with depression, loneliness, and loss (e.g., death of spouse, retirement)
3. A focus on rebuilding the patient's social-support network
4. A pace and content of treatment appropriate for the older person
5. Staff members who are interested and experienced in working with older adults
6. Linkages with medical services, services for the aging, and institutional settings for referral into and out of treatment, as well as case management

Although the older adult with alcohol or substance abuse issues is difficult to treat, the prognosis for a person who has lived to this point without recourse to substances—and their use being precipitated by losses and stressors—is excellent. This individual often responds very positively to a recovery program, especially if it is accompanied by environmental interventions

## BOX 30-4   MICHIGAN ALCOHOLISM SCREENING TEST—GERIATRIC VERSION (MAST-G)

Please answer "Yes" or "No" to each question by marking the line next to the question. When you finish answering the questions, please add up how many "Yes" responses you checked, and put that number in the space provided at the end.

1.  After drinking, have you ever noticed an increase in your heart rate or beating in your chest? ____ Yes ____ No

2.  When talking to others, do you ever underestimate how much you actually drank? ____ Yes ____ No

3.  Does alcohol make you sleepy so that you often fall asleep in your chair? ____ Yes ____ No

4.  After a few drinks, have you sometimes not eaten or been able to skip a meal because you didn't feel hungry? ____ Yes ____ No

5.  Does having a few drinks help you decrease your shakiness or tremors? ____ Yes ____ No

6.  Does alcohol sometimes make it hard for you to remember parts of the day or night? ____ Yes ____ No

7.  Do you have rules for yourself that you won't drink before a certain time of the day? ____ Yes ____ No

8.  Have you lost interest in hobbies or activities you used to enjoy? ____ Yes ____ No

9.  When you wake up in the morning, do you ever have trouble remembering part of the night before? ____ Yes ____ No

10. Does having a drink help you sleep? ____ Yes ____ No

11. Do you hide your alcohol bottles from family members? ____ Yes ____ No

12. After a social gathering, have you ever felt embarrassed because you drank too much? ____ Yes ____ No

13. Have you ever been concerned that drinking might be harmful to your health? ____ Yes ____ No

14. Do you like to end an evening with a nightcap? ____ Yes ____ No

15. Did you find your drinking increased after someone close to you died? ____ Yes ____ No

16. In general, would you prefer to have a few drinks at home rather than go out to social events? ____ Yes ____ No

17. Are you drinking more now than in the past? ____ Yes ____ No

18. Do you usually take a drink to relax or calm your nerves? ____ Yes ____ No

19. Do you drink to take your mind off your problems? ____ Yes ____ No

20. Have you ever increased your drinking after experiencing a loss in your life? ____ Yes ____ No

21. Do you sometimes drive when you have had too much to drink? ____ Yes ____ No

22. Has a doctor or nurse ever said they were worried or concerned about your drinking? ____ Yes ____ No

23. Have you ever made rules to manage your drinking? ____ Yes ____ No

24. When you feel lonely, does having a drink help? ____ Yes ____ No

**TOTALS:** ____ **Yes** ____ **No**

*Scoring:* A score of 3 points or less is considered to indicate no alcoholism; a score of 4 points is suggestive of alcoholism; a score of 5 points or more indicates alcoholism.
**Source:** Blow, F., & Brower, K, et al. (1992). The Michigan Alcoholism Screening Test-Geriatric Version: A new elderly specific screening instrument. Alcoholism: Clinical and Experimental Research, 16, 372. Michigan Alcoholism Screening Test-Geriatric Version (MAST-G). © The Regents of the University of Michigan, 1991.

(Salisbury, 1999). It is important that health care providers recognize this recovery potential. Proper education and awareness of a positive outcome for the older-adult problem drinker can increase the availability of resources; if the prognosis is good, providers and agencies should be more willing to spend resources on treatment. Nurses can be pioneers in the developing need for substance abuse rehabilitation focused on older adults.

### Trauma

Older adults are also susceptible to the effects of psychological trauma. Chapter 27 discusses interpersonal violence in more detail. Refer to Chapter 28 for more information regarding the consequences of sexual assault.

## HEALTH CARE CONCERNS OF OLDER ADULTS

### Pain

Pain is common among older adults and affects their sense of well-being and quality of life. Up to 85% of the older population is thought to have conditions that predispose them to pain, such as arthritis, peripheral vascular disease, and diabetic neuropathy (Luggen, 2000).

## RESEARCH HIGHLIGHT

### *Trauma—The Potential Impact of Canadian Residential Schools Among Canadian First Nations People*

**Source:** Elais, B., Mignone, J., Hall, M., et al. (2012). Trauma and suicide behaviour histories among a Canadian indigenous population: An empirical exploration of the potential role of Canada's residential school system. *Social Science & Medicine, 74*(10), 1560–1569. doi:10.1016/j.socscimed.2012.01.026.

**Problem**

Currently, four generations of Canadians have been exposed to the Canadian residential school system. All of these individuals are First Nations. Tens of thousands of Canadian indigenous children were sent to residential schools, whose primary mandate was to Christianize, civilize, and resocialize these children. The last Canadian residential school closed in 1996. The residential school children experienced a loss of culture, language, traditional values, family bonding, parenting skills, and community connections. The residential school survivors may have transmitted the trauma that they experienced to their own children and their grandchildren and to other community members by indirect trauma effects.

**Purpose of Study**

The purpose of the study was to investigate if direct or indirect exposure to the mass trauma linked to being in a residential school was associated with trauma and suicidal behaviour of the residential school survivors, their offspring, and broader community members.

**Methods**

Ethical approval for the study was obtained from a research ethics board at the University of Manitoba. A multistage stratified random sampling method was used to identify potential participants. An in-person interview was used to collect information on the lifetime history of abuse, suicidal thoughts and behaviour, relationship status, residential school attendance, and general health and well-being. Bivariate testing was conducted, with all covariate explanatory variables using logistic regression modelling.

**Key Findings**

- Residential school experiences have resulted in multigenerational trauma that has had a negative impact on these individuals, their family members, and their communities.
- Older adults who were the first generation to attend residential schools and who do not have a complex trauma history appear to be more resilient.
- The chronic stress experienced by older Canadian indigenous people may predispose them to ineffectively cope (i.e., experience suicidal ideation) as they age.
- Some residential school survivors have been resilient to the effects of the trauma they experienced.

**Implications for Nursing Practice**

- The experience of trauma can have multigenerational effects.
- When providing nursing care to Canadian First Nations people, assessment of the individual, family, and community is needed to determine the direct and indirect effects of historical trauma. Useful frameworks to conceptualize the traumas experienced include describing the trauma in terms of connectedness, collectivity, and relationships.
- People who have experienced historical and contemporary trauma have increased rates of suicidal thoughts and attempts; therefore, thorough risk assessments are required.
- Although mental and emotional support services are provided to residential school survivors and their families through Health Canada First Nations and Inuit Health's Indian Residential Schools Resolution Health Support Program, the effects of this multigenerational trauma need to be recognized when and where Canadian indigenous people access health services.

---

Pain is often associated with depression. Jann and Slade (2007) describe three categories of depressive symptoms: emotional (mood, motivation, apathy, anxiety), cognitive (concentration, memory), and physical (insomnia, fatigue, headache, and stomach, back, and neck pain).

The older adult's functioning and ability to perform activities of daily living such as walking, toileting, and bathing can be affected by pain, especially pain from musculoskeletal disease. Pain can lead to increased stress, delayed healing, decreased mobility, disturbances in sleep, decreased appetite, and agitation with accompanying aggressive behaviours. Chronic pain can cause depression, low self-esteem, social isolation, and feelings of hopelessness (Wynne, Ling, & Remsburg, 2000).

### Principles of Pain Management

***Assessment tools.*** When pain is suspected, the nurse begins with a physical assessment for medical origins of the pain and assesses characteristics of the pain itself. To aid older adults who may have sensory deficits or cognitive impairments, simply worded questions and simple drawings may be necessary. The Wong-Baker FACES Pain Rating Scale (Figure 30-1) is an assessment instrument currently in use. The FACES scale shows facial expressions on a scale from 0 (a smile) to 5 (crying grimace). Respondents are asked to choose the face that depicts the pain they feel. Studies have shown that 86% of long-term care residents can successfully use the FACES scale (Flaherty, 2000).

**FIGURE 30-1** Wong-Baker FACES Pain Rating Scale. **Source:** Hockenberry, M.J., & Wilson, D. (2009). *Wong's essentials of pediatric nursing* (8th ed., p. 1301). St. Louis: Mosby. Used with permission. Copyright Mosby.

| 0 | 1 | 2 | 3 | 4 | 5 |
|---|---|---|---|---|---|
| NO HURT | HURTS LITTLE BIT | HURTS LITTLE MORE | HURTS EVEN MORE | HURTS WHOLE LOT | HURTS WORST |

| | 0 | 1 | 2 | Score |
|---|---|---|---|---|
| **Breathing** Independent of vocalization | Normal | Occasional laboured breathing; short period of hyperventilation | Noisy, laboured breathing; long period of hyperventilation; Cheyne-Stokes respirations | |
| **Negative Vocalization** | None | Occasional moan or groan; low-level speech with a negative or disapproving quality | Repeated troubled calling out; loud moaning or groaning; crying | |
| **Facial Expression** | Smiling or inexpressive | Sad; frightened; frown | Facial grimacing | |
| **Body Language** | Relaxed | Tense; distressed pacing; fidgeting | Rigid; fists clenched; knees pulled up; pulling or pushing away; striking out | |
| **Consolability** | No need to console | Distracted or reassured by voice or touch | Unable to console, distract, or reassure | |
| | | | **TOTAL** | |

FIGURE 30-2 Pain Assessment in Advanced Dementia (PAINAD) scale. **Source:** Reprinted from Warden, V., Hurley, A.C., & Volicer, L. (2003). Development and psychometric evaluation of the Pain Assessment in Advanced Dementia [PAINAD] scale. *Journal of the American Medical Directors Association*, 4(1), 9–15. Copyright 2003, with permission from Elsevier.

The present pain intensity (PPI) rating from the McGill Pain Questionnaire (MPQ) (Davis & Srivastana, 2003) is another tool accepted for use with older patients. Patients are asked to respond by selecting the description (from "no pain" [0] to "excruciating pain" [5]) that they believe identifies the pain they feel. Wynne, Ling, and Remsburg (2000) found that the PPI rating of the MPQ was the most useful instrument for pain assessment in long-term care residents, including both the cognitively intact and cognitively impaired.

The Pain Assessment in Advanced Dementia (PAINAD) scale is used to evaluate the presence and severity of pain in patients with advanced dementia who no longer have the ability to communicate verbally (Figure 30-2). The scale evaluates five domains: breathing, negative vocalization, facial expression, body language, and consolability (Box 30-5). The score guides the caregiver in the appropriate pain intervention (Lane, Kuntupis, MacDonald, et al., 2003; Warden, Hurley, & Volicer, 2003).

***Barriers to accurate pain assessment.*** Binaso (2002) identifies beliefs and misconceptions held by older adults about pain that may interfere with appropriate assessment and treatment. Older adults may believe that pain is a punishment for past behaviours, an inevitable part of aging, indicative of pending death, related to serious illness, or a sign of weakness. External obstacles include inadequate assessment by health care providers, complicated clinical presentation, assumptions by health care providers that pain is part of aging, and communication deficits due to cognitive impairment.

Changes in behaviour may indicate pain and should be assessed, especially in people who have difficulty verbally communicating their needs (e.g., those with dementia). Unlike younger adults, older adults may understate their pain using words such as *discomfort*, *hurting*, or *aching*. Multiple painful problems may occur together, making differentiation of new pain from pre-existing pain difficult. Sensory impairments, memory loss, dementia, and depression can add to the difficulty of obtaining an accurate pain assessment. An interview with family members, caregivers, or friends is vital.

***Pain treatment.*** There are three essential features of treating pain:

1. Do a thorough assessment and establish an accurate diagnosis.
2. Recognize that pain reduction may be the treatment goal, rather than complete elimination of pain.
3. Treat symptoms of coexisting disorders, such as depression, anxiety, or other physical conditions that exacerbate the pain.

**Pharmacological pain treatments.** The cause of the pain should be addressed along with treatment of the pain itself. Pain should be managed with pharmacological or alternative measures. Pharmacological pain management relies on the use of prescription and nonprescription medications, frequently based on the recommendation of the health care provider. These include analgesics, opioid analgesics, and adjuvant medications. When administering and teaching patients about these types of medication, information should be provided

## BOX 30-5 THE FIVE ELEMENTS OF THE PAIN ASSESSMENT IN ADVANCED DEMENTIA (PAINAD) SCALE

1. **Breathing**

*Normal breathing* is effortless breathing characterized by quiet, rhythmic respirations.

*Occasional laboured breathing* is characterized by episodic bursts of harsh, difficult, or wearing respirations.

*Short period of hyperventilation* is characterized by intervals of rapid, deep breaths lasting a short period of time.

*Long period of hyperventilation* is characterized by excessive rate and depth of respirations lasting a considerable time.

*Cheyne-Stokes respirations* are characterized by rhythmic waxing and waning of breathing from very deep to shallow respirations with periods of apnea.

2. **Negative Vocalization**

*None* is characterized by speech or vocalization that has a neutral or pleasant quality.

*Occasional moan or groan:* Occasional moaning is characterized by mournful or murmuring sounds, wails, or laments. Occasional groaning is characterized by louder than usual inarticulate involuntary sounds, often abruptly beginning and ending.

*Low-level speech with negative or disapproving quality* is characterized by muttering, mumbling, whining, grumbling, or swearing in a low volume with a complaining, sarcastic, or caustic tone.

*Repeated, troubled calling out* is characterized by phrases or words being used over and over in a tone that suggests anxiety, uneasiness, or distress.

*Loud moaning or groaning:* Loud moaning is characterized by mournful or murmuring sounds, wails, or laments in a much louder than usual volume. Loud groaning is characterized by louder than usual inarticulate involuntary sounds, often abruptly beginning and ending.

*Crying* is characterized by an utterance of emotion accompanied by tears. There may be sobbing or quiet weeping.

3. **Facial Expression**

*Smiling or inexpressiveness:* Smiling is characterized by upturned corners of the mouth, brightening of the eyes, and a look of pleasure or contentment. Inexpressiveness refers to a neutral, at ease, relaxed, or blank look.

*Sad* is characterized by an unhappy, lonesome, sorrowful, or dejected look. Eyes may be teary.

*Frightened* is characterized by a look of fear, alarm, or heightened anxiety. Eyes may appear wide open.

*Frowning* is characterized by a downward turn of the corners of the mouth. Increased facial wrinkling in the forehead and around the corners of the mouth may appear.

*Facial grimacing* is characterized by a distorted, distressed look. The brow is more wrinkled, as is the area around the mouth. Eyes may be squeezed shut.

4. **Body Language**

*Relaxed* is characterized by a calm, restful, mellow appearance. The person seems to be taking it easy.

*Tense* is characterized by a strained, apprehensive, or worried appearance. The jaw may be clenched.

*Distressed pacing* is characterized by activity that seems unsettled. There may be a fearful, worried, or disturbed element present. The rate may be faster or slower.

*Fidgeting* is characterized by restless movement. Squirming about or wiggling in the chair may occur. The person might be hitching a chair across the room. Repetitive touching, tugging, or rubbing body parts can also be observed.

*Rigid* is characterized by stiffening of the body. The arms and/or legs are tight and inflexible. The trunk may appear straight and unyielding (exclude contractures).

*Fists clenched* is characterized by tightly closed hands. They may be opened and closed repeatedly or held tightly shut.

*Knees pulled up* is characterized by flexing the legs and drawing the knees upward toward the chest (exclude contractures).

*Pulling or pushing away* is characterized by resistiveness upon approach or to care. The person is trying to escape by yanking or wrenching himself or herself free or by shoving you away.

*Striking out* is characterized by hitting, kicking, grabbing, punching, biting, or other forms of personal assault.

5. **Consolability**

*No need to console* is characterized by a sense of well-being. The person appears content.

*Distracted or reassured by voice or touch* is characterized by a disruption in the behaviour when the person is spoken to or touched. The behaviour stops during the period of interaction, with no indication that the person is at all distressed.

*Unable to console, distract, or reassure* is characterized by the inability to soothe the person or stop a behaviour with words or actions. No amount of verbal or physical comforting will alleviate the behaviour.

***Scoring:*** (See Figure 30-3 for point allocation.)

**0–1** = No significant pain
**2–3** = Mild to moderate pain
**4–6** = Moderate to severe pain
**7–10** = Severe to very severe pain

**Source:** Lane, P., Kuntupis, M., MacDonald, S., et al. (2003). A pain assessment tool for people with advanced Alzheimer's and other progressive dementias. *Home Healthcare Nurse, 21*(1), 36.

about their potentially addictive nature. Consultation with a pain-management specialist is often helpful with chronic pain syndromes. Some considerations for pharmacological pain management in older adults are listed in Box 30-6.

As an individual ages, the body's ability to eliminate drugs via the kidney decreases. Nurses must be aware of this change, which can result in overdosing. On the other hand, fear of narcotic overmedication, which can cause respiratory depression and falls, may lead the nurse to give out less pain medication to

older adults than is needed for effective treatment (Celia, 2000). It is critical for nurses to evaluate the effectiveness of pain interventions at regular intervals and to be attentive to behavioural changes or verbal responses that indicate that the patient is experiencing pain. It is a common misconception that the ability to perceive pain decreases with aging. No physiological changes in pain perception in older adults have been demonstrated. In fact, older adults may feel pain even more keenly than younger persons do. Careful and continuing assessments and

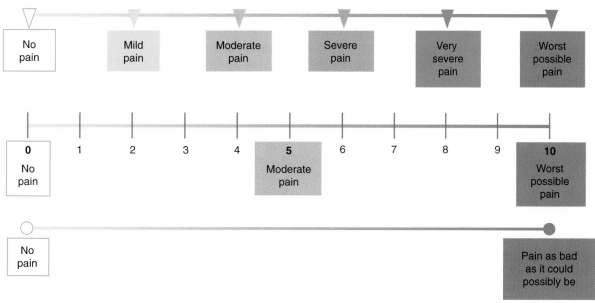

**FIGURE 30-3**  Visual analogue scales used in the management of cancer pain. **Source:** Jacox, A., Carr, D.B., Payne, R., et al. (1994, March). *Management of cancer pain (Clinical Practice Guideline No. 9, AHCPR Publication No. 94-0952)*. Rockville, MD: U.S. Department of Health and Human Services, Public Health Service, Agency for Health Care Policy and Research.

---

## BOX 30-6    TIPS FOR PHARMACOLOGICAL PAIN MANAGEMENT IN OLDER ADULTS

- Remember that many older adults receive pain medication less often than younger adults because their pain is often considered a natural part of aging. As a result, many older adults receive inadequate pain relief.
- Safe administration of analgesics is complicated because of possible interactions with drugs used to treat certain chronic disorders, as well as because of nutritional alterations and altered pharmacokinetics in older adults.
- Analgesics reach a higher peak and have a longer duration of action in older adults than in younger individuals. Start with one-fourth to one-half the adult dose, and titrate up carefully.
- Give oral analgesics around the clock at the beginning. Administer on an as-needed basis later on, as indicated by the patient's pain status.
- If acute confusion occurs, assess for other contributing factors before changing the medication or stopping analgesic use. Confusion in postoperative patients has been found to be associated with unrelieved pain rather than with opiate use.

- Acetaminophen is an effective analgesic in older adults. Although there is an increased risk of end-stage renal disease with long-term use, it does not produce the gastrointestinal bleeding seen with nonsteroidal anti-inflammatory drugs (NSAIDs).
- Analgesics and adjuvants, such as anticholinergics and pentazocine, may produce increased confusion in older adults. NSAIDs can have the same effect during their initial period of administration.
- Opiates have a greater analgesic effect and longer duration of action than nonopioid analgesics. Avoid the use of meperidine, whose active metabolite may stimulate the central nervous system and lead to confusion, seizures, and mood alterations. If this drug is selected, do not use it for more than 48 hours. Avoid intramuscular administration in the older adult because of tissue irritation and poor absorption. Morphine is a safer choice than meperidine because its duration of action is longer, so a smaller overall dose is required.
- Assess bowel function daily, because constipation can be a frequent adverse effect of opiates.

**Source:** Davis, M., & Srivastava, M. (2003). Demographics, assessment and management of pain in the elderly. *Drugs & Aging, 20*(1), 23–35.

---

an understanding of pain physiology are necessary for effective pain management of older adults.

**Nonpharmacological pain treatments.** Nonpharmacological treatments for pain include vagal nerve stimulation, exercise, hydrotherapy, heat and cold packs, chiropractics, and transcutaneous electrical nerve stimulation (TENS). Yoga, biofeedback, hypnosis, acupuncture, massage, shiatsu, reiki, guided imagery, reflexology, and therapeutic touch are integrative therapies for managing pain. Herbal remedies include cayenne, capsaicin, ginger extract, echinacea, kava kava, and willow bark. It is

important to ask older adults if they are using any alternative treatments for pain relief. Pain-management education is important for both the patient and caregivers. The key to successful pain management lies in the application of a variety of techniques that the patient must learn and practise. See Chapter 37 for a full discussion of integrative therapies.

### Caregiver Burden

Another phenomenon with the aging population is the increase in caregiver burden. Although there is not a consistent definition of caregiver burden, most researchers and clinicians view this concept as the physical, psychological, emotional (e.g., increased depression, increased stress, increased fatigue), social, and financial (e.g., increased costs associated with caring, decreased work hours) stresses that individuals experience as a result of providing care (Bastawrous, 2013; Black, Gauthier, Dalziel, et al., 2012). A common scenario would be the two-income family in the middle of raising children and planning for their future retirement, who are now faced with aging parents in need of help. Shorter lengths of stay for hospitalization, limited home care options, and complicated procedures to access care have increased the need for adult children to advocate for and provide care to aging parents. Unfortunately, this scenario is different for older adults who have lived with a chronic mental illness. Schizophrenia and bipolar disorders take a toll on family members and intimate relationships, and it is not uncommon for those with severe mental illness to have no family support available as they age. Grown children may be estranged because of a parent's frequent hospitalization, poor parenting ability, or paranoid symptoms. The support system of those aging with chronic mental illness often becomes case managers, community nurses, and mental health care providers.

### Access to Care

The disparity of mental health services in Canada has developed into a fragmented system of care so complicated that some patients become resigned to go without care (Horgan, LeClair, Donnelly, et al., 2009). Nurses may feel powerless to change shortfalls in the health care system; however, they can take advantage of their numbers and the respect given to the profession to be strong advocates for improving health care.

Access to care is also impacted by the availability of financial resources. Although every Canadian has access to all medically necessary services, regardless of ability to pay, "all medically necessary services" is typically interpreted within an illness- or disease-focused paradigm. As a result, health promotion activities and many factors associated with the social determinants of health—for example, housing—are not included within the delivery of "all medically necessary services." People, therefore, are individually responsible for the costs associated with meeting their overall health care needs.

### Ageism

In Western culture, growing older is not viewed as a privilege, and old age does not tend to confer a revered social status upon those who have attained it. Ageism has been defined as a bias against older people because of their age. It is based on erroneous beliefs that older adults are unattractive, unintelligent, asexual, unemployable, and senile. Ageism impacts not only employment opportunities for the older population but also the quality of health care this population receives (Stall, 2012). For example, most older people present with several co-morbid conditions, yet the Canadian health care system is organized into single diagnostic specialties (e.g., psychiatry, endocrinology, hematology, surgery). This division poses the risk that patients with diagnoses in several areas may not receive the best possible care because of the complexity of their presentation.

Additionally, there are a decreasing number of health care providers choosing geriatrics as a specialty area (Eymard & Douglas, 2012).

Ageism is not limited to the way the young view the old, though; it can also be exhibited by older adults themselves. Indeed, the attitudes of older adults toward their contemporaries, particularly those with mental disabilities, are often negative—perhaps because the threat of contagion by association with the frail and infirm raises feelings of vulnerability. Ageism differs from other forms of discrimination in that it cuts across gender, race, religion, and socioeconomic status to reach the majority of those over age 65.

### Ageism and Public Policy

The results of ageism can be observed in every level of society. Financial and political support for programs for older adults is difficult to obtain. The needs of this population often are addressed only after those of younger, albeit smaller, population groups. However, the Canadian Association for Retired Persons (CARP), a powerful lobbying group, is fighting to change this trend.

### Ageism and Drug Testing

Clinical drug trials often exclude people over the age of 65 on the assumption that they already take multiple medications or have an existing chronic illness. Information about medications for the general population has to be generalized for older adults, and appropriate (generally lower) doses may not have been tested or even be available (Rochon, 2008).

## NURSING CARE OF OLDER ADULTS

Nurses encounter older adults in a variety of settings, and in each of these settings, the nurse is responsible for applying the nursing process to the individual patient's situation.

Studies suggest that because nursing students are not given enough information about older adults and often are not exposed to older patients, they may hold ageist views when they begin their nursing careers. Such biases have significant implications for practice, education, and research (Lueckenotte, 2000). Morris and Mentes (2006) discussed the challenges of geropsychiatric nursing education, citing the lack of standardized curriculum and credentialling. It is important for all nurses to gain a better understanding of the aging process. Adequate theory and principles of practice are needed to provide safe and excellent care for older adults. The Canadian Gerontological Nursing Association (2010) has developed practice standards to define the uniqueness and scope of gerontological nursing. The standards are organized into six categories: (1) physiological health, (2) optimizing functional health, (3) responsive care, (4) relationship care, (5) health system, and (6) safety and security.

Positive attitudes toward older adults and their care need to be instilled during basic nursing education. Education programs must include the following:
- Information about the aging process
- Discussion of attitudes relating to the care of older adults

- Sensitization of participants to their patients' needs
- Exploration of the dynamics of nurse–patient and staff–patient interactions
- Respect for older patients and appreciation of their wisdom and life experience

## Assessment Strategies

Nurses who work with older adults benefit from specific knowledge about normal aging, drug interactions, and chronic disease. Those who work with older patients who have mental health problems need to have specific skills in interviewing and assessing and special knowledge of effective treatment modalities. The Canadian Gerontological Nursing Association (2010) has recommended a comprehensive geriatric assessment, which includes the following areas: physiological, functional, cognitive, psychological, sociocultural, spiritual, environmental, risk factors, response to pharmacological intervention and drug use patterns, and diagnostic results and implications related to treatment. Specific assessment questions should also be asked related to assessing pain in older adults. Figure 30-4 shows what is considered in a comprehensive geriatric assessment.

A thorough assessment, including a physical assessment and diagnostic testing, must precede any treatment or diagnosis of a mental illness in older adults. Common tests include thyroid, kidney, and liver function; complete blood count; comprehensive metabolic panel; vitamin $B_{12}$, folic acid, and therapeutic drug levels; urinalysis; syphilis serology (RPR); B-type natriuretic peptide (BNP); and computed tomography (CT) of the head. A review of current medications and possible adverse reactions or drug–drug interactions must also occur (Rochon, 2008). Confusion can be caused by anticholinergics, antihistamine, and benzodiazepines. Psychosis has been linked to steroids and even cholesterol-lowering medications, and depression has been linked with beta blockers, alpha adrenergics, and opiates. Serious medical conditions such as cancer, anemia, diabetes, infections, electrolyte imbalance, malnutrition, dehydration, and cardiac disease can manifest in symptoms such as fatigue or anorexia before more specific physical manifestations occur. Nurses are in a unique position to advocate for and coordinate appropriate medical evaluation for older adults.

An examination and interview of an older adult conducted in unfamiliar surroundings can produce anxiety. Unlike younger patients, who may be comfortable discussing personal issues—family conflicts, feelings of sadness, sexual practices, finances, and bodily functions—older adults may view such topics as private or taboo and be uncomfortable discussing them. It is important to respect these feelings while reviewing essential history by doing the following:

- Conducting the interview in a private area
- Introducing oneself and asking the patient what he or she would like to be called (use of the first name is rarely appropriate unless one is invited to use it)
- Establishing rapport and putting the patient at ease by sitting or standing at the same level as the patient
- Ensuring that lighting is adequate and noise level is low in recognition of the fact that hearing and vision may be impaired

- Using touch (with permission) to convey warmth, while at the same time respecting the patient's comfort level with personal touch
- Summarizing the interaction, inviting feedback and questions, and thanking the patient for giving his or her time and information

Assessment of the cognitive, behavioural, and emotional status of the older adult is very important in managing the nursing care of the patient and is particularly vital for detecting dementia, delirium, and depression, whose prevalence increases with age (Dharmarajan & Norman, 2003). The Geriatric Depression Scale (Short Form) (Box 30-7) is a subjective questionnaire (Sheikh & Yesavage, 1986), and the Cornell Scale for Depression in Dementia is an objective screening tool for caregivers to help identify the presence of depressive symptoms (Alexopoulos, Abrams, Young, et al., 1988). The periodic repetition of these assessments serves to evaluate the effectiveness of intervention.

It is also essential to assess for suicidal thoughts and suicidal intent by asking specific questions such as these:
- Have you ever thought about killing yourself?
- Have you ever felt that life is not worth living?
- Have you ever tried to hurt yourself in the past?

Thoughts of harming others also must be assessed. Interventions for the prevention of suicide in older adults are discussed in greater depth later in this chapter. Also see Chapter 25 for a more detailed discussion of suicide assessment and intervention.

Older adult abuse is another area to explore during a nursing assessment and is discussed in depth in Chapter 27.

### BOX 30-7 GERIATRIC DEPRESSION SCALE (SHORT FORM)

1. Are you basically satisfied with your life? Yes/No
2. Have you dropped many of your activities and interests? Yes/No
3. Do you feel that your life is empty? Yes/No
4. Do you often get bored? Yes/No
5. Are you in good spirits most of the time? Yes/No
6. Are you afraid that something bad is going to happen to you? Yes/No
7. Do you feel happy most of the time? Yes/No
8. Do you often feel helpless? Yes/No
9. Do you prefer to stay at home rather than going out and doing new things? Yes/No
10. Do you feel you have more problems with memory than most? Yes/No
11. Do you think it is wonderful to be alive now? Yes/No
12. Do you feel pretty worthless the way you are now? Yes/No
13. Do you feel full of energy? Yes/No
14. Do you feel that your situation is hopeless? Yes/No
15. Do you think that most people are better off than you are? Yes/No

**Source:** Sheikh, J.I., & Yesavage, J.A. (1986). Geriatric Depression Scale (GDS): Recent evidence and development of a shorter version. In T.L. Brink (Ed.), *Clinical gerontology: A guide to assessment and intervention* (pp. 165–173). New York: Hawthorn Press.

| COMPREHENSIVE GERIATRIC ASSESSMENT | | | | | |
|---|---|---|---|---|---|
| Name: | | Date of birth: | | Gender: | |

**Physical Health**

| | | | | | |
|---|---|---|---|---|---|
| *Chronic disorder* | | | | | |
| *Vision* | Adequate | Inadequate | Eyeglasses: Y  N | | Needs evaluation |
| *Hearing* | Adequate | Inadequate | Hearing aids: Y  N | | |
| *Mobility* | Ambulatory: Y  N | | Assistive device: | | |
| | Falls: Y  N | | | | Needs evaluation |
| *Nutrition* | Albumin: | TLC: | HCT: | | |
| | Weight: | Weight loss or gain: Y  N | | | Needs evaluation |
| *Incontinence* | Y  N | Treatment: | Y  N | | Needs evaluation |
| *Medications* | Total number: | Reviewed & revised: Y  N | | | |
| | Adverse effects/allergy: | | | | |
| *Screening* | Cholesterol: | TSH: | B12: | Folate: | |
| | Colonoscopy: Date: | | N/A | | |
| | Mammogram: Date: | | N/A | | |
| | Osteoporosis: Date: | | N/A | | |
| | Pap smear: Date: | | N/A | | |
| | PSA: Date: | | N/A | | |
| *Immunization* | Influenza: Date: | | | | |
| | Pneumonia: Date: | | | | |
| | Tetanus: Date: | | Booster: | | |
| *Counselling* | Diet | Exercise | Calcium | Vitamin D | |
| | Smoking | Alcohol | Driving | Injury prevention | |

**Mental Health**

| | | | | | |
|---|---|---|---|---|---|
| *Dementia* | Y  N | MMSE score: | Date: | Cause (if known): | |
| *Depression* | Y  N | GDS score: | Date: | Treatment: Y  N | |

**Functional Status**

| | | | | | |
|---|---|---|---|---|---|
| *ADL* | Bathing: I  D | | Dressing: I  D | | Toileting: I  D |
| | Transferring: I  D | | Feeding: I  D | | Continence: Y  N |

**FIGURE 30-4** Comprehensive geriatric assessment. *ADL*, activities of daily living; *B12*, vitamin B12; *D*, dependent; *GDS*, Geriatric Depression Scale; *HCT*, hematocrit; *I*, independent; *MMSE*, Mini-Mental State Examination; *N*, no; *PSA*, prostate-specific antigen; *TLC*, total lymphocyte count; *TSH*, thyroid-stimulating hormone; *Y*, yes.

Questions about being hit, pushed, kicked, and slapped are important, but it is also imperative to inquire about care being withheld. Not being fed, cleaned, helped, or cared for are critical issues. Asking initially, "How are you being treated at home?" or "Are you afraid of anyone?" may encourage further exploration. Financial exploitation is another issue that is difficult to uncover. Older adults may feel ashamed or embarrassed to admit they have been taken advantage of by family, friends, or strangers (Spangler & Brandl, 2007). Box 30-8 provides helpful interview techniques to use with older adults.

| BOX 30-8 | HELPFUL TECHNIQUES FOR INTERVIEWING OLDER ADULTS |
|---|---|

- Gather preliminary data before the session, and keep questionnaires relatively short.
- Ask about often-overlooked problems, such as difficulty sleeping, incontinence, falling, depression, dizziness, and loss of energy.
- Pace the interview to allow the patient to formulate answers; resist the tendency to interrupt prematurely.
- Use yes-or-no or simple-choice questions if the older patient has trouble coping with open-ended questions.
- Begin with general questions such as "How can I help you most at this visit?" or "What's been happening?"
- Be alert for information about the patient's relationships with others, thoughts about families or co-workers, typical responses to stress, and attitudes toward aging, illness, occupation, and death.
- Assess mental status for deficits in recent or remote memory, and determine if confusion exists.
- Be aware of all medications the patient is taking, and assess for adverse effects, efficacy, and possible drug interactions.
- Determine how fast the condition of the patient has been changing to assess the extent of the patient's concerns.
- Include the family or significant other in the interview process for added input, clarification, support, and reinforcement.

**Source:** National Institute on Aging. (2008). *Talking with your older patient: A clinician's handbook.* Retrieved from http://www.nia.nih.gov/health/publication/talking-your-older-patient-clinicians-handbook/keeping-door-open.

## Intervention Strategies

Certain psychotherapeutic methods are especially useful for older adults:

- Applying crisis intervention techniques (see Chapter 24)
- Providing empathic understanding and active listening
- Encouraging ventilation of feelings and normalizing emotional responses
- Re-establishing emotional equilibrium when anxiety is moderate to severe
- Providing health education and explaining alternative solutions
- Assisting in the use of problem-solving approaches
- Allowing adequate time to process information
- Ensuring hearing aids are working or using an amplifier to facilitate good communication

An older adult may require acute inpatient mental health care for signs and symptoms of severe psychiatric conditions, such as nondementia psychiatric illnesses, major depression with suicidal thoughts, bipolar disorder, and schizophrenia (Hoover, Akincigil, Prince, et al., 2008). The number of patients with nondementia psychiatric illnesses treated on an inpatient basis is declining. Regardless of the person's age, inpatient treatment is recommended when the patient is at high risk for self-harm (whether intentional or unintentional) or poses a risk for harm to other people.

Specialized geropsychiatric units provide a comprehensive and specialized approach to care. These units use a multidisciplinary approach to assessment, treatment planning, implementation, and evaluation of care. Ideally, the team consists of a geriatric psychiatrist, geriatrician, social worker, nurses, a pharmacist, psychologist, dietitian, occupational therapist, physiotherapist, and other specialists as indicated. Nurses play the major role in providing continuous care from admission to discharge.

### Psychosocial Interventions

The basic-level nurse uses counselling skills to assist the patient in talking about present problems, examining his or her present situation, looking at alternatives, and planning for the future. Sometimes counselling is provided through group therapy, which helps to decrease the sense of disorientation and isolation. Remotivation therapy (Box 30-9) and reminiscence therapy are also appropriate interventions for the basic-level nurse.

The advanced-practice nurse may provide individual or group psychotherapy to older adults with depression. Groups are useful because they can diminish social isolation and loneliness and help the members understand that they are not alone in their situation. Group members can learn creative ways to improve their mood and increase quality of life (Yalom, 2005). Table 30-1 outlines the purpose, format, and desired outcomes for each type of psychotherapeutic group. Individual therapies, specifically cognitive-behavioural, interpersonal, and psychodynamic therapy, are also useful. The best outcomes result from combining some kind of therapy with medication. Primary care providers, therefore, must acquire the skills to enable sensitive assessment for depression and suicide risk and must be knowledgeable about methods of intervention. Collaboration with other mental health care providers is best practice.

### Pharmacological Interventions

Evidence about the biology of mental illness and the discovery of new psychotropic medications have expanded the role of the geropsychiatric nurse. Nurses play a vital role in monitoring, reporting, and managing medication adverse effects such as acute dystonia, akathisia, pseudoparkinsonism, neuroleptic malignant syndrome (NMS), serotonin syndrome, and anticholinergic effects. Physical assessment of response to medication is also important and includes monitoring vital signs, pain, lab work, elimination (bowel and bladder), changes in gait, prevention of falls, and neurological checks when appropriate. The nurse assesses for underlying medical problems. Often, patients with chronic persistent mental illnesses, such as schizophrenia, misinterpret or do not report visceral cues, pain, and vital symptoms of illness (Reeves & Torres, 2003).

### Health Teaching and Health Promotion

The nurse provides health teaching to both patient and caregiver on a variety of issues, including the nature of the patient's illness, symptom management, maintenance of safety, self-care strategies, management of medications (see Patient and Family Teaching box), coping skills, steps necessary for recovery, and resources that will support recovery. When information is printed, providing a large print version is often helpful.

## BOX 30-9  EXAMPLE OF REMOTIVATION SESSION (BODIES OF WATER)

**Step 1: Climate of Acceptance**
The leaders personally welcomed each participant as he or she arrived at the group session. After the leaders introduced themselves, each group member made a self-introduction. The leader used a calendar to orient the members to the date and time of the current remotivation session. The theme for session four was introduced by the leader as "Bodies of Water—Rivers, Lakes, and Oceans." All group members had some familiarity with bodies of water because of their residence in Seattle.

**Step 2: Creating a Bridge to Reality**
The world globe was used as a visual aid to stimulate discussion on bodies of water. The leader asked questions such as "How are bodies of water formed from glaciers?" Pictures of glaciers, rivers, and lakes were shown.

The leader read poems about tide pools, seashells, and fishing written by anonymous grade-school children. Discussion was stimulated by the leader's asking, "What can we do at the ocean?" Visual aids and props were provided for direct sensory stimulation. Some examples of these aids and props were (1) different types of seashells, (2) fishing tackle and bait, (3) suntan lotion, (4) sun hat, and (5) sunglasses.

An anonymous author's poem about fishing was read to the group, followed by recorded music with lyrics about fishing experiences.

**Step 3: Sharing the World We Live In**
Group discussion focused on jobs related to bodies of water. Topics the participants discussed in regard to self or others included crabbing, clamming, shrimping, and fishing. Visual aids, such as pictures of river rafting, canoeing, scuba diving, and sailing, stimulated further discussions of past related experiences involving bodies of water.

**Step 4: An Appreciation of the World of Work**
This time was used for the members to think about work in relation to others. More experiences in past work roles, as well as hobbies and pastimes, were discussed. The group then participated in singing a familiar old song, "Love Letters in the Sand," written in 1931 by J. Fred Coots and revived in 1957, when sung by Pat Boone.

**Step 5: Climate of Appreciation**
The leaders thanked the group members individually for coming to the group and sharing their experiences. The next remotivation session theme and meeting date were announced prior to terminating the session.

**Group Response to Session Four**
Most members of the group appeared to enjoy discussing their experiences in relation to bodies of water. Many members recalled fishing and boating experiences. Other members expressed interest in this topic by their nonverbal participation in touching and smelling some physical props and observation of visual aids. All but two participants touched the seashells and smelled the fish eggs. One lady in the group stood up and modelled the sun hat and glasses, while a man demonstrated how to reel in the line on a fishing pole. Several participants remarked on how beautiful the pictures of the glaciers were. All but a couple of group members sang to the recorded lyrics on fishing. One member stood up and danced to the music while many others clapped to her movements.

**Source:** Reprinted with permission from SLACK Incorporated: Janssen, J.A., & Giberson, D.L. (1988). Remotivation therapy. *Journal of Gerontological Nursing, 14*(6), 31–34.

## PATIENT AND FAMILY TEACHING: DRUG SAFETY

- Learn about your medicines:
  - Read medicine labels and package inserts, and follow the directions.
  - If you have questions, ask your doctor or other health care providers.
- Talk to your team of health care providers about your medical conditions, health concerns, and all the medicines you take (both prescription and over-the-counter), as well as dietary supplements, vitamins, and herbal supplements.
  - The more they know, the more they can help.
  - Do not be afraid to ask questions.
- Keep track of adverse effects or possible drug interactions, and let your doctor know right away about any unexpected symptoms or changes in the way you feel.
- Make sure to go to all doctor appointments and to any appointments for monitoring tests done by your doctor or at a laboratory.
- Use a calendar, pillbox, or something to help you remember what medications you need to take and when.
- Write down information your doctor gives you about your medicines or your health condition.
- Take a friend or relative to your doctor's appointments if you think you need help to understand or remember what the doctor tells you.
- Have a "medicine checkup" at least once a year.
  - Go through your medicine cabinet to get rid of old or expired medicines.
  - Ask your doctor or pharmacist to go over all the medicines you now take. Remember to include all the over-the-counter medicines, vitamins, dietary supplements, and herbal supplements you take.
- Keep all medicines out of the sight and reach of children.

| TABLE 30-1 | **USEFUL GROUP THERAPY MODALITIES FOR OLDER ADULTS** | |
|---|---|---|
| **REMOTIVATION THERAPY** | **REMINISCENCE THERAPY (LIFE REVIEW)** | **PSYCHOTHERAPY** |
| **PURPOSE OF GROUP** | | |
| Resocialize regressed and apathetic patients<br>Reawaken interest in the environment | Share memories of the past<br>Increase self-esteem<br>Increase socialization<br>Increase awareness of the uniqueness of each participant | Alleviate psychiatric symptoms<br>Increase ability to interact with others in a group<br>Increase self-esteem<br>Increase ability to make decisions and function more independently |
| **FORMAT** | | |
| Groups are made up of 10 to 15 people.<br>Meetings are held once or twice a week.<br>Meetings are highly structured in a classroomlike setting.<br>Group uses props.<br>Each session discusses a particular topic.<br>See Box 30-9 for the five basic steps used in each session. | Groups are made up of 6 to 8 people.<br>Meetings are held once or twice weekly for 1 hour.<br>Topics include holidays, major life events, birthdays, travel, and food. | Group size is 6 to 12 members.<br>Group members should share similar:<br>• Problems<br>• Mental status<br>• Needs<br>Groups should be mixed (both men and women).<br>Group meets at regularly scheduled times (certain number of times a week, specific duration of session) and place. |
| **DESIRED OUTCOMES** | | |
| Increases participants' sense of reality<br>Offers practice of health roles<br>Realizes more objective self-image | Alleviates depression in institutionalized older adults<br>Through the process of reorganization and reintegration, provides avenue by which members:<br>• Achieve a new sense of identity<br>• Achieve a positive self-concept | Decreases sense of isolation<br>Facilitates development of new roles and re-establishes former roles<br>Provides information for other types of groups<br>Provides group support for effecting changes and increasing self-esteem |

**Source:** Matteson, M.A., & McConnell, E.S. (Eds.). (1988). *Gerontological nursing: Concepts and practice* (p. 80). Philadelphia: Saunders.

## Promotion of Self-Care Activities

Hospitalization may result in regression that ranges from needing assistance to requiring total care in accomplishing the activities of daily living. A goal for nurses is to encourage the patient to regain independence in the realm of personal care. Hospitalization may be an opportunity for the patient to receive much-needed assessment of the skin, feet, hair, mouth, and perineal areas. These assessments can often uncover hidden infections, unhealed wounds, and growths that may otherwise have been missed and lead to needed medical attention.

## Milieu Management

The major roles of the nurse in terms of milieu management are to assist the patient in adjusting to the environment, keep the patient safe at all times (e.g., make sure roommates are compatible, call lights are within reach, patients at risk for falling are placed close to the nurses' station), minimize the adverse effects of hospitalization on functional capacity (e.g., encourage patients to walk and to do so as independently as possible), provide reality orientation, and engage in therapeutic communication with the patient. It helps to know that reorienting a patient is not always therapeutic, especially if the patient

has dementia and reorientation causes agitation. Using distraction techniques is often the intervention of choice.

Another vital aspect of milieu management is the prevention and reduction of agitation by maintaining a visible presence on the unit and anticipating the patient's needs (Johnson & Delaney, 2007). Crisis intervention techniques may be used if an agitated patient does not respond to redirection or verbal attempts to de-escalate agitation. As a crisis situation unfolds, staff response will largely determine the outcome, and a well-trained crisis team improves these outcomes. The crisis team leader is usually a nurse for several reasons:

- Nurses provide professional care 24 hours a day, 7 days a week and have detailed knowledge of patients.
- The nurse is aware of the patient's medical condition.
- The nurse is able to guide the team and help prevent injury of a patient who needs physical restraint but has osteoporosis.

After the crisis has been de-escalated, the team leader, the team, and other patients (as indicated) help restore a sense of safety and calm. As the agitated patient gains control, it is important to help the individual ease back into the milieu with dignity.

## Care Settings

### Skilled Nursing Facilities

As acute hospital care of older adults with nondementia psychiatric illnesses is decreasing, the use of long-term skilled nursing facilities is increasing (Hoover, Akincigil, Prince, et al., 2008). The use of these facilities to treat older adults with severe mental illness is controversial, and opponents fear that "nursing homes" will become the mental institutions of the twenty-first century, providing little more than custodial care.

Whereas some long-term care settings provide specialized psychiatric mental health care, most do not. There may be little consistency in the education of nurses and nursing assistants in appropriate psychiatric assessment and intervention. Clinicians may believe that patients who refuse personal hygiene, medication, or wound care are exercising their rights to refuse care, rather than recognizing the negative symptoms of schizophrenia. Nurses who accept these refusals may inadvertently contribute to a patient's deterioration.

The skilled nursing facility setting can be a stabilizing environment for a person with severe mental illness who thrives within the structure of a therapeutic environment. Providing a documented plan of care and intervening when behavioural symptoms increase are as important as monitoring and intervening when a resident has signs of infection.

There now is much greater awareness and focus on the use of nonpharmacological interventions for the treatment of agitation, wandering, confusion, yelling, and aggression. Drugs often deemed "unnecessary" are generally antipsychotics, anti-anxiety agents, and sedatives. Patients with a history of depression, schizophrenia, obsessive-compulsive disorder, generalized anxiety disorder, or bipolar disorder need ongoing treatment to prevent relapse and re-emergence of symptoms. Nurses can play an important role in advocating for psychiatric evaluation and intervention to assist with (1) managing medications, (2) monitoring and documenting behavioural changes, (3) notifying the physician of behavioural changes, and (4) planning care for the needs of those residents with mental illness.

### Residential Care Settings

Older adults with chronic and persistent mental illness (e.g., schizophrenia) are increasingly difficult to place in residential care settings. As discussed in Chapters 5 and 6, the mental health system has increasingly become focused on the goal of community living rather than institutional living, but resources necessary to meet this goal have been chronically underfunded. Patients who would benefit from residential care are often moved from the most structured environment (inpatient care) to unstructured and unsupervised living situations in the community.

### Partial Hospitalization

Partial hospitalization, or acute psychiatric day hospital programs, are sometimes recommended for ambulatory patients who do not need 24-hour nursing care but require and would benefit from intensive, structured psychiatric treatment. A review of acute psychiatric day hospitals in the United Kingdom found that patients who received care in partial hospitalization programs showed a more rapid improvement in mental status than patients randomly assigned to inpatient care; this type of care also led to cost reductions ranging from 20.9% to 36.9%, as compared to inpatient care (Marshall, 2003).

Health services provided in these programs include symptom monitoring and management, medication education and management, relapse and stress prevention, and problem solving of health maintenance issues to enable the patient to adapt to active functioning in the community. The nurse also reviews with the team, in collaboration with the patient and family or caregiver, additional referrals for needed services (e.g., Meals on Wheels, transportation services, church activities, and home care services).

### Day Treatment Programs

Multipurpose centres for older adults provide a broad range of services, including (1) health promotion and wellness programs; (2) health screening; (3) social, educational, and recreational activities; (4) meals; and (5) information and referral services. For those in need of nursing care and custodial care services, an adult support program is an appropriate choice. There are three types of adult support programs: (1) social care, (2) adult health or medical treatment programs, and (3) maintenance care. In each type, older adults are cared for during the day and stay in a home environment at night. The boundaries of these programs blend and overlap. All three models are meant to provide a safe, supportive, and nonthreatening environment and fulfill a vital function for older adults and their families. The programs allow older adults to continue their present living arrangements and maintain their social ties to the community; they also relieve families of the burden of 24-hour-a-day care for older adult dependents. If institutionalization becomes necessary, adult day care staff can work with patients and their families to assess the situation and make recommendations for placement.

### Behavioural Health Home Care

Older adults typically prefer the continuum of services to be delivered in the least restrictive setting, which is usually their homes. Home-based behavioural health care is particularly recommended to assist the homebound older adult adjust to and manage illness and disability either before or after hospitalization. It is often the role of the behavioural health home care nurse to help a person affected by a cognitive brain disorder or a severe and persistent mental illness remain in the home or to facilitate a transfer to a temporary or permanent facility, if necessary. Local home care agencies can assist with providing nursing and rehabilitation services; home health care aide services to provide assistance with activities of daily living; homemaking services, such as housekeeping and meal preparation (although many provincial health care plans do not cover homemaking costs); or a combination of services. The goal of all of these services is to increase the older adult's ability to live independently.

The target population for behavioural health home care includes older adults who need help with activities of daily living, have behavioural issues related to their physical illness, or have an enduring mental illness. Nursing services are usually provided by a basic-level practitioner, a certified generalist nurse in community health or home health care, or an advanced-practice registered nurse certified in adult psychiatric mental health nursing. Chapter 6 discusses home psychiatric mental health care in greater detail.

### Community-Based Programs

The hazards of institutionalization are numerous: increased risk for nosocomial infections, which may result in increased mortality; injuries may occur due to initial disorientation to a new setting; and patients may develop learned helplessness, losing interest in self-care activities. (Chapter 2 provides the historical overview of deinstitutionalization.) There also may be fewer opportunities for socialization. In contrast, community-based programs aim to promote the older adult's independent functioning and reduce the stress on the family system.

Community-based programs that provide specialized case-management services assist older adults with coordination of care and assistance (e.g., Meals on Wheels, transportation). Constant assessment of the changing needs of older adults requires frequent contact and rapid intervention when they become sick or need additional services. Hospitalization can be averted if aggressive and skilled case management is in place, and nurses are uniquely qualified to fulfill the role of case manager.

Older adults living in the community may still be driving, which can become a safety concern for caregivers, family, and the public. If there is evidence that the older adult can no longer safely drive a vehicle (e.g., failing visual acuity, hearing loss, memory deficits, impaired mobility, movement disorders such as Parkinson's disease), or there have been occurrences of frequent small collisions, it is appropriate to notify the provincial or territorial ministry of motor vehicles for a driving evaluation to determine the capacity for safe operation of a vehicle.

## ■ KEY POINTS TO REMEMBER

- The older-adult population continues to increase exponentially.
- The increase in the number of older adults poses a challenge not only to nurses but to the entire health care system to be prepared to respond to the special needs of this population.
- Attitudes toward older adults are often negative, reflecting ageism—a bias against older adults based solely on age.
- Ageism is found at all levels of society and even among health care providers and can affect the quality of care of older patients.
- Nurses who care for older adults in various settings may function at different levels. All should be knowledgeable about the process of aging and be cognizant of the differences between normal and abnormal aging changes.

- Older adults face increasing problems of substance abuse and suicide.
- Adequate pain assessment is important, and the nurse must bear in mind that older adults tend to understate their pain. Sufficient pain medication should be administered and the drugs carefully titrated.
- Nurses working with mentally ill patients must know psychotherapeutic approaches relevant for the older adult. Advanced-practice nurses may offer psychotherapy groups geared toward the special needs of this population.

## ■ CRITICAL THINKING

1. Mr. Abbott has received treatment for alcohol withdrawal. He is a very quiet, religious man who refuses to eat, does not sleep at night, admits to thoughts of desperation, and wishes he could die. He also confides that he attempted suicide when his wife died five years earlier, which is when he started drinking heavily.
   a. What cultural considerations may be helpful to know about religious people's response to depression?
   b. Which depression assessment tool is appropriate to use in assessing the severity of Mr. Abbott's condition? Explain your answer.

2. Mrs. Bélanger is 75 years old and lives with her daughter's family. She has moderate to advanced Alzheimer's disease. Although Mrs. Bélanger's family wants to keep her at home for as long as possible, they are overwhelmed by her needs and by being unable to leave her alone. What community placements might be best for Mrs. Bélanger? Explain your answer.

3. How should the nurse frame the multigenerational effects of historical trauma among Canadian First Nations people?
   a. Useful frameworks should describe the trauma in terms of connectedness, collectivity, and relationships.

## CHAPTER REVIEW

1. The nurse is caring for an older-adult patient. Which symptom should the nurse recognize as a normal part of aging?
   1. Depression
   2. Memory loss
   3. Situational grieving
   4. Dementia

2. The nurse is caring for an older-adult patient with depression. Which nursing response is appropriate when the patient's daughter asks, "Will he ever stop acting like this?"
   1. "I'm sorry, your father will likely be in this state from now on."
   2. "Although older adults have a high incidence of depression, it is treatable and your father will improve on the antidepressants."
   3. "Depression is caused by infections or electrolyte imbalances, and the damage is permanent."
   4. "A benzodiazepine will help alleviate the depression."

3. The nurse is caring for an older adult patient with pain. What is one myth about pain held by health care providers?
   1. Pain is an inevitable part of aging.
   2. Older adults may understate their pain using words such as *discomfort*, *hurting*, or *aching*.
   3. Dementia and depression can add to the difficulty of obtaining an accurate pain assessment.
   4. An interview with family members, caregivers, or friends is vital.

4. An older-adult patient experiencing pain states that she is going to use kava kava, which she has heard provides pain relief. Which nursing response is appropriate?
   1. "Kava kava is an appropriate herb to use for pain relief."
   2. "Older adults should not use herbal preparations."
   3. "Willow bark would be a better herbal supplement to use."
   4. "Are you using any other treatments for pain relief?"

## ℮volve WEBSITE

Post-Test interactive review

*Visit the Evolve Web site for Chapter Review Answers and Rationales, Critical Thinking Answer Guidelines, and additional resources related to the content in this chapter: http://evolve.elsevier.com/Canada/Varcarolis/psychiatric/*

## REFERENCES

Alexopoulos, G.S., Abrams, R.C., Young, R.C., et al. (1988). Cornell scale for depression in dementia. *Biological Psychiatry*, 23, 271–284. doi:10.1016/0006-3223(88)90038-8.

Bastawrous, M. (2013). Caregiver burden: A critical discussion. *International Journal of Nursing Studies*, 50(3), 431–441. doi:10.1016/j.ijnurstu.2012.10.005.

Binaso, K. (2002, December). *Pain management for the geriatric patient.* Presented at the 37th Annual American Society of Health System Pharmacists Midyear Clinical Meeting, Atlanta, GA.

Black, S., Gauthier, S., Dalziel, W., et al. (2012). Canadian Alzheimer's disease caregiver survey: Baby-boomer caregivers and burden of care. *International Journal of Geriatric Psychiatry*, 25(8), 807–813. doi:10.1002/gps.2421.

Canadian Coalition for Seniors' Mental Health. (2006). *National guidelines for seniors' mental health: The assessment of suicide risk and prevention of suicide.* Toronto: Author.

Canadian Gerontological Nursing Association. (2010). *Gerontological nursing competencies and standards of practice 2010.* Vancouver: Author.

Cassidy, K., & Rector, N. (2008). The silent geriatric giant: Anxiety disorders in late life. *Geriatrics and Aging*, 11(3), 150–156.

Celia, B. (2000). Age and gender differences in pain management following coronary artery bypass surgery. *Journal of Gerontological Nursing*, 26(5), 7–13.

Cremens, M.C. (2008). Geriatric psychiatry. In T.A. Stern, J.F. Rosenbaum, M. Fava, et al. (Eds.), *Massachusetts General Hospital comprehensive clinical psychiatry* (pp. 963–971). St. Louis: Mosby.

Davis, M., & Srivastana, M. (2003). Demographics, assessment and management of pain in the elderly. *Drugs & Aging*, 20(1), 23–35.

Dharmarajan, T., & Norman, R. (2003). *Clinical geriatrics.* New York: Parthenon.

Ebersole, P., Hess, P., & Luggen, A. (2004). *Toward healthy aging: Human needs and nursing response* (6th ed.). St. Louis, MO: Mosby.

Eymard, A., & Douglas, D. (2012). Ageism among health care providers and interventions to improve their attitudes toward older adults: An integrative review. *Journal of Gerontological Nursing*, 38(5), 26–35. doi:10.3928/00989134-20120307-09.

Fandrey, S. (2007). The essentials of … Seniors and substance abuse. Ottawa: Canadian Centre on Substance Abuse.

Flaherty, E. (2000). Assessing pain in older adults. *Journal of Gerontological Nursing*, 26(3), 5–6.

Health Canada. (2011). *Canadian alcohol and drug use monitoring survey: Summary of results for 2011.* Ottawa: Author.

Hoover, D.R., Akincigil, A., Prince, J.D., et al. (2008). Medicare inpatient treatment of elderly non-dementia psychiatric illnesses 1992–2002: Length of stay and expenditures by facility type. *Administration and Policy in Mental Health*, 35(4), 231–240.

Horgan, S., LeClair, K., Donnelly, M., et al. (2009). Developing a national consensus on the accessibility needs of older adults with concurrent and chronic, mental and physical health issues: A preliminary framework informing collaborative mental health care planning. *Canadian Journal on Aging*, 28(2), 97–105. doi:10.1017/S0714980809090175.

Jann, M.W., & Slade, J.H. (2007). Antidepressant agents for the treatment of chronic pain and depression. *Pharmacotherapy*, 27(11), 1571–1587.

Johnson, M.E., & Delaney, K.R. (2007). Keeping the unit safe: The anatomy of escalation. *Journal of the American Psychiatric Nurses Association*, 13, 42–52. doi:10.1177/1078390307301736

Karlamangla, A., Zhou, K., Reuben, D., et al. (2006). Longitudinal trajectories of heavy drinking in adults in the United States of America. *Addiction (Abingdon, England)*, 101(1), 91–99.

Lane, P., Kuntupis, M., MacDonald, S., et al. (2003). A pain assessment tool for patients with advanced Alzheimer's and other progressive dementias. *Home Healthcare Nurse*, 21(1), 30–37.

Lueckenotte, A. (2000). Gerontologic assessment. In A. Lueckenotte (Ed.), *Gerontologic nursing*. St. Louis, MO: Mosby.

Luggen, A. (2000). Pain. In A. Lueckenotte (Ed.), *Gerontologic nursing*. St. Louis, MO: Mosby.

Luggen, A. (2004). Mental wellness and disturbances. In P. Ebersole, P. Hess, & A.S. Luggen (Eds.), *Toward healthy aging: Human needs and nursing response*. St. Louis, MO: Mosby.

Marshall, M. (2003). Acute psychiatric day hospitals. *British Medical Journal, 327*, 116–117. doi:10.1136/bmj.327.7407.116.

Mental Health Commission of Canada. (2012). Changing directions, changing lives: The mental health strategy for Canada. Calgary: Author.

Morris, D., & Mentes, J. (2006). Geropsychiatric nursing education: Challenge and opportunity. *Journal of the American Psychiatric Nurses Association, 12*(2), 105–115.

Reeves, R.R., & Torres, R.A. (2003). Exacerbation of psychosis by misinterpretation of physical symptoms. *Southern Medical Journal, 96*(7), Retrieved from http://www.medscape.com/viewarticle/459197_print.

Rochon, P.A. (2008). *Drug prescribing for older adults. UpToDate*. Retrieved from http://www.uptodate.com/contents/drug-prescribing-for-older -adults.

Salisbury, S. (1999). Alcoholism. In J. Stone (Ed.), *Clinical gerontological nursing* (p. 537). Philadelphia: Saunders.

Sheikh, J.I., & Yesavage, J.A. (1986). Geriatric Depression Scale (GDS): Recent evidence and development of a shorter version. In T.L. Brink (Ed.), *Clinical gerontology: A guide to assessment and intervention* (pp. 165–173). New York: Haworth Press.

Spangler, D., & Brandl, B. (2007). Abuse in later life: Power and control dynamics and a victim-centered response. *Journal of the American Psychiatric Nurses Association, 12*, 322–331. doi:10.1177/ 1078390306298878.

Stall, N. (2012). Time to end ageism in medical education. *Canadian Medical Association Journal, 184*(6), 728. doi:10.1503/cmaj.112179/-/DC1.

Statistics Canada. (2010a). *Projected population by age according to three projection scenarios for 2006, 2011, 2016, 2021, 2026, 2031 and 2036, at July 1* (Table 052-005, Cat. no. 91-520-X). Retrieved from http://www.statcan .gc.ca/tables-tableaux/sum-som/l01/cst01/demo23a-eng.htm.

Statistics Canada. (2010b). *Suicide and suicide rate, by sex and by age group (Both sexes no.)* (Table 102-0551, Cat. no. 84F0209X). Retrieved from http://www.statcan.gc.ca/tables-tableaux/sum-som/l01/cst01/hlth66a -eng.htm.

Statistics Canada. (2010c). *Suicide and suicide rate, by sex and by age group (Female rate)* (Table 102-0551, Cat. no. 84F0209X). Retrieved from http:// www.statcan.gc.ca/tables-tableaux/sum-som/l01/cst01/hlth66c-eng.htm.

Statistics Canada. (2010d). *Suicide and suicide rate, by sex and by age group (Males no.)* (Table 102-0551, Cat. no. 84F0209X). Retrieved from http:// www.statcan.gc.ca/tables-tableaux/sum-som/l01/cst01/hlth66b-eng.htm.

Wagenaar, D., Mickus, M., & Wilson, J. (2001). Alcoholism in late life: Challenges and complexities. *Psychiatric Annals, 31*(11), 665–672.

Warden, V., Hurley, A.C., & Volicer, L. (2003). Development and psychometric evaluation of the Pain Assessment in Advanced Dementia (PAINAD) scale. *Journal of the American Medical Directors Association, 4*, 9–15. doi:10.1097/00130535-200301000-00002.

Wynne, C., Ling, S.M., & Remsburg, R. (2000). Comparison of pain assessment instruments in cognitively intact and cognitively impaired nursing home residents. *Geriatric Nursing, 21*(1), 20–23. doi:10.1067/ mgn.2000.105793.

Yalom, I.D. (2005). *The theory and practice of group psychotherapy* (5th ed.). Cambridge, MA: Basic Books.

# 31

# Living With Recurrent and Persistent Mental Illness

*Edward A. Herzog, Nancy Christine Shoemaker*
*Adapted by Catherine A. Thibeault*

## KEY TERMS AND CONCEPTS

community treatment orders (CTOs), 642
institutionalized, 633
psychoeducation, 637
rehabilitation, 634
social skills training, 639

stigma, 635
supported-employment model, 640
supportive psychotherapy, 639
vocational rehabilitation, 639

## OBJECTIVES

1. Discuss the effects of serious mental illness on daily functioning, interpersonal relationships, and quality of life.
2. Describe three common problems associated with serious mental illness.
3. Discuss five evidence-informed practices for the care of the person with serious mental illness.
4. Explain the role of the nurse in the care of the person with serious mental illness.
5. Develop a nursing care plan for a person with serious mental illness.
6. Discuss the causes of treatment nonadherence, and plan interventions to support treatment adherence.

## evolve WEBSITE

*Visit the Evolve website for Flashcards, Case Studies, and additional testing resources related to the content in this chapter:* http://evolve.elsevier.com/Canada/Varcarolis/psychiatric/    Pre-Test   interactive review

The term *mental illness* encompasses a wide range of human illness experience, from acute and time-limited reactions to stress to severe disruptions in cognitive functioning. The terms *serious mental illness* and *biologically based mental illness* refer to a small but significant group of mental illnesses. In Canada, there is no uniform definition of serious mental illness (SMI) or *serious and persistent mental illness* (SPMI), but many Canadian researchers and clinicians use *serious mental illness* to refer to schizophrenia, mood disorders, and other psychotic disorders. In the United States, categorizing mental illnesses according to levels of severity has tremendous implications for setting mental health policy and facilitating access to appropriate care. In Canada, where health care is funded through a comprehensive government-sponsored health insurance plan, strict categorization of levels of severity is less critical. That said, in Canada, there is considerable variation in spending on mental health services among the provinces (Jacobs, Yim, Ohinmaa, et al., 2008); the understanding that mental illness exists on a continuum of severity can help clinicians and policymakers as they work to develop a national and comprehensive mental health policy.

SMI is a significant health care challenge: the prevalence of depression is 4.8%, the prevalence of mania is 1.0%, and the prevalence of schizophrenia is 0.9% (Goeree, Fanahati, Burke, et al., 2005). Individuals with SMI usually have difficulties in multiple areas, including activities of daily living, relationships, social interaction, task completion, communication, leisure activities, safe movement about the community, finances and budgeting, health maintenance, vocational and academic activities, and coping with stressors.

SMIs are chronic or recurrent. Some patients experience remissions interrupted by exacerbations of varying lengths; the remissions may be essentially symptom-free but in most cases involve some degree of residual symptoms. Other patients experience illness as a chronic and sometimes deteriorating experience, during which symptoms wax and wane but never remit.

People with SMI are at risk for multiple physical, emotional, and social problems: they are more likely to be victims of crime, be medically ill, have undertreated or untreated physical illnesses, die prematurely, be homeless, be incarcerated, be unemployed or underemployed, engage in binge substance abuse, live in poverty, and report lower quality of life than persons without such illnesses (Aquila & Emanuel, 2003; Glied, 2007).

The impairments associated with SMI, along with related factors such as poverty, stigma, unemployment, and inadequate housing, can significantly impact quality of life and can cause persons with SMI to live in a "parallel universe" separate from persons who do not have SMI (Fitch, 2007). Symptoms or socially inappropriate behaviour caused by SMIs can cause others to reject the patient and refuse friendship, housing, or employment.

## SERIOUS MENTAL ILLNESS ACROSS THE LIFESPAN

SMI occurs in persons of any gender, age, culture, or geographical location. However, the population of people currently living with SMIs can be separated into two groups who have had different experiences with the mental health care system: (1) those old enough to have experienced long-term institutionalization and (2) those young enough to have been hospitalized only for acute care during exacerbations of their disorders.

### Older Adults

Until the second half of the twentieth century, most psychiatric inpatient treatment took place in large institutions uniquely dedicated to the care of the severely mentally ill. During this time, psychiatric hospitals were the long-term residences for many people (see Chapter 5). Medical paternalism, in which the health care provider made all decisions for patients with SMIs, was a pervasive philosophical stance at that time. Thus, patients became institutionalized (i.e., they became dependent on the services and structure of institutions and unable to function independently outside such institutions). It was difficult to distinguish whether behaviours were the result of the disease process or altered responses that resulted from institutionalization.

Some of today's older adults with SMI have experience with this system of care. They have learned that they are just to accept the treatment team's decisions. Today's emphasis on patient-centred care, which requires the patient to express his or her opinions and wishes, challenges some older adults who grew up in the paternalistic institutions of the past.

It was between 1960 and 1980 that all Canadian provinces began to make changes in the inpatient treatment of SMI by closing beds in large mental hospitals and opening inpatient units in general hospitals (Sealy & Whitehead, 2004). The 1990s heralded further deinstitutionalization of psychiatric services as

the total number of inpatient days for mental health care in psychiatric hospitals and general hospitals declined (Sealy & Whitehead, 2004).

> **VIGNETTE**
> At the age of 19, Marian was admitted to a facility that cares for people with serious mental illnesses. She is now 79, and, with the exception of living in a group home for two years in her 30s, she has been an inpatient at the SMI facility. Marian's symptoms have been stable, and the treatment team discusses discharge with her. She accepts their recommendations that she no longer needs inpatient treatment. She is discharged to a community supportive-living home. At her new home, she spends long periods sitting in front of the living room window. Marian does not ask to go out into the garden she watches for so many hours. Indeed, she rarely asks for anything, including snacks or recreational activities. The caregivers work with Marian for several months to help her to recognize her needs of the moment and then to articulate or act on them. There is a major celebration the day she walks into the kitchen and makes a peanut butter sandwich of her own volition. Some of the dependency caused by the institutionalization is being positively altered.

### Younger Adults

People young enough never to have been institutionalized usually do not have problems of passivity and dependency. However, treatment via a series of short-term hospitalizations has given them limited experience with formal treatment and has contributed to some patients' not truly believing a problem exists. Individuals who do not understand that they are ill, perhaps because of the impairment of the illness itself (*anosognosia*), are at particular risk for additional problems. Young adults with SMI, for example, are at particular risk for additional problems such as legal difficulties, substance abuse, and unemployment.

> **VIGNETTE**
> After graduating from high school, Christopher enlists in the armed forces and serves for five years. He settles in Nova Scotia and takes a job in a security firm. In his first psychotic break, Christopher becomes paranoid and threatening at work and is hospitalized briefly. Upon discharge, Christopher refuses aftercare and will not take medication. He quits his job and moves to another city. For the next 15 years, Christopher works intermittently, is homeless off and on, and drinks heavily whenever he has money. He is hospitalized only when his behaviour is threatening to others. He consistently resists aftercare recommendations, showing no insight into his illness. One day, Christopher simply disappears.

## DEVELOPMENT OF SERIOUS MENTAL ILLNESS

SMI has much in common with chronic physical illness: the original problem increasingly overwhelms and erodes basic coping mechanisms and increases the use of compensatory processes. As the disorder extends beyond the acute stage, more and more of the neighbouring systems are involved. For example, a person with schizophrenia may experience disturbed thought processes and social skills, which cause interactions with others to become increasingly awkward and anxiety provoking for both parties. This awkwardness, in turn, results in others' becoming increasingly hesitant to interact with the affected person and in the affected person's self-esteem weakening.

## REHABILITATION VERSUS RECOVERY: TWO MODELS OF CARE

For many years, the concept of rehabilitation, which focused on managing patients' deficits and helping patients learn to live with their illnesses, dominated psychiatric care. Staff directed the treatment and concentrated on helping patients function in their daily roles. Advocates for improved mental health care and people with SMI (many of whom prefer to call themselves *consumers* to emphasize the choices they have, or seek to have, over their treatment) have increasingly sought a different treatment approach.

The recovery model developed out of the consumer movement. The recovery model is patient- or consumer-centred and involves active partnership with care providers (Fisher & Ahern, 2002). It is a hopeful, empowering, strengths-focused model whereby staff assist the consumer to achieve the highest quality of life possible (Mulligan, 2005). This model of care encourages a high degree of patient independence and self-determination focusing on achieving goals of the patient's choosing and leading increasingly productive and meaningful lives (Resnick & Rosenheck, 2006). The emphasis is on the person and the future rather than on the illness and the present. A patient in recovery stated, "Slowly I accepted my illness but wanted to live a full life in spite of it. I was desperate to succeed in the real world, and I entered college. There I expanded my social ties so I wouldn't have to be forced into the identity of schizophrenia. My teachers gave me courage and respect" (Group for the Advancement of Psychiatry, 2000, p. 22).

Although it has been suggested that the recovery philosophy has been slower to take hold in Canada (Piat, Lesage, Boyer, et al., 2008), the Mental Health Commission of Canada (MHCC) (2012) identified recovery as central to mental health care reform. According to the MHCC, a recovery-oriented system creates the possibility for people with severe mental illness to gain more control over their lives and make choices about treatments, while being supported by professionals, families, and other people who are significant in their lives.

## ISSUES CONFRONTING THOSE WITH SERIOUS MENTAL ILLNESS

### Establishing a Meaningful Life

Finding meaning in life and establishing goals can be difficult for people living with SMI, particularly if they also experience

 **RESEARCH HIGHLIGHT**

### The Meaning of Recovery

**Source:** Piat, M., Sabetti, J., & Bloom, B. (2009). The importance of medication in consumer definitions of recovery from serious mental illness: A qualitative study. *Issues in Mental Health Nursing, 30,* 482–490. doi:10.1080/01612840802509452.

**Problem**

Persons with SMI who are being cared for within a recovery model face many complex choices in relation to medication treatment.

**Purpose of Study**

Nurses need to understand the personal meanings that consumers attach to the concept of recovery with respect to medication treatment.

**Methods**

In this Canadian multisite qualitative study, 60 consumers with SMI who had been receiving treatment from mental health services for at least six months were asked about the meaning of recovery. Themes and patterns were identified in consumer responses.

**Key Findings**

Many consumers valued the experience of stability and balance that medication seemed to provide. Participants also placed considerable value on the support they received from health care providers and mental health services in general. Participants understood recovery to be a realization of their hopes and dreams and considered both medication and therapeutic relationships important factors in helping them work toward their recovery goals.

**Implications for Nursing Practice**

Nurses and other health team members need to understand the experience of recovery from consumers' perspectives, so that they can develop collaborative, patient-centred relationships with consumers.

poor self-esteem or apathy. Patients may struggle with the possibility that they may never be the person they once expected to be. Finding a way to "reset" one's goals so that meaning can be found in new ways (e.g., helping others, volunteering, or simply surmounting a significant illness) is important to achieving a satisfactory quality of life and avoiding despair.

Those who cannot work or attend school have a significant amount of free time to be filled. If these people do not own a car or have easy access to public transit, lack money for movies or other pastimes, are afraid to go outside, or do not have enough confidence to join peers, options can be very limited.

### Co-Morbid Conditions
#### Physical Disorders

One of the strategic directions of the MHCC is to achieve an "increase [in] the life expectancy of people living with severe mental illnesses" (Mental Health Commission of Canada, 2012, p. 129). People with SMI are at greater risk for co-occurring physical illnesses, particularly hypertension, obesity, cardiovascular disease, and diabetes (Nitkin & Gastaldo, 2010). The risk for premature death is 1.6 to 2.8 times greater than that for the general population, and on average patients with SMI die 28 years prematurely (Miller, Paschall, & Svendsen, 2007). Contributing factors include failing to provide for their own health needs, inability to access or pay for care, and other obstacles, such as stigma or stereotyping. Expressing health care needs in an eccentric or unclear manner, for example, can influence the quality of care received. One patient with schizophrenia experienced a detached retina and sought assistance at a local health clinic. She told the nurse that she had "the sun in (her) eye." Because the nurse knew the patient's history, she decided that the patient was hallucinating and delusional and did not perform any physical examination. It wasn't until the next morning, after an antipsychotic had been administered and the patient reported that the visual disturbance persisted, that the nurse examined the patient's eye more carefully. Staff bias or inadequate understanding of mental illness had resulted in a less thorough evaluation and a delay in treatment. Inequalities in access and delivery of health care may also be related to the separation of mental health programs from other health care programs (Lawrence & Kisely, 2010).

## Depression and Suicide

Persons with SMI may experience a profound sense of loss. This loss can lead to acute or chronic grief, which, along with the chronicity of the illness and its demands and impact on daily life, can contribute to despair, depression, and risk for suicide, which occurs in 5% to 10% of persons with schizophrenia (Palmer, Pankratz, & Bostwick, 2005); however, it is estimated that 50% of people with SMI engage in self-harming behaviours as a means of ending their hopelessness (Besnier, Gavaudan, Navez, et al., 2009). In a survey of persons who had suffered depression within the previous 12 months, 28.7% reported that they had suicidal ideation (Rhodes, Bethell, & Bondy, 2006).

## Substance Abuse

People who experience SMI are at much higher risk for substance abuse than people in the general population (National Institute on Drug Abuse, 2010). A person who experiences both a mental disorder and a substance use disorder is said to have a *concurrent disorder*; in Canada, the prevalence of concurrent disorders ranges from 20% to 80% (Centre for Addiction and Mental Health, 2009). It has been reported that 65.2% of persons with schizophrenia abuse nicotine, 47.3% abuse alcohol, and 20% have abused at least one drug in the previous 30 days (Margolese, Malchy, Negrete, et al., 2004). Substance abuse may be a form of self-medication, countering the dysphoria or other symptoms caused by illness or its treatment (e.g., the sedation caused by one's medications). Nicotine use has always been higher in the population of those with SMI and is not declining as it has been in the general population. Substance abuse contributes to co-morbid physical health problems, reduced quality of life, incarceration, relapse, and reduced effectiveness of medications (McCloughen, 2003).

## Social Problems
### Stigma

Stigma has been described as negative attitudes or behaviours toward a person or group based on a belief that they possess negative traits (Gonzalez, Perlick, Miklowitz, et al., 2007). The Mental Health Commission of Canada (2012) reported that stigma and discrimination of all kinds "are the major reasons that mental health issues have remained in the shadows for so long" (pp. 22–23). Stigma stems from a lack of understanding of mental illness that causes others to make assumptions about those with SMI. Stigma can result in discrimination and cause shame, anger, and further isolation (Stuart, 2006). It is perpetuated by stereotypical images in North American culture. Meeting and talking with someone with an SMI can help the general public reduce their stigmatizing behaviours and attitudes toward people with SMIs. A member of the public stated:

> People assume that an oddly behaving person sitting on a street corner has to be on drugs or is some crazy loser that is a discard of our society: someone that cannot get better. Next time you look at a young person on the street or an older adult, think of them as your son or daughter, or maybe your sister or brother. They could be. (Mental Health Commission of Canada, 2009, p. 84)

Initiatives such as the *Opening Minds* project seek to improve understanding and acceptance through education and reduction of stigma (Mental Health Commission of Canada, 2009).

## Isolation and Loneliness

Social isolation and loneliness are concerns of many people with chronic illnesses, not just those with SMI. Stigma reduces the social contact of persons with SMI, and individual factors such as poor self-image, poverty (which interferes with recreational and social activities), passivity, and impaired hygiene also interfere with relationships. Romantic relationships and opportunities for sexual expression, usually desired among persons with SMI just as in any population, are also affected by isolation (and often by sexual dysfunction from medications). In response to this challenge, dating services specifically for persons with disabilities or mental illness have been created.

## Victimization

Stereotypes would have us believe that people with SMI are more likely to be violent than people who do not have mental illness. But the reverse is actually true: mentally ill people are more likely to be victims of violence than perpetrators of it (Schanda, 2005; White, Chafetz, Collins-Bride, et al., 2006). Sexual assault or coerced sexual activity also commonly occurs within this vulnerable population. Impaired judgement, impaired interpersonal skills (e.g., unknowingly acting in ways that might provoke others, such as standing too close or not leaving when told to), passivity, poor self-esteem, dependency, residence in high-crime neighbourhoods, and an appearance of vulnerability may contribute to this significant problem.

## Economic Challenges

### Unemployment and Poverty

Most people derive at least part of their identity and sense of value from the work they do. Many people with SMI would like to work, but symptoms such as cognitive slowing or disorganization interfere with obtaining or succeeding at work. According to the Mental Health Commission of Canada (2013), between 70% and 90% of people with SMI are unemployed, and 50% of those with SMI do not receive sufficient income from their disability entitlements. It can be difficult to find an employer open to hiring a person with SMI, and laws to prevent discrimination do not guarantee a job.

Atypical antipsychotic medications can be extremely expensive. Each province administers its own prescription drug plan, and patients with SMI may be able to obtain coverage under these plans. However, not every medication is covered. Because people with SMI are less likely to be employed, they are less likely to have private insurance coverage to cover the additional costs of medication. In addition to the challenges of obtaining pharmacological treatment, in many cases, those with SMI do not have private or public insurance to cover treatment from other mental health care providers (e.g., psychologists), which may be a significant barrier to mental health treatment in Canada (Mulvale & Hurley, 2008).

### Housing Instability

Even though safe and affordable housing is very important for people living with SMI (Piat, Lesage, Boyer, et al., 2008), homelessness is unfortunately prevalent (Montgomery, Forchuk, Duncan, et al., 2008). Many people with SMI have limited funds, which equates to limited options for housing. Obtaining an affordable apartment may require one to live far from needed resources (e.g., stores, health care centres, support persons) or in unsafe neighbourhoods. An episode of inappropriate behaviour could lead to eviction and a negative reputation among landlords, closing doors to future housing. Living with family can produce interpersonal strains and conflict about patient behaviour (e.g., nonadherence, impaired self-care), which, in turn, often lead to estrangement and loss of housing with family.

Symptoms can cause behaviour that leads to police arrest. For example, one patient asked a store clerk if he could pay him later for a bottle of pop and, thinking concretely, mistook the clerk's sarcastic "Oh, sure" as genuine approval, only to leave with the pop and find himself charged with theft an hour later. A single bad decision caused an arrest that could leave the person ineligible for housing subsidies or public housing. Even with a subsidy, however, waiting lists can be up to two years long. Finding and keeping good housing can be very challenging for these patients.

### Caregiver Burden

Caregivers, particularly family members, provide important support for people with SMI. However, coping with the persistent and challenging needs of people with SMI can be extremely challenging and requires significant emotional, physical, and, at times, financial resources. Caregivers also age, become ill, and may require care themselves, depleting their ability to provide support for the person with SMI. When caregivers are no longer able to provide the needed support for the person with SMI, a very difficult adjustment can result, leading to crises such as homelessness, conflict between caregiver and patient, and even exacerbation of the SMI symptoms.

## Treatment Issues

### Nonadherence

At any point in time, nearly half of all people with mental illness are not receiving treatment or are nonadherent to treatment, thereby potentially doubling the likelihood of relapse (Amador, 2007). Most health care providers address this problem with medication education, but patients faced with repetitive medication groups and exhortations to take medications often become more resistant rather than insightful. Other obstacles, such as adverse effects, drug costs, interruptions in treatment, and rotating treatment providers, increase the risk for nonadherence and threaten stability and prognosis. Box 31-1 describes nursing interventions that promote adherence.

### Anosognosia

Many people assume that people with mental illness who do not understand that they are mentally ill must be in denial (i.e., they know they are ill but cannot accept it). Although denial is a possibility, another is *anosognosia* (ă-nō′sog-nō′sē-ă), the inability to recognize one's deficits due to one's illness. Individuals who do not understand that their symptoms are illness-related will find it difficult to recognize that they have an illness. Others believe that the illness will go away on its own (Vasiliadis, Lesage, Adair, et al., 2005). People who do not perceive themselves to be mentally ill are unlikely to seek or accept treatment, resulting in a common impediment for treatment adherence (Amador, 2007). It can take months or years for a person with SMI to acknowledge having a mental illness.

### Medication Adverse Effects

Psychotropic medications, especially antipsychotic agents, can produce a range of distressing adverse effects, from involuntary movements to increased risk for diabetes. Some adverse effects are treatable; others may diminish over time or can be compensated for via behavioural changes (e.g., changing position slowly to reduce dizziness from hypotension). Addressing adverse effects is essential to preventing nonadherence and maximizing quality of life. See Chapter 4 for a detailed discussion of antipsychotic drugs.

### Treatment Inadequacy

It has been suggested that there are significant gaps between the quality of mental health care provided and optimal care (Addington, Kyle, Desair, et al., 2010). Patients must be informed and diligent in ensuring that they are receiving the most effective treatment, and agencies and staff must be diligent in updating their programs and practice.

## BOX 31-1 INTERVENTIONS TO IMPROVE ADHERENCE TO TREATMENT

- Select treatments and dosages that are most likely to be effective and well tolerated by each patient.
- Actively manage adverse effects to avert or minimize patient distress, which could result in nonadherence.
- Simplify treatment regimens to make them more acceptable and understandable to the patient (e.g., once-a-day dosing instead of twice-daily dosing).
- Tie treatment adherence to achieving the patient's goals to increase motivation. Point out and reinforce improvements, connecting them to treatment adherence.
- To improve patient insight and motivation, provide psycho-education (an approach to care that emphasizes helping a person gain knowledge necessary to manage the illness) about SMI and the role of treatment in recovery. Take care not to assume that nonadherence means the patient does not understand. There are many reasons for nonadherence; applying psychoeducation when the problem is something other than a lack of knowledge is unlikely to succeed.
- Assign consistent, committed caregivers who have (or are skilled at building) positive therapeutic bonds with the patient and who will be able to work with the patient for extended periods of time.
- Involve the patient in support groups with members who have greater insight and first-hand experience with illness and treatment—people whose viewpoints the patient may be more likely to accept.
- Provide culturally sensitive care. Cultural beliefs and practices (e.g., suspicious attitudes toward health care and authority figures, valuing self-sufficiency or privacy above health care) can be a barrier to therapeutic relationships and result in rejection of treatment (Lutz & Warren, 2001).
- Carefully monitor medication decreases or changes to control adverse effects and improve the therapeutic effect (Wieden, 2007).
- When other interventions have not been successful, use medication monitoring, long-acting forms of medication (depot injections or sustained-release formats), and other techniques as indicated to increase the likelihood that needed medication will be in the patient's system.
- Never reject, blame, or shame the patient when nonadherence occurs. Instead, label it as simply an issue for continuing focus, often requiring numerous tries.

**Sources:** Lutz, W.J., & Warren, B.J. (2001). Symptomatology and medication monitoring for public mental health consumers: A cultural perspective. *Journal of the American Psychiatric Nurses Association, 7,* 115–124. doi:10.1067/mpn.2001.117879; and Wieden, P.J. (2007). Discontinuing and switching antipsychotic medications: Understanding the CATIE schizophrenia trial (Supplemental material). *Journal of Clinical Psychiatry, 68,* 12–19.

## Residual Symptoms

Residual symptoms are those that do not improve completely or consistently with treatment. They can be very frustrating, and patients may feel that these symptoms mean they will not get better or that treatments are not working (promoting help-lessness and hopelessness). The patient may then discontinue treatment, worsening the illness. Residual symptoms can also cause or worsen associated issues (e.g., inappropriate social behaviour and impulsiveness that can add to stigmatization and isolation).

### Relapse, Chronicity, and Loss

The majority of patients with SMI face the possibility of relapse even when adhering to treatment, which may contribute to hopelessness and helplessness. Living with SMI paradoxically requires more effort and emotional resources from people less able to cope with such demands. Each relapse can cause loss of relationships, employment, and housing, adding that much more loss to the patient's life and making discharge planning significantly more complicated.

## RESOURCES FOR PEOPLE WITH SERIOUS MENTAL ILLNESS

### Comprehensive Community Treatment

Community services, particularly for those with serious mental illness, have been described as fragmented and inefficient, with blurring of responsibility among agencies, programs, and levels of government (Mental Health Commission of Canada, 2009). Ideally, the community-based mental health care system provides comprehensive, coordinated, and cost-effective (from the perspective of the government) care for the patient with mental illness.

The overall goal of community psychiatric treatment is to improve the patient's ability to function independently in the community. Community services vary according to local needs and resources. Patients sometimes find that needed services are not locally available or have long wait lists, and they may have difficulty identifying the best programs for their needs amid the maze of agencies and services. When people with SMI are unable to access community-based services, they are often forced to rely on institution-based care (Standing Senate Committee on Social Affairs, Science and Technology, 2006).

### Community Services and Programs

A case-management program is a comprehensive service provided by a multidisciplinary team. The team coordinates the patient's overall care, brokers access to services, and provides psychosocial education, guidance, and support (Aquila & Emanuel, 2003; O'Brien, MacFarland, Kealy, et al., 2012). Case managers can provide medication monitoring, wherein they observe and facilitate the patient's use of medications. Intensive case management has been strongly linked to improved consumer engagement, psychological functioning, and adaptation to the demands of everyday living (O'Brien, MacFarland, Kealy, et al., 2012). Assertive community treatment (ACT), discussed later in this chapter, is one model of case management. Other community services and programs that may be available include social skills training, crisis intervention services, emergency psychiatric services, and community outreach programs.

**VIGNETTE**

After three years of living on his own, Christopher returns home to his parents. He is soon arrested for threatening a police officer with a steel pipe, is found "not criminally responsible," and is released on the condition that he receive psychiatric treatment. Because of his history of nonadherence, he goes to a clinic and receives intramuscular depot medication. He is also enrolled in a day program and is assigned a case manager, who helps him apply for income assistance and refers him to a group home when his aging parents state that he can no longer live with them. Because he wants to work, he is referred to a supported-employment program. He gets a job unloading delivery trucks and stays in that job for the next five years. When the requirements of his conditional release are completed, he continues in treatment and continues working nearly full time. Because he is stable, his medication is changed to an oral atypical antipsychotic, and he continues to receive supervision in his group home.

## Substance Abuse Treatment

A variety of services exist for those who have a concurrent diagnosis of SMI and alcohol- or drug-related problems. Chemical-dependency clinics provide therapeutic and rehabilitative services, including medical and psychosocial assessment, detoxification, crisis intervention, and medication such as methadone. Most clinicians endorse treatment that is integrated (i.e., delivered by a single provider rather than split between a mental health agency and a drug or alcohol agency), using personnel with dual areas of expertise, but this standard has not yet been met in some settings (Centre for Addiction and Mental Health, 2009; Ziedonis, Smelson, Rosenthal, et al., 2005). See Chapter 19 for a detailed discussion of treatment settings for patients with substance abuse issues.

## EVIDENCE-INFORMED TREATMENT APPROACHES

### Assertive Community Treatment

Assertive community treatment (ACT) is an approach to caring for the person with severe mental illness in the community. ACT teams provide multidisciplinary, comprehensive, and, in some cases, intensive treatment services. The ACT model of care is a structure of treatment and rehabilitative and supportive services that enhance the ability of the person with SMI to live successfully in the community. ACT serves individuals who have not been able to successfully manage their illnesses in traditional outpatient or rehabilitation services. Key principles of ACT include maintaining small patient-to-staff ratios, engaging in a proactive approach, and establishing highly individualized treatment plans. ACT has been shown to improve symptoms of SMI and reduce inpatient admissions, incarceration, and homelessness among persons with mental illness (Coldwell & Bender, 2007; Government of Ontario, 2005; Lamberti, Weisman, & Faden, 2004; Yang, Law, Chow, et al., 2005).

 **RESEARCH HIGHLIGHT**

*Assertive Community Treatment (ACT)*

**Source:** Shattell, M., Donnelly, N., Scheyett, A., et al. (2011). Assertive community treatment and the physical health needs of persons with severe mental illness: Issues around integration of mental health and physical health. *Journal of the American Psychiatric Nurses Association, 17*(1), 57–63. doi:10.1177/1078390310393737.

**Problem**

Many people with an SMI have higher rates of other chronic health conditions (e.g., cancer, diabetes) and a reduced life expectancy than the general population. An ACT multidisciplinary treatment team seems to be well suited to overcome some of the obstacles to providing physical care to people with SMI; however, this theory has not been investigated.

**Purpose of Study**

As little is known about how assertive community treatment teams address the physical needs of people with SMI, the intent of this study was to explore the successes and challenges of providing physical care to people with SMIs within an ACT treatment model.

**Methods**

The researchers used a qualitative design to explore how ACT teams in the Midwestern United States integrated physical health care into their programs. Representatives of five ACT teams participated in focus group interviews. The research team used coding strategies to identify relevant themes, arriving at the final themes by consensus.

**Key Findings**

The researchers identified three major themes: (1) ACT teams recognized serious physical health problems and illnesses in their clients; (2) ACT nurses assumed a wide range of care roles, including providing health education and health assessment, to help clients meet their physical health needs; other team members shared in some of these activities; and (3) ACT team members found that it was challenging but critical to help clients meet their physical health needs.

**Implications for Nursing Practice**

- There is a significant need to integrate physical health with mental health care in programs directed at persons with severe mental illness.
- ACT team members must have the knowledge and skills to work with clients' physical health challenges.
- Nurses, as members of the ACT team with extensive knowledge of integrated, whole-person care, play a critical role in providing physical health care to this population.

### Cognitive-Behavioural Therapy

Cognitive-behavioural therapy (CBT) has been shown to be effective in helping patients with SMI reduce and cope with symptoms such as auditory hallucinations (England, 2007). The cognitive component of CBT focuses on patterns of thinking and "self-talk" (i.e., what one says to oneself internally). It identifies cognitive distortions and guides patients to substitute

Christopher, now age 50, has schizophrenia. He has lived in a group home since his late 20s. He has been stable for the past ten years and has had a steady girlfriend for the past three years. He announces that he wants to move out on his own and maybe get married. Despite respectful disagreement from his nurse therapist, he finds himself a room to rent. Over the next two months, his mental status remains stable: he is polite, quiet, and guarded as usual. However, his psychiatrist, who weighs him monthly, notices that he has lost 20 pounds. Christopher cannot identify any change in his eating habits, and he is referred to his primary care provider for an evaluation. He does not follow up with the primary care provider, and over the next four weeks, he loses another ten pounds. His nurse therapist calls his work supervisor, who reports that Christopher is behaving differently: he is talking out loud to himself, becoming more isolated, and, one morning, smelled of alcohol. She is supportive of Christopher and hopes he will get treatment. At his next clinic appointment, the psychiatrist and therapist discuss these changes and recommend that Christopher go into the partial hospital program for medication re-evaluation. He reluctantly agrees, denying that he has any problem.

more effective forms of thinking. The behavioural component of CBT uses natural consequences and positive reinforcers to shape the person's behaviour in a more positive or adaptive manner.

## Cognitive Enhancement Therapy

Cognitive enhancement therapy (CET) is based on the principle that the brain is able to change and that compromised neurological functions can be assumed by healthier areas of the brain. CET involves many hours (i.e., 60 or more) of computer-based drills and exercises that incrementally challenge functions, such as focusing attention, processing and recalling information, and interpreting social and emotional information (e.g., inferring a person's mood from his or her expression or tone of voice). Research has shown that CET leads to sustained improvement in these functional areas and improves social and vocational functioning (Eack, Greenwald, Hogarty, et al., 2009; Hogarty, Flesher, Ulrich, et al., 2004).

## Family Support and Partnerships

Families and significant others can face considerable stresses related to the mental illness of a loved one and may suffer from insufficiencies in empathy and understanding (Chan, 2011). Having sound family support and partnerships is one of the strongest predictors of recovery; treatment is enhanced, and conflict is reduced when treatment providers work as empathic partners with both patients and their significant others. The Canadian Mental Health Association (CMHA) partners with a variety of public and private agencies to provide family support programs that are tailored to the specific needs of a community or region. Provincial branches of the CMHA serve as an excellent source of information, support, and practical guidance for patients and their significant others.

## Social Skills Training

Social skills training focuses on the teaching of a wide variety of social and activities of daily living (ADL) skills. People with SMI often have social deficits that cause functional impairment; for example, those unable to respond assertively may respond aggressively instead. Complex interpersonal skills, such as negotiating or resolving a conflict, are broken down into subcomponents, which are then taught in a step-by-step fashion.

## Supportive Psychotherapy

Although definitions vary, supportive psychotherapy is generally understood to be an approach that stresses empathic understanding, a nonjudgemental attitude, and the development of a therapeutic alliance (Brenner, 2012). Supportive psychotherapy has been shown to enhance the therapeutic alliance and improve long-term recovery prospects in patients with serious mental illness (Hellerstein, Rosenthal, Pinsker, et al., 1998; Penn, Mueser, Tarrier, et al., 2004).

**VIGNETTE**
Christopher attends the partial hospital program for four weeks. In the first week, the nurse calls the therapist to report that he is severely paranoid: he will not eat or drink out of any open containers and is observed spitting out his pills. His medication is changed to a quickly disintegrating tablet form. He attends groups that focus on education about medication, chronic illness, substance use, and healthy habits. He begins to eat normally, gaining five pounds in two weeks. Finally, he admits that he had not taken any medication since he moved out of his group home.

The discharge plan is referral to the psychosocial program again for structure and case management to assist with finding a new home, medical care, and eventual return to work, with a biweekly medication injection and supportive group therapy. Over the next three months, Christopher gradually returns to his baseline level of functioning. His case manager finds him another group home with his previous caregiver. He returns to work two days per week and still attends the day program for three days. Christopher never is able to identify the trigger for his relapse, but his nurse therapist now observes his physical status more closely and inquires specifically about his work and social activities at each session.

## Vocational Rehabilitation and Related Services

Vocational rehabilitation and related services vary widely but can include vocational training, financial support for attaining employment, or supported-employment services. Like most people, those with SMI want to feel as though they contribute and, therefore, want to be engaged in meaningful employment (Crain, Penhale, Newstead, et al., 2009; Drake, Becker, & Bond, 2003). The benefits of employment (or volunteer work) are enhanced self-esteem, improved organizational abilities, and increased socialization and income.

Vocational rehabilitation programs using a clubhouse model, in which patients jointly run their own business, such as a coffee shop or housekeeping service, teach all members to perform a job in order to make the business work. Such programs have led to the supported-employment model, which has been shown to be one of the most effective evidence-informed interventions for helping people with SMI achieve employment (Crain, Penhale, Newstead, et al., 2009). The model includes rapid job placement, on-the-job support, and provision of a job coach who is linked to the mental health team (Cook, Leff, Blyler, et al., 2005; Mueser, Aalto, Becker, et al., 2005).

 **RESEARCH HIGHLIGHT**

### Supported Employment

**Source:** Drake, R., Xie, H., Bond, G., et al. (2013). Early psychosis and employment. *Schizophrenia Research, 146*(1–3), 111–117. doi:10.1016/j.schres.2013.02.012.

**Problem**
Employment has many benefits (e.g., provides structure, meaning, friendships, increased self-esteem) for people with mental health disorders. However, it is not clear how employment affects the use of mental health services and the use of disability and welfare programs for people who experience early psychosis either from a primary psychosis or a substance-induced psychosis.

**Purpose of Study**
This study examined the employment outcomes in a large and diverse sample of patients with early psychosis who presented to a large urban emergency department.

**Methods**
Following assessment, treatment, and stabilization, 351 people experiencing early psychosis were interviewed when they sought mental health services at a large urban emergency department. Patients were asked a variety of questions regarding their current competitive-employment status, quality of life, level of education, degree of substance use, and the severity of their symptoms. Follow-up interviews were conducted at 6, 12, 18, and 24 months after the initial interview. At the follow-up appointments, interviewers asked the participants about their current competitive-employment status, quality of life, degree of substance use, and the severity of their symptoms.

**Key Findings**
* People experiencing early psychosis who have better education and work histories are more likely to have better psychosocial adjustment to their illness.
* People who experience substance-induced psychosis rather than primary psychosis generally experience fewer negative symptoms.
* Individuals who have competitive employment take fewer medications, use mental health services less frequently, and rely less on disability or welfare for financial support.

**Implications for Nursing Practice**
* Because people with early psychosis who are employed show several signs of better adjustment, it is important that nurses contribute to employment success by connecting unemployed or underemployed patients to supported-employment services.
* The delay of competitive employment contributes to disability and impacts the individual's self-esteem, support networks, and positive and negative symptoms.

## OTHER POTENTIALLY BENEFICIAL SERVICES OR TREATMENT APPROACHES

While not yet evidence-informed practices, research to date supports use of the following services and treatment approaches.

### Consumer-Run Programs

The CMHA and other organizations offer training that enables consumers to assist peers in the recovery process. Consumer-run programs range from informal "clubhouses," which offer socialization, recreation, and sometimes other services, such as educational programs, to competitive businesses, which are often part of a vocational rehabilitation program.

### Wellness and Recovery Action Plans

Wellness and recovery action plans (WRAPs) and similar programs are psychoeducational programs that empower and train patients in skills that promote recovery and prepare them to deal with stressors and crises (Copeland, 2007). Training focuses on daily maintenance plans (i.e., things that must be done and resources needed to maintain wellness), identification and management of triggers that could provoke a relapse, early identification of impending relapse, and crisis plans (i.e., plans for managing crises or impending relapse). Typically, a wide variety of useful tools, templates, and techniques are provided, and the programs lead to developing practical and concrete action plans for promoting recovery.

### Exercise

Exercise holds many benefits for persons with SMI, including improved activity tolerance and ability to cope with symptoms, reduced anxiety and depression, enhanced self-esteem, weight control or loss (important for patients with weight-related co-morbidities, such as diabetes and hypertension), and cost-effectiveness (Beebe, Tian, Morris, et al., 2005; Erdner & Magnusson, 2012).

## NURSING CARE OF PATIENTS WITH SERIOUS MENTAL ILLNESS

Nurses encounter patients with SMI in a variety of inpatient and community settings. All roles and techniques used by psychiatric mental health nurses in inpatient psychiatric settings also apply in the community and other settings.

### Assessment Strategies

Important assessments include the following:
* Signs of risk to self or others (suicidality or homicidality)
* Depression or hopelessness
* Signs of relapse (especially increased impulsivity or paranoia, diminished reality testing, increased delusional thinking or command hallucinations)
* Inadequate attention to proper nutrition, adequate clothing or medical care, and carelessness while driving, smoking, or cooking (e.g., leaving pots on the stove and becoming distracted or falling asleep)

## TABLE 31-1 POTENTIAL NURSING DIAGNOSES FOR THE PATIENT WITH SERIOUS MENTAL ILLNESS

| SIGNS AND SYMPTOMS | NURSING DIAGNOSES |
|---|---|
| Speaking too softly to be heard | Communication, impaired verbal |
| Verbalization incongruent with the setting | Social interaction, impaired |
| Silence in groups or withdrawal when approached | Social isolation |
| Failure to keep appointments Admitted missing of medication or observed return of symptoms | Noncompliance |
| Self-negating verbalization | Chronic low self-esteem |
| Fear of trying new things or situations Nonassertiveness or passivity | Powerlessness |
| Distortion of patient's health problem, often denial Neglect of other members of family Excessive concern for and supervision of patient | Disabled family coping Caregiver role strain |

## TABLE 31-2 NOC OUTCOMES RELATED TO SERIOUS MENTAL ILLNESS

| NURSING OUTCOME AND DEFINITION | INTERMEDIATE INDICATORS | SHORT-TERM INDICATORS |
|---|---|---|
| Self-care: Instrumental activities of daily living (IADL): Ability to perform activities needed to function independently in the home or community, with or without assistive device | Manages medications Manages money | Shops for groceries Prepares meals Uses phone Travels on public transportation |
| Family coping: Family actions to manage stressors that tax family resources | Uses available social support Cares for needs of all members | Involves family members in decision making Establishes family priorities Plans for emergencies |

**Source:** Moorhead, S., Johnson, M., Maas, M., et al. (2008). *Nursing outcomes classification (NOC)* (4th ed.). St. Louis, MO: Mosby.

- Signs of treatment nonadherence or impending relapse (early detection and correction of relapse reduces its intensity and duration and prevents hospitalization, loss of housing, arrest, and loss of entitlements)
- Physical health problems, such as brain tumours or drug toxicity, which can cause psychiatric symptoms and be mistaken for mental illness or relapse
- Co-morbid illnesses (ensuring that the patient provides appropriate self-care and receives adequate health care)

Table 31-1 lists potential nursing diagnoses that apply to the patient with SMI. Table 31-2 lists examples of specific nursing outcomes.

### Intervention Strategies

Basic nursing interventions for patients with serious mental illness include the following:
- Empowering the patient by involving him or her in goal setting and treatment selection increases the likelihood of treatment adherence and success.
- Emphasizing quality-of-life issues conveys an interest in the person (rather than in the illness) and reflects the patient's best interests (rather than the staff's preferences).
- Developing and maintaining relationships are keys to overcoming anosognosia and achieving treatment adherence. People with SMI often require extended periods of working with staff to form these connections.

- Supportive psychotherapy aids in maintaining therapeutic rapport and helps the patient maintain positive self-esteem and cope effectively.
- Impaired reality testing is the hallmark of SMI and contributes to hallucinations and delusional thinking. Encouraging the patient to seek independent information on whether experiences are real or not can help the patient identify these experiences as part of the illness and respond accordingly.
- SMIs predispose people to isolation due to stigma, impaired social skills, and social discomfort. Isolation contributes to loneliness and reduces access to support. Activities that increase skill and comfort with interaction, reduce aloneness, or provide opportunities for socialization (especially with supportive persons and positive role models, such as other patients who are further along in recovery) contribute to improved functioning and a higher quality of life.
- Support groups such as the Schizophrenia Society of Canada expose the patient to members who "have been there." In addition to providing support and socialization opportunities, such groups often have practical suggestions for issues and problems patients and significant others face. Involvement in support groups is often empowering for the patient.
- Education and reinforcement are essential since SMI may result in impaired judgement, desperation for connectedness, or other vulnerabilities that increase the risk for victimization, sexually transmitted infections, and undesired pregnancies.
- Care for the whole person is especially important with SMI patients, who have higher burdens of physical illness, poorer hygiene and health practices, less access to effective medical

## BOX 31-2  *NIC* INTERVENTIONS FOR SERIOUS MENTAL ILLNESS

### *Self-Care Assistance: IADL*

*Definition of* self-care assistance: IADL: Assisting and instructing a person to perform instrumental activities of daily living (IADL) needed to function in the home or community

*Activities:*
- Instruct individual on appropriate and safe storage of medications.
- Instruct individual on alternative methods of transportation (e.g., buses and bus schedules, taxis, city or county transportation for disabled people).
- Assist individual in establishing methods and routines for cooking, cleaning, and shopping.

### Family Support

*Definition of* family support: Promotion of family values, interests, and goals

*Activities\*:*
- Listen to family concerns, feelings, and questions.
- Accept the family's values in a nonjudgemental manner.
- Identify congruence between patient, family, and health professional expectations.

\*Partial list.
**Source:** Bulechek, G.M., Butcher, H.K. & Dochterman, J.M. (2008). *Nursing interventions classification (NIC)* (5th ed.). St. Louis, MO: Mosby.

treatment, and more premature mortality than the general population. Averting or reducing obesity through good nutritional and health practices can reduce the risk of co-morbidities such as metabolic syndrome; sound physical health conserves energy and resources for use in coping with SMI (Thomas, 2007).

- Involving people with co-occurring substance abuse in Alcoholics Anonymous or Narcotics Anonymous and other services for people with concurrent disorders is important since substance abuse rates are high in SMI populations, and such abuse increases relapse and interferes with recovery.

Box 31-2 outlines two relevant *Nursing Interventions Classification (NIC)* interventions for the management of serious mental illness (Bulechek, Butcher, & Dochterman, 2008).

## Evaluation

Identified outcomes serve as the basis for evaluation. Each *NOC* outcome has a built-in rating scale (immediate, short-term, and potentially long-term indicators) that helps the nurse to measure improvement.

## CURRENT ISSUES

### Involuntary Treatment

Involuntary treatment involves treatment mandated by a court and delivered without the patient's consent. Traditionally, this situation involved involuntary inpatient admissions, but beginning in the 1990s, provinces began to experiment with community treatment orders (CTOs), which provide mandatory treatment in a less restrictive setting. It has been suggested that implementation of a CTO may facilitate patient engagement with community services and improve access to supportive housing (O'Brien, Farrell, & Faulkner, 2009). One difficulty in implementing CTOs is determining how to respond if the person does not follow the ordered outpatient treatment: rehospitalization is an expensive option and may not have any

positive impact on a patient's desire to participate in treatment (Allen & Smith, 2001; Segal & Burgess, 2006).

### Criminal Offences and Incarceration

In Canada, the number of incarcerated offenders with mental illness continues to increase; it is now estimated that 25% of newly admitted offenders have a mental illness (Office of the Correctional Investigator, 2010). People with SMIs may commit crimes out of desperation, impaired judgement, or impulsivity; most often they are nonviolent crimes, such as disorderly conduct. Police may also become involved with patients who seem unable to care for themselves and cannot be persuaded to accept treatment but do not meet criteria for involuntary treatment (usually imminent danger to self or others). Consider a patient with impaired judgement who does not dress adequately for cold weather and spends time in laundromats and libraries for warmth, causing disruption. When expelled, the individual is at risk for hypothermia. In such cases, the risk to self may not be "imminent," and hospitalization may not be possible. Loved ones or police may then seek arrest simply to get the person off the street for his or her own safety.

Many advocates for the mentally ill feel that incarceration, even if considered "for the patient's own good," is harmful. Imprisonment can lead to victimization, increased hopelessness, relapse due to increased stress and isolation, or overstimulation. Also, mental health care in correctional settings is usually both expensive and inadequate, and a criminal record can reduce future access to housing or employment. Advocates instead seek diversion from jail to clinical care. Two interventions to achieve this end are these:

1. Educating police so they can identify mental illness, distinguish it from criminal intent, and connect persons with SMI to help instead of jailing them
2. Establishing mental health courts that are designed to intercept persons whose crimes are secondary to mental illness and that feature specially trained officials with authority to order treatment instead of imprisonment

## KEY POINTS TO REMEMBER

- Patients with SMI suffer from multiple impairments in thinking, feeling, and interacting with others.
- The course of SMI involves exacerbations and remissions, as do many chronic medical illnesses.
- Coordinated, comprehensive community services help the SMI patient to function at his or her optimal level.
- People with SMI often suffer complications due to insufficient housing, nonadherence to treatment, co-morbid medical or substance use problems, and the stigma of mental illness.
- The family and support systems play a major part in the care of many persons with SMI and should be included as much as possible in planning, education, and treatment activities.
- The recovery model stresses hope, strengths, quality of life, patient involvement as an active partner in treatment, and eventual recovery.

## CRITICAL THINKING

1. John Yang, 42, concurrently diagnosed with schizophrenia and alcohol and marijuana abuse, is brought to the clinic by his mother, Mrs. Yang. During this initial assessment, Mrs. Yang reports that she has been caring for her son at home since he was 15; however, since recently moving to town, she is at a loss about what is available in the community. John has been prescribed haloperidol (Haldol), but Mrs. Yang says he rarely takes it because of muscle rigidity and sexual adverse effects. They have tried many of the traditional antipsychotic drugs without success.
   a. Given your understanding of the problems faced by a person with a severe mental illness, what are some areas of John's life you might want to explore in your assessment? Consider relationships, employment history, cognitive abilities, social skills, and behaviour. How would knowledge in these areas help your long-term planning?
   b. After you assess John's medication history, how can you be an advocate in terms of his nonadherence to traditional antipsychotics? What are some of the obstacles to adherence for a person with a concurrent disorder? What approach or change in treatment would offer the best chance of success?
   c. Of the resources mentioned in this chapter, which might be appropriate for John?
   d. Identify three basic aims of psychoeducation for John and his mother.
   e. What would recovery mean to John?

2. You are doing your psychiatric rotation in a psychiatric inpatient unit where many of the patients are diagnosed with schizophrenia. Although you had been apprehensive about this rotation, you are surprised to realize that patients respond well to you and that you are fascinated by this specialty area and may consider it as a career. A fellow student remarks, "You must be crazy to want to work with these people."
   a. What social problem is represented by this student's remark?
   b. Identify other social prejudices that have been significant problems in Canada. What responses were effective in reducing and eliminating their impact?

3. During your mental health rotation, you notice that there are several patients with other chronic physical illnesses. When assessing a person with SMI, why is it important to include a comprehensive physical assessment?

4. Competitive employment is an important factor in recovering from a psychotic episode. Identify the factors related to work that contribute to its importance in recovering from mental illness.

## CHAPTER REVIEW

1. A patient with schizophrenia does not feel that he needs medication because "there is nothing wrong with me." This response is most likely an example of:
   1. Denial
   2. Projection
   3. Anosognosia
   4. Paranoid ideation

2. Sarah, a young woman with schizophrenia who has struggled with hygiene and other activities of daily living, has been on a four-hour pass. She is tearful and reports that when she sat down on the bus to return to the hospital, the woman she sat next to immediately moved to another seat. Which response(s) would most likely be therapeutic? Select all that apply.
   1. Acknowledge Sarah's distress, and remind her that dinner will be ready in 30 minutes so she has time to settle in before eating.
   2. State, "You sound discouraged. Sometimes people who do not understand mental illness can be hurtful," and offer to sit with her.
   3. Advise Sarah that the woman's behaviour was simply rude and can be ignored because it is something people with mental illness have to get used to.

4. Suggest to Sarah that perhaps her hygiene would benefit from improvement, and offer to help her improve her hygiene so that others will be less likely to reject her.

3. Christopher is a 25-year-old male who has been hospitalized three times for exacerbations of schizophrenia. Each time he was discharged, he became homeless and relapsed. Typically, he is very disorganized, does not spend his money responsibly, loses his housing when he does not pay the rent, and, in turn, cannot be located by his case manager, leading to treatment nonadherence and relapse. Which response would be most therapeutic in this situation?
   1. Advise Christopher that if he does not pay his rent, he will be placed in a group home instead of independent housing.
   2. Discuss with Christopher the option of having a guardian who will ensure that the rent is paid and that his money is managed to meet his basic needs.
   3. Suggest to Christopher's prescribing clinician that he be placed on a long-acting injectable form of antipsychotic medication to address the issue of treatment nonadherence.
   4. Encourage Christopher's case manager to hold him responsible for the outcomes of his poor decisions by allowing such periods of homelessness to serve as a natural consequence.

4. Pia has experienced repeated episodes of severe depression and mania. These episodes and related hospitalizations have disrupted her full-time employment and created discord within her marriage. She argues with the outpatient staff about medications, does not believe she has a mental illness, and—although she takes her medications while hospitalized—she stops taking them after discharge. She will be discharged in two weeks. Which intervention is most likely to increase her adherence to medications?
   1. Advise Pia that she will be assigned to new outpatient staff to reduce the conflicts she is experiencing with her current providers.
   2. Explain to Pia that the medications will help her and that all medications have adverse effects she can learn to live with in time.
   3. Involve her in a medication education group that will help her learn the types and names of psychotropic medications, their purpose, and possible adverse effects.
   4. Explore with Pia her perceptions of the medications and her experiences with them, and guide her to connect use of the medications with achieving her goals.

5. Which intervention(s) would be appropriate to promote recovery for persons with serious mental illness who live in the community? Select all that apply.
   1. Meet regularly with the patients, and encourage them to make steady progress toward complete independence.
   2. Introduce patients to others with similar illnesses, and encourage participation in social activities with peers.
   3. Support the development of advance directives and involvement in social and employment activities run by other patients.
   4. Use public transportation to take patients to a museum, and share a nutritious dinner with them at an inexpensive restaurant.
   5. Instruct them to develop written plans that identify resources to maintain stability and steps to take when faced with unusual stressors.
   6. Over time, guide the patients to identify and switch to sources of support outside the family to reduce dependence on their loved ones as their primary support resource.

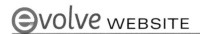 WEBSITE

Post-Test interactive review

*Visit the Evolve Web site for Chapter Review Answers and Rationales, Critical Thinking Answer Guidelines, and additional resources related to the content in this chapter: http://evolve.elsevier.com/Canada/Varcarolis/psychiatric/*

## REFERENCES

Addington, D., Kyle, T., Desair, S., et al. (2010). Facilitators and barriers to implementing quality treatment in primary mental health care. *Canadian Family Physician, 56*, 1322–1331.

Allen, M., & Smith, V.F. (2001). Opening Pandora's box: The practical and legal dangers of involuntary outpatient commitment. *Psychiatric Services, 52*(3), 342–346.

Amador, X. (2007). *I am not sick, I don't need help!* Peconic, NY: Vida Press LLC.

Aquila, R., & Emanuel, M. (2003). *Managing the long-term outlook of schizophrenia.* Retrieved from http://www.medscape.com/viewprogram/2680_pnt2003.

Beebe, L.H., Tian, L., Morris, N., et al. (2005). Effects of exercise on mental and physical health parameters of persons with schizophrenia. *Issues in Mental Health Nursing, 26*(6), 661–676. doi:10.1080/01612840590959551.

Besnier, N., Gavaudan, G., Navez, A., et al. (2009). Clinical features of suicide occurring in schizophrenia: (I) Risk factors identification. *Encephale, 35*, 176–181. doi:10.1016/j.encep.2008.02.009.

Brenner, A. (2012). Teaching supportive psychotherapy in the twenty-first century. *Harvard Review of Psychiatry, 20*(5), 259–267. doi:10.3109/10673229.2012.726526.

Bulechek, G.M., Butcher, H.K., & Dochterman, J.M. (2008). *Nursing interventions classification (NIC)* (5th ed.). St. Louis, MO: Mosby.

Centre for Addiction and Mental Health. (2009). *Partnering with families affected by concurrent disorder: Facilitators guide.* Retrieved from http://www.camh.net/Publications/Resources_for_Professionals/Partnering_with_families/app1_references.html.

Chan, S. (2011). Global perspective of burden of family caregivers for persons with schizophrenia. *Archives of Psychiatric Nursing, 25*(5), 339–349. doi:10.1016/j.apnu.2011.03.008.

Coldwell, C.M., & Bender, W.S. (2007). The effectiveness of assertive community treatment for homeless populations with severe mental illness: A meta-analysis. *American Journal of Psychiatry, 164*, 393–399. doi:10.1176/appi.ajp.164.3.393.

Cook, J.A., Leff, H.S., Blyler, C., et al. (2005). Results of a multisite randomized trial of supported employment interventions for individuals with severe mental illness. *Archives of General Psychiatry, 62*(5), 505–512.

Copeland, M.E. (2007). *About mental health recovery and WRAP.* Retrieved from http://mentalhealthrecovery.com/aboutus.php.

Crain, M., Penhale, C., Newstead, C., et al. (2009). The contribution of IPS to recovery from serious mental illness: A case study. *Work, 33*, 459–464. doi:10.3233/WOR-2009-0894.

Drake, R.E., Becker, D.R., & Bond, G.R. (2003). Recent research on vocational rehabilitation for persons with severe mental illness. *Current Opinions in Psychiatry, 16*(4), 451–455.

Eack, S., Greenwald, D., Hogarty, D., et al. (2009). Cognitive enhancement therapy for early-course schizophrenia: Effects of a two-year randomized controlled trial. *Psychiatric Services, 60*, 1468–1476. doi:10.1176/appi.ps.60.11.1468.

England, M. (2007). Efficacy of cognitive nursing intervention for voice hearing. *Perspectives in Psychiatric Care, 43*, 69–76. doi:10.1111/j.1744-6163.2007.00114.x.

Erdner, A., & Magnusson, A. (2012). Physical activities and their importance to the health of people with severe mental illness in Sweden. *Issues in Mental Health Nursing, 33*(10), 676–679.

Fisher, D.B., & Ahern, L. (2002). Evidence-based practices and recovery. *Psychiatric Services, 53*(5), 632–633.

Fitch, B. (2007, March). *Growing through psychosis: The patient's journey toward mental health.* Presentation at the Eighth Annual All-Ohio Institute on Community Psychiatry, Beachwood, OH.

Glied, S. (2007, March). *Better, but not well: Mental health policy in the United States.* Presentation at the Eighth Annual All-Ohio Institute on Community Psychiatry, Beachwood, OH.

Goeree, R., Fanahati, F., Burke, N., et al. (2005). The economic burden of schizophrenia in Canada in 2004. *Current Medical Research and Opinion, 21*, 2017–2028. doi:10.1185/030079905x75087.

Gonzalez, J.M., Perlick, D.A., Miklowitz, D., et al. (2007). STEP-BD family experience study group. Factors associated with stigma among caregivers of patients with bipolar disorder in the STEP-BD study. *Psychiatric Services, 58*, 41–48. doi:10.1176/appi.ps.58.1.41.

Government of Ontario, Ministry of Health and Long Term Care. (2005). *Ontario program standards for assertive community treatment (ACT) teams* (2nd ed.). Retrieved from http://www.health.gov.on.ca/en/common/ministry/publications/reports/mentalhealth/act_standards.pdf.

Group for the Advancement of Psychiatry. (2000). *Now that we are listening.* Dallas, TX: Committee on Psychiatry and the Community Group for the Advancement of Psychiatry.

Hellerstein, D.J., Rosenthal, R.D., Pinsker, H., et al. (1998). A randomized prospective study comparing supportive and dynamic therapies: Outcome and Alliance. *Journal of Psychotherapy Practice and Research, 7*(4), 261–271.

Hogarty, G.E., Flesher, S., Ulrich, R., et al. (2004). Cognitive enhancement therapy for schizophrenia: Effects of a 2-year randomized trial on cognition and behaviour. *Archives of General Psychiatry, 61*(9), 866–876.

Jacobs, P., Yim, R., Ohinmaa, A., et al. (2008). Expenditures on mental health and addictions for Canadian provinces in 2003/04. *Canadian Journal of Psychiatry, 53*(5), 306–313. Retrieved from http://publications.cpa-apc.org/browse/documents/339.

Lamberti, J.S., Weisman, R., & Faden, D.I. (2004). Forensic assertive community treatment: Preventing incarceration of adults with severe mental illness. *Psychiatric Services, 55*(11), 1285–1293.

Lawrence, D., & Kisely, S. (2010). Inequalities in health care provision for people with severe mental illness. *Journal of Psychopharmacology, 24*(11), Suppl. 4, 61–68. doi:10.1177/1359786810382058.

Margolese, H., Malchy, L., Negrete, J., et al. (2004). Drug and alcohol use among patients with schizophrenia and related psychoses: Levels and consequences. *Schizophrenia Research, 67*, 157–166. doi:10.1016/S0920-9964(02)00523-6.

McCloughen, A. (2003). The association between schizophrenia and cigarette smoking: A review of the literature and implications for mental health nursing practice. *International Journal of Mental Health Nursing, 12*, 119–129. doi:10.1046/j.1440-0979.2003.00278.x.

Mental Health Commission of Canada. (2009). *Toward recovery and well-being: A framework for a mental health strategy for Canada.* Ottawa: Author.

Mental Health Commission of Canada. (2012). *Changing directions, changing lives: The mental health strategy for Canada.* Calgary: Author.

Mental Health Commission of Canada. (2013). *The aspiring workforce: Employment and income for people with serious mental illness.* Calgary: Author.

Miller, B.J., Paschall, C.B., & Svendsen, D.P. (2007). *Mortality and medical co-morbidity in patients with serious mental illness.* Poster presentation at the Eighth Annual All-Ohio Institute on Community Psychiatry, Beachwood, OH.

Montgomery, P., Forchuk, C., Duncan, C., et al. (2008). Supported housing programs for persons with serious mental illness in rural northern communities: A mixed method evaluation. *BMC Health Services Research, 8*, 156. doi:10.1186/1472-6963-8-156.

Mueser, K.T., Aalto, S., Becker, D.R., et al. (2005). The effectiveness of skills training for improving outcomes in supported employment. *Psychiatric Services, 56*, 1254–1260. doi:10.1176/appi.ps.56.10.1254.

Mulligan, K. (2005). Recovery model seeks more than symptom relief. *Psychiatric News, 40*(18), 6–36.

Mulvale, G., & Hurley, J. (2008). Insurance coverage and treatment of mental illness: Effect on medication and provider use. *Journal of Mental Health Policy and Economics, 11*(4), 177–199. Retrieved from http://www.researchgate.net/journal/1091-4358_The_Journal_of_Mental_Health_Policy_and_Economics.

National Institute on Drug Abuse. (2010). *Comorbidity: Addiction and other mental illnesses* (NIH Publication 10-5771). Retrieved from http://www.drugabuse.gov/publications/research-reports/comorbidity-addiction-other-mental-illnesses.

Nitkin, D., & Gastaldo, D. (2010). Addressing physical health problems experienced by people with schizophrenia in Canada: A critical literature review. *Canadian Journal of Nursing Research, 42*(3), 124–140. Retrieved from http://cjnr.mcgill.ca.

O'Brien, A., Farrell, S., & Faulkner, S. (2009). Community treatment orders: Beyond hospital utilization rates examining the association of community treatment orders with community engagement and supportive housing. *Community Mental Health Journal, 45*(6), 415–419. doi:10.1007/s10597-009-9203-x.

O'Brien, S., MacFarland, J., Kealy, B., et al. (2012). A randomized-controlled trial of intensive case management emphasizing the recovery model among patients with severe and enduring mental illness. *Irish Journal of Medical Sciences, 181*(3), 301–308. doi:10.1007/s11845-011-0795-0.

Office of the Correctional Investigator, Government of Canada. (2010). *Annual report of the office of the correctional investigator.* Retrieved from http://www.oci-bec.gc.ca/cnt/rpt/annrpt/annrpt20092010-eng.aspx.

Palmer, B., Pankratz, V., & Bostwick, J. (2005). The lifetime risk of suicide in schizophrenia: A reexamination. *Archives of General Psychiatry, 62*(3), 247–253. Retrieved from http://archpsyc.ama-assn.org/content/vol62/issue3/index.dtl.

Penn, D., Mueser, K., Tarrier, N., et al. (2004). Supportive therapy for schizophrenia: Possible mechanisms and implications for adjunctive psychotherapy. *Schizophrenia Bulletin, 30*, 101–112.

Piat, M., Lesage, A., Boyer, R., et al. (2008). Housing for persons with serious mental illness: Consumer and service provider preferences. *Psychiatric Services, 59*, 1011–1017. doi:10.1176/appi.ps.59.9.1011.

Resnick, S.G., & Rosenheck, R.A. (2006). Recovery and positive psychology: Parallel themes and potential synergies. *Psychiatric Services, 57*, 120–122. doi:10.1176/appi.ps.57.1.120.

Rhodes, A., Bethell, J., & Bondy S.J. (2006). Suicidality, depression and mental health service use in Canada. *Canadian Journal of Psychiatry, 51*(1), 35–41.

Schanda, H. (2005). Psychiatry reforms and illegal behaviour of the severely mentally ill. *Lancet, 365*, 367–369. doi:10.1016/S0140-6736(05)17843-X.

Sealy, P., & Whitehead, P. (2004). Forty years of deinstitutionalization of psychiatric services in Canada: An empirical assessment. *Canadian Journal of Psychiatry, 49*(4), 249–257. Retrieved from http://ww1.cpa-apc.org:8080/publications/archives/cjp/2004/april/sealy.asp.

Segal, S.P., & Burgess, P.M. (2006). Conditional release: A less restrictive alternative to hospitalization? *Psychiatric Services, 57*, 1600–1606. doi:10.1176/appi.ps.57.11.1600.

Standing Senate Committee on Social Affairs, Science and Technology. (2006). *Out of the shadows at last: Transforming mental health, mental illness and addiction services in Canada.* Retrieved from http://www.parl.gc.ca/content/sen/committee/391/soci/rep/rep02may06-e.htm.

Stuart, H. (2006). Mental illness and employment discrimination. *Current Opinion in Psychiatry, 19*, 522–526.

Thomas, P. (2007). The stable patient with schizophrenia—From antipsychotic effectiveness to adherence. *European Neuropsychopharmacology, 17*, S115–S122. doi:10.1016/j.euroneuro.2007.02.003.

Vasiliadis, H., Lesage, A., Adair, C., et al. (2005). Service use for mental health reasons: Cross-provincial differences in rates, determinants and equity of access. *Canadian Journal of Psychiatry, 50*(10), 614–619. Retrieved from https://ww1.cpa-apc.org/Publications/Archives/CJP/2005/september/vasiliadis.asp.

White, M.C., Chafetz, L., Collins-Bride, G., et al. (2006). History of arrest, incarceration, and victimization in community-based severely mentally ill. *Journal of Community Health, 31*, 123–135. doi:10.1007/s10900-005-9005-1.

Yang, J., Law, S., Chow, W., et al. (2005). Assertive community treatment for persons with severe and persistent mental illness in ethnic minority groups. *Psychiatric Services, 56*, 1053–1056. doi:10.1176/appi.ps.56.9.1053.

Ziedonis, D.M., Smelson, D., Rosenthal, R., et al. (2005). Improving the care of individuals with schizophrenia and substance use disorders: Consensus recommendations. *Journal of Psychiatric Practice, 11*(5), 315–339.

# Psychological Needs of Patients With Medical Conditions

*Roberta Waite, Elizabeth M. Varcarolis*
*Adapted by Sandra Mitchell*

## KEY TERMS AND CONCEPTS

coping skills, 654

holistic approach, 647

psychiatric consultation liaison nurse (PCLN), 655

stigmatized persons with medical conditions, 655

## OBJECTIVES

1. Describe the influence of stress on general medical conditions.
2. Construct a nursing diagnosis for an individual who has HIV and depression.
3. Explain the importance of nurses' teaching relaxation techniques and coping skills to patients with medical illnesses.
4. Perform a comprehensive nursing assessment for a patient with a medical illness.
5. Assess the patient's coping skills by identifying (a) areas for psychoeducation teaching and (b) areas of strength.
6. Identify two instances in which a consultation with a psychiatric consultation liaison nurse might have been useful for your medical-surgical patients.

## evolve WEBSITE

*Visit the Evolve website for Flashcards, Case Studies, and additional testing resources related to the content in this chapter:* http://evolve.elsevier.com/Canada/Varcarolis/psychiatric/   Pre-Test   interactive review

There are two separate though related classifications of the relationship between physical conditions and psychological factors. Somatic symptom disorders—psychological problems that manifest themselves through physical symptoms such as chronic pain or preoccupation with illnesses—were discussed in Chapter 23. Now we turn our attention to people who have diagnosed or diagnosable general medical conditions that are influenced by psychological factors or psychiatric disorders.

Psychological factors have been found to influence a variety of physical illnesses. Stressful life events may result in further health risk and increase disability through stress-related physiological responses (Fava & Wise, 2007). The presence of psychiatric disorders along with general medical conditions may increase the likelihood of adverse events, length of stay, and cost; they also may negatively impact outcomes and increase morbidity and mortality (Levenson, 2008).

This chapter helps to prepare nurses to use a holistic approach, which addresses both the psychological and

physiological needs of patients. Despite the reality that the health care delivery system is fragmented for people with both medical and mental health problems, psychiatric mental health nurses must provide holistic care for patients with physical illnesses and nurses who work outside of psychiatric settings must be aware of the influence of psychological factors and psychiatric disorders on the course of general medical conditions and plan for care accordingly.

## PSYCHOLOGICAL FACTORS AFFECTING MEDICAL CONDITIONS

Both the medical and mental health communities recognize the interrelationships between psychiatric and medical co-morbidities. Psychological factors may present a risk for medical disease, or they may magnify or adversely affect a medical condition.

Researchers have gained an increased understanding of the basic physiological responses to stress (see Chapter 12), and

**647**

## BOX 32-1 PATIENT-SPECIFIC OUTCOMES OF PRIMARY CARE–PSYCHIATRY COLLABORATION

- Accuracy of diagnosis
- Retention in care
- Adherence with the treatment plan
- Decreased medication problems
  - Adverse or toxic effects
  - Drug–drug interactions
- Stabilization on long-term care plan
- Attainment of remission
  - Symptom control
  - Functional improvement
- Improved medical outcomes
  - Preventive measures
  - Chronic disease management
- Improved care of family
- Decreased suicidal behaviours

**Source:** Culpepper, L. (2003, May). The successful intervention: Management of the patient with medical comorbidities. In G. Jayaram (Scientific Program Chair), *Psychiatry and medicine: Common patients, different perspectives.* Symposium conducted at the 156th Annual Meeting of the American Psychiatric Association, San Francisco, CA.

there is deep interest in improving both the outcomes and the efficiency of health care delivery. Collaboration among providers of primary health care and mental health care can lead to more accurate diagnoses. Furthermore, treatment adherence for psychiatric disorders can be improved by addressing both psychiatric and physical problems, thereby reducing the stigma of seeking mental health care and making care more convenient. Obtaining remission, improving care of the family, and decreasing suicidal behaviour are major points of focus (Culpepper, 2003) (Box 32-1).

Stress is certainly a psychological factor. Important psychosocial and contextual factors can be identified as stressors in an individual's life and might become a primary focus of treatment. Hans Selye (1956) was the first to introduce the concept of stress into the fields of medicine and physiology. Stress can lead to changes in physical and mental health in many ways (see Chapter 12). Cannon's (1914) identification of the fight-or-flight response and Selye's description of the general adaptation syndrome provided insight into the biological and molecular reactions to stressors in the sympathetic nervous system, the pituitary–adrenocortical axis, and the immune system. Chronic stressors can have detrimental effects on components of the immune system. Extensive studies have left little doubt that psychosocial stress can affect the course and severity of illness.

Various medical disorders have been studied with regard to the effects of stress on the course of the illness. Table 32-1 identifies some common medical conditions that are negatively affected by stress and would benefit from stress reduction and support. However, anyone experiencing a serious medical condition needs a variety of psychological supports and may benefit from learning new coping skills.

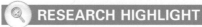

## RESEARCH HIGHLIGHT

### *The Intersecting Risks of Violence and HIV for Rural Aboriginal Women*

**Source:** Varcoe, C., & Dick, S. (2008). The intersecting risks of violence and HIV for rural Aboriginal women in a neo-colonial Canadian context. *Journal of Aboriginal Health, 4*(1), 42–52.

**Problem**
Aboriginal and rural women face multiple barriers to their health and safety, and their rates of human immunodeficiency virus (HIV) infection are rising more quickly than those of other women.

**Purpose of Study**
To identify strategies to minimize the interacting risks of violence and HIV infection among women in rural communities. It also aimed to improve understanding of the relationship between violence against women and their risk for exposure to HIV, as well as the impact of social and economic factors on risk for HIV for women living in rural communities.

**Methods**
An ethnographic design was used, and data were collected through individual interviews with women who had experienced intimate partner violence (IPV) and thought they were at risk for HIV.

**Key Findings**
Both the Aboriginal and non-Aboriginal women had endured harsh life experiences, including multiple experiences of abuse. These experiences were compounded by poverty, substance use, and limited access to support services, all of which put them at significant risk for exposure to HIV and other sexually transmitted infections (STIs).

**Implications for Nursing Practice**
Nurses need to attend to the complex intersections between violence and HIV and the multiple health risks that are worsened by broader inequities related to gender, rural living, and poverty, as well as the downsizing of social services.

## PSYCHOLOGICAL RESPONSES TO SERIOUS MEDICAL CONDITIONS

The diagnosis of a medical problem or condition is stressful for nearly everyone. However, the degree of stress is dependent upon the person's perception of the illness. People's questions can be many and varied when they find themselves faced with a serious medical problem:

- Will I be disfigured?
- Will I have a long-term disability?
- Will I be able to function as a wife or husband, parent, and member of society?
- Will I be able to continue to work?
- Will I suffer pain?
- Will I be stigmatized?

People who face the crisis of a serious medical diagnosis need the kind of emotional support that allows them to face their burdens without censure or fear of judgement (Jenkins, 2006).

| MEDICAL CONDITION | INCIDENCE | GENETIC AND BIOLOGICAL CORRELATES | COMMON PRECIPITATING FACTORS | HOLISTIC THERAPIES IN ADDITION TO MEDICAL MANAGEMENT |
|---|---|---|---|---|
| **TABLE 32-1** | **COMMON MEDICAL CONDITIONS NEGATIVELY AFFECTED BY STRESS** | | | |
| Cardiovascular disease (e.g., coronary heart disease) | Rates are higher in women of all ages than in men (Heart and Stroke Foundation, 2011) | Family history of cardiac disease a risk factor; other risk factors include hypertension, increased serum lipid levels, obesity, sedentary lifestyle, and cigarette smoking. Psychosocial risk factors: stress, depression, loneliness. High anxiety risk in patients with prior cardiac events | Often, myocardial infarction occurs after sudden stress preceded by a period of losses, frustration, and disappointments | Relaxation training, stress management, group social support, and psychosocial intervention. Support groups for type-A personalities and type-A modification helpful. Antianxiety agents (benzodiazepines) and antidepressants when indicated |
| Peptic ulcer (caused by *Helicobacter pylori* infection) | Men have a higher rate of *H. pylori* infection than women. About 10–15% of adults infected with *H. pylori* develop ulcers. Approximately 75% of people in First Nations communities infected with *H. pylori* (Canadian Digestive Health Foundation, 2011) | Infection with *H. pylori* associated with 95–99% of peptic ulcers. Both peptic and duodenal ulcers cluster in families, but separately from each other | Periods of social tension and increased life stress. After losses; often after menopause | Biofeedback can alter gastric acidity; cognitive-behavioural approaches for stress management |
| Cancer | In Canada, 40% of women and 45% of men will develop cancer. In men, the most common cancers are prostate, colorectal, bladder, and lung. In women, the most common cancers are breast, colorectal, uterine, and lung (Canadian Cancer Society, 2011) | Genetic evidence suggests dysfunction of cellular proliferation. Familial patterns for breast cancer, colorectal cancer, stomach cancer, melanoma | Prolonged and intensive stress. Stressful life events (e.g., separation from or loss of significant other two years before diagnosis). Feelings of hopelessness, helplessness, and despair (depression) may precede the diagnosis of cancer | Relaxation (e.g., meditation, autogenic training, self-hypnosis). Visualization. Psychological counselling. Support groups. Massage therapy. Stress management |
| Tension headache | Occurs in 80% of population when under stress. Begins at end of workday or early evening | | Associated with anxiety and depression | Psychotherapy usually prescribed for chronic tension headaches. Learning to cope or avoiding tension-creating situations or people. Relaxation techniques, stress-management techniques, cognitive-restructuring techniques |
| Essential hypertension | Females more likely than males to have hypertension. High blood pressure rates increase with age (Statistics Canada, 2009) | Family history of cardiac disease and hypertension | Life changes and traumatic life events. High-stress job (e.g., air traffic controller). Hypothesized to be found more in areas of social stress and conflict | Behavioural feedback, stress reduction techniques, meditation, yoga, hypnosis. *Note:* Pharmacological treatment considered primary for treatment of hypertension |

**Sources:** Canadian Cancer Society's Steering Committee on Cancer Statistics. (2011). *Canadian cancer statistics 2011.* Toronto: Canadian Cancer Society. Retrieved from http://www.cancer.ca/cancer-information/cancer-101/what-is-cancer; Canadian Digestive Health Foundation. (2011). *Peptic ulcer.* Retrieved from http://www.cdhf.ca/en/disorders/details/id/16; Heart and Stroke Foundation. (2011). *Statistics.* Retrieved from http://www.heartandstroke.com/site/c.ikIQLcMWJtE/b.3483991/k.34A8/Statistics.htm; and Statistics Canada. (2009). High blood pressure. Retrieved from http://www.statcan.gc.ca/pub/82-625-x/2010002/article/11262-eng.htm.

When strong emotional supports and social ties are not available, other questions may arise:

- How will I cope?
- How will this affect my life?
- Will I retain a reasonable quality of life?

The psychological impact of medical illness can be severe and can account for a higher rate of disruption in functional ability than just the medical illness alone would indicate. Among the most common psychological responses to physical illness are depression, anxiety, substance use, denial, hopelessness, and anger (Dunn, 2005). A psychological condition, however, may supersede or be co-morbid with a medical condition. In general, individuals with medical disorders and psychological symptoms have poorer outcomes than those with the same medical disorders but without psychological problems (Levenson, 2008).

## Depression

Among individuals with a serious medical illness, the risk of a major depressive disorder is high—thought to be as high as 20% to 50% (Jiang, 2008). Often, depression is masked by the medical condition itself and goes unrecognized and thus untreated. Just a few of the medical illnesses that typically are associated with depression are cancer (depression rate as high as 50%), HIV (depression rate of 41%), diabetes (depression rate of 9% to 27%), and stroke (depression rate of 20% to 30%) (Gaynes, Pence, Eron, et al., 2008; Herrmann, 2006; Pirl, 2004). Depression can amplify the pathophysiology of endocrine and cardiac disease and diminish functional ability (Jiang, 2008).

It is important to note that depression is also a risk factor for nonadherence to medication and treatment regimen. Patients with depression have been found to be three times more likely to be nonadherent to medical treatment than are patients without depression (Culpepper, 2003). If not recognized and treated, depression can affect the severity of the medical disorder, increase personal distress, impair functioning, and interfere with adherence to a prescribed medical regimen. However, people with medical conditions who get treatment for co-occurring depression often experience improvement in their overall medical condition, show better adherence to recommendations for general medical care, and experience a better quality of life (Simon, Von Korff, & Lin, 2005).

A possible nursing diagnosis for Candace in the vignette above is the following: *Severe anxiety* related to declining health status as evidenced by verbal comments, insomnia, and depression related to financial implications of health condition as evidenced by excessive crying, insomnia, and irritability.

## Anxiety

Anxiety disorders are among the most common mental health problems seen in primary health care settings, with as many as one third of patients displaying significant symptoms (Weisberg, Dyck, Culpepper, et al., 2007). Anxiety disorders and medical illnesses are commonly co-morbid, especially when pain, disability, hospitalization, economic loss, or fear of death is present (Katon, Lin, & Kroenke, 2007). Psychological and social factors and the severity and presence of co-morbid medical conditions play an important role in the level of anxiety experienced (Cohen, Batista, & Gorman, 2007).

Acute anxiety can influence a person's coping capacity, defensive structure, adaptive capacity, and resilience. Anxiety may also lead to heightened awareness of physical symptoms, as well as physiologically causing medical symptoms because of increased muscle tension and autonomic nervous system and hypothalamic–pituitary axis dysregulation. The burden of physical symptoms and resulting functional impairment caused by complications of medical illness are likely to worsen episodes of anxiety (Katon & Roy-Byrne, 2007). Recognizing treatable anxiety disorders that are highly concurrent with medical co-morbid conditions is important in alleviating distress and improving the course of the illness.

Verbalization can be an effective outlet for anxiety. However, the ability to effectively communicate one's feelings may be compromised by cultural expectations, disability, or lack of a listener. A sense of helplessness often accompanies anxiety in the person who feels a loss of control over events, such as when awaiting surgery or undergoing invasive treatments. In this case, defence mechanisms (e.g., denial or regression) may be used with greater frequency, or compulsive behaviours may surface. Unreasonable requests of caregivers (e.g., demanding that the

---

**VIGNETTE**

Candace is a single, 61-year-old head administrative paralegal who was recently hospitalized for congestive heart failure. She is referred by her physician because of excessive crying, insomnia, and irritability. Candace complains of waking up at night obsessing about small details and having chest pain. She states, "I feel very scared and alone, and I worry about my health and having to retire. I don't know where I would get the money to live or to pay for my medications if I get sick again. I am too old, and it is just too difficult to go on." These observations were reported to the nurse practitioner. After a thorough assessment and medical workup, it is determined that Candace is experiencing depression and severe anxiety, which precipitated physiological symptoms.

---

**VIGNETTE**

At 27 years of age, Manjeet tests positive for HIV infection. During the post-test counselling session, the public health nurse at the community health centre gives him referrals and information regarding the virus. The nurse notes that Manjeet is having difficulty focusing on details and needs to have information repeated several times. The nurse gives him the opportunity to explore his feelings aloud, but Manjeet has difficulty doing so because he was raised to believe that it is a strength to deal with crises alone. Manjeet is also experiencing a great deal of denial in this initial period of loss. For these reasons, the nurse anticipates the most common and immediate concerns that might be facing a person who has just discovered that he is HIV positive and gently leads Manjeet into discussion of these concerns over a period of several weeks, with the use of reflective statements and silence. This approach gives Manjeet the opportunity to verbalize his feelings and begin to unburden himself in a safe environment.

nurse sit with a patient throughout the night) may be a cover for feelings of inadequacy.

Possible nursing diagnoses for Manjeet in the vignette above include the following:

- *Risk for ineffective coping* related to inability to ask for help as evidenced by his belief that it is a strength to deal with crises alone
- *Ineffective denial* related to recent diagnosis of HIV as evidenced by inability to express his feelings

## Substance Abuse

Long-term abuse of various substances can lead to a variety of medical complications; for example, alcohol use is associated with hepatic conditions, marijuana use with lung disease, cocaine use with cardiac toxicity, and use of ecstasy (3,4-methylenedioxymethamphetamine, or MDMA) with neurotoxicity (e.g., problems with memory, reasoning, impulse control). However, patients who are diagnosed with serious medical conditions often turn to alcohol or other substances to cope with overwhelming feelings of hopelessness, fear, anxiety, depression, or pain.

Linking medical and mental health services with addiction services is important because substance abuse is a concurrent diagnosis in large numbers of medical and mental health patients (Weisner & Matzger, 2003). Untreated substance abuse can increase the number of hospitalizations and the severity of the illness (whether medical, mental health, or both) in patients with a concurrent disorder (Rosack, 2003). Thus, relevant research indicates that health care providers need to be diligent in their initial assessments and identify any coexisting or resulting psychological responses or disorders. In most cases of physical illness, the focus is on the complaints of physical symptoms, and minimal attention is given to the psychological responses of the patient.

## Grief and Loss

Serious medical illnesses are nearly always accompanied by grief. As well, any type of treatment or procedure intended to treat a physical illness that creates a major permanent change is accompanied by feelings of loss. The dynamics involved in coping with these feelings are similar to those in a person who is dealing with his or her own impending death or the death of a loved one. The person must grieve for the loss, just as the dying person must work through the confusion and darkness until a degree of acceptance and relative peace is achieved. Negotiating the loss of physical well-being involves movement through feelings of frustration, vulnerability, and sadness to become a whole person once again. This journey encompasses both spiritual and emotional changes and, for this reason, requires spiritual assessment of the patient, as well as a focus on psychosocial issues.

Possible nursing diagnoses for Lillian in the next vignette include the following:

- *Hopelessness* related to chronic illness as evidenced by verbal comments and feelings of resentment toward others who are healthy
- *Ineffective individual coping* related to chronic illness as evidenced by expressions of anger and feelings of hopelessness.

**VIGNETTE**

Lillian is a 47-year-old woman being treated with hemodialysis. She has been complaining of frequent tension headaches and occasional stomach upsets before her treatment appointments. The hemodialysis nurse has always been impressed by Lillian's patience and compliant attitude in spite of her debilitating illness, which has robbed her of a normal family life. For this reason, the nurse suspects that Lillian's physical complaints could be a way of dealing with emotions, so the nurse makes a point of spending more time with Lillian to allow her to talk about her frustrations. Lillian expresses anger and some feelings of hopelessness. She resents others who are healthy, including the people who care for her. Frequent opportunities to verbalize these feelings gradually result in the lessening of her somatic complaints and a decrease in her sense of powerlessness and isolation.

## Denial

Common responses to the initial symptoms of illness, the diagnosis, and functional limitations and impairments evoke the complicated process of denial, acceptance, and adaptation (although not necessarily in that order). Denial, an unconscious defence mechanism, may be evident when the diagnosed person and the family seem to have little knowledge or interest in learning about the condition or define the illness as acute rather than chronic. Nurses and other health care providers may actually foster such beliefs by withholding information about the meaning and likely consequences of a particular problem. Initial illness crises support explanations of the illness as acute and can be so overwhelming for patients and families as to prevent consideration of a long-term course.

As symptoms and acute crises repeat over time, individuals begin to accept the chronicity of their illnesses and the effects of the illness on their daily lives. People begin to experience their bodies as altered and come to think of illness as real in ways that allow them to relate symptoms and the changes in their lives. They compare their present condition with that of the past, weighing the risks of continuing their regular activities and activity levels and then adapting those activity levels. Patients may feel estranged from the person they have become,

**VIGNETTE**

After a car accident, Katya is being assessed by the triage nurse in the emergency department for possible injuries. She complains of a slight headache and dizziness but denies having any other pain or symptoms. Katya is preoccupied with seeing that her 2-year-old son, who was also in the car, is being examined, so she denies her own need for medical attention. Katya's blood pressure is 86/50 mm Hg and her body posture indicates that she is guarding her abdomen. These observations are reported to the examining physician immediately because they indicate possible internal bleeding and danger of shock. Katya is eventually taken to the operating room so the bleeding may be stopped.

betrayed by their own bodies, or guilty for not meeting standards of activity levels, functioning, and appearance. Patients can also distance themselves from their illness, diagnosis, and bodies, objectifying their symptoms as a way of coping. Bodily changes affect individuals' identities in important ways, and some chronically ill patients work very hard at maintaining their pre-illness identity, sometimes to the detriment of their health (Green, 2004).

Possible nursing diagnoses for Katya in the vignette above include the following:

- *Acute pain* related to recent car accident as evidenced by headache, dizziness, and body posture indicating she is guarding her abdomen
- *Anxiety* related to concern for her child as evidenced by being preoccupied with seeing her 2-year-old son.

### Fear of Dependency

Responses to being dependent might be exhibited as the inability to accept warmth, nurturing, or tenderness from caregivers or as a refusal to accept treatment or medical advice. This reaction is strongest in those who have unmet dependencies and those who have had negative experiences when seeking help in the past. Anger may mask acute embarrassment over being in a dependent position or may be used by the patient who feels the need to project an independent image. Others are fearful of not having their dependency needs met and do not express any negative feelings to caregivers. These people strive to be "good" patients out of fear that they will be abandoned if they are perceived to be difficult. Suppressed anxiety or anger, however, could be exhibited through increased somatic complaints.

---

**VIGNETTE**

Rebecca, a 50-year-old woman with HIV, worked as a home attendant until she fractured her leg and sustained a severe elbow injury when a patient she was assisting fell on her. The resultant disabilities prevented her from resuming her job as a home attendant. Prior to this incident, she was independent, hard working, self-supporting, and was able to manage a mild anxiety disorder through cognitive reframing and controlled breathing. Her injury forced her to apply for financial support and rely on her son for assistance with transportation and care of her apartment. She began to experience shortness of breath, palpitations, and impaired concentration.

---

A possible nursing diagnosis for Rebecca in the vignette above is the following:

*Anxiety* related to recent change in health status as evidenced by impaired concentration and palpitations.

## NURSING CARE OF PATIENTS WITH MEDICAL CONDITIONS

### Psychosocial Assessment

Psychosocial factors are relevant to the course of an illness, and the way a person thinks and feels can have a profound effect on how the disease progresses. Struggling with illness evokes a range of difficult emotions such as fear, anger, sadness, confusion, and guilt. Patients may feel overwhelmed and alone, while family members may feel helpless and at a loss emotionally (Meyerstein, 2005). How can a health care provider know what a patient thinks or feels unless the patient's psychosocial situation is assessed?

The elements of a thorough psychosocial assessment are described in detail in Chapter 9. The following are some highlights that can help the nurse plan necessary interventions. When working with someone who is medically ill, it is important to know if the person has:

- Someone who can share his or her concerns and who cares for him or her
- Friends and supports in the community
- Any coexisting conditions that could negatively affect adjustment to the illness, the course of the illness, adaptation to the illness, or ability to heal (e.g., depression; personality disorder; substance abuse; compulsive behaviours such as gambling, eating, or cybersex)
- Risky health behaviours (e.g., sedentary lifestyle, smoking, engaging in unsafe sex practices, abusing alcohol or drugs)
- A cultural view of health and illness that helps or impedes the process of seeking adequate care

Table 32-2 provides an outline for a psychosocial assessment of a patient with a medical condition. A psychosocial assessment is performed in tandem with a thorough physical workup and mental status examination.

### Quality of Life

For interventions to be most effective, the nurse must understand how a person's medical condition affects his or her quality of life. For example, how is the medical illness affecting the ability to function in the home, at work, or in school? How are the patient's feelings about the illness (e.g., depression, anxiety, hopelessness) affecting his or her relationships and ability to function? The World Health Organization's (2004) Quality of Life—BREF (WHOQOL-BREF) tool can be used to examine an individual's perceptions about quality of life in the context of culture, value systems, and personal goals, standards, and concerns. The development of this tool was based on statements made by patients from a variety of cultures and with a range of diseases.

### Coping Skills

Assessing how a patient has dealt with adversity in the past provides information about the person's coping skills available for use now and in the future. Health care providers can also support the patient in gaining additional coping skills that may help him or her better manage a serious medical or surgical situation.

A person who has a life-threatening disease or chronic illness often deals with distressing physical adverse effects and changes in body image. For example, a patient who is given a colostomy to avoid death from cancer or ulcerative colitis is left with complex emotional as well as physical issues, especially true for women. The patient must learn techniques for dealing with not only the stoma but also the lifelong consequences and their

| TABLE 32-2 | PSYCHOSOCIAL ASSESSMENT OF PATIENTS WITH MEDICAL CONDITIONS |
|---|---|
| **AREAS TO ASSESS** | **SPECIFIC QUESTIONS TO ASK** |
| | **SOCIAL SUPPORTS AND CULTURAL ISSUES** |
| Family | What were the effects of the patient's illness, treatments, and recovery on the family in the past? |
| Friends | Who can the patient share painful feelings with?<br>Does the patient have friends to joke and laugh with?<br>Are there people the patient believes would stand by him or her? |
| Religious or spiritual beliefs | Does the patient find comfort and support in spiritual practices?<br>Is the patient a member of a spiritual or religious group in the community (e.g., church, temple, other place of worship)?<br>Does the patient find inner peace and strength in religious or spiritual practices?<br>The following statements may be used in performing a spiritual assessment of a patient:<br>• I [often/sometimes/seldom] believe that life has value, meaning, and direction.<br>• I [often/sometimes/seldom] feel a connection with the universe.<br>• I [often/sometimes/seldom] believe in a power greater than myself.<br>• I [often/sometimes/seldom] believe that my actions make a difference.<br>• I [often/sometimes/seldom] believe that my actions express my true self. |
| Cultural beliefs | Does the patient use specific culture-oriented treatments or remedies for his or her condition?<br>Do the patient's cultural beliefs allow for adequate treatment by Western medical standards? |
| Work | Are there colleagues at work the patient can count on for support? |
| | **CONCURRENT PHYSICAL CONDITIONS AFFECTING PSYCHOSOCIAL WELL-BEING** |
| Physical pain | Is the patient in pain? If yes:<br>• How does the patient cope with it?<br>• Is the pain disabling?<br>• Are there pain-reducing techniques that might help? |
| Major illness | Does the patient have a co-occurring major illness that will negatively affect his or her current condition?<br>Is the patient undergoing treatments that are affecting daily life more than expected?<br>Are there interventions that would help the patient better cope with the sequelae of the illness and treatments?<br>Has the patient been hospitalized in the past? If yes:<br>• How many times?<br>• For what?<br>• How did the patient cope? |
| Addictions and mental health | Does the patient have a co-occurring mental health problem (e.g., depression, anxiety, compulsions)?<br>Has the patient suffered a mental illness in the past?<br>Does the patient participate in any compulsive behaviour (e.g., smoking, overworking, excessive spending, gambling, cybersex)?<br>Does the patient abuse substances (i.e., alcohol, drugs [illicit, over-the-counter, prescription])? |

effects on body image, appearance, and relationships. Concerns such as the following may arise (Manderson, 2005):

• Will my partner still be attracted to me?
• Will I continue to be interested in sexual relationships?
• Will I be embarrassed by my friends' reactions to my situation?
• Will people still think of me and relate to me the way they did before this illness?

Breast cancer survivors, for example, have been helped by camaraderie with other survivors who openly share their techniques for dealing with appliances or prostheses. Other survivors can also show patients how to respond to well-intended but probing or embarrassing questions. Women who have previously travelled the same path are the best resources for helping those newly diagnosed establish how to manage inevitable questions about their illness.

Table 32-3 highlights some of the characteristics that allow people to cope well and some of the characteristics that may be changed or improved through psychosocial interventions or cognitive-behavioural approaches.

### Spirituality and Religion

Nurses and other health care workers are becoming increasingly aware of the role spirituality or religion plays in many patients' lives and its importance as a source of peace. Support from a priest, pastor, rabbi, or other religious leader may be indicated, especially in a case of spiritual distress. Beliefs and practices are forces that promote resilience; practising healthy coping

| TABLE 32-3 | ASSESSMENT OF COPING SKILLS | |
|---|---|
| **EFFECTIVE COPING SKILLS** | **INEFFECTIVE COPING BEHAVIOURS** |
| Has optimistic attitude (sees glass as half full) | Has pessimistic attitude (sees glass as half empty) |
| Confronts the issues; acts accordingly | Minimizes critical health status or signals |
| Seeks information; gets guidance | Shows tendency to escape or withdraw |
| Shares concerns; finds consolation | Blames someone or something else |
| Has capacity for healthy denial | Denies as much as possible; shows prolonged denial |
| Redefines the situation, reviews alternatives, examines consequences | Feels things are hopeless, were meant to be; has attitude of "What's the use?" |
| Constructively uses distractions: keeping busy; maintaining positive emotional ties with family, friends, community | Withdraws; broods; is overwhelmed with self-pity, anger, envy, guilt about having caused the illness |

depends upon the capacity to create meaning from experiences (Meyerstein, 2005).

### Social Support

Medical conditions initially may elicit strong support from friends and family, but as time wears on, this support may begin to wane. Knowing who is there for the patient will be helpful in planning for later interventions. Does the patient have sufficient social supports (e.g., family, friends, elders, religious or spiritual help) to enable him or her to share thoughts and feelings? Would the patient benefit from a medical support group?

### General Interventions

In an ideal situation, a multidisciplinary team of health care providers, including a psychiatric consultation liaison nurse (see page 655), would be involved in the treatment of patients with serious medical illness. Using the data from the holistic assessment, clinicians can provide useful and effective interventions.

People who have a medical condition are vulnerable to a variety of psychosocial stresses. How they cope with these stresses may make the difference between living with an acceptable quality of life and giving in to despair, withdrawal, helplessness, or hopelessness. Nurses are in a position to assess and understand patients' psychosocial stressors, identify needed coping skills, and teach stress-management techniques. Nurses can play an important role not only in providing and managing patients' immediate medical care but also in helping patients to improve their ability to cope and increase their quality of life during the course of a chronic medical illness.

Effective coping skills are healthier ways of looking at and dealing with illness (e.g., assertiveness training, cognitive reframing, problem-solving skills, social supports). They are many and varied and can be taught. A nurse is in a key position to assess patients' ability to cope, educate patients about coping skills, or provide referrals to patients to learn healthier ways of looking at and dealing with illness. Consider referring the patient for instruction in a variety of relaxation techniques, such as meditation, guided imagery, or breathing exercises,

or teach the patient such techniques yourself. Behavioural techniques are useful, and nurses with special training can offer their patients progressive muscle relaxation or biofeedback. Relaxation techniques, stress management, and supportive education should be part of the care of the patient with a medical condition, regardless of the medical diagnosis.

Although medical procedures may extend or promote life, they often take a toll on the patient's physical state because of the high degree of anxiety they evoke. Research has shifted the focus from patients' knowledge of the disease and its treatment to their confidence and skills in managing their condition. Interventions now support patients' and their support system's being active participants in managing their condition (Wagner, Austin, Davis, et al., 2001). The following have all been shown to affect a patient's recovery positively:

- Educating the patient regarding the specific medical treatment
- Referring the patient to community support groups (or systems)
- Teaching patients more effective coping skills that take into consideration patients' values, preferences, and lifestyle
- Focusing on a patient's strengths and reinforcing coping skills that work (e.g., prayerfulness, participation in hobbies, relaxation techniques)

There is growing evidence that psychotherapy can help people endure medical illness (Turvey & Klein, 2008). Beneficial psychotherapy approaches include:

- Cognitive-behavioural psychotherapy
- Guided imagery, biofeedback, acupressure, and hypnosis
- Psychodynamic psychotherapy

The Patient and Family Teaching box provides guidelines for teaching patients and their families how to adapt to a major medical illness.

## HUMAN RIGHTS ABUSES OF STIGMATIZED PERSONS WITH MEDICAL CONDITIONS

Some consumers of health care and some health care providers have voiced the need for examination of human rights abuses

## PATIENT AND FAMILY TEACHING: COPING WITH A MAJOR MEDICAL ILLNESS

**Learn all you can about your illness.** Knowledge can help reduce anxiety. Keeping your anxiety at manageable levels helps you understand your options and helps you make decisions you believe are right for you.

**Practise healthy behaviours.** Good sleep hygiene, diet, and exercise are good policies. Even if you are physically limited, exercise promotes a positive state of well-being. Lack of sleep can increase pain, irritability, and fatigue. Proper nutrition in the face of a medical illness can preserve or promote a healthy immune system.

**Take advantage of support groups that help you manage your medical condition.** Support groups that focus on your medical issue can provide you with information, help you learn how to handle difficult situations related to your illness, reduce isolation, and offer a safe place to share difficult thoughts and feelings.

**Consider entering psychotherapy.** There is growing evidence that psychotherapy helps people endure medical illness. Benefits include less pain, better coping skills, and even longer survival in some situations.

**Find a way to express your feelings.** Studies have examined the profound healing power of putting upsetting experiences into words (e.g., writing them down, keeping a journal). Acknowledging thoughts and feelings can help your nervous system relax.

**Seek additional help if you become depressed, demoralized, anxious, or panicky or have unremitting pain.** Your clinician might not be aware of these changes, and there are approaches (e.g., acupuncture, acupressure, biofeedback) that can give people control over their physiological responses and reduce the need for higher doses of medication.

**Find a creative outlet.** Doing anything creative—writing poetry or prose, painting or making collages, playing an instrument or singing—is a powerful tool in working with the feelings of fear, anger, and loss that are stirred up by illness.

**If you are a caregiver, do not neglect your own self-care.** Take time for rest and restoration and time to renew important life interests and activities. If you become depleted, you cannot give to another what is depleted and you no longer possess.

**Sources:** Adapted from Zerbe, K.J. (1999). *Women's mental health in primary care.* Philadelphia: Saunders.

in the health care system—specifically, the inadequate care of people who are stigmatized by health care providers, leading to their undue stress, worsening of physical illness, and even death. These stigmatized persons with medical conditions are assumed by health care providers to be bad, disgusting, or even just unusual and often include those who have mental illnesses, those who are HIV positive, and those who have undergone transgender surgeries or treatments. The abuses many of these

patients endure can result in inadequate care and lead to undue stress, worsening of physical illness, and even death. By making assumptions about these patients, health care workers fail to acknowledge and understand that their psychosocial issues are similar to those of others and that the same nursing interventions for anger, anxiety, and grief are applicable. Examples of human rights abuse include:

- Failure to fully investigate somatic complaints made by emergency-department patients with a history of psychiatric illness
- Avoidance of contact with, or refusal to care for, persons who are stigmatized, which results in worsening illness or death
- Hastily labelling with a psychiatric diagnosis and giving a prescription of antipsychotic drugs to persons who are experiencing normal emotional responses (e.g., sadness, anger) to chronic physical illness
- Inappropriate psychiatric admission of persons who are on medical units or in nursing homes, based on the financial needs of the institution or on the staff's inability to manage emotional responses to physical illness or the aging process

Such situations may occur more frequently to individuals who lack family support or the personal resources to advocate for themselves (e.g., those from the lower socioeconomic classes, newly arrived immigrants, those living socially "unacceptable" lifestyles). The key to increasing awareness of human rights issues in psychiatric mental health care may be the integration of these concepts into nursing curricula. Humanitarian values are at the very heart of our profession and practice. Nurses are in a unique position to advocate for equal patient treatment, but many hesitate to confront employers about violations of basic patient rights, fearing reprisal. A committee composed of nurses and other hospital employees could be formed to review such cases and make recommendations to the hospital administration. In this age of managed care and cuts in hospital budgets, upholding human rights is one of nursing's greatest challenges.

## PSYCHIATRIC CONSULTATION LIAISON NURSE

A psychiatric consultation liaison nurse (PCLN) functions as a consultant to other nurses in managing psychological concerns and symptoms of psychiatric disorders and also works directly with patients as a clinician to help them deal more effectively with physical and emotional problems. The PCLN is a resource for members of a nursing staff who feel unable to intervene therapeutically with a patient who presents a management problem or has problems that impede care. The PCLN first meets with the nurse who initiated the consultation and then reviews the patient's medical records, talks with the physicians, and interviews the patient. After the patient interview, the PCLN discusses the assessment and suggestions for care with the referring nurse.

## KEY POINTS TO REMEMBER

- There is irrefutable evidence that psychiatric disorders and psychological responses influence general medical conditions.
- A bidirectional effect exists between physical and emotional states of health. Physical illnesses are often accompanied by a spectrum of emotional responses, particularly anxiety and depression. Likewise, adverse emotional states often increase the severity of physical symptoms.
- The holistic philosophy of nursing dictates that all nurses, regardless of their roles or specialties, assess patients' psychosocial needs as well as their strengths.
- Health care personnel in the medical and mental health communities recognize the need to target both the psychological and physical problems of a patient to increase adherence to the care regimen, maximize quality of life, and promote healing.
- Understanding a patient's psychosocial needs and knowing when to intervene and where to refer the patient are essential for the nurse who practises holistic care and more effectively promotes health.
- Identifying the existence of depression, anxiety, and substance abuse and getting the patient treatment can help promote a positive outcome of the medical disorder and improve the patient's quality of life.
- A holistic approach to patient care includes assessment of physical, psychosocial, social, and spiritual needs.
- A growing concern about patients is the state of their spiritual lives. Including this dimension in the holistic nursing assessment allows nurses to see inner strengths in their patients that might be overlooked by a more traditional approach.
- The psychiatric consultation liaison nurse is a nurse clinician who is in the key position of being able to help other health care personnel look at their patients in a holistic manner and to help those who care for these patients understand nonmedical issues that are impeding medical progress.

## CRITICAL THINKING

1. Marie Vaudrie is a 45-year-old woman who has had a partial hysterectomy. Although she is asymptomatic and has a normal physical examination, her lab results indicate that she is HIV positive. Marie was unaware that her boyfriend of two years was engaging in unprotected sex with men. She and her ex-husband have been divorced for five years but maintain a good relationship and share custody of their three teenage children. Marie has a supportive extended family and several close friends, and she belongs to a church. After her diagnosis, Marie is encouraged to talk about her feelings and see a therapist. Marie states, "I will be able to do everything I did before. I feel healthy." The nurse has several concerns, including Marie's focus on self-care, her acceptance and understanding of her HIV-positive status, and her willingness to disclose her status to sexual or intimate partners.
   a. How would you evaluate Marie's social support system?
   b. What other information about her situation would be helpful in your assessment (e.g., cultural beliefs about illness)?
   c. What recommendations or referrals could you make to Marie, and how would you approach her with these recommendations? Would you include contact data for any medically related or HIV-related support groups in the information you would give her?

2. Discuss how you would approach the physician regarding Marie's need to be evaluated for depression. What are some of the compelling reasons depression (and any coexisting mental condition) should be treated in any and all seriously ill medically patients?

3. What cognitive-behavioural coping skills have been proven useful for a patient who is HIV-positive?

4. What important areas should the nurse assess with an Aboriginal woman attending an outpatient clinic with a past history of intimate partner violence and expressing a fear that she may have HIV?

## CHAPTER REVIEW

1. Which statement about the psychological impact of medical illnesses is accurate?
   1. An experience of grief and loss is not typical of most serious medical illnesses.
   2. Depression is a significant issue in over 60% of persons with cancer or heart disease.
   3. Psychological responses to medical illnesses can delay recovery but do not worsen the outcome.
   4. Patients often have significant concerns regarding the impact a medical illness can have on their ability to function.

2. While taking the vital signs of a patient about to undergo surgery, you notice she is tearful. When asked, she tells you that her mother had the same surgery and later died of a postoperative infection. Which response is most likely to be therapeutic?
   1. Ask the patient if she would like to speak with the chaplain before surgery.
   2. Reassure the patient that she has an excellent surgeon and that complications for her surgery are rare.
   3. State, "Surgery can be very frightening," and sit down next to the patient to convey your availability to talk.
   4. State, "Many people become anxious before surgery, but this is a normal reaction. You will be fine."

3. An older-adult male with heart disease feels both angry and guilty about his illness, blaming himself for becoming obese and inactive and feeling anger toward tobacco and fast-food companies. He presented in the emergency department today four hours after the onset of unrelenting chest pain, reporting that it "didn't hurt that much" and that, given his prior experiences with chest pain, he "did not think it would matter much" whether he came in quickly or tried to "wait it out." Now awaiting the results of his ECG, he is reading magazines and talking about the likelihood that a new stent will again give him a new lease on life. Based on this information, how well would you expect this patient to be able to cope with his illness?
   1. Poorly
   2. Inadequately
   3. Adequately
   4. Exceptionally

4. A nurse on a medical-surgical unit is admitting a patient with a history of bipolar disorder and alcohol abuse. Which action would be most appropriate for assuring that this patient receives the best possible nursing care?
   1. Consult with the psychiatric consultation liaison nurse regarding assessment skills and interventions likely to benefit this patient.
   2. Review Internet, textbook, or journal resources pertaining to the patient's mental health and substance abuse disorders.
   3. Consult more experienced colleagues and the head nurse for tips on assessing and caring for persons with co-morbid psychiatric disorders.
   4. Focus primarily on the patient's physical health needs, and refer the patient for outpatient psychiatric care at discharge if the patient requests it.

5. Which statements about persons with mental illness who present with serious medical conditions are most accurate? Select all that apply.
   1. Such patients are at higher risk for receiving inadequate care, owing to failure to fully assess somatic complaints.
   2. Patients who have a medical and a mental illness tend to receive more care and more costly care because of their concurrent disorders.
   3. Staff are more likely to minimize their time with such patients compared to medically ill patients without mental illness.
   4. Such patients risk being admitted to psychiatric settings instead of needed medical-surgical units, owing to staff's anxiety about caring for them.
   5. Emotional responses to medical conditions may be mistakenly attributed to psychiatric illness rather than being addressed as normal responses to medical conditions.

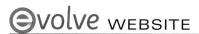 **WEBSITE**

Post-Test interactive review

*Visit the Evolve Web site for Chapter Review Answers and Rationales, Critical Thinking Answer Guidelines, and additional resources related to the content in this chapter: http://evolve.elsevier.com/Canada/Varcarolis/psychiatric/*

## REFERENCES

Cannon, W.B. (1914). The emergency function of the adrenal medulla in pain and the major emotions. *American Journal of Physiology, 33*, 356–372.

Cohen, M., Batista, S., & Gorman, J. (2007). In M. Cohen & J. Gorman (Eds.), *Comprehensive textbook of AIDS psychiatry.* New York: Oxford University Press.

Culpepper, L. (2003, May). The successful intervention: Management of the patient with medical comorbidities. In G. Jayaram (Chair), *Psychiatry and medicine: Common patients, different perspectives.* Symposium conducted at the 156th Annual Meeting of the American Psychiatric Association, San Francisco, CA.

Dunn, S. (2005). Hopelessness as a response to physical illness. *Journal of Nursing Scholarship, 37*, 148–155. doi:10.1111/j.1547-5069.2005.00027.x.

Fava, G.A., & Wise, T.N. (2007). Issues for *DSM-V:* Psychological factors affecting either identified or feared medical conditions: A solution for somatoform disorders. *American Journal of Psychiatry, 164*, 1002–1003. doi:10.1176/appi.ajp.164.7.1002.

Gaynes, B., Pence, B., Eron, J., et al. (2008). Prevalence and comorbidity of psychiatric diagnoses based on reference standard in an HIV+ patient population. *Psychosomatic Medicine, 70*, 505–511. doi:10.1097/PSY.0b013e31816aa0cc.

Green, C. (2004). Fostering recovery from life-transforming mental health disorders: A synthesis and model. *Social and Health Theory, 2*(4), 293–314. doi:10.1057/palgrave.sth.8700036.

Herrmann, N. (2006). Post-stroke depression. *Brain and Cognition, 63*, 195. doi:10.1016/j.bandc.2006.08.015.

Jenkins, A. (2006). Face the feelings: Patients may need emotional support to cope with life-threatening illness. *Nursing Standard, 20*(24), 31.

Jiang, W. (2008). Impacts of depression and emotional distress on cardiac disease. *Cleveland Clinic Journal of Medicine, 75*(Suppl.), S20–S25. doi:10.3949/ccjm.75.Suppl_2.S20.

Katon, W., Lin, E., & Kroenke, K. (2007). The association of depression and anxiety with medical symptom burden in patients with chronic medical illness. *General Hospital Psychiatry, 29*, 147–155. doi:10.1016/j.genhosppsych.2006.11.005.

Katon, W., & Roy-Byrne, P. (2007). Anxiety disorders: Efficient screening is the first step in improving outcomes. *Annals of Internal Medicine, 146*(5), 390–392.

Levenson, J.L. (2008). Psychological factors affecting medical conditions. In R.E. Hales, S.C. Yudofsky, & G.O. Gabbard (Eds.), *Textbook of psychiatry* (5th ed., pp. 999–1024). Washington, DC: American Psychiatric Publishing.

Manderson, L. (2005). Boundary breaches: The body, sex and sexuality after stoma surgery. *Social Science & Medicine, 61*, 405–415. doi:10.1016/j.socscimed.2004.11.051.

Meyerstein, I. (2005). Sustaining our spirits: Spiritual study/discussion groups for coping with medical illness. *Journal of Religion and Health, 44*, 207–225. doi:10.1007/s10943-005-2778-9.

Pirl, W.F. (2004). Evidence report on the occurrence, assessment, and treatment of depression in cancer patients. *Journal of National Cancer Institute Monographs, 32*, 32–39. doi:10.1093/jncimonographs/lgh026.

Rosack, J. (2003). Comorbidity common in addicts, but integrated treatment rare. *Psychiatric News, 38*(2), 30.

Selye, H. (1956). *The stress of life.* New York: McGraw-Hill.

Simon, G., Von Korff, M., & Lin, E. (2005). Clinical and functional outcomes of depression treatment in patients with and without chronic medical illness. *Psychological Medicine, 35*, 271–279. doi:10.1017/S0033291704003071.

Turvey, C., & Klein, D. (2008). Remission from depression comorbid with chronic illness and physical impairment. *American Journal of Psychiatry, 165*, 569–575. doi:10.1176/appi.ajp.2007.07081224.

Wagner, E., Austin, B., Davis, C., et al. (2001). Improving chronic illness care: Translating evidence into action. *Health Affairs, 20*, 64–78. doi:10.1377/hlthaff.20.6.64.

Weisberg, R.B., Dyck, I., Culpepper, L., et al. (2007). Psychiatric treatment in primary care patients with anxiety disorders: A comparison of care received from primary care providers and psychiatrists. *American Journal of Psychiatry, 164*, 276–283. doi:10.1176/appi.ajp.164.2.276.

Weisner, C., & Matzger, H. (2003). Missed opportunities in addressing drinking behaviour in medical and mental health services. *Alcoholism: Clinical & Experimental Research, 27*, 1132–1141. doi:10.1097/01.ALC.0000075546.38349.69.

World Health Organization. (2004). *World Health Organization Quality of Life—BREF.* Retrieved from http://www.who.int/substance_abuse/research_tools/en/english_whoqol.pdf.

# Care for the Dying and for Those Who Grieve

*Cyndee L. MacPhee*

## KEY TERMS AND CONCEPTS

## OBJECTIVES

1. Compare and contrast specific goals of end-of-life care inherent in the hospice palliative care model with those of the medical model.
2. Analyze the effects of specific interventions nurses can implement when working with a dying person and his or her family and loved ones.
3. Analyze how the Four Gifts of Resolving Relationships (forgiveness, love, gratitude, and farewell) can be used to help people respond to a dying loved one.
4. Explain the distinction between the terms *grief* and *mourning* as presented in this chapter and how the

effectiveness of a holistic approach can be beneficial to the person.
5. Differentiate among some of the characteristics of normal bereavement and complicated grieving.
6. Explain how various models of understanding grieving (dual process, four tasks of mourning) can enhance your care of those who grieve.
7. Discuss at least five guidelines for dealing with catastrophic loss, and identify appropriate support for someone in acute grief.

## ⊖volve WEBSITE

*Visit the Evolve website for Flashcards, Case Studies, and additional testing resources related to the content in this chapter:* http://evolve.elsevier.com/Canada/Varcarolis/psychiatric/   Pre-Test  interactive review

Caring for patients who have terminal illnesses or are near death due to other conditions challenges and rewards nurses in deep and personal ways. In caring for the dying, nurses may grow personally, both by accepting their patients' deaths and by developing a richer understanding of their own mortality. Nurses also have an opportunity to bring dignity to the dying and help shape an enduring positive memory for family members and caregivers.

Nurses continue to provide care for dying patients primarily in medical institutions, despite evidence supporting care in the home (Stajduhar, Roberts, McLeod, et al., 2010). Although 70%

of Canadian deaths occur in hospital (Canadian Hospice Palliative Care Association, 2010a), most Canadians prefer to die at home, surrounded by loved ones (Canadian Institute for Health Information, 2007), which decreases health care costs and improves patient and family satisfaction (Candy, Holman, Leurent, et al., 2011). Patient-centred palliative care is an interdisciplinary and collaborative effort aimed at relieving pain and suffering and involving various health care providers (Canadian Hospice Palliative Care Association, 2013; Pellett, 2009) and in which nurses play an integral and important role. In addition to using the necessary assessment and management skills, nurses are often the entry point into the system for patients and their families.

Health care providers in all settings must be advocates for the chronically and terminally ill and their often overburdened caregivers. The Canadian hospice palliative care treatment model (Ferris, Balfour, Bowen, et al., 2002) and the advanced-care-planning national framework (Canadian Hospice Palliative Care Association, 2010b) provide tools that promote patient- and family-centred care for people facing potentially life-threatening situations. The tools support basic human rights, including having control over decisions affecting health and living situations; having advance directives completed and followed, such as instructions to suspend or withhold curative efforts; and receiving excellent palliative care that promotes optimum comfort.

## HOSPICE PALLIATIVE CARE

In 1967, in response to a system in which dying people were often neglected, isolated, and left to die in pain, Dame Cicely Saunders, a nurse, social worker, and physician, established St. Christopher's Hospice in London (Clarke, 2010; Richmond, 2005). Dame Cicely received universal recognition as the founder of the modern hospice movement. Central to her work was an aggressive pursuit of effective pain management that contributed to optimal quality of life (Richmond, 2005).

During the same time period, in the United States, Dr. Elisabeth Kübler-Ross, also a nurse, began actively listening to the terminally ill. In her groundbreaking work, Kübler-Ross (1969) identified distinctive phases, or cycles, in people's responses to terminal illness: denial, anger, bargaining, depression, and acceptance. She also realized that personal growth actually accelerated in the last stages of life. Encouraged by the work of Kübler-Ross, those working with the dying adapted the St. Christopher's comprehensive model, and the multidisciplinary care team evolved to include a physician, a nurse, a social worker, a pastor or chaplain, and an aide.

The term *palliative care* was first coined in the mid-1970s by Canadian physician Balfour Mount, who was inspired by the work of Kübler-Ross and Dame Cicely Saunders (Cahill, 2010). Like those before him, Dr. Mount found that treatments for the terminally ill were abysmally inadequate, so he set up a hospital-based palliative care unit at the Royal Victoria Hospital in Montreal, taking the name *palliative* from its meaning, "to improve the quality of something" (Duffy, 2005). Dr. Balfour is known as "the father of palliative care," an approach that evolved into a pan-Canadian movement, with goals of relieving suffering and improving quality of life for those who are living with or dying from an illness (Ferris, Balfour, Bowen, et al., 2002). This movement eventually led to the development of the Canadian Hospice Palliative Care Association (CHPCA), established in 1991 (Ferris, Balfour, Bowen, et al., 2002), which is the national voice for hospice palliative care (HPC) in Canada. HPC is defined as whole-person health care aimed at relieving suffering and improving quality of life rather than aiming for a cure (Canadian Hospice Palliative Care Association, 2013).

Death is considered a natural and inevitable part of life. Using an interdisciplinary approach, the national HPC model is appropriate for patients and families of all ages living with or at risk for developing a life-threatening illness of any kind or magnitude, for whom HPC may complement therapy or be the total focus of care (Ferris, Balfour, Bowen, et al., 2002). The goals of HPC are to address all needs (physical, psychological, social, cultural, spiritual, and practical), prepare for and manage self-determined life closure and the dying process, and help with coping with loss and grief during illness and bereavement (Canadian Hospice Palliative Care Association, 2013). Historically, the terms *hospice* and *palliative care* were often used interchangeably; however, the CHPCA has brought the two terms together to form HPC. One of the central themes of HPC in Canada is the belief that each of us has the right to die pain-free and with dignity (Canadian Hospice Palliative Care Association, 2013).

> **VIGNETTE**
>
> Mr. Spence contracted amyotrophic lateral sclerosis (ALS) at the age of 52. He lived at home until his care overwhelmed his family, and he has now been in a care centre for nine months. He is almost completely paralyzed but can still use a letter board with a head-mounted laser pointer. He has a warm smile and a pleasant gaze. He is experiencing shooting pains in his legs and has increasing difficulty with swallowing and breathing. Despite being barely able to eat, he has refused a feeding tube. The staff feel helpless. How can they just stand by while he starves to death? Will he starve to death? One of the aides has decided to quit working with him because caring for Mr. Spence has become so emotionally difficult for her.
>
> An HPC referral was made. A nurse and social worker visited the care facility and offered practical help and guidance for staff, patient, and family in treating Mr. Spence. They talked with him about what to expect as his condition declines. Comfort-oriented medication and nonpharmacological care were reviewed, and Mr. Spence was offered as many choices as possible. Emotional, spiritual, and educational support were offered to the family and staff concerning the course of the illness, anticipatory grieving, and ways of using the remaining time to meet goals and nurture relationships. Mr. Spence, assisted by his family and an HPC volunteer, chose to work on a memoir about his illness and its impact on his growth as a person.

Quality palliative care is the right of every Canadian (Carstairs, 2010). Although palliative care is widely available to all Canadians, regardless of age or diagnosis, access to high-quality integrated care is not the same across the county. Despite the progressive move toward an integrated, streamlined system, many Canadians, unlike Mr. Spence, are still dying without adequate supports (Carstairs, 2010; Canadian Hospice Palliative Care Association, 2010c). Among the reasons for this lack of supports are geography, lack of patient-centred care, lack of knowledge and policy leadership, cultural diversity, and funding.

Although HPC grew from the concept of caring for the dying, it is now used to guide care at any point during an acute, chronic, or life-threatening illness or bereavement (Ferris, Balfour, Bowen, et al., 2002).

Carstairs (2010) suggested that because Canadians are living longer with chronic health conditions, access to quality care is required at an earlier point in the continuum of life and not just at the end of life. Patients can receive HPC in hospital, at home, in community care homes (e.g., long-term care), or in hospice programs. Respite beds are also available. However, Collier (2011) said that serving marginalized populations, particularly the homeless, is problematic. Recently, CMA president, Dr. Jeffrey Turnbull, helped establish a palliative hospice in an Ottawa homeless shelter, with successful outcomes for patients, even saving substantial government health care dollars (Podymow, Turnbull, & Coyle, 2006). Several factors need to be considered when determining the best place for providing care, such as personal choice, a balance between patient and family needs, and the availability of resources to meet those needs.

Regardless of setting, the HPC approach is multidisciplinary. In addition to access to health care providers, this approach also requires spiritual care, volunteer services, bereavement services, medical equipment, medications, and supplies related to the illness. A personalized plan of care is developed with the patient, reflected in the care, and regularly reviewed and updated.

## NURSING CARE AT THE END OF LIFE

*End-of-life (EOL) care* is a term adopted to make it clear that a person dying from any cause, other than sudden and unexpected death, might benefit from HPC services (Ministry of Health, 2006). Providing nursing care for those at the end of life, and supporting their families in any setting, calls for a holistic approach, assisting people as they progress through the final stage of life.

### Hospice Palliative Care Nursing

While nurses are educated to provide holistic care, few are prepared to deal with the death and dying trajectory they will ultimately face at some point in their career. A survey by the Canadian Association Schools of Nursing (CASN) demonstrated the need for enhanced preparation for new graduate nurses when dealing with death and dying experiences (Canadian Association Schools of Nursing, 2008), prompting the development of an educational resource (Jacono, Cable-Williams, Foster, et al., 2009). In addition to providing practical care, nurses need to demonstrate enhanced communication, coordination, and management skills, self-care, and the ability to "recognize and attend to the meaning in suffering" (Vogel, 2011, p. 418). Nurses working in HPC settings should pursue additional certification.

### The Art, Presence, and Caring of Nursing

Caring for patients at the end of life requires a shift in professional expectations. It involves not only curing but also healing concepts of care (Hutchinson, Hutchinson, & Arnaert, 2009),

the demand for genuine human presence toward the patient while using evidence-informed knowledge, the management of pain and symptom control, and other technical aspects of care. "Whole-person care" involves seeing the patient first as a human being while being attentive to all aspects of suffering. The Canadian Hospice Palliative Care Association (2006) developed gold standards for nurses providing HPC and EOL care, with the following five dimensions of nursing to help guide their work in any setting.

- **Valuing**—believing in the intrinsic value of others, in the value of life, and that death is a natural process
- **Connecting**—establishing a therapeutic relationship with the person and the family through making, sustaining, and closing the relationship
- **Empowering**—providing care that is empowering for the person and the family
- **Doing for**—providing care based on best practice in pain and symptom management, coordination of care, and advocacy
- **Finding meaning**—helping the person and family find meaning in their lives and their experiences of illness

Inherent in these dimensions is the ability to engage in therapeutic relationships with people who are grounded in the *art*, *presence*, and *caring* concepts of nursing. Previously, these three were considered individual concepts, but Finfgeld-Connett (2008a) proposed their convergence into one theoretical framework based on their similarities. Interactions with patients are characterized by openness and honesty, while demonstrating vulnerability, kindness, compassion, and empathy (Finfgeld-Connett, 2006; 2008b; 2008c). Positive outcomes are experienced by the nurse as well as the patient, with enhanced physical well-being for the patient and enhanced emotional well-being for both (Finfgeld-Connett, 2008a).

To approach nursing work with art, presence, and caring, two essential skills you can practise are listening and observing (see Chapters 10 and 11). Reflect back to the speaker what you heard by restating or summarizing the message. Observe the patient's nonverbal communications. Do you sense well-being? Sorrow? Suffering? Ask the patient and family open-ended questions like the following:

- Would you tell me what this is like for you?
- How do you see your condition right now?
- Where do you see things going?
- Are you worried about anything?
- What are you hoping for?

Practise staying silent and giving the patient or family member all the time needed to respond. Offer a reassuring touch. The artful, present, and caring nurse can invite and permit the patient to discover new dimensions of his or her own experiences, bringing greater wholeness.

### Assessment for Spiritual Issues

Spirituality, the dimension of human experience that can provide meaning for life, is integral to EOL care. Conducting a comprehensive spiritual assessment is important to understanding how a patient's spirituality may enhance comfort. Edwards, Pang, Shiu, and colleague (2010) found that, much like physical care, spiritual care was something felt by patients. They want to feel genuinely cared about and have the opportunity to talk about their fears, hopes, issues, and despair. Nurses must focus on presence, listening, connecting, creating openings, and engaging in reciprocal sharing as they make the journey with their patients. Time spent with the patient and family is considered essential for successful outcomes (Bailey, Moran, & Graham, 2009; Edwards, Pang, Shiu, et al., 2010). Assessment of spirituality is best guided by an appropriate spirituality assessment tool such as SHARE (Kramer-Howe & Huls, 2004), FICA (Puchalski, 2007), or HOPE (Anandarajah & Hight, 2001). Regardless of the tool used, it is important to use unbiased, open language and ensure appropriate timing in the relationship, having already established trust and rapport (Dameron, 2005). Some examples of questions may be, Tell me how you are doing spiritually. What gives your life meaning? What role do your beliefs play in regaining your health? Spiritual caring is a huge part of holistic care and can be interwoven with the nurse's daily work through the process of self-awareness, empathy, and commitment to EOL care (Bailey, Moran, & Graham, 2009). In addition to thoroughly assessing connections to a specific religion, nurses can become skilled at listening for the patient's intrinsic spirituality. For many patients, religion provides context, community, and comfort when facing EOL challenges.

## Awareness and Sensitivity of Cultural Contexts

Spiritual and cultural contexts and care are often inextricably intertwined. While it is impossible for the nurse to know all things about all cultures, it is imperative as professionals to be aware of the need to explore cultural practices impacting care at all times across the health care continuum (see Chapter 7). Canada is a multicultural nation, but in particular, it has a growing older adult Aboriginal population (Bourassa, Hampton, Baydala, et al., 2010; Prince & Kelley, 2010). As Aboriginals age, they suffer even higher burdens of chronic disease and illness than non-Aboriginal Canadians. In addition, many Aboriginal people live in rural communities, which often do not have the same access to health care services (palliative care among these) as their urban counterparts. Like other Canadians, the majority of Aboriginal people living in remote First Nations communities would prefer to die at home (Wilson, Justice, Sheps, et al., 2006; McGrath, 2007). However, unlike many other Canadians, they are not often given this opportunity, due to a lack of services and resources (Prince & Kelley, 2010). In addition to this difference, even when HPC is available, it is often not safe for or sensitive to Aboriginal or other cultures. Bourassa, Hampton, Baydala, and colleagues (2010) developed a curriculum for health care providers that is inclusive of culturally sensitive and appropriate protocols for providing support to Aboriginal families in need of HPC services. Many cultural practices of Aboriginals (e.g., respect for elders, the special gifts of elders, the role of sacred items such as feathers, ceremonies) are rooted in culture and grounded in spirituality (Bourassa, Hampton, Baydala, et al., 2010). Research on palliative care for First Nations communities is a priority (see Research Highlight Box).

 **RESEARCH HIGHLIGHT**

### First Nations Communities and Palliative Care

**Source:** Prince, H., & Kelley, M.L. (2010). An integrative framework for conducting palliative care research with First Nations communities. *Journal of Palliative Care, 26*(1), 47–53.

**Problem**

Many elders were dying in hospital and long-term care homes outside their communities due to a lack of palliative care programs for First Nations.

**Purpose of Study**

The purpose of the study was to develop a framework to help guide the development and implementation of palliative care programs in twelve First Nations communities in northwestern Ontario and to evaluate the interventions and resources used.

**Methods**

Partnerships were formed with Aboriginal health organizations; 12 First Nations communities composed of elders, chiefs, and residents; and the researchers. A needs assessment—including questionnaires, interviews, and focus groups—helped identify values and beliefs related to death and dying and EOL care issues. Each community then identified and developed culturally appropriate educational materials.

**Key Findings**

The integrative palliative care framework included the development of strong partnerships, using a participatory action research approach that adhered to research ethics, embraced ownership and control, and celebrated cultural competence and safety across all cultural groups encountered, including the research team. Three of the 12 communities involved in the study followed up by developing local palliative care teams, and regional palliative care experts further supported the development of protocols for home death.

**Implications for Nursing Practice**

Nurses can and should be a part of culturally sensitive palliative care research. Strategies from the framework provide useful approaches for nurses, who—as part of their professional practice competencies—are responsible for demonstrating sensitivity to and respect for diversity in health practices and beliefs (e.g., spirituality, culture) and for advocating for improved services.

## Palliative Symptom Management

Excellent symptom management is a hallmark of HPC nursing (Canadian Hospice Palliative Care Association, 2008). The patient or substitute decision maker has the right to be informed and make decisions about all aspects of care, including the right to a dignified and comfortable death (Canadian Hospice Palliative Care Association, 2008; Canadian Nurses Association, 2008). Nurses can offer a wide spectrum of interventions to alleviate symptoms, guided by patients' own reports and careful assessment. The most commonly reported EOL symptoms are pain, constipation, dyspnea, fatigue, depression, and delirium (Lee & Washington, 2008). It is gratifying to relieve pain or

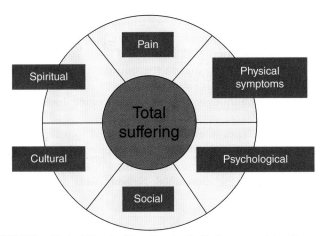

FIGURE 33-1 Woodruff's Total Suffering model. **Source:** Woodruff, R. (2004). *Palliative medicine: Evidence-based symptomatic and supportive care for patients with advanced cancer* (4th ed.). New York: Oxford University Press.

| BOX 33-1 | GUIDELINES WHEN CARING FOR THE DYING |
|---|---|

***Pain***—Remember that patients' pain is what they say it is, and they have the right to have their pain needs met effectively, using the simplest route. Reassure them that you will provide relief from their pain to help decrease their anxiety.

***Physical***—Intervene quickly to manage symptoms that may affect other organ systems (e.g., nausea, constipation or diarrhea, incontinence, air hunger, inadequate nutrition) in order to promote and maintain the highest level of comfort possible.

***Psychological***—Keep patients and their families informed about the disease and its symptoms. Invite them to deal with their emotions, acknowledging the losses and changes in their lives. Practise the art of presence and caring through active listening, genuine empathy, and personal sharing.

***Social***—Many people at the end of life are afraid of dying alone and need reassurance that they are not alone. Promote this sense of security by verbalizing this reassurance, and demonstrate it by responding to their needs quickly and spending time with them. Provide companionship for them by supporting their visitors, engaging in conversations with them and their families, and providing privacy when appropriate or when requested.

***Cultural***—Ask questions to discover the person's cultural background and meaningful practices used during EOL care to promote a peaceful journey. Explore appropriate language used (are there any taboo words?), and inquire about whom to share information with first. Explore the role of the family in care, and explore care practices other than science-based medicine, such as alternative medicines or other therapies.

***Spiritual***—By asking appropriate questions, offer the opportunity to patients to discuss what is meaningful in their lives, such as relationships, any faith or spiritual practices they use to keep themselves calm, and who or what they turn to when dealing with the challenges of life. Exploring spirituality can offer the opportunity to assess and promote effective coping skills based on past behaviours.

nausea or to give patients control over bowel medications and breathing treatments. For symptoms such as worry, fear, sadness, and low energy, however, better approaches might include education, normalization, counselling, integrative therapies (e.g., massage, music), and stress-reduction practices.

Each symptom should be assessed individually. Treatable, reversible, and temporary conditions can be mistakenly attributed to the terminal diagnosis. For example, if a patient reports feeling depressed, it is important not to assume that the feelings are due to the dying process. If the patient becomes confused or lethargic, it is essential to rule out causes such as medication effects, dehydration, delirium, urinary tract infections, and constipation before attributing the symptom to terminal decline.

Care of the patient and family can be viewed from the lens of Roger Woodruff's Total Suffering model. See Figure 33-1. This model can also be used to describe guidelines when caring for the dying (see Box 33-1). The use of such a model can help guide the practice of nurses throughout the nursing process when working with palliative care patients.

## The Importance of Effective Communication

Nurses need excellent communication skills when working in all settings, at all times, and with all members involved in the HPC experience (Heyland, Dodek, Rocker, et al., 2006; Heyland, Cook, Rocker, et al., 2010; Reinke, Shannon, Engelberg, et al., 2010). Nurses have a role even at the beginning of the EOL continuum. The value of simply asking patients and their families, "Do you have any concerns?" followed by strong encouragement to seek out their support system while waiting for news (Brown, 2011) cannot be understated.

Having information about the patient's condition in preparation for the death has been shown to improve both bereavement outcomes and family satisfaction (Rhodes, Mitchell, Miller, et al., 2008). During stressful periods, two factors seem to make things more bearable: (1) the ability to have—or believe

one can have—some control over the situation and (2) the ability to predict changes. Information and education from nurses can improve a family's sense of control. Information should be conveyed slowly, given repeatedly, written down, and reviewed often. People tend to need several reiterations of information when under stress (see Chapter 12).

Effective communication skills are at the heart of developing a therapeutic relationship, assessing the patient, and providing holistic care to the patient and family. A strong therapeutic relationship will guide discussions and decision making for patients and families in times of loss (see Chapter 10). In addition, effective communication helps decrease distress and total pain and suffering (Canadian Hospice Palliative Care Association, 2009b).

The following vignette illustrates the confusion and misery that can result from lack of information, the desire to take control of one's life situation, and the inadequacy of the term *dying* to describe living with a terminal disease.

## Anticipatory Grief

Patients and families can experience "grief ahead of time," known as anticipatory grief, when they receive a life-limiting diagnosis (Nelson, 2011) or when threatened with loss of ability to function independently, loss of identity, and changes in role definition (Hottensen, 2010). Future loss is mourned as people acknowledge the importance of the impending loss, adjust their lives to accommodate the intervening time, and anticipate how their futures will be altered by the loss (Hottenson, 2010). Sensitive communication and support can help family members process this information.

The experience of anticipatory grief varies by individual, family, and culture (see Box 33-2). Clukey (2007) described anticipatory grieving as adjusting one's own life to meet caregiving demands ..., "doing it all" and being overwhelmed at times, and finalizing the connection with the dying person. A common emotional experience is anger (e.g., at the disease, at the medical community), in addition to sadness, hurt, fear,

**VIGNETTE**

Susan, a 74-year-old divorced woman living alone, is told by her doctor that she is dying of liver cancer. Upon hearing that she cannot be cured, she assumes she will die in a few days or weeks. She goes home, settles all her affairs, calls everyone she cares about and says goodbye, accepts hospice care, and begins to await death. As weeks and then months go by, Susan feels betrayed by her doctor, embarrassed to be alive, unsure how to behave, and uncomfortable with her friends and relatives. She has time to begin worrying about how her death will be, how much control she will lose, and how she can afford care at the end. She is confused and even disoriented by the unexpected apparent improvement in her symptoms.

Susan shares her feelings with the nurse. The nurse educates Susan about her cancer and how to interpret her symptoms. The HPC team addresses her emotions and needs in many ways. They encourage her to take a trip she had postponed and to begin seeing friends again. They educate her on the concept of "living with terminal illness" rather than dying from it. Susan needs to learn new approaches to living meaningfully with an uncertain future. When Susan finally enters the end stage of her disease, she is comfortable and cared for by her relatives at home.

### BOX 33-2   SIGNS OF ANTICIPATORY GRIEF

- Feelings of emptiness or of being lost
- A sense of being numb and fatigued
- A feeling of unreality and disbelief
- Periods of weeping or raging
- The desire to run away from the situation
- The need to protect the patient from suffering or death by overseeing every detail of care
- Worry about the future and the unknown
- Anger at the patient, health care providers, or both
- Pronounced clinging to or dependency on the patient or other family members
- Fear of going crazy

anxiety, and hidden grief. Nurses can help patients and loved ones understand that their feelings are common and assist them with developing coping strategies and with redefining their roles within the family and in the outside world (Hottenson, 2010). Nurses must also remind those in their care to keep in mind that, although they are experiencing loss, there is always hope.

As with all types of grieving, nurses need to recognize that people can experience symptoms of grief physically, cognitively, emotionally, socially, and spiritually (Canadian Hospice Palliative Care Association, 2008; Nelson, 2011) and intervene appropriately.

### The Four Gifts of Resolving Relationships

An important role of the nurse during EOL care is to invite families to accept the dying of their loved one and say goodbye. Taking the opportunity to say goodbye has been correlated with more positive bereavement outcomes (Gamino & Sewell, 2004). The Four Gifts of Resolving Relationships is one means of opening conversations about the coming separation. The concept of the *Four Gifts* was interpreted from the writings of Elisabeth Kübler-Ross and used with her permission by Beverly Ryan of the Hospice of the Twin Cities in Minnesota. In her workshops for the terminally ill, Dr. Kübler-Ross witnessed many couples and families shift from being distant, cold, or angry to becoming warm, loving, and close. She observed that this change resulted from a predictable sequence of communications, which were later formulated into the Four Gifts. People often intuitively recognize the gifts as processes they have already been experiencing. Perhaps these processes are innate within human relationships, but anxiety, sorrow, and denial can obstruct their expression.

The nurse can describe the gifts in simple terms and encourage families and patients to express them in their own ways. The gifts—forgiveness, love, gratitude, and farewell—can work for both giver and receiver. When given with sincerity and simplicity, they can precipitate a healing shift in relationships.

*Forgiveness.* The first step in forgiveness is to admit to wrongs and hurts experienced in the relationship. The intention is to forgive, seek forgiveness, and release the hurt so healing can occur. Sometimes a face-to-face encounter is not possible (e.g., when the patient is sedated, comatose, or experiencing dementia), and sometimes it is not advisable (e.g., when it would cause more distress than it would relieve). Reconciliation requires two people who wish to heal a broken relationship. Forgiveness is a one-sided act, which can be given unilaterally. Granting forgiveness does not mean condoning or accepting a truly injurious or abusive action. It does not make a wrong right. What it does is signal a desire to let go of blame and anger, to release one's own heart from the chains of resentment. As such, it is a gift to the one who offers forgiveness, whether reconciliation is possible or not.

*Love.* The second gift is to express love to each other. Many adult children wish to hear their parent say, "I love you, and I am proud of you." Between spouses, in some long-term marriages, these words have faded away to be replaced by daily togetherness and the practical caring of a shared life. It is not uncommon in bereavement for survivors to regret that they did not hear or say the words, "I love you," and long for that final recognition of the relationship's value. Ultimately, the message we need to hear at the end of life is that we are loved for being who we are, not for what we have done or achieved.

*Gratitude.* Expressions of love naturally flow into gratitude for what each has been in the other person's life. People look back over life together and remember the good times and the tough times. They can take out photograph albums, show videotapes, reminisce, and listen again to favourite stories. It is especially gratifying to acknowledge the things that were taken for granted. Parents or caregivers may never have been thanked for going to work every day for 30 or 40 years, caring for the home, or offering nurturance, support, or guidance. Similarly, acknowledgement of the love and attention of caregivers or dependents can be important expressions of gratitude. Many exhausted caregivers weep when they are told they really are doing a good job and are appreciated.

*Farewell.* Many people say they hate goodbyes because they bring up feelings of grief at the finality of parting. Also, it is awkward to say goodbye before someone is actually leaving. It may appear to be rushing the person or even causing the departure. Yet when the final separation of death awaits us, the act of saying goodbye is deeply appropriate and meaningful. In cases when there is no chance to say goodbye, or when the opportunity to say goodbye is not taken, survivors may express long-term regret. The words or gestures used do not matter as long as the meaning is adequately expressed.

---

**VIGNETTE**

Trent is a 28-year-old man with developmental disabilities and bipolar disorder. He arrives at his dying father's home to see him for the last time. Trent lives in a group home and has not seen his family for many months. The last time he visited, he had not taken his medication, and his behaviour caused his family to avoid him. The HPC nurse tells Trent his father is dying and explains the Four Gifts. The young man sadly enters his father's bedroom and sits on the bed. He says, "Dad, I know you are going to die, and I want you to know that I am so sorry for the ways I have acted and the trouble I have caused. Please forgive me, Dad. You have always looked out for me, and I shouldn't have gone off my meds. I love you, Dad. You've never given up on me. Thank you for finding me the place where I live and people to love me and look after me. Thanks for being my dad. I know I have to say goodbye. I promise I will keep taking my meds so I will behave right. I promise I'll listen to my counsellors and have a good life. I love you so much, Dad. Goodbye." He weeps with his father, who holds him for a little while. Then he comes out of the room with a tear-streaked face, knowing he will never see his father alive again. He feels complete, however. He has said the important things with courage and taken proper leave of his father.

---

In the preceding vignette, Trent did not rehearse, resist, or complicate the Four Gifts but used the sequence to express the full range of his feelings. His story illustrates how simple and natural this process can be. Many families need no encouragement to forgive, cherish, thank, and release a loved one. The

Four Gifts can be a helpful contribution, however, to families whose members are overwhelmed, cling to false hope, or are emotionally reticent.

### Self-Care

As front-line medical caregivers, nurses are educated to help patients get better, stronger, and more independent. Supporting patients at the end of life, as they grow weaker, sicker, and ultimately die, can be overwhelming, challenging the nurse's sense of competency and professionalism. The demands inherent in EOL nursing lead to increased vulnerability to emotional attachments and compassion fatigue. These experiences, along with daily exposure to grief and dying, require nurses to practise conscious self-care in both their professional and private lives. Health care providers naturally grow attached to some patients and may experience both anticipatory grieving and bereavement. To maintain emotional balance and health, it is essential to rely on the support of others and practise good self-care. This is a journey that promotes greater self-understanding, wisdom, and compassion (Bailey, Murphy, & Porock, 2011). The multidisciplinary team approach of supportive supervision is helpful in this process.

Caring for patients who are dying and those who grieve can bring up personal reactions, which may be triggered by a patient who is younger than the nurse, one who resembles a significant person in the nurse's own life, one who is experiencing symptoms reminiscent of other difficult deaths, or one who offends the nurse's sense of fairness or acceptability. Workplace conditions such as complex caseloads, rapid turnover in office staff, several losses in a short period of time, or too many demands for on-call time or overtime can intensify a nurse's vulnerability to feeling overwhelmed (Pereira, Fonseca, & Carvalho, 2011). Box 33-3 provides guidelines to help the health care provider maintain emotional health when working with death and the dying.

## NURSING CARE FOR THOSE WHO GRIEVE

Loss is part of the human experience, and grieving is the response that enables people to accept and reconcile the loss and adapt to change. We grieve the commonplace losses in our lives, be they loss of a relationship (e.g., divorce, separation, death, abortion); health (e.g., a body function or part, mental or physical capacity); friendship, status, or prestige; security (e.g., occupational, financial, social, cultural); or a dream. Other normal losses include changes in circumstances, such as retirement, promotion, marriage, and aging. These losses can promote growth through adaptation or may result in apathy, anger, and resentment.

Losing a significant person through death is a major life crisis. Long-term relationships deeply bond us to each other, shaping our world and our identity in it. Their loss can diminish aspects of our own self-concept and tear apart our assumptive world. Grief is experienced holistically, affecting us emotionally, cognitively, spiritually, and physically. Those who grieve sometimes describe the death of a loved one as an amputation.

## GRIEF REACTIONS, BEREAVEMENT, AND MOURNING

Grief encompasses all of an individual's reactions to loss and is defined as sorrow experienced in anticipation of, during, and after a loss (Ferris, Balfour, Bowen, et al., 2002). Normal grief reactions include depressed mood, insomnia, anxiety, poor appetite, loss of interest, guilt, dreams about the deceased, and poor concentration. Psychological states include shock, denial, and yearning or searching for the deceased. Bereavement, derived from the Old English word *berafian*, meaning "to rob," is the period of grieving following a death. Mourning refers to things people do to cope with their grief, including shared, social expressions of grief, such as attending funerals and participating in bereavement groups. Everyone grieves, but not everyone engages in the work of mourning. The length of time, degree, and rituals for mourning are often typically determined by cultural, religious, and familial factors. Despite a wide variation in experiences of duration and intensity, grief becomes a serious physical and mental health concern for relatively few people (Prigerson, Horowitz, Jacobs, et al., 2009).

The study of human grief and bereavement has evolved over the past 40 years. Research examines questions such as, What constitutes normal, healthy grieving? What are predictors of complicated grief? What interventions, if any, benefit different populations of grieving people? When is medication useful for the bereaved person? What is the impact of losses on family systems? What are cultural mediators of delivering grief support? How does complicated or unresolved grief affect public and private health care usage? What are best practices to intervene in special types of loss, such as traumatic loss, genocidal loss, societal loss, and wartime losses?

### Types of Grief

Grief is a multifaceted, deeply personal human response to loss. The time it takes to grieve is individual and unique to each person. Even each family member affected grieves differently. Many variables affect how people grieve, such as how the death occurred, coping skills, previous losses, other life stressors, and support systems. The nature of the relationship with the person who has died is of particular importance (Nelson, 2011). Nurses are in a position to provide appropriate assessment to help differentiate disenfranchised grief, anticipatory grief, and complicated grief from the normal grieving process (Canadian Hospice Palliative Care Association, 2008).

Disenfranchised grief can occur when losses are not always openly acknowledged, supported, or recognized as significant, such as a loss through suicide, the loss of a friend, the loss of a pet, or the grief of someone thought incapable of grieving (e.g., a child, a person with dementia) (Nelson, 2011). A sense of isolation can occur, and nurses need to recognize the grief as real and intervene by acknowledging the loss, supporting feelings, and encouraging the person grieving to reach out to supportive networks.

Nurses also need to recognize when grief becomes complicated grief, a term applied to severe (prolonged, dysfunctional, or maladaptive) reactions after the loss of a loved one. In the past, there was debate about how best to recognize and manage more severe reactions to grief, with some supporting the need to consider complicated grief a separate entity under the *Diagnostic and Statistical Manual of Mental Disorders*, and others arguing the need to stop trying to pathologize varied grief experiences (Collier, 2011; Harris, 2010; & Worden, 2009). The newly revised *DSM-5* has addressed this debate and cautions clinicians to differentiate normal grieving from a mental health diagnosis of major depressive or adjustment disorders, following clear criteria for these distinct disorders. The goal is to ensure that those who need intervention receive an accurate diagnosis.

With appropriate supports, patients should be allowed to experience grief as a normal process of life in their own unique and personal way. Nurses should consider *Chronic sorrow* as a potential nursing diagnosis, defined as "the presence of pervasive, grief-related feelings that have been found to occur periodically throughout the lives of individuals with chronic health conditions, their family caregivers and the bereaved" (as cited in Alligood & Thomey, 2010, p. 656). A Theoretical Model of Chronic Sorrow was developed by Eakes, Burke, and Hainsworth (1998) and can be used by nurses to help understand the reactions to loss and as a tool to view the experience of bereavement (see Figure 33-2). *Chronic sorrow* is also defined

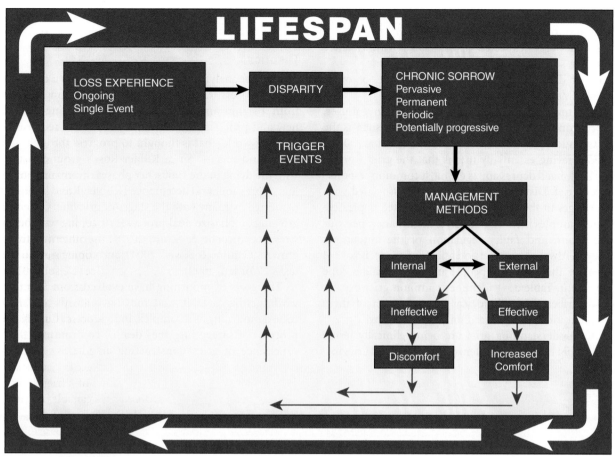

**FIGURE 33-2**  Theoretical Model of Chronic Sorrow. **Source:** Eakes, G.G., Burke, M.L., & Hainsworth, M.A. (1998). The middle-range theory of chronic sorrow (Figure 1). *The Journal of Nursing Scholarship, 30*(2), 179–184. Copyright © 2007, John Wiley and Sons.

as "the periodic recurrence of permanent, pervasive sadness or other grief-related feelings associated with ongoing disparity resulting from a loss experience" (Eakes, Burke, & Hainsworth, 1998, p. 180). That "chronic sorrow is viewed as a normal response to an abnormal situation" (p. 180) is a key premise of the model. These nurse theorists recognize that people may periodically re-experience initial grief-related feelings cyclically, precipitated by triggers. The model allows for coping strategies used by the person with chronic sorrow (internal) and for interventions provided by professionals (external). External interventions nurses may employ include the use of appropriate communication skills and education, such as teaching appropriate ways of coping.

Nurses are expected to identify those at risk for complicated grieving and differentiate between grief and depression (Canadian Hospice Palliative Care Association, 2009a), intervening in timely and appropriate ways, such as providing counselling and coordinating referrals.

Careful assessment must be done to determine the potential for complicated grieving. Factors that can complicate bereavement have been identified by Prigerson, Horowitz, Jacobs, and colleagues (2009) and include:

- Heavy emotional dependence on the deceased
- Unresolved conflicts between the bereaved person and the deceased

**VIGNETTE**

On a large, extended-family picnic, Mr. and Mrs. Doiron's youngest child was accidently crushed by the tires of a relative's truck as it backed up. The three-year-old died in her mother's arms on the way to the hospital. Many family members, including the older siblings of the toddler, witnessed the event. After six months, the Doiron family was still in chaos and shock. Mrs. Doiron, especially, was unable to resume normal responsibilities. Her husband had returned to work and did his best to support her. The surviving children were exhibiting behavioural problems. The Doirons sought out a grief counsellor and attended support groups. The mixture of horror, shock, anger, disbelief, grief, and senselessness that engulfed them complicated their mourning. Gradually, some of the feelings softened, and the family began to regain some stable routines. After two years, Mrs. Doiron had progressed to the point of organizing support networks in her daughter's name for parents whose children had suffered similar deaths.

- Young age of the deceased (often the most profound loss) or of the bereaved person
- Lack of a surviving meaningful relationship or support system
- A history of losses
- A lack of sound coping skills

- A death that was associated with a cultural stigma (e.g., acquired immune deficiency syndrome [AIDS], suicide)
- A death that was unexpected or associated with violence (e.g., murder, suicide)
- A history of depression, drug or alcohol abuse, or other psychiatric illness

Assessment may include validated screening inventories, such as depression and other specific grief measures such as the Brief Grief Questionnaire (Ito, Nakajima, Fujisawa, et al., 2012). Complicated grieving essentially means that the grief work is unresolved. Prolonged depression is the most common response to unresolved grief. Disturbances in mood are associated with biological changes in the body during stress-related depressive illness. Some examples include electrolyte disturbance, nervous system alterations, and faulty regulation of the autonomic nervous system. Always assess the potential for suicide. Box 33-4 offers guidelines that can help people and their families cope with bereavement. Table 33-1 identifies common grief experiences and describes the pathological intensification of these phenomena that indicates the need for psychotherapy.

Models for understanding grief are being clinically tested and refined so that health care systems can understand grieving, best utilize limited health care resources, and relieve suffering whenever possible.

## Theories

The psychoanalytic model of grieving posits a distinct psychological process that involves disengaging strong emotional ties from a significant relationship and reinvesting those ties in a new and productive direction. This process requires engaging in "grief work" that is thought to progress through predictable stages and phases. Since Kübler-Ross's groundbreaking work with the dying in the 1960s, her phases of denial, anger, bargaining, depression, and acceptance (Kübler-Ross, 1969) have been identified by many with the stages of grieving. Other models of grieving emphasize dual processes of coping with bereavement stressors (Stroebe & Schut, 2010), the potential for personal growth (Gamino & Sewell, 2004), and coping skills and adaptive tasks (Worden, 2009).

The goals of mourning have evolved from "doing the grief work, getting over it, and moving on with life." Many now regard mourning as a complex, individual, culturally embedded process of accepting the death, confronting the painful experience of grief, constructing an identity and a life in a

---

### BOX 33-4 GUIDELINES FOR DEALING WITH BEREAVEMENT

**Global effect of loss.** The death of someone close can be life-changing, affecting all areas of your life. It can feel as though your world has shattered. Grieving is a journey between how things were and how they will be. It is your personal journey.

**Grief as a natural process.** The grief you feel is because of living, loving, and having a connection with your loved one. Grief is a normal response to loss. Understanding how you respond can help.

**Individual differences in grieving styles.** How you grieve is a reflection of your personality, past losses, and the relationship you had with the person who died. Each person grieves in his or her own way and with his or her own timetable. Some people openly express their emotions, while others control their thoughts and emotions. Neither is right or wrong; each can be effective.

**Children and grief.** Children look to the adults in their lives to learn how to grieve. They are sensitive to the moods and behaviour of adults and will not talk about their thoughts and feelings unless the adults do. Children are frightened by what they do not know or understand. Simple information about death and grief is most helpful.

**Social connections and support.** You want and need support from others now more than ever. Some people may not be able to provide the understanding and caring you expect from them because of their own experience with grief or for other reasons. Because all of the relationships in your life will be altered in some way, it is normal to look at, change, or sometimes even end certain relationships. You may find the company of other bereaved people particularly comforting.

**Experiences you might have in grief.** You may feel very different from your usual self as your emotions, mind, and reactions seem unreliable. You may feel intense pain and emotions not felt before. You are not going crazy; these feelings are natural. Symptoms and emotions like fatigue, forgetfulness, and irritability are common.

**Fluctuations in the grief process.** As you journey through grief, your feelings and responses will vary at different times. There will be ups and downs; there may be good days and bad days. Understand and value the good days as a rest in your journey.

**Self-care and what helps.** There are things you can do to help yourself. Information about grief can help you understand. Be gentle, patient, and forgiving with yourself. Do what you can to keep some normal routine for health and social contact. Support may come from different sources (e.g., family, friends, bereavement groups, chat rooms). If you are concerned about yourself and your grief, seek professional help.

**Time for grief.** Despite what you may hear about "getting over it" or "the first year," there are no timelines for grief; it takes as long as it takes. Often the journey is longer than you or others expected, and you may feel pressured to "move on." This loss will continue to be part of your life, and you will always have times when you think about, miss, and grieve for your loved one.

**Grief as a spiritual journey of healing.** Your life has changed, putting you on a different path. Nothing will ever be the same, yet you must somehow go on and find meaning in your changed life. As the journey continues, you may experience healing and personal growth as a result of the suffering you have endured and the lessons you have learned about what you truly value.

**Source:** Adapted from Victoria Hospice Bereavement Services. (2011). *Ten things to know about grief.* Retrieved from http://www.victoriahospice.org/sites/default/files/imce/VicHospTenThings.pdf.

| TABLE 33-1 | COMMON EXPERIENCES DURING GRIEF AND THEIR PATHOLOGICAL INTENSIFICATION | |
|---|---|---|
| **PHENOMENON** | **TYPICAL RESPONSE** | **PATHOLOGICAL INTENSIFICATION** |
| Dying | Emotional expression and immediate coping with the dying process | Avoidance; feeling of being overwhelmed, dazed, confused; self-punitive feelings; inappropriately hostile feelings |
| Death and outcry | Outcry of emotions with news of the death and turning to others for help or isolating self with self-soothing | Panic; dissociative reactions, reactive psychoses |
| Warding off (denial) | Avoidance of reminders and social withdrawal, focusing elsewhere, emotional numbing, not thinking of implications to self or of certain themes | Maladaptive avoidance of confronting the implications of death, drug or alcohol abuse, promiscuity, fugue states, phobic avoidance, feeling of being dead or unreal |
| Re-experience (intrusion) | Intrusive experiences, including recollections of negative experiences during relationship with the deceased, bad dreams, reduced concentration, compulsive re-enactments | Flooding with negative images and emotions; uncontrolled ideation, self-impairing compulsive re-enactments, night terrors, recurrent nightmares, distraught feelings resulting from the intrusion of anger, anxiety, despair, shame, or guilt; physiological exhaustion resulting from hyperarousal |
| Working through | Recollection of the deceased and a contemplation of self with reduced intrusiveness of memories and fantasies and with increased rational acceptance, reduced numbness and avoidance, more "dosing" of recollections, and a sense of working through it | Feeling of inability to integrate the death with a sense of self and continued life; persistent warding-off of themes that may manifest as anxious, depressed, enraged, shame-filled, or guilty moods and psychophysiological syndromes |
| Completion | Reduction in emotional swings and a sense of self-coherence and readiness for new relationships; ability to experience positive states of mind | Failure to complete mourning, which may be associated with inability to work or create or to feel emotion or positive states of mind |

**Source:** Horowitz, M.J. (1990). A model of mourning: Change in schemas of self and others. *Journal of the American Psychoanalytic Association, 38*(2), 297–324. doi:10.1177/000306519003800202. Copyright © 1990 by SAGE. Reprinted by Permission of SAGE Publications.

transformed environment, and finding an enduring relationship with the deceased, based not on physical presence but on accurate memory. Depending on many factors, this process can take many months to a number of years. Our losses transform our lives, and we are never quite the same person again. Over time, people move from pain defining who they are, and constant preoccupation with their loss, to living with the residual pain and forever carrying the memory of the loved one.

### Dual Process Model of Coping With Bereavement

Bereavement is an enormously challenging life stressor (Table 33-2). Healthy adaptation is crucial for long-term health and re-engagement in life. In a review of the dual process model (DPM), Stroebe and Schut (2010) identify adaptive versus maladaptive coping activities using three central constructs: loss-oriented coping, restoration-oriented coping, and oscillation (Richardson, 2010). The DPM attempts to address inadequacies in the "grief work" concept, such as a lack of specificity about grief stressors, cultural bias, the favouring of intuitive or female expressions of grief over instrumental styles (Stroebe & Schut, 2010), and the discounting of the value of denial and distraction in grieving.

Using the DPM as a guide, Stroebe & Schut (2010) identified *loss-oriented stressors*, which include concentrating on the loss experience, feeling the pain of grief, remembering, and longing. *Restoration-oriented stressors* re-engage the mourner with the outer world, as in overcoming loneliness (seeking social support), mastering skills and roles once performed by the deceased person, finding a new identity, and facing many practical details of life. By identifying specific coping activities on both sides of the model, the nurse can strengthen a grieving person's skills and reinforce positive meanings.

Both orientations assert that denial, avoidance, and distraction from grief are beneficial, as long as they are not excessive. The process of alternating between the two spheres of coping results in the third construct called *oscillation*, wherein confronting and avoiding various stressors of bereavement are an indication of healthy adaptation. However, a prolonged moving back and forth between these poles can be seen as an indication of complicated grieving (Stroebe & Schut, 2010).

### Four Tasks of Mourning

Many theorists who have studied the grief process, including George Engel, Colin Parkes, Erich Lindemann, John Bowlby, and J. William Worden, have identified similar, commonly

| TABLE 33-2 | PHENOMENA EXPERIENCED DURING BEREAVEMENT |
|---|---|
| **SYMPTOMS** | **EXAMPLES** |

### SENSATIONS OF SOMATIC DISTRESS

| | |
|---|---|
| The bereaved person may experience tightness in the throat, shortness of breath, sighing, mental pain, or exhaustion; food may taste like sand; things may feel unreal. Pain or discomfort may be identical to the symptoms experienced by the dead person. Normally, symptoms are brief. | A woman whose husband died of a stroke complains of weakness and numbness on her left side. |

### PREOCCUPATION WITH THE IMAGE OF THE DECEASED

| | |
|---|---|
| The bereaved person brings up and thinks and talks about numerous memories of the deceased. The memories are positive. This process goes on with great sadness. The idealization of the deceased lets the bereaved person relive the gratifications associated with the deceased and helps resolve any guilt she or he feels concerning the deceased. The bereaved person may also take on many of the mannerisms of the deceased through identification—identification serves the purpose of holding on to the deceased. Preoccupation with the dead person can continue for many months before it lessens. | A man whose wife recently died states, "I just can't stop thinking about my wife. Everything I see reminds me of her. We picked up this seashell on our honeymoon. I remember every wonderful moment we had together. The pain is so great, but the memories just keep coming." His friends notice that when he talks, his hand gestures and expressions are like those of his recently deceased wife. |

### GUILT

| | |
|---|---|
| The bereaved person reproaches himself or herself for real or fancied acts of negligence or omissions in the relationship with the deceased. | "I should have made him go to the doctor sooner." "I should have paid more attention to her, been more thoughtful." |

### ANGER

| | |
|---|---|
| The anger the bereaved person experiences may not be toward the object that gives rise to it. Often, the anger is displaced onto the medical or nursing staff. Other times, it is directed toward the deceased. The anger is at its height during the first month but is often intermittent throughout the first year. The overflow of hostility disturbs the bereaved person, resulting in the feeling that he or she is "going insane." | "The doctor didn't operate in time. If he had, Mary would be alive today." "How could he leave me like this ... how could he?" |

### CHANGE IN BEHAVIOUR: DEPRESSION, DISORGANIZATION, RESTLESSNESS

| | |
|---|---|
| The bereaved person may exhibit marked restlessness and an inability to organize his or her behaviour. A depressive mood during routine activities is common, decreasing as the year passes and the intensity of the grief declines. Absence of depression is more abnormal than its presence. Loneliness and aimlessness are most pronounced 6 to 9 months after the death. | Six months after her husband died, Mrs. Faye states, "I just can't seem to function. I have a hard time doing the simplest tasks. I can't be bothered with socializing. I feel so down ... so, so empty." |

### REORGANIZATION OF BEHAVIOUR DIRECTED TOWARD A NEW OBJECT OR ACTIVITY

| | |
|---|---|
| Gradually, the bereaved person renews his or her interest in people and activities. The grieving thus releases him or her from one interpersonal relationship, and new ones are free to take its place. | Twenty months after her husband's death, Mrs. Faye tells a friend, "I'll be away this weekend. I am going fishing with my brother and his friend. This is the first time I've felt like doing anything since Harry died." |

experienced psychological and behavioural phenomena, including the following:

- Shock and disbelief
- Sensation of somatic distress
- Preoccupation with the image of the deceased
- Guilt
- Anger
- Change in behaviour (e.g., depression, disorganization, restlessness)
- Reorganization of behaviour directed toward a new object or activity

Worden organizes aspects of mourning into four tasks: (1) accept the reality of the loss, (2) experience the pain of grief, (3) adjust to an environment without the loved one (externally, internally, and spiritually), and (4) relocate and memorialize the loved one. He emphasizes that every loss must be assessed according to mediating factors such as the nature of the person who died, the nature of the attachment, the circumstances of the death, personality factors, family history, social circumstances, and concurrent changes resulting from the death (Worden, 2009). His model can be readily understood by the mourner as empowering and hopeful and serves

## TABLE 33-3  GUIDELINES FOR HELPING PEOPLE IN ACUTE GRIEF

| INTERVENTION | RATIONALE |
|---|---|
| Give your full presence: Use appropriate eye contact, attentive listening, and appropriate touch. | Talking is one of the most important ways of dealing with acute grief. Listening patiently helps the bereaved person express all feelings, even ones he or she feels are "negative." Appropriate eye contact helps to convey that you are there and are sharing the person's sadness. Suitable human touch can express warmth and nurture healing. Inappropriate touch can leave a person confused and uncomfortable. |
| Be patient with the bereaved person in times of silence. Do not fill silence with empty chatter. | Sharing painful feelings during periods of silence is healing and conveys your concern. |
| Know about and share with the bereaved person information about the phenomena that occur during the normal mourning process because they may concern some people (e.g., intense anger at the deceased, guilt, symptoms the deceased had before death, unbidden floods of memories). Give the bereaved person support during the occurrence of these phenomena and a written handout to refer to. | Although the knowledge will not eliminate the emotions, it can greatly relieve a person who is thinking there is something wrong with having these feelings. |
| Encourage the support of family and friends. If no supports are available, refer the person to a community bereavement group. (Bereavement groups are helpful even when a person has many friends or much family support.) | Friends can help with routine matters—for example: • Bringing food into the house • Making phone calls • Driving to the funeral home • Taking care of the bereaved person's children or other family members |
| Offer spiritual support and referrals when needed. | Dealing with an illness or catastrophic loss can cause the most profound spiritual anguish. |
| When intense emotions are in evidence, show understanding and support (see Guidelines for Communication box). | Empathic words that reflect acceptance of a bereaved individual's feelings are healing. |

as a specific guide for the nurse providing counselling or therapy.

## Helping People Cope With Loss

The majority of people who suffer bereavement are resilient and recover from the experience. However, Stroebe (2009) is concerned that the emphasis on understanding the consequences of bereavement and the protective qualities that help people cope with loss has shifted focus from early interventions for those at risk for mental health problems or complicated grief. Van der Houwen, Stroebe, Stroebe, and colleagues (2010) assert that many risk factors for mental health problems associated with grief cannot be changed (e.g., gender, unexpected death) or might be difficult to change (e.g., a negative change in finances), but it is important to identify those risk factors that can be changed with appropriate interventions. Some people who are grieving are resilient, and limited counselling support, focusing on grief education, normalizing of experiences, and skilled supportive presence, seems to be helpful for them (Grimby & Johansson, 2008). As well, a deeper understanding of the grief process can provide reassurance for those grieving (Baier & Buechsel, 2012). Other helpful interventions include writing letters (both to and from the deceased), performing simple rituals and ceremonies, "dosing" times of grieving throughout the day or week, working on projects to

memorialize the deceased (e.g., planting a tree, creating a Web site), and planning ahead for holidays and anniversary dates. Table 33-3 provides guidelines for helping people grieve, and the Guidelines for Communication box offers advice for communicating with a person suffering a profound loss.

## Palliative Care for Patients With Dementia

The incidence of Alzheimer's disease and related dementias in Canada continues to grow at a staggering rate (Alzheimer Society, 2010), a trend that is expected to continue. It is difficult to determine survival or time until death (Lee & Chodosh, 2009), often leaving those with dementia to die without appropriate palliative care services (Mitchell, Kiely, & Hamel, 2004) or, as some researchers suggest, to receive aggressive interventions to the detriment of their quality of life (Ryan, Ingleton, Gardiner, et al., 2009). As with other chronic illnesses, HPC should be considered at the time of a dementia diagnosis and assessed regularly for changes in status. Enhanced educational opportunities for nurses and other caregivers about the unique elements of palliative dementia care are essential to promote increased comfort and enhanced quality of life for this population. The Registered Nurses' Association of Ontario (2004) best practice guideline for older adults with dementia, although not specifically from an HPC perspective, can help guide nursing practice.

## GUIDELINES FOR COMMUNICATION WITH A BEREAVED PERSON

| SITUATION | SAMPLE RESPONSE |
|---|---|
| When you sense an overwhelming sorrow | "This must hurt terribly." |
| When you hear anger in the bereaved person's voice | "I hear anger in your voice. Most people go through periods of anger when their loved one dies. Are you feeling angry now?" |
| If you discern guilt | "Are you feeling guilty? This is a common reaction many people have. What are some of your thoughts about this?" |
| If you sense a fear of the future | "It must be scary to go through this." |
| When the bereaved person seems confused | "This can be a bewildering time." |
| In almost any painful situation | "This must be very difficult for you." |

**Source:** Adapted from Robinson, D. (1997). *Good intentions: The nine unconscious mistakes of nice people* (p. 249). New York: Warner Books.

People with advanced dementia experience significant impairments in insight, language, and judgement, limiting their ability to communicate unmet needs and desires. Difficult behaviours such as irritability or refusal to cooperate with care are often a form of communication, indicating discomfort in body, mind, or spirit. Caregivers who use an anticipatory approach to care can frequently prevent or reduce behaviours that result when a person with dementia is unable to communicate important unmet needs. Caregivers must remember to focus on the person, rather than the disease, and recognize the numerous opportunities that arise with every interaction to affirm the meaning of the individual's life, uphold dignity, and provide pleasurable sensory and spiritual experiences. The goal is to create meaningful connections for these patients. One effective method for customizing care that honours the unique preferences and lifelong interests of the patient is to use some form of life story or About Me form (Dougherty, Gallagher, Cabral, et al., 2007). This abbreviated biography guides and informs care to enhance the patient's enjoyment of life's simple pleasures.

Best practice recommendations for palliative care in dementia are to ensure that people with advanced dementia are included in the provision of palliative care; they remain in familiar surroundings whenever possible; restraint-free policy and staff education programs are developed; and quality of EOL experiences for those with dementia and their families are evaluated (Joanna Briggs Institute, 2011). More specifically, it is also important to address health care decisions for those with advanced dementia, such as resuscitation, hospitalizations, antibiotics, and nutrition and hydration. Health care providers should (1) identify the patient's goals for care and consider educating the family to minimize aggressive medical interventions, (2) eliminate medications that may detract from safety or quality of life, and (3) proactively manage issues such as pain and depression. Families and friends spend a significant amount of time, finances, and emotions caring for a loved one with dementia. It is important to recognize and support the role of family caregivers as they navigate the day-to-day challenges and cope with many losses.

## IMPLICATIONS FOR FURTHER STUDY

We are emerging from a time when many people who are grieving have been pathologized and treated with psychotropic drugs for depression, anxiety, and sleep disorders. A recent study found that compassionate primary caregivers, seeing symptoms of acute grief such as crying and sleep disturbances in their older-adult patients, spontaneously prescribed benzodiazepines, contrary to all major guidelines on the subject (Cook, Marshall, Masci, et al., 2007). On the other end of the spectrum, grief has been overlooked by many health care providers as a possible underlying contributor to their patients' presenting problems. Internationally, grief recovery models are being adapted to diverse cultures to assist traumatized people, especially children and youth, to begin to heal and re-engage with life, hope, and the future. There is a growing urgency for practitioners to become knowledgeable and skilled at supporting human mourning in all health care settings. The realization of full human health and happiness may depend on it.

## KEY POINTS TO REMEMBER

- The HPC movement offers compassionate care for those who are dying. HPC focuses on patients' physical and emotional comfort and offers holistic support for people who are dying and their families.
- More hospitals are offering palliative expertise for EOL care, but in many hospitals, conflict continues to exist between the wishes of people who are dying and their families and the medical model of treatment that focuses on the prolongation of life.
- In work with HPC patients, nursing goals include providing physical, emotional, cultural, and spiritual support and helping with adjustments in lifestyle and relationships. Nurses need to see the value of providing a caring human presence even in the face of helplessness.
- People with dementia may exhibit challenging behaviours during EOL care that may communicate discomfort in mind, body, or spirit. Care should focus on providing meaningful connections with patients and between family members and patients.
- Those who work with people who are dying need to maintain their own emotional health. EOL care is usually delivered by multidisciplinary teams so that no one discipline

bears too much responsibility. Nurses need to learn to draw on team support, protect their private lives by setting clear personal boundaries, and recognize their human and professional limitations.

- Providing timely and ongoing information about the disease and its effects and about physical and psychological signs of death can help the family deal with anticipatory mourning.
- Health care workers involved in care of the dying can teach families communication skills, such as the Four Gifts of Resolving Relationships, that will help them to express love, share memories, say goodbye, and provide a sense of peace.
- Family members may experience anticipatory grief, and it is helpful for them to understand that this grief is normal, although difficult.

- Common phenomena are evident during the experience of grief, and mourning is greatly influenced by cultural norms. However, everyone's experience of grieving is shaped by many mediating factors, such as the relationship to the person who died and the capacities of the mourner.
- Indicators of the potential for complicated grief include social isolation, extensive dependency on the deceased person, unresolved interpersonal conflicts, loss of a child, violent and senseless death, and catastrophic loss.
- Grief work is successful when the relationship to the deceased person has been restructured, energy is available for new relationships and life pursuits, and the mourner can remember realistically both the pleasures and the disappointments of the lost relationship. Outcomes for successful grief work have been identified.

## CRITICAL THINKING

1. George is dying of pancreatic cancer. His wife and adult children are asking about using HPC services. Help George's family to make an informed decision by comparing and contrasting the HPC model of care with the medical model of care for someone who is dying.

2. How can you use the Four Gifts of Resolving Relationships in working with the families of dying people in your practice of nursing? Do you think you would find this tool useful for a personal family member in the future?

3. What are some concrete ways in which you can help another person to cope with a loss? Identify specific components in the following areas:

a. How can you let the person tell his or her story, and what is the potential therapeutic value of doing so?

b. Avoiding banal (overused or trite) advice, what are some things you might say that could offer comfort? Use the guidelines in Table 33-3 and the Guidelines for Communication box to describe how you would help a person who is suffering a profound loss.

4. What practices would demonstrate a culturally safe and sensitive approach for Aboriginal Canadian people seeking palliative care?

## CHAPTER REVIEW

1. The nurse is caring for a patient who is grieving. The patient has stated she is angry that she has been diagnosed with terminal cancer. Which behaviour should the nurse anticipate next as the patient reconciles her anger?
   1. Denial that she has cancer
   2. Depression over the diagnosis of cancer
   3. Acceptance that her cancer is a reality
   4. Begging God to remove the cancer from her body

2. The nurse is planning hospice palliative care for a dying patient. Which outcome is most appropriate?
   1. Patient will regain health
   2. Patient will remain pain-free
   3. Patient will not fear death
   4. Patient will decline all medications

3. Which patient statement regarding spirituality would require further nursing teaching?
   1. "I am not religious, so therefore I am not spiritual."
   2. "Death scares me."
   3. "My family is what gives my life meaning."
   4. "I believe in a higher power."

4. The nurse identifies that a patient is experiencing complicated grieving related to the loss of her spouse. Which evaluation finding would indicate that a treatment plan is appropriate? The patient:
   1. No longer thinks of her spouse
   2. Copes without the need for a support system
   3. States she should have taken her spouse to the doctor more often
   4. Laughs occasionally with her grandchildren

5. The nurse is caring for a patient whose partner—with whom she was having an affair—died suddenly after a myocardial infarction. The patient had told no one about the affair, so no friends or family were aware that she experienced a loss. How should the nurse document the patient's grieving?
   1. Disenfranchised grief
   2. Dysfunctional grief
   3. Maladaptive grief
   4. Normal bereavement

# Ⓔvolve WEBSITE

Post-Test interactive review

*Visit the Evolve Web site for Chapter Review Answers and Rationales, Critical Thinking Answer Guidelines, and additional resources related to the content in this chapter: http://evolve.elsevier.com/Canada/Varcarolis/psychiatric/*

## REFERENCES

Alligood, M.R., & Thomey, A.M. (2010). *Nursing theorists and their work* (7th ed.). St. Louis, MO: Mosby Elsevier.

Alzheimer Society. (2010). *Rising tide: The impact of dementia on Canadian society*. Retrieved from http://www.alzheimer.ca/en/Get-involved/Raise-your-voice/Rising-Tide.

Anandarajah, G., & Hight, E. (2001). Spirituality and medical practice: Using the HOPE questions as a practical tool for spiritual assessment. *American Family Physician*, 63(1), 81–88. Retrieved from http://www.aafp.org/afp/2001/0101/p81.pdf.

Baier, M., & Buechsel, R. (2012). A model to help bereaved individuals understand the grief process. *Mental Health Practice*, 16(1), 28–32.

Bailey, M., Moran, S., & Graham, M. (2009). Creating a spiritual tapestry: Nurses' experiences of delivering spiritual care to patients in an Irish hospice. *International Journal of Palliative Nursing*, 15(1), 42–48.

Bailey, C., Murphy, R., & Porock, D. (2011). Professional tears: Developing emotional intelligence around death and dying in emergency work. *Journal of Clinical Nursing*, 20(23/24), 3364–3372.

Bourassa, C., Hampton, M., Baydala, A., et al. (2010). Completing the circle: End of life care with aboriginal families. Canadian Virtual Hospice. Retrieved from http://www.virtualhospice.ca/en_US/Main+Site+Navigation/Home/For+Professionals/For+Professionals/The+Exchange/Current/Completing+the+Circle_++End+of+Life+Care+with+Aboriginal+Families.aspx.

Brown, L.P. (2011). From the other side of the curtain: The nurse as patient. *The ABNF Journal*, 22(1), 13–14.

Cahill, G. (2010, August 25). Whole person care: The legacy of Balfour Mount [Web log post]. *Social innovation generation*. Retrieved from http://sigeneration.ca/blog/?p=52.

Canadian Association of Schools of Nursing. (2008). *Final report: Competencies for palliative and end-of-life care* (Contract Reference Number: 4500171593). Retrieved from http://casn.ca/vm/newvisual/attachments/856/Media/FinalReporttoHealthCanada.pdf.

Canadian Hospice Palliative Care Association. (2006). *The pan-Canadian gold standard for palliative home care*. Ottawa: Author. Retrieved from http://www.chpca.net/media/7652/Gold_Standards_Palliative_Home_Care.pdf.

Canadian Hospice Palliative Care Association. (2008). *Certification examination: List of assumptions and competencies*. Ottawa: Author. Retrieved from http://www.chpca.net/media/7511/Canadian_HPC_Nursing_Assumptions_and_Competencies.pdf.

Canadian Hospice Palliative Care Association. (2009a). *Canadian hospice palliative care nursing standards of practice*. Ottawa: Author. Retrieved from http://www.chpca.net/media/7505/Canadian_Hospice_Palliative_Care_Nursing_Standards_2009.pdf.

Canadian Hospice Palliative Care Association. (2009b). *Nursing competencies case examples*. Ottawa: Author. Retrieved from http://www.chpca.net/media/7502/Canadian_Hospice_Palliative_Care_Nursing_Competencies_Case_Examples_Revised_Feb_2010.pdf.

Canadian Hospice Palliative Care Association. (2010a). *Fact sheet: Hospice palliative care in Canada*. Ottawa: Author. Retrieved from http://www.chpca.net/media/7622/fact_sheet_hpc_in_canada_may_2012_final.pdf.

Canadian Hospice Palliative Care Association. (2010b). *Advance care planning in Canada: A national framework*. Ottawa: Author. Retrieved from http://www.chpca.net/media/7449/acp_synopsis_of_the_framework_sept_16_10.pdf.

Canadian Hospice Palliative Care Association. (2010c). *Policy brief on hospice palliative care. Quality end-of-life care? It depends on where you live and where you die*. Ottawa: Author. Retrieved from http://www.chpca.net/media/7682/HPC_Policy_Brief_-_Systems_Approach_-_June_2010.pdf.

Canadian Hospice Palliative Care Association. (2013). *About the Canadian Hospice Palliative Care Association*. Ottawa: Author. Retrieved from http://www.chpca.net/Home.

Canadian Institute for Health Information. (2007). *Health care use at the end of life in Western Canada*. Ottawa: Author.

Canadian Nurses Association. (2008). *Code of Ethics for Registered Nurses*. Ottawa: Author.

Candy, B., Holman, A., Leurent, B., et al. (2011). Hospice care delivered at home, in nursing homes and in dedicated hospice facilities: A systematic review of quantitative and qualitative evidence. *International Journal of Nursing Studies*, 48(1), 121–133. doi:10.1016/j.ijnurstu.2010.08.003.

Carstairs, S. (2010). *Raising the bar: A roadmap for the future of palliative care in Canada*. Ottawa: Senate of Canada.

Clarke, D. (2010). Dame Cicely Biography. *Cicely Saunders International*. Retrieved from http://www.cicelysaundersfoundation.org/about-us/dame-cicely-biography.

Clukey, L. (2007). Just be there: Hospice caregivers' anticipatory mourning experience. *Journal of Hospice and Palliative Nursing*, 9, 150–158. doi:10.1097/01.NJH.0000269992.13625.00.

Collier, R. (2011). Bringing palliative care to the homeless. *Canadian Medical Association Journal*, 183(6), E317–8. Retrieved from http://www.cmaj.ca/content/183/6/E317.full.pdf+html.

Cook, J.M., Marshall, R., Masci, D., et al. (2007). Physicians' perspectives on prescribing benzodiazepines for older adults: A qualitative study. *Journal of General Internal Medicine*, 22(3), 303–307.

Dameron, C. (2005). Spiritual assessment made easy … with ACRONYMS! *Journal of Christian Nursing*, 22(1), 14–16. doi:10.1097/01.CNJ.0000262323.59843.2e.

Dougherty, J., Gallagher, M., Cabral, D., et al. (2007). About me: Knowing the person with advanced dementia. *Alzheimer's Care Quarterly*, 8(1), 12–16.

Duffy, A. (2005, April 23). A moral force: The story of Dr. Balfour Mount. *The Ottawa Citizen*. Retrieved from http://www.virtualhospice.ca/Assets/Bal%20Mount%20article_20090310154705.pdf.

Eakes, G.G., Burke, M.L., & Hainsworth, M.A. (1998). The middle-range theory of chronic sorrow. *The Journal of Nursing Scholarship*, 30(2), 179–184.

Edwards, A., Pang, N., Shiu, V., et al. (2010). Review: The understanding of spirituality and the potential role of spiritual care in end-of-life and palliative care: A meta-study of qualitative research. *Palliative Medicine*, 24, 753–770. doi:10.1177/0269216310375860.

Ferris, F.D., Balfour, H.M., Bowen, K., et al. (2002). *A model to guide hospice palliative care*. Ottawa: Canadian Hospice Palliative Care Association. Retrieved from http://www.chpca.net/media/7422/a-model-to-guide-hospice-palliative-care-2002-urlupdate-august2005.pdf.

Finfgeld-Connett, D. (2006). Meta-synthesis of presence in nursing. *Journal of Advanced Nursing*, 55, 708–714. doi:10.1111/j.1365-2648.2006.03961.x.

Finfgeld-Connett, D. (2008a). Qualitative convergence of three nursing concepts: Art of nursing, presence and caring. *Journal of Advanced Nursing*, 63, 527–534. doi:10.1111/j.1365-2648.2008.04622.x.

Finfgeld-Connett, D. (2008b). Qualitative comparison and synthesis of nursing presence and caring. *International Journal of Nursing Terminologies and Classifications*, 19, 111–119. doi:10.1111/j.1744-618X.2008.00090.x.

Finfgeld-Connett, D. (2008c). Meta-synthesis of caring in nursing. *Journal of Clinical Nursing*, 17, 196–204. doi:10.1111/j.1365-2702.2006.01824.x.

Gamino, L.A., & Sewell, K.W. (2004). Meaning constructs as predictors of bereavement adjustment: A report from the Scott and White Grief Study. *Death Studies*, 28, 397–421. doi:10.1080/07481180490437536.

Grimby, A., & Johansson, A.K. (2008). Does early bereavement counseling prevent ill health and untimely death? *American Journal of Hospice and Palliative Medicine, 24,* 475–478. doi:10.1177/1049909107305651.

Harris, D. (2010). Oppression of the bereaved: A critical analysis of grief in Western society. *Omega: Journal of Death & Dying, 60,* 241–253. doi:10.2190/OM.60.3.c.

Heyland, D.K., Cook, D.J., Rocker, G.M., et al. (2010). Defining priorities for improving end-of-life care in Canada. *Canadian Medical Association Journal, 182,* E747–E752. doi:10.1503/cmaj.100131.

Heyland, D.K., Dodek, P., Rocker, G., et al. (2006). What matters most in end-of-life care: Perceptions of seriously ill patients and their family members. *Canadian Medical Association Journal, 174,* 627–633. doi:10.1503/cmaj.050626.

Hottensen, D. (2010). Anticipatory grief in patients with cancer. *Clinical Journal of Oncology Nursing, 14,* 106–107. doi:10.1188/10.CJON.106-107.

Hutchinson, T.A., Hutchinson, N., & Arnaert, A. (2009). Whole person care: encompassing the two faces of medicine. *Canadian Medical Association Journal, 180,* 845–846. doi:10.1503/cmaj.081081.

Ito, M., Nakajima, S., Fujisawa, D., et al. (2012). Brief measure for screening complicated grief: Reliability and discriminant validity. *PLoS ONE, 7*(2), e31209. doi:10.1371/journal.pone.0031209.

Jacono, B., Cable-Williams, B., Foster, C., et al. (2009). *The principles and practice of palliative care nursing and palliative care competencies for Canadian nurses.* Retrieved from http://casn.ca/vm/newvisual/attachments/856/Media/CompetenciesDocumentFinalupdated.pdf.

Joanna Briggs Institute. (2011). Palliative approach to care for people with advanced dementia. Best Practice: evidence-based information sheets for health professionals. *Best Practice, 15*(5):1–4. Retrieved from http://connect.jbiconnectplus.org/ViewSourceFile.aspx?0=7116.

Kramer-Howe, K., & Huls, P.T. (2004). *A spiritual assessment tool.* Phoenix: Hospice of the Valley.

Kübler-Ross, E. (1969). *On death and dying.* New York: Macmillan.

Lee, M., & Chodosh, J. (2009). Dementia and life expectancy: What do we know? *Journal of the American Medical Directors Association, 10,* 466–471. doi:10.1016/j.jamda.2009.03.014.

Lee, N.P., & Washington, G. (2008). Management of common symptoms at end of life in acute care settings. *The Journal for Nurse Practitioners, 4,* 610–615. doi:10.1016/j.nurpra.2008.05.007.

McGrath, P. (2007). "I don't want to be in that big city; this is my country here": Research findings on Aboriginal peoples' preference to die at home. *Australian Journal of Rural Health, 15,* 264–268. doi:10.1111/j.1440-1584.2007.00904.x.

Ministry of Health (British Columbia). (2006). *A provincial framework for end-of-life care.* Retrieved from http://www.health.gov.bc.ca/library/publications/year/2006/framework.pdf.

Mitchell, S.L., Kiely, D.K., & Hamel, M.B. (2004). Dying with advanced dementia in the nursing home. *Archives of Internal Medicine, 164*(3), 321–326. Retrieved from http://archinte.ama-assn.org/cgi/reprint/164/3/321.

Nelson, F. (2011). What is grief? *Canadian Virtual Hospice.* Retrieved from http://www.virtualhospice.ca/en_US/Main+Site+Navigation/Home/Topics/Topics/Emotional+Health/Grief+Work.aspx.

Pellett, C. (2009). Provision of end of life care in the community. *Nursing Standard, 24*(12), 35–40.

Pereira, S.M., Fonseca, A.M., & Carvalho, A.S. (2011). Burnout in palliative care: A systematic review. *Nursing Ethics, 18*(3), 317–326. doi:10.1177/0969733011398092.

Podymow, T., Turnbull, J., & Coyle, D. (2006). Shelter-based palliative care for the homeless terminally ill. *Palliative Medicine, 20,* 81–86. doi:10.1191/0269216306pm1103oa.

Prigerson, H.G., Horowitz, M.J., Jacobs, S.C., et al. (2009). Prolonged grief disorder: Psychometric validation of criteria proposed for *DSM-V* and *ICD-11. Plos Medicine, 6*(8), 1–12. doi:10.1371/journal.pmed.1000121.

Prince, H., & Kelley, M.L. (2010). An integrative framework for conducting palliative care research with First Nations communities. *Journal of Palliative Care, Special Edition, 26*(1), 47–53.

Puchalski, C.M. (2007). Spirituality and the care of patients at the end-of-life: An essential component of care. *OMEGA: Journal of Death and Dying, 56*(1), 33–46.

Registered Nurses' Association of Ontario (RNAO). (2004). *Caregiving strategies for older adults with delirium, dementia and depression.* Retrieved from http://rnao.ca/bpg/guidelines/caregiving-strategies-older-adults-delirium-dementia-and-depression.

Reinke, L.F., Shannon, S.E., Engelberg, R., et al. (2010). Nurses' identification of important yet under-utilized end-of-life care skills for patients with life-limiting or terminal illnesses. *Journal of Palliative Medicine, 13,* 753–759. doi:10.1089/jpm.2009.0423.

Rhodes, R.L., Mitchell, S.L., Miller, S.C., et al. (2008). Bereaved family members' evaluation of hospice care: What factors influence overall satisfaction with services? *Journal of Pain and Symptom Management, 35,* 365–371. doi:10.1016/j.jpainsymman.2007.12.004.

Richardson, V.E. (2010). The dual process model of coping with bereavement: A decade later. *OMEGA: Journal of Death & Dying, 61*(4), 269–271. doi:10.2190/OM.61.4.a.

Richmond, C. (2005). Dame Cicely Saunders: Founder of the modern hospice movement [Obituary]. *British Medical Journal, 331.* doi:10.1136/bmj.331.7510.238.

Ryan, T., Ingleton, C., Gardiner, C., et al. (2009). Supporting people who have dementia to die with dignity. *Nursing Older People, 21*(5), 18–23.

Stajduhar, K., Roberts, D., McLeod, B., et al. (2010). *Access to care at the end of life: Encounters between home care nurses and family caregivers.* Retrieved from http://www.coag.uvic.ca/eolcare/documents/Access%20to%20Care%20at%20the%20End%20of%20Life%20Final%20Report.pdf.

Stroebe, M. (2009). From vulnerability to resilience: Where should research priorities lie? *Bereavement Care, 28,* 18–24. doi:10.1080/02682620902996020.

Stroebe, M., & Schut, H. (2010). The dual process model of coping with bereavement: A decade on. *OMEGA: Journal of Death & Dying, 61,* 273–289. doi:10.2190/OM.61.4.b.

van der Houwen, K., Stroebe, M., Stroebe, W., et al. (2010). Risk factors for bereavement outcome: A multivariate approach. *Death Studies, 34,* 195–220. doi:10.1080/07481180903559196.

Vogel, L. (2011). Nursing schools to teach new ways to cope with death. *Canadian Medical Association Journal, 183,* 418. doi:10.1503/cmaj.109-3788.

Wilson, D., Justice, C., Sheps, S., et al. (2006). Planning and providing end-of-life care in rural areas. *The Journal of Rural Health, 22,*174–181. doi:10.1111/j.1748-0361.2006.00028.x.

Worden, J.W. (2009). *Grief counseling and grief therapy* (4th ed.). New York: Springer.

# Forensic Psychiatric Nursing

*Wendy Stanyon*

## KEY TERMS AND CONCEPTS

correctional nursing, 681
forensic nursing, 677
forensic psychiatric mental health nurse, 679

## OBJECTIVES

1. Define forensic nursing, forensic psychiatric mental health nursing, and correctional nursing.
2. Identify the functions of forensic nurses.
3. Describe three subspecialties of forensic nursing.
4. Identify three roles of psychiatric mental health nurses in the specialty of forensic nursing.
5. Describe clinical competencies associated with forensic psychiatric mental health nursing.

6. Compare and contrast the roles of forensic psychiatric mental health nurses and correctional nurses.
7. Describe the health care needs of incarcerated individuals.
8. Discuss the challenges or issues associated with being a nurse in a correctional facility.

## evolve WEBSITE

*Visit the Evolve website for Flashcards, Case Studies, and additional testing resources related to the content in this chapter: http://evolve.elsevier.com/Canada/Varcarolis/psychiatric/*    Pre-Test  interactive review

According to the *World Report on Violence and Health* (World Health Organization, 2002), over 1.6 million people worldwide lose their lives annually to self-directed (suicide), interpersonal, or collective (societal) violence. Of the 2.2 million Criminal Code incidents reported by police services in Canada in 2008, one in five was violent. Across the country, the highest crime rates were in the territories and Western Canada, with the highest overall crime rate in Saskatchewan. Ontario and Quebec had the lowest rates according to the *2009 Canada Year Book, Crime and Justice* (Statistics Canada, 2009).

Individuals living with mental health challenges are over-represented in the Canadian criminal justice system (Mental Health Commission of Canada, 2012). It is estimated that the rates of serious mental health issues among individuals in federal correctional facilities have increased by 60% or 70% since 1997 (Parliament of Canada, 2010). More than 45% of the total male inmate population and 69% of the female inmate

population received mental health care services in 2010 and 2011 (Office of the Correctional Investigator, 2012). In particular, Aboriginal people are significantly over-represented in the Canadian criminal justice system. Incarceration rates of Aboriginal people are five to six times higher than the national average. Statistics show that while Aboriginal people represent only 2.8% of the Canadian population, they account for 18% of those who are incarcerated in federal institutions (Correctional Service of Canada, 2010). One in three women incarcerated in a federal facility is Aboriginal. Trevethan, Moore, Auger, and colleagues (2002) note that Aboriginal offenders are more likely than non-Aboriginal offenders to have experienced poverty, family violence, and substance abuse in their home environment, and as children, they were more likely to have been involved with child welfare services.

A number of factors have contributed to the over-representation of all people with mental health and addictions problems in the criminal justice system, including the deinstitutionalization of people challenged by mental illness without adequate community mental health services, a lack of affordable housing, and inadequate income-support programs. These factors increase the vulnerability of individuals with mental illnesses, leading to greater victimization of this population. The media often portrays individuals living with mental illness as violent and unpredictable; however, the reality is people who have a mental illness are much more likely to be the victims of violence than are people in the general population (Canadian Mental Health Association, 2013). In fact, one in four individuals with a mental illness is likely to be a victim of violence in a given year (Hiday, Swanson, Swartz, et al., 2001; Teplin, McClelland, Abram, et al., 2005). Experiencing victimization intensifies feelings of anxiety and vulnerability and can lead to an exacerbation of one's illness and a lower quality of life (Teplin, McClelland, Abram, et al., 2005).

This increased risk of victimization continues during incarceration. Both male and female inmates with a mental illness are more likely than other inmates to have been physically assaulted by their peers or correctional staff (Blitz, Wolff, & Shi, 2008). In addition, individuals with a mental illness may be more likely to engage in acts of self-harm while incarcerated. The Office of the Correctional Investigator of Canada (2009) has found that self-harm behaviour among federal inmates is increasing, as individuals struggle with a stressful and often dehumanizing environment and limited assistive services.

In Canada, the 2007 death of teenager Ashley Smith led to a greater interest in, and ultimately a formal investigation into, the treatment of correctional inmates experiencing mental illness and engaging in self-harming behaviours. Ashley Smith, who had ongoing mental health challenges while incarcerated in a number of facilities over a period of 11 months, had repeatedly engaged in self-harming behaviours, specifically strangulation using handmade ligatures, before her suicide on October 19, 2007. A coroner's inquest was launched, with formal hearings beginning in January 2013, for the purpose of determining how correctional institutions may better address the needs of inmates with mental illness and reduce the incidence of death and self-harm within the prison population (CBC News, 2013).

Mental health support must not end when a person is released from incarceration, however. The transition back into society is difficult for many individuals, who often receive little to no support in obtaining housing, employment, and other services upon their release (BearPaw Media Productions, 2009). Individuals with a mental illness who have been involved in the criminal justice system tend to have higher rates of homelessness, difficulty adhering to treatment, lower rates of social support, and greater incidence of substance abuse in comparison to other adults with a mental illness (Canadian Institute for Health Information, 2008). Without adequate services and a treatment plan in place, the likelihood of further victimization and recidivism among this population is high. Mental health care in the criminal justice system serves, in this way, as a crime-prevention strategy.

Canada's National Crime Prevention Strategy (NCPS) is based on the premise that well-designed interventions can have

---

**BOX 34-1 KEY ELEMENTS OF CANADA'S NATIONAL CRIME PREVENTION STRATEGY**

- Expand the knowledge base of risk factors associated with the likelihood that individuals will engage in criminal activity.
- Identify individuals at different stages of development who exhibit or are exposed to these risk factors.
- Build on the body of knowledge on effective interventions for addressing these risk factors.

**Source:** Public Safety Canada. (2010). Supporting the successful implementation of the National Crime Prevention Strategy (NCPS). Retrieved from http://publications.gc.ca/pub?id=353274&sl=0.

---

a positive influence on behaviours: by addressing risk factors associated with offending, crimes can be reduced or prevented. Successful interventions have been shown to reduce not only victimization but also the social and economic costs that result from criminal activities and the costs related to processing cases in the criminal justice system. In its 2008 budget, the Government of Canada provided $30 million in ongoing funding for crime prevention, effectively doubling the strategy's permanent funding base to $63 million per year (Public Safety Canada, 2010). Box 34-1 outlines the key elements of the NCPS.

*Forensics* (an abbreviation derived from *forensic science*) is an umbrella term that refers to legal issues or working with the courts. In recent years, nurses formalized a broad category called *forensic nursing*, which brings together components of traditional nursing care and legal issues to serve victims of violence and individuals who have committed acts that have brought them into contact with the criminal justice system. In this chapter, we will explore a variety of roles that registered nurses assume within the legal system, identify competencies and challenges associated with the forensic nursing role, and profile the priority health care needs of patients who have committed an offence.

## FORENSIC NURSING

Forensic nursing is the application of nursing science to public or legal proceedings and the combination of the forensic and biopsychosocial aspects of health care in the scientific investigation of trauma or death of victims and perpetrators of abuse, violence, criminal activity, and traumatic accidents (International Association of Forensic Nurses, 2006b). Unlike most nursing specialties, forensic nursing includes several different areas of nursing practice: *forensic nurse examiners* work with sexual assault survivors; *forensic nurse death investigators* work with the deceased; *forensic psychiatric mental health nurses* work with mentally ill offenders; *clinical forensic nurses* work with victims of interpersonal violence; *forensic correctional nurses* work with offenders; and *forensic geriatric* or *pediatric nurses* work with victims of abuse and neglect (Kent-Wilkinson, 2008). Forensic nurses provide direct services to victims of crime and individuals who have committed crimes; consultation services to colleagues in nursing-, medical-, and law-related agencies;

and expert court testimony in cases of trauma or questioned death, adequacy of service delivery, and specialized diagnoses of specific conditions related to nursing. Forensic nurses also work with families or significant others and the community (International Association of Forensic Nurses, 2006a).

The International Association of Forensic Nurses (IAFN), formed in 1992 by 74 nurses, most of whom were sexual assault nurse examiners (SANEs), represents nurses whose practice overlaps with key areas of forensic science and law (International Association of Forensic Nurses & American Nurses Association, 2009). The group currently represents nurses who are forensic nurse generalists, SANEs, forensic psychiatric nurses, death investigators, coroners, correctional nurse specialists, and those in other forensic nursing specialties that continue to evolve. A year after its creation, the organization had more than tripled in size, and by 2008, the IAFN's membership had grown to more than 3000 nurses (International Association of Forensic Nurses, 2006a). The American Nurses Association (ANA) officially recognized forensic nursing as a specialty practice area in 1995 and combined efforts with the IAFN to develop the *Scope and Standards of Forensic Nursing* in 1997. This document was updated in July 2009. While these standards may be useful guidelines for forensic nursing practice, they may not be directly applicable in Canada. Each provincial or territorial practice site and the federal Correctional Service of Canada has unique guidelines that nurses in Canada must follow.

The goals of the IAFN (2006a) are paraphrased as follows:

- To incorporate primary prevention strategies into nurses' work at every level in an attempt to eliminate violence
- To establish and improve standards and ethics for forensic nursing practice
- To promote and encourage the exchange of ideas and the transmission of knowledge among members and related disciplines
- To create and facilitate educational opportunities for forensic nurses and related disciplines

While the Canadian Nurses Association (CNA) has endorsed psychiatric mental health nursing as a specialty area of practice and offers certification for nurses who meet the criteria, it has not yet recognized forensic nursing as a distinct specialty area of practice. However, in July 2007, the CNA did approve the Forensic Nurses' Society of Canada (FNSC) as an emerging special interest group. The goal of the FNSC is to provide a network for forensic nurses and a platform for sharing ideas and discussing evidence-informed practice in the area of forensics (Forensic Nurses' Society of Canada, 2012).

## Education

In 2001, certification in forensic nursing became available for the subspecialty of sexual assault nurse examiners. At the same time, the IAFN called for the incorporation of forensic content at all levels of nursing education. In Canada, however, many nurses are involved in forensic nursing without having any specialized training. Some topics relevant to forensic nursing may be covered at the undergraduate level as part of psychiatric mental health nursing or community nursing courses; however, more often, forensic nursing is taught as a certificate program

following the completion of a basic nursing program or as a course at the postgraduate level, where the core fundamentals of nursing are already established. Canada was first in the world to offer an online forensic studies certificate program. Currently, Canada does not offer forensic nursing master's or doctoral programs (Kent-Wilkinson, 2008).

## Roles and Functions

In forensic nursing, it is not the role of the forensic nurse to make a decision as to guilt or innocence or to determine whether a victim is being candid in his or her reporting of what happened. The roles of the forensic nurse centre on the identification of victims, creation of appropriate treatment plans, and collection, documentation, and preservation of potential evidence. The forensic nurse possesses expertise in assessment and treatment roles related to competency, risk, and danger. Forensic nurses are educated in nursing science and may have taken additional courses in theories of violence and victimology and legal issues, enabling them to objectively assess the circumstances of the case.

An understanding of both the victim and the offender enhances evidence collection. Forensic nurses may apply medical-surgical knowledge to the care of victims and offenders, and they may function in a legal role as they collect evidence, testify in court, or collaborate with law practitioners with relation to a forensic patient.

### Nurse Examiner/Sexual Assault Nurse Examiner

The sexual assault nurse examiner (SANE) was the first specialized forensic role for nurses that required advanced education. The largest group of self-identified forensic nurses, SANEs are registered nurses who seek training in the care of adult and pediatric victims of sexual assault (*SANE-A* and *SANE-P* respectively).

The IAFN has established clear guidelines for the preparation of SANEs and provides SANE certification for nurses, although not all nurses who work in this capacity have certification. The training is relatively brief: the course is typically five days and 40 contact hours and is available online or in a classroom setting. The course may also include a clinical component. Currently, seven of the ten provinces in Canada offer SANE programs.

Nurses recognize the need to provide consistent care for all victims; therefore, nurses and leaders in many communities in Canada have set standards for educating the public on sexual assault prevention techniques and establishing comprehensive care for victims through sexual assault response teams (SARTs), which use a multidisciplinary model in providing care. SANEs are involved in the formation of SARTs in many communities across Canada. Along with SANEs, members of a SART may include representatives from the health department, police services, advocacy groups, the local department of children and family services, Crown attorneys' offices, local hospitals, victim assistance programs, and other service areas, as pertinent (Sekula, 2006). The multidisciplinary approach provides a standard of care that includes expert care in the acute setting, advocacy for the acute and long-term needs of the victim, and referral for counselling for survivors in an effort to decrease long-term effects resulting from the assault.

### Nurse Coroner or Death Investigator

This forensic nursing subspecialty is recognized internationally as having its historical roots in Alberta, Canada. Passage of the *Fatalities Inquiries Act* led to the formation of the Medical Examiners' Office in 1977 in Alberta. Subsequently, the medical examiners' system for investigation of all deaths (unnatural, unexpected, or unexplained) was adopted, and nurses were hired as death investigators or medical examiner's nurse investigators (Stewart, 1984). Currently, the medical examiner system operates in Alberta, Manitoba, Nova Scotia, and Newfoundland. Other provinces have a coroner system or a combination of both system types (Kent-Wilkinson, 2008). Over the years, registered nurses have also held the position of coroner in some territories and provinces. This nursing role involves assessing the deceased through understanding, discovery, preservation, and use of evidence.

As a representative of the medical examiner's or coroner's office, the forensic nurse death investigator is in charge of the body at a scene and works in collaboration with police services and other officials involved in the case. This nurse interviews witnesses, collects evidence, and documents findings. He or she may also notify the next of kin of the death (Romano, 2011). Such nurses are able to expand the role of the coroner and improve services provided to families, health care agencies, and communities by employing the basic principles of holistic nursing care.

### The Forensic Mental Health System in Canada

An increasing number of individuals struggling with mental illness and living in the community without adequate mental health services and resources are coming into contact with the law. This phenomenon is frequently referred to as the *criminalization of the mentally ill*. According to Crocker and Côté (2009), the psychiatric deinstitutionalization movement, which started in the 1960s, and changes to civil law that rendered involuntary treatment and hospitalization more difficult (both part of the movement toward the promotion of the self-determination of individuals with mental illness) have contributed to the criminal justice system's becoming the new entry point to mental health services for many individuals with mental illness. Peternelji-Taylor (2008) points to the continuing lack of adequate mental health policies for individuals living with chronic mental illness and the lack of community-based services, resulting in a fragmented mental health care system.

The Canadian forensic mental health system provides mental health services (inpatient and community) to individuals who have a mental illness and have come into contact with the justice system. While health care in Canada receives financial support from the federal government and the Criminal Code dictates some degree of consistency, the forensic mental health systems in the provinces and territories have evolved separately because the Constitution grants each jurisdiction authority over health matters (Constitution Act, 1982, s. 92). The provincial and territorial forensic mental health systems, therefore, reflect the uniqueness of each jurisdiction—geography, climate, existing services, population needs, and available resources and expertise (Livingston, 2006).

## FORENSIC PSYCHIATRIC NURSING

A forensic psychiatric mental health nurse "integrates nursing philosophy and theory with knowledge and skill of mental health and potentially dangerous behaviours, and where the location contains enhanced security, for patients held under the authority of the criminal justice system" (Devnick, 2010, p. 17). Devnick (2010, p. 48) describes forensic mental health nursing as multifaceted, calling for the balancing of competing philosophies of caring and containment; inciting contradictory emotions in response to possibly heinous behaviours and trauma; and requiring complex skills of collaborating with interdisciplinary health, legal, and security staff in the management of clinical interventions to address potentially dangerous behaviours. This specialty requires skills in psychiatric mental health nursing assessment, evaluation, and treatment of forensic clients diagnosed with a mental illness.

Evidence collection is central to the role of the forensic psychiatric nurse. For example, evidence is collected by a careful evaluation of a forensic patient's mental status at the time of an offence. This evaluation aids in determining the individual's fitness to stand trial and may later influence the sentence. Forensic psychiatric nurses may spend many hours with an accused individual collecting evidence and carefully documenting the dialogue. In this capacity, the role of the forensic psychiatric nurse is not to determine guilt or innocence but to provide assessment data that can help make a final diagnosis within the multidisciplinary forensic team (Sekula & Burgess, 2006).

### Roles and Functions

The role of the forensic psychiatric nurse formally began in Canada in the 1970s, when mentally disordered offenders were separated from the general inmate population and forensic psychiatric services were provided federally by the Correctional Service of Canada. The role subsequently evolved with the establishment of forensic psychiatric inpatient units (Kent-Wilkinson, 2008). The role has continued to evolve, and forensic psychiatric nurses may now function as forensic nurse examiners, expert witnesses, and consultants to the criminal justice system, law enforcement, or health care agencies. These roles may involve providing nursing services to forensic clients and victims of violence, expert court testimony, and services to a Crown attorney or defence lawyer.

Roles of the forensic psychiatric nurse may be examined in relationship to the settings in which the nurse is employed. The forensic psychiatric nurse, as a member of an interprofessional team, may work on a forensic assessment unit in a mental health facility, conducting court-ordered evaluations of criminal responsibility and court-ordered treatment to determine if individuals are fit to stand trial, or on a forensic rehabilitation unit providing treatment, care, and rehabilitation for patients who have been found to be unfit or not criminally responsible on account of a mental disorder (NCRMD).

Canadian law specifies that a person cannot be tried for a criminal offence if, because of a mental disorder, he or she is unable to provide a defence. The Criminal Code defines "unfit to stand trial" as unable on account of mental disorder to conduct a defence at any stage of the proceedings before a verdict is rendered or to instruct counsel to do so, and, in particular, unable on account of mental disorder to:

1. understand the nature or object of the proceedings,
2. understand the possible consequences of the proceedings, or
3. communicate with counsel. (Canadian Criminal Code, 1985, s. 2)

It is the accused individual's capacity *at the time of trial* that is in question in determining fitness to stand trial. The court may decide that an individual found unfit to stand trial is to be treated for the purpose of making the individual fit to do so. Before rendering this decision, the court must be satisfied, based on medical evidence, that the proposed treatment is likely to make the individual fit to stand trial and that without treatment the individual is likely to remain unfit; that any potential harm associated with the treatment does not outweigh the anticipated benefits; and that the specified treatment is the least restrictive and least intrusive given the circumstances. Then every two years, until the person is either acquitted or tried, a review board holds a hearing to determine if the person has become fit to stand trial (Department of Justice Canada, 2009). Although there continues to be much debate, Canadian law currently requires only that individuals be able to provide a factual account to their lawyers but not necessarily an analytical or rational analysis.

*Criminal responsibility* refers to the mental state of a defendant at the time of the offence. A person is not criminally responsible (NCR) if he or she has a mental disorder that makes him or her unable to judge the nature or quality of the criminal act or to understand that the act was wrong at the time it was committed (Canadian Criminal Code, s. 16). Merely having a mental disorder does not automatically exempt a person from criminal responsibility. The courts make the decision based on a thorough legal and psychiatric review to determine the person's state at the time of the offence. If the person is tried, the verdict will then be guilty, not guilty, or not criminally responsible on account of mental disorder.

A literature review of the role of the forensic psychiatric mental health nurse identified a series of competencies (see Box 34-2).

The forensic psychiatric nurse must be highly skilled in interpersonal communications and able to develop collegial relationships with those in other disciplines. The ability to be self-reflective and objective is also critical (Lyons, 2009).

One of the most challenging aspects of forensic psychiatric nursing is balancing the custodial role with the therapeutic role. The forensic psychiatric nurse must be able to look beyond the index offence and see forensic patients as human beings with specific needs (Volstad, 2008).

The following Research Highlight box describes the findings of a research study that explored how nurses working with

---

**BOX 34-2** **COMPETENCIES ASSOCIATED WITH THE ROLE OF A FORENSIC PSYCHIATRIC MENTAL HEALTH NURSE**

**Specific Task-Oriented Areas**
- Safety and security
- Assessment and management of risk
- Monitoring of patients and their property
- Management of violent and aggressive behaviour
- Therapies
- Practical skills (e.g., first aid)
- Escorting patients within and outside of the secure environment
- Visitor-related issues (e.g., observation, communication)
- Management of hostage situations and other security breaches
- Report writing

**Knowledge**
- Mental health and criminal justice systems
- Appreciation of physical, legal, emotional, and spiritual consequences of being legally detained
- Mental health wellness and illness
- Public attitudes, moral values, ignorance and stigma, empowerment, and paternalism

**Skills**
- Self-awareness, reflection, and honesty
- Therapeutic use of self
- Clinical risk assessment and management
- Planning of therapeutic interventions
- Development and maintenance of independent living skills
- Facilitation of meaningful relationships
- Help in the identification of behavioural boundaries and the development of self-control
- Addressing of socially unacceptable behaviours

**Personal Qualities (Values and Attitudes)**
- Ability to be nonjudgemental (e.g., ensuring principles of equality, fairness, and confidentiality are maintained)
- Ability to be detached (i.e., not personalizing negative events)
- Ability to appear calm and relaxed (i.e., never being threatening)
- Understanding and setting boundaries in therapeutic relationships
- Ability to make decisions effectively

**Source:** Adapted from Bowering-Lossock, E. (2006). The forensic mental health nurse: A literature review. *Journal of Psychiatric & Mental Health Nursing, 13,* 780–785. doi:10.1111/j.1365-2850 .2006.00993.x. Copyright © 2006, John Wiley and Sons.

---

patients in medium security forensic psychiatric units understand and demonstrate the concept of respect.

Forensic psychiatric nursing appeals to a particular type of nurse, one who thrives in a stimulating intellectual environment, seeks out opportunities to apply clinical skills to complex legal problems, and enjoys pushing the limits of traditional boundaries. Because of the value placed on tradition by the nursing profession, the forensic psychiatric nurse is sometimes

## RESEARCH HIGHLIGHT

### Respect in Forensic Psychiatric Nurse–Patient Relationships

**Source:** Rose, D.N., Peter, E., Gallop, R., et al. (2011). Respect in forensic psychiatric nurse–patient relationships: A practical compromise. *Journal of Forensic Nursing, 7*, 3–16. doi:10.1111/j.1939-3938.2010.01090.x.

#### Problem

Respect is considered essential within the nurse–patient relationship. However, nurses often morally struggle with respecting patients who have committed horrific offences. The forensic psychiatric setting is a particularly challenging environment for nurses, and there is a need for further research in this area.

#### Purpose of Study

The study explored the concept of respect as understood and enacted by nurses working in a forensic psychiatric setting.

#### Methods

It was a focused ethnographic study.

#### Key Findings

- Forensic psychiatric nurses strike a practical compromise in their understanding and enactment of respect in therapeutic relationships with forensic psychiatric patients.
- Kantian-like respect (a minimum level of respect that acknowledges patient autonomy and noninterference) is the most prevalent form of respect articulated by forensic nurses.
- Caring respect (positive attitude toward a patient; valuing a patient's individuality) is enacted by forensic nurses if they are able to discover forensic patients' individuality and perceive them as being remorseful.

#### Implications for Nursing Practice

Based on their findings, the researchers recommended teaching forensic psychiatric nurses about the philosophy of respect and providing them with the vocabulary to engage in discussions with each other and other professionals.

viewed with scepticism in nursing and with caution in the legal system. These responses must be met with professionalism by forensic psychiatric nurses in their practice, research, and education.

## Correctional Nursing in Canada

The number of incarcerated individuals (both men and women) in Canada has increased significantly over the past two decades. Currently, the Correctional Service of Canada (CSC) oversees approximately 22 000 incarcerated individuals: 13 280 are in prison and 8720 are being supervised in the community (Kearley & Steeves, 2010). Incarcerated individuals are 20 times more likely than those in the general public to have been infected with the hepatitis C virus; 10 times more likely to have been infected with human immunodeficiency virus (HIV); more than twice as likely to have had a mental disorder; and more likely to have been treated for chronic conditions such as diabetes, cardiovascular conditions, and asthma (Bouchard, 2004).

Offenders are guaranteed the right to treatment as well as the right to refuse treatment (Constitution Act, 1982). Therefore, correctional facilities are required to provide "adequate and reasonable" health services to inmates, either directly or through community health services organizations. Correctional nursing is defined by the location of the work or the legal status of the patient, rather than by the role or functions being performed. In fact, the role of nurses in correctional settings involves all aspects of nursing practice, including emergency care, medication administration, comprehensive mental and physical health assessments, infection control, health teaching, provision of treatments such as wound care, management of acute and chronic mental and physical illnesses, and collaboration with other health care providers (Doran & Almost, 2010).

As mentioned, today's inmates experience a disproportionately greater number of chronic illnesses and infectious diseases than the general population. Treatment and services for inmates with chronic mental health diagnoses are a significant part of the job for nurses working in correctional facilities. Between 1997 and 2005, the number of offenders identified as having a mental disorder on admission increased by 71% (Kearley & Steeves, 2010). Approximately one in ten male inmates (12%) and one in five female inmates (21%) is experiencing a serious mental disorder upon admission to a federal correctional institution (Parliament of Canada, 2010). This rate of mental illness is several times higher than the rate of mental health disorders in the general Canadian population.

Box 34-3 highlights the health profile of individuals incarcerated in federal correctional institutions in Canada.

Correctional nurses provide care for many individuals with serious mental illness who are caught in a cycle of homelessness, psychiatric hospitals, and prison. Unfortunately, only some will end up being admitted to either a regional hospital or regional mental health treatment centre, where they can receive comprehensive psychiatric mental health services. Frequently, these individuals instead become incarcerated as a result of psychiatric emergencies that generally include threats made to others. Because psychiatric resources to help manage such emergencies are scarce, these individuals often end up in prison instead of in a hospital. Once they are in a correctional facility, their psychiatric condition often worsens because of the lack of adequate psychiatric intervention.

Another issue that must be considered in the treatment of those who are incarcerated is substance use and abuse. In Canada, some 80% of offenders serving prison sentences of two years or more have problems with drugs, alcohol, or both (Parliament of Canada, 2012). Drug courts, mandatory drug treatment, and drug or alcohol treatment within correctional facilities have all been shown to decrease the likelihood of recidivism and increase the likelihood of abstinence from drugs or alcohol after release.

Because of the impacts of mental health and addiction problems on recidivism (repeat offences) and on resource allocation, policymakers and legislators are beginning to recognize the importance of providing treatment for individuals who are

## BOX 34-3 HEALTH PROFILE OF INDIVIDUALS INCARCERATED IN CANADIAN FEDERAL INSTITUTIONS IN COMPARISON TO THE GENERAL POPULATION

**Socioeconomic Measures**
- Twice as likely not to have finished high school
- Nine times more likely to have been unemployed

**Health Behaviours**
- More than twice as likely to smoke
- Thirty times more likely to inject drugs
- Two to ten times more likely to have an alcohol or substance abuse disorder

**Chronic Conditions**
- Males 40% more likely to be treated for diabetes; females three times more likely
- Males 68% more likely to be treated for cardiovascular conditions; females over two times more likely
- Males 43% more likely to be treated for asthma; females almost three times more likely
- 50% more likely to need mechanical aids

**Infectious Diseases**
- More than twice as likely to have been infected with hepatitis B virus
- More than 20 times more likely to have been infected with hepatitis C virus
- More than ten times more likely to have been infected with HIV
- Much more likely to be infected with tuberculosis

**Mental Health Disorders**
- More than twice as likely to have had any mental disorder
- Males three times more likely to have schizophrenia; females 20 times more likely
- Four times more likely to have a mood disorder

**Mortality**
- At a 45% increased risk for death
- Eight times more likely to die by homicide
- Almost four times more likely to die by suicide

**Source:** Bouchard, F. (2004). A health care needs assessment of federal inmates in Canada. *Canadian Journal of Public Health*, *95*(Suppl. 1), S49.

## BOX 34-4 TYPES OF HEALTH CARE SETTINGS IN THE CORRECTIONAL SERVICE OF CANADA

**Institutional Health Units (Ambulatory Care Centres)**
Every CSC institution has a health services centre with varying hours of operation based on factors such as level of security and proximity to community services. The primary care providers in these units are nurses. Each institution provides a variety of routine and emergency psychology services to offenders.

**CSC Regional Hospital**
Each region has a hospital located within the compound of a multilevel or maximum security level institution that provides more specialized or comprehensive health care services on a 24-hour basis. Services include but are not limited to postoperative care, trauma care, observation, dialysis, palliative care, and any condition requiring 24-hour nursing services.

**CSC Reception Centre**
Each region has at least one reception centre that conducts the CSC standardized admission process (both health and security) for all newly sentenced federal offenders. The admission process involves various health assessments, such as a mental status assessment, comprehensive health assessment, and tuberculosis assessment.

**CSC Regional Treatment Centre (Mental Health)**
An inpatient mental health treatment facility is located in each region to provide treatment to inmates with psychiatric disorders that are too severe to allow them to remain in the general inmate population.

There are over 700 nurses at CSC working in a variety of settings, including correctional remand, psychiatric assessment, and prison facilities; regional hospitals; mental health treatment centres; and Aboriginal healing lodges (see Box 34-4). They can specialize in a wide range of areas, from mental disorders to substance abuse to chronic care (Correctional Service of Canada, 2011).

The Correctional Service of Canada has recognized that correctional nurses face a number of challenges, including a high level of stress associated with the correctional environment, demanding work hours, caring for individuals who have a substance use disorder, and concerns for personal safety expressed by family and friends. In response to these challenges, CSC has implemented extensive education and training for newly hired nurses as well as those who have been working in corrections for a number of years (Correctional Service of Canada, 2011).

Correctional nurses perform psychiatric mental health nursing role functions, including completing comprehensive mental status examinations and implementing psychiatric care plans. The following vignette illustrates a challenging situation facing a nurse working in the health services centre of a correctional facility.

incarcerated. In Canada, the *Corrections and Conditional Release Act* (1992) actually references the fact that inmates receiving mental health treatment alongside correctional programming (in prison and in the community) demonstrate functional improvement. The correctional setting, however, is not conducive to the intensive therapy required to adequately treat mental health issues; therefore, the needs of the vast majority of people with mental illnesses or concurrent disorders in the correctional system are not appropriately addressed.

**VIGNETTE**

Suzanne is a 45-year-old woman incarcerated at a federal institution in the general inmate population. She was convicted of assault with a deadly weapon following a confrontation with a "friend." Her psychiatric diagnoses include major depression and PTSD (resulting from severe abuse in her childhood and from an intimate partner during her early 20s). Although she is not in a locked forensic unit, she is being treated with medication and seen by one of the institution's nurses for medication management.

While watching television in the common area one morning, Suzanne attacked a fellow inmate for no apparent reason, screaming and clawing at anyone who approached her. The staff was unable to control her physically. She was placed in solitary confinement with mechanical restraints; these actions did nothing to control her screaming. She was seen by the nurse on call, who reported that Suzanne was having a flashback related to her PTSD. The solitary confinement and mechanical restraints were only worsening her flashbacks. The staff and the nurse were facing a common dilemma in correctional health care: custody versus caring. While the nurse was focusing on the needs of the individual inmate, the correctional staff was focused on the goals of the correctional facility related to custody of violent offenders and protection of the environment. The successful correctional treatment team seeks to balance the two sides of this debate: creating an environment in which the potential rehabilitation of offenders is possible without compromising the compulsory "punitive" aspects of incarceration.

# KEY POINTS TO REMEMBER

- Forensic nursing is an emerging specialty area of practice that combines elements of traditional nursing, forensic science, and criminal justice.
- The IAFN was established in 1992 as the professional association representing this specialty internationally.
- Forensic nurses fulfill a variety of roles, including that of sexual assault nurse examiner, nurse coroner or death investigator, forensic psychiatric mental health nurse, and correctional nurse.
- Incarcerated individuals have higher rates of serious and chronic physical and mental illnesses than the general population.

# CRITICAL THINKING

1. How would you describe the nurse–patient relationship in forensic nursing? In what ways does it differ from the nurse–patient relationship in other areas of nursing?

2. Respect is an essential component of any therapeutic nurse–patient relationship; however, nurses often find it challenging to respect patients who have committed serious offences. Is it possible for nurses working in a forensic or correctional setting to respect every patient? Explain your answer.

# CHAPTER REVIEW

1. Which statement regarding forensic nursing is accurate?
   1. Forensic nurses must all be prepared at the doctoral level.
   2. Forensic nurses perform only sexual assault examinations.
   3. Forensic nurses may participate in death investigations.
   4. Forensic psychiatric mental health nurses work only in correctional facilities.

2. What is one of the most challenging aspects of forensic psychiatric nursing?
   1. Working independently instead of as a member of an interdisciplinary team
   2. Balancing the custodial role with the therapeutic role
   3. Spending time in maximum security settings
   4. Determining the guilt or innocence of forensic patients

3. What does it mean for an individual to be found unfit to stand trial?
   1. The individual is unable to understand the court proceedings.
   2. The individual has a life-threatening physical illness.
   3. The individual has a chronic mental illness.
   4. The individual does not demonstrate insight into his or her mental illness.

4. Which type of patients would a correctional nurse typically see?
   1. Students
   2. Police officers
   3. Teachers
   4. Inmates

5. The nurse is caring for an incarcerated patient. Based on an understanding of the health profile of incarcerated individuals, what health care challenge may the nurse most anticipate working on with this patient?

1. Drug or alcohol issues
2. Autoimmune diseases
3. Eating disorders
4. Anxiety

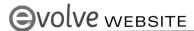 WEBSITE

Post-Test interactive review

*Visit the Evolve Web site for Chapter Review Answers and Rationales, Critical Thinking Answer Guidelines, and additional resources related to the content in this chapter: http://evolve.elsevier.com/Canada/Varcarolis/psychiatric/*

## REFERENCES

BearPaw Media Productions. (2009). *The BANG you feel.* Retrieved from http://www.bearpaweducation.ca/publications/bang-you-feel.

Blitz, C.L., Wolff, N., & Shi, J. (2008). Physical victimization in prison: The role of mental illness. *International Journal of Law and Psychiatry, 31,* 385–393. doi:10.1016/j.ijlp.2008.08.005.

Bouchard, F. (2004). A health care needs assessment of federal inmates in Canada. *Canadian Journal of Public Health, 95*(Suppl. 1), S1–S63.

Canadian Institute for Health Information. (2008). *Improving the health of Canadians: Mental health, delinquency and criminal activity.* Retrieved from https://secure.cihi.ca/free_products/mh_crime_full_report_apr11_08_e.pdf.

Canadian Mental Health Association. (2013). *Violence and mental illness.* Retrieved from http://www.cmha.ca/mental_health/violence-and-mental-illness/.

CBC News. (2013). *Ashley Smith coroner calls inquest a "memorial" to teen.* Retrieved from http://www.cbc.ca/news/canada/story/2013/01/14/ashley-smith-coroner-inquest-begins.html.

Constitution Act, 1982, c. 11.

Correctional Service of Canada. (2010). *Quick facts: Health services sector, types of health care settings.* Retrieved from http://www.csc-scc.gc.ca/text/pblct/qf/15-eng.shtml.

Correctional Service of Canada. (2011). *Changing lives, protecting Canadians: A career in nursing.* Retrieved from http://www.csc-scc.gc.ca/text/pblct/hsbroch/nur.pdf.

Corrections and Conditional Release Act, S.C. 1992, c. 20.

Criminal Code, R.S.C. 1985, c. C-46.

Crocker, A.G., & Côté, G. (2009). Evolving systems of care: Individuals found not criminally responsible on account of mental disorder in custody of civil and forensic services. *European Psychiatry, 24,* 356–364. doi:10.1016/j.eurpsy.2009.07.008.

Department of Justice Canada. (2009). *Review of the mental disorder provisions of the Criminal Code.* Response to the 14th report of the Standing Committee on Justice and Human Rights. Retrieved from http://www.parl.gc.ca/HousePublications/Publication.aspx?DocId=557270&Language=E&Mode=1&Parl=37&Ses=1.

Devnick, B.R. (2010). *The forensic mental health nurse: Confusion, illusion, or specialization? A scoping literature review* (Master's project). University of Victoria, Victoria, B.C.

Doran, D., & Almost, J. (2010). *Exploring worklife issues in provincial correctional settings: Final report to the nursing secretariat, Ontario Ministry of Health and Long Term Care.* Retrieved from http://www.nhsru.com/wp-content/uploads/2010/11/Exploring-Worklife-Issues-in-Provincial-Correctional-Settings-201011.pdf.

Forensic Nurses Society of Canada. (2012). *About.* Retrieved from http://forensicnurse.ca/about.

Hiday, V.A., Swanson, J.W., Swartz, M.S., et al. (2001). Victimization: A link between mental illness and violence? *International Journal of Law and Psychiatry, 24*(6), 559–572.

International Association of Forensic Nurses. (2006a). *About IAFN.* Retrieved from http://www.iafn.org/displaycommon.cfm?an=3.

International Association of Forensic Nurses. (2006b). *What is forensic nursing.* Retrieved from http://www.iafn.org/displaycommon.cfm?an=1&subarticlenbr=137.

International Association of Forensic Nurses & American Nurses Association. (2009). *Scope and standards of forensic nursing practice.* Washington, DC: American Nurses Publishing.

Kearley, C., & Steeves, S. (2010). Caring in corrections. *Canadian Nurse, 106*(4), 23–29. Retrieved from http://www.canadian-nurse.com/.

Kent-Wilkinson, A. (2008). *Forensic nursing education in North America: An exploratory study* (Doctoral dissertation). Department of Educational Administration, University of Saskatchewan, Saskatoon, SK. Retrieved from http://library2.usask.ca/theses/available/etd-08262008-171000/.

Livingston, J.D. (2006). A statistical survey of Canadian forensic mental health inpatient programs. *Healthcare Quarterly, 6*(2), 56–61.

Lyons, T. (2009). The role of the forensic psychiatric nurse. *Journal of Forensic Nursing, 5,* 53–57. doi:10.1111/j.1939-3938.2009.01033.x.

Mental Health Commission of Canada. (2012). *Changing directions, changing lives: The mental health strategy for Canada.* Calgary: Author.

Office of the Correctional Investigator Canada. (2009). *Annual report of the Office of the Correctional Investigator, 2008–2009.* Retrieved from http://www.oci-bec.gc.ca/cnt/rpt/pdf/annrpt/annrpt20082009-eng.pdf.

Office of the Correctional Investigator Canada. (2012). *Annual report of the Office of the Correctional Investigator, 2011–2012.* Retrieved from http://www.oci-bec.gc.ca/cnt/rpt/annrpt/annrpt20112012-eng.aspx.

Parliament of Canada. (2010). *Mental health and drug and alcohol addiction in the federal correctional system: Report of the Standing Committee on Public Safety and National Security.* Retrieved from http://www.parl.gc.ca/HousePublications/Publication.aspx?DocId=4864852&Language=E&Mode=1&Parl=40&Ses=3.

Parliament of Canada. (2012). *Drugs and alcohol in federal penitentiaries: An alarming problem: Report of the Standing Committee on Public Safety and National Security.* Retrieved from http://www.parl.gc.ca/content/hoc/Committee/411/SECU/Reports/RP5498869/securp02/securp02-e.pdf.

Peternelji-Taylor, C. (2008). Criminalization of the mentally ill. *Journal of Forensic Nursing, 4,* 185–187. doi:10.1111/j.1939-3938.2008.00031.x.

Public Safety Canada. (2010). *Supporting the successful implementation of the National Crime Prevention Strategy.* Retrieved from http://www.publicsafety.gc.ca/cnt/rsrcs/pblctns/spprtng-mplmtn/index-eng.aspx.

Romano, C. (2011). Examining the role of the forensic nurse death investigator. *Nursing, 111,* 20–21. doi:10.1097/01.NAJ.0000392855.52189.ce.

Sekula, L.K. (2006). Forensic nursing in the 21st century (5, supplemental issue ed.). In C.H. Wecht (Ed.), *Forensic Sciences* (5th ed.). Albany, NY: Matthew Bender.

Sekula, L.K., & Burgess, A.W. (2006). *Forensic and legal nursing* (Vol. 1). Boca Raton, FL: CRC Press.

Statistics Canada. (2009). *Canada Year Book: Crime and justice.* Retrieved from http://www41.statcan.gc.ca/2009/2693/cybac2693_000-eng.htm.

Stewart, K. (1984). Work in the chief medical examiner's office. *Alberta Association of Registered Nurses Newsletter, 40*(7), 13. Retrieved from http://www.ncbi.nlm.nih.gov/pubmed/6564830.

Teplin, L.A., McClelland, G.M., Abram, K.M., et al. (2005). Crime victimization in adults with severe mental illness. *Archives of General Psychiatry, 62*, 911–921. doi:10.1001/archpsyc.62.8.911.

Trevethan, S., Moore, J.-P., Auger, S., et al. (2002). Childhood experiences affect Aboriginal offenders. *FORUM on Corrections Research, 14*(3), 7–9. Retrieved from http://www.csc-scc.gc.ca/text/pblct/forum/e143/143c_e.pdf.

Volstad, C.M.S. (2008). An RN shares her perspective on forensic psychiatric nursing. *Alberta RN, 64*(4), 12–13.

World Health Organization. (2002). *World report on violence and health: Summary.* Geneva, Switzerland: World Health Organization.

# Advanced Intervention Modalities

# Therapeutic Groups

*Karyn I. Morgan, Nancy Christine Shoemaker*
*Adapted by Wilma Schroeder*

## KEY TERMS AND CONCEPTS

conflict, 688
group, 687
group content, 688
group norms, 688
group process, 688
group psychotherapy, 694

group themes, 688
group work, 687
psychoeducational groups, 692
self-help groups, 694
support groups, 694
therapeutic factors, 688

## OBJECTIVES

1. Identify basic concepts related to group work.
2. Describe the phases of group development.
3. Define task and maintenance roles of group members.
4. Discuss the therapeutic factors that operate in all groups.

5. Discuss four types of groups commonly led by nurses.
6. Describe a group intervention for (1) a member who is silent or (2) a member who is monopolizing the group.

## €volve WEBSITE

*Visit the Evolve website for Flashcards, Case Studies, and additional testing resources related to the content in this chapter:* http://evolve.elsevier.com/Canada/Varcarolis/psychiatric/   Pre-Test   interactive review

We all live and interact among groups throughout our lives. We are born into a family group and grow up with various peer groups, such as those at school, at work, within religious or spiritual affiliations, and so on. As adults, we establish our own family group. A group consists of two or more people who come together for the purpose of pursuing common goals, interests, or both. A group's progress and outcomes are influenced by the group's characteristics, including the following:

- Size
- Defined purpose
- Degree of similarity among members
- Rules
- Boundaries
- Content (what is said in the group)
- Process (underlying dynamics among group members)

Box 35-1 defines terms related to types of groups and group work. Group work is a method whereby individuals with a

common purpose come together and benefit by giving and receiving feedback within the context of group life.

There are advantages and disadvantages of the group approach for people living with mental illness. Advantages include the following:

- Engaging multiple people in treatment at the same time, thereby saving costs
- Enabling participants to benefit from the feedback not only of the nurse leader but also of peers, who may possess a unique understanding of the issues
- Providing a relatively safe setting to try out new ways of relating to other people and practising new communication skills
- Promoting a feeling of belonging
  Disadvantages include the following:
- Time constraints in which an individual member may feel cheated for floor time, particularly in large groups

**TERMS CENTRAL TO THERAPEUTIC GROUPS**

**Terms Describing Group Work**

Group content—all that is said in the group

Group process—the dynamics of interaction among the members (e.g., who talks to whom, facial expressions, body language)

Group norms—expectations for behaviour in the group that develop over time and provide structure for members (e.g., starting on time, not interrupting)

Group themes—members' expressed ideas or feelings that recur and have a common thread (The leader can clarify a theme to help members recognize it more fully.)

Conflict—open disagreement among members (Positive conflict resolution within a group is key to successful outcomes.)

**Terms Describing Types of Groups**

*Heterogeneous group*—a group in which there is a range of differences among members

*Homogeneous group*—a group in which all members share central traits (e.g., men's group, group of people with bipolar disorder)

*Closed group*—a group in which membership is restricted; no new members are added when others leave

*Open group*—a group in which new members are added as others leave

*Subgroup*—an individual or a small group that is isolated within a larger group and functions separately (Members of a subgroup may have greater loyalty, more similar goals, or more perceived similarities to one another than they do to the larger group.)

**THERAPEUTIC FACTORS IN GROUPS**

*Instillation of hope*—The leader shares optimism about group treatment, and members share their improvements.

*Universality*—Members realize that they are not alone in their problems, feelings, or thoughts.

*Imparting of information*—Participants receive formal teaching by the leader or advice from peers.

*Altruism*—Members feel a reward from giving support to others.

*Corrective recapitulation of the primary family group*—Members repeat patterns of behaviour in the group that they learned in their families; with feedback from the leader and peers, they learn about their own behaviour.

*Development of socializing techniques*—Members learn new social skills based on feedback from others.

*Imitative behaviour*—Members may copy behaviour from the leader or peers and can adopt healthier habits.

*Interpersonal learning*—Members gain insight into themselves based on feedback from others. This process is complex and occurs later in the group, after trust is established.

*Group cohesiveness*—This powerful factor arises in a mature group, when each member feels connected to the other members, the leader, and the group as a whole; in a cohesive group, members can accept positive feedback and constructive criticism.

*Catharsis*—Intense feelings, as judged by the member, are shared.

*Existential resolution*—Members learn to accept painful aspects of life (e.g., loneliness, death) that affect everyone.

**Source:** Data from Yalom, I.D. (2005). *The theory and practice of group psychotherapy* (5th ed.). New York: Basic Books.

- Concerns that private issues may be shared outside the group
- Disruptive member behaviour during an emotionally vulnerable point

Not everyone benefits from group treatment. People who are acutely psychotic, acutely manic, or intoxicated have difficulty interacting effectively in groups and may interfere with other members' ability to remain focused on group goals and progress.

## THERAPEUTIC FACTORS COMMON TO ALL GROUPS

Irvin D. Yalom (2005), one of the most noted researchers on group psychotherapy, is credited with identifying the factors that make groups therapeutic (Box 35-2). Therapeutic factors are aspects of the group experience that facilitate therapeutic change. For example, as group members begin to share life experiences, feelings, and concerns, they may recognize for the first time that they are not "alone in the world"—their experiences may be more universal than they initially thought, allowing them to connect with others. Yalom calls this factor *universality*—the recognition that other people feel the same way or have had the same experiences. Recognizing universality can provide a validation of the person's experiences and, subsequently, a profound sense of relief. Different therapeutic factors operate at different phases of a group, and during the

initial phase, the leader may role-model several behaviours, such as instilling hope and imparting information. Just as with other types of treatment, each person's response to a group is highly individualized, based on past experiences and level of participation.

## PLANNING A GROUP

Planning a group should include developing a description of its specific characteristics—for example:

- Name and objectives of the group
- Common concerns or diagnoses of members
- Group schedule (frequency, times of meetings, etc.)
- Descriptions of leader's and members' responsibilities
- Methods or means of evaluating outcomes of the group

Planning and structure is especially important when group leaders are likely to change (e.g., in inpatient settings, where staffing patterns change) or when several groups are running at the same time with a common goal (e.g., in a research study).

## PHASES OF GROUP DEVELOPMENT

All groups go through developmental phases similar to those identified for individual therapeutic relationships (see

Chapter 10). In each phase, the group leader has specific roles and challenges to address in support of positive interaction, growth, and change.

In the *orientation phase*, the group leader's role is to structure an atmosphere of respect, confidentiality, and trust. The purpose of the group is stated, and members are encouraged to get to know one another. Group rules such as confidentiality or avoidance of potentially inflammatory topics such as politics are reviewed. Initially, members may be overly silent or overbearing because they have not yet established trust with one another. Therapeutic interaction is supported when the group leader points out similarities between members, encourages them to talk directly to each other rather than to the leader, and reminds members about ground rules for respectful interaction.

In the *working phase*, the group leader's role is to encourage focus on problem solving consistent with the purpose of the group. As group members begin to feel safe within the group, conflicts may be expressed, which should be viewed by the group leader as a positive opportunity for group growth. It is important for the leader to guide and support conflict resolution. Through successful resolution of conflicts, group members are empowered to develop confidence in their problem-solving abilities and better support one another in their individual efforts to grow and change.

In the *termination phase*, the group leader's role is to encourage members to reflect on progress they have made and identify post-termination goals. Members may experience feelings of loss or anger about the group ending; at times, these feelings can be directed toward other group members or the leader. It is important to openly address such feelings as part of the group's work toward successful termination.

## GROUP MEMBER ROLES

We each have a unique style of interacting with others, and we gravitate toward specific comfort zones within groups. Consider your own behaviours within groups. You may tend to sit back and mainly observe, giving your opinion only after careful consideration. Or perhaps you feel it is important to keep everyone moving in a common direction or help maintain order and actively urge people to continue working. The way we behave in groups is a function of our innate personalities, socialization, and the specific context of the group.

Studies of group dynamics have identified informal roles that group members often assume and that may or may not be helpful in the group's development. The classic descriptive categories for these roles are *task*, *maintenance*, and *individual* roles (Benne & Sheats, 1948). Task roles serve to keep the group focused on its main purpose and get the work done. Maintenance roles function to help each person feel worthwhile and create a sense of group cohesion. Individual roles have nothing to do with helping the group but instead relate to specific personalities, personal agendas, and a desire to have needs met by shifting the group's focus to them. Awareness of roles can assist the group leader to identify behaviours that need to be confronted or reinforced. Table 35-1 describes the informal roles of group members.

## GROUP LEADERSHIP

### Responsibilities

The group leader has multiple responsibilities in initiating, maintaining, and terminating a group.

The first responsibility is to determine the purpose, parameters, and membership of the group. Will the group be open, accepting new members regularly, or closed to new members after it begins? How often will the group meet, where, and for how long? It is also advisable in many instances to choose a co-leader to help facilitate the group and, especially on inpatient units, one or more observers.

The leader and co-leader should base selection of group members on clear criteria, depending on the type of group. Group members need to have a certain degree of cognitive functioning in order to participate in an insight-oriented psychotherapy group.

The styles of group leadership vary depending on the type of group and on the stage of group development. For example, the leader is often most direct in the orientation phase. During this phase, the structure, size, composition, purpose, and timing of the group are defined. Task and maintenance functions may be discussed and demonstrated. During the working phase, the leader facilitates communication and ensures that meetings begin and end on time. In the termination phase, the leader ensures that each member summarizes individual accomplishments and gives positive and negative feedback regarding the group experience.

Maintenance of cultural safety for individual members is a key responsibility of the group leader. The leader initially sets a foundation for open communication by defining the importance of mutual respect and rules for group conduct. As group members begin to engage with one another, the leader's sensitivity to issues that may have a cultural basis can be pivotal in facilitating efforts to maintain open communication and mutual respect.

Diversity may exist in many forms, including racial, ethnic, economic, and sexual orientation. Encouraging members to share and explore their cultural foundations and beliefs promotes genuine communication and provides the group with the opportunity to share similarities and differences in an environment of mutual respect.

Consider the example of a woman who came to group after seriously harming herself. She remained silent and withdrawn until the leader encouraged her to explore her feelings about the group. The woman revealed that she "wasn't smart like everyone else" and that she was "basically just trailer trash." Other group members began to share their similarities and differences in backgrounds, with a focus on their common needs, fears, and insecurities. When this woman finished the group, she acknowledged having learned an important lesson: she could give and get help from people she saw as different from her, and not everyone would treat her as though she was "less than them."

### Styles of Leadership

There are three main styles of group leadership, and a leader selects the style that is best suited to the therapeutic needs of a

| TABLE 35-1 | INFORMAL ROLES OF GROUP MEMBERS | |
|---|---|---|
| | ROLE | FUNCTION |
| Task roles | Coordinator | Tries to connect various ideas and suggestions |
| | Elaborator | Gives examples and follows up meaning of ideas |
| | Energizer | Encourages group to make decisions or take actions |
| | Evaluator | Measures the group's work against a standard |
| | Information giver | Shares facts or own experience as an authority figure |
| | Information seeker | Tries to clarify the group's values |
| | Initiator–contributor | Offers new ideas or a new outlook on an issue |
| | Opinion giver | Shares opinions, especially to influence group values |
| | Orienter | Notes the progress of the group toward goals |
| | Procedural technician | Supports group activity by distributing papers, arranging seating, etc. |
| | Recorder | Keeps notes and acts as the group's memory |
| Maintenance roles | Compromiser | In a conflict, yields to preserve group harmony |
| | Encourager | Praises and seeks input from others |
| | Follower | Agrees with the flow of the group |
| | Gatekeeper | Monitors the participation of all members to keep communication open |
| | Group observer | Keeps records of different aspects of group process and reports to the group |
| | Harmonizer | Tries to mediate conflicts between members |
| | Standard setter | Verbalizes standards for the group |
| Individual roles | Aggressor | Criticizes and attacks others' ideas and feelings |
| | Blocker | Disagrees with group issues; oppositional |
| | Dominator | Tries to control other members of the group with flattery or interruptions |
| | Help seeker | Asks for sympathy of group excessively |
| | Playboy | Acts uninterested in group process |
| | Recognition seeker | Seeks attention by boasting and discussing achievements |
| | Self-confessor | Verbalizes feelings or observations unrelated to group |
| | Special-interest pleader | Advocates for a special group, usually with own prejudice or bias |

**Source:** Data from Benne, K., & Sheats, P. (1948). Functional roles of group members. *Journal of Social Issues, 4,* 41–49. doi:10.1111/j.1540-4560.1948.tb01783.x.

particular group—the therapeutic needs of the group are determined by the type of group and by the stage of group development. The *autocratic leader* exerts control over the group and does not encourage much interaction among members. For example, staff leading a community meeting with a fixed, time-limited agenda may tend to be more autocratic. In contrast, the *democratic leader* supports extensive group interaction in the process of problem solving. Psychotherapy groups most often employ this leadership style. In this style, the leader and co-leader take a facilitative role, redirecting questions or issues to group members, rather than providing answers or solutions. A *laissez-faire leader* allows the group members to behave in any way they choose and does not attempt to control the direction of the group. In a creative group, such as an art or horticulture group, the leader may choose a laissez-faire style.

In any group, the leader must be thoughtful about communication techniques since these can have a tremendous impact on group content and process. Table 35-2 describes communication techniques frequently used by group leaders. It is also important to note that inpatient groups have significant differences from outpatient groups (Table 35-3), and consequently the role of the leader must be adapted accordingly.

## Clinical Supervision

Clinical supervision, sometimes referred to as *peer supervision* or *clinical consultation*, is important for group leaders as it provides feedback about performance and enhances professional growth of the nurse. Transference and counter-transference issues occur in groups just as in individual treatment (see Chapter 10), and a more objective input supports a focus on therapeutic goals. Feedback related to the functioning of the group and the leadership style being used can also help further develop the skills related to respect and engagement. Another strategy used to support group leader development is co-leadership. Co-leadership is a common practice and has several benefits, including (1) providing training for less experienced staff, (2) allowing for immediate feedback between leaders after each session, and (3) offering two role models for teaching communication skills to members.

## Group Observation

In some groups, it is useful—and even essential—to assign staff as observers. In some cases, the use of an observer may occur for the purpose of clinical supervision. Another reason would

## TABLE 35-2 GROUP LEADER COMMUNICATION TECHNIQUES

| TECHNIQUE | EXAMPLE |
|---|---|
| Giving information—provides resources and information that support treatment goals | "Antidepressants may take as long as 4 weeks or more to show real therapeutic effects." |
| Clarification—asks group members to expand and clarify what they mean | "What do you mean when you say 'I can't go back to work'?" |
| Confrontation—encourages group members to explore inconsistencies in their communication or behaviour | "Jane, you're saying 'nothing's wrong,' but you're crying." |
| Reflection—encourages group members to explore and expand on feelings (rather than on thoughts or events) | "I noticed you're clenching your fists. What are you feeling right now?"<br>"It sounds like that really upset you." |
| Summarization—closes a discussion or group session by pointing out key issues and insights | "We've talked about different types of cognitive distortions, and everyone identified at least one irrational thought that has influenced his or her behaviour in a negative way. In the next group, we'll explore some strategies for correcting negative thinking." |
| Support—gives positive feedback and acknowledgement | "It took a lot of courage to explore those painful feelings. You're really working hard on resolving this problem." |

## TABLE 35-3 COMPARISON OF OUTPATIENT AND INPATIENT GROUPS

| OUTPATIENT GROUPS | INPATIENT GROUPS |
|---|---|
| The group has a stable composition. | The group is rarely made up of the same members for more than one or two meetings. |
| Members are carefully selected and prepared. | Members are admitted to the group with little prior selection or preparation. |
| The group is homogeneous with regard to ego function. | The group has a heterogeneous level of ego function. |
| Motivated, self-referred people make up the group; therapy is growth oriented. | Members are ambivalent, and, often, therapy is compulsory; therapy is relief oriented. |
| Treatment proceeds as long as required; it may continue for one to two years. | Treatment is limited to the hospital period, with rapid member turnover. |
| The boundary of the group is well maintained, with few external influences. | Whatever happens on the unit affects the group. |
| Group cohesion develops normally, given sufficient time in treatment. | There is no time for cohesion to develop spontaneously; group development is limited to the initial phase. |
| The leader allows the process to unfold; there is ample time to set up group norms. | The group leader structures time and is not passive. |
| Members are encouraged to avoid extra-group contact. | Members eat, sleep, and live together outside of the group; extra-group contact is endorsed. |

**Source:** Adapted from Mackenzie, K.R. (1997). *Time-managed group psychotherapy: Effective clinical applications.* Washington, DC: American Psychiatric Press.

be for staff to observe how group members interact and then share their observations with the leaders in order to assess and plan for modifications to the group or individual patient care plans. In inpatient groups or day programs, there may be concern about patients leaving the group in a fragile emotional state; one role of the observer is to maintain safety. The observer follows and tends to the needs of any group member who left the session before it was over.

It is useful for the group observer to monitor not just content but process—that is, not only *what* is talked about but *how* it is talked about. A simple method is to draw a diagram of who is sitting where and, while observing, draw lines between members to indicate who speaks to whom. This diagram can give instant feedback as to patterns of behaviour in group members.

## NURSE AS GROUP LEADER

Psychiatric mental health nurses are involved in a variety of therapeutic groups in acute care and long-term treatment settings. Nurses are able to provide strong leadership skills in a variety of basic groups, such as activity, psychoeducational, task, and support groups, and, with support, they may co-lead more advanced groups, such as cognitive-behavioural therapy or counselling groups. More complex skills are necessary for leading psychotherapy groups, and only advanced-practice nurses or nurse therapists are qualified to lead these and other specialized groups.

For all group leaders, a clear theoretical framework is necessary to provide a foundation for analyzing the group interaction. Table 35-4 describes several theoretical frameworks commonly used in group work.

### Basic Groups
#### Psychoeducational Groups
Psychoeducational groups aim to increase knowledge or skills about a specific subject and allow members to communicate emotional concerns. These groups may be time limited or may be supportive for long-term treatment. Generally, written handouts or audiovisual aids are used to focus on specific teaching points. Nurses are prepared to teach a variety of health subjects.

*Medication Education.* The most common psychoeducational group led by a nurse is the medication education group. These groups are designed to teach patients about their medications, answer their questions, and prepare them for self-management. When patients have concerns about taking medications, it is often the group members themselves who are in the position to respond to these questions: "Yes, I got a dry mouth when I first started taking that, but it got better. Hang in there." Box 35-3 outlines an example of a medication education group protocol, and Figure 35-1 shows a tool used to evaluate a medication group.

*Health Education.* Nurses also frequently lead health education groups, including groups on sex education. For instance, people who have used poor judgement in sexual behaviour because of mental illness are at high risk for sexually transmitted infections.

*Family Education.* Nurses may also facilitate family psychoeducational groups, usually as part of an interdisciplinary team. Individual relapse rates decrease significantly when families are

| TABLE 35-4 | THEORETICAL FOUNDATIONS FOR GROUP THERAPY | |
| --- | --- | --- |
| **THEORY** | **CONCEPTS** | **ROLE OF THERAPIST** |
| Psychodynamic/ psychoanalytic | Applies Freud's concepts of psychoanalysis to individual members and to the group itself; focus is on unconscious conflicts and transference; goal is insight | Helps members to recognize unconscious conflicts and encourages peer feedback |
| Interpersonal | Applies Sullivan's theories about interpersonal learning; focus is on understanding how current relationships repeat early significant relationships; goal is to rebuild individual's personality | Helps to reduce anxiety and encourages members to validate feelings and thoughts with each other |
| Communication | Applies a systems model, holding that the whole (group) is greater than the sum of its parts (members); focus is on subgroups and communication, both verbal and nonverbal; goal is to learn clear, congruent communication skills | Helps point out confusing or contradictory messages; acts as a role model for clear communication |
| Group process | Analyzes the group with a focus on individual roles and group patterns of behaviour (phases, norms, etc.); goal is to resolve authority and intimacy issues | Helps develop a mature group in which members trust each other and give supportive feedback |
| Existential/gestalt | Applies theories of Maslow and Rogers to encourage individuals to develop to full potential; focus is on the here and now to increase members' awareness of feelings; goal is self-actualization, in which individual takes full responsibility for choices | Helps focus members on here-and-now experiences to promote self-learning; promotes emphasis on the "what" of behaviours, not the "why" |
| Cognitive-behavioural | Applies concepts of learning theory and Ellis's cognitive therapy; focus is on behaviour and thinking patterns, with the group used to reinforce adaptive behaviour and extinguish maladaptive patterns; usually time limited; goal is to change behaviour or thinking patterns | Helps develop a trusting group in which members give supportive feedback to reinforce healthier behaviour; may provide formal teaching, including homework assignments |

**Source:** Data from Dies, R. (1992). Models of group psychotherapy: Sifting through confusion. *International Journal of Group Psychotherapy, 42*(1), 1–17; and Scheidlinger, S. (1997). Group dynamics and group psychotherapy revisited: Four decades later. *International Journal of Group Psychotherapy, 47*(2), 141–159.

## BOX 35-3   EXAMPLE OF MEDICATION EDUCATION GROUP PROTOCOL

**Description of Group**
A group for all patients, regardless of level of concentration, that prepares them for self-management of medication on discharge

**Criteria for Member Selection**
Open to all inpatients except those who are displaying suicidal or homicidal behaviours or the potential for assault

**Visual Aids**
PowerPoint slides, transparencies, flip charts, films, patient medication education sheets

**Purpose**
1. To educate members on the primary function of their medications
2. To provide information on adverse effects (that benefits can outweigh risks)
3. To describe a mechanism to negotiate relationships with health care workers
4. To enhance a sense of self-control over treatment

**Procedure**
1. Orientation and introduction to the group
2. Brief description of major symptoms in a diagnosis
3. Overview of antipsychotic drugs or antidepressants
4. Use of medication education sheets
5. Specific open question period

**Behavioural Objectives**
At the end of the 45-minute session, members will be able to:
1. State one of their symptoms that is treated by their medication
2. Be able to ask at least one question about their medication
3. Identify one mechanism that helps in adhering to the medication regimen

**Theoretical Justification**
Even people who think they are adherent take only 80% of doses. Counselling and therapy are always adjuncts to drug therapy.

**Source:** Adapted from Ott, C.A. (2000). *Pediatric psychopharmacology*. South Easton, MD: American Healthcare Institute.

| Criteria | Strongly Agree | Somewhat Agree | Agree | Disagree | Strongly Disagree |
|---|---|---|---|---|---|
| 1. I know the name(s) of the medication(s) I am taking. | | | | | |
| 2. I know what symptoms the medication(s) can help me with. | | | | | |
| 3. I know the common adverse effects of my medication(s). | | | | | |
| 4. I feel comfortable talking to my prescriber if I am having problems with my medication(s). | | | | | |
| 5. It is important to take my medication(s) at the same time every day. | | | | | |

**FIGURE 35-1** Medication group evaluation tool.

educated about mental illness, treatments, and recovery, as well as strategies for interacting with an ill family member and managing crises. Family psychoeducation is a recognized evidence-informed practice in psychosocial rehabilitation (Bond & Campbell, 2008).

***Concurrent Disorders.*** Concurrent disorder groups integrate learning about co-existing mental illnesses and substance abuse. Since treatment issues for people with a concurrent disorder can be complex, group leaders must have demonstrated competency in both mental health and chemical dependence treatment. The goal is to engage people in treatment and decrease their use of substances in a step-by-step process. Research has shown that combined treatment for people with serious mental illness produces improved outcomes (Drake, Essock, Shaner, et al., 2001).

***Symptom Management.*** For people with a common symptom such as anger or anxiety, symptom management

groups are ideal. The focus is on sharing positive and negative experiences so that members learn coping skills from each other. A primary goal is to increase self-control or prevent relapse by helping members develop an individualized plan for action at the first appearance of symptoms.

***Stress Management.*** Often, time-limited stress management groups teach members about various relaxation techniques, including deep breathing, exercise, music, and spirituality. One such technique that is increasingly demonstrating efficacy in stress management is mindfulness (Chadwick, Taylor, & Abba, 2005). Mindfulness groups focus on developing awareness of the present moment, with the intent to induce relaxation and promote insight into thoughts, emotions, and physical responses. Although much of the research has focused on the use of this technique in outpatient settings, one study by York (2007) reports the benefits of this technique for acutely ill patients on an inpatient unit.

***Support and Self-Help Groups.*** Support groups (often facilitated by a professional) and self-help groups (facilitated by the group itself) are structured for the purpose of providing members with the opportunity to maintain or enhance personal and social functioning through cooperation and shared understanding of life's challenges (Hayes, Hope, Terryberry-Spohr, et al., 2006; Yalom, 2005). Examples include support groups for survivors of cancer, bereavement support, or support groups for families who have lost a loved one to suicide. Hayes and colleagues (2006) present evidence of the benefits of supportive group therapy for severe mental illness as well. Their findings indicated that adding structured cognitive exercises enhanced the overall improvement in this population over supportive group therapy alone.

The nurse may serve as a resource for individuals and families and must be aware of the wide array of self-help groups available. One of the most important functions of such groups is to demonstrate to individuals and families that they are not alone in having a particular problem. Participants in these types of group report feeling as though their experiences and feelings have been validated. Thus, these groups provide members with support, and their members help each other by telling their stories and providing alternative ways to view and to resolve problems. Box 35-4 describes characteristics of support and self-help groups.

## Advanced-Practice Nurse or Nurse Therapist
### Group Psychotherapy

Group psychotherapy is a specialized treatment intervention in which a trained leader (or co-leaders) establishes a group for the purpose of treating people with psychiatric disorders. Expertise is necessary since the group is used as a tool to bring about personality change (Sadock & Sadock, 2008). Often, group psychotherapy is done in conjunction with individual psychotherapy as part of an ongoing plan. The Canadian Group Psychotherapy Association provides standards and training for mental health professionals, including nurses, to develop skills in this specialty.

***Psychodrama Groups.*** Psychodrama groups are specialized groups in which members are encouraged to act out life experiences or situations for the purpose of learning and insight. Leaders should have graduate-level education and training specific to this approach.

***Dialectical Behaviour Treatment.*** Dialectical behaviour treatment (DBT) is a type of group psychotherapy in which people are seen each week with the goal of improving interpersonal, behavioural, cognitive, and emotional skills and reducing self-destructive behaviours (Sadock & Sadock, 2008). Unlike in other types of group therapy, DBT group members are discouraged from making observations about others in the group. This treatment also requires specialized training and advanced education.

***Integrative Groups.*** An integrative group program consists of a number of sessions with a particular theme or purpose, in which individual group sessions may draw from any of the aforementioned approaches. An example is a group for treatment of binge eating behaviour, which is reported in the

---

## BOX 35-4    SUPPORT AND SELF-HELP GROUPS

**Target Population**
- People who have shared the experience of a common problem, illness, crisis, or tragedy

**Group Leader Activities**
- May or may not be defined; may rotate among members
- Role is often more task oriented

**Examples of Support Groups**
- Bereavement groups for those who have experienced the loss of a loved one
- Suicide survivor groups for those who have lost a loved one to suicide
- Canadian Mental Health Association (CMHA) groups for patient or family support (or both), education, and advocacy
- Cancer support groups for families and individuals coping with the ramifications of this illness
- Internet support groups for a growing number of people, providing online, real-time interaction and support

**Examples of Self-Help Groups and Resources**
- Twelve-step groups that use a common model for recovery:
  - Alcoholics Anonymous (AA)—the prototype for other 12-step groups
  - Gamblers Anonymous (GA)
  - Overeaters Anonymous (OA)
  - Narcotics Anonymous (NA)
  - Co-Dependents Anonymous
  - Adult Children of Alcoholics (ACOA)
- Online listings of self-help resources in Canada:
  - eMentalHealth.ca (listing of national self-help and mutual aid groups): http://www.ementalhealth.ca/canada/en/_Selfhelp_mutual_aid_and_support_groups_a1_b44.html?filterLocalOnly=1
  - National Network for Mental Health (NNMH): http://www.nnmh.ca/Home/tabid/380/language/en-CA/Default.aspx
  - Self Help Connection: http://www.selfhelpconnection.ca
  - Canadian Coalition of Alternative Mental Health Resources: http://ccamhr.ca/memberslist.html

**Goals of Support and Self-Help Groups**
- To provide health education and networking for resources
- To reduce anxiety and decrease feelings of isolation
- To provide support and encouragement of positive coping behaviours:
  - Decrease feelings of isolation
  - Provide mutual support
  - Provide psychoeducation and health education
  - Reduce stress
  - Help people cease self-destructive behaviours or come to terms with an overwhelming event or situation

**Frequency and Duration**
- Meets one or more times per week for an indefinite period of time
- Ongoing and open membership

Research Highlight box. Integrative groups may also be used to support and treat psychological symptoms that survivors of interpersonal trauma or abuse may experience. Chapter 27 further describes support and treatment approaches for people who have experienced interpersonal trauma.

## Dealing With Challenging Member Behaviours

Research has identified certain behaviours of individual members that are challenging to manage within a group. Defensive behaviours interfere with people's ability to function or achieve satisfaction in their lives. Group therapy is about working through problem behaviours, but some behaviours can be especially disruptive to the group process and difficult for the leader to manage. The person who monopolizes the group, the person who complains but continues to reject help, the demoralizing person, and the silent person are examples (Yalom, 2005).

In dealing with any problematic behaviours in groups, members may appreciate help disclosing their own feelings and responses. The leader encourages the use of statements such as "When you speak this way, I feel . . ." The leader helps by noting that feelings are not right or wrong but simply exist. People tend to feel less defensive when "I feel" statements rather than "you are" statements are used. This approach helps members feel like part of the group, not alienated from it.

### Monopolizing Member

The person who monopolizes the group may be attempting to deal with anxiety. As group tension grows, the person's level of anxiety rises, and the tendency to speak increases. Some people are just extremely talkative or may be hypertalkative due to hypomania or mania. In any case, no one else gets a chance to be heard, and other group members eventually lose interest and begin to withdraw.

---

**VIGNETTE**

Holly is the most talkative member of the group until the nurse intervenes. Initially, Holly talks at length about her early experiences related to losing both of her parents and having to live with her grandparents. The other members of the group become bored with the same old story, and they drift off. They have heard these stories many times, not only in group therapy but also during other activities.

---

There are several useful strategies for dealing with an overly talkative group member. One strategy is to request a response from group members who have not had a chance to talk about the day's topic. If the behaviour continues, it may be necessary to speak directly to the monopolizing group member, either privately or in the group setting. In private, you can share your observations and suggest that perhaps nervousness may be a factor causing the talkativeness. Asking for clarification may lead to a greater understanding of what the group member is experiencing. You may then ask him or her to limit contributions to a specific number of times (e.g., two or three). In the

## RESEARCH HIGHLIGHT

### Integrative Group Therapy for Binge Eating Behaviour

**Source:** Seamoore, D., Buckroyd, J., & Stott, D. (2006). Changes in eating behaviour following group therapy for women who binge eat: A pilot study. *Journal of Psychiatric and Mental Health Nursing, 13*(3), 337–346. doi:10.1111/j.1365-2850.2006.00960.x.

**Problem**

Although there have been a number of studies that support the effectiveness of group therapy for eating disorders, there is a gap in knowledge about the effectiveness of group therapy for obese women who experience binge or compulsive eating patterns. Additionally, few studies have evaluated the effectiveness of integrating nutritional, behavioural, and psychological interventions within one therapeutic treatment group.

**Purpose of Study**

The goal of this study was to determine if a group intervention could reduce episodes of binge eating or compulsive eating and address personal factors that contribute to eating pathology.

**Methods**

A single group before-and-after mixed-methods design was used to collect evaluative data. Effectiveness of the group was evaluated using the Binge Eating Scale, Clinical Outcomes in Routine Evaluation Measure, and personal interviews that focus on perceived changes in body image, self-concept, eating behaviours, and relationship to food. In this study, nine people between the ages of 24 and 56 participated in treatment (attended a group once a week for 24 sessions over a period of six months). Sessions were 90 minutes long and semi-structured, introducing themes relevant to group members and relevant experiential activities. The group progressed through stages based on a variety of therapeutic models. The first stage explored personal history and weight history. The next stage was psychoeducational, covering a variety of related topics. Following stages were based on a cognitive-behavioural approach. As well as cognition, food and behaviour, body image, confidence, and relationships, the group explored family and sociocultural influences, self-image, and self-agency.

**Key Findings**

At 26 weeks postgroup, all participants had made changes in eating behaviour and reduced binge eating. Follow-up at week 52 found that five of the nine participants had maintained changes in eating behaviour, and four had made considerable improvement.

**Implications for Nursing Practice**

Nurses encounter obese patients in a variety of clinical settings. These settings include but are not limited to surgery, medicine, home care, and psychiatry. The shame and personal distress that accompanies binge and compulsive eating disorders, and the assumptions about health care worker perceptions, may create difficulties for the sufferers to self-disclose these illnesses. Working with people who have binge or compulsive eating disorders requires use of an integrated approach (nutritional, behavioural, and psychological). Changing dichotomous thinking, exploring personal issues, and clarifying the role that food plays in dealing with stress are paramount in successful treatment plans.

group setting, the leader may ask the group if they would like to share observations or feedback about other members, thereby offering a chance for growth. This strategy is probably the most challenging but potentially the most rewarding in that members feel empowered, and the real therapeutic forces of groups are realized.

***Complaining Member Who Rejects Help.*** The person who complains but continues to reject help brings problems to the group, often describing them in a manner that makes the problems seem insurmountable. In fact, the person appears to take pride in the insolubility of his or her problems. He or she comes across as entirely self-centred, and the group's attempts to help are continually rejected.

The person who uses these tactics generally has highly conflicting feelings about his or her own dependency; any notice from the leader temporarily increases the person's self-esteem. On the other hand, the person has a pervasive mistrust of all authority figures. Most people who complain but continue to reject help have been subjected to severe deprivation early in their lives and may have experienced emotional or physical abuse or both.

> **VIGNETTE**
> Shamaila is always complaining about how horrible her relationship with her boyfriend is, and she manages to get the entire group worked up over the situation. Members tell her to leave him, not to spend all her time with him, and not to spend all her money on him, but each week she reports a new incident or crisis. In every session, the group members become concerned and offer encouragement, advice, and solutions. Each time, the group becomes angry at her lack of change, and she is frustrated by her own inability to change. She asserts that the group is not helpful.

The leader should acknowledge the person's pessimism but maintain a neutral affect. If the person stays in the group long enough, and the group develops a sense of cohesion, this individual can be helped to recognize relationship patterns. The leader should encourage the person to look at the habitual "yes . . . but" behaviour objectively.

### Demoralizing Member

Some people whose behaviour is self-centred, angry, or depressed may lack empathy or concern for other members of the group. They refuse to take any personal responsibility and can challenge the group leader and negatively affect the group process.

In this case, the group leader should listen to the comments objectively. Again, the leader may choose to speak to the group member in private and ask what is causing the anger. Sometimes this simple exchange can make the person feel a greater connection with the nurse and more important as a member of the group, which likely will decrease hostile behaviour and increase the group's benefit. In the group setting, the leader can focus on positive group members, whose comments may reduce the hostility of the negative group member.

> **VIGNETTE**
> Dina comes to the support group on the inpatient psychiatric unit. She is very angry, stating, "I don't know why I come to these groups anyway! They don't help." Dina is to be discharged the next day to a 28-day alcohol rehabilitation program. She has a previously scheduled dental appointment before the rehabilitation intake interview, and she is being strongly encouraged by her therapist to reschedule the appointment. The therapist fears Dina is at high risk for drinking again, because she states that she constantly has the urge to drink. When a group member who is an addictions therapist confronts Dina about not being flexible and prioritizing her need for alcohol treatment, she explodes. "I thought this group was for support. This is outrageous!" Group members are obviously uncomfortable with her anger.

Remember that angry people may be extremely vulnerable, and devaluing or demoralizing keeps others at a distance and maintains the person's own precarious sense of safety. Leaders must empathize with the member in a matter-of-fact manner, such as "You seem angry that the group wants to support you in putting sobriety ahead of your dental needs."

### Silent Member

Members who are silent in the group may be observing intently until they decide the group is safe for them, or they may believe they are not as competent as other, more assertive group members. Silence does not mean that the member is not engaged or involved, but it should be addressed, for several reasons. The person who does not speak cannot benefit from others' feedback, and other group members are deprived of this group member's valuable insights. Furthermore, a silent group member may make others uncomfortable and create a sense of mistrust.

> **VIGNETTE**
> Anne has attended three group sessions for survivors of childhood sexual abuse. While she appears to be listening, she rarely makes eye contact with the leader or other group members. She responds to yes or no questions, but when it comes to open-ended questions such as "What do you think, Anne?" she tends to shrug her shoulders and respond with "I don't know." Other group members have tried to draw Anne out, as has the leader. Katia, another group member, is beginning to exhibit frustration with Anne: "Look, I have shared some of the most private and painful memories of my childhood. I feel like you think you're too good to share what happened to you."

There are several techniques that may help in this case, including allowing the person to have extra time to formulate his or her thoughts before responding. Saying, "I'll give you a moment to think about that," and waiting or coming back to the group member later is often helpful. Another tactic is to make an assignment that every person in the group respond to a certain topic or question. For example, "Let's all think of a positive and assertive response to something that you generally feel helpless about. I'll give you a minute or so to think this topic over, and then I'm going to ask each of you to share."

Sometimes partnering with another group member will give the silent member the courage she or he needs to participate. You may break the group into pairs and ask them to discuss a certain topic and then each report back to the group what they heard the other person say.

## EXPECTED OUTCOMES

Expected outcomes of group participation will vary, depending on the type and purpose of the group. For education groups, such as a medication education group, the expected outcome would be demonstration of knowledge. For therapy groups, the expected outcomes will focus more on insights, behaviour changes, and reduction in symptoms. For example, in an alcohol treatment group, an expected outcome might be that the person develops insight into the connection between drinking and negative consequences. An expected behavioural outcome could be abstinence from alcohol use. In groups that focus primarily on emotional issues such as depression or anxiety, standardized tests can be used to measure symptom reduction as an outcome of group participation.

## ▌ KEY POINTS TO REMEMBER

- Research has identified 11 therapeutic factors that operate in groups and lead to therapeutic change for members. Yalom's therapeutic factors identify specific positive aspects of groups, such as universality of experience, imparting information, altruism, corrective recapitulation of the primary family group, development of socializing techniques, imitative behaviour, interpersonal learning, group cohesiveness, catharsis and existential resolution, and the instillation of hope.
- When a new group is formed, similarities and differences in many dimensions, including diagnosis, age, gender, and culture, must be considered.
- A group format has advantages over individual therapy, including cost savings, increased feedback, an opportunity to practise new skills in a relatively safe environment, and instillation of a sense of belonging.
- Groups develop through predictable phases over time.
- For a group to continue and be productive, members must fulfill specific functions known as *task* or *maintenance roles*. Individual roles are not productive and are based on individual personalities and needs.

- Clinical supervision is important so that group leaders can objectively analyze group interactions and leadership techniques.
- Nurses have opportunities to lead or co-lead therapeutic groups, some in the hospital but primarily in community settings.
- Psychoeducational groups, activity groups, task groups, and support groups are often led by nurses and provide significant treatment as part of the multidisciplinary treatment plan.
- Advanced-practice nurses and nurse therapists may lead psychotherapy groups based on various theoretical models.
- Challenging member behaviours, such as silence, complaining, or demoralizing, can be especially difficult. A variety of interventions are recommended to minimize the disruption to the group and maximize the benefit to the person engaging in these behaviours.

## ▌ CRITICAL THINKING

1. You are assigned to work with Malia, a 30-year-old woman who was admitted to the psychiatric unit with major depression after recently harming herself. Her nurse has told her she needs to attend group therapy. While lying in bed and staring at the ceiling, Malia tells you that she is a private person and that listening to other people's problems won't help and will only make her more depressed.
   a. How would you describe the benefits of group therapy to Malia?
   b. What intervention(s) might make it easier for Malia to attend group therapy?

2. Construct an outline for a medication teaching group that would cover information useful for your patients. If possible, co-lead this group with a staff member, with guidelines from your instructor.

3. Ms. Joseph is a 22-year-old Haitian-born nursing student admitted to the psychiatric unit after a nearly lethal overdose of acetaminophen (Tylenol). She admits to drinking excessively for the past six months. She is at risk of failing school. She complains of depressed mood, a loss of interest in her studies, decreased concentration, and social isolation. In the concurrent disorders group, she has been silent for the past two sessions and sits staring at the floor.
   a. What is your evaluation of Ms. Joseph's situation?
   b. What might Ms. Joseph's nonverbal behaviour mean?
   c. What approach would you use to involve her more in the group?
   d. What criteria could you use to evaluate the effectiveness of your intervention?
   e. What cultural implications should you consider?

## CHAPTER REVIEW

1. The nurse is caring for four patients. Which patient would not be appropriate to consider for group therapy?
   1. The patient with limited financial resources
   2. The patient who is acutely manic
   3. The patient who has few friends on the unit
   4. The patient who does not speak up often, yet listens to others

2. The nurse tells group members that they will be working on expressing conflicts during the current group session. Which phase of group development is represented?
   1. Formation phase
   2. Orientation phase
   3. Working phase
   4. Termination phase

3. Group members are having difficulty deciding what topic to cover in today's session. Which nurse leader response reflects autocratic leadership?
   1. "We are talking about fear of rejection today."
   2. "Let's go around the room and make suggestions for today's topic."
   3. "I will let you come to a conclusion together about what to talk about."
   4. "I'll work with you to find a suitable topic for today."

4. The nurse is planning care that includes a concurrent disorders group. A patient with which of the following disorders would be appropriate for this group?
   1. Depression and suicidal tendencies
   2. Anxiety and frequent migraine headaches
   3. Bipolar disorder and anorexia nervosa
   4. Schizophrenia and alcohol abuse

5. A member continues to dominate the group conversation despite having been asked to allow others to speak. What is the most appropriate nursing response to address this behaviour?
   1. "You are monopolizing the conversation."
   2. "When you talk constantly, it makes everyone feel angry."
   3. "You are supposed to allow others to talk also."
   4. "When you speak out of turn, I feel concerned that others cannot participate equally."

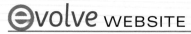 WEBSITE

Post-Test   interactive review

*Visit the Evolve Web site for Chapter Review Answers and Rationales, Critical Thinking Answer Guidelines, and additional resources related to the content in this chapter:* http://evolve.elsevier.com/Canada/Varcarolis/psychiatric/

## REFERENCES

Benne, K.D., & Sheats, P. (1948). Functional roles of group members. *Journal of Social Issues, 4,* 41–49. doi:10.1111/j.1540-4560.1948.tb01783.x.

Bond, G.R., & Campbell, K. (2008). Evidence-based practices for individuals with severe mental illness. *Journal of Rehabilitation, 74*(2), 33–44.

Chadwick, P., Taylor, K.N., & Abba, N. (2005). Mindfulness groups for people with psychosis. *Behavioural & Cognitive Psychotherapy, 33,* 351–359. doi:10.1017/S1352465805002158.

Drake, R.E., Essock, S.M., Shaner, A., et al. (2001). Implementing dual-diagnosis services for clients with severe mental illness. *Psychiatric Services, 52*(4), 469–476.

Hayes, S.A., Hope, D.A., Terryberry-Spohr, L.S., et al. (2006). Discriminating between cognitive and supportive group therapies for chronic mental illness. *Journal of Nervous & Mental Disease, 194,* 603–609. doi:10.1097/01.nmd.0000230635.03400.2d.

Sadock, B.J., & Sadock, V.A. (2008). *Kaplan & Sadock's concise textbook of clinical psychiatry* (3rd ed.). Philadelphia: Lippincott Williams & Wilkins.

Yalom, I.D. (2005). *The theory and practice of group psychotherapy* (5th ed.). New York: Basic Books.

York, M. (2007). A qualitative study into the experience of individuals involved in a mindfulness group within an acute inpatient mental health unit. *Journal of Psychiatric & Mental Health Nursing, 14,* 603–608. doi:10.1111/j.1365-2850.2007.01148.x.

# Family Interventions

*Sylvia Stevens, Verna Benner Carson*
*Adapted by Elaine M. Mordoch*

## KEY TERMS AND CONCEPTS

behavioural family therapy, 707
boundaries, 702
clear boundaries, 703
enmeshed boundaries, 703
family systems theory, 706
family triangle, 705
flexibility, 707

genogram, 709
insight-oriented family therapy, 707
intergenerational issues, 708
nuclear family, 705
psychoeducational family therapy, 713
rigid boundaries, 703
sociocultural context, 707

## OBJECTIVES

1. Define the concept of family.
2. Differentiate between functional and dysfunctional family patterns of behaviour as they relate to the five family functions.
3. Compare and contrast insight-oriented family therapy and behavioural family therapy.
4. Identify family theorists and their contributions to the family therapy movement.
5. Incorporate the family's sociocultural context when assessing and planning intervention strategies.
6. Construct a genogram using a three-generation approach.
7. Formulate outcome criteria that a nurse counsellor and family might develop together.
8. Identify strategies for family intervention in specific psychiatric clinical situations.
9. Distinguish between the nursing intervention strategies of a basic-level nurse and those of an advanced-practice nurse with regard to counselling and psychotherapy and psychobiological issues.
10. Explain the importance of the nurse's role in psychoeducational family therapy.

## ⊖volve WEBSITE

*Visit the Evolve website for Flashcards, Case Studies, and additional testing resources related to the content in this chapter: http://evolve.elsevier.com/Canada/Varcarolis/psychiatric/* `Pre-Test` `interactive review`

While family structure and function have changed dramatically over the years, the Canadian family remains central to the fabric of Canadian society. Same-sex marriages, recognition of common-law relationships, and blended families have influenced family structure and roles. In addition, Canada is a multicultural society with diverse cultural expectations of family roles, all of which are subject to societal influences. For example, during World War II, women undertook tasks that were previously assigned to men, changing women's perceptions of their roles. However, during the 1950s, the predominant family formation in mainstream society reverted to a heterosexual married couple—a breadwinner husband and homemaker wife—with children and a commitment to a lifelong marriage. As the second-wave feminist movement of the 1960s advocated for gender equality, more women began working outside the family home, moving toward emancipation (Wollstonecraft,

1975). As a result, today's family frequently consists of two income earners, with women often being the higher wage earner.

As another example of societal influence on Canadian families, in the late nineteenth century, the Canadian government's assimilation policies toward Aboriginal peoples significantly influenced the erosion of Aboriginal traditional family structure and values (Miller, 1996). The residential school system policies severely affected family structure, parenting roles, and traditions, which contributed to intergenerational trauma and cultural loss. Children were removed from their homes and lost their culture, language, and connection to family and the land (Kirmayer, Simpson, & Cargo, 2003). Furthermore, adoption policies allowed for the removal of Aboriginal children from their homes to be adopted by white families. This practice is regarded by some Aboriginal communities as a form of genocide from which communities are still recovering (Kirmayer, Simpson, & Cargo, 2003). These nineteenth-century Canadian policies caused intergenerational conflict still apparent today due to missed opportunities to learn traditional parenting practices, contributing to significant past and current psychosocial problems (Miller, 1996).

There has been a steady increase in the number of children living in care (e.g., Children's Aid Society) over the past decade, with 67 000 Canadian children in care, 27 000 of whom are Aboriginal children. Unfortunately, existing services have not kept up with the needs of these children, positioning them for additional life burdens and obstacles (Vanier Institute of the Family, 2013).

Canadian families are experiencing rapid change and growing diversity in family configurations. While previous laws prevented interracial adoptions, families of mixed race are more visible in Canadian society today. Canadians often opt to adopt children from Asia or South America, where more infants are available for adoption (Adoptiveparents.ca, n.d.). Today, in contrast to the experience of adopted Aboriginal children of the past, many adoptive parents work toward helping their children identify with both their ethnic and Canadian cultures.

Other ways in which the composition of families may differ from that of the past include parental genders (e.g., two dads, a transgendered parent), parental numbers (e.g., lone-parent families), and blended families (e.g., with stepsiblings) (Vanier Institute of the Family, 2013). As well, many families, including those of immigrants, refugees, and Aboriginal peoples, may belong to groups that they regard as family but that may not be legally, biologically, and socially regarded as such (Weiman, 2009).

While there is a shift from the traditional married nuclear family to alternative family structures, the majority of Canadian families remain married couples (70%), with 13.8% common-law couples and the remaining 15.5% lone-parent families. The average size of the Canadian family is decreasing and is reported to be 3.0 persons (Canadian Council on Social Development, 2011). Nunavut has the largest average family size, with 4.4 persons, and a high percentage of the First Nations population is under the age of 6 (Canadian Council on Social Development, 2011). Other trends affecting the Canadian family are an increasing aging population and decreasing workforce; immigration policies resulting in diversity in family structure and roles; the phenomenon of "boomerang kids," young adults who return home or stay home longer than those in previous generations; and multiple demands on time and increased stress in dual-income families (Vanier Institute of the Family, 2013).

Our relationships with family are significant and emotionally charged, but the parent–child relationship is one of the most important in Canadian society. Parents are expected to raise their children and provide for them until they are adults. The Vanier Institute of the Family (2013) suggests that families provide for the physical care of family members, socialization of children, production and consumption of goods (electronics, clothes, etc.), and affective nurturance and love. When meeting these demands, families are considered to function well. Dysfunctional families, however, experience difficulty in meeting these obligations, and discord among family members may result or the family may become trapped in behaviours that do not benefit it or its members.

Family intervention may assist such families to gain a more healthy way of being. Children growing up in families in which there is mental illness, high stress, historical oppression, or intergenerational trauma may have emotional problems both in childhood and in their adult lives (Kirmayer, Simpson, & Cargo, 2003; Mordoch & Hall, 2002, 2008). Some families may need psychotherapeutic intervention during the early years of a child's development to assist the child and family to correct maladaptive patterns. This intervention may minimize psychological impairment and build on the strengths of the family. During times of crisis, inclusive of health crises, families require psychological, emotional, and practical supports to restore their equilibrium.

Family in its ideal form may provide security, kinship, a means to maintain traditions and culture, and a place of belonging. As such, family is a positive force in assisting its members through crises and the life cycle. Alternatively, family experiences may include difficulties such as mental illness, abuse, poverty, or violence (Canadian Centre for Justice Statistics, 2009). The United Nations Children's Fund (2005) noted, for example, that a higher number of Canadian children are living in poverty (14.9%) as compared to Scandinavian children (4.8%). This statistic is partially attributed to differences in taxes and social benefits and is significant for child and family health outcomes due to the chronic stress of living in poverty. As well, one in five Canadians is expected to suffer from a mental illness at some point, and 80% of Canadians will experience the effects of mental illness through a colleague, friend, or family member. A secondary analysis of national survey data (Statistics Canada, 2003) identified that (1) 12.1% of Canadian children under 12 years of age live in households in which one or more psychiatric disabilities (mood, anxiety, or substance abuse disorders) have been diagnosed; (2) 17% of these children live in lone-parent households, which present an increased risk for adverse events (Bassani, Padoin, Phillip, et al., 2008); and (3) three quarters of the parents with mental illnesses had received no treatment in the previous 12 months. To facilitate nonjudgemental and sensitive practice to assist families to heal from such overwhelming circumstances, nurses require education in and understanding of diverse family experiences, economics, emotions, and context (Doane & Varcoe, 2006).

## FAMILY

What is a family? The Registered Nurses' Association of Ontario (2012) and Wright and Leahey (2013) state that families are self-defined—in other words, the family is made up of the people the patient identifies as family and can include neighbours and significant people in the community. For example, young, male, inner-city Aboriginal youth counted as family nonrelatives, including friends with whom they had relationships that were among the most stable in their lives (Brown, Higgitt, Wingert, et al., 2005). When working with families, nurses must be sensitive about and honour the patient's identification of family (Wright & Leahey, 2013).

The family is the primary system to which a person belongs. Birth, puberty, marriage, and death occur within the context of the family experience. The family can be the source of love or hate, pride or shame, security or insecurity. Although individual family members have roles and functions, the overriding value in families lies in the relationships among family members. It is these family relationships that provide the primary context of human development. Many family theorists consider the intergenerational connectedness of the family to be one of our greatest human resources.

---

**VIGNETTE**

Anna Lowen is a 54-year-old Hutterite Canadian woman who has been admitted to the acute psychiatric ward for an episode of mania. She had been diagnosed with bipolar disorder several years before and has had two previous episodes of mania. Anna lives in a Hutterite colony with her three children and her husband, Jake, and is respected for her hard work and good nature with older adults and children.

Before being admitted to the hospital, she had been unable to sleep or eat for one week. In the mornings she was loud and irritable in the community kitchen and insisted on serving all of the children large bowls of porridge with eggs that she had collected from the henhouse. Currently, she is on a medication to stabilize her mood and help her to sleep and eat.

Her husband, sisters, and several community members are visiting her at the hospital. The children have been left at the colony and do not understand what has happened to their mother. The nurse assesses the situation and adopts a family-centred nursing care approach inclusive of the community members. First, he identifies his own need to increase his understanding of the Hutterite culture, adapts psychoeducational materials to meet the family's needs, and encourages the family to bring the children to a meeting to have their questions about their mother answered.

---

## Family Functions

The Vanier Institute of the Family (2013) identified the following as functions of a Canadian family:

- Provision of love and nurturance
- Socialization of children
- Social control of members
- Production and consumption of goods and services
- Addition of new family members through birth or adoption
- Physical care and maintenance of family members

These functions take place within a societal context, which also influences family members.

Families play a significant and often underacknowledged role as caregivers (Canadian Institute for Health Information, 2011). The *Caregiver Recognition Act of Manitoba* (2011) recognizes caregivers and their contributions to society and posits an emerging framework to provide guidance for caregivers. However, not all caregivers are adults. Approximately 15% of Canadian children are potentially affected by growing up with a parent with a mental illness (Bassani, Padoin, Phillip, et al., 2008). These children are often invisibly caregivers of their parents. Based on the Children's Society National Young Carers Initiative in the United Kingdom, which identifies children who care for their ill parents and siblings, a Young Carers Initiative has begun in Canada with pilot projects in Ontario and British Columbia. Assuming too much responsibility in childhood could interfere with attainment of children's developmental needs. These groups acknowledge the role children play in caretaking and recognize that they may need respite from these duties (Young Carers Initiative, 2012). Children of parents with mental illness could benefit from a family approach in health, social, and educational services, which could assist them to know other children in the same situation and gain understanding and respite from their responsibilities (Mordoch & Hall, 2008; Ostman, 2008).

### Families and Mental Illness

Historically, when mental illness occurred, health care providers often cast blame on the family. Blame was particularly predominant in the mental illness of children, especially those with autism, eating disorders, or schizophrenia. Theories charged that mothers' ways of interacting with their children were the root cause of child disturbance. "Cold" parenting was identified in the etiology of children with autism and "controlling" parenting in the development of eating disorders. Today, theories suggest holistic, complex explanations for illness (Mental Health Commission of Canada, 2010; Schoen-Johnson & Pearson, 2003). Nurses need to be aware of this history of parental blame as remnants of these ideas may exist in practice settings. Parental blame has propelled families to advocate for health care services, acknowledgement of parents' knowledge about their children, and research in mental health (Hinshaw, 2005).

An important component of nursing practice is to advise family members of appropriate support groups. Those experiencing a first psychotic break of a child are particularly vulnerable to being overwhelmed by the situation. Parental support groups such as the Prevention and Early Intervention in Psychosis Program (www.PEPP.ca) in London, Ontario, were founded to assist such families.

The Effective Family Program, which focuses on mental health promotion and intervention for families and children, has been implemented in Finland to address the issues children of parents with mental illness have raised (Solantaus & Toikka, 2006). See the Research Highlight.

 **RESEARCH HIGHLIGHT**

### How Children Understand Parental Mental Illness

**Source:** Mordoch, E. (2010). How children understand parental mental illness: "You don't get life insurance. What's life insurance?" *Journal of the Canadian Academy of Child and Adolescent Psychiatry, 19*(1). 19-25.

**Problem**
There is a need to know how children understand parental mental illness so that they can be assisted in dealing with and responding to the illness.

**Purpose of Study**
To identify how children living with parental mental illness (PMI) understand mental illness (MI) and what they want to tell other children.

**Methods**
The study design was a secondary analysis of a grounded theory study exploring Canadian children's perceptions of living with PMI. Interviews with 22 children, aged 6 to 16, living with a parent receiving treatment for depression, bipolar disorder, or schizophrenia were reread, coded, and analyzed along with data categories, their properties, field notes, and memos from the original data.

**Key Findings**
Children revealed that they had limited understanding of MI and received few factual explanations of what was happening. Limited information on MI caused undue hardship. Younger children worried about their parent dying while older children were concerned about also developing MI. Children offered suggestions for other children in similar circumstances.

**Implications for Nursing Practice**
This study raises awareness of children living with PMI and identifies them as a population requiring assistance to understand and to respond to PMI. Mental health and primary health care clinicians have opportunities to assist these children within collaborative care models developed in conjunction with school services.

## CANADIAN MODELS OF FAMILY NURSING CARE AND ASSESSMENT

Three esteemed Canadian models of family care are the McGill Model of Nursing developed by Dr. Moyra Allan and the Calgary Family Assessment Model and Calgary Intervention Model, both based on the work of Wright and Leahey (2013). These models guide both beginning and advanced-level nurses to practise from a family nursing perspective.

### McGill Model of Nursing

The McGill Model of Nursing (http://www.mcgill.ca/nursing/about/model/) focuses on family health, collaboration, learning, and health promotion. It was developed in response to

health care system changes when universal health care was introduced in Canada. It has been widely adopted in Canada within many diverse nursing areas. Its main assumption is that families possess strengths, motivations, and resources. These serve to assist families to move toward health promotion, which will result in improved health outcomes. Because health behaviour is predominantly learned within the family context, it is imperative that nurses focus on working with the family by setting goals and establishing learning environments to share knowledge, build on existing knowledge, and assist in making changes in behaviours. Family members become active learners in the implementation phase of the nursing process. The processes of coping and development are dynamic (i.e., they occur in any phase). Family health is achieved by building on the strengths of the family and its individual members and using external resources, such as nurses and other health care providers (Feeley & Gottlieb, 2000).

### Calgary Family Assessment Model (CFAM) and Calgary Family Intervention Model (CFIM)

The basic assumptions underlying CFAM and CFIM are derived from systems, cybernetics, communication, differing views of reality, and change theories. The models are multidimensional and consider structure, development, and function (Robinson & Wright, 1995). These models are built on processes of engagement wherein the nurse welcomes the family, focuses on building trust in relationships, and identifies the problems that led to the need for medical intervention, which helps to put illness and problems in their place (Robinson & Wright, 1995).

## FAMILY THERAPY

Family therapy is a psychotherapeutic process that focuses on changing the interactions among the people who make up the family or marital unit. It serves to improve the family, the subsystems within the family, and the individuals who make up the family. It focuses on evaluating these relationships and the communication patterns, structure, and rules that govern the family interactions (Sadock & Sadock, 2008). While novice nurses do not engage in family therapy, nurses may take additional educational courses to develop family therapy skills.

Every day in every family, decisions are made regarding the functions of power, rule making, provision of financial support, future planning, and goods allocation. Families may address these functions in a variety of ways, but most commonly, the adults in the family determine how these functions are to be performed. In lone-parent families, these functions may sometimes become overwhelming, highlighting the need for additional supports. In chaotic families, a member not well prepared to make decisions, such as a teenager, may be the decision maker. Although children learn decision-making skills as they mature and increasingly make choices about their own lives, they should not be expected to take on responsibility for the family. Cultural expectations and norms affect the allocation of roles and perspectives on how families negotiate these tasks.

Boundaries are the distinctions made between individuals in the family. Boundaries may be clear, enmeshed, rigid, or inconsistent (see Box 36-1). Most families exhibit several

## BOX 36-1 TYPES OF BOUNDARIES

- **Clear boundaries**: Boundaries that are well understood by all members of the family and give family members a sense of "*I*-ness" and also "*we*-ness." They help define family members' roles and allow members to function without unnecessary interference from other members. However, they are not so rigid as to restrict contact among family members. For example, a mother tells her 14-year-old daughter, "You don't need to worry whether your little brother eats his breakfast. Your father and I will handle that." This boundary may be redefined: "I want you to make sure that your little brother gets his homework done while your father and I are at the movies."
- **Enmeshed boundaries** (also called *diffuse boundaries*): Boundaries that result from a blending together of the roles, thoughts, and feelings of the individual family members so that clear distinctions fail to emerge. The members of a family that operates with enmeshed boundaries are more prone to psychological or psychosomatic symptoms. A common phenomenon within families with enmeshed boundaries is that individuals expect other members of the family to know what they are thinking (e.g., "Why did you take that? You know I wanted it!") and believe they know what other family members are thinking (e.g., "I know exactly why you did that!").
- **Rigid boundaries** (also called *disengaged boundaries*): Boundaries in which the rules and roles are consistently adhered to no matter what; thus, rigid boundaries prevent family members from trying out new roles or, in some cases, from taking on more mature functions as time goes on. In families in which rigid boundaries predominate, isolation may be marked. Family members are often cut off from the community and outside influences and even from each other.

combinations of the various boundary types (Goldenberg & Goldenberg, 2008). When boundaries are functioning properly, family members work out arrangements by compromise based on understanding of appropriate roles. Each generation is made aware of how decisions will be made and clearly understands who is in charge and when. Blurred boundary function results in family members interfering with each other's goals, creating tension and anxiety between family members. Children in these families may become confused, manipulative, and insecure.

## Issues Associated With Family Therapies
### Communication
Communication patterns are important in family life. Healthy communication patterns are characterized by clear and comprehensible messages (e.g., "I would like to go now"; "I don't like it when you interrupt what I'm saying"). Families with healthy communication are encouraged to ask for what they want and to express their feelings appropriately. In these families, both affection and conflict are openly expressed, and members have no need to resort to manipulation. When communication is unclear, solving problems or resolving conflicts becomes difficult; therefore, the cardinal rule for effective and functional communication is "Be clear and direct in saying what you want and need."

As simple as this concept may seem, it may be difficult to activate in a family system. To be direct, individuals must first have a sense that the self is respected and loved; they then will be confident to set healthy boundaries with others. The consequences of being clear and direct may be unpleasant when boundaries are enmeshed and confusion is the norm. Changing a family pattern will cause discomfort in the system. Explicitly stating what one wants and needs is especially difficult when one believes that family members should already know—especially if the family member is a spouse, a parent, or a close sibling. No one is able to mind-read, but emotionally undifferentiated members may believe family members can. The following vignette describes a spousal situation that shows how easily communication can be misunderstood when clear and direct messages are not sent. See Box 36-2 for examples of unhealthy communication patterns.

## BOX 36-2 EXAMPLES OF DYSFUNCTIONAL COMMUNICATION

**Manipulating:** Instead of asking directly, family members manipulate others to get what they want. A family member makes requests with "strings attached" so that the other person has a difficult time refusing the request: "If you do this for me, I won't tell Daddy you are getting poor grades in school."

**Distracting:** To avoid functional problem solving and resolve conflicts within the family, family members introduce irrelevant details into problematic issues (e.g., asking who picked up the dry cleaning when discussing communication problems).

**Generalizing:** When dealing with problematic family issues, members use global statements like *always* and *never* instead of dealing with specific problems and areas of conflict. Family members may say "Adem is always angry" instead of "Adem, what is upsetting you?"

**Blaming:** Family members blame other family members for failures, errors, or negative consequences of an action to keep the focus away from themselves. Blaming is a response to fear of being blamed by others.

**Placating:** Family members pretend to be inadequate but well meaning to keep peace in the family at any price: "Don't yell at the children, dear. I'll put the shoes on the stairs."

## VIGNETTE
Liz would like to spend more time on the weekends with her husband, Michael; however, Michael always seems to be busy around the house or talking with friends on the telephone. Liz feels that he does not notice her or maybe is not interested in her, so she spends a lot of time working out. Michael figures that Liz is doing what she wants to do and that it makes her happy, so he contents himself with finding things to do alone. The result is that Liz and Michael spend little time together. Liz finally confronts Michael clearly and directly about his "lack of interest" in her and tells him what she wants and needs—to spend more time together on the weekends. Michael replies that he had no idea she felt that way. He had thought she enjoyed the way things were, and he would like to have more time together too.

## Emotional Support

All families encounter conflicts during their life journeys. However, in a healthy family, feelings of affection are generally uppermost, and anger and conflict do not dominate the family's pattern of interaction. Healthy families are concerned about each other and consistently meet family members' emotional and physical needs. Members feel supported and free to grow and explore new roles and facets of their personalities. A family that is dominated by conflict and anger alienates its members, leaving them isolated, fearful, and emotionally fragile. It is important for the nurse to note that patterns of abuse and addictions may have underlying links to historical oppression and colonization. For example, the abuse and addiction problems that plague some First Nations families and communities can be linked to historical oppression that has contributed to intergenerational trauma (Miller, 1996). An Aboriginal approach to helping in these situations would be based on sharing circles; concepts of harmony; and emotional, physical, spiritual, and psychological balance (Hart, 2002).

## Socialization

Within families, each member learns socialization skills. People learn coping skills and how to interact, negotiate, and plan for the future. Children learn to socialize effectively within the family, and then apply their skills in society.

## Family Life Cycle

The life cycle of individuals takes place within the family life cycle, the primary context of human development. Family life takes place within relationships, and changes within the relationships affect the roles of the parents. For example, as children mature and leave home, parents may renegotiate the pattern of their lives together. "Boomerang children" may unexpectedly return home, causing yet another change in family roles. Later, parents may need their adult children's help as they become less able to care for themselves. As the Canadian population ages, more family members will be providing care to older-adult parents.

The family system moves through time, with potential for family stress at transition points (e.g., birth of a child, employment changes, children leaving home, retirement) or during an interruption in the life cycle (e.g., untoward events such as an unexpected suicide, first psychotic break of a young adult, imprisonment, divorce). At these times, therapeutic efforts may be required to assist family members to proceed in the life cycle. For family members who feel trapped within a dysfunctional family system, extreme pressures can lead to mental illness or suicide. Symptoms can be perceived as a response to an interruption in the family life cycle. This family life cycle assumes a traditional family organization and requires modification for nontraditional family structures, as in, for example, a male lone-parent family, the number of which has increased significantly in Canada over the past decade (Canadian Council on Social Development, 2011).

In the traditional Canadian family type, there are six main phases of the family life cycle: (1) launching the single young adult, (2) joining families through couple formation, (3) becoming parents and caring for young children, (4) parenting adolescents, (5) launching children and moving on, and (6) experiencing later life, often encompassing the role of grandparent. Families may experience some of the phases and not others. In addition, with the increased cultural diversity of Canadian society, nurses may expect to see diverse interpretations of family tasks.

In Canada, people are marrying at a later age, with the average bride and groom respectively being 31.5 and 34 years of age. Divorce rates have been relatively stable over the past decade (Canadian Council on Social Development, 2011).

## Working With the Family

Many concepts are used when working with families. The concepts of the *identified patient*, the *family triangle*, and the *nuclear family emotional system* are discussed here. Box 36-3 describes other concepts relevant to family work.

---

**BOX 36-3  CENTRAL CONCEPTS OF FAMILY SYSTEMS THEORY**

**Triangulation:** The tendency, when two-person relationships are stressful and unstable, to draw in a third person to stabilize the system through the formation of a coalition in which the two join the third. Triangles often occur with low differentiation and high anxiety and tend to draw in the third person but freeze the conflict as irresolvable.

**Scapegoating:** A form of displacement in which a family member (usually the least powerful) is blamed for another family member's distress. The purpose is to keep the focus off the painful issues and problems of the blamers. In a family, the blamers are often the parents, and the scapegoat a child.

**Double bind:** A situation in which a positive command (often verbal) is followed by a negative command (often nonverbal), which leaves the recipient confused, trapped, and immobilized because there is no appropriate way to act. A double bind is a "no win" situation in which you are "darned if you do, darned if you don't."

**Hierarchy:** The function of power and its structures in families, differentiating parental and sibling roles and generational boundaries.

**Family life cycle:** The family's developmental process over time; refers to the family's past course, its present tasks, and its future course.

**Differentiation:** The ability to develop a strong identity and sense of self while at the same time maintaining an emotional connectedness with one's family of origin.

**Sociocultural context:** The framework for viewing the family in terms of the influence of gender, race, ethnicity, religion, economic class, and sexual orientation.

**Mino-Pimatisiwin** (an Aboriginal approach to helping): Seeking the good life with focus on the interconnections between individual, family, community and nations. Key concepts are wholeness, balance, harmony, and healing (Hart, 2002).

**Intergenerational issues:** The continuation and persistence from generation to generation of certain emotional interactive family patterns. Various patterns of behaviour (e.g., involving geographical distance between members, suicide, divorce, addiction, affairs, grief, triangles, historical colonization, loss) that continue to impact successive generations.

## The Identified Patient

The *identified patient* is the individual in the family whom everyone regards as "the problem." A descriptive term for this person is the "family symptom-bearer." This family member is generally the focus of most of the family system's anxiety. She or he may serve to divert the attention from other more serious and debilitating problems within the family, such as a crumbling marriage, substance abuse, or infidelity. Furthermore, the symptoms of the identified patient may serve as a stabilizing mechanism to bring about customary behaviour in a distressed family (Goldenberg & Goldenberg, 2008). The identified patient may even be aware at some level of the role he or she serves in "saving" the family. For example, adult children may sacrifice their autonomy by staying in the home to hold the parents together.

When a family comes for treatment, the presenting problem, which is usually related to one member of the family, must be addressed before the underlying systemic problem. The family member who is the identified patient may or may not be the one who initially seeks help from inpatient or outpatient services.

When working with families, it is important to consider not only the family as a system in a particular stage of life-cycle development but also the individual developmental stage of each member. For example, a family may present with parents in Erikson's stage of generativity vs. stagnation, adolescent children dealing with identity vs. role confusion issues, a school-age child facing challenges of industry vs. inferiority, and grandparents dealing with ego integrity vs. despair. Thus, there is more than one perspective to be considered when looking at the identified patient in terms of the family system. The focus is on the family system's anxiety.

## Family Triangles

Bowen (1985) described an important and common relationship process in families; it can be seen as a system of interlocking triangles. When tension in a family is low, the dyad or two-person system may interact comfortably, although some tension lies in the struggle between closeness and independence. When the tension in a close twosome builds, a third person (child, friend, or parent) may be brought in to help lower the tension. The family triangle (Figure 36-1) then becomes the basic building block of interpersonal relationships. All triangles contain a close side, a distant side, and a side in which conflict or tension exists between two people (Nelson, 2003).

The intensity of the triangling process varies among families and within the same family over time because triangles create emotional instability. The lower the level of differentiation in a family, the higher the tension is and the more important the role of triangling is to the lowering of tension and the preservation of emotional stability. As the family becomes stressed for whatever reasons, the anxiety in the system is triggered, and the triangles become more active.

A common problem that occurs in families is the setting up of a triangle among two parents and a child; one parent is overinvolved with the child, and the other plays a more peripheral role. In this situation, the child eventually becomes the means by which the parents communicate with each other about issues they cannot deal with directly. In other words, spousal conflicts may be brought into the parental arena, where they do not belong.

---

**VIGNETTE**

Six-year-old Kamilah is having trouble making friends. Her mother, Makayla, has been feeling anxious and helpless as she tries to find ways to engage Kamilah with other youngsters. Makayla develops an overprotectiveness that further inhibits Kamilah from making friends. Makayla feels that her husband, Leon, is uncaring and disinterested because he thinks that she should be more relaxed about Kamilah's social life and let things develop naturally. Leon's job requires that he travel most of the week, so he is not involved with Makayla's daily experiences and struggles with Kamilah.

Makayla and Leon have been avoiding intimacy for almost a year. Makayla is angry with Leon for spending so much time with his parents, which further casts him in a peripheral role in their nuclear family, and Leon is angry with Makayla, sensing her rejection of him. Both are feeling isolated and alienated and are consequently angry with each other. Neither Leon nor Makayla addresses this issue directly. Instead, they play out their anger in the parental arena as they battle over how to handle Kamilah's social isolation.

---

***The Nurse's Response to Triangulation.*** Although basic-level nurses do not provide family therapy, they do interact with patients and families. Nurses should be aware of their own differentiation process and family-of-origin issues, which may affect their responses. When personal reactions interfere, the nurse may become "triangled" into the family's system. The nurse's continued self-assessment is necessary to maintain emotional stability in the face of a chaotic family situation, in which the nurse's own issues may arise.

For advanced-practice nurses who engage in family therapy, holding family members accountable for themselves—making clear that the responsibility for change is theirs and not the nurse's—is a way of remaining clear of triangles. For example, the nurse therapist could become triangled into a family system in any number of ways: perhaps the nurse recently experienced the loss of a family member; the nurse may belong to an enmeshed family system, in which the children are regularly drawn into spousal arguments; or perhaps stubbornness is an unresolved issue for the nurse. Any of these possibilities could allow the nurse to become triangled into a family system, making therapeutic intervention difficult. Engaging in personal family-of-origin therapy and regular supervision are recommended when nurse therapists work with individuals, couples, or families. Supervision can be conducted with peer professionals, in groups, or privately with a more experienced clinician. One indication that a nurse is being triangled is that his or her level of anxiety is greater than the situation warrants.

## The Nuclear Family Emotional System

The term nuclear family refers to parents and the children under the parents' care. Bowen (1985) developed the concept

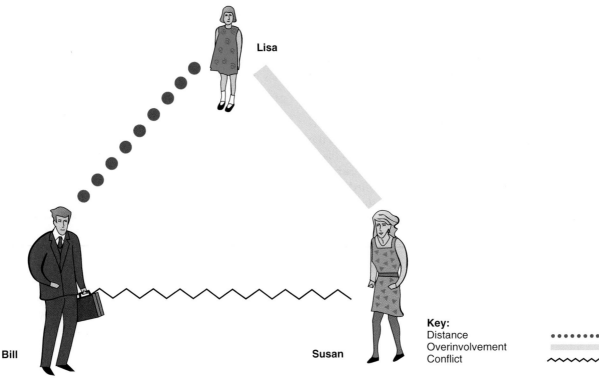

**FIGURE 36-1** Example of a family triangle.

Key:
Distance ••••••••
Overinvolvement
Conflict ∿∿∿∿

of a *nuclear family emotional system*, defined as the flow of emotional processes within the nuclear family. This concept views symptoms as belonging to the nuclear family emotional system rather than to an individual. Bowen made a distinction between conventional medical (psychiatric) diagnosis and family diagnosis: rather than viewing a symptom as reflecting a disease that is confined to a patient, Bowen identified an emotional process that transcends the boundaries of a patient and encompasses the family relationship system. The example in the vignette (page 707) of 8-year-old Luca, whom family and others believed had ADHD, illustrates how Luca's symptoms could be viewed as reflecting the family's conflicts and changes.

Refer to Box 36-3 for a summary of concepts central to family life.

## FAMILY THERAPY THEORY

Family therapy emerged from the early child guidance clinics and marriage counselling efforts in the early twentieth century, stemming from social work movements in the United Kingdom and the United States. Psychotherapists began to consider the effects of the social milieu on their patients and included the family in clinical observations and practice. The formal development of family therapy occurred in the 1940s and 1950s and was propelled by a focus on communication, which shifted the previous focus on individual pathology to a more systemic perspective (Becvar & Becvar, 2008). An *interactive* (interpersonal) rather than *indwelling* (intrapsychic Freudian) model of mental

illness was becoming more widely accepted. These influences paved the way for an interest in the family system as it related to psychiatric disorders.

Leading theorists such as Virginia Satir (1972, 1983) and Jay Haley (1980, 1996), shifted the focus from the patient's symptoms (*indwelling*) to the patient's position and relationships within the family (*interactive*). Further work by Salvador Minuchin (1974, 1996), a structural therapist, established the legitimacy of family therapy within psychiatry. Bowen (1975, 1985) was a leading proponent of the family systems theory, a theory that downplays problem resolution, focusing instead on the long-term differentiation of individual family members. *Differentiation* is a term introduced by Bowen (1975) that describes the ability of an individual to make autonomous choices while separating out feelings and cognitions. Decisions are not driven by emotionality, but the individual remains emotionally connected to a significant relationship system (e.g., the family). Extreme lack of differentiation and rigid cultural expectations are reflected in honour killings, in which young women, average age of 21, are killed by family members—usually fathers or brothers—because of dishonouring the family. Canadian cases generally result from these girls engaging in "inappropriate" relationships and dressing and behaving in ways that male members of their families consider disrespectful (Galloway, 2010).

The aims of the family systems theory are to decrease emotional reactivity and encourage differentiation among individual family members. Parents or adults in the system are encouraged to recognize emotional patterns from their family of origin and to use resources from members of the extended family to re-engage in more mature interaction patterns. Children who are identified as the "problem" receive counselling and behavioural therapy but are not the focus of the therapy. Instead, parents are encouraged to consider system factors contributing to the child's emotional or behavioural problems.

The terms *strategic* and *structural* are used to identify the frameworks adopted by specific therapists. A *strategic model of family therapy* assumes that change in any single element in the family system will bring about change in the entire system. The aim of strategic therapy is to change the patterns, rules, and meaning of family interactions.

---

**VIGNETTE**

Eight-year-old Luca De Santis, who is hyperactive and disruptive at school and at home, is brought to the community mental health clinic to be evaluated for attention deficit–hyperactivity disorder (ADHD). The nurse clinician performs an assessment and finds that a great deal of turmoil exists within the De Santis family. The family is composed of Luca's married parents, their other two children, and a grandmother. Luca's father has just lost his job, and his grandmother was recently diagnosed with bladder cancer. Luca's mother is considering filing for separation because of constant, unresolved arguments with her husband. She was raised a strict Roman Catholic and is unsure of this plan. Because of the family's communication patterns and cultural background, none of these issues have been discussed with Luca. Viewing this family from a strategic model, the nurse clinician sees Luca's symptoms as a function of many difficult losses and transitions that are stressing the entire family's coping mechanisms.

The nurse considers the multiple family stressors and their potential influence on Luca's symptoms of acting out and hyperactivity. Once the family issues are addressed, perhaps Luca's symptoms will subside. She refers the couple to a family therapist and, in the meantime, encourages them to focus more on their own issues and less on Luca's behaviour. An appointment is made to return to the clinic in one month, at which time Luca will be re-evaluated.

---

In the vignette above, the family's communication patterns and decision making, partly for cultural reasons, exclude any discussion with the children. Children in such families often feel powerless and act out. Using the strategic model, the family therapist works with the family to change rigid communication patterns so that children are informed earlier in the decision-making process and so as to ease the emotional turmoil of the parents. This change provides children an opportunity to comment or offer suggestions about how issues could be resolved. Being given a sense of control over some aspects of one's life can alleviate anxiety and reduce behavioural problems. This intervention would result in a systemic change in the way the family communicates.

The *structural model of family therapy* explains family problems from the perspective of dysfunctional boundary and role structure. These problems become evident when the family is exposed to a stressor or a transition point and is unable to adapt to the changing conditions (Goldenberg & Goldenberg, 2008). A therapist using the structural model with the De Santis family in the vignette, rather than focusing on changing a specific pattern, would highlight the importance of boundaries between the parental and sibling (child) subsystems. At the same time, the therapist would emphasize the importance of flexibility, which would allow for the changes inherent in normal growth and development.

In family therapy, there is no single accepted model for treating families. Not all techniques are applicable to all problems, so the experienced clinician must be discerning. Most of the theoretical schools of marital and family therapy fall into two broad classifications: insight-oriented family therapy (a combination of behavioural therapy and education of families in better understanding their power struggles, defence mechanisms, and other negative behaviours) and behavioural family therapy (a collection of psychological techniques for modifying maladaptive behaviours). Table 36-1 summarizes some of the types of therapy in each classification, describes their basic concepts and approaches, and lists the major theorists.

## The Family as a System

Every family can be viewed as a unique system with its own structure, rules, and history of handling life problems and crises. Focusing on family patterns and interactions is fundamental to marital family therapy. The focus is *not* on an individual, as it is in traditional therapy, but rather on the interpersonal process of the family group (Nichols, 2004).

# APPLICATION OF THE NURSING PROCESS

## ASSESSMENT

Intervention is designed based on the initial assessment of family issues and adjusted with ongoing assessment throughout the nursing process. The Calgary Family Assessment Model (CFAM) (see Figure 36-2) has multiple focuses including but not limited to the following (Nichols, 2004):

- Family system
- Family subsystems
- Individual members of the family
- Sociocultural context of family
- Past medical and mental health illness
- Family interactions and communication styles
- Stressors within the family system

Doane and Varcoe (2006) identified a number of issues that should be assessed in family therapy, nursing practice, and counselling environments:

- Phases of the family life cycle
- Sociocultural context, beliefs
- Multigenerational issues, inclusive of historical oppression
- Relational practice

### Sociocultural Context

Rather than as an isolated unit, the family is viewed in a sociocultural context, wherein issues of gender, race, ethnicity, class,

## TABLE 36-1    INSIGHT-ORIENTED AND BEHAVIOURAL FAMILY THERAPIES

| TYPE OF THERAPY | CONCEPTS | MAJOR THEORISTS |
|---|---|---|
| **INSIGHT-ORIENTED FAMILY THERAPY** | | |
| Psychodynamic therapy | Problems arise from:<br>• Developmental arrest<br>• Current interactions<br>• Projections<br>• Current stresses<br>Improvement through insight into problematic relationships originating in the past | Nathan Ackerman<br>James Framo<br>Ivan Boszormenyi-Nagy |
| Family-of-origin therapy | Family viewed as an emotional relationship system:<br>• Goal of fostering differentiation and decreasing emotional reactivity<br>• Concept of triangulation<br>• Emphasis on the family of origin | Murray Bowen |
| Experimental–existential therapy | Goal of therapy is to encourage the growth of family:<br>• Symptoms express family pain<br>• Family is responsible for its own solutions<br>• Therapist uses nurturing and identifies dysfunctional communication patterns | Carl Whitaker<br>Virginia Satir<br>Leslie Greenberg<br>Susan Johnson |
| **BEHAVIOURAL FAMILY THERAPY** | | |
| Structural therapy | Focus is on organizational patterns, boundaries, systems and subsystems, and use of scapegoating:<br>• Restructures dysfunctional triangles<br>• Clarifies boundaries<br>• Looks at enmeshment and disengagement (excessive distance) issues | Salvador Minuchin |
| Strategic therapy | Goal is to change repetitive and maladaptive interaction patterns:<br>• Identifies inequality of power, life-cycle perspectives, and use of double-bind messages<br>• Uses paradox<br>• Prescribes rituals | Jay Haley<br>Chloe Madanes<br>Milan group (Mara Palazzoli, Gianfranco Cecchin, Giuliana Prata) |
| Cognitive-behavioural therapy | Based on learning theory; focuses on changing cognition and behaviour:<br>• Problem solving and solutions focused on present situations<br>• Skills training emphasized | Gerald Patterson<br>Richard Stuart<br>Robert Liberman |

sexual orientation, and religion are considered equally. Each of these contextual issues affects the family's values, norms, traditions, roles, and rules. For example, the way the family relates to a terminally ill family member may be decidedly different in a first-generation Filipino Canadian Catholic family than in a traditional First Nations family. The nurse assesses how the family's cultural and religious beliefs affect acceptable care options.

Gender is often related to status and diverse cultural perspectives. In addition, beliefs about mental illness and their etiology and treatment have culturally diverse family interpretations. Cultural sensitivity prepares the nurse to provide culturally competent family intervention in all nursing practice settings. A holistic assessment will include pertinent information on sexual orientation, religious and spiritual beliefs, and trauma histories so as to provide an understanding of influencing factors on the current situation.

### Intergenerational Issues

The influence of family is not restricted to the immediate family. Family is composed of the entire emotional system of at least three, and sometimes four generations, meaning that the family is affected by intergenerational issues. Various patterns of behaviour (e.g., involving geographical distance between members, suicide, divorce, addiction, affairs, grief, triangles, historical colonization, loss) may impact successive generations. The legacy of the multigenerational family may relate to the patient's presenting problem. For example, in working with a First Nations family of a teenager who has engaged in self-harming behaviours, nurses will consider the historical and current context of the family life. A history of residential school attendance may contribute to the family's current parenting problems due to the lack of culturally appropriate role models, loss of identity, and loss of traditional way of life (Niezen, 2009). An astute nurse will also be aware of the potential for mistrust

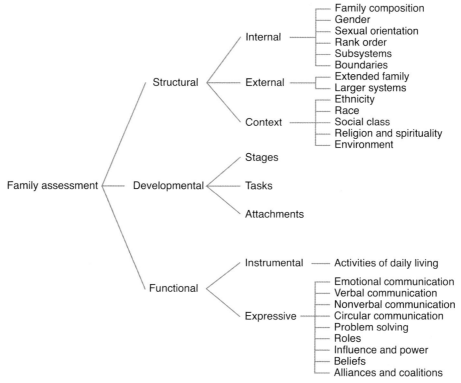

**FIGURE 36-2** Calgary Family Assessment Model **Source:** Wright, L.M., & Leahey, M. (2009). *Nurses and families: A guide to family assessment and intervention* (5th ed., p. 48, Fig. 3-1). Philadelphia: F.A. Davis with permission.

of health care providers and authority figures related to historical oppression and incorporate this knowledge into management of the current situation. This family may deal with grief by using silence and little outward expression of painful feelings. The nurse would respect the family's way of expressing feelings. First Nations families often bring extended family to the hospital to support the ill family member. Accommodation for this cultural expression of support is helpful for the family to resolve hospitalization issues. More important, Aboriginal people are seeking to understand colonialism and history through their own perspectives and interpretation of current problems of poverty, suicide, addictions, and injustice. Currently, Canadian society is working toward truth about and reconciliation of past abuses of First Nations peoples. Nurses must be aware of the potential to misappropriate or use token aspects of cultural knowledge and encourage authentic incorporation of Aboriginal perspectives (Hart, 2002).

### Constructing a Genogram

The genogram is a tool for efficiently providing a clinical summary of information and relationships across generations of a family. It provides a graphic display of complex patterns and serves as a source of hypotheses as to how the presenting problem connects to the family context and the evolution of the family. It may help the family understand patterns of behaviours.

Information for the genogram should be gathered in an empathic and caring manner. Bowen (1985) provided the conceptual framework for the analysis of genogram patterns. He

proposed that the family is organized according to generation, age, sex, roles, functions, and interests and suggested that where each individual fits into the family structure influences the family functioning, relational patterns, and type of family formed in the next generation. Sex and birth order shape sibling relationships and characteristics. Some issues are played out from generation to generation through persisting interactive emotional patterns (Bowen, 1975).

By using a genogram, nurses may map family structure and record family information inclusive of location, occupation, and educational level; functional information regarding medical, emotional, and behavioural status; and critical events such as moves, job changes, separations, abortions, imprisonment, illnesses, and deaths. Figure 36-3 provides an example of a genogram derived from data about the family in the vignette on page 711.

### Self-Awareness

Nurses frequently interact with families in hospital and community-based settings. Nurses who are aware of their personal family-of-origin issues and who practise ongoing self-awareness are most effective. Common defence mechanisms of nurses may contribute to issues in nurse–family relationships: the formation of triangles to reduce anxiety, defensive reactions when personal family-of-origin issues arise, and role blurring when sensitive personal issues and conflicts are triggered. Inexperienced nurses without supervision are particularly at risk for boundary violations.

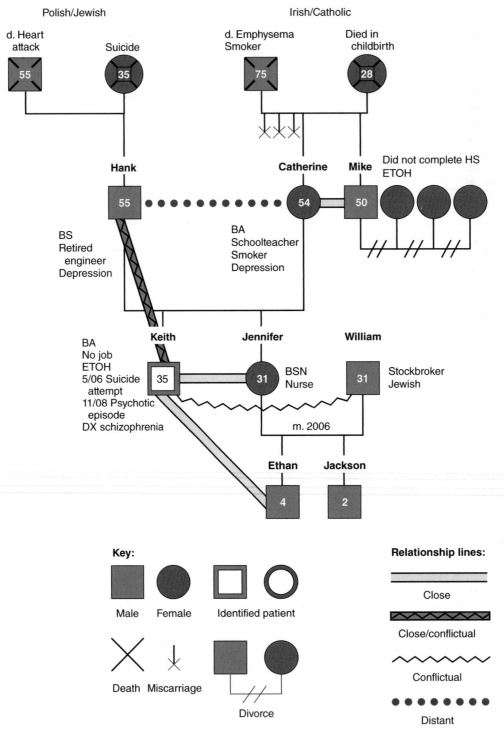

**FIGURE 36-3** Genogram of the Schneider family. *DX,* Diagnosis; *ETOH,* alcohol; *HS,* high school; *m.,* married; *d.,* deceased.

An advanced-practice nurse educated at the master's level, with special training in family work, is best qualified to conduct family therapy. Nurses may experience intense reactions to alcohol or drug use, family abuse, codependency, rescue fantasies, and lifestyles choices. Clinical supervision is necessary to ensure the nurse remains neutral and is not drawn into the client–family dynamics.

## DIAGNOSIS

Families have unique needs at different times in their developmental stages. Family life involves new members, deaths, mental and physical illnesses, economic challenges, developmental crises, and unanticipated blows of life. Severe dysfunctional patterns (e.g., marked relational conflict, sexual misconduct,

Hank (of Polish Jewish descent) and Catherine Schneider (of Irish Catholic descent) are both university educated, and each suffers from intermittent depression. Hank is an only child whose father died of a heart attack at age 55, Hank's present age. Hank's mother committed suicide at age 35. This is a toxic subject in Hank's family of origin. In Catherine's family of origin, she is the eldest, born after three miscarriages. Much pressure and many expectations were placed on her. Catherine's brother, Mike, was born four years after Catherine, and their mother died during Mike's birth. Mike never finished high school. He is now 50 years old, has a serious alcohol addiction, and has had three marriages that ended in divorce. One can speculate about the level of guilt Mike may feel regarding the loss of his mother.

Hank and Catherine have two children, Keith and Jennifer. Keith, the identified patient, is 35 years old, has a university degree, but has not been able to hold down a job. He has an addiction to alcohol. In 2006, Keith made a suicide attempt. In November 2008, Keith experienced a psychotic episode for which he was hospitalized, and he was diagnosed as having schizophrenia. His younger sister, Jennifer, 31, has a university degree and is a practising pediatric nurse. She married William, a Jewish stockbroker the same age as she, in 2006, the year Keith attempted suicide. Jennifer and William have two young children, Ethan and Jackson, ages 4 and 2 respectively.

abuse, violence, suicide) exist within many families that cause significant physical or mental anguish to family members. Upon entering into a therapeutic relationship with a family, to promote health and wellness, nurses need to consider the economic, social, historical, and geographical context of the family. As well, nurses must understand how their own views were formed, consider their position in society and the privilege associated with that position, and then begin to understand how other people may be in different positions (Doane & Varcoe, 2006). In context with the above, words such as *dysfunctional* need to be carefully considered prior to use. Nursing diagnoses useful in working with families are identified in Box 36-4.

## BOX 36-4 POSSIBLE NURSING DIAGNOSES FOR FAMILY INTERVENTIONS

- (Risk for) Caregiver role strain
- Sexual dysfunction
- Interrupted family processes
- Altered family processes
- Spiritual distress
- Risk for compromised resilience
- Ineffective denial
- Deficient knowledge
- Impaired verbal communication
- Defensive coping
- Relocation stress syndrome
- (Risk for) Impaired parenting

## OUTCOMES IDENTIFICATION

Different therapists adhere to various theories and use a wide variety of methods; however, the goals of family therapy are basically the same (Nichols, 2004):

- To reduce *dysfunctional* behaviour of individual family members (Recognize the power of language and recall that families also have strengths. Root causes of dysfunction may be related to circumstances that are difficult to rise above.)
- To resolve or reduce intra-family relationship conflicts
- To mobilize family resources and encourage adaptive family problem-solving behaviours
- To improve family communication skills
- To heighten awareness of other family members' emotional needs and help family members meet those needs
- To strengthen the family's ability to cope with major life stressors and traumatic events, including chronic physical or psychiatric illness
- To improve integration of the family system into the societal system (i.e., especially the extended family but also school, medical facilities, workplace, and so on)
- To promote appropriate individual psychosocial development of each member of the family
- Family psychoeducational teaching is often provided by nurses. Goals for the family include these:
  - Learning to accept a family member's illness
  - Learning to deal effectively with an ill member's symptoms (e.g., hallucinations, delusions, poor hygiene, physical limitations, paranoia, aggression)
  - Understanding the role of medications and when to seek medical advice
  - Learning about community resources and how to access them
  - Feeling less anxiety and regaining control and balance in family life

## PLANNING

The immediate and long-term needs of the family should be determined. For example, is the family in crisis—related to a member being severely ill, homicidal, suicidal, abusive, or a victim of abuse? Is hospitalization necessary to protect the family member? What are the family's coping mechanisms? What new skills can be used to help the family facilitate resolution of normal life-cycle crises? Is there a need for psychoeducational family interventions? Nurses are adept at educating family about the illness of one of the members (e.g., severe mental illness, dementia), providing information about medications and potential adverse effects, and identifying support groups and community resources to help the family cope with the crisis and improve the quality of life for family members.

A careful analysis of assessment data helps the nurse and other health care team members identify the most appropriate family interventions.

## IMPLEMENTATION

Family therapy has been applied to virtually every type of disorder among children, adolescents, and adults and has demonstrated efficacy for each population studied (Liddle & Rowe, 2004; Pinsof & Wynne, 2000). Family therapy appears to be effective in the treatment of substance abuse disorders, child behavioural problems, marital relationship distress, and as an element of the treatment plan for schizophrenia (Liddle & Rowe, 2004).

### Counselling and Communication Techniques

The basic-level nurse may provide counselling through the use of a problem-solving approach to address an immediate-family difficulty related to health. Developing and practising strong listening skills and viewing family members in a positive, nonjudgemental way are critically important qualities for nurses.

Nurses respond to family members' cues that indicate the degree and amount of stress the family system is experiencing. Indicators of stress in a family system include the following:

- Inability of the family or a family member to understand and act on certain recommended treatment directives
- Various somatic complaints among family members
- High degree of anxiety
- Depression
- Problems in school
- Drug use

Promoting and monitoring a family's mental health can occur in any setting and often requires maximizing an opportune moment, rather than a formal meeting. Sometimes an informal conversation (*therapeutic encounter*) can have a significant effect on the family.

Nurses can convey a nonjudgemental approach by the way information is presented, their tone of voice, and how they ask questions. For example, the question "Don't you think you should at least try to comply with your medical regimen?" would probably cause the patient to become defensive, whereas the invitation statement "Tell me what your medical regimen is like" invites collaborative problem solving.

This nonjudgemental approach promotes open communication among professionals and family members and respects everyone's viewpoint. Information imparted in a clear, understandable manner to all family members assists discussion and decision making regarding the patient's care. Family decision making empowers families by indicating that they are accountable and responsible for how they choose to use the information. Families also possess strengths that may be manifested in forms of resilience. Families use their skills to prevent the deterioration of their family units, oppose threats to the family, and keep their families intact (Cadell, Karabanow, & Sanchez, 2008). Refugee and immigrant families often provide examples of extraordinary efforts to keep their families together. First Nations families who have lost children and family members to the 1960s "Sixties Scoop," a public policy that placed Aboriginal children in foster care and resulted in some children being adopted by families in the United States, have also demonstrated resilience in finding their missing family members

(Kirmayer, Tait, & Simpson, 2009). Currently, Aboriginal children continue to be overly represented in child and family services agencies. The perspective of each family member must be elicited and heard. Often, family members hear another member's view for the first time and may be surprised (e.g., "I didn't know you felt that way"). This approach defines the family as the central psychosocial unit of care. The following vignette provides an example of maintaining neutrality and hearing from all members.

---

**VIGNETTE**

Ms. Chang, the head nurse on the adolescent psychiatric unit, is concerned about the negative comments staff members are making regarding the fact that none of Aaron's family has visited him for 10 days. Ms. Chang is concerned that Aaron is picking up the staff's feelings as well. After many attempts, Ms. Chang reaches Aaron's mother by telephone and begins to assess the situation. She discovers that Aaron's mom is divorced and is working double shifts to meet the family's expenses. There is a 2-year-old at home and a set of twins in grade four.

Aaron's mother had been planning to visit on the weekend, but her babysitter cancelled.

Once Ms. Chang understood the situation from another perspective and learned that this family has young children and is struggling to make ends meet, she called a staff meeting to address the situation.

---

Further possible interventions for the situation in the vignette above would be to problem-solve with Aaron and his mother what is realistic for each of them regarding visiting and to organize regular telephone contact. Perhaps an extended family member or a friend can visit when the mother cannot. Long-range discharge planning for Aaron will include the identification of family supports.

Unfortunately, negative comments about family members by staff occur all too often. Hearing these comments can present a difficult situation for the nursing student, who is entering the unit as an outsider and who realizes the negative effect this behaviour has on family members. The student should seek supervision from the instructor so that the most effective approach can be planned. One useful technique is for the student to ask questions of the head nurse and staff in such a manner that alternative ways of viewing the family are embedded in the questions. An example of this is "Has anyone had a chance to contact Aaron's mother to see if there are any problems?" or "I wonder what it's like for Aaron's mother to have her son in a psychiatric unit."

### Family Therapy

The advanced-practice nurse who has graduate or postgraduate training in family therapy may conduct private family therapy sessions. Family therapy is viewed by professionals as appropriate for most situations, although it may be contraindicated in the following circumstances (Nichols, 2004):

- The therapeutic environment is unsafe, and harm results from information, anxiety, or hostility.

- Family members demonstrate an unwillingness to be honest.
- Family members demonstrate an unwillingness to maintain confidentiality.
- A parental conflict involves issues of sexuality that are inappropriate for the children.

In most other situations, traditional family therapy is useful, especially when combined with psychopharmacology in the treatment of bipolar disorder, depression, or schizophrenia. Other options that may be less costly and time consuming are psychoeducational family therapy and self-help groups.

## Traditional Family Therapy

Family therapists use diverse theoretical philosophies and techniques to bring about change in dysfunctional behaviours and interactions. Some therapists focus on the here and now; others rely more heavily on a family's history and reports of happenings between sessions. Most family therapists use an eclectic approach, drawing on a variety of techniques to fit the particular personality and strengths of the family.

Multiple-family group therapy is used with families who have a family member in an inpatient setting. These groups can help family members gain insight into their problems, as they are reflected in the problems of other families. Several families meet in one group with one or more therapists, usually once a week until their ill family member is discharged; these groups often continue for a specific period of time after discharge.

## Psychoeducational Family Therapy

**Psychoeducational family therapy** provides families with the information they need about mental illness and the coping skills that will help them deal with their family member's psychiatric disorder. Psychoeducational family training has been applied successfully in treatment of patients with schizophrenia. Family work supports families in coping with a family member with a severe mental illness.

The primary goal of psychoeducational family therapy is the sharing of mental health information. Family education groups help family members understand their member's illness, prodromal symptoms (symptoms that may appear before a full relapse), medications, and ways to access community resources. Psychoeducational family meetings encourage the expression of feelings and identify strategies to manage problems. For example, parents may learn how to work with a child with a conduct disorder. Feelings of anger, loss, stigmatization, sadness, and helplessness can be shared and put in a perspective that the family and individual members can more satisfactorily manage.

## Self-Help Groups

Self-help groups are led by laypeople who have the illness or a family member of someone who has the illness. They assist people with a personal problem or social deprivation and families with a member who has a specific diagnosis. Some groups focus on families with healthy members, whereas others offer assistance to families whose members are experiencing a health disorder or crisis. Nurses help patients and their families find appropriate support groups. For many people, self-help groups provide healing and ongoing therapeutic support.

## Case Management

Case managers coordinate services for patients and families and monitor the patient's condition. The patient's and family's culture, ethnicity, socioeconomic status, stage of family life cycle, and beliefs about illness combine to affect an individual's response to case management. Case management entails teaching, giving appropriate referrals, and offering emotional support.

---

**VIGNETTE**

David Gilbert, age 21 years, is leaving the hospital after experiencing his first psychotic episode while taking his final examinations before graduation from university. David is being discharged back to his family, consisting of his mother and father; his maternal grandfather, who is bedridden; and a younger brother, Louis, who is 17 years of age. David's diagnosis is paranoid schizophrenia.

While David is hospitalized and later, in postdischarge family therapy, the nurse meets with the family and takes a psychoeducational approach with them. Through reading materials and discussion, initial interventions convey information about David's mental illness and recovery. The nurse identifies psychosocial support groups and how to access them. The nurse performs ongoing assessment of the family's strengths and weaknesses, including community support. She identifies areas that require discussion. Issues include the following:

- Reorganizing family roles related to a newly diagnosed serious mental illness
- Managing the bedridden grandfather
- Attending to Louis's probable fears that he may develop this illness
- Dealing with potential parental guilt feelings
- Planning how to mobilize should David experience another psychotic episode
- Managing medication and adherence
- Dealing with concerns about David's future
- Formulating realistic expectations
- Coping with feelings of loss for what was and what was hoped for
- Maintaining the spousal subsystem

The nurse discusses these issues with the family and how they can best be addressed. For example, a visiting nurse will evaluate the grandfather's situation and need for home care, and a multiple-family psychoeducation group is contacted to increase the family's understanding of David's illness, help the family learn to cope with common problems, and provide a safe place for family members to share feelings of loss and grief.

---

## Pharmacological Interventions

The nurse is often the first to explain to the family the purpose of a prescribed medication, the desired effects, and potential adverse reactions. Generally, the more information family members have, the less likely that anxiety will distort their observations and decision making after discharge. The nurse reviews David's medication with him and his family during his hospitalization and before discharge. The nurse monitors David to determine if adverse effects are interfering with his functioning. The nurse may consult with a physician to titrate medications based on the efficacy of the medications and David's toleration of any adverse effects.

## EVALUATION

Evaluation focuses on whether family members have improved functioning, reduced or resolved conflicts, improved communication skills, and strengthened coping and whether the family is more integrated into the societal system.

## KEY POINTS TO REMEMBER

- Family therapy is based on a variety of theoretical concepts.
- Family therapy aims to decrease emotional reactivity and to encourage differentiation among family members.
- The primary characteristics of healthy family functioning are flexibility and clear boundaries.
- Family-oriented approaches that help family gain insight and make behavioural changes are most successful.
- The genogram is an efficient clinical summary for providing information and defining relationships across at least three generations.

- The family's culture, ethnicity, socioeconomic status, and life-cycle phase, as well as its unique beliefs about illness, affect the individual patient's progress and response to case management.
- Assessment of the family includes a focus on the family life-cycle phase, multigenerational issues, the individual's developmental stage, and the family's sociocultural status.
- Nurses with basic education frequently conduct psychoeducation with families.
- Nurses with specialized education and certification provide family therapy using diverse theoretical approaches.

## CRITICAL THINKING

1. Select a family with whom you've worked during your clinical experience. Evaluate this family's status in terms of functionality or dysfunctionality with reference to the family functions described in the text (i.e., provision of love and nurturance, socialization of children, social control of members, production and consumption of goods and services, addition of new family members through birth or adoption, and physical care and maintenance of family members).

2. Create your own personal genogram, including at least three generations.
   a. Be sure to include the following:
      - Location, occupation, and educational level
      - Critical events such as births, marriages, moves, job changes, separations, divorces, illnesses, deaths
      - Relationship patterns, if possible, such as emotional cutoffs, distancing, overinvolvement, and conflict

   b. Analyze and reflect on patterns of behaviour that may have been transmitted through the generations within your family. These may be positive patterns or more painful patterns.

3. A family has just found out that their young son is going to die. The parents have been fighting and blaming each other for ignoring the child's ongoing symptom of leg pain, which was eventually diagnosed as advanced cancer. There are two other siblings in the family.
   a. How would you apply family concepts to help this family?
   b. What would be your outcome criterion?

4. A mother of a 6-year-old girl has recently been diagnosed with schizophrenia. How would you address her mother's diagnosis with the 6-year-old?

## CHAPTER REVIEW

1. Jeff is a single, noncustodial parent recently divorced. He will be hospitalized for several days following surgery. Which primary concern of Jeff's should the nurse anticipate during this time?
   1. Mourning the loss of his nuclear family
   2. Wondering how to deal with his spouse's extended family
   3. Attempting to restructure the relationship with his former spouse
   4. Finding ways to continue to effectively parent his child

2. While the nurse works with a family, the father—with a smirk on his face—states, "I love my wife, and she's a good woman who would do anything for her family," and rolls his eyes. Which behaviour should the nurse recognize?
   1. Triangulation
   2. Scapegoating
   3. Double-binding
   4. Differentiation

3. Which family member should the nurse refer to individual therapy rather than family therapy?
   1. The mother who has anxiety controlled by medication
   2. The father who is questioning his sexual orientation
   3. The brother who is verbally angry with his parents
   4. The sister who has consented to maintaining confidentiality

4. The nurse is evaluating the family therapy experience. Which behaviour would indicate that further family therapy is indicated?
   1. The wife has set aside 15 minutes daily to connect with her husband.
   2. The son's grades have risen from a "D" average to a "C" average.
   3. The daughter's headaches have subsided.
   4. The mother has stopped using illicit substances, and the father's use has decreased.

5. The nurse is conducting family therapy. Which nursing intervention would be appropriate for an advanced-practice nurse?
   1. Mobilizing family resources and encouraging adaptive family problem-solving behaviours
   2. Improving family communication skills
   3. Explaining what medications can and cannot do
   4. Working with the underlying dynamics and structure of the family group

## ⊖volve WEBSITE

**Post-Test** interactive review

*Visit the Evolve Web site for Chapter Review Answers and Rationales, Critical Thinking Answer Guidelines, and additional resources related to the content in this chapter:* http://evolve.elsevier.com/Canada/Varcarolis/psychiatric/

## REFERENCES

Adoptiveparents.ca. (n.d.). *An adoptive resources guide for Canadians.* http://www.adoptiveparents.ca/on_intadoption.shtml.

Bassani, D.G., Padoin, C.V., Phillip, D., et al. (2008). Estimating the number of children exposed to parental psychiatric disorders through a national health survey. *Child and Adolescent Psychiatry and Mental Health, 3*(6). doi:10.1186/1753-2000-3-6.

Becvar, D.S., & Becvar, R.J. (2008). *Family therapy: A systematic integration* (7th ed.). Boston, MA: Allyn & Bacon.

Bowen, M. (1975). Family therapy after 20 years. In S. Ariti, D. Freedman, & J. Dyrud (Eds.), *American Handbook of Psychiatry* (2nd ed., pp. 379–391). New York: Gardner Press.

Bowen, M. (1985). *Family therapy in clinical practice.* New York: Jason Aronson.

Brown, J., Higgitt, N., Wingert, S., et al. (2005). Challenges faced by Aboriginal youth in the inner city. *Canadian Journal of Urban Research, 14*(1), 81–106.

Cadell, S., Karabanow, J., & Sanchez, M. (2008). Community, empowerment and resilience: Pathways to wellness. *Canadian Journal of Community Mental Health, 20*(1), 21–35.

Canadian Centre for Justice Statistics. (2009). *Family violence in Canada: A statistical profile.* Ottawa: Statistics Canada.

Canadian Council on Social Development. (2011). *Stats and facts.* Retrieved from http://www.ccsd.ca/factsheets/family/.

Canadian Institute for Health Information. (2011). *Health care in Canada: A focus on seniors and aging.* Ottawa: Author.

*Caregiver Recognition Act of Manitoba.* (2011). Retrieved from http://web2.gov.mb.ca/bills/39-5/b042e.php.

Doane, G., & Varcoe, C. (2006). The hard spots of family nursing: Connecting across difference and diversity. *Journal of Family Nursing, 12*(1), 7–21.

Feeley, N., & Gottlieb, L. (2000). Nursing approaches for working with family strengths and resources. *Journal of Family Nursing, 6*(1), 9–24.

Galloway, G. (2010). Women's minister warns against "honour killings." *Globe and Mail.* Retrieved from http://www.theglobeandmail.com/news/politics/ottawa-notebook/womens-minister-warns-against-honour-killings/article1390510/.

Goldenberg, H., & Goldenberg, I. (2008). *Family therapy: An overview* (7th ed.). Belmont, CA: Thomson.

Haley, J. (1980). *Leaving home.* New York: McGraw-Hill.

Haley, J. (1996). *Learning and teaching therapy.* New York: Guilford.

Hart, M.A. (2002). *Seeking mino-pimatisiiwin: An Aboriginal approach to helping.* Halifax: Fernwood Publishing.

Hinshaw, S. (2005). The stigmatization of mental illness in parents and children: Developmental issues, family concerns and research needs. *Journal of Child Psychology and Psychiatry, 46*(7), 714–734.

Kirmayer, L., Simpson, C., & Cargo, M. (2003). Healing traditions: Culture, community and mental health promotion with Canadian Aboriginal people. *Australian Psychiatry, 11*(suppl.), 15s–23s.

Kirmayer, L., Tait, C., & Simpson, C. (2009). The mental health of Aboriginal peoples in Canada: Transformations of identity and community. In L.K. Kirmayer & G. Guthrie Valaskakis (Eds.), *Healing traditions: The mental health of Aboriginal peoples in Canada* (pp. 3–35). Vancouver: UBC Press.

Liddle, H.A., & Rowe, C.L. (2004). Advances in family therapy research. In M.P. Nichols (Ed.), *Family therapy: Concepts and methods* (6th ed.). New York: Pearson Education.

Mental Health Commission of Canada. (2010). *Development for mental health strategy for Canada, phase 11. Roundtable meeting on family involvement and support. Round table highlights report.* Retrieved from http://www.mentalhealthcommission.ca/English/node/713?terminitial=52.

Miller, J.R. (1996). *Shingwauk's vision: A history of native residential schools.* Toronto: University of Toronto Press.

Minuchin, S. (1974). *Families and family therapy.* Cambridge, MA: Harvard University Press.

Minuchin, S. (1996). *Mastering family therapy.* New York: John Wiley & Sons, Inc.

Mordoch, E., & Hall, W. (2002). Children living with a parent who has a mental illness: A critical analysis of the literature and research implications. *Archives of Psychiatric Nursing, 16*, 208–216. doi:10.1053/apnu.2002.36231.

Mordoch, E., & Hall, W. (2008). Children's perceptions of living with a parent with a mental illness: Finding the rhythm and maintaining the frame. *Qualitative Health Research, 18*, 1127–1144. doi:10.1177/1049732308320775.

Nelson, T.S. (2003). Transgenerational family therapies. In L.L. Hecker & J.L. Wetchler (Eds.), *An introduction to marriage and family therapy*. New York: Haworth Clinical Practice Press.

Nichols, M.P. (2004). *Family therapy: Concepts and methods* (6th ed.). New York: Pearson Education.

Niezen, R. (2009). Suicide as a way of belonging: Causes and consequences of cluster suicides in Aboriginal communities. In L.J. Kirmayer & G. Valaskakis (Eds.), *Healing traditions: The mental health of Aboriginal peoples in Canada* (pp. 178–194). Vancouver: UBC Press.

Ostman, M. (2008). Interviews with children of persons with a severe mental illness: Investigating their everyday situation. *Niforma UK Limited, 62*(5), 354–359. doi:10.1080/08039480801960065.

Pinsof, W.M., & Wynne, L.C. (2000). Toward progress research: Closing the gap between family therapy practice and research. *Journal of Marital and Family Therapy, 26*, 1–8.

Registered Nurses' Association of Ontario. (2012). *Supporting and strengthening families through expected and unexpected life events.* Retrieved from http://rnao.ca/resources/my/back-issues.

Robinson, C.A., & Wright, L.M. (1995). Family nursing intervention: What families say makes a difference. *Journal of Family Nursing, 1*(3), 327–345.

Sadock, B.J., & Sadock, A. (2008). *Kaplan & Sadock's concise textbook of clinical psychiatry* (3rd ed.). Philadelphia: Lippincott.

Satir, V. (1972). *Peoplemaking.* Palo Alto, CA: Science and Behaviour Books.

Satir, V. (1983). *Conjoint family therapy.* Palo Alto, CA: Science and Behaviour Books.

Schoen-Johnson, B., & Pearson, G.S. (2003). The client with a thought disorder. In W.K. Mohr (Ed.), *Johnson's Psychiatric Mental Health Nursing* (5th ed., pp. 521–533). New York: Lippincott.

Solantaus, T., & Toikka, S. (2006). The effective family program: Preventative services for children of mentally ill parents in Finland. *International Journal of Mental Health Promotion, 1*(3), 37–44.

Statistics Canada. (2003). *Canadian community health survey.* Ottawa: Author.

United Nations Children's Fund. (2005). Childhood under threat. *The State of the World's Children.* New York: Author.

Vanier Institute of the Family. (2013). *Definition of family.* Retrieved from http://www.vanierinstitute.ca/definition_of_family#.

Weiman, C. (2009). Six Nations mental health services: A model of care for Aboriginal communities. In L.J. Kirmayer & G. Valaskakis (Eds.), *Healing traditions: The mental health of Aboriginal peoples in Canada* (pp. 401–412). Vancouver, BC: UBC Press.

Wollstonecraft, M. (1975). *A vindication on the rights of women (1792).* Baltimore: Penguin.

Wright, L.M., & Leahey, M. (2013). *Nurses and families: A guide to family assessment and intervention* (6th ed.). Philadelphia: F.A. Davis.

Young Carers Initiative. (2012). *What is new?* Retrieved from http://youngcarers.ca/pages.php?page=news.

## KEY TERMS AND CONCEPTS

acupuncture, 723
aromatherapy, 728
chiropractic medicine, 729
conventional health care, 717
healing touch, 730
holistic nurse, 722
homeopathy, 723
integrative health care, 717

natural health products (NHP), 718
naturopathy, 723
reflexology, 729
Reiki, 730
therapeutic touch, 730
traditional, complementary, and alternative medicine
  (TCAM), 718

## OBJECTIVES

1. Define the terms integrative, traditional, complementary, and alternative health care.
2. Identify trends in integrative health care.
3. Discuss how to help educate the public in the safe use of integrative modalities.
4. Explore information resources available through literature and online sources.

5. Explore five aspects of integrative care: whole medical systems, mind–body–spirit approaches, biologically based interventions, manipulative approaches, and energy therapies.
6. Discuss the techniques used in major traditional, complementary, and alternative modalities and potential applications to psychiatric mental health nursing practice.

## ⊖volve WEBSITE

*Visit the Evolve website for Flashcards, Case Studies, and additional testing resources related to the content in this chapter:* *http://evolve.elsevier.com/Canada/Varcarolis/psychiatric/*   Pre-Test  interactive review

This chapter considers *integrative care* as part of a holistic nursing philosophy. Integrative health care is a model of health care with the intent to synergistically blend the best of all evidence-informed healing practices to provide relationship-based, holistic care. It focuses on the least invasive, least toxic, and least costly methods to help facilitate health (Rakel & Weil, 2007, 2012). Canadian authors Boon, Verhoef, O'Hara, and colleagues (2004) define *integrative health care* as an interdisciplinary, nonhierarchical blending of both conventional health care and traditional, complementary, or alternative health care.

In Western countries, conventional health care is also referred to as *biomedicine, allopathic medicine,* or *mainstream*

*medicine* and is based largely on highly controlled, evidence-informed scientific research (Rakel & Weil, 2012). Meanwhile, *traditional medicine (TM)* is defined by the World Health Organization (WHO) as the treatment and maintenance of physical and mental illness with practices informed by the knowledge and beliefs of specific cultures (Bodeker, Ong, Grundy, et al., 2005). In many Western countries, the term *traditional medicine* is used interchangeably with *complementary and alternative medicine (CAM)* and refers to a broad set of health care practices that are not integrated into the dominant or conventional health care system (Bodeker, Ong, Grundy, et al., 2005). This chapter will use the WHO terminology of traditional, complementary, and alternative medicine (TCAM). The term *TCAM* recognizes that many of the philosophical underpinnings for the approaches presented are derived from both non-Western cultural traditions and newer concepts from quantum physics and studies in the nature of energy and reality, which have not historically been a part of conventional health care delivery. However, TCAM will be discussed in the broader context of integrative health care. Integrative mental health care is increasingly being promoted as the preferred model of mental health services (Lake, 2007, 2008, 2009).

## INTEGRATIVE HEALTH CARE IN CANADA

A 2006 Fraser Institute survey revealed much about the Canadian context for integrative health care. The survey found that more than half (54%) of Canadians used at least one alternative therapy the year prior, an increase from the rate of use in 1997 (50%) (Esmail, 2007). Seventy-three percent of Canadians had used at least one alternative therapy at some time in their lives and had used alternative therapies an average of 8.6 times the year prior. During the latter half of 2005 and the first half of 2006, Canadians spent more than $5.6 billion out of pocket on visits to providers of alternative medicine. The five most commonly used modalities were massage, spiritual practice, chiropractic, relaxation, and herbal therapies. Table 37-1 details use of CAM therapies in Canada in 1997 and 2006.

Thirty-two percent of Canadians surveyed indicated that they sought assistance from alternative and conventional providers at the same time (up from 26% in 1997) and 74% reported the belief that using both conventional and alternative therapies is better than using either one alone, reflecting the movement toward integrative health care.

The term natural health products (NHP) is used in Canada to describe substances such as vitamins and minerals, herbal medicines, homeopathic preparations, energy drinks, probiotics, and many alternative and traditional medicines (Health Canada, 2012b). A Health Canada consumer survey in relation to NHPs also suggests an attitudinal trend toward integration of conventional care and TCAM (Health Canada, 2012c). A majority of Canadians agreed that NHPs can be used to maintain or promote health (77%) or to treat illness (68%). Fewer (43%) agreed that NHPs were better than conventional medicine. At the same time, 81% of Canadians thought it was important to respect the role that NHPs play in some cultures. Eighty-one percent also thought the use of NHPs would increase over the next ten years, and 72% expressed the belief that Canadians have the right to use any NHP they choose.

Health Canada responded to integrative health care trends by establishing the Natural Health Products Directorate (NHPD) in 1999. The NHPD's mandate is "to ensure that Canadians have ready access to natural health products that are safe, effective and of high quality while respecting freedom of choice and philosophical and cultural diversity" (Natural Health Products Directorate in Ramsey, 2009). The directorate's Natural Health Products Regulations (NHPR) came into effect January 1, 2004. Under the NHPR, NHPs require a product licence to be legally sold in Canada. To receive a licence to be sold as an NHP, products must be appropriate for consideration as over-the-counter products and not need a prescription. Products needing a prescription are regulated as drugs (Health Canada, 2012b). Controversy has been associated with the NHPR in relation to concerns of increased cost and decreased access to NHPs (Health Canada, 2012d; Ramsay, 2009).

Jurisdiction over Canadian practitioners of TCAM is currently at the provincial and territorial level, resulting in a mosaic of relevant registrations, certifications, and licensures (Ramsay, 2009). In this context, various TCAM practitioners are working toward achieving professional status for their respective modalities and practices (Welsh, Kelner, Wellman, et al., 2004). Those who have been successful, such as massage therapists, chiropractors, and naturopathic doctors (NDs), are increasingly becoming part of mainstream health care (Canadian Association of Naturopathic Doctors, 2011; Canadian Chiropractic Association, 2011; Massage.ca, 2011; Welsh, Kelner, Wellman, et al., 2004). For example, legislation requiring licensure for naturopathic doctors currently exists in British Columbia, Saskatchewan, Manitoba, Ontario, and Nova Scotia, while new regulations for NDs in Alberta have been prepared and await government approval; all other provinces and territories are actively pursuing regulation (Canadian Association of Naturopathic Doctors, 2011). Many conventional health care practitioners, including those in mental health services, are integrating evidence-informed TCAM practices into their professional practice (Canadian Holistic Nurses Association, 2011; Willison, 2008). For example, acupuncture is being integrated by a variety of health care providers as an adjunct to the other techniques and treatments within their scopes of practice (Acupuncture Foundation of Canada Institute, 2011). These practitioners are not called acupuncturists but rather use acupuncture as a tool and are regulated accordingly by their professional regulating body (Acupuncture Foundation of Canada Institute, 2011). Further information about the current status of regulation across provinces and territories for various integrative modalities can be obtained by contacting applicable professional associations. (Box 37-1 highlights several national associations; numerous related provincial and territorial associations also exist.)

Because of the growing interest in and use of TCAM, the United States government's National Institute of Health (NIH) established the National Center for Complementary and Alternative Medicine (NCCAM) in 1998. Since no equivalent Canadian organization has been established to date, NCCAM is an essential resource for Canadian health care providers and patients. The NCCAM supports fair and scientific evaluation of integrative therapies and dissemination of information that allow health care providers and patients to make good choices regarding the safety and appropriateness of various TCAM modalities (National Center for Complementary and Alternative Medicine, 2011g). The World Health Organization (2004) also offers guidelines to support safe, informed choices in relation to TCAM, drawing on syntheses of current research on TCAM for mental health concerns and other conditions. In addition, a variety of emerging Canadian and international

| TABLE 37-1 | USE OF COMPLEMENTARY AND ALTERNATIVE THERAPIES IN CANADA IN THE 12 MONTHS PRECEDING THE SURVEY, BY REGION, 1997 AND 2006 (%)[1] | | | | | | | | | | | | | | | |

| THERAPY | CANADA* | | CANADA** | | BC** | | AB** | | SK & MB** | | ON** | | QC** | | ATLANTIC CANADA** | |
|---|---|---|---|---|---|---|---|---|---|---|---|---|---|---|---|---|
| Year | 1997 | 2006 | 1997 | 2006 | 1997 | 2006 | 1997 | 2006 | 1997 | 2006 | 1997 | 2006 | 1997 | 2006 | 1997 | 2006 |
| Used at least one therapy in past 12 months* (%) | 50 | 54 | — | — | 60 | 64 | 54 | 68 | 58 | 59 | 50 | 55 | 44 | 45 | 45 | 39 |
| Massage (%) | 12 | 19 | 51 | 55 | 52 | 52 | 42 | 57 | 62 | 59 | 51 | 56 | 52 | 58 | 46 | 30 |
| Prayer or spiritual practice (%) | 18 | 16 | 85 | 87 | 93 | 94 | 81 | 92 | 84 | 93 | 83 | 86 | 85 | 83 | 87 | 81 |
| Chiropractic care (%) | 13 | 15 | 36 | 37 | 39 | 35 | 41 | 52 | 42 | 36 | 39 | 33 | 27 | 39 | 24 | 26 |
| Relaxation techniques (%) | 17 | 14 | 72 | 71 | 81 | 81 | 73 | 72 | 81 | 74 | 72 | 71 | 69 | 59 | 47 | 64 |
| Herbal therapies (%) | 12 | 10 | 71 | 63 | 78 | 50 | 65 | 72 | 88 | 56 | 71 | 66 | 46 | 71 | 80 | 63 |
| Yoga (%) | 4 | 9 | 37 | 57 | 47 | 53 | 30 | 51 | 34 | 67 | 38 | 66 | 22 | 48 | 42 | 45 |
| Aromatherapy (%) | 5 | 5 | 81 | 58 | 82 | 61 | 95 | 67 | 85 | 55 | 73 | 52 | 77 | 73 | 100 | 19 |
| Energy healing (%) | 3 | 5 | 50 | 49 | 72 | 50 | 57 | 60 | 46 | 47 | 48 | 44 | 28 | 46 | 39 | 68 |
| Acupuncture (%) | 2 | 4 | 22 | 25 | 31 | 32 | 28 | 30 | — | 17 | 20 | 23 | 20 | 25 | 24 | 18 |
| Folk remedies (%) | 6 | 4 | 50 | 47 | 46 | 46 | 67 | 63 | 51 | 49 | 57 | 44 | 23 | 39 | 61 | 44 |
| Special diet programs (%) | 3 | 4 | 27 | 40 | 9 | 53 | 33 | 38 | 25 | 22 | 29 | 43 | 41 | 35 | 19 | 26 |
| Naturopathy (%) | 3 | 4 | 46 | 44 | 37 | 35 | 54 | 54 | 41 | 43 | 54 | 42 | 37 | 53 | 100 | 57 |
| Lifestyle diet (%) | 5 | 4 | 64 | 53 | 68 | 47 | 66 | 58 | 47 | 54 | 65 | 57 | 62 | 41 | 60 | 67 |
| Imagery techniques (%) | 5 | 4 | 67 | 59 | 59 | 50 | 80 | 75 | 86 | 66 | 73 | 54 | 69 | 50 | 35 | 81 |
| Homeopathy (%) | 5 | 4 | 54 | 42 | 31 | 50 | 57 | 41 | 23 | 14 | 64 | 42 | 53 | 39 | 85 | 58 |
| Self-help group (%) | 3 | 3 | 41 | 36 | 57 | 41 | 8 | 39 | 42 | 50 | 43 | 36 | 42 | 27 | 11 | 35 |
| Spiritual or religious healing by others (%) | 2 | 2 | 54 | 48 | 45 | 53 | 51 | 57 | 19 | 48 | 89 | 47 | 52 | 58 | 35 | — |
| High-dose or mega vitamins (%) | 3 | 2 | 61 | 60 | 45 | 47 | 30 | 59 | 100 | 56 | 78 | 64 | 41 | 88 | 31 | 31 |
| Osteopathy (%) | <1 | 1 | 28 | 36 | — | 18 | — | — | — | — | 46 | 56 | 36 | 32 | — | 59 |
| Biofeedback (%) | 1 | 1 | 25 | 32 | 31 | 37 | 45 | 35 | — | 35 | 15 | 35 | — | — | 27 | — |
| Hypnosis (%) | <1 | 1 | 10 | 16 | 5 | 28 | 45 | — | — | 11 | 10 | 19 | 8 | 19 | — | — |
| Chelation (%) | <1 | <1 | 30 | 33 | 58 | 64 | — | 47 | — | — | 25 | — | 53 | — | — | — |

[1]In instances where a positive percentage would have rounded to 0, "<1" has been substituted.
*Base: total population
**Base: those who have used therapies in their lifetimes
Note: Due to rounding, percentages do not always sum to total.
**Source:** Esmail, N. (2007). Complementary and alternative medicine in Canada: Trends in use and public attitudes, 1997–2006. *Fraser Institute Public Policy Sources, 87*, 19–22 (Table 5, p. 18).

## BOX 37-1  INTEGRATIVE HEALTH CARE RESOURCES

- Acupuncture Foundation of Canada Institute: http://www.afcinstitute.com/Home/tabid/36/Default.aspx
- Canadian Association of Naturopathic Doctors: http://www.naturopathicassoc.ca/
- Canadian Chiropractic Association: http://www.chiropracticcanada.ca/en-us/Home.aspx
- Canadian Federation of Aromatherapists: http://cfacanada.com/
- Canadian Foundation for Trauma Research & Education: http://www.cftre.com/
- Canadian Holistic Nurses Association (CHNA): http://www.chna.ca/
- Canadian Interdisciplinary Network for Complementary & Alternative Research (IN-CAM): http://www.incamresearch.ca/index.php?home&lng=en
- Canadian Research Institute of Spirituality & Healing: http://www.crish.org/
- The Center for Contemplative Mind in Society: http://www.contemplativemind.org/
- Health Canada: Natural Health Products: http://www.hc-sc.gc.ca/dhp-mps/prodnatur/index-eng.php
- Integrative Mental Health (Dr. James Lake): http://progressivepsychiatry.com/
- International Network of Integrative Mental Health: http://www.inimh.org/
- Massage.ca: http://massage.ca/
- National Center for Complementary and Alternative Medicine (NCCAM) (American/International): http://www.nccam.nih.gov/
- Native Mental Health Association of Canada (NMHAC): http://www.nmhac.ca/
- Natural Standard: The Authority on Integrative Medicine: http://www.natural standard.com
- Reflexology Association of Canada: http://www.reflexolog.org/index.html
- The Role of the Registered Psychiatric Nurse in Relation to Complementary and Alternative Healing: http://rpnascom.jumpstartdev.com/alternative%20healing
- Somatic Experiencing Trauma Institute: http://www.traumahealing.com/somatic-experiencing/index.html
- Spiritual Directors International: http://www.sdiworld.org/
- World Health Organization (WHO): http://www.who.int/en (Search "Traditional, Complementary, and Alternative Healing" for various guidelines and updates.)

## BOX 37-2  TCAM RESEARCH CHALLENGES

- Individual, cultural, and environmental variables
- Lack of or limited funding sources
- Time as a variable to measure change
- Interpretation and meaning of an experience
- Impact of other intervening life experiences
- Effect and timing of a specific intervention or approach on a particular problem, specifically placebo and experimental effects
- Personality, belief systems, spiritual practices, and temperament of both the researcher and participants
- Difficulty trying to standardize modalities; variations in methods, approaches, and skill of the researcher
- Influence of studying a phenomenon or person within a naturalistic setting
- Interpretation of results
- The recognized value of both qualitative and quantitative results
- Acknowledgement of the importance of the relationship between the healer and the person being healed

**Source:** Zahourek, R. (2005). Intentionality: Evolutionary development in healing. *Journal of Holistic Nursing, 23,* 89–109. doi:10.1177/0898010104272026. Copyright © 2005 by SAGE. Reprinted by Permission of SAGE Publications.

financial incentive to support the research, and (3) the difficulties encountered when researching these modalities (Box 37-2). Still, as evident in Box 37-1, an increasing number of governmental and private sources of research funding are emerging, particularly as the emphasis shifts from a "mainstream versus alternative" mentality to one of promoting evidence-informed integrative health care (Lake, 2007, 2008; Rakel & Wiel, 2012).

In any case, it is important for health care providers to remember that evidence-informed practice relies on much more than the results of randomized controlled trials (RCTs); the integration of clinical expertise with the best evidence available is also essential (Lloyd & Dunn, 2007, p. 32).

## PATIENTS AND INTEGRATIVE CARE

Patients are attracted to integrative care for a variety of reasons, including the following:

- A desire to be an active participant in their health care and to engage in holistic practices that can promote health and healing
- A desire to find therapeutic approaches that seem to carry lower risks than medications
- A desire to find less expensive alternatives to high-cost conventional care
- Positive experiences with holistic, integrative TCAM practitioners, who tend to spend more time with and learn about their patients as a whole
- Dissatisfaction with the practice style of conventional medicine (e.g., rushed office visits, short hospital stays)
- A need to find modalities and remedies that provide comfort for chronic conditions for which no conventional medical cure exists, such as anxiety, chronic pain, and depression

organizations offer ongoing information and research updates (Box 37-1).

### Research

Research on the efficacy of TCAM is increasing in the field of mental health, most notably concerning anxiety and depression (Sarris, Moylan, Camfield, et al., 2012). Studies in the field are, however, minimal when compared to those of conventional medicine (Khorsan, Coulter, Crawford, et al., 2011). Reasons for this lack of research include (1) the relatively recent use of some of these therapies in Western countries, (2) the lack of

(Bodeker, Kronenberg, & Burford, 2007; Koopsen & Young, 2009; Young & Koopsen, 2011)

The knowledgeable patient, relying on health information available through public libraries, at popular bookstores, and on the Internet, may question conventional health care. It is essential that nurses maintain up-to-date knowledge of these modalities, continue to evaluate the evidence supporting the effectiveness and safety of TCAM, and be able to help patients make safe choices about the use of these treatments for their mental health and recovery.

## Safety and Efficacy

People who use TCAM therapies often do so without informing their conventional health care providers, which poses some risk. In a 2010 survey, 15% of Canadians who used NHPs reported that they had experienced unwanted adverse effects; this number is up from 12% in a 2005 survey (Health Canada, 2012c). Some patients may believe that a natural substance from a health food store must be safe and effective; however, "natural" does not mean "harmless." Herbal products and supplements may contain powerful active ingredients that can cause damage if taken inappropriately or in combination with pharmaceutical preparations (Ulbricht, 2011). Health Canada (2012a) consumer guidelines for safe use of NHPs are listed in Box 37-3.

Nurses have a professional responsibility to provide patient education that protects patients from unscrupulous practices. The Registered Psychiatric Nurses Association of Saskatchewan's *Position Statement on the Role of the Registered Psychiatric Nurse in Relation to Complementary and Alternative Healing* (2011) recommends that the patient choosing TCAM be encouraged to select practitioners who address the following:

- Can provide documentation regarding their credentials, educational preparation, and experience that demonstrate that they have the necessary qualifications to practise the modality professionally

- Can identify whether or not their modality is regulated by a professional organization and, if so, can provide documentation of membership in that organization and show that they practise in accordance with its code of ethics, standards of practice, and any other appropriate guidelines
- Facilitate informed consent by outlining potential risks, benefits, and limitations of the modality
- Support a multidisciplinary approach

Another concern regarding TCAM therapies that nurses need to address with their patients is that diagnosis and treatment may be delayed while patients try alternative interventions, which is common with mental health disorders such as major depression and anxiety. On the other hand, many TCAM and conventional health care practitioners are aware of patients who have been injured by an uncaring conventional medical system or have suffered consequences from the use of conventional pharmaceuticals. Nurses, in consultation with all relevant practitioners, can play a key role in assisting patients to carefully and safely weigh the risks and benefits of all treatments under consideration.

## Cost

The growth in use of TCAM therapies is also linked to the rising cost of conventional medical care. There is mounting pressure to control health care spending; therefore, efforts are focused on the development of less expensive treatments (Esmail, 2007). Before we can adopt alternative methods of treatment—even those that are less expensive—it is essential to have reliable information about the clinical effectiveness of integrating these treatment methods into care (Khorsan, Coulter, Crawford, et al., 2011).

### Reimbursement

Payment for TCAM services comes from a wide array of sources, although third-party coverage is still the exception rather than the rule (Esmail, 2007). Some health insurance companies and employee benefits plans include coverage for certain modalities (Esmail, 2007; Khorsan, Coulter, Crawford, et al., 2011).

### Placebo Effect

Some people make the claim that integrative therapies work through a mechanism known as the *placebo effect*. The term *placebo effect* refers to a treatment that actually does nothing, yet the condition for which it is used improves (Caspi, 2007; Rakel & Jonas, 2012); the improvement comes about because of the power of suggestion and a belief that the treatment works. Research on this phenomenon continues and is necessary to deepen our understanding of it. In the meantime, it is known that integrative care is based on optimism; a positive approach and the use of positive suggestion, no matter what treatment modality is being implemented, offer a greater chance of success than does communication that is negative or fosters a poor response. The placebo effect can be most powerful when the need is greatest and a trusting relationship has been established between patient and health care provider. In fact, the literature on integrative health care increasingly refers to this positive placebo effect as "the healing response" that should

---

**BOX 37-3  HOW CAN I USE HEALTH PRODUCTS SAFELY?**

- Talk to a health care professional like a doctor, pharmacist, or naturopath before choosing a product. This is especially important for children, pregnant or breastfeeding women, older adults, and people with serious medical conditions.
- To prevent interactions, make sure your health care provider knows what other drugs and natural health products you are using.
- Use approved products. Look for NPN/DIN-HM numbers that identify licensed products.
- Be sceptical of health-related claims that seem too good to be true. Don't rely on ads: do your own research and talk to your health care provider.
- Read and follow all instructions on the product label.
- Report unwanted side effects (adverse reactions) to your health care provider and Health Canada.

**Source:** Health Canada. (2012). *About natural health products: How can I use natural health products safely?* Retrieved from http://www.hc-sc.gc.ca/dhp-mps/prodnatur/about-apropos/cons-eng.php#a3. Reproduced with permission from the Minister of Health, 2013.

intentionally be activated within holistic care to enhance healing outcomes (Caspi, 2007; Rakel & Jonas, 2012).

## INTEGRATIVE NURSING CARE

The Canadian Holistic Nurses Association (CHNA) recognizes holistic nursing as a specialty that supports holistic health and a philosophy of holistic nursing encompassing self-care and responsibility, humanizing health care, and wellness promotion (Canadian Holistic Nurses Association, 2011). The CHNA is affiliated with the American Holistic Nurses Association (AHNA), which defines the holistic nurse as one who recognizes and integrates body–mind–emotion–spirit–environment principles into practice; attends to self-awareness and personal healing; removes barriers to the healing process; facilitates growth in others; and assists illness recovery or transition to a peaceful death (Mariano, 2013, pp. 60–61).

Regardless of their practice philosophy, nurses need to have a basic knowledge of treatments used in integrative care since they care for patients who increasingly use a variety of unconventional modalities to meet their health needs. In addition, nurses need to respond to the reality that patients are looking to nurses and other health care providers to offer holistic health care (Willison, 2008). Nursing education programs are beginning to include basic integrative modalities such as relaxation, imagery, and contemplative practices in their curricula, and some may include energy-based approaches such as therapeutic touch (Canadian Holistic Nurses Association, 2011; Barrere, 2013; Young & Koopsen, 2011).

To fully understand and respond to the needs of patients, nurses must ask questions about the use of TCAM as part of a holistic assessment (Mariano, 2013; Registered Psychiatric Nurses Association of Saskatchewan, 2011). Such inquiry can be naturally integrated into holistic exploration of the mental, emotional, physical, spiritual, social, and cultural dimensions of the person's life and healing process.

## CLASSIFICATION OF INTEGRATIVE CARE

NCCAM has developed a system of classification for TCAM therapies. These classifications are adapted in this chapter to include the following: (1) whole medical systems, (2) mind–body–spirit approaches, (3) biologically based practices, (4) manipulative approaches, and (5) energy therapies. It is important for readers to keep in mind that these classifications are interrelated; many of the modalities discussed could fit into more than one such classification. Furthermore, many modalities are increasingly being classified as "conventional" in light of ever-expanding research and usage. It is essential for nurses to regularly revisit the literature on the effectiveness of a given modality in relation to a specific mental health issue.

### Whole Medical Systems

NCCAM defines a whole medical system as a complete system of theory and practice that has evolved over time in a variety of cultures and apart from biomedical and allopathic medicine. Whole medical systems addressed in this chapter are traditional Aboriginal medicine, Ayurvedic medicine, traditional Chinese medicine, homeopathy, and naturopathy.

### Traditional Aboriginal Medicine

Traditional Aboriginal medicine is central to integrative health care in Canada, given the large number of Canadians who are of First Nations or Aboriginal ancestry. In this healing system, mental, emotional, spiritual, social, cultural, and physical health are inseparable (Binda, 2011; McAdam, 2009; Mehl-Madrona, 2008). Discussed in more detail in Chapter 7, Aboriginal medicine wheel teachings are increasingly being integrated into mental health treatment approaches for those from Aboriginal and non-Aboriginal ancestry. Specific teachings vary, depending on the affiliation of Aboriginal peoples. Traditional Aboriginal elders and healers combine such narrative with a variety of spiritual and healing practices such as ceremonies (e.g., sweat lodges), vibrational medicine (e.g., chanting and drumming), and use of traditional medicines (e.g., native herbs) to restore balance and harmony (Binda, 2011; McAdam, 2009; Mehl-Madrona, 2008, 2010). Further information about Aboriginal mental health and healing, as well as practices to acknowledge the elders and keepers of traditional knowledge, can be obtained from the Native Mental Health Association of Canada (2008).

### Ayurvedic Medicine

Ayurvedic (pronounced i•yur•vay•dik) medicine originated in India around 5000 BC and is one of the world's oldest medical systems. *Ayurveda* means "the science of life" and is a philosophy that emphasizes individual responsibility for health. It is holistic, promotes prevention, and recognizes the uniqueness of the individual. Ayurvedic practitioners offer a variety of natural treatments such as herbs, dietary adjustments, contemplative practices, cleansing techniques, and ways of balancing the individual's *chakras*. According to Jackson and Keegan (2013), a chakra is the "specific centre of consciousness in the human energy system that allows for the inflow and directing of energy from outside, as well as for outflow from the individual's energy field" (p. 347). Seven major chakras relate to the spine, alongside many minor energy systems throughout the body.

Ayurvedic treatments aim to eliminate impurities and balance the individual's unique constitution (*prakriti)* and life forces (*doshas)* (National Center for Complementary and Alternative Medicine, 2011a).

### Traditional Chinese Medicine

Traditional Chinese medicine (TCM) provides the basic theoretical framework for many TCAM therapies, including acupuncture, acupressure, herbs, transcendental meditation, tai chi, and qigong (Koopsen & Young, 2009). TCM is derived from the philosophy of Taoism and emphasizes the need to promote harmony (health) or bring order out of chaos (illness). TCM is a vast medical system based on a constellation of concepts, theories, laws, and principles of energy movement within the body (Koopsen & Young, 2009). Therapy is aimed at addressing the patient's illness in relation to the complex interaction of mind, body, and spirit. As such, various aspects of TCM may be helpful in reducing symptoms of anxiety and depression

(National Center for Complementary and Alternative Medicine, 2011h).

Adherents of TCM say that it addresses not only symptoms but also what they call "cosmologic" events—events that relate to the dynamics of the universe. According to Taoists, the life force (*qi* or *chi*) is a two-part force (*yin* and *yang*); these parts are complementary and equally important. The goal of life is *transformation*—returning to and being reabsorbed into the qi, which circulates throughout the universe and in our bodies in precise channels called *meridians* (Koopsen & Young, 2009). These meridians become significant in the practice of acupuncture, touch therapy, and energy-based therapies more recently used to treat emotional symptoms and promote mental health.

Health is viewed as the balance between yin and yang, and illness as emanating from imbalances. TCM practitioners use the patient's history and physical examination to understand the imbalances of mind, body, and spirit that have contributed to the patient's illness. Diagnosis involves both questioning and observing body structure, skin colour, breath, body odours, nail condition, voice, gestures, mood, and pulse. Treatment includes an individualized blend of TCM modalities aimed at restoring harmony within the patient's entire being and environment and reawakening the spirit to its possibilities and purpose. Active participation in associated lifestyle changes is essential to successful therapy (Koopsen & Young, 2009, pp. 137–165).

***Acupuncture.*** Given that acupuncture is an integral part of TCM, it is discussed within this context, although it has also become an increasingly popular therapy in Western countries as a healing modality in and of itself. Acupuncture involves the placement of needles into the skin at meridian points to modulate the flow of energy (qi). Sometimes acupuncture needles are inserted and removed immediately, and at other times they are twirled, attached to electrodes for stimulation, or allowed to remain in place for a time. Sensations are described as rushing, warm, tingling, or, occasionally, painful. Acupuncture is thought to stimulate physical changes such as in brain activity, blood chemistry, endocrine functions, blood pressure, heart rate, and immune-system response. Acupuncture can play a role in regulating blood cell counts and in relieving pain and emotional distress by triggering endorphin production (National Center for Complementary and Alternative Medicine, 2011c).

Acupuncture has been used to manage symptoms of withdrawal from substances, reduce hallucinations in schizophrenia, and treat mood disorders and post-traumatic stress disorder (PTSD), with mixed results according to the literature to date (Cheng, Wang, Xiao, et al., 2009; Lee, Shin, Ronan, et al., 2009; National Center for Complementary and Alternative Medicine, 2011c; Rathbone & Xia, 2009; Zhang, Chen, Yip, et al., 2010). A 2009 systematic review suggests that acupuncture is effective in the treatment of insomnia (Cao, Pan, Li, et al., 2009). Risks identified relate to improper technique in sterilization or placement of needles (National Center for Complementary and Alternative Medicine, 2011c).

## Homeopathy and Naturopathy

Homeopathy and naturopathy are examples of Western whole medical systems. Developed in Germany over 200 years ago, homeopathy uses small doses (dilutions) of specially prepared plant extracts, herbs, minerals, and other materials to stimulate the body's defence mechanisms and healing processes. Infinitesimally small doses of diluted preparations that produce symptoms mimicking those of an illness are used to help the body heal itself. Homeopathy is based on the Law of Similars ("like cures like"), and dilutions are prescribed to match the patient's illness or symptom (or both) and personality profile (National Center for Complementary and Alternative Medicine, 2011d).

Homeopathy has been difficult to study using current scientific methods because its highly diluted solutions cannot be readily measured and homeopathic treatments are highly individualized (National Center for Complementary and Alternative Health, 2011d). A systematic review found that homeopathic remedies in high dilution, taken under the supervision of trained professionals, are generally considered safe and unlikely to cause severe adverse reactions. They are not known to interact with conventional drugs. Patients with addictions should be informed that some homeopathic remedies contain alcohol. Patients should also be informed that there may be a temporary worsening of symptoms before they improve (National Center for Complementary and Alternative Medicine, 2011d).

There is mixed evidence on the effectiveness of homeopathic treatments for different mental illnesses. For instance, the breadth of evidence does not currently support homeopathic treatments for anxiety disorders (Sarris, Moylan, Camfield, et al., 2012).

Naturopathy emphasizes health restoration rather than disease treatment and combines nutrition, homeopathy, herbal medicine, hydrotherapy, light therapy, massage therapy, therapeutic counselling, and other treatments. It is a whole medical system that has evolved from a combination of traditional practices and health care approaches popular in Europe during the nineteenth century. Naturopathic practitioners, guided by a philosophy that emphasizes the healing power of nature, now use a variety of traditional and modern therapies. Practitioners view their role as supporting the body's inherent ability to maintain and restore health, and prefer to use treatment approaches they consider the most natural and least invasive. Such holistic concepts are useful in considering the body–mind–spirit nature of mental health and illness (National Center for Complementary and Alternative Medicine, 2011f).

## Mind–Body–Spirit Approaches

Mind–body–spirit (MBS) approaches make use of the continuous interaction between mind, body, and spirit (Lloyd & Dunn, 2007). Most of these techniques emphasize facilitating the mind and spirit's capacity to affect bodily function and symptoms; however, a reciprocal relationship is also part of the equation (i.e., physical illness affects mental and spiritual health). These approaches are based on the recent research advances in psychoneuroimmunology and psychoneuroendocrinology (Lloyd & Dunn, 2007).

The MBS relationship is well accepted in conventional medicine and likely to be the domain most familiar to psychiatric mental health nurses and nurses in general. Many of the MBS interventions, such as cognitive-behavioural therapy, relaxation techniques, guided imagery, hypnosis, and support groups, are now considered mainstream and have been the subject of considerable research. Research substantiates that these approaches dampen the parasympathetic responses in trauma that can lead to chronic health problems, PTSD, anxiety, and depression (Anselmo, 2013; Schaub & Burt, 2013b). Meditation, prayer, spiritual healing, and therapies using creative outlets such as dance, music, and art have been researched less and often continue to be categorized as TCAM.

### Guided Imagery

The use of guided imagery has been in nursing literature for at least three decades. In her seminal work, Zahourek describes imagery as a holistic phenomenon that is a "multidimensional mental representation of reality and fantasy that includes not only visual pictures, but also remembrance of situations and experiences such as sound, smell, touch, movement and taste" (2002, p. 113). As such, it can be used to promote the healing response in all dimensions of health. The clinical effectiveness of imagery has been well documented in the treatment of anxiety, depression, and a variety of stress-related illnesses (Schaub & Burt, 2013b). Nurses can actively assist patients to explore what health-promoting images they can integrate into their self-care practices (Schaub & Burt, 2013b).

Principles of imagery have been integrated with new expressions of mind–body–spirit therapy, such as somatic experiencing (SE) and self-regulation therapy (SRT), as a way of holistically processing and releasing trauma (Canadian Foundation for Trauma Research & Education, 2010; Levine, 2010). Specialized preparation is required for practice of these modalities.

### Biofeedback

Biofeedback is the use of some form of external equipment or method of feedback (some as simple as a handheld thermometer; others as complex as cardiac monitoring) that informs a person about his or her psychophysiological processes and state of arousal (Anselmo, 2013). This process enables the person to begin to voluntarily control reactions that were previously outside conscious awareness. Biofeedback has been extensively practised and researched since the 1960s to treat anxiety, substance abuse, and a variety of stress-related health challenges (Anselmo, 2013; Schaub & Burt, 2013a).

### Hypnosis and Therapeutic Suggestion

Hypnosis is both a state of awareness (consciousness) and an intervention. As a state of consciousness, hypnosis is a natural focusing of attention that may range in susceptibility to suggestion. In stress states, people are more susceptible to suggestion because their focus of attention is narrowed. People who dissociate in traumatic situations are in a trancelike state. When relaxation and imagery techniques are used, individuals frequently will enter a similarly altered state of awareness, or trancelike state, that can promote a healing response (Gurgevich, 2012).

### Meditation

Several forms of meditation have become popular self-help methods to reduce stress and promote wellness. Meditation practices include such simple behaviours as consciously breathing and focusing attention while walking, sitting, or engaging in other contemplative activity such as yoga (Fortney & Bonus, 2012; Srivastava, Talukdar, & Lahan, 2011). Other forms of meditation have arisen from scientifically based work such as that done by Benson in relation to "the relaxation response" and by Kabat Zinn in relation to mindfulness-based stress reduction (MBSR) (Anselmo, 2013; Plante, 2010). Whatever its origins, meditation practice cultivates a contemplative state of mind that can induce an experience of deep relaxation and calm (Anselmo, 2013; Plante, 2010). Nurses may guide patients toward individual teachers, meditation books, audio recordings, or group classes, with religious (e.g., Hindu, Buddhist) or non-religious (e.g., MBSR) approaches, depending on patients' preferences and interests.

Recent meta-analyses have demonstrated the effectiveness of meditation, in particular in the treatment of anxiety (Chen, Berger, Manheimer, et al., 2012; Sedlmeier, Eberth, Schwartz, et al., 2012). A literature review by Hofmann, Sawyer, Witt, and colleague (2010) suggests that mindfulness-based therapy is a particularly promising intervention for treating anxiety and mood problems (see the Research Highlight). An Australian research synthesis showed strong evidence for moderate exercise and mindfulness meditation in the management of anxiety disorders. The trials reviewed found significant oxygenation and neurochemical changes as a result of even brief meditation practices (Sarris, Moylan, Camfield, et al., 2012).

Such meditative practices are increasingly being integrated with neuroscience by such pioneers as University of Toronto psychiatrist Dr. Norman Doidge, who has pioneered their use in promotion of brain neuroplasticity and "re-wiring" in relation to anxiety, mood symptoms, and other mental health challenges (Doidge, 2007). Numerous recent studies featured by NCCAM reveal that meditation is, indeed, associated with structural changes in the brain, opening the door to further study of specific applications to treat specific mental health challenges (National Center for Complementary and Alternative Medicine, 2011d).

### Rhythmic Breathing

While breathing is an integral part of meditation practice, Kitko (2007) describes rhythmic breathing as an easy-to-learn and easy-to-implement MBS intervention in its own right. The nurse helps the patient focus on purposeful breath and usually breathes alongside the patient. This activity enhances the relaxation response in both nurse and patient and has implications for psychiatric mental health nurses working with agitated patients.

### Spirituality

Historically, there are many precedents for the inclusion of spirituality in mental health care (Koenig, 2009, 2011). Today, there is increasing interest in the use of spiritual interventions

**RESEARCH HIGHLIGHT**

### How Do We Know It Works?: Mindfulness-Based Therapy for Anxiety and Depression

**Source:** Adapted from Hofmann, S.G., Sawyer, A.T., Witt, A.A., et al. (2010). The effect of mindfulness-based therapy on anxiety and depression: A meta-analytic review. *Journal of Consulting and Clinical Psychology, 78*, 169–183. doi:10.1037/a0018555.

**Problem**

There is a growing body of evidence on the effectiveness of mindfulness-based therapy for anxiety and depression; however, different variables and methods of study make it difficult to determine the strength of the effect of mindfulness-based therapy on outcomes.

**Purpose of Study**

The purpose of this study was to conduct an effect-size analysis of mindfulness-based therapy for anxiety and mood symptoms in clinical samples.

**Methods**

An effect-size analysis of mindfulness-based therapy for anxiety and mood symptoms in clinical samples was conducted using a systematic review of the literature. A meta-analysis of 39 studies was ultimately explored, totalling 1140 participants receiving mindfulness-based therapy for a range of conditions, including cancer, generalized anxiety disorder, depression, and other psychiatric or medical conditions.

**Key Findings**

Effect-size estimates suggested that mindfulness-based therapy was moderately effective for improving anxiety and mood symptoms from pre- to post-treatment in the overall sample. In patients with anxiety and mood disorders, this intervention was associated with effect sizes of 0.97 and 0.95 for improving anxiety and mood symptoms, respectively. These robust effect sizes were unrelated to publication year or number of treatment sessions, and were maintained over follow-up.

**Implications for Nursing Practice**

These results suggest that mindfulness-based therapy is a promising intervention for treating anxiety and mood problems in clinical populations. Nurses are advised to be aware of the approaches, referral sources, and basic techniques for mindfulness-based interventions.

in all aspects of health (Kalish, 2012; Olson & Clark, 2010). Their positive influence on mental health has been well documented in the interdisciplinary literature in terms of enhanced coping, improved quality of life, and faster recovery (Balbuena, Baetz, & Bowen, 2013; Koenig, 2011). Integration of spiritual care has been associated with fulfilled spiritual needs (such as connectedness, trust, hope, meaning, mastery, and calm), which are observed to promote enhanced overall physiological functioning and openness to mental, emotional, spiritual, and relational transformation, whether or not chronic psychiatric

symptoms persist (Clarke, Watson, & Brewer, 2009; Hood, Olson, & Allen, 2007; Kalish, 2012; Pike, 2011; Rakel & Jonas, 2012; Tarko, 2002; Wright & Bell, 2010).

One challenge in meeting the spiritual needs of psychiatric patients is maintaining appropriate boundaries. Patients may experience difficulty in knowing where their own beliefs stop and those of the health care provider begin. Patients are in a vulnerable position of potentially being unfairly influenced by someone with strong beliefs, particularly if their functioning is compromised by psychiatric symptoms (Baetz & Toews, 2009; Koenig, 2009). In meeting the spiritual needs of psychiatric patients, it is imperative that nurses be continually aware and respectful of boundary issues and never impose their beliefs on patients. This awareness is particularly important in the pluralistic Canadian context, wherein a great diversity of spiritual world views coexist (Bibby, 2011; Pesut, 2010). For example, Koenig reported in 2009 that 12.5% of Canadians describe themselves as nonreligious and 1.9% as atheist. As such, it is important for the nurse to avoid the assumption that tending to spiritual needs involves connection to religious activity.

To address the spiritual needs of patients, we explore their spiritual practices, concerns, beliefs, questions, and resources. The assessment itself is a powerful intervention. When we ask patients about the importance of spirituality in their lives, we are helping them to mobilize their spiritual resources to promote healing (Young & Koopsen, 2011). In the mental health setting, such inquiry must always be done in a way that does not reinforce any religious delusions that may be present (Baetz & Toews, 2009).

The Canadian-based T.R.U.S.T. Model for Inclusive Spiritual Care draws upon the interdisciplinary literature to offer guidelines for a nonintrusive, integrative approach to spiritual assessment and intervention in a pluralistic context (Scott Barss, 2012) (Figure 37-1). Inclusive spiritual care is defined as relevant, nonintrusive care that tends to the spiritual dimension of health by addressing universal spiritual needs, honouring unique spiritual world views, and helping individuals to explore and mobilize factors that can help them gain or regain a sense of trust in order to promote optimal healing. The spiritual dimension of health is defined as the dimension of health associated with "matters of the spirit," as ultimately defined by each individual (Scott Barss, 2012). The spiritual dimension may or may not involve a sense of connection to a divine presence or to religious structures or traditions, and it is associated with universal spiritual needs such as trust, hope, meaning, purpose, interconnection, reconciliation, inspiration, and creativity (Kalish, 2012; Scott Barss, 2012; Young & Koopsen, 2011). Box 37-4 includes sample questions to inform patient-centred spiritual exploration should patients wish to have it included in their holistic health care (Scott Barss, 2012). The table highlights initial assessment questions to help nurses to meet minimum standards for spiritual care that emphasize that all patients are to be invited to receive spiritual care in keeping with their individual world view (Pinto, March, & Pravikoff, 2008). The initial assessment questions are closed-ended to ensure such inquiry is nonintrusive. They need to be accompanied by explicit statements establishing their relevance and affirming

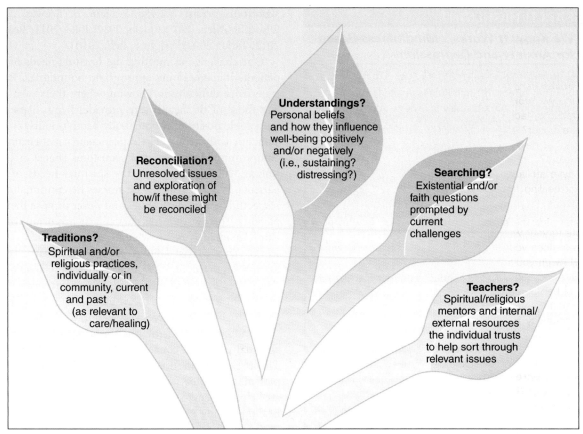

**FIGURE 37-1** T.R.U.S.T. Model for Inclusive Spiritual Care. **Source:** Scott Barss, K. (2011). T.R.U.S.T.: An affirming model for inclusive spiritual care. *Journal of Holistic Nursing, 30* (1), 24–34. doi: 10.1177/ 0898010111418118. Copyright © 2011 by SAGE. Reprinted by Permission of SAGE Publications.

the availability of related exploration at a later time if the patient is not currently interested. Any such inquiry may need to be postponed if the patient is actively psychotic or unable to focus on such exploration (Koenig, 2009). Deep listening is essential for health care providers to be able to discern which, if any, questions are currently relevant to explore with the patient; of course, such questions are just one dimension of the therapeutic dialogue (Scott Barss, 2012). In the process, patients can integrate spiritual and cultural practices and resources to support their healing. Those individuals specifically trained to offer therapy and counselling from a religious and spiritual perspective (e.g., leaders with Shamanic training, Islamic imams, Christian pastors or priests, spiritual or cultural care leaders or hospital chaplains, Catholic or Buddhist nuns) may be an important resource at times of illness and crisis. Certain religious communities offer informal or formal community outreach and events that may be an important part of ongoing recovery and inclusion into community life for patients as well as families (Young & Koopsen, 2011).

## Biologically Based Therapies

Biologically based therapies include the use of dietary supplements such as vitamins, minerals, herbs, or other botanicals; amino acids; and substances such as enzymes, organ tissues, and metabolites (National Center for Complementary and Alternative Medicine, 2011g). With the proliferation of literature on

natural health products, many people are purchasing over-the-counter products and bypassing a visit to a health care provider (Esmail, 2007). Open discussions and ongoing literature reviews on the associated risks and benefits are a must within the nurse–patient relationship. The NCCAM and Natural Standard Web sites and publications offer ongoing research updates in this rapidly expanding area (National Center for Complementary and Alternative Medicine, 2011b; Natural Standard, 2011; Ulbricht, 2011). This chapter briefly introduces dietary and herbal supplements that have been used in relation to various mental health challenges and directs readers to engage in additional ongoing research in order to promote patient safety. Consultation with all relevant members of the patient's integrative health care team is also essential in accessing accurate, up-to-date information.

## Diet and Nutrition

It is essential that nurses assess the patient's nutritional status and practices and address this area in health teaching. Assess for the use of nutrients such as vitamins, protein supplements, herbal preparations, enzymes, and hormones that are considered dietary supplements. Since some nutritional supplements interact with medications, nurses should specifically ask about the use of supplements during the assessment and should not expect patients to share this information without being asked (Ulbricht, 2011). Nurses can review the use of the supplements

## BOX 37-4   T.R.U.S.T. MODEL FOR SPIRITUAL ASSESSMENT AND CARE

### Traditions and Practices

- **Are there things about your spiritual, religious, cultural, and/or healing traditions/practices/experiences you would like the health care team to be aware of? How might these affect how we work together?**
- What practices, activities, or issues are you inspired by/passionate about? How can these be integrated into your healing? What new practices, activities, or issues might you like to explore?
- Do you have affiliation with any particular spiritual, religious, cultural or healing traditions? If so, do you see it/them as a current source of strength? Of distress? How so? Are there aspects of or experiences with your tradition(s) that you feel contribute to your well-being? Compromise your well-being?
- What do or does your tradition(s) say about the nature of suffering? How do you feel about that?
- What gives you hope? How can we help you connect to your sources of hope?
- How are you creative in your daily life? In your coping? How can this creativity be applied to your current challenges? To your life in general?

### Reconciliation

- **Are there any unresolved issues you would like support in exploring at this time?**
- Are there situations, choices, or actions of others in your life with whom you cannot currently make peace? How does this influence your sense of well-being? What do you wish to do with this awareness?
- Do you find yourself focusing on past choices or actions that you regret? How does this focus influence your sense of well-being? What do you wish to do with this awareness?
- What does "reconciliation" mean to you? What would "reconciliation" look and feel like to you? What might be the benefits of reconciliation?
- Do your current spiritual/religious/cultural traditions play a role in finding reconciliation? What do their teachings say about "reconciliation," "forgiveness," "non-attachment," or "rebalancing"? Do they assist/interfere? How so?
- Have you found anything positive arising from your painful experiences? (e.g., development of inner strengths you didn't know you had; closer relationships; deeper trust; lessons learned; deeper appreciation for the good times; a sense of purpose or meaning, more creative coping?) If so, how does/can this enhance your daily life amidst the difficulties you face? If not, does it feel okay, for now, to grieve the losses associated with your difficulties?
- What/who can sustain you until you feel more hopeful/peaceful? Do you see yourself being able to feel more hopeful/peaceful?

### Understandings

- **Are there particular personal beliefs or practices sustaining you/offering you comfort at this time? How can we help you draw upon these for strength?**

- Are you aware of any beliefs or questions that are distressing/compromising your well-being? If so, how do you wish to address these? Do you see it as possible to eventually transform them into ones that promote wellness?
- Are there particular spiritual, religious, or cultural influences that influence or inform your understandings? How do you feel about these influences?
- What do you believe about the nature of suffering? How do you think these beliefs are influencing your current healing process?
- What gives your life meaning? Is there any meaning that you make in relation to your current difficulties? If so, what? How does this influence the way you navigate your circumstances?
- Has this experience prompted you to ponder your overall life's purpose(s)? If so, what is your sense about it/them? How does this influence your well-being/your approach to life/your healing process?

### Searching

- **Are there spiritually oriented questions about your current difficulties that you would like an opportunity to explore?**
- How have your current difficulties influenced your beliefs? Are there any of your previously held beliefs that you are currently questioning? How do you feel about questioning these beliefs? Does this type of questioning feel safe/unsafe? What/who contributes to this sense of safety/risk?
- What answers about life/death/spirituality are you currently seeking? How difficult is this searching?
- What/who is a source of disillusionment for you? Have you had an opportunity to grieve associated losses? If not, how might you do so?
- Has the imposition of others' beliefs added to your distress? If so, how? How can you gain protection from these intrusions?

### Teachers

- **Are there people/groups/resources you find helpful in exploring spiritual questions? How can they be involved in your healing process?**
- Who do you consider to be your spiritual teachers/mentors/leaders/companions?
- What readings and activities do you find personally inspiring or comforting? How might they contribute to your healing? How can you draw these resources into your regular routine?
- What new mentors, readings, activities, and events would you like to access?
- What resources within yourself can you name and draw upon? What new internal resources would you like to develop?

*Note:* Bolded questions have been identified as suitable for initial assessment/trust-building.

**Source:** Scott Barss, K. (2012). T.R.U.S.T.: An affirming model for inclusive spiritual care. *Journal of Holistic Nursing, 30*(1), 24–34. doi:10.1177/0898010111418118. Copyright © 2011 by SAGE. Reprinted by Permission of SAGE Publications.

and the potential interactions with foods, drugs, and other supplements to reduce risks and maximize benefits.

Nutritional therapies are used to treat a variety of mental health disorders, including depression, anxiety, ADHD, menopausal symptoms, dementia, and addictions (National Center for Complementary and Alternative Medicine, 2011e). The efficacy of omega-3 fatty acids continues to be studied in the treatment of mood, impulse control, and psychotic disorders (Chiu, Liu, & Su, 2008; National Center for Complementary and Alternative Medicine, 2011e). B vitamins, especially vitamin $B_6$ and folic acid, appear to improve anxiety and depression (Schneider & Lovett, 2007). According to Lake (2009), these vitamins often augment conventional care with antipsychotic, antidepressant, and mood-stabilizing medications. The literature supports combining such approaches with exercise and meditative practices (Chiu, Liu, & Su, 2008; Lake, 2009; National Center for Complementary and Alternative Medicine, 2011e; Schneider & Lovett, 2007).

Megavitamin therapy, also called *orthomolecular therapy*, is a specific approach to nutritional therapy used in integrative mental health care that involves taking large amounts of vitamins, minerals, and amino acids. The theory is that the inability to absorb nutrients from a proper diet alone may lead to the development of different illnesses (Ford, Flicker, Thomas, et al., 2008). The earliest use of megavitamin therapy was for the treatment of schizophrenia, for which a high dosage of niacin was recommended. Canadian psychiatrist Dr. Abram Hoffer pioneered this controversial approach in 1952 and continued to study and promote it throughout his career (Hoffer, 1999; Hoffer & Prousky, 2008).

## Herbal Therapy

As with dietary and nutritional supplements, health care providers need to be aware of their patients' use of herbal therapies and any potential adverse effects, interactions, and benefits. Related information can be obtained through NCCAM & Natural Standard Web sites and publications. Increasingly, pharmacists are able to provide additional information and resources. Each herbal preparation needs to be researched in the same manner as a medication in order to provide safe care. To facilitate this process, it is helpful for nurses to be aware of herbal therapies most frequently used in relation to mental health challenges.

St. John's wort has been used for centuries to improve mood and alleviate pain. It has been extensively researched and generally found to be as effective as antidepressants in the treatment of mild to moderate depression (National Center for Complementary and Alternative Medicine, 2011b). Results are inconclusive in relation to severe depression, prompting ongoing research (National Center for Complementary and Alternative Medicine, 2011b). St. John's wort should not be taken in tandem with antidepressant pharmaceuticals due to its serotonergic effects. Caution is also warranted with bipolar disorder as cases of mania have been reported with its use (Ulbricht, 2011).

Ginkgo biloba has been used and studied in relation to prevention and treatment of cognitive decline, depression, and memory loss associated with electroconvulsive therapy. Overall, results are inconclusive, and studies are ongoing (National

Center for Complementary and Alternative Medicine, 2011b; Ulbricht, 2011).

Kava kava is an herb from the South Pacific taken for anxiety. Kava was considered both safe and effective until 2002, when at least 25 cases of liver toxicity—including hepatitis, cirrhosis, and liver failure—were linked to its use. In the United States, the Food and Drug Administration (FDA) issued a consumer advisory based on this potential risk, and NCCAM discontinued its research (National Center for Complementary and Alternative Medicine, 2011b). According to Lake (2009), the cases of liver failure were associated with a processing error in the production of a single batch of kava. In response to the above controversial information, much confusion has arisen as to its legal status in Canada. However, kava kava is currently not legal for sale through Canadian businesses.

Valerian is used as an antianxiety agent and has also been reported to have antidepressant and sedative properties (National Center for Complementary and Alternative Medicine, 2011b). Results about its efficacy are mixed, but it is generally recognized as safe for the short-term treatment of insomnia when taken at the recommended dosages and not taken in combination with other sedative medications (National Center for Complementary and Alternative Medicine, 2011b).

Herbal teas have long been used for their sedative–hypnotic effects. Common ingredients in these teas (in addition to valerian) are hops, lemon balm, chamomile, and passionflower. The most studied of these is chamomile, a tea widely used as a folk remedy. Chamomile extract has been found to bind with gamma-aminobutyric acid (GABA) receptors. These teas, along with improving sleep hygiene, may be part of a set of interventions for insomnia; they are generally safely recommended but should be used with awareness of their individual potential effects, adverse effects, and interactions (National Center for Complementary and Alternative Medicine, 2011b; Ulbricht, 2011).

## Aromatherapy

Aromatherapy, the use of essential oils for enhancing physical and mental well-being and healing, is a popular therapy. Essential oils, often derived from herbs and plants, may be applied directly to the skin by carrier oil or diffused into the atmosphere through a diffuser. Essential oils are believed to stimulate the release of neurotransmitters in the brain. The sense of smell connects with the part of the brain that controls the autonomic (involuntary) nervous system. Depending on the essential oil used, the resulting effects are calming, pain reducing, stimulating, sedating, or euphoria producing (Smith & Kyle, 2008).

Smith and Kyle (2008, p. 7) provide a convenient chart on how various classifications of oils affect people:
- Rooty oils such as patchouli and valerian affect calming, grounding, and stabilizing.
- Floral oils such as ylang-ylang and jasmine create mood uplifting, relaxation, and sensuality.
- Green herbaceous oils such as lavender and chamomile create balance, regulation, and clarification.

Aromatherapy has been used to treat anxiety and mood disorders. Several recent research studies featured by NCCAM report positive results in this regard (National Center for Complementary and Alternative Medicine, 2011e). Some individuals, particularly those with pulmonary disease, may be sensitive or allergic to essential oils when they come into contact with the skin or are inhaled. To prevent an allergic reaction, always dilute oils, administer a small amount, and perform a 24-hour skin patch test before massaging any essential oil into the skin. Ongoing consultation with a trained aromatherapist is essential, keeping in mind that the training and practice of aromatherapists currently remains unregulated (Canadian Federation of Aromatherapists, 2011).

## Manipulative Practices

Manipulative practices are based on physically touching another person. (Therapeutic touch is included among the energy therapies since it technically does not involve physical touching of a patient.) The use of any physical touch in psychiatric mental health nursing practice continues to be controversial. Some believe it is not used enough, but most believe it should be used sparingly, with clear intent, recognizing that maintenance of therapeutic boundaries is extremely important, particularly with patients who have psychiatric disorders and might misinterpret touch (Jackson & Latini, 2013; Weze, Leathard, Grange, et al., 2007).

## Chiropractic Medicine

Chiropractic medicine is one of the most widely used integrative therapies. The term *chiropractic* comes from the Greek words *praxix* and *cheir*, meaning "practice" or "treatment by hand." Chiropractic medicine focuses on the relationship between the body's structure (mainly the spine) and function and the way that relationship affects the preservation and restoration of health, using manipulative therapy as a treatment tool. Many chiropractors treat patients with depression, anxiety, and chronic pain (National Center for Complementary and Alternative Medicine, 2011i). Limited formal research is evident in this regard.

## Massage Therapy

Massage therapy includes a broad group of practices and techniques that press, rub, and manipulate muscles and soft tissues of the body. There are over 80 different types of massage therapy (Esmail, 2007). It is intended to promote relaxation and circulation in order to promote healing. Massage has been used in the mental health context to enhance mood and reduce anxiety associated with a variety of diagnoses; as such, it is considered an appropriate adjuvant therapy for those who are so inclined (Schneider & Lovett, 2007). Shiatsu massage, which stimulates similar points to those in acupuncture, may be a favourable alternative to acupuncture for patients with an aversion to the use of needles. Shiatsu has shown promise in reducing both psychopathology and pharmaceutical adverse effects in schizophrenia when used as an adjuvant therapy (Lichtenberg, Vass, Ptaya, et al., 2009).

## Reflexology

Reflexology is a type of manipulative practice that focuses on the feet, hands, or ears. This approach is based on the understanding that zones and points on these areas of the body (most commonly the feet) correspond to other parts of the body. The purpose of treatments is to improve circulation in the feet to promote optimal function elsewhere in the body (Jackson & Latini, 2013; Koopsen & Young, 2009). Research on this intervention is sparse at present. Morris (2006) completed a pilot study with peri- and postmenopausal women using hand, ear, and foot reflexology. Results indicated that women were more relaxed and had more sleep after a 50-minute reflexology session once a week.

## Energy Therapies

Energy therapies are based on the belief that nonphysical bioenergy forces pervade the universe and people. Explanations vary as to the nature of this energy, the form of the therapies, and the rationale for how healing is believed to occur, depending on the affiliated world view. The energy is referred to as *qi* in TCM, *prana* in Indian Ayurvedic medicine, *ki* in Japanese medicine, and a variety of other names in other cultures, including *biofield energy* in contemporary Western cultures (Esmail, 2007; Slater, 2013). This energy takes a particular form in each person, called the *human energy field* or *aura*. This energy field is said to contain a number of layers, each with energy of different frequencies. Energy is transferred between layers and eventually into the physical body through *chakras*. Disturbances of the energy field are seen as the cause of illness, and healing is understood to occur when the human energy field is balanced and energy is flowing freely (Anderson & Taylor, 2011; Esmail, 2007; Koopsen & Young, 2009; Slater, 2013).

Practitioners of energy medicine believe that they are able to increase their awareness of the human energy field and enhance healing through meditation and centring (or other practice to access a sense of inner calm) (Zahourek, 2005). Practitioners believe they can then detect problems in others' energy fields and adjust the quality or create balance. This detection is accomplished by placing one's hands in or through these fields to direct the energy through visualized or actual pressure or manipulation (or both) of the body. Energy-based modalities currently have uncertain biomedical research support (Anderson & Taylor, 2011; National Center for Complementary and Alternative Medicine, 2011e). Engebretson and Wardell (2007) explain that such research on energy therapies presents particular challenges. First, determining a method to measure the success of energy therapies is difficult since their success is based on restoring balance and total healing, which are not easily quantified. Further, establishing the appropriate time for an intervention to take effect and the dosage of an energy therapy are currently impossible. Finally, establishing control groups and dealing with personality variables with individual healers and patients confound results. Still, several recent qualitative studies report positive results of the biofield therapies in terms of patients' self-reported sense of well-being, specifically in relation to reduced anxiety, depression, and pain. In addition, no adverse effects have been documented, warranting ongoing investigation and use as relevant to patients' world views and preferences (Anderson & Taylor, 2011; Jackson & Latini, 2013; Slater, 2013).

Therapeutic touch, healing touch, and Reiki are the most common energy therapies practised by nurses, and in many provinces and territories, the integration of such therapies into nursing practice is regulated by standards of nursing practice, alongside institutional guidelines, and always with patient consent. The CHNA, the AHNA, and Healing Touch International offer certificate courses in therapeutic touch and healing touch (College & Association of Registered Nurses of Alberta, 2011; College of Nurses of Ontario, 2009; Jackson & Latini, 2013; Slater, 2013). These modalities are sometimes blended with thought field therapy (TFT) and emotional freedom technique (EFT), which are discussed below.

### Therapeutic Touch

Therapeutic touch was developed in the 1970s by Dolores Krieger, a nursing professor at New York University, and Dora Kunz, a Canadian healer. The premise for therapeutic touch is that healing is promoted by balancing the body's energies. In preparation for a treatment session, practitioners focus completely on the person receiving the treatment, without any other distraction. Practitioners then assess the energy field, clear and balance it through hand movements, and direct energy in a specific region of the body. The therapist does not physically touch the patient. After undergoing a session of therapeutic touch, patients report a sense of deep relaxation (Jackson & Latini, 2013).

### Healing Touch

Healing touch is a derivative of therapeutic touch developed by a registered nurse, Janet Mentgen (Anderson & Taylor, 2011). Healing touch combines several energy therapies and is based on the belief that the body is a complex energy system that can be influenced by another through that person's intention for healing and well-being. Healing touch is related to therapeutic touch in the belief that working energetically with people to achieve their highest level of well-being, and not necessarily relieving a specific symptom, is the goal. Healing touch involves gentle "laying of the hands" on a clothed body or moving over the body in the energy field. The practitioner may focus on a specific problem area or the full body (Jackson & Latini, 2013).

### Reiki

The Japanese spiritual practice of Reiki has become an increasingly popular modality for nurses to learn and practise. Reiki is an energy-based therapy in which the practitioner's energy is connected to a universal source (chi, qi, prana, and ki) and is transferred to a recipient for physical or spiritual healing (National Center for Complementary and Alternative Medicine, 2011h). Numerous hospitals, hospices, cancer support groups, and clinics are now offering Reiki in complementary programs. Research has been conducted on such topics as reducing anxiety, depression, and pain and on promoting self-care for caregivers (Brathovde, 2006; vanderVaart, Gijsen, de Wildt, et al., 2009; Vitale, 2007). It has thus been used as an adjunct in psychotherapy (Jackson & Latini, 2013; LaTorre, 2005).

### Thought Field Therapy and Emotional Freedom Technique

Thought field therapy (TFT) was first developed by Roger Callahan in the 1980s and then modified in the 1990s by Gary Craig, who called his version the *emotional freedom technique* (EFT). The basis for these interventions is the idea that negative emotions are the result of energy imbalances and blocks in the body. The goal is to release these blocks and view the problem with less distress by tapping specific acupuncture points and meridians and repeating a positive mantra (Borgatti, 2008).

### Bioelectromagnetic-Based Therapies

In contrast, bioelectromagnetic-based therapies involve the unconventional use of electromagnetic fields, such as pulsed fields, magnetic fields, or alternating-current or direct-current fields. Transcranial magnetic stimulation (TMS) and vagus nerve stimulation (VNS) treatments for depression are in this category (Carlat, 2008). Pulsating magnetic fields are sent through a metal coil attached to the person's scalp using these techniques (see Chapter 14, Figure 14-4). High-frequency pulses stimulate, and low-frequency pulses dampen, neural impulses. TMS has been used to treat depression and to decrease auditory hallucination in schizophrenia (see Chapter 14). Vagus nerve stimulation was originally developed for epilepsy and showed some promise in treating medication-resistant depression. Its effectiveness is still being evaluated (see Chapter 14). Similarly, transcutaneous electric acupoint stimulation is being evaluated as an adjunctive treatment for opioid detoxification (Meade, Lukas, McDonald, et al., 2010).

*Note:* The NCCAM Web site (http://nccam.nih.gov) provides detailed information, reviews, and updates about the above and other traditional, complementary, and alternative modalities.

## ▊ KEY POINTS TO REMEMBER

- A philosophy of holism and the promotion of a therapeutic relationship are at the heart of psychiatric mental health nursing and are important no matter what healing modality is used.
- Traditional, complementary, alternative, and integrative approaches are in demand as patients seek a broader range of therapies than those offered by biomedical approaches.
- With the availability of online information, patients are more likely to have researched their symptoms or condition and identified potential TCAM treatments.

- Nurses are in an ideal position to guide patients to reliable resources, such as NCCAM, that provide up-to-date information for health care providers and patients.
- Nurses need to keep abreast of current research about major TCAM therapies so that they can (1) identify those that could be beneficial, affordable, and safe; (2) help patients avoid incurring unnecessary costs on ineffective therapies; (3) guide patients in discerning which therapies could be harmful; and (4) assist patients to maximize the benefits of TCAM therapies.

# CRITICAL THINKING

1. As a nurse, you may have patients who use integrative therapies in conjunction with the conventional therapies prescribed by the health care provider. Identify issues that are important to assess, and discuss how you would ask about the use of these nonconventional practices.

2. By visiting the Web sites listed in Box 37-1, determine how these informational resources can be used in your nursing practice.

3. By reviewing the chapter's list of references, identify the recent studies that have implications for your current nursing practice.

4. Choose and research a healing modality that you would like to use for self-care. Reflect upon your experience of accessing evidence-informed studies and how they improve your nursing practice.

5. Since mindfulness-based approaches demonstrate good effects for patients with anxiety and depression, consider what the nurse can do to support the patient's efforts in using these strategies.

# CHAPTER REVIEW

1. A patient has questioned the nurse about the safety of a herbal supplement. Which nursing response is most appropriate?
   1. "Herbal supplements are regulated by the provinces and territories."
   2. "Since they are natural products, herbal supplements are harmless."
   3. "I know of a couple of Web sites and a pharmacist that can help us address your question."
   4. "If your supplement was available over the counter, it should be safe."

2. Which of the following is true of integrative health care?
   1. It is synonymous with complementary and alternative healing.
   2. It is being widely offered in the Canadian health care system.
   3. It requires nurses to focus solely on the patient.
   4. It encourages nurses to adopt an overall holistic lifestyle.

3. A patient with schizophrenia has asked the nurse about replacing prescribed antipsychotic medications with meditation and shiatsu massage. Which nursing response is most appropriate?

   1. "Both modalities may have benefits as adjuncts to your antipsychotic medication, but likely not as replacements. How can I help you find out more?"
   2. "You shouldn't even consider it. They're not safe."
   3. "I'm concerned that your illness is affecting your judgement. I think we should talk with your doctor about a medication adjustment."
   4. "I've read that they're very promising. It's worth a try."

4. In facilitating spiritual care in a mental health setting, it is important for nurses to do which of the following:
   1. Avoid facilitating spiritual care with patients who are psychotic
   2. Explicitly share personal beliefs so patients know where they stand
   3. Address spiritual needs without reinforcing any delusional thinking present
   4. Rely on referral to clergy since their expertise is needed to approach the topic

5. Contemplative practices are an important aspect of integrative mental health care because of which of the following:
   1. They have the potential to positively enhance brain structure and function.
   2. They promote a sense of calm and trust.
   3. They reduce symptoms of anxiety and depression.
   4. All of the above are important aspects of integrative mental health care.

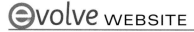 WEBSITE

Post-Test interactive review

*Visit the Evolve Web site for Chapter Review Answers and Rationales, Critical Thinking Answer Guidelines, and additional resources related to the content in this chapter:* http://evolve.elsevier.com/Canada/Varcarolis/psychiatric/

# REFERENCES

Acupuncture Foundation of Canada Institute. (2011). *Regulation in Canada.* Retrieved from http://www.afcinstitute.com/AboutAcupuncture/RegulationinCanada/tabid/78/Default.aspx.

Anderson, J., & Taylor, A. (2011). Effects of healing touch in clinical practice: A systematic review of randomized clinical trials. *Journal of Holistic Nursing, 29*(3), 221–228. doi:0898010110393353.

Anselmo, J. (2013). Relaxation. In B. Dossey & L. Keegan (Eds.), *Holistic nursing: A handbook for practice* (6th ed., pp. 327–361). Sudbury, MA: Jones and Bartlett.

Baetz, M., & Toews, J. (2009). Clinical implications of research on religion, spirituality and mental health. *Canadian Journal of Psychiatry, 54*(5), 292–301.

Balbuena, L., Baetz, M., & Bowen, R. (2013). Religious attendance, spirituality, and major depression in Canada: A 14-year follow-up study. *Canadian Journal of Psychiatry, 58*(4), 225–232.

Barrere, C. (2013). Teaching future holistic nurses: Integrating holism into an undergraduate nursing curriculum. In B. Dossey & L. Keegan (Eds.), *Holistic nursing: A handbook for practice* (6th ed., pp. 815–824). Sudbury, MA: Jones and Bartlett.

Bibby, R. (2011). *Beyond the gods and back: Religion's demise and rise and why it matters.* Lethbridge, AB: Project Canada Books.

Binda, J. (2011). *The renaissance of native spirituality: The journey of the spiritual seeker and traditional healing practices.* Bloomington, IN: iUniverse Books.

Bodeker, G., Kronenberg, F., & Burford, B. (2007). Policy and public health perspectives on traditional, complementary and alternative medicine: An overview. In G. Bodeker & G. Burford (Eds.), *Traditional, complementary, and alternative medicine: Policy and public health perspectives.* London, UK: Imperial College Press.

Bodeker, G., Ong, C., Grundy, C., et al. (2005). *WHO global atlas of traditional, complementary, and alternative medicine: Text volume.* Kobe, Japan: World Health Organization.

Boon, H., Verhoef, M., O'Hara, D., et al. (2004). Integrative healthcare: Arriving at a working definition. *Alternative Therapies in Health and Medicine, 10*(5), 48–56.

Borgatti, J.C. (2008). Tap your way to fast relief. *American Nurse Today, 3*(1), 32–33.

Brathovde, A. (2006). A pilot study of Reiki for self-care of nurses and healthcare providers. *Holistic Nursing Practice, 20*(2), 95–100.

Canadian Association of Naturopathic Doctors. (2011). *Education & regulation.* Retrieved from http://www.cand.ca/index.php?40 http://www.cand.ca/index.php?40.

Canadian Chiropractic Association. (2011). *Chiropractic and you.* Retrieved from http://www.chiropracticcanada.ca/en-us/about-chiropractic/chiropractic-and-you.aspx.

Canadian Federation of Aromatherapists. (2011). *About us.* http://cfacanada.com/about/.

Canadian Foundation for Trauma Research & Education. (2010). *Self regulation therapy.* Retrieved from http://www.cftre.com/courses-seminars/what-is-self-regulation-therapy/.

Canadian Holistic Nurses Association. (2011). *Specialization program in holistic nursing.* Retrieved from http://www.chna.ca/Specialization.

Cao, H., Pan, X., Li, H., et al. (2009). Acupuncture for treatment of insomnia: A systematic review of randomized controlled trials. *Journal of Alternative and Complementary Medicine, 15*, 1171–1186. doi:10.1089/acm.2009.0041.

Carlat, D.J. (2008). Transcranial magnetic stimulation: The saga continues. *The Carlat Report, 6*(1), 1, 3. Retrieved from http://www.thecarlatreport.com/sites/default/files/TCPR%20Jan%2008%20Brain%20Devices.pdf.

Caspi, O. (2007). Activating the healing response. In D. Rakel (Ed.), *Integrative medicine* (2nd ed., pp. 1073–1080). Toronto: Saunders.

Chen, K.W., Berger, C.C., Manheimer, E., et al. (2012). Meditative therapies for reducing anxiety: A systematic review and meta-analysis of randomized controlled trials. *Depression and Anxiety, 29*(7), 545–562. doi:10.1002/da.21964.

Cheng, J., Wang, G., Xiao, L., et al. (2009). Electro-acupuncture versus sham acupuncture for auditory hallucinations in patients with schizophrenia:

A randomized controlled trial. *Clinical Rehabilitation, 23*, 579–588. doi:10.1177/0269215508096172.

Chiu, C.C., Liu, J.P., & Su, K.P. (2008). The use of omega-3 fatty acids in the treatment of depression: The lights and shadows. *Psychiatric Times, 25*(9), 76–80.

Clarke, P., Watson, J., & Brewer, B.B. (2009). From theory to practice: Caring science according to Watson and Brewer. *Nursing Science Quarterly, 22*, 339–345. doi:10.1177/0894318409344769.

College & Association of Registered Nurses of Alberta. (2011). *Complementary and/or alternative therapy and natural health products: Standards for registered nurses.* Retrieved from http://www.nurses.ab.ca/Carna-Admin/Uploads/Complementary_Alternative_Therapy.pdf.

College of Nurses of Ontario. (2009). *Practice guideline: Complementary therapies.* Retrieved from http://www.cno.org/Global/docs/prac/41021_CompTherapies.pdf.

Doidge, N. (2007). *The brain that changes itself: Stories of personal triumph from the frontiers of brain science.* New York: Viking.

Engebretson, J., & Wardell, D.W. (2007). Energy-based modalities. *Nursing Clinics of North America, 42*, 243–259. doi:10.1016/j.cnur.2007.02.004.

Esmail, N. (2007). Complementary and alternative medicine in Canada: Trends in use and public attitudes, 1997–2006. *Fraser Institute Public Policy Sources, 87*, 19–22.

Ford, A.H., Flicker, L., Thomas, J., et al. (2008). Vitamins $B_{12}$, $B_6$, and folic acid for onset of depressive symptoms in older men: Results from a 2-year placebo-controlled trial. *Journal of Clinical Psychiatry, 69*(8), 1203–1209.

Fortney, L., & Bonus, K. (2012). Recommending meditation. In D. Rakel (Ed.), *Integrative Medicine* (3rd ed., pp. 873–881). Toronto: Saunders.

Gurgevich, S. (2012). Self-hypnosis techniques. In D. Rakel (Ed.), *Integrative Medicine* (3rd ed., pp. 836–842). Toronto: Saunders.

Health Canada. (2012a). *Drugs and health products: About natural health products: How can I use natural health products safely?* Retrieved from http://www.hc-sc.gc.ca/dhp-mps/prodnatur/about-apropos/cons-eng.php.

Health Canada. (2012b). *Drugs and health products: Natural health products.* Retrieved from http://www.hc-sc.gc.ca/dhp-mps/prodnatur/index-eng.php.

Health Canada. (2012c). *Natural health product tracking survey—2010 final report.* Retrieved from http://epe.lac-bac.gc.ca/100/200/301/pwgsc-tpsgc/por-ef/health/2011/135-09/report.pdf.

Health Canada. (2012d). *The regulation of natural health products (NHPs) in Canada: Myths and facts.* Retrieved from http://www.hc-sc.gc.ca/dhp-mps/prodnatur/about-apropos/nhp-myth-psn-eng.php.

Hoffer, A. (1999). *Orthomolecular treatment for schizophrenia: Megavitamin supplements and nutritional strategies for healing and recovery.* Lincolnwood, IL: Keats.

Hoffer, A., & Prousky, J. (2008). Successful treatment of schizophrenia requires optimal daily doses of vitamin B3. *Alternative Medicine Review, 13*(4), 287–291.

Hofmann, S., Sawyer, A., Witt, A., et al. (2010). The effect of mindfulness-based therapy on anxiety and depression: A meta-analytic review. *Journal of Consulting and Clinical Psychology, 78*(2), 169–183. doi:10.1037/a0018555.

Hood, L.E., Olson, J., & Allen, M. (2007). Learning to care for spiritual needs: Connecting spiritually. *Qualitative Health Research, 17*, 1198–1206. doi:10.1177/1049732307306921.

Jackson, C., & Keegan, L. (2013). Touch. In B.M. Dossey & L. Keegan (Eds.), *Holistic nursing: A handbook for practice* (6th ed., pp. 347–366). Sudbury, MA: Jones & Bartlett.

Jackson, C., & Latini, C. (2013). Touch and hand-mediated therapies. In B.M. Dossey & L. Keegan (Eds.), *Holistic nursing: A handbook for practice* (6th ed., pp. 417–437). Sudbury, MA: Jones & Bartlett.

Kalish, N. (2012). Evidence-based spiritual care: A literature review. *Current Opinions & Support in Palliative Care, 6*(2), 242–246.

Khorsan, R., Coulter, I.D., Crawford, C., et al. (2011). Systematic review of integrative health care research: Randomized control trials, clinical controlled trials, and meta-analysis. *Evidence-Based Complementary and Alternative Medicine, 1*–10. doi:10.1155/2011/636134.

Kitko, J. (2007). Rhythmic breathing as a nursing intervention. *Holistic Nursing Practice*, 21, 85–88. doi:10.1097/01.HNP.0000262023.27572.65.

Koenig, H. (2009). Research on religion, spirituality, and mental health: A review. *Canadian Journal of Psychiatry*, 54(5), 283–291.

Koenig, H. (2011). *Spirituality & health research*. West Conshohocken, PA: Templeton.

Koopsen, C., & Young, C. (2009). *Integrative health: A holistic approach for health professionals*. Toronto: Jones & Bartlett.

Lake, J. (2007). Integrative mental health care: From theory to practice, Part 1. *Alternative Therapies in Health & Medicine*, 13(6), 50–56.

Lake, J. (2008). Integrative mental health care: From theory to practice, Part 2. *Alternative Therapies in Health & Medicine*, 14(1), 36–42.

Lake, J. (2009). *Integrative mental health care: A therapist's handbook*. New York: W.W. Norton.

LaTorre, M.A. (2005). The use of Reiki in psychotherapy. *Perspectives in Psychiatric Care*, 41(4), 184–187.

Lee, M., Shin, B., Ronan, P., et al. (2009). Acupuncture for schizophrenia: A systematic review and meta-analysis. *International Journal of Clinical Practice*, 63, 1622–1633. doi:10.1111/j.1742-1241.2009.02167.x.

Levine, P. (2010). *An unspoken voice: How the body releases trauma and restores goodness*. Berkeley, CA: North Atlantic Books.

Lichtenberg, P., Vass, A., Ptaya, H., et al. (2009). Shiatsu as an adjuvant therapy for schizophrenia: An open-label pilot study. *Alternative Therapies in Health and Medicine*, 15(5), 44–46.

Lloyd, L., & Dunn, L. (2007). Mind–body–spirit medicine: Interventions and resources. *JAAPA: Official Journal of the American Academy of Physician Assistants*, 20(10), 31–35.

Mariano, C. (2013). Holistic nursing: Scope and standards of practice. In B. Dossey & L. Keegan (Eds.), *Holistic nursing: A handbook for practice* (6th ed., pp. 59–84). Sudbury, MA: Jones & Bartlett.

Massage.ca. (2011). *Professional development*. Retrieved from http://massage.ca/professional_development.html.

McAdam, S. (2009). *Cultural teachings: First Nations protocols and methodologies*. Saskatoon, SK: Saskatchewan Indian Cultural Centre.

Meade, C., Lukas, S., McDonald, L., et al. (2010). A randomized trial of transcutaneous electric acupoint stimulation as adjunctive treatment for opioid detoxification. *Journal of Substance Abuse Treatment*, 38, 12–21. doi:10.1016/j.jsat.2009.05.010.

Mehl-Madrona, L. (2008). What traditional indigenous elders say about cross-cultural mental health training. *Explore*, 5, 20–29. doi:10.1016/j.explore.2008.10.003.

Mehl-Madrona, L. (2010). *Healing the mind through the power of story: The promise of narrative psychiatry*. Rochester, VT: Bear & Co.

Morris, D. (2006). Pilot study using reflexology. *Beginnings*, 26(5), 28–29.

National Center for Complementary and Alternative Medicine. (2011a). *Ayurvedic medicine: An introduction*. Retrieved from http://nccam.nih.gov/health/ayurveda/introduction.htm.

National Center for Complementary and Alternative Medicine. (2011b). *Herbs at a glance*. Retrieved from http://nccam.nih.gov/health/herbsataglance.htm.

National Center for Complementary and Alternative Medicine. (2011c). *Highlighted research results—acupuncture*. Retrieved from http://nccam.nih.gov/health/357/research.

National Center for Complementary and Alternative Medicine. (2011d). *Homeopathy: An introduction*. Retrieved from http://nccam.nih.gov/health/homeopathy/.

National Center for Complementary and Alternative Medicine. (2011e). *Mental health*. Retrieved from http://nccam.nih.gov/health/mentalhealth.htm.

National Center for Complementary and Alternative Medicine. (2011f). *Naturopathy*. Retrieved from http://nccam.nih.gov/health/naturopathy/.

National Center for Complementary and Alternative Medicine. (2011g). *NCCAM facts-at-a-glance and mission*. Retrieved from http://nccam.nih.gov/about/ataglance/.

National Center for Complementary and Alternative Medicine. (2011h). *Reiki information*. Retrieved from http://nccam.nih.gov/health/reiki/.

National Center for Complementary and Alternative Medicine. (2011i). *Spinal manipulation*. Retrieved from http://nccam.nih.gov/health/chiropractic/.

Native Mental Health Association of Canada. (2008). *Charting the future of native mental health in Canada: Ten-year strategic plan 2008–2018*. Chilliwack, BC: Author. Retrieved from http://www.nmhac.ca/documents/Final_NMHAC_STRATEGIC_PLAN_April_07[1].pdf.

Natural Standard: The Authority on Integrative Medicine. (2011). *Homeopathy*. Retrieved from http://naturalstandard.com/search.asp?text=homeopathy.

Olson, J., & Clark, M. (2010). Spirituality. In B.J. Kozier, G. Erb, A.J. Berman, et al. (Eds.), *Fundamentals of nursing* (2nd Can. ed., pp. 1471–1488), Toronto: Pearson Education Canada.

Pesut, B. (2010). Ontologies of nursing in an age of spiritual pluralism: Closed or open worldview? *Nursing Philosophy*, 11, 15–23. doi:10.1111/j.1466-769X.2009.00420.x.

Pike, J. (2011). Spirituality in nursing: A systematic review of the literature from 2006–2010. *British Journal of Nursing*, 20(12), 743–749.

Pinto, S., March, P., & Pravikoff, D. (2008). *Evidence-based care sheet: Spiritual needs of hospitalized patients*. Glendale, CA: Cinahl Information Systems.

Plante, T. (Ed.) (2010). *Contemplative practices in action: Spirituality, meditation and health*. Santa Barbara, CA: Praeger.

Rakel, D., & Jonas, W. (2012). Creating optimal healing environments. In D. Rakel (Ed.), *Integrative medicine* (3rd ed., pp. 12–19). Philadelphia: Saunders.

Rakel, D., & Weil, A. (2007). Philosophy of integrative medicine. In D. Rakel (Ed.), *Integrative medicine* (2nd ed., pp. 3–13). Philadelphia: Saunders.

Rakel, D., & Weil, A. (2012). Philosophy of integrative medicine. In D. Rakel (Ed.), *Integrative medicine* (3rd ed., pp. 2–22). Philadelphia: Saunders.

Ramsay, C. (2009). *Unnatural regulation: Complementary and alternative medicine policy in Canada*. Retrieved from http://www.fraserinstitute.org/research-news/display.aspx?id=13571.

Rathbone, J., & Xia, J. (2009). Acupuncture for schizophrenia: Review. *Cochrane Library*, 1–26. doi:10.1002/14651858.CD005475.

Registered Psychiatric Nurses Association of Saskatchewan. (2011). *Position statement: The role of the RPN in relation to complementary and alternative healing*. Retrieved from http://rpnascom.jumpstartdev.com/alternative%20healing.

Sarris, J.J., Moylan, S.S., Camfield, D.A., et al. (2012). Complementary medicine, exercise, meditation, diet, and lifestyle modification for anxiety disorders: A review of current evidence. *Evidence-Based Complementary and Alternative Medicine*, 1–20. doi:10.1155/2012/809653.

Schaub, B., & Burt, M. (2013a). Addiction and recovery counseling. In B.M. Dossey & L. Keegan (Eds.), *Holistic nursing: A handbook for practice* (6th ed., pp. 539–562). Sudbury, MA: Jones & Bartlett.

Schaub, B., & Burt, M. (2013b). Imagery. In B.M. Dossey & L. Keegan (Eds.), *Holistic nursing: A handbook for practice* (6th ed., pp. 363–396). Sudbury, MA: Jones & Bartlett.

Schneider, C., & Lovett, E. (2007). Depression. In D. Rakel (Ed.), *Integrative medicine* (2nd ed., pp. 73–83). Toronto: Saunders.

Scott Barss, K. (2012). T.R.U.S.T.: An affirming model for inclusive spiritual care. *Journal of Holistic Nursing*, 30(1), 24–34. doi:10.1177/0898010111418118.

Sedlmeier, P., Eberth, J., Schwartz, M., et al. (2012). The psychological effects of meditation: A meta-analysis. *Psychological Bulletin*, 138(6), 1139–1171. doi:10.1037/a0028168.

Slater, V. (2013). Energy healing. In B.M. Dossey & L. Keegan (Eds.), *Holistic nursing: A handbook for practice* (6th ed., pp. 752–774). Sudbury, MA: Jones & Bartlett.

Smith, M.C., & Kyle, L. (2008). Holistic foundations of aromatherapy for nursing. *Holistic Nursing Practice*, 22, 3–9. doi:10.1097/01.HNP.0000306322.03590.e9.

Srivastava, M., Talukdar, U., & Lahan, V. (2011). Meditation for the management of adjustment disorder anxiety and depression. *Complementary Therapies in Clinical Practice*, 17(4), 241–245.

Tarko, M. (2002). *A grounded theory study of the experience of spirituality among persons living with schizophrenia* (Doctoral dissertation). University of British Columbia, Vancouver, BC.

Ulbricht, C. (2011). *Davis's pocket guide to herbs and supplements.* Philadelphia: Natural Standard Research Collaboration/F.A. Davis.

vanderVaart, S., Gijsen, V., de Wildt, S., et al. (2009). A systematic review of the therapeutic effects of Reiki. *Journal of Alternative and Complementary Medicine, 15*(11), 1157–1169. doi:10.1089/acm.2009.0036.

Vitale, A. (2007). An integrative review of Reiki touch therapy research. *Holistic Nursing Practice, 21,* 167–179. doi:10.1097/01.HNP.0000280927 .83506.f6.

Welsh, S., Kelner, M., Wellman, B., et al. (2004). Moving forward? Complementary and alternative practitioners seeking self-regulation. *Sociology of Health & Illness, 26*(2), 216–241.

Weze, C., Leathard, H., Grange, J., et al. (2007). Healing by gentle touch ameliorates stress and other symptoms in people suffering with mental health disorders or psychological stress. *Evidence-Based Complementary and Alternative Medicine, 4,* 115–123. doi:10.1093/ecam/nel052.

Willison, K.D. (2008). Advancing integrative medicine through interprofessional education. *Health Sociology Review, 17*(4), 342–352. doi:10.5172/hesr.451.17.4.342.

World Health Organization. (2004). *Guidelines on developing consumer information on proper use of traditional, complementary and alternative medicine.* Geneva, Switzerland: Author. Retrieved from http://apps.who .int/medicinedocs/en/d/Js5525e/.

Wright, L., & Bell, J. (2010). *Beliefs and illness: A model for healing.* Calgary: 4th Floor Press.

Young, C., & Koopsen, C. (2011). *Spirituality, health, and healing: An integrative approach* (2nd ed.). Toronto: Jones & Bartlett.

Zahourek, R. (2002). *Imagery in holistic health and healing.* Philadelphia: F.A. Davis Co.

Zahourek, R. (2005). Intentionality: Evolutionary development in healing: A grounded theory study for holistic nursing. *Journal of Holistic Nursing, 23,* 89–109. doi:10.1177/0898010104272026.

Zhang, Z., Chen, H., Yip, K., et al. (2010). The effectiveness and safety of acupuncture therapy in depressive disorders: Systematic review and meta-analysis. *Journal of Affective Disorders, 124,* 9–21. doi:10.1016/ j.jad.2009.07.005.

# Psychiatric Mental Health Nursing Standards of Practice, Code of Ethics, Beliefs, and Values

## CANADIAN FEDERATION OF MENTAL HEALTH NURSES STANDARDS OF PRACTICE

Psychiatry/mental health is a specialized area of nursing practice, education, and research. The psychiatric mental health (PMH) nurse uses evidence-informed and experiential knowledge from nursing and related health sciences. This practice is grounded in the values as stated in the Canadian Nursing Association Code of Ethics (CNA, 2002a). Practice involves the promotion of mental health and the prevention, treatment, and management of mental disorders.

### Standard I:

Provides Competent Professional Care Through the Development of a Therapeutic Relationship

### Standard II:

Performs/Refines Client Assessments Through the Diagnostic and Monitoring Function

### Standard III:

Administers and Monitors Therapeutic Interventions

### Standard IV:

Effectively Manages Rapidly Changing Situations

### Standard V:

Intervenes Through the Teaching–Coaching Function

### Standard VI:

Monitors and Ensures the Quality of Health Care Practices

### Standard VII:

Practices Within Organizational and Work-Role Structure

### Beliefs/Values

Psychiatric and mental health nurses believe:
- The therapeutic nurse–client relationships, based on trust and mutual respect, are central to practice.
- In the alleviation of the stigma and discrimination.
- In the conduct and utilization of research for improvement in care.
- In social action to promote political and social awareness to influence health and organizational policy.
- In working in collaborative relationships with the individual, family, community, populations, and social agencies.
- In a holistic approach that is essential to understanding the unique experience of the client.
- In equitable access to culturally competent care.
- In reflective ethical practice and a commitment to continuous learning.
- In the protection of human rights in context to civil commitment and relevant aspects of jurisprudence.
- In advocating for practice environments that facilitate and ensure safe and positive work relationships.
- In fostering a legacy of moral and visionary psychiatric mental health nursing leaders.

**Source:** Canadian Federation of Mental Health Nurses. (2006). Canadian standards for psychiatric-mental health nursing (3rd ed.). Toronto: Author. Retrieved from http://cfmhn.ca/sites/cfmhn.ca/files/CFMHN%20standards%201.pdf.

# REGISTERED PSYCHIATRIC NURSES OF CANADA

## Standards of Psychiatric Nursing Practice

Psychiatric nursing, as a distinct profession, provides service to individuals whose care needs relate to mental, physical, and developmental health. Registered psychiatric nurses engage in various roles providing health services to individuals, families, groups, and communities. The practice of psychiatric nursing occurs within the domains of direct practice, education, administration, and research.

## Standard 1: Therapeutic Interpersonal Relationships

Registered psychiatric nurses establish professional, interpersonal, and therapeutic relationships with individuals, groups, families, and communities.

## Standard 2: Application and Integration of Theory-Based Knowledge

Registered psychiatric nurses apply and integrate theory-based knowledge relevant to professional practice derived from psychiatric nursing education and continued lifelong learning.

## Standard 3: Professional Responsibility

Registered psychiatric nurses are accountable to the public for safe, competent, and ethical psychiatric nursing practice.

## Standard 4: Professional Ethics

Registered psychiatric nurses understand, promote, and uphold the ethical values of the profession.

### The Code of Ethics

Through the *Code of Ethics*, registered psychiatric nurses uphold the values of:
- Safe, competent, and ethical practice to ensure the protection of the public;
- Respect for the inherent worth, right of choice, and dignity of persons;
- Health, mental health, and well-being; and,
- Quality practice.

**Source:** Registered Psychiatric Nurses of Canada. (2010). *Code of ethics & standards of psychiatric nursing practice*. Edmonton: Author. Retrieved from http://www.crpnbc.ca/wp-content/uploads/2011/02/2010_Code_Standards.pdf.

# NANDA-I Nursing Diagnoses 2012–2014

## Domain 1: Health Promotion

Class 1: Health Awareness
  Deficient Diversional Activity (00097)
  Sedentary Lifestyle (00168)
Class 2: Health Management 153
  Deficient Community Health (00215)
  Risk-Prone Health Behaviour (00188)
  Ineffective Health Maintenance (00099)
  Readiness for Enhanced Immunization Status (00186)
  Ineffective Protection (00043)
  Ineffective Self-Health Management (00078)
  Readiness for Enhanced Self-Health Management (00162)
  Ineffective Family Therapeutic Regimen Management (00080)

## Domain 2: Nutrition

Class 1: Ingestion
  Insufficient Breast Milk (00216)
  Ineffective Infant Feeding Pattern (00107)
  Imbalanced Nutrition: Less Than Body Requirements (00002)
  Imbalanced Nutrition: More Than Body Requirements (00001)
  Readiness for Enhanced Nutrition (00163)
  Risk for Imbalanced Nutrition: More Than Body Requirements (00003)
  Impaired Swallowing (00103)
Class 2: Digestion
Class 3: Absorption
Class 4: Metabolism
  Risk for Unstable Blood Glucose Level (00179)
  Neonatal Jaundice (00194)
  Risk for Neonatal Jaundice (00230)
  Risk for Impaired Liver Function (00178)
Class 5: Hydration
  Risk for Electrolyte Imbalance (00195)
  Readiness for Enhanced Fluid Balance (00160)
  Deficient Fluid Volume (00027)
  Excess Fluid Volume (00026)
  Risk for Deficient Fluid Volume (00028)
  Risk for Imbalanced Fluid Volume (00025)

## Domain 3: Elimination and Exchange

Class 1: Urinary Function
  Functional Urinary Incontinence (00020)
  Overflow Urinary Incontinence (00176)
  Reflex Urinary Incontinence (00018)
  Stress Urinary Incontinence (00017)
  Urge Urinary Incontinence (00019)
  Risk for Urge Urinary Incontinence (00022)
  Impaired Urinary Elimination (00016)
  Readiness for Enhanced Urinary Elimination (00166)
  Urinary Retention (00023)
Class 2: Gastrointestinal Function
  Constipation (00011)
  Perceived Constipation (00012)
  Risk for Constipation (00015)
  Diarrhea (00013)
  Dysfunctional Gastrointestinal Motility (00196)
  Risk for Dysfunctional Gastrointestinal Motility (00197)
  Bowel Incontinence (00014)
Class 3: Integumentary Function
Class 4: Respiratory Function
  Impaired Gas Exchange (00030)

## Domain 4: Activity/Rest

Class 1: Sleep/Rest
  Insomnia (00095)
  Sleep Deprivation (00096)
  Readiness for Enhanced Sleep (00165)
  Disturbed Sleep Pattern (00198)
Class 2: Activity/Exercise
  Risk for Disuse Syndrome (00040)
  Impaired Bed Mobility (00091)
  Impaired Physical Mobility (00085)
  Impaired Wheelchair Mobility (00089)
  Impaired Transfer Ability (00090)
  Impaired Walking (00088)

Class 3: Energy Balance
  Disturbed Energy Field (00050)
  Fatigue (00093)
  Wandering (00154)
Class 4: Cardiovascular/Pulmonary Responses
  Activity Intolerance (00092)
  Risk for Activity Intolerance (00094)
  Ineffective Breathing Pattern (00032)
  Decreased Cardiac Output (00029)
  Risk for Ineffective Gastrointestinal Perfusion (00202)
  Risk for Ineffective Renal Perfusion (00203)
  Impaired Spontaneous Ventilation (00033)
  Ineffective Peripheral Tissue Perfusion (00204)
  Risk for Decreased Cardiac Tissue Perfusion (00200)
  Risk for Ineffective Cerebral Tissue Perfusion (00201)
  Risk for Ineffective Peripheral Tissue Perfusion (00228)
  Dysfunctional Ventilatory Weaning Response (00034)
Class 5: Self-Care
  Impaired Home Maintenance (00098)
  Readiness for Enhanced Self-Care (00182)
  Bathing Self-Care Deficit (00108)
  Dressing Self-Care Deficit (00109)
  Feeding Self-Care Deficit (00102)
  Toileting Self-Care Deficit (00110)
  Self-Neglect (00193)

## Domain 5: Perception/Cognition

Class 1: Attention
  Unilateral Neglect (00123)
Class 2: Orientation
  Impaired Environmental Interpretation Syndrome (00127)
Class 3: Sensation/Perception
Class 4: Cognition
  Acute Confusion (00128)
  Chronic Confusion (00129)
  Risk for Acute Confusion (00173)
  Ineffective Impulse Control (00222)
  Deficient Knowledge (00126)
  Readiness for Enhanced Knowledge (00161)
  Impaired Memory (00131)
Class 5: Communication
  Readiness for Enhanced Communication (00157)
  Impaired Verbal Communication (00051)

## Domain 6: Self-Perception

Class 1: Self-Concept
  Hopelessness (00124)
  Risk for Compromised Human Dignity (00174)
  Risk for Loneliness (00054)
  Disturbed Personal Identity (00121)
  Risk for Disturbed Personal Identity (00225)
  Readiness for Enhanced Self-Concept (00167)
Class 2: Self-Esteem
  Chronic Low Self-Esteem (00119)
  Situational Low Self-Esteem (00120)
  Risk for Chronic Low Self-Esteem (00224)
  Risk for Situational Low Self-Esteem (00153)

Class 3: Body Image
  Disturbed Body Image (00118)

## Domain 7: Role Relationships

Class 1: Caregiving Roles
  Ineffective Breastfeeding (00104)
  Interrupted Breastfeeding (00105)
  Readiness for Enhanced Breastfeeding (00106)
  Caregiver Role Strain (00061)
  Risk for Caregiver Role Strain (00062)
  Impaired Parenting (00056)
  Readiness for Enhanced Parenting (00164)
  Risk for Impaired Parenting (00057)
Class 2: Family Relationships
  Risk for Impaired Attachment (00058)
  Dysfunctional Family Processes (00063)
  Interrupted Family Processes (00060)
  Readiness for Enhanced Family Processes (00159)
Class 3: Role Performance
  Ineffective Relationship (00223)
  Readiness for Enhanced Relationship (00207)
  Risk for Ineffective Relationship (00229)
  Parental Role Conflict (00064)
  Ineffective Role Performance (00055)
  Impaired Social Interaction (00052)

## Domain 8: Sexuality

Class 1: Sexual Identity
Class 2: Sexual Function
  Sexual Dysfunction (00059)
  Ineffective Sexuality Pattern (00065)
Class 3: Reproduction
  Ineffective Childbearing Process (00221)
  Readiness for Enhanced Childbearing Process (00208)
  Risk for Ineffective Childbearing Process (00227)
  Risk for Disturbed Maternal–Fetal Dyad (00209)

## Domain 9: Coping/Stress Tolerance

Class 1: Post-Trauma Responses
  Post-Trauma Syndrome (00141)
  Risk for Post-Trauma Syndrome (00145)
  Rape-Trauma Syndrome (00142)
  Relocation Stress Syndrome (00114)
  Risk for Relocation Stress Syndrome (00149)
Class 2: Coping Responses
  Ineffective Activity Planning (00199)
  Risk for Ineffective Activity Planning (00226)
  Anxiety (00146)
  Defensive Coping (00071)
  Ineffective Coping (00069)
  Readiness for Enhanced Coping (00158)
  Ineffective Community Coping (00077)
  Readiness for Enhanced Community Coping (00076)
  Compromised Family Coping (00074)
  Disabled Family Coping (00073)
  Readiness for Enhanced Family Coping (00075)
  Death Anxiety (00147)

Ineffective Denial (00072)
Adult Failure to Thrive (00101)
Fear (00148)
Grieving (00136)
Complicated Grieving (00135)
Risk for Complicated Grieving (00172)
Readiness for Enhanced Power (00187)
Powerlessness (00125)
Risk for Powerlessness (00152)
Impaired Individual Resilience (00210)
Readiness for Enhanced Resilience (00212)
Risk for Compromised Resilience (00211)
Chronic Sorrow (00137)
Stress Overload (00177)
Class 3: Neurobehavioural Stress
Autonomic Dysreflexia (00009)
Risk for Autonomic Dysreflexia (00010)
Disorganized Infant Behaviour (00116)
Readiness for Enhanced Organized Infant Behaviour (00117)
Risk for Disorganized Infant Behaviour (00115)
Decreased Intracranial Adaptive Capacity (00049)

## Domain 10: Life Principles
Class 1: Values
Readiness for Enhanced Hope (00185)
Class 2: Beliefs
Readiness for Enhanced Spiritual Well-Being (00068)
Class 3: Value/Belief/Action Congruence
Readiness for Enhanced Decision-Making (00184)
Decisional Conflict (00083)
Moral Distress (00175)
Noncompliance (00079)
Impaired Religiosity (00169)
Readiness for Enhanced Religiosity (00171)
Risk for Impaired Religiosity (00170)
Spiritual Distress (00066)
Risk for Spiritual Distress (00067)

## Domain 11: Safety/Protection
Class 1: Infection 417
Risk for Infection (00004)
Class 2: Physical Injury 421
Ineffective Airway Clearance (00031)
Risk for Aspiration (00039)
Risk for Bleeding (00206)
Impaired Dentition (00048)
Risk for Dry Eye (00219)
Risk for Falls (00155)
Risk for Injury (00035)
Impaired Oral Mucous Membrane (00045)

Risk for Perioperative Positioning Injury (00087)
Risk for Peripheral Neurovascular Dysfunction (00086)
Risk for Shock (00205)
Impaired Skin Integrity (00046)
Risk for Impaired Skin Integrity (00047)
Risk for Sudden Infant Death Syndrome (00156)
Risk for Suffocation (00036)
Delayed Surgical Recovery (00100)
Risk for Thermal Injury (00220)
Impaired Tissue Integrity (00044)
Risk for Trauma (00038)
Risk for Vascular Trauma (00213)
Class 3: Violence 447
Risk for Other-Directed Violence (00138)
Risk for Self-Directed Violence (00140)
Self-Mutilation (00151)
Risk for Self-Mutilation (00139)
Risk for Suicide (00150)
Class 4: Environmental Hazards 454
Contamination (00181)
Risk for Contamination (00180)
Risk for Poisoning (00037)
Class 5: Defensive Processes 461
Risk for Adverse Reaction to Iodinated Contrast Media (000218)
Latex Allergy Response (00041)
Risk for Allergy Response (00217)
Risk for Latex Allergy Response (00042)
Class 6: Thermoregulation 467
Risk for Imbalanced Body Temperature (00005)
Hyperthermia (00007)
Hypothermia (00006)
Ineffective Thermoregulation (00008)

## Domain 12: Comfort
Class 1: Physical Comfort
Class 2: Environmental Comfort
Class 3: Social Comfort
Impaired Comfort (00214)
Readiness for Enhanced Comfort (00183)
Nausea (00134)
Acute Pain (00132)
Chronic Pain (00133)
Social Isolation (00053)

## Domain 13: Growth/Development
Class 1: Growth
Risk for Disproportionate Growth (00113)
Class 2: Development
Delayed Growth and Development (00111)
Risk for Delayed Development (00112)

Nursing Diagnoses Retired from the NANDA-I Taxonomy 2009–2014:
Health-Seeking Behaviours (00084) Retired 2009–2011
Disturbed Sensory Perception (Specify: Visual, Auditory, Kinesthetic, Gustatory, Tactile, Olfactory) (00122) Retired 2012–2014

# GLOSSARY

## A

**abandonment** The relinquishment of responsibilities.

**abnormal motor behaviour** Alterations in behaviour, including bizarre and agitated behaviours. Grossly disorganized behaviours may include mutism, stupor, or catatonic excitement.

**Aboriginal peoples** The descendants of the original inhabitants of Canada; First Nations, Inuit, and Métis.

**abuse** The stage of addiction when the problems resulting from misuse of a substance or behaviour become much more regular and disabling.

**acculturation** The process by which members of one cultural group adopt the behaviours of another cultural group, generally due to close, prolonged contact with the other group.

**action phase** A stage of change during which the patient is actively working toward the desired change, including modifying his or her environment, experiences, or behaviour.

**active listening** Awareness of the patient's verbal and nonverbal communications and the monitoring of personal verbal and nonverbal communications.

**acupuncture** A method of traditional Chinese medicine that involves the placement of needles into the skin at meridian points to modulate the flow of energy and stimulate physical changes such as in brain activity, blood chemistry, endocrine functions, blood pressure, heart rate, and immune-system response.

**acute dystonia** Acute sustained contraction of muscles, usually of the head and neck.

**acute phase** The earliest of three phases of mania, during which the person experiences poor judgement, excessive and constant motor activity, probable dehydration, and difficulty evaluating reality. The overall outcome of the acute phase is injury prevention.

**acute stress disorder** A short-term reaction to a highly traumatic event. Occurs within one month of event and resolves within four weeks.

**addiction** The persistent, compulsive dependence on or use of a substance or behaviour despite its negative consequences and the increasing frequency of those consequences.

**admission criteria** Factors that justify the hospitalization of an individual. Admission criteria must include evidence of one or more of the following: (1) imminent danger of harming self, (2) imminent danger of harming others, (3) inability to care for basic needs, placing individual at imminent risk of harming self.

**adult support program** There are three types of adult support programs: (1) social care, (2) adult health or medical treatment programs, and (3) maintenance care. In each type, older adults are cared for during the day and stay in a home environment at night.

**advance directives** Documents that express patients' treatment choices.

**advanced-practice nursing (APN)** Includes the roles of nurse practitioner and clinical nurse specialist. Clinical nurse specialists work as consultants, educators, and clinicians in inpatient and outpatient psychiatry throughout Canada. Nurse practitioners work as consultants or collaborative team members who can diagnose, prescribe and manage medications, and provide psychotherapy.

**adventitious crisis** A state of imbalance that results from events not part of everyday life, such as a natural disaster, a national disaster, or the results of crime.

**affect** The outward representation of a person's internal state of being, manifested in facial expression, tone of voice, and body language.

**affective symptoms** Symptoms involving emotions and their expression.

**ageism** A bias against older adults based solely on age.

**aggravated sexual assault** A legal term used when, during a sexual assault, the life of the survivor is endangered or the assault results in injury.

**aggression** An emotion that results in a verbal or physical attack. Aggression is not always inappropriate.

**agnosia** Loss of sensory ability to recognize objects.

**agonist** An agent that interacts with a specific receptor and enhances the normal response for that receptor.

**agoraphobia** Fear of being in an open, crowded, or public place, such as a field, tunnel, bridge, congested street, or busy department store, where escape is perceived as difficult or help as not available in the case of a sudden incapacitation.

**agraphia** Inability to read or write.

**akathisia** Psychomotor restlessness evident as pacing or fidgeting, sometimes pronounced and very distressing.

**Al-Anon** A self-help group that offers support and guidance for adult family members and friends of people who have problems with alcohol use.

**Alateen** A self-help group that offers support and guidance for adolescent family members and friends of people who have problems with alcohol use.

**Alcoholics Anonymous (AA)** A 12-step program (the prototype for all that were subsequently developed for various types of addiction) that offers the behavioural, cognitive, and dynamic structure needed by those in recovery from alcohol addiction.

**alcohol poisoning** A state of toxicity that results when an individual has consumed large amounts of alcohol either quickly or over time.

**alcohol withdrawal** A physical reaction to the cessation or reduction of alcohol (ethanol) intake that develops within a few hours of the last intake.

**alcohol withdrawal delirium** An altered level of consciousness, presenting with seizures, following acute alcohol withdrawal. Alcohol withdrawal delirium is a medical emergency and can result in death even if treated.

**alternate personality (alter)** Also called *supersonality*. An additional personality within a single individual that has its own pattern of perceiving, relating to, and thinking about the self and the environment.

**Alzheimer's disease (AD)** A form of degenerative dementia.

**anergia** Lack of energy or passivity.

**anger** A strong feeling of displeasure or hostility.

**anhedonia** The loss of ability to experience joy or pleasure in living.

**anorexia nervosa** An eating disorder characterized by a refusal to maintain a minimally normal weight for height and by an intense fear of gaining weight.

**anosognosia** An inability to recognize illness in oneself, which is caused by the illness itself.

**antagonist** An agent that interacts with a specific receptor site and blocks or depresses the normal response for that receptor.

**antianxiety (anxiolytic) drugs** Drugs that enhance $GABA_A$ receptors or increase 5-HT, norepinephrine, or both.

**anticholinergic-induced delirium** A potentially life-threatening medical emergency secondary to use of anticholinergic drugs and characterized by dry mucous membranes; reduced or absent peristalsis; mydriasis; nonreactive pupils; hot, dry, red skin; hyperpyrexia without diaphoresis; tachycardia; agitation; unstable vital signs; worsening of psychotic symptoms; delirium; urinary retention; seizure; and repetitive motor movements.

**anticholinesterase drugs** Drugs that interfere with the action of acetylcholinesterase with the result of elevated levels of the neurotransmitter acetylcholine.

**anticipatory grief** A patient's or loved one's experience of grief ahead of time, after a life-limiting diagnosis or when threatened with loss of ability to function independently, loss of identity, or changes in role definition.

**anticonvulsant drugs** A group of drugs (e.g., carbamazepine, valproic acid) used especially in treating people with mania that has been refractory to lithium therapy. These drugs are also useful in treating people who need rapid de-escalation and do not respond to other treatment approaches.

**antisocial personality disorder** A personality disorder in which the main pathological features are antagonistic behaviours such as deceit, manipulativeness for personal gain, and hostility if the person's needs are blocked. People with this disorder also display disinhibited behaviours such as high risk-taking, disregard for responsibility, and impulsivity.

**anxiety** A feeling of apprehension, uneasiness, uncertainty, or dread resulting from a real or perceived threat.

**aphasia** Loss of language ability.

**apraxia** Loss of purposeful movement in the absence of motor or sensory impairment.

**aromatherapy** The use of essential oils for enhancing physical and mental well-being and healing.

**assault** Reasonable belief that a person means to cause one harm.

**assent** Expressed agreement to participate in health care or research.

**assertive community treatment (ACT)** An intensive type of case management developed in response to the community-living needs of people with serious, persistent psychiatric symptoms.

**assimilation** The process by which different cultural groups come to share a culture; generally, when a minority group adapts to the dominant culture and loses its uniqueness.

**associative looseness** Disorganized thinking, manifested as jumbled and illogical speech and impaired reasoning (also known as *looseness of association*).

**asylums** Retreats from society designed with the hope that, with early intervention and several months of rest, people with mental illness could be cured.

**attention deficit–hyperactivity disorder (ADHD)** A disorder that causes an inappropriate degree of inattention, impulsiveness, and hyperactivity, all of which interfere with functioning or development.

**atypical antipsychotics** Drugs that are predominantly dopamine and serotonin antagonists. Also known as *second-generation antipsychotics*.

**automatic thoughts** Rapid, unthinking, often irrational responses based on schemata. These responses are particularly intense and frequent in psychiatric disorders such as depression and anxiety. Also called **cognitive distortions**.

**autonomy** the rights of others to make their own decisions

**avoidant personality disorder** A personality disorder in which the main pathological features are an extreme sensitivity to rejection and robust avoidance of interpersonal situations.

**B**

**barriers to treatment** Factors that impede access to psychiatric care, including stigma, geographic challenges, financial limitations, policy issues, and system shortcomings.

**battery** Harmful or offensive touching.

**Beck's cognitive triad** Three thoughts that perpetuate depression: (1) a negative, self-deprecating view of self; (2) a pessimistic view of the world; and (3) the belief that negative reinforcement (or no validation for the self) will continue in the future.

**behavioural family therapy** A collection of psychological techniques for modifying maladaptive behaviours.

**behavioural therapy** A treatment method that is concerned with patterns of behaviour rather than inner motivations. Behavioural therapy is effective in treating people with phobias, alcoholism, schizophrenia, and many other conditions.

**beneficence** The duty to act to benefit or promote the good of others.

**Benson's relaxation technique** A method, influenced by Eastern practices, for switching from the fight-or-flight response to a state of relaxation; achieved by adopting a calm and passive attitude and focusing on a pleasant mental image in a calm and peaceful environment.

**bereavement** The period of grieving following a death.

**bibliotherapy** The use of literature for children or adolescents to help the individual express feelings in a supportive environment, gain insight into feelings and behaviour, and learn new ways to cope with difficult situations.

**binge eating disorder** An eating disorder characterized by repeated episodes of binge eating, after which patients experience significant distress but, in most cases, do not use compensatory behaviours.

**bioethics** Deontological principles that are irreducible and must be balanced in clinical situations.

**biofeedback** A form of behavioural therapy, especially effective in stress management, that uses sensitive instrumentation to provide immediate and exact information about physiological responses.

**biopsychiatry** A theoretical approach to understanding mental health disorders as biological malfunctions of the nervous system.

**biopsychosocial model** A model that takes a holistic view of the client, including the person's biology, social environment and skills, and psychological characteristics.

**bipolar I disorder** A chronic, recurrent illness marked by shifts in mood, energy, and ability to function and in which at least one episode of mania alternates with major depression. Psychosis may accompany the manic episode.

**bipolar II disorder** A chronic, recurrent illness marked by shifts in mood, energy, and ability to function and in which hypomanic episode(s) alternate with major depression. Psychosis is not present. Hypomania tends to be euphoric and often increases functioning; depression in this disorder tends to put people at particular risk for suicide.

**blame** Attachment of personal responsibility for the assault onto the victim.

**blood alcohol level (BAL)** A measure (by urinalysis or Breathalyzer) of the level of alcohol in the blood.

**borderline personality disorder** The most well-known and dramatic of the personality disorders, characterized by patterns of marked instability in emotion regulation, unstable interpersonal relationships, impulsivity, identity or self-image distortions, and unstable mood.

**boundaries** Distinctions made between individuals in the family. Boundaries may be clear, enmeshed, rigid, or inconsistent.

**boundary impairment** An impaired ability to sense where one's self ends and others' selves begin.

**bulimia nervosa** An eating disorder characterized by repeated episodes of binge eating followed by compensatory behaviours, such as

self-induced vomiting; misuse of laxatives, diuretics, or other medications; fasting; or excessive exercise.

**bullying** A repetitive behaviour that sustains an imbalance of power.

**C**

**Canadian Federation of Mental Health Nurses** An organization of registered nurses across Canada who specialize in psychiatric mental health nursing. Under the umbrella of the Canadian Nurses Association and with consumer input, this organization set the standards of practice for psychiatric mental health nursing for registered nurses.

**caregiver burden** The physical, psychological, emotional, social, and financial stresses that individuals experience as a result of providing care.

**case management** Care coordination activities the nurse does with or for the patient; includes referrals, assistance with paperwork applications, connection to resources, and overall navigation of the health care system.

**catastrophic reactions** Overreactions to a seemingly normal, nonthreatening situation, commonly experienced in Alzheimer's disease.

**chiropractic medicine** A system of medicine based on the relationship between the body's structure (mainly the spine) and function and its relationship to the preservation and restoration of health, using manipulative therapy as a treatment tool.

**circadian rhythms** The fluctuation of various physiological and behavioural parameters over a 24-hour cycle.

**circumstantiality** The inclusion of unnecessary and often tedious details in one's conversation.

**clang associations** The stringing together of words because of their rhyming sounds, without regard to their meaning.

**classical conditioning** Bringing about involuntary behaviour or reflexes through conditioned responses to stimuli.

**clear boundaries** Boundaries that are well understood by all members of the family and that give family members a sense of both "I-ness" and "we-ness."

**clinical epidemiology** A broad field that addresses what happens after people with illnesses are seen by clinical care providers.

**clinical pathway** A guideline that is used to describe and implement clinical standards. It helps to provide quality and efficient patient care.

**clinical supervision** A mentoring relationship characterized by evaluation and feedback and a gradual increase in autonomy and responsibility.

**closed-ended questions** Questions that elicit a "yes" or "no" response. They are useful for getting information efficiently, as in an assessment, but do little to encourage the sharing of feelings.

**codependence** A cluster of behaviours and psychological characteristics of overdependence on meeting the needs of others.

**cognitive-behavioural therapy (CBT)** A commonly employed, effective, and well-researched therapeutic tool based on both cognitive psychology and behavioural theory that is used to treat a variety of psychiatric disorders (e.g., depression, anxiety, phobias, and pain problems).

**cognitive disorders** Disorders resulting from changes in the brain and marked by disturbances in orientation, memory, intellect, judgement, and affect.

**cognitive distortions** Rapid, unthinking, often irrational responses based on schemata. Prevalent in many forms of mental illness. Also called **automatic thoughts**.

**cognitive reframing** The changing of an individual's perceptions of stress through the reassessment of a situation and the replacing of irrational beliefs ("I can't pass this course") with more positive self-statements ("If I choose to study for this course, I will increase my chances of success").

**cognitive symptoms** Difficulty with attention, memory, information processing, cognitive flexibility, and executive functions (e.g., decision making, judgement, planning, problem solving).

**colonization** The process whereby a people are overcome by a more powerful group and the views, philosophies, values, and beliefs of the powerful group are imposed on the original inhabitants of the land.

**command hallucinations** "Voices" that direct the person to take an action.

**community treatment orders (CTOs)** Mandatory treatment provided in a less restrictive community setting.

**co-morbid condition** Having more than one mental disorder at a time.

**competency** The capacity to understand the consequences of one's decisions.

**complicated grief** Grief that is prolonged, maladaptive, and dysfunctional, experienced after the loss of a loved one.

**compulsions** Ritualistic behaviours or thoughts an individual feels compelled to perform in an attempt to reduce anxiety.

**concrete thinking** An impaired ability to think abstractly. The person interprets statements literally.

**concurrent disorder** The complex combination of a diagnosis of mental illness and a substance abuse disorder or addiction.

**conditioning** The pairing of a behaviour with a condition that reinforces or diminishes the behaviour's occurrence.

**conduct disorder** A disorder characterized by a persistent pattern of behaviour in which the rights of others are violated and age-appropriate societal norms or rules are disregarded.

**confabulation** The creation of stories or answers in place of actual memories to maintain self-esteem.

**confidentiality** A person's right to privacy of information.

**conflict** Open disagreement among members. Positive conflict resolution within a group is key to successful outcomes.

**confusional arousal disorders** Recurrent episodes of incomplete waking from sleep with or without terror or movement, usually occurring during the first third of the major sleep episode and contributing to impaired nighttime and daytime safety or functioning.

**conscious** One of Freud's levels of awareness. It contains all the material a person is aware of at any one time, including perceptions, memories, thoughts, fantasies, and feelings.

**consent** A person's capacity to understand information and voluntarily to act on this information.

**consequentialist theory** The belief that every person in society has the right to be happy and that we have an obligation to make sure happiness results from our actions.

**contemplation phase** A stage of change when a person is thinking about but is ambivalent about change and likely not considering change within the next month.

**continuation phase** The second of three phases of bipolar disorder, lasting four to nine months, during which the overall outcome is relapse prevention. Many other outcomes must be accomplished to achieve this outcome.

**continuum of psychiatric mental health treatment** The range of psychiatric services, from higher to lower levels of intensity, that people might receive care from over the course of a mental illness.

**contract** An agreement, either stated or written, that contains the place, time, date, and duration of the meetings between nurse and patient.

**controlled style of coping** A contained response to an event that may be ambiguous in appearance and reactions and exhibited by a lack of affective response or even calm or subdued behaviours.

**conventional antipsychotics** Drugs that are strong antagonists at the $D_2$ dopamine receptors. Also known as *first-generation antipsychotics*.

**conventional health care** A system of medicine based largely on highly controlled, evidence-informed scientific research. Also known as *biomedical, allopathic,* or *mainstream* medicine.

**conversion disorder** Also called *functional neurological disorder*. An illness in the absence of a neurological diagnosis that presents with neurological symptoms such as deficits in voluntary motor or sensory functions, including paralysis, blindness, movement disorder, gait disorder, numbness, paresthesia (tingling or burning sensations), loss of vision or hearing, or episodes resembling epilepsy.

**coping** Navigating through challenges using skills, either learned or natural, to meet goals.

**coping methods** The thinking, behavioural, and emotional processes individuals use to support functioning in the face of stressors.

**coping skills** Healthier ways of looking at and dealing with illness (e.g., assertiveness training, cognitive reframing, problem-solving skills, social supports).

**coping styles** Personal attributes people develop to help manage stress.

**copycat suicide** A suicide that follows that of a public figure, an idol, or a peer in the community—usually someone with whom the individual identified.

**correctional nursing** Nursing practice organized by the location of the work or the legal status of the patient, rather than by the role or functions being performed. The role involves all aspects of nursing practice.

**counter-transference** The health care worker's unconscious personal response to the patient.

**crisis** An acute state of psychological imbalance resulting in poor coping with evidence of distress and functional impairment.

**crisis intervention** A process focused on resolution of the immediate problem through personal, social, and environmental resources.

**crisis situation** A situation that puts stress on a family that includes a violent member.

**critical incident stress debriefing (CISD)** A group-level crisis intervention carried out very soon following a traumatic event.

**cultural competence** The ability of nurses to apply knowledge and skill appropriately in cross-cultural situations and to adapt care delivery to meet the patient's cultural needs and preferences.

**cultural filters** Filters through which each of us interprets ourselves, others, and the world.

**culture** The shared beliefs, values, and practices of a group that shapes members' thinking and behaviour in patterned ways. Culture can also be viewed as a blueprint for guiding actions that impact care, health, and well-being.

**culture-bound syndromes** Sets of signs and symptoms that are common in a limited number of cultures but virtually nonexistent in most other cultural groups.

**custodial care** Assistance in performing the basic daily necessities of life, such as dressing, eating, using a toilet, walking, and so on.

**cyclothymia** Hypomanic episodes that alternate with minor depressive episodes of at least two years' duration. Individuals with cyclothymia tend to have irritable hypomanic episodes.

## D

**death by suicide** The act of taking one's own life. Also called *suicide*.

**decompensation** Deterioration of mental health.

**de-escalation techniques** Methods and tools, including advanced communication skills, used to defuse any incident of acting out, anger, aggression, or violence.

**defence mechanisms** Innate, unconscious means of preventing conscious awareness of threatening feelings or of denying or distorting reality to ward off anxiety.

**deinstitutionalization** The shift from caring for people with mental illness in institutions to caring for them in communities.

**delirium** A neurocognitive disturbance characterized by inattention, disorganized thinking, altered consciousness, and fluctuations in mental status.

**delusions** Alterations in *thought content* (what a person thinks about). Delusions are false fixed beliefs that cannot be corrected by reasoning.

**dementia** Global deterioration of cognitive functioning (e.g., memory, judgement, ability to think abstractly, and orientation). Often progressive and irreversible, depending on the underlying cause.

**deontology** Duty-based ethics with the central concepts of reason and duty.

**dependency** The stage of addiction when a person loses the ability to choose to use or not to use a substance or engage in a behaviour.

**depersonalization** A nonspecific feeling that a person has lost his or her identity, that the self is different or unreal, or that the person is an observer of his or her own body or mental processes. An aspect of depersonalization/derealization disorder.

**derealization** An aspect of depersonalization/derealization disorder that results in individuals' experiencing a recurring feeling that their surroundings are unreal or distant—an external or outside feeling of disconnect.

***Diagnostic and Statistical Manual of Mental Disorders*, fifth edition (*DSM-5*)** The official guideline for diagnosing psychiatric disorders.

**dialectical behaviour therapy (DBT)** Evidence-informed therapy used to treat chronically suicidal people with borderline personality disorder.

**diathesis–stress model** A general theory that explains psychopathology using a systems approach. This theory helps us understand how personality disorders emerge from the multifaceted factors of biology and environment.

**diathesis–stress model of depression** A theory that depression results from a dynamic interplay of biology and the environment.

**disasters** Events that threaten the well-being of citizens.

**disenfranchised grief** Grief that can promote a sense of isolation and occurs when losses are not always openly acknowledged, supported, or recognized as significant, such as a loss through a suicide, the loss of a friend, the loss of a pet, or the grief of someone thought incapable of grieving (e.g., a child, a person with dementia).

**disorganized thinking** The loosening of associations, manifested as jumbled and illogical speech and impaired reasoning.

**dissent** Expressed refusal to participate in health care or research.

**dissociative amnesia** An inability to recall important autobiographical information, often of a traumatic or stressful nature, that is too pervasive to be explained by ordinary forgetfulness.

**dissociative disorders** A group of illnesses in which mind–body connections are unconsciously altered.

**dissociative fugue** A subtype of **dissociative amnesia**, characterized by sudden, unexpected travel away from the customary locale and an inability to recall one's identity and information about some or all of the past.

**dissociative identity disorder (DID)** An illness in which a person experiences two or more distinct personality states that alternately and recurrently take control of the person's behaviour.

**distress** A negative, draining energy that results in anxiety, depression, confusion, helplessness, hopelessness, and fatigue.

**Dorothea Dix** A passionate social reformer, she advocated for improved treatment and public care of people with mental illness and was influential in lobbying for the first public mental hospital in the United States and for reform in institutions in Britain and Canada.

**double-bind messages** Communication that contains two contradictory messages given by the same person at the same time, to which the receiver is expected to respond, putting the receiver in "a bind," or an impossible conflict. Constant double-bind situations result in feelings of helplessness, fear, and anxiety in the recipient of such messages.

**double messages** Conflicting messages (also known as *mixed messages*).

**duty to protect** responsibility of the nurse when the nurse determines—or, pursuant to professional standards, should have determined—that the patient presents a serious danger to another.

**duty to warn** Responsibility to notify potential victim of a threat to his or her well-being or to notify authorities of such a threat.

**dyspareunia** Painful coitus that can affect men or women. Potential causes in women include estrogen deficiency, vaginal infections, and vaginal lesions.

**dyssomnias** Sleep disturbances associated with the initiation and maintenance of sleep or of excessive sleepiness.

**dysthymic disorder (DD)** A chronic depressive syndrome that is usually present for most of the day, more days than not, for at least two years.

## E

**echolalia** The pathological repeating of another's words, often seen in catatonia.

**echopraxia** The mimicking of the movements of another.

**ecological model** An analytical tool that identifies personal (victim or perpetrator) characteristics, family members, the immediate social context (often referred to as *community factors*), and the characteristics of the larger society to help understand the multilevel, multifaceted nature of violence.

**economic abuse** The withholding of financial support or the illegal or improper exploitation of funds or other resources for one's personal gain.

**ego** One of three psychological processes that make up the Freudian system of personality (id, ego, superego). The ego is one's sense of self and provides such functions as problem solving, mobilization of defence mechanisms, reality testing, and the capability of functioning independently. The ego is said to be the mediator between one's primitive drives (the id) and internalized parental and social prohibitions (the superego).

**electroconvulsive therapy (ECT)** A procedure in which electric currents are passed through the brain, intentionally triggering a brief seizure.

**electronic health care** Health care services provided from a distance through the Internet.

**elopement** Absence from unit without leave.

**emotional abuse** The infliction of mental anguish (e.g., threatening, humiliating, intimidating, isolating).

**empathy** The ability of one person to imagine him- or herself inside another's world and see things from the other person's perspective and to communicate this understanding to the other person.

**enabling** Denying or rationalizing the abuse problem instead of confronting it. Enabling allows for abuse to continue and for harmful consequences of addiction to persist.

**enculturation** The learning, usually passed from parents, about which behaviours, beliefs, values, and actions are "right" and which are "wrong."

**engagement** The connection between the self and another. It is through this connection that nurses can develop a meaningful understanding of another person's experience, perspective, and vulnerability.

**enmeshed boundaries** A blending together of the roles, thoughts, and feelings of the individual family members so that clear distinctions fail to emerge. Also called *diffuse boundaries*.

**epidemiology** The quantitative study of the distribution of mental disorders in human populations.

**ethical dilemmas** Situations in which there are two choices to be made, neither of which resolves the situation in an absolutely ethical way. Weighing of the ethical principles and contextual issues is necessary.

**ethics** An expression of the values and beliefs that guide practice.

**ethnicity** The sharing of common traits, customs, and race. Ethnic groups have a common heritage, history, and world view.

**ethnic psychopharmacology** A field of study that examines the effects of culture, environment, genetics, biophysiology, and psychosocial factors on the prescribing and metabolism of and the response to psychotherapeutic medications.

**ethnocentrism** A perception that one's own values, beliefs, and behaviours are superior.

**ethnopharmacology** A relatively new field that investigates the genetic and ethnic variations in drug pharmacokinetics.

**euphoric mood** When associated with mania, unstable mood during which the patient may describe an intense feeling of well-being. The overly joyous mood may seem out of proportion to the situation, and cheerfulness may be inappropriate for the circumstances, considering that the person is full of energy but has had little or no sleep.

**eustress** A positive, beneficial energy that motivates and results in feelings of happiness, hopefulness, and purposeful movement.

**evidence-informed practice** Care based on the collection, interpretation, and integration of valid, important, and applicable patient-reported, clinician-observed, and research-derived evidence.

**excessive sleepiness (ES)** At least one month of prolonged sleep episodes or daytime sleep episodes that occur almost daily and cause significant distress and social and vocational impairment.

**exhibitionism** The intentional—and illegal—display of the genitals in a public place.

**expressed style of coping** An outwardly expressed behavioural response to an event—for example, crying, withdrawing, smoking, abusing alcohol and drugs, talking about the traumatic event.

**extinction** The absence of reinforcement through the withholding of a reward that has become habitual.

**extrapyramidal side effects (EPS)** Adverse effects, including akathisia, acute dystonias, pseudoparkinsonism, and tardive dyskinesia, caused by blockage of $D_2$ dopamine receptor sites in the motor areas.

## F

**factitious disorders** Disorders in which patients intentionally and consciously feign illnesses.

**false imprisonment** Detention of a voluntarily admitted patient, with no agency or legal policies to support detaining.

**family systems theory** A theory of family therapy that downplays problem resolution, focusing instead on the long-term ability of family members to make autonomous choices. Its goals are to decrease emotional reactivity and encourage differentiation among individual family members.

**family triangle** A basic building block of interpersonal relationships; a third person is brought into a dyad to lower tensions once they build. All triangles contain a close side, a distant side, and a side in which conflict or tension exists between two people.

**family violence** Abuse within a family, including child abuse, intimate partner abuse, and older adult abuse.

**fear** A reaction to a specific danger.

**feedback** Communication of one person's impressions of and reactions to another person's actions or verbalizations.

**fetishism** Intense sexually arousing fantasies, urges, or behaviours in which the individual uses a nonliving object (e.g., woman's highheeled shoe, stockings) in a sexual manner.

**fight-or-flight response** The body's way of preparing for a situation perceived as a threat to survival; this response results in increased blood pressure, heart rate, and cardiac output.

**flashbacks** Dissociative experiences during which the event is relived, and the person behaves as though he or she is experiencing the event in the present.

**flexibility** Allowance for the changes inherent in normal growth and development.

**flight of ideas** A nearly continuous flow of accelerated speech, with abrupt changes from topic to topic that are usually based on understandable associations or plays on words.

**forensic nursing** The application of nursing science to public or legal proceedings. The practice combines the forensic and biopsychosocial aspects of health care in the scientific investigation of trauma or death of victims and perpetrators of abuse, violence, criminal activity, and traumatic accidents.

**forensic psychiatric mental health nurse** A nurse who integrates nursing philosophy and theory with knowledge of and skill in mental health care and legal proceedings in the investigation or treatment of the trauma of victims and perpetrators of criminal activity.

**Four Gifts of Resolving Relationships** A predictable sequence of communications about four processes that can be shared with a person who is dying (forgiveness, love, gratitude, farewell).

**frotteurism** Rubbing or touching a nonconsenting person.

## G

**GABA–benzodiazepine theory** One of various theories regarding the causes of anxiety disorders. This theory proposes that abnormalities of the benzodiazepine receptors lead to unregulated anxiety levels.

**gender dysphoria** Feelings of unease about one's maleness or femaleness.

**gender identity** A person's sense of maleness or femaleness. Gender identity is not inborn but is usually established by the age of 3 years.

**general adaptation syndrome (GAS)** A three-stage theory of stress proposed by Hans Selye: (1) the *alarm* stage, the initial, brief, and adaptive response (fight or flight) to the stressor; (2) the *resistance* stage, during which sustained and optimal resistance to the stressor occurs; (3) the *exhaustion* stage (occurring only when attempts to resist the stressor prove futile)—resources are depleted, and the stress may become chronic, producing a wide array of psychological and physiological responses and even death.

**generalized anxiety disorder (GAD)** An anxiety reaction characterized by persistent and exaggerated apprehension and tension.

**genogram** A tool for efficiently providing a clinical summary of information and relationships across generations of a family.

**genuineness** Self-awareness of one's feelings as they arise within the nurse–patient relationship and the ability to communicate them when appropriate.

**grandiosity** A state in which people with mania may exaggerate their achievements or importance, say that they know famous people, or believe they have great powers. Grandiosity is also apparent in behaviour. Boasts of exceptional powers and status can take delusional proportions. Also called *inflated self-regard.*

**grief** All of an individual's reactions to loss (e.g., depressed mood, insomnia, anxiety, poor appetite, shock, denial, guilt); sorrow experienced in anticipation of, during, and after a loss.

**group** Two or more people who come together for the purpose of pursuing common goals, interests, or both.

**group content** All that is said in the group.

**group norms** Expectations for behaviour in the group that develop over time and provide structure for members (e.g., starting on time, not interrupting).

**group process** The dynamics of interaction among the members (e.g., who talks to whom, facial expressions, body language).

**group psychotherapy** A specialized treatment intervention in which a trained leader (or coleaders) establishes a group for the purpose of treating people with psychiatric disorders.

**group themes** Members' expressed ideas or feelings that recur and have a common thread. The leader can clarify a theme to help members recognize it more fully.

**group work** A method whereby individuals with a common purpose come together and benefit by giving and receiving feedback within the context of group life.

**guardianship** An involuntary trust relationship in which one party, the guardian, acts on behalf of an individual, the ward.

**guided imagery** A process whereby a person is led to envision images that are both calming and health enhancing; can be used in conjunction with Benson's relaxation technique.

## H

**hallucinations** The perception of a sensory experience for which no external stimulus exists (e.g., hearing a voice when no one is speaking).

**healing touch** A therapeutic modality related to therapeutic touch that combines several energy therapies and is based on the belief that the body is a complex energy system that can be influenced by another, through that person's intention for healing and well-being.

**health teaching** Includes identifying the health education needs of the patient and teaching basic principles of physical and mental health, such as giving information about coping, interpersonal relationships, social skills, mental health disorders, the treatments for such illnesses and their effects on daily living, relapse prevention, problem-solving skills, stress management, crisis intervention, and self-care activities.

**holistic approach** An approach to care that addresses both the psychological and physiological needs of the patient.

**holistic nurse** A nurse who recognizes and integrates body–mind–emotion–spirit–environment principles and modalities in daily life and clinical practice.

**homeopathy** A system of treatment of disease that uses small doses (dilutions) of specially prepared plant extracts, herbs, minerals, and other materials to stimulate the body's defence mechanisms and healing processes.

**hospice palliative care** Whole-person health care aimed at relieving suffering and improving quality of life rather than at a cure; grounded in the belief that each of us has the right to die pain-free and with dignity.

**hypermetamorphosis** A compulsion to touch everything in sight.

**hyperorality** The need to taste and chew, resulting in putting everything in one's mouth.

**hypersomnia** Excessive daytime sleep.

**hypersomnia disorder** Excessive sleepiness that occurs three or more times per week for three or more months despite a main sleep lasting seven hours or longer.

**hypnotic** An effect, produced by drugs, of blunting the degree to which a person feels alert and focused, often resulting in drowsiness.

**hypoactive sexual desire disorder** is characterized by a deficiency or absence of sexual fantasies or desire for sexual activity.

**hypomania** State in which people have voracious appetites for social engagement, spending, activity, and even indiscriminate sex. During hypomania, constant activity and a reduced need for sleep prevent proper rest.

## I

**id** One of three psychological processes that make up the Freudian system of personality (id, ego, and superego). The id is the source of all primitive drives and instincts.

**ideal body weight** A weight that is believed to be maximally healthful for a person, based chiefly on height but modified by factors such as gender, age, build, and degree of muscular development.

**ideas of reference** The giving of personal significance to trivial events; the perception that events relate to one when they do not.

**illness anxiety disorder** An illness that results in the misinterpretation of physical sensations as evidence of a serious illness.

**illusions** Misperceptions or misinterpretations of a real experience.

**implied consent** Nonwritten consent.

**incidence** The number of new cases of mental disorders in a healthy population within a given period of time.

**informed consent** A patient's approval of recommended treatment with the knowledge of the potential positive and adverse effects of treatment; based on a person's right to self-determination and the ethical principle of **autonomy**.

**insight-oriented family therapy** A combination of behavioural therapy and education of families in better understanding their power struggles, defence mechanisms, and other negative behaviours.

**insomnia disorder** A state of constant hyperarousal, involving biological, psychological, and social factors, that disrupts sleep and impairs daytime functioning for three or more nights per week for three or more months.

**institutionalized** Dependent on the services and structure of institutions and therefore unable to function independently outside such institutions.

**integrative health care** An interdisciplinary, nonhierarchical blending of both conventional health care and traditional, complementary, or alternative health care, with the intent to synergistically blend the best of all evidence-informed healing practices to provide relationship-based, holistic care.

**intentional torts** Voluntary acts intended to bring about a physical or mental consequence.

**intergenerational issues** Various patterns of behaviour (e.g., involving geographical distance between members, suicide, divorce, addiction, affairs, grief, triangles, historical colonization, loss) that impact successive generations.

**interpersonal psychotherapy** An effective short-term therapy that is predicated on the notion that disturbances in interpersonal relationships can play a role in initiating or maintaining clinical depression. The goal of interpersonal psychotherapy is to reduce or eliminate psychiatric symptoms (particularly depression) by improving interpersonal functioning and satisfaction with social relationships.

**intrusive thoughts** Thoughts about the sexual assault that break into the survivor's conscious mind during the day and during sleep. May include flashbacks (re-experiencing of the traumatic event) or dreams with violent content.

## J

**journaling** The keeping of an informal diary of daily events and activities; journaling can reveal surprising information on sources of daily stress.

**justice** The duty to distribute resources or care equally, regardless of personal attributes.

## L

**la belle indifférence** Lack of emotional concern about the symptoms.

**learned helplessness** Seligman's (1973) theory of depression in which individuals perceive a lack of control over a situation

**lethality** The degree of suicidal risk.

**light therapy** A treatment used in seasonal affective disorder (SAD) consisting of 30 to 45 minutes of exposure daily to a 10,000-lux light source.

**limbic system** Complex set of brain structures, including the hypothalamus, the amygdala, and the hippocampus, that plays a crucial role in emotional status and psychological function.

**lithium carbonate** Mood stabilizer drug used in patients with bipolar disorder.

**locus of control (LOC)** An inherent factor in our experience and expression of mood.

## M

**maintenance phase** A stage of change during which the patient focuses on actively working to maintain changes made and prevent relapse. Also, the final phase of bipolar disorder, the focus of which is prevention of relapse and limitation of the severity and duration of future episodes.

**major depressive disorder (MDD)** A history of one or more major depressive episodes without a history of manic or hypomanic episodes.

**malingering** A consciously motivated act to deceive for material gain.

**malpractice** An act or omission of an act that breaches the duty of due care and results in or is responsible for a person's injuries.

**mania** An exaggerated euphoria or irritability.

**maturational crisis** A critical period of increased vulnerability and heightened potential—a turning point.

**medicine wheel** An ancient symbol that can be interpreted in many ways—the four directions, the four grandfathers, the four components of human nature (physical, mental, spiritual, and emotional)—and that represents the interrelatedness of all aspects of the person, a holistic world view of health and illness based on deep personal connections to the natural world and the tribe.

**meditation** A discipline for training the mind to develop greater calm and then using that calm to bring penetrative insight into one's experience.

**mental health** A state of well-being in which the individual is able to realize his or her potential, cope with the normal stresses of life, work productively and fruitfully, and make a contribution to the community. Psychiatry's definition is continually evolving since it is shaped by the prevailing culture, societal values, and political climate.

**mental health emergency** A state of overwhelming anxiety that can lead to serious personality disorganization, depression, confusion, and behavioural disturbances.

**mental health first aid (MHFA)** The help provided to a person developing a mental health problem or experiencing a mental health crisis.

**mental illness** Alterations in cognition, mood, or behaviour that are coupled with significant distress and impaired functioning.

**mental status examination (MSE)** Analogous to the physical examination in general medicine. The purpose is to evaluate an individual's current cognitive, affective (emotional), and behavioural functioning.

**metabolic syndrome** A set of metabolic abnormalities (e.g., weight gain, hypertension, hyperlipidemia) indicative of increased risk for heart disease and diabetes.

**metabolites** The products that result from the body's breaking down a drug.

**mild anxiety** The level of anxiety that occurs in the normal experience of everyday living and that allows an individual to perceive reality in sharp focus. A person experiencing a mild level of anxiety sees, hears, and grasps more information, and problem solving becomes more effective.

**milieu therapy** The use of a living, learning, or working environment, including people, setting, structure, and emotional climate, to treat psychiatric patients. Milieu therapy uses naturally occurring events in the environment as rich learning opportunities for patients.

**mindfulness** A centuries-old form of meditation that is based on the premise that we are not aware of ourselves moment-to-moment but operate on a sort of mental autopilot. Being mindful requires observing and monitoring the content of our consciousness and recognizing that thoughts are just thoughts and that negative interpretations can become positive.

**misuse** The stage of addiction when people begin to experience problems associated with their use of alcohol, other drugs, or other behaviours.

**moderate anxiety** A level of anxiety that interferes with what a person sees, hears, and grasps—the perceptual field narrows, and some details are excluded from observation.

**monoamine oxidase inhibitors (MAOIs)** Group of antidepressant drugs that prevent the destruction of monoamines by inhibiting the action of monoamine oxidase.

**mood disorders** A group of diagnoses related to disturbances in mood.

**mood stabilizer** Drug used to treat mood disorders by balancing brain neurotransmitters.

**moral agent** A person who has the power and capacity to do what is good and right.

**moral distress** A response to one's values and commitments being compromised.

**moral residue** Feelings that are carried forward from situations that resulted in moral distress or uncertainty.

**moral treatment** Social and psychological approaches to treatment that included retreats from society, calm environments, and several months of rest.

**moral uncertainty** An uneasy feeling that results from a person's being unable to make an ethical decision.

**motivational interviewing** An approach to both assessment and treatment whereby nurses and other practitioners work with patients to facilitate movement through fluctuations between the stages of change.

**mourning** Things people do to cope with their grief, including shared, social expressions of grief, such as attending funerals and participating in bereavement groups.

**multiculturalism** The presence of diverse racial and ethnic minorities who identify themselves as different and wish to remain so; a set of ideals celebrating the cultural diversity of Canada adopted at the federal, provincial, and municipal levels.

**multidisciplinary treatment plan** A plan of care that has been developed with input from all the treatment team members, including the patient.

**Munchausen's syndrome** A factitious disorder whereby the person self-inflicts injury or illness or fabricates symptoms of physical or mental illness in order to receive medical care or hospitalization.

**Munchausen's syndrome by proxy** An illness in which a caregiver deliberately feigns illness in a vulnerable dependent.

**mutual storytelling** A psychodramatic technique developed to help young children express themselves verbally.

## N

**narcissistic personality disorder** A personality disorder in which the primary feature is arrogance with a grandiose view of self-importance. The individual with this disorder has a need for constant admiration, along with a lack of empathy for others, which strains most relationships.

**natural health products (NHP)** Substances such as vitamins and minerals, herbal medicines, homeopathic preparations, energy drinks, probiotics, and many alternative and traditional medicines.

**naturopathy** A system guided by a philosophy emphasizing the healing power of nature and restoring the body's natural ability to maintain and restore health using a variety of traditional and modern therapies.

**negative reinforcement** The removal of an unpleasant consequence of a behaviour; it is not the same as **punishment**. This concept is related to **positive reinforcement**.

**negative symptoms** The absence of something that should be present but is not (e.g., apathy, lack of motivation, anhedonia, poor thought processes).

**neglect** Failure to provide basic needs for a dependant. Includes physical neglect (failure to provide for basic needs or to protect from harm), emotional neglect (failure to attend to basic emotional needs and nurturing), educational neglect (failure to provide a child with experiences, including formal education necessary for intellectual growth and development), and medical neglect (failure to provide basic medical, dental, or psychiatric care).

**negligence** Carelessness.

**neologisms** Made-up words (or idiosyncratic uses of existing words) that have meaning for the person but a different or nonexistent meaning to others. This eccentric use of words represents disorganized thinking and interferes with communication.

**neurodevelopmental disorders** Disorders characterized by developmental deficits in the young (i.e., preschool-aged) child that produce impairments in social skills, intelligence, academic and occupational functioning, and communication skills.

**neuroleptic malignant syndrome (NMS)** A potentially fatal reaction to antipsychotic medications. Symptoms include muscular rigidity, hyperpyrexia, and sometimes oculogyric crises.

**neurons** Specialized nerve cells that process and transmit information through electrical and chemical signals.

**neurotransmitters** Chemicals that transmit signals from one neuron to the next across synapses.

**nonmaleficence** The duty to minimize harm and do no wrong to the patient.

**nontherapeutic communication techniques** Any method of communication that detracts from the therapeutic relationship.

**nonverbal behaviours** Behaviours such as body language, the crossing of arms or tapping of the foot or fingers on a surface, tone of voice, and other expressions other than the content of speech.

**nonverbal communication** Interpersonal communication conveyed through such nonverbal behaviours as body language, eye contact, facial expressions, tone of voice, or gestures.

**norepinephrine** A neurotransmitter in the brain believed to alter mood states.

**normal anxiety** A healthy reaction necessary for survival, providing the energy needed to carry out everyday tasks and strive toward goals.

**nuclear family** Parents and the children under their care.

***Nursing Interventions Classification (NIC)*** A tool used to standardize, define, and measure nursing care.

***Nursing Outcomes Classification (NOC)*** A reference that provides a comprehensive list of standardized outcomes, definitions, and measures to describe client outcomes influenced by nursing practice.

## O

**obsessions** Thoughts, impulses, or images that persist and recur and cannot be dismissed from the mind. Obsessions often seem senseless to the individual who experiences them (*ego-dystonic*), and their presence causes severe anxiety.

**obsessive-compulsive personality disorder** A personality disorder in which the main pathological traits are rigidity and inflexible standards of self and others, along with persistence to goals long after it is necessary, even if it is self-defeating or harmful to relationships.

**open-ended questions** Questions that encourage lengthy responses and information about experiences, perceptions, or responses to a situation and cannot be answered by a simple "yes" or "no" response.

**operant conditioning** A type of behaviour modification in which voluntary behaviours are increased or decreased through reinforcement or punishment.

**oppositional defiant disorder** A recurrent pattern of negativistic, disobedient, hostile, defiant behaviour toward authority figures without going so far as to seriously violate the basic rights of others.

**orientation phase** The phase during which the nurse conducts the initial interview; can last for a few meetings or extend over a longer period.

**outcome criteria** The hoped-for outcomes that reflect the maximal level of patient health that can realistically be achieved through nursing interventions.

## P

**palliative care** An interdisciplinary and collaborative approach to care for the treatment of pain and suffering of chronically and terminally ill patients.

**panic** The most extreme level of anxiety, marked by an inability to process the meaning of activity in the environment, noticeably disturbed behaviour, and, sometimes, a lost sense of reality.

**panic attack** The sudden onset of extreme apprehension or fear, usually associated with feelings of impending doom. The feelings of terror present during a panic attack are so severe that normal function is suspended, the perceptual field is severely limited, and misinterpretation of reality may occur.

**panic disorder (PD)** An anxiety disorder characterized by recurring severe panic attacks. It may also effect significant behavioural changes lasting at least a month and ongoing worry about having other attacks.

**paranoia** Any intense and strongly defended irrational suspicion.

**paraphilias** Distressing and repetitive sexual fantasies, urges, or behaviours.

**paternalism** An approach to care under which patients are told what to do rather than being active participants in their treatment.

**pedophilia** Sexual activity with a prepubescent child (generally 13 years or younger). The most common paraphilia.

**perpetrators** Those who initiate violence. Perpetrators often consider their own needs to be more important than anyone else's and look to others to meet their needs.

**perseveration** The repetition of phrases or behaviour.

**persona** Latin word meaning *mask* and the origin of the word *personality*. May refer to the person as other people see him or her.

**personality** The combination of qualities or characteristics that makes a person a distinct individual. Personality determines the quality of experiences among people and serves as a guide for one-to-one interaction and in social groups.

**personality disorders** Disorders that cause significant challenges in self-identity or self-direction and problems with empathy or intimacy within relationships.

**pharmacodynamics** Biochemical and physiological effects of drugs on the body, which include the mechanisms of drug action and its effect.

**pharmacogenetics** An approach to treatment that takes into consideration individual genetic differences when determining which and how much medication to prescribe.

**pharmacokinetics** The study of the action of drugs within the body; used to determine the blood level of a drug and to guide the dosage schedule.

**phases of crisis** Four distinct phases of physical and psychological experiences in response to a crisis as identified by Caplan.

**Philippe Pinel** Eighteenth-century reformer who, along with William Tuke, introduced the moral treatment era of psychiatry, which attempted to focus on providing peaceful, nurturing environments for people with mental illness.

**physical abuse** The infliction of physical pain or bodily harm (e.g., slapping, punching, hitting, choking, pushing, restraining, biting, throwing, burning).

**physical stressors** Negative changes to our environment (e.g., trauma, excessive cold or heat) or physical beings (e.g., infection, hemorrhage, hunger, pain).

**pica** The persistent eating of nonnutritive substances without an aversion to eating food. Infants and toddlers may eat paint, plaster, string, or cloth.

**play therapy** Usually, a one-to-one session the therapist has with a child in a playroom. The therapist offers a choice of play materials to the child to aid self-expression, assess developmental and emotional status, determine diagnosis, and institute therapeutic interventions.

**positive reinforcement** The presentation of a reward immediately following a behaviour, making the behaviour more likely to occur in the future.

**positive symptoms** The presence of something that is not normally present (e.g., hallucinations, delusions, bizarre behaviour, paranoia).

**post-traumatic stress disorder (PTSD)** An acute emotional response to a traumatic event or situation involving severe environmental stress.

**postvention** Interventions with the family and friends of a person who has died by suicide. Postvention aims to both reduce the traumatic after-effects and explore effective means of addressing survivor problems using primary and secondary interventions.

**preconscious** One of Freud's levels of awareness. Just below the surface of awareness, it contains material that can be retrieved rather easily through conscious effort.

**precontemplation phase** A stage of change during which a person is not currently considering changing behaviour or intending to take action in the foreseeable future (usually in the next six months).

**premature ejaculation** The persistent or recurrent achievement of orgasm and ejaculation before intended.

**preorientation phase** The phase of the therapeutic relationship during which the nurse prepares for the orientation phase—for instance, familiarizing him- or herself with the patient's background or engaging in self-reflection.

**preparation phase** A stage of change during which a person is ready to change, may have had some experience with change, and is actively making attempts at change or has plans to take action within the month.

**prevalence** The total number of cases, new and existing, in a given population during a specific period of time, regardless of when the subjects became ill.

**primary care** In terms of mental health care, care that promotes mental health and reduces mental illness to decrease the incidence of crisis.

**primary dementia** An irreversible, progressive dementia that is not secondary to any other disorder.

**primary intervention** In relation to suicide, activities that provide support, information, and education to prevent suicide.

**primary prevention** In regard to abuse, measures taken to prevent the occurrence of abuse.

**principle of least restrictive intervention** This principle requires that more restrictive interventions be used only after less restrictive interventions to manage the behaviour have been attempted.

**progressive muscle relaxation (PMR)** A stress relaxation technique performed by tensing groups of muscles (beginning with feet and ending with face) as tightly as possible for eight seconds and suddenly releasing them.

**pseudodementia** A disorder that mimics dementia.

**pseudoparkinsonism** A medication-induced, temporary constellation of symptoms associated with Parkinson's disease: tremor, reduced accessory movements, impaired gait, and stiffening of muscles.

**psychiatric consultation liaison nurse (PCLN)** A nurse who functions as a consultant to other nurses in managing psychological concerns and symptoms of psychiatric disorders and who works directly with patients as a clinician to help them deal more effectively with physical and emotional problems.

**psychodynamic therapy** A therapy focused on the present that uses many of the tools of psychoanalysis, such as free association, dream analysis, transference, and countertransference, but in which the therapist has increased involvement and interacts with the patient more freely.

**psychoeducation** An approach to care that emphasizes helping a person gain knowledge necessary to manage the illness.

**psychoeducational family therapy** Therapy that provides families with the information they need about mental illness and the coping skills that will help them deal with their loved one's psychiatric disorder.

**psychoeducational groups** Groups that aim to increase knowledge or skills about a specific subject and allow members to communicate emotional concerns.

**psychological stressors** Changes that are cognitive- or emotion-based (e.g., divorce, loss of a job, unmanageable debt, the death of a loved one, retirement, fear of a terrorist attack); psychological stressors also include changes we might consider positive (e.g., marriage, the arrival of a new baby, unexpected success).

**psychomotor agitation** The need to fidget (e.g., constant pacing and wringing hands).

**psychomotor retardation** The slowing of physical movements and, often, of thoughts.

**psychoneuroimmunology** An area of study focused on the relationship between the mind, the nervous system, and the immune system.

**psychosocial assessment** An evaluation of the person's social functioning and the systems in which the person operates.

**psychosocial rehabilitation** Treatment that moves the mentally ill patient beyond stabilization toward recovery and a higher quality of life.

**punishment** An unpleasant consequence of a behaviour.

## R

**rage** An uncontrollable, violent state of anger that prevents a person from thinking clearly or logically, impeding psychosocial or cognitive-behavioural interventions.

**rape-trauma syndrome** A variant of post-traumatic stress disorder that consists of an acute phase and a long-term reorganization process that occurs after an actual or attempted sexual assault.

**rapid cycling** Four or more mood episodes in a 12-month period. The term is used to indicate more severe symptoms, such as poorer global functioning, high recurrence risk, and resistance to conventional somatic treatments.

**rapport** A relationship characterized by trust, support, and understanding.

**reality testing** The ability to determine accurately whether or not an experience is based in reality.

**receptors** Protein molecules, embedded in a cell, to which one or more specific kinds of signaling molecules may attach.

**recovery** The ability of a patient to work, live, and participate in the community after an illness.

**recovery model** A patient-centred approach that stresses hope, living a full and productive life, and eventual recovery. Patients partner with health care providers and aim to extend their improvement beyond stability.

**reflexology** A form of manipulative therapy based on the understanding that zones and points of the body relate to one another. Focuses primarily on the feet to improve circulation and promote optimum function elsewhere in the body.

**refugee** A person who is seeking asylum in a new country due to threat of trauma or actual trauma and violation of human rights.

**Registered Psychiatric Nurses of Canada** An organization representing the four Western provincial associations for registered psychiatric nurses.

**rehabilitation** A program focused on managing patients' deficits and helping patients learn to live with their illnesses.

**Reiki** An energy-based therapy in which the practitioner's energy is connected to a universal source and is transferred to a recipient for physical or spiritual healing.

**reinforcement** An outcome that causes a behaviour to occur more frequently.

**relapse** A return to an earlier stage of change, toward old behaviours, after going through later stages of change.

**relational ethics** A developing ethical theory with the core elements of mutual respect, engagement, embodied knowledge, interdependent environment, and uncertainty.

**resilience** A characteristic of mental health that aids people to recognize stressors and negative emotions, deal with them, and learn from the experience.

**respect for autonomy** Respecting the rights of others to make their own decisions (e.g., acknowledging the patient's right to refuse medication promotes autonomy).

**reticular activating system (RAS)** Part of the brain that helps control sleep, motivation, and breathing.

**reuptake** Reabsorption of a neurotransmitter by a neuron following impulse transmission across a synapse.

**right to privacy** The assurance that only people with a right to know will have access to privileged information.

**right to refuse treatment** A person's ability to understand and appreciate his or her condition and determine if he or she will accept treatment.

**rigid boundaries** Boundaries in which the rules and roles are consistently adhered to no matter what. Rigid boundaries prevent family members from trying out new roles or, in some cases, from taking on more mature functions as time goes on. Also called *disengaged boundaries*.

**rumination disorder** The repeated regurgitation and rechewing of food without apparent nausea, retching, or gastrointestinal problems.

**S**

**SAD PERSONS scale** A simple and practical guide for triaging potentially suicidal patients.

**safety plan** A plan for a rapid escape when abuse recurs.

**schizotypal personality disorder** A personality disorder in which the main pathological features are expressed in strikingly odd characteristics, including magical thinking, derealization, perceptual distortions, and rigid, peculiar ideas.

**seclusion protocol** An outline of the proper reporting procedure, through the appropriate channels, to be used when seclusion is used as a treatment.

**secondary care** In terms of mental health, care that includes intervention during an acute crisis to prevent prolonged anxiety from diminishing personal effectiveness and personality organization.

**secondary dementia** A form of dementia that occurs as a result of some other pathological process (e.g., metabolic, nutritional, or neurological).

**secondary gains** Benefits derived from the symptoms alone.

**secondary intervention** In relation to suicide, a treatment of the actual suicidal crisis. It is practised in clinics, hospitals, and jails and on telephone hotlines.

**secondary prevention** In regard to abuse, early intervention in abusive situations to minimize their disabling or long-term effects.

**secondary victimization** The sexual assault survivor's experiencing further stress or trauma when seeking help.

**selective inattention** An impairment in the ability to see or hear everything in the environment.

**selective serotonin reuptake inhibitors (SSRIs)** Medications that increase both serotonin and norepinephrine.

**self-care activities** Personal responsibility for activities of daily living (ADL).

**self-help groups** Groups (often run by the members themselves) that are structured for the purpose of providing members with the opportunity to maintain or enhance personal and social functioning through cooperation and shared understanding of life's challenges. See also *support groups*.

**serious mental illness** Chronic and recurrent mental illness (e.g., schizophrenia, mood disorders, and other psychotic disorders) in which the person experiences severe challenges in multiple areas of functioning.

**serotonin** A neurotransmitter that regulates sleep, appetite, and libido.

**serotonin syndrome** A potentially life-threatening reaction caused by concurrently taking two medications that increase the level of serotonin.

**severe anxiety** A level of anxiety that seriously impairs the person's ability to notice his or her environment, even when it is pointed out by another. A person with severe anxiety may instead focus on one particular detail or many scattered details.

**sex** The mix of chromosomes (XX or XY) that identify a person as biologically female or male.

**sexual abuse** Any form of sexual contact or exposure without consent or in circumstances in which the victim is incapable of giving consent.

**sexual assault** Any sexual activity for which consent is not obtained or freely given. Also called *sexual violence*.

**sexual assault nurse examiners (SANEs)** Nurses who are specially trained in the care and assessment (including of psychological and emotional trauma) of adult and pediatric victims of sexual assault (*SANE-A* and *SANE-P* respectively).

**sexual disorders** Psychiatric disorders in which sexual problems are considered to be socially atypical, have the potential to disrupt meaningful relationships, and may result in insult or even significant injury to other people.

**sexual dysfunction** A diminished or absent feeling of sexual interest or desire, absence of sexual thoughts or fantasies, and a lack of responsive desire.

**sexuality** The ways in which people experience and express themselves as sexual beings.

**situational crisis** Acute imbalance that arises from events that are extraordinary, external rather than internal, and unanticipated.

**sleep architecture** The structural organization of non–rapid eye movement and rapid eye movement sleep.

**sleep continuity** The distribution of sleep and wakefulness across the sleep period.

**sleep deprivation** The discrepancy between hours of sleep obtained and hours of sleep required for optimal functioning.

**sleep efficiency** Ratio of sleep duration to time spent in bed.

**sleep fragmentation** Disruption of sleep stages as indicated by excessive amounts of stage 1 sleep, multiple brief arousals, and frequent shifts in sleep staging.

**sleep hygiene** Conditions and practices that promote continuous and effective sleep.

**sleep latency** The time it takes to go to sleep.

**sleep restriction** Limiting the total sleep time to create a temporary, mild state of sleep deprivation and strengthen the sleep homeostatic drive.

**social determinants of health** Elements of one's lifestyle that affect health, including economic status, genetics, job security, employment opportunities, access to safe and affordable housing, child care availability, food security, and inclusion and exclusion from society.

**social phobia** Also called *social anxiety disorder (SAD)*. Severe anxiety or fear provoked by exposure to a social or performance situation (e.g., fear of being scrutinized, saying something that sounds foolish in public, not being able to answer questions in a classroom, eating in public, performing on stage).

**social relationship** A relationship that is initiated primarily for the purpose of friendship, socialization, enjoyment, or accomplishment of a task. Mutual needs are met during social interaction (e.g., participants share ideas, feelings, and experiences).

**social skills training** The teaching of a wide variety of social and activities of daily living (ADL) skills.

**sociocultural context** The equal consideration of issues of gender, race, ethnicity, class, sexual orientation, and religion.

**somatic symptom disorders** Thoughts, feelings, and behaviours caused by excessive worry about physical signs and symptoms.

**somatization** Emotional or psychological distress expressed as physical pain.

**specific phobias** High levels of anxiety or fear in response to specific objects or situations (e.g., an animal or dirt), activities (e.g., meeting strangers or leaving the familiar setting of a home), or physical situations (e.g., heights and open or closed spaces).

**splitting** A primary defence or coping style used by people with borderline personality disorder. Splitting makes the person unable to incorporate positive and negative aspects of people (self or others), into a whole image.

**standards of nursing practice** Authoritative statements that promote, guide, direct, and regulate professional nursing practice.

**stereotyped behaviours** Repeated motor behaviours that do not presently serve a logical purpose.

**stereotyping** A generalized conscious or unconscious conceptualization of a group of people that does not allow for individual differences with the group.

**stigma** Negative attitudes or behaviours toward a person or group based on a belief that they possess negative traits.

**stigmatized persons with medical conditions** Patients assumed by health care workers to be bad, disgusting, or even just unusual; often include those who have mental illnesses, those who are HIV positive, and those who have undergone transgender surgeries or treatments.

**stimulus control** A strategy of adherence to five basic principles that decrease negative associations with the bed and bedroom and strengthen the stimulus for sleep.

**stressors** Psychological or physical stimuli that are incompatible with current functioning and require adaptation.

**subpersonality** Also called *alternate personality (alter)*. An additional personality within a single individual that has its own pattern of perceiving, relating to, and thinking about the self and the environment.

**substance-abuse intervention** A useful strategy for helping patients resistant to seeking help or engaging in treatment. Significant others arrange for a meeting with the person experiencing an addiction to point out current problems and offer treatment alternatives.

**substance-induced anxiety disorder** The onset of symptoms of anxiety, panic attacks, obsessions, or compulsions that develop with the use of a substance or within a month of discontinuing use of the substance.

**suicidal behaviour** Actions that cause self-harm (also referred to as self-injury) initiated with a clear intent to cause bodily harm or death by suicide.

**suicidal ideation** Also known as *suicidal thoughts*. These thoughts can range from a fleeting idea about one's own death (or about not being here) that does not include the act of killing oneself to a detailed plan, including the final act of killing oneself.

**suicide** The act of taking one's own life. Also called *death by suicide*.

**sundowning** Also known as *sundown syndrome*. Symptoms become more pronounced in the evening. This symptom-exacerbation pattern may occur in people who have either delirium or dementia.

**superego** One of three psychological processes that make up the Freudian system of personality (id, ego, superego). The superego consists of the conscience and the ego ideal. The superego represents the ideal rather than the real and seeks perfection rather than pleasure or reason.

**supported-employment model** A model of care that includes rapid job placement, on-the-job support, and provision of a job coach who is linked to the mental health team.

**support groups** Groups (usually facilitated by a professional) that are structured for the purpose of providing members with the opportunity to maintain or enhance personal and social functioning through cooperation and shared understanding of life's challenges. See also *self-help groups*.

**supportive psychotherapy** An approach that stresses empathic understanding, a nonjudgemental attitude, and the development of a therapeutic alliance.

**survivor** A person who has endured abuse and recovered. This term recognizes the recovery and healing process that follows victimization.

**survivors of suicide** Family and friends of a person who has died by suicide.

**synapse** Structure that permits a neuron (or nerve cell) to pass an electrical or chemical signal to another cell.

**T**

**tangentiality** A departure from the main topic to talk about less important information; going off on tangents in a way that takes the conversation off-topic.

**tardive dyskinesia (TD or TDK)** A persistent extrapyramidal side effect that usually appears after prolonged treatment and persists even after the medication has been discontinued. TD consists of involuntary tonic muscular contractions that typically involve the tongue, fingers, toes, neck, trunk, or pelvis.

**temperament** The style of behaviour habitually used to adapt to the demands and expectations of the environment. This style is present in the infant, is modified by maturation, and develops in the context of the social environment.

**termination phase** The final, integral phase of the nurse–patient relationship, during which the patient and nurse summarize the achievement of goals and discuss the continued implementation by the patient of strategies learned.

**tertiary care** In terms of mental health care, provision of support for those who have experienced a severe crisis and are now recovering from a disabling mental state.

**tertiary intervention** In relation to suicide, interventions with the family and friends of a person who has died by suicide. Tertiary interventions aim to both reduce the traumatic after-effects and explore effective means of addressing survivor problems using primary and secondary interventions.

**tertiary prevention** In regard to abuse, the facilitating of the healing and rehabilitative process through counselling of individuals and families, provision of support for groups of survivors, and provision of assistance to survivors of violence to achieve their optimal level of safety, health, and well-being.

**therapeutic communication skills and strategies** Communication that reflects the use of skills such as warmth, respect, and empathy and strategies such as using silence, recognizing strengths, and making observations.

**therapeutic communities** An ongoing treatment and recovery community (offering a choice of inpatient or outpatient support) accessed after detoxification or rehabilitation programs.

**therapeutic encounter** A brief, informal meeting between nurse and patient that is useful and important for the patient.

**therapeutic factors** Aspects of the group experience that facilitate therapeutic change.

**therapeutic games** Specific games played with children that elicit children's fears and fantasies and help with assessment and treatment.

**therapeutic index** The ratio of the lethal dose to the effective dose; a measure of overall drug safety regarding the possibility of overdose or toxicity.

**therapeutic relationship** A relationship in which the nurse maximizes his or her communication skills, understanding of human behaviours, and personal strengths to enhance the patient's growth.

**therapeutic touch** A healing modality based on the premise that healing is promoted by balancing the body's energies through hand movements and direct energy (but no physical touch) to the energy field of the body.

**therapeutic use of self** One's individual, genuine ways of being with another person based upon one's personal values and beliefs of humanity and enhanced by the application of microcommunication skills to guide the process of developing, maintaining, and terminating a therapeutic relationship.

**tolerance** A physiological experience that occurs when a person's reaction to a substance decreases with repeated administrations of the same dose.

**tort law** Law developed from obligations to another.

**traditional, complementary, and alternative medicine (TCAM)** A system of medicine that recognizes that many of the philosophical underpinnings for different approaches are derived from both non-Western cultural traditions and newer concepts from quantum physics and studies in the nature of energy and reality, which have not historically been a part of conventional health care delivery.

**transcranial magnetic stimulation (TMS)** A noninvasive treatment modality that uses MRI-strength magnetic pulses to stimulate focal areas of the cerebral cortex.

**transference** The patient's experience of feelings toward the nurse or therapist that were originally held toward significant others in his or her life.

**transsexualism** An extreme case of gender dysphoria in which a person wishes to change his or her anatomical sexual characteristics to those of the opposite sex.

**Transtheoretical Model of Change** A behaviour change model that is the basis for developing effective interventions to promote health behaviour change in addictions services.

**trauma** Experiencing or witnessing events that threaten an individual's very survival (physical or psychological).

**trauma-informed care** Care focused on patients' past experiences of violence or trauma and the role it currently plays in their lives.

**tricyclic antidepressants** Drugs that block the reuptake of norepinephrine for the secondary amines and both norepinephrine and serotonin for the tertiary amines.

**typology of interpersonal violence** Four modes in which the abuse of power may be inflicted: physical abuse, sexual abuse, psychological or emotional abuse, and deprivation or neglect. (Economic abuse is another mode in which violence can be inflicted.)

**U**

**unconscious** One of Freud's levels of awareness. The unconscious includes all repressed memories, passions, and unacceptable urges lying deep below the surface. The unconscious exerts a powerful yet unseen effect on the conscious thoughts and feelings of the individual.

**unintentional torts** Unintentional acts that produce injury or harm to another person.

**utilitarianism** Bringing about the greatest good and the least harm for the greatest number of people.

## V

**vaginismus** Involuntary constriction of the muscles that close the vagina, potentially caused by estrogen deficiency, vaginal infections, or vaginal lesions.

**vagus nerve stimulation (VNS)** Electrical stimulation of the vagus nerve to increase the level of neurotransmitters and improve mood.

**values** Abstract standards that represent an ideal, either positive or negative.

**vegetative signs of depression** Alterations in those activities necessary to support physical life and growth (e.g., change in bowel movements and eating habits, sleep disturbances, disinterest in sex).

**verbal communication** All the words a person speaks.

**violence** Any action that has the intent to harm. It can be directed at self, others, or objects.

**virtue ethics** An ethical theory that espouses that good people will make good decisions.

**virtues** Attitudes, dispositions, or character traits that enable us to be and to act in ways that develop ethical potential and ensure ethical outcomes.

**vocational rehabilitation** A program providing vocational training, financial support for attaining employment, or supported-employment services.

**voyeurism** The (illegal) seeking of sexual arousal through viewing, usually secretly, other people in intimate situations (e.g., naked, in the process of disrobing, engaging in sexual activity).

**vulnerable person** An adult or child who, as a result of illness, physical condition, or experiences, is at greater risk than the general population for being harmed.

## W

**Weir Report** A report released in 1932 by the Canadian Medical Association and the Canadian Nurses Association. It concluded that drastic changes to nursing education programs were needed, including the standardization of curriculum, work hours, and instructor training, and that the care of people with mental illnesses needed to be integrated into all generalist programs.

**Western tradition** A world view based on the scientific biomedical model and aligned with values of autonomy, individualization, and independence.

**William Tuke** Eighteenth-century reformer who, along with Philippe Pinel, introduced the moral treatment era of psychiatry, which attempted to focus on providing peaceful, nurturing environments for people with mental illness.

**withdrawal** The experiences and physiological changes that occur when blood and tissue concentrations of a drug decrease in individuals who have maintained heavy and prolonged use of a substance.

**word salad** A jumble of words that is meaningless to the listener—and perhaps to the speaker as well—because of an extreme level of disorganization.

**working phase** The phase of the nurse–patient relationship during which the nurse and patient identify and explore areas that are causing problems in the patient's life.

**world view** A major paradigm that is used to explain the world and its mysteries, including beliefs about health, illness, and the hereafter. The major world views used to explain health and illness phenomena are attributed to the paradigms of magic and religion, empirical science, and holistic health.

Page numbers followed by "f" indicate figures, "t" indicate tables, and "b" indicate boxes.